Compendium of 3D Bioprinting Technology

Editor

P.V. Mohanan

Sree Chitra Tirunal Institute for Medical Sciences and Technology
(Government of India), Kerala, India

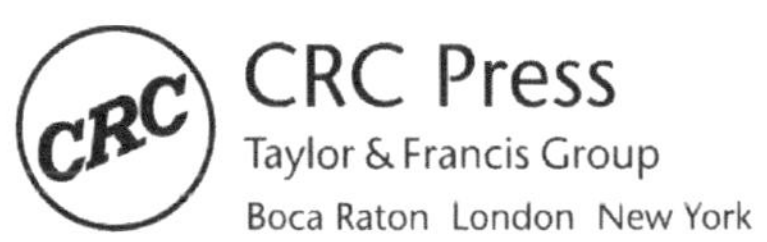

CRC Press

Taylor & Francis Group

Boca Raton London New York

CRC Press is an imprint of the
Taylor & Francis Group, an **informa** business

A SCIENCE PUBLISHERS BOOK

First edition published 2025
by CRC Press
2385 NW Executive Center Drive, Suite 320, Boca Raton FL 33431

and by CRC Press
4 Park Square, Milton Park, Abingdon, Oxon, OX14 4RN

Library of Congress Cataloging-in-Publication Data (applied for)

ISBN: 978-1-032-81833-7 (hbk)
ISBN: 978-1-032-82575-5 (pbk)
ISBN: 978-1-003-50519-8 (ebk)

DOI: 10.1201/9781003505198

Typeset in Times New Roman
by Prime Publishing Services

Preface

3D bioprinting is an emerging innovative technology that includes the fabrication of essential 3D functional biomedical constructs by the combination of cells, and biomaterials with vital growth and differentiation factors. This technology aims to recapitulate the natural tissue milieu. This advanced approach holds great promise in various fields, especially in tissue engineering, regenerative medicine, drug development and testing, and precision medicine. The 3D functional tissue construct can address the need for tissues and organs that are suitable for transplantation to overcome the organ shortage and the risk of transplant rejection. The technique can replace the need for animal experimentation and improve the accuracy of preclinical studies for testing the safety and efficacy of new drugs in bioprinted tissues. To gain more insights into disease mechanisms, the 3D bioprinted disease-specific models help to study, screen the treatment methods, and understand the mechanism of action. In personalized medicine, patient-specific tissue and organ constructs can be developed for specific surgeries and treatments tailored to patient's unique anatomy and genetics.

Several challenges are associated with bioprinting. The primary concern is the maintenance of cell viability and functionality within the bioprinted construct to ensure biocompatibility with the human body and prevent an immune response. Additionally, developing vascularization within tissue construct is crucial to supply nutrients and oxygen to cells. Lastly, meeting regulatory standards for safety and efficiency is essential for tissue and organ transplantation. However, further remarkable research advances and innovations are expected to seal these limitations for an outstanding transformation in this area. 3D bioprinting is a rapidly evolving field with the potential to revolutionize healthcare. As the research advances, it is expected to become more common in clinical practices contributing to functional replacement of organs and personalized medical treatments. It promises advancement in tissue regenerative medicine, improved patient care, and reduction in animal testing.

The book aims to provide a comprehensive idea of the application of 3D bioprinting technology. The knowledge detailed in the proposed book will be highly useful for pharma companies, product developers, students, researchers, academicians, and practitioners. The book 'Compendium of 3D Bioprinting Technology' is a collection of contributions from different authors who have several years of experience in their chosen areas. This will be highly useful for pharma companies, CROs, product developers, students, researchers, academicians, policymakers, and practitioners. This book is focused on the technology of 3D bioprinting and is a collection of contributions from different authors who have several years of experience in their chosen areas. The book has 28 chapters consisting of the latest information on the status and methodologies of 3D Bioprinting Technology and its applications. The key focus features of this book are;

- Advances in 3D bioprinting
- Bioinks for 3D bioprinting
- 3D printing in medicine, food technology, tissue engineering
- Bioprinting of prosthetic devices, scaffolds, and microfluidic devices
- Bioprinting of liver, lungs, skin, eye, ovary, kidney, cartilage, bone
- Safety/toxicity of 3D printed medical products

- Ethics associated with 3D printed organs
- Challenges in 3D bioprinting techniques
- Advantages and disadvantages of 3D bioprinting

It has been a great pleasure to work with multidisciplinary researchers/scientists/professors, who have several years of experience in their chosen areas. Without their cooperation, it would not have been possible to bring out this book, focusing on the compendium of 3D bioprinting technology. Furthermore, I wish to express my sincere gratitude to the Director and Head, of the Biomedical Technology Wing, Sree Chitra Tirunal Institute for Medical Sciences and Technology (Department of Science and Technology, Government of India), Trivandrum, Kerala for their phenomenal support and advice throughout this work. The support and encouragement from family and friends is greatly acknowledged.

Editor
P.V. Mohanan

Contents

Part III: Medical Applications of Bioprinting

List of Contributors

Aashwini Bhavsar
Centre for Interdisciplinary Programs, Indian Institute of Technology Hyderabad, Kandi, India.

Abhirami Dinesan
Amrita School of Nanosciences and Molecular Medicine, Amrita Institute of Medical Sciences and Research Centre, Amrita Vishwa Vidyapeetham, Ernakulam, India.

Ahmed Fatimi
Chemical Science and Engineering Research Team (ERSIC), Department of Chemistry, Polydisciplinary Faculty of Beni Mellal (FPBM), Sultan Moulay Slimane University (USMS), Mghila, Morocco.

Alfonso Carlos Marcos Romero
Department of Graphic Expression, University of Extremadura, Spain.

Amit Ghosh
Department of Biomedical Engineering, Indian Institute of Technology Hyderabad, Kandi, India.

Amit Kumar Jaiswal
Centre for Biomaterials Cellular and Molecular Theranostics (CBCMT), Vellore Institute of Technology (VIT) Vellore, Vellore, India.

Amit Panwar
School of Biological Sciences, Amity University Punjab, Mohali, India.

Ana Isabel Rodríguez Cendal
Biomedical Research Institute of A Coruña (INIBIC). Building attached to the Hospital Materno Infantil Teresa Herrera, 1st floor. Carretera As Xubias, A Coruña, Spain.

Anastasia Kirillova
The Royal Women's Hospital, Locked Bag 300, Grattan St and Flemington Rd, Parkville.

Antonio Macías García
Department of Mechanical, Energy and Materials Engineering. School of Industrial Engineering. University of Extremadura. Avenida de Elvas, Badajoz. Spain.

Anwesha Ghosh
Department of Biomedical Engineering, Indian Institute of Technology Hyderabad, Kandi, India.

Aravind Kumar Rengan
Department of Biomedical Engineering, Indian Institute of Technology Hyderabad, Kandi, India.

Arunkumar Palaniappan
Human Organ Manufacturing Engineering (HOME) Lab, Centre for Biomaterials, Cellular and Molecular Theranostics, Vellore Institute of Technology, Vellore, India.

Ashis Kumar Bera
Department of Biomedical Engineering, Indian Institute of Technology Hyderabad, Kandi, India.

Ashish Kumar
Nalanda College of Engineering, Bihar Engineering University, Science, Technology and Technical Education Department, Government of Bihar, Bihar, India.

Ashtami J
Division of Toxicology, Biomedical Technology Wing, Sree Chitra Tirunal Institute of Medical Science and Technology, Thiruvananthapuram, Kerala, India.

Beyza Topcu
Center for Nanotechnology & Biomaterials Application and Research (NBUAM), Marmara University, Istanbul, Turkey.

Canan Dogan
Center for Nanotechnology & Biomaterials Application and Research (NBUAM), Marmara University, Turkey.

Chandra Lekha Putta
Department of Biomedical Engineering, Indian Institute of Technology Hyderabad, Kandi, India.

Deepan Karuppan
School of Mechanical Engineering. Vellore Institute of Technology, Vellore.

Dheeraj D
Department of Oral surgery, Century Dental College, Poinachi, India.

Dilruba Baykara
Center for Nanotechnology & Biomaterials Application and Research (NBUAM).

Drishya Prakashan
DBT-National Institute of Animal Biotechnology (NIAB), Hyderabad, India.

Elif Ilhan
Center for Nanotechnology & Biomaterials Application and Research (NBUAM).

Esra Pilavci
Center for Nanotechnology & Biomaterials Application and Research (NBUAM), Marmara University, Turkey.

Falguni Pati
Department of Biomedical Engineering, Indian Institute of Technology Hyderabad, Kandi, India.

Gaddam Kiranmai
Department of Biomedical Engineering, Indian Institute of Technology Hyderabad, Kandi, India.

Greeshma N
Department of Biomedical Engineering, Indian Institute of Technology Hyderabad, Sangareddy, Telangana.

Haleema Sabia
Department of Zoology, Institute of Science, Banaras Hindu University, Varanasi, India.

Haneen Moustafa
Department of Chemistry, Manipal Institute of Technology, Manipal Academy of Higher Education, Manipal, India.

Harshada M. Adhyapak
Department of Chemistry, Manipal Institute of Technology, Manipal Academy of Higher Education, Manipal, India.

Humira Assad
Department of Chemistry, School of Chemical Engineering and Physical Sciences, Lovely Professional University, India.

Jayantha Saha
DBT-National Institute of Animal Biotechnology (NIAB), Hyderabad, India.

Jesús Manuel Rodríguez Rego
Department of Graphic Expression, University of Extremadura, Spain.

Juan Pablo Carrasco Amador
Department of Graphic Expression, University of Extremadura, Spain.

Jyotirmayee Sahoo
Department of Physiology, SBIMS, University of Health Sciences, Raipur, India.

Kirthanashri S Vasanthan
Manipal Centre for Biotherapeutics Research, Manipal Academy of Higher Education, Manipal, India.

Krithaksha V
Georgian National University SEU, Tbilisi, U.S.A.

Laura Mendoza Cerezo
Department of Graphic Expression, University of Extremadura, Spain.

Lubna Zeenat
Centre for Interdisciplinary programs, Indian Institute of Technology Hyderabad, Kandi, India

Manisha Sonthalia
School of Bio-Sciences and Technology (SBST).

Manjoosha RY
Department of Biomedical Engineering, Indian Institute of Technology Hyderabad, Sangareddy, Telangana.

MD Abdullah
Department of Biomedical Engineering, Indian Institute of Technology Hyderabad, Kandi, India.

Mansi Dixit
Department of Biomedical Engineering, Indian Institute of Technology Hyderabad, Kandi, India.

Meenu T S
Department of Biomedical Engineering, Indian Institute of Technology Hyderabad, Kandi, India.

Megha KB
Division of Toxicology, Sree Chitra Tirunal Institute of Medical Science and Technology, Thiruvananthapuram, India.

Mehmet Bozdag
Center for Nanotechnology & Biomaterials Application and Research (NBUAM), Marmara University, Turkey.

Mereena George Ushakumary
Biological Sciences Division, Pacific Northwest National Laboratory, Richland, U.S.A.

Mohanan PV
Division of Toxicology, Biomedical Technology Wing, Sree Chitra Tirunal Institute of Medical Science and Technology, Thiruvananthapuram, Kerala, India.

Mrunmayi Gadre
Manipal Centre for Biotherapeutics Research, Manipal Academy of Higher Education, Manipal, India.

Musa Ayran
Center for Nanotechnology & Biomaterials Application and Research (NBUAM), Marmara University, Turkey.

Namratha B
Department of Chemistry, The Yenepoya Institute of Arts, Science, Commerce and Management, Mangaluru, India.

Oguzhan Gunduz
Center for Nanotechnology & Biomaterials Application and Research (NBUAM), Marmara University, Turkey.

Prakash Srinivasan Timiri Shanmugam
Global Product Safety & Toxicology, Avanos medical Inc, Alpharetta, USA.

Priyanshu Shukla
Department of Biomedical Engineering, Indian Institute of Technology Hyderabad, Kandi, India.

Purnimajayasree Ramesh
Human Organ Manufacturing Engineering (HOME) Lab, Centre for Biomaterials, Cellular and Molecular Theranostics, Vellore Institute of Technology, Vellore, India.

Radha Chaube
Department of Zoology, Institute of Science, Banaras Hindu University, India.

Rahul Sayal
UC Davis Center for Surgical Bioengineering, University of California Davis, U.S.A.

Rashmi Ramakrishnan
CÚRAM, Science Foundation Ireland Research Centre for Medical Devices, University of Galway, Galway, Ireland.

Renold Elsen Selvam
School of Mechanical Engineering. Vellore Institute of Technology, Vellore.

Renu John
Department of Biomedical Engineering, Indian Institute of Technology Hyderabad, Sangareddy, Telangana.

Rohin Shyam
Human Organ Manufacturing Engineering (HOME) Lab, Centre for Biomaterials, Cellular and Molecular Theranostics, Vellore Institute of Technology, Vellore, India.

Rounik Karmakar
Department of Biomedical Engineering, Indian Institute of Technology Hyderabad, Kandi, India.

Sandhiya Thamizharasan
The Tooth Doctor, Advanced Implant Centre, Vellapanchavadi, Chennai, India.

Sandhya Sharma
Department of Zoology, Institute of Science, Banaras Hindu University, India.

Santosh L. Gaonkar
Department of Chemistry, Manipal Institute of Technology, Manipal Academy of Higher Education, Manipal, India.

Santosh LG
Department of Chemistry, Manipal Institute of Technology, Manipal Academy of Higher Education, Manipal, India.

Saumya S K
Department of Pharmacology, VMCGH, Dr. YRS University of Health Sciences, Andhra Pradesh, India.

Silvia María Díaz Prado
Biomedical Research Institute of A Coruña (INIBIC). Building attached to the Hospital Materno Infantil Teresa Herrera, 1st floor. Carretera As Xubias, A Coruña, Spain.

Soham Ghosh
Department of Biomedical Engineering, Indian Institute of Technology Hyderabad, Kandi, India.

Songul Ulag
Department of Metallurgical and Materials Engineering, Faculty of Technology, Marmara University, Istanbul, Turkey.

Sonu Gandhi
DBT-National Institute of Animal Biotechnology (NIAB), Hyderabad, India.

Sourita Ghosh
Department of Biomedical Engineering, Indian Institute of Technology Hyderabad, Kandi, India.

Sule Ilgar
Center for Nanotechnology & Biomaterials Application and Research (NBUAM), Marmara University, Istanbul, Turkey.

Sumeyye Cesur
Center for Nanotechnology & Biomaterials Application and Research (NBUAM), Marmara University, Turkey.

Suresha KR
Department of Pharmacology, VMCGH, Dr. YRS University of Health Sciences, AP, India.

Thamizharasan Sampath
Department of Pharmacology & Toxicology, VMCGH, Dr. YRS University of Health Sciences, Kurnool, India.

Umanath Puthillam
School of Mechanical Engineering. Vellore Institute of Technology, Vellore.

Vidhi Mathur
Manipal Centre for Biotherapeutics Research, Manipal Academy of Higher Education, Manipal, India.

Yofiel Wyle
UC Davis Center for Surgical Bioengineering, University of California Davis, U.S.A.

Bio Sketch of Editor

Dr. P.V. Mohanan

Dr. Mohanan is a Fellow of the National Academy of Science, India, and the Royal Society of Biologists, UK. He was a JSPS Postdoctoral Fellow at the University of Tsukuba, Japan in the field of Neurotoxicity. As a toxicologist, he has been intimately associated with all the medical devices/technologies developed at SCTIMST (Govt. of India). Currently, he heads both the Division of Toxicology and Dept. of Applied Biology. Dr. Mohanan is a member of the Empowered Committee on the 'Rapid Response Regulatory Framework for COVID-19 to deal with applications for the development of vaccines, diagnostics, prophylactics, and therapeutics and an expert member in the statutory Committee, RCGM, DBT, New Delhi. Mohanan is also serving as an expert member at the DST, SERB, DBT, ICMR, CSIR, and FSSAI Scientific committees. He is an Expert member at the Joint Food and Agriculture Organization of the United Nations and the World Health Organization (JECFA), USA. Mohanan is a member of the Scientific Advisory Committee of ICMR-NARFBR, Hyderabad. He was a Visiting Professor and Visiting Researcher at Toyo University, Japan, and a Certified Biological Safety Specialist. Mohanan is an Adjunct Professor at the Indian Institute of Technology, Hyderabad, Jamia Hamdard University, New Delhi, and at K.S Hegde Medical Academy, Mangalore. He received a lifetime achievement award from the Society of Toxicology India, for his outstanding contribution in the field of toxicology. He patented an ELISA kit for the measurement of pyrogenicity. Mohanan made significant contributions to the development of medical device regulations in India. He received a certificate of appreciation from the Hon. Minister of Science and Technology, Govt. of India for the contribution to India getting full adherent status on GLP from OECD. He has authored more than 300 publications and 10 books, 5 filed patents, and 9 design registrations. Presently he is the Secretary General of the Society of Toxicology, India and Vice President Kerala Academy of Sciences, India.

Dr. PV. Mohanan, PhD, FNASc, FRSB(UK), FST, FASc(Aw), FAS, FSAB
Scientist-G & Head, Toxicology Division, Head, Dept. of Applied Biology, Biomedical Technology Wing, Sree Chitra Tirunal Institute for Medical Sciences and Technology (Govt. of India), Poojapura, Trivandrum, India.

1

The History of 3D Bioprinting

Ahmed Fatimi[1]*

1. Introduction

Three-dimensional (3D) bioprinting is a biomedical application of additive manufacturing processes for the artificial production of tissue (Agarwal et al., 2020; Fatimi et al., 2022; Li et al., 2016; Vanaei et al., 2021). It involves the creation of cellular structures in a confined space using 3D printing techniques while retaining cellular function and viability in the bioprinted construction (Zhang et al., 2023). This technology uses the layer-by-layer principle of 3D printing and is defined as a disruptive technology resulting from the combination of knowledge in chemistry, physics, biology, mechanics, and computer science (Yu et al., 2018). 3D bioprinting has many innovative potential applications, although its current applications are limited due to its recent discovery. Since the first experiments, 3D bioprinting has developed, and new bioprinting techniques have been developed, such as extrusion-based and droplet-based bioprinting (Tripathi et al., 2023). The arrival of commercial bioprinters has rapidly advanced the tissue engineering field. In the past few years, new bioprinting approaches and novel bioink formulations have emerged, enabling several research groups to demonstrate the use of such technology to fabricate functional and relevant tissue models. Further, several companies have launched bioprinters, pushing for early adoption and democratization of bioprinting (Choudhury et al., 2018a).

3D bioprinting has a fascinating history dating back to the 1980s. Based on a structured and comprehensive approach, this chapter, composed of four sections, is a look at its evolution over time. The first section of this historical exploration of 3D bioprinting highlights the potential impact of this technology on regenerative medicine, pharmaceutical research, and other related fields. With a thorough understanding of the subject, we begin by defining 3D bioprinting as a revolutionary technology, introducing the ability to fabricate complex biological structures on a microscopic scale using a 3D printer. This section covers the different printing methods, such as extrusion-based, droplet-based, laser-assisted, and vat polymerization-based bioprinting, highlighting the advantages and limitations of each approach over time. A deep dive into the evolution of bioprinter technologies from early prototypes to today's state-of-the-art models is presented in the second

[1] Chemical Science and Engineering Research Team (ERSIC), Department of Chemistry, Polydisciplinary Faculty of Beni Mellal (FPBM), Sultan Moulay Slimane University (USMS), Mghila, Morocco.

* Corresponding author: a.fatimi@usms.ma

section. Additionally, this section gives a tour of current applications for 3D bioprinting, focusing on its use in regenerative medicine, the creation of artificial organs, and other emerging fields such as tissue production for *in vitro* drug testing. The third section of this chapter explores the work of the pioneers who laid the foundations for 3D bioprinting. A detailed profile of companies that helped advance the technology is included. Finally, the fourth section analyzes the current challenges of 3D bioprinting, whether technical, ethical, or regulatory. Then it explores future prospects, including anticipated technological advances, new potential applications, and ethical implications as the technology continues to develop.

2.   3D bioprinting: Definition and Background

3D bioprinting is a technology that constructs biological cells or tissues in a 3D structure using viable cells, biomaterials, and biological molecules (Kačarević et al., 2018). It is based on the precise layer-by-layer positioning of these components, allowing for the fabrication of complex 3D structures. This technology has shown great potential in tissue engineering and regenerative medicine, as it can fabricate individualized biological constructs with precise geometric designability, bridging the gap between engineered tissue constructs and natural tissues (Tan et al., 2021).

There are several advantages to 3D bioprinting over conventional tissue engineering methods. These include rapid prototyping of customized structures, high precision in spatial cell delivery, and the engineering of highly controllable microenvironments (Tan et al., 2021). Furthermore, the majority of structures undergo crosslinking to achieve full stability, typically achieved through treatment of the construct. Following the bioprinting process, the resulting tissues are scrutinized using microscopy and imaging techniques. These techniques provide insights into the *in vivo* distribution of cells within tissue or organs. Additionally, the assessment includes examining whether the dispersed cells establish connections and perform specific functions similar to those of natural tissue or organs through physical and chemical stimulation, as per the proposed objectives (Gu et al., 2020 not found in refs). Subsequently, the cell-filled constructs that meet these criteria are placed in an incubator or bioreactor for cultivation and maturation, a phase lasting from a few days to a couple of weeks. Depending on the intended application, the tissue constructs are then utilized for either *in vivo* implantation or *in vitro* testing (Figure 1). Further, some of the current applications of 3D bioprinting in tissue engineering include bone tissue, cartilage tissue, vascular grafts, skin, neural tissue, heart tissue, liver tissue, and lung tissue (Fatimi et al., 2022; Zandrini et al., 2023).

The 3D bioprinting techniques used in most cases include extrusion-based (e.g., pneumatic, piston), droplet-based (e.g., inkjet bioprinting, electro-hydrodynamic jetting), laser-assisted (e.g., laser-induced forward transfer, laser-guided direct write), and vat polymerization-based (e.g., stereolithography, digital light processing) bioprinting (Figure 2). On the other hand, bioinks are the materials used in 3D bioprinting. They contain living cells, bioactive molecules, and biomaterials that mimic the extracellular matrix environment, supporting cell adhesion, proliferation, and differentiation after printing. Biomaterials that qualify as bioinks (i.e., cell-laden inks) must serve as a cell-delivery medium during formulation and bioprinting processing (Levato et al., 2017). Nevertheless, biomaterials suitable for bioprinting, which can be seeded with cells after the bioprinting process rather than being directly formulated with cells, meet the criteria for biomaterial inks (i.e., cell-free inks) (Levato et al., 2017). In such instances, these biomaterials do not fall under the classification of bioink. Instead, cells are introduced within the bioprinted biomaterial scaffold, alleviating the biological constraints on the inks (Figure 3).

Bioinks must be biocompatible, allow for network remodeling post-printing, and have tunable substrate stiffness (Fatimi et al., 2022). The commonly used bioink materials include hydrogels (e.g., gelatin methacryloyl, collagen, alginate, poly(ethylene glycol)), cell aggregates, microcarriers, and decellularized matrix components (Fatimi et al., 2022). However, each of these bioinks has its own advantages and disadvantages, and the choice could depend on the specific requirements of the tissue or organ being 3D bioprinted (Fatimi et al., 2022).

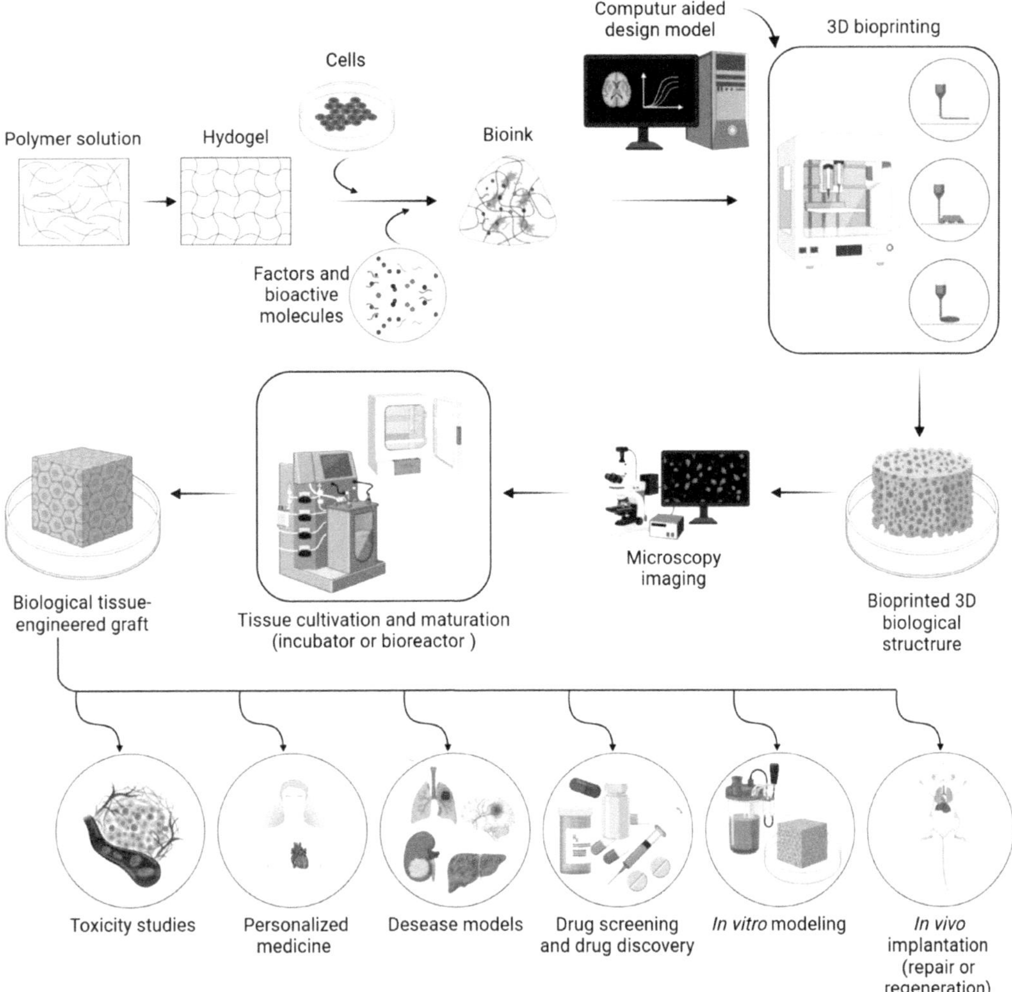

Fig. 1 Schematic illustration of the 3D bioprinting process using hydrogel-based bioinks and the bioprinted tissue as well as applications (Created by Ahmed Fatimi in BioRender.com)

3. Evolution of Bioprinter Technologies

The history of 3D bioprinting is punctuated by several key dates that have marked important milestones in its development. A detailed history of bioprinting evolution is shown in Table 1. Moreover, Figure 4 displays a brief timeline of different key events in the bioprinting evolution.

3.1 1981-1990

3D bioprinting was first demonstrated in 1984 using the conventional stereolithography method. The patented technology allowed 3D object printing from digital data (Hull, 1986). Four years later, inkjet printing converted digital data of an image or character from a computer and reproduced it on a material or substrate using ink drops in a noncontact mode (Mohebi and Evans, 2002). In early 1988, Klebe presented a method of micro-positioning cells to create synthetic tissues in 2D or 3D. A graphics plotter for specific positioning of cells, a commercially available Hewlett-Packard thermal drop-on-demand inkjet printer, and a hydrogel as bioink were used to deposit cells by the cytoscribing process (Klebe, 1988).

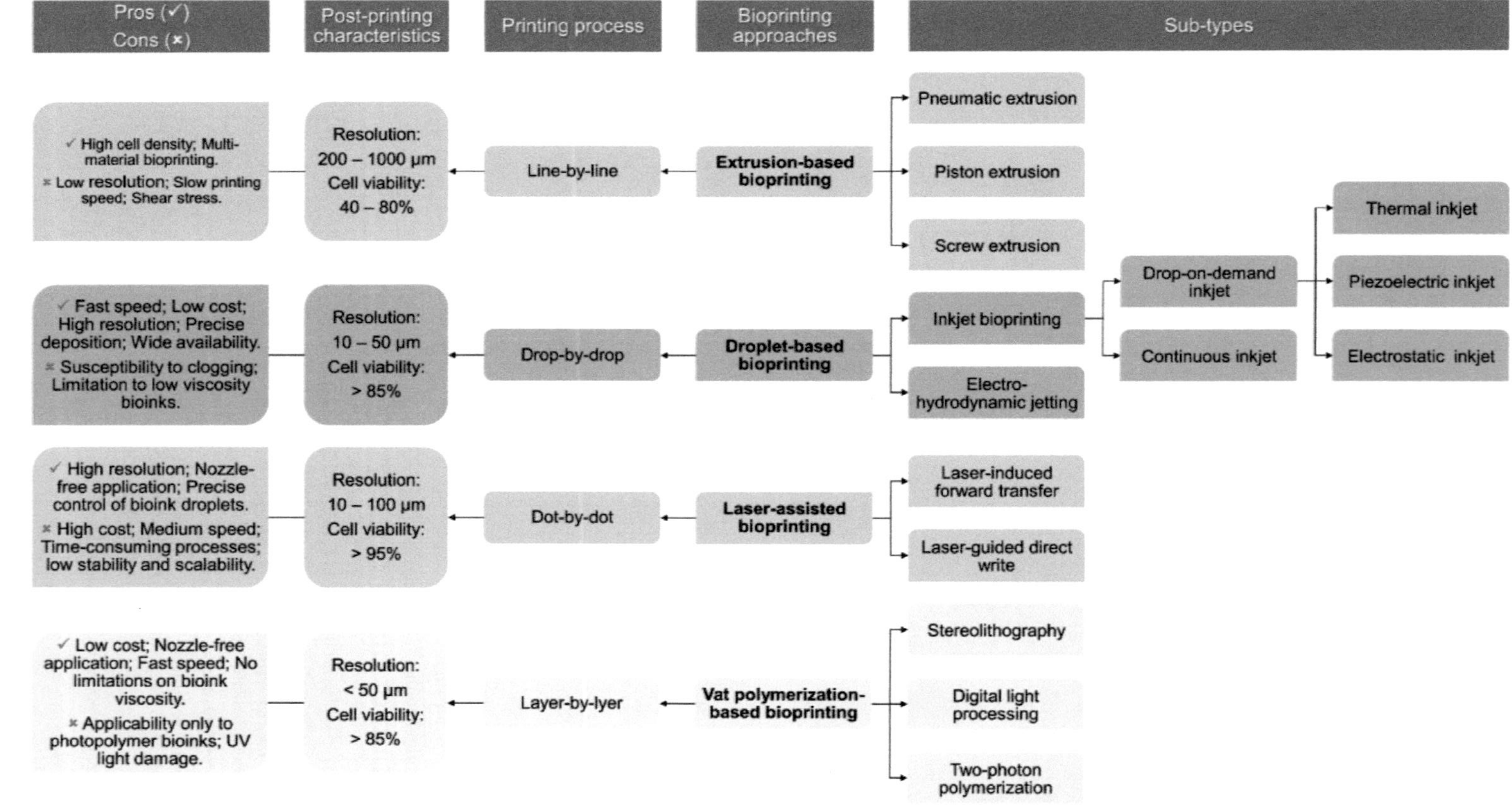

Fig. 2   Schematic illustration of the 3D bioprinting techniques.

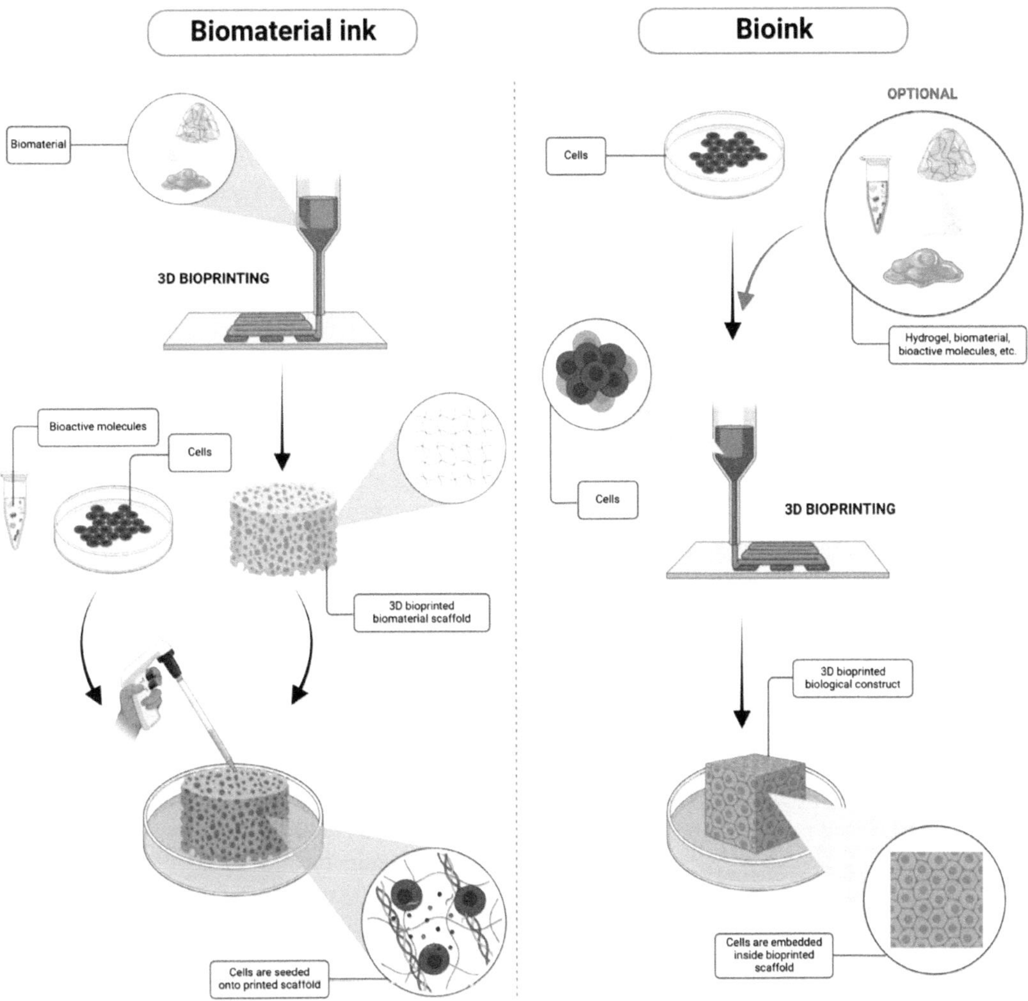

Fig. 3 Comparison of biomaterial inks (i.e., cell-free inks) vs. bioinks (i.e., cell-laden inks) for 3D bioprinting: In biomaterial inks (left image), cells are introduced within the 3D bioprinted biomaterial scaffold, reducing the biological constraints on the inks. In bioinks (right image), cells are intrinsic components of the printing formulation (Created by Ahmed Fatimi in BioRender.com)

3.2 1991-2000

In 1996, Foty et al. discovered that individual cellular aggregates can be arranged and could form, by self-organizing and self-assembling, new combined structures into completely new 3D scaffolds (e.g., biomaterials) (Foty et al., 1996). A year later, the development of the first human stem cell lines took place. Results suggest that peripheral blood progenitor cell transplantation is a procedure that allows the collection of large numbers of circulating white blood cells and progenitor cells, which can be used for autologous transplants (Jansen et al., 2002). In 1999, Odde and Renn described the use of laser-induced optical forces to guide and deposit particles onto solid surfaces, a process referred to as "laser-guided direct writing" (Odde and Renn, 1999). This first use of laser technology demonstrated 2D patterning of living cells. The technology has potential applications in 3D cell patterning for tissue engineering, hybrid biological-electronic device construction, and biochip-array fabrication.

3.3   2001-2010

In 2002, the first extrusion-based bioprinter was used for rapid prototyping to create scaffolds for tissue engineering applications (Landers et al., 2002). The rapid prototyping technology used in the study was a significant advancement in the field of tissue engineering, as it enables the creation of customized scaffolds for various applications. The technology was rapid, inexpensive, reproducible, and scalable, making it an ideal approach for both research and clinical applications. In 2003, the first inkjet technology for bioprinting viable cells was patented. Boland et al. invented the concept of cell and organ printing, which involves the use of protein and cell printers to create stable, functional protein arrays and cell libraries (Boland et al.*2006*). The technology was based on inkjet printing and has the potential to advance various fields, including tissue engineering, drug discovery, and fundamental research (Wilson Jr. and Boland, 2003). A year later, a cell-loaded bioprinting system with a commercially available stereolithography printer was proposed (Dhariwala et al., 2004). The study introduced a novel approach to fabricating 3D scaffolds for tissue engineering applications using poly(ethylene oxide) and poly(ethylene glycol) dimethacrylate photopolymerizable hydrogels (Dhariwala et al., 2004). In the same year, Forgacs et al. described and claimed through a patent a bioprinting apparatus comprising, among other things, a cartridge comprising one or more cell aggregates. The concept of bioprinting a fused ring structure was then demonstrated by the inventors using cell aggregates and poly (N-(hydroxypropyl) methacrylamide)-based hydrogels (Forgacs et al., 2012). This invention, which claimed for the first time the first patented hydrogel-based bioink formulation, confirmed that 2004 is considered the starting year of the patenting of hydrogel-based bioinks (Fatimi, 2022).

In 2005, a self-assembling cell aggregate system was patented. The invention by Forgacs et al. described a method for creating 3D tissue constructs using self-assembling cell aggregates, which can be used in tissue engineering applications. The patent recognizes that cell aggregates, such as bioink particles, have the ability to fuse into 3D organotypic structures upon contact and that this process can be used to create complex tissue structures (Forgacs et al., 2012).

In 2006, Jayasinghe et al. successfully bioprinted cells for the first time, marking the start of practical experiments in the field (Jayasinghe et al., 2006). An advanced electric-field-driven jetting phenomenon called electrohydrodynamic jet processing was applied to deposit living cells (Jayasinghe et al., 2006). This technology has potential applications in cell manipulation, cell patterning, and tissue engineering. In the same year, Atala et al. demonstrated the use of tissue engineering techniques to generate bladders that can be implanted in patients requiring cystoplasty (Atala et al., 2006). The engineered bladder tissues were created with autologous urothelial and muscle cells seeded on collagen-polyglycolic acid scaffolds and wrapped in omentum after implantation. The study proved the creation and implantation of the first synthetic lab-grown organ that was successfully implanted in patients (Atala et al., 2006).

The year 2009 was marked by the successful bioprinting of vascular tissue, overcoming one of the main challenges of bioprinting linked to vascularization (Norotte et al., 2009). Fully cellular blood vessels using only primary human cells without scaffolds were 3D bioprinted (Norotte et al., 2009). In the same year, Lee et al. proposed a method to create multi-layered engineered tissue composites consisting of human skin fibroblasts and keratinocytes, which mimic skin layers (Lee et al., 2009). The technique involves using a 3D freeform fabrication technique based on direct cell dispensing on a robotic platform that prints collagen hydrogel precursor, fibroblasts, and keratinocytes. The process is repeated in a layer-by-layer, resulting in two distinct cell layers of inner fibroblasts and outer keratinocytes. The results suggest that organotypic skin tissue culture is feasible using on-demand cell printing techniques, with future potential applications in creating skin grafts tailored for wound shape or artificial tissue assays for disease modeling and drug testing (Lee et al., 2009).

A year later, the biofabrication of a 3D liver micro-organ as an *in vitro* drug metabolism model was realized by Chang et al. (Chang et al., 2010). The published study presents a technique that involves using a 3D bioprinting method to create a 3D liver tissue construct consisting of hepatocytes and non-parenchymal cells. The resulting 3D liver micro-organ was capable of mimicking the *in vivo* liver microenvironment and can be used as an *in vitro* model for drug metabolism studies. The conclusion suggests that the 3D liver micro-organ has the potential to be used as a tool for drug screening and toxicity testing (Chang et al., 2010).

3.4 2011-2020

Related to the history of 3D bioprinting, three events took place in 2012. Firstly, Koch et al. demonstrated the use of laser-assisted bioprinting for the generation of multicellular 3D constructs mimicking tissue functions, specifically focusing on skin tissue generation (Koch et al., 2012). The research investigated the arrangement of living cells in predefined patterns to create skin tissue substitutes and the formation of skin-like structures in the dorsal skinfold chamber in mice (Koch et al., 2012). Secondly, Skardal et al. investigated the use of bioprinted amniotic fluid-derived stem cells for wound healing in a mouse model of skin regeneration (Skardal et al., 2012). The research used bioprinting technology to treat full-thickness skin wounds, and the results showed that bioprinted structures accelerated wound healing and improved skin regeneration in the mouse model (Skardal et al., 2012). Thirdly, to demonstrate the importance of direct cartilage repair and promising anatomic cartilage engineering using 3D bioprinting technology Cui et al. presented for the first time a method for direct human cartilage repair using 3D bioprinting technology (Cui et al., 2012). The research used a bioprinting system with simultaneous photopolymerization. The bioink was composed of poly (ethylene glycol) dimethacrylate loaded with human chondrocytes, and it was printed to repair defects in osteochondral plugs in layer-by-layer assembly. The results showed that the bioprinted cartilage constructs have good cell viability, extracellular matrix composition, and mechanical properties (Cui et al., 2012).

In 2013, Duan et al. demonstrated the use of 3D bioprinting to fabricate living heterogeneous aortic valve conduits using alginate/gelatin hydrogels. The research successfully bioprinted the aortic valve conduits with the direct encapsulation of smooth muscle cells in the valve root and valve interstitial cells in the leaflets (Duan et al., 2013).

In 2015, Gao et al. presented a novel 3D bioprinting method based on hollow calcium alginate filaments using a coaxial nozzle (Gao et al., 2015). The studied method enabled the creation of high-strength cell-laden hydrogel 3D structures with built-in microchannels for nutrient delivery. The microchannels within the bioprinted structures were designed to have the potential to enhance the viability and functionality of bioprinted tissues by providing a means for efficient nutrient delivery and waste removal (Gao et al., 2015). In the same year, the company POIETIS (Pessac, France) developed Poieskin®, a human full-thickness skin model entirely produced by 3D bioprinting, showcasing the company's advancements in tissue models and biofabrication (Cadau et al., 2017).

A year later, six events took place. Firstly, a study by Nguyen et al. demonstrated the use of 3D bioprinted primary liver tissues as an *in vitro* model for assessing organ-level responses to clinical drug-induced toxicity (Nguyen et al., 2016). The results suggested that the 3D liver tissues could be a valuable addition to the pre-clinical toxicity pipeline and could help reduce the need for animal testing in drug development (Nguyen et al., 2016). Secondly, Colosi et al. presented a novel 3D bioprinting method using a low-viscosity bioink and a coaxial extrusion needle to produce highly defined 3D biostructures (Colosi et al., 2016). The technique incorporated a microfluidic device to control the bioink arrangement deposition, demonstrating the versatility of the bioprinting technique. The results emphasized the potential of this technique for creating heterogeneous 3D tissue constructs with tailored biological and mechanical properties, which are needed in regenerative medicine and tissue engineering (Colosi et al., 2016). Thirdly, Mandrycky et al. proposed the use of an integrated tissue-organ printer (ITOP) for fabricating human-scale tissue constructs from living cells with or without a carrier material in a layer-by-layer manner (Mandrycky et al., 2016). This technology enables the fabrication of scaffolds, devices, and tissue models with high complexity, and it allows the construction of tissues from commonly used medical images using computer-aided design, including its potential applications in high-throughput predictive drug screening and regenerative therapies (Mandrycky et al., 2016).

The same ITOP technology has been used by Kang et al. to produce 3D vascularized cellular constructs of clinically relevant size, shape, and structural integrity (Kang et al., 2016). In this study, the system demonstrated its capabilities by fabricating mandible and calvarial bone, cartilage, and skeletal muscle. The ITOP system, as described in the study, consists of three major units: a 3-axis stage/controller, a dispensing module including a multi-cartridge and pneumatic pressure controller, and a closed acrylic chamber with a temperature controller and humidifier (Kang et al., 2016). A little further, in the same year, O'Connell et al. developed for the first time a handheld biofabrication tool (i.e., the "Biopen") that enables the deposition of living cells and biomaterials in a manual and direct-write manner (O'Connell et al., 2016). The system was designed to print stem cells in 3D constructs directly into damaged cartilage during surgery *in situ*. The gelatin-methacrylamide/hyaluronic acid-methacrylate hydrogel was UV-crosslinked during the deposition process to generate surgically sculpted 3D structures. The device has the potential for *in situ* surgical cartilage engineering and paves the way for the use of 3D bioprinting during the surgical process (O'Connell et al., 2016). Finally, a major breakthrough in 3D bioprinted medicine has brought hope to patients with cardiovascular disease. As a result of research and development, the company REVOTEK successfully 3D-bioprinted blood vessels and implanted them in rhesus monkeys in 2016 (Reeser and Doiron, 2019). It was a major step on the road to mass bioprinting human organs for transplants and the first to have maintained the viability of the cells with the 3D bioprinting technology. The bioink used for the bioprinting process was made from stem cells derived from the fat tissue of monkeys in a microenvironment of growth factors and nutrients that can stimulate the cells to grow into the types of cells needed to form a functioning blood vessel (Kang and Zuo, 2016).

In 2017, the world's first 3D-printed organ transplant was successfully biofabricated, marking a crucial step towards the clinical viability of bioprinting. Bulanova et al. demonstrated the bioprinting of a functional vascularized mouse thyroid gland construct from embryonic tissue spheroids (Bulanova et al., 2017). The research utilized tissue spheroids capable of self-assembly as building blocks to create the thyroid tissue. The bioprinted construct was found to be functional, as it could normalize blood thyroxine levels and body temperature after grafting under the kidney capsule of hypothyroid mice (Bulanova et al., 2017). The concept of the "Biopen" was again proven in 2017 by Duchi et al. (Duchi et al., 2017). The "Biopen" was designed to print stem cells in 3D constructs directly into damaged cartilage during surgery *in situ*. The study demonstrated again that co-axial bioprinting has great potential for *in vivo* application directly at the surgical point of cartilage repair, particularly in the field of musculoskeletal tissue regeneration and repair (Duchi et al., 2017). In the same year, human kidney tissue was 3D bioprinted by King et al. (King et al., 2017). More specifically, a 3D bioprinted model of the proximal tubule interstitial interface has been developed, comprising renal fibroblasts, endothelial cells, and primary human renal proximal tubule epithelial cells. This model aimed to enable more accurate prediction of tissue-level clinical outcomes and to serve as a test bed for the mechanistic assessment of human nephrotoxicity (King et al., 2017).

In 2018, Choudhury et al. used a decellularized extracellular matrix (dECM) as a bioink for 3D bioprinting. The study explored the use of dECM as a biomimetic bioink derived from different decellularized organs (Choudhury et al., 2018b). The results suggested that dECM bioinks have emerged as arguably the most biomimetic bioinks and have the potential to revolutionize bioink manufacturing (Choudhury et al., 2018b). For another biomedical application, Ng et al. presented a two-step bioprinting method to produce pigmented human skin constructs (Ng et al., 2018). The study discussed the fabrication of 3D pigmented human skin constructs using a 3D bioprinting approach, which involves the use of three different types of skin cells: keratinocytes, melanocytes, and fibroblasts. The 3D bioprinted pigmented skin constructs are compared to those fabricated by a conventional manual-casting approach, and in-depth characterization indicates that the 3D bioprinted skin constructs have a higher degree of resemblance to native skin tissue. This approach has the potential to facilitate the development of 3D bioprinting *in vitro* pigmented human skin constructs for potential toxicology testing and fundamental cell biology research (Ng et al., 2018).

In 2019, the first 3D-engineered vascularized human heart was bioprinted, opening up new prospects for the biofabrication of vital organs. This innovation had significant implications for the fields of regenerative medicine and personalized healthcare. Noor et al. addressed the challenge of generating thick, vascularized tissues that fully match the patient in cardiac tissue engineering (Noor et al., 2019). The study focused on the 3D printing of personalized, thick, and perfusable cardiac patches and hearts, aiming to create patient-specific cardiac tissue constructs (Noor et al., 2019). Always in the area of 3D printing technology, with the goal of addressing the unmet challenge of generating vascularized tissues that match the patient's specific needs in cardiac tissue engineering. Lee et al. presented a method to 3D bioprint collagen using freeform reversible embedding of suspended hydrogels to engineer components of the human heart at various scales, from capillaries to the full organ (Lee et al., 2019a). This method provided a porous microstructure that enables rapid cellular infiltration and microvascularization, as well as mechanical strength for the fabrication and perfusion of multiscale vasculature and tri-leaflet valves (Lee et al., 2019a).

In 2020, a handheld 3D bioprinter for printing biocompatible biomaterials including, stem cells, for performing *in situ* surgical repairs was patented (Thorpe et al., 2020). The inventors, Thorpe et al., claimed a handheld 3D printing apparatus for printing biocompatible materials, including stem cells, for in-situ surgical repairs, potentially offering new possibilities for on-demand tissue engineering and regenerative medicine (Thorpe et al., 2020). In the same year, the company ASPECT BIOSYSTEMS made significant strides in the creation and validation of bioprinted tissues for preclinical drug testing and transplantation. The creation of the 3DBioRing™ AIRWAY was the first bioprinted tissue capable of faithfully reproducing acute bronchoconstriction events observed during an asthma attack (Dickman et al., 2020).

3.5 2021-2023

In 2021, the cosmetic company L'Oreal (Aulnay-sous-Bois, France) created a reconstructed epidermis using 3D printing with two distinct halves in a single insert, each composed of a different keratinocyte sub-population. The resulting model exhibited a well-organized epidermal structure, with each half possessing the phenotypic characteristics of its constituent cells, indicating successful and stable tissue reconstruction. The patterned skin model aims to mimic the edges of lesions as seen in certain skin conditions, as well as replicate the complex and heterogeneous nature of native human skin in *in vitro* models (Madiedo-Podvrsan et al., 2021). In the same year, the bioprinting company ADVANCED SOLUTIONS (Louisville, KY, United States) launched the BioAssemblyBot® 200, a versatile four-axis robotic 3D bioprinter, and the BioAssemblyBot® 500, a six-axis biosafety cabinet bioprinter. These innovations were the results of the awarded patent for BioAssemblyBot® in 2018 (Golway et al., 2018).

In 2022, the bioprinting company REVOTEK (Chengdu, China) announced that it had received clearance to begin a clinical study with its first stem cell 3D bioprinting product for patients with peripheral artery diseases. The clearance concerns the world's first universal bioink that allows scaffold-free bioprinting products using the 3D blood vessel bioprinter (T-Series™) (Ilic and Liovic, 2022). In the same year, Moss et al. realized the automated fabrication of a cell-dense human vascularized liver tissue model. The biofabrication of the tissue involved 3D bioprinting and the incorporation of primary human hepatocytes, primary human non-parenchymal cells, and isolated fragments of intact human microvessels as vascular precursors. As conclusions suggest, the inclusion of adipose-derived human microvessels enhanced functional gene expression, including an enhanced response to a drug challenge. Finally, this research has implications for liver disease modeling, infectious agent studies, and cancer investigations (Moss et al., 2022).

In recent months, Jafari et al. employed 3D printing technology to produce a living and operational heart valve (Jafari et al., 2023). The used inks were based on poly(vinyl alcohol), gelatin, and carrageenan. This significant advancement presents considerable potential for addressing congenital heart defects in children. Further, the remarkable aspect of the developed heart valve lies in its exceptional capacity to undergo development and synchronize growth with the surrounding cardiac tissue compared to traditional methods (Jafari et al., 2023).

Table 1   A detailed history of 3D bioprinting evolution.

Year	*Events*	*References*
1984	A stereolithography method was patented that allowed 3D objects to be printed from digital data.	(Hull, 1986)
1988	A standard Hewlett-Packard inkjet printer was transformed and used to deposit cells using cytoscribing technology using hydrogel biomaterials.	(Klebe, 1988)
1996	Discovery that individual cellular aggregates can be arranged and could form, by self-organizing and self-assembling, new combined structures into completely new 3D scaffolds (e.g., biomaterials).	(Foty et al., 1996)
1998	Development of the first human stem cell lines.	(Jansen et al., 2002)
1999	The first use of laser technology demonstrated 2D patterning of living cells.	(Odde and Renn, 1999)
2002	The first extrusion-based bioprinter was used.	(Landers et al., 2002)
2003	The first inkjet technology for bioprinting viable cells was patented.	(Boland et al., 2006) (Wilson Jr. and Boland, 2003)
2004	A cell-loaded bioprinting system with a commercial stereolithographic printer was proposed.	(Dhariwala et al., 2004)
2004	The first bioink formulation, using cell aggregates and poly (N-(hydroxypropyl) methacrylamide)-based hydrogels, for bioprinting a fused ring structure was patented.	(Forgacs et al., 2012) (Fatimi, 2022)
2005	A self-assembling cell aggregate system was patented.	(Forgacs et al., 2012-Not found in refs)
2006	The first electrohydrodynamic jet was applied to deposit living cells.	(Jayasinghe et al., 2006)
2006	Creation and implantation of the first synthetic lab-grown organ (engineered bladder tissue) that was successfully implanted in patients.	(Atala et al., 2006)
2009	Fully cellular blood vessels using only primary human cells without scaffolds were 3D bioprinted.	(Norotte et al., 2009)
2009	Multi-layered engineered tissue composites mimic skin layers and were 3D bioprinted.	(Lee et al., 2009)
2010	A cell-writing biofabrication process was developed, and a 3D liver micro-organ was bio fabricated.	(Chang et al., 2010)
2012	Cells embedded in collagen were 3D bioprinted for skin tissue generation by using a laser-assisted bioprinter.	(Koch et al., 2012)
2012	*In situ* bioprinting was attempted on mouse models to accelerate the healing of large skin wounds.	(Skardal et al., 2012)
2012	The first articular cartilage was developed using a 3D bioprinting system with simultaneous photopolymerization.	(Cui et al., 2012)
2013	Heterogeneous aortic valve conduits were 3D bioprinted using alginate/gelatin hydrogels.	(Duan et al., 2013)
2015	A tubular structure for nutrient delivery was 3D bioprinted by coaxial technology.	(Gao et al., 2015)
2015	The company POIETIS (Pessac, France) developed Poieskin®, a human full-thickness skin model entirely produced by 3D bioprinting, showcasing the company's advancements in tissue models and biofabrication.	(Cadau et al., 2017)

Contd.

Table 1   *Contd.*

Year	Events	References
2016	Human liver tissue models were 3D bioprinted.	(Nguyen et al., 2016)
	The concept of microfluidic bioprinting was approved and took center stage.	(Colosi et al., 2016)
	Integrated tissue-organ printer (ITOP) for fabricating human-scale tissue constructs.	(Mandrycky et al., 2016)
	The cartilage model was manufactured by the ITOP system.	(Kang et al., 2016)
	A handheld biofabrication tool (Biopen) for direct deposition of living cells and biomaterials was developed.	(O'Connell et al., 2016)
	3D bioprinting of blood vessels and implantation in rhesus monkeys. The first implant to have maintained the viability of the cells with the 3D bioprinting technology developed by the company REVOTEK (Chengdu, China).	(Reeser and Doiron, 2019) (Kang and Zuo, 2016)
2017	The world's first animal thyroid gland was 3D-bioprinted and successfully transplanted into a living mouse.	(Bulanova et al., 2017)
	Application of handheld bioprinting (Biopen) to in situ surgical cartilage repair.	(Duchi et al., 2017)
	A human kidney tissue was 3D bioprinted.	(King et al., 2017)
2018	New dECM-based bio-ink formulations were introduced for 3D bioprinting.	(Choudhury et al., 2018b)
	3D *in vitro* pigmented human skin constructs have been fabricated using a 3D bioprinting approach.	(Ng et al., 2018)
2019	The first 3D-engineered vascularized human heart was bioprinted.	(Noor et al., 2019)
	Collagen in the human heart at various scales was engineered by 3D bioprinting.	(Lee et al., 2019a)
2020	A handheld 3D bioprinter for printing biocompatible materials, including stem cells, for performing in situ surgical repairs was patented.	(Thorpe et al., 2020)
	The company ASPECT BIOSYSTEMS created the first bioprinted tissue (3DBioRing™ AIRWAY) capable of accurately replicating the acute bronchoconstriction events witnessed during an asthma attack.	(Dickman et al., 2020)
2021	The cosmetic company L'Oreal (Aulnay-sous-Bois, France) developed 3D-printed skin tissues. The created tissues replicated the complex and heterogeneous nature of native human skin in in vitro models for product testing.	(Madiedo-Podvrsan et al., 2021)
	The bioprinting company ADVANCED SOLUTIONS (Louisville, KY, United States) launched the series of BioAssemblyBot® bioprinters that were already patented in 2018.	(Golway et al., 2018)
2022	The world's first universal bioink allows scaffold-free bioprinting products for patients with peripheral artery diseases.	(Ilic and Liovic, 2022)
	The use of an automated fabrication of a 3D human liver model supplemented with human adipose microvessels.	(Moss et al., 2022)
2023	The 3D printing of a living and operational heart valve with the capacity to undergo development and synchronize growth with the surrounding cardiac tissue.	(Jafari et al., 2023)

4.   The Pioneers of 3D Bioprinting

In the last decade, many companies have developed bioprinters based on different bioprinting technologies. Hereinafter, the pioneering bioprinters are presented according to different

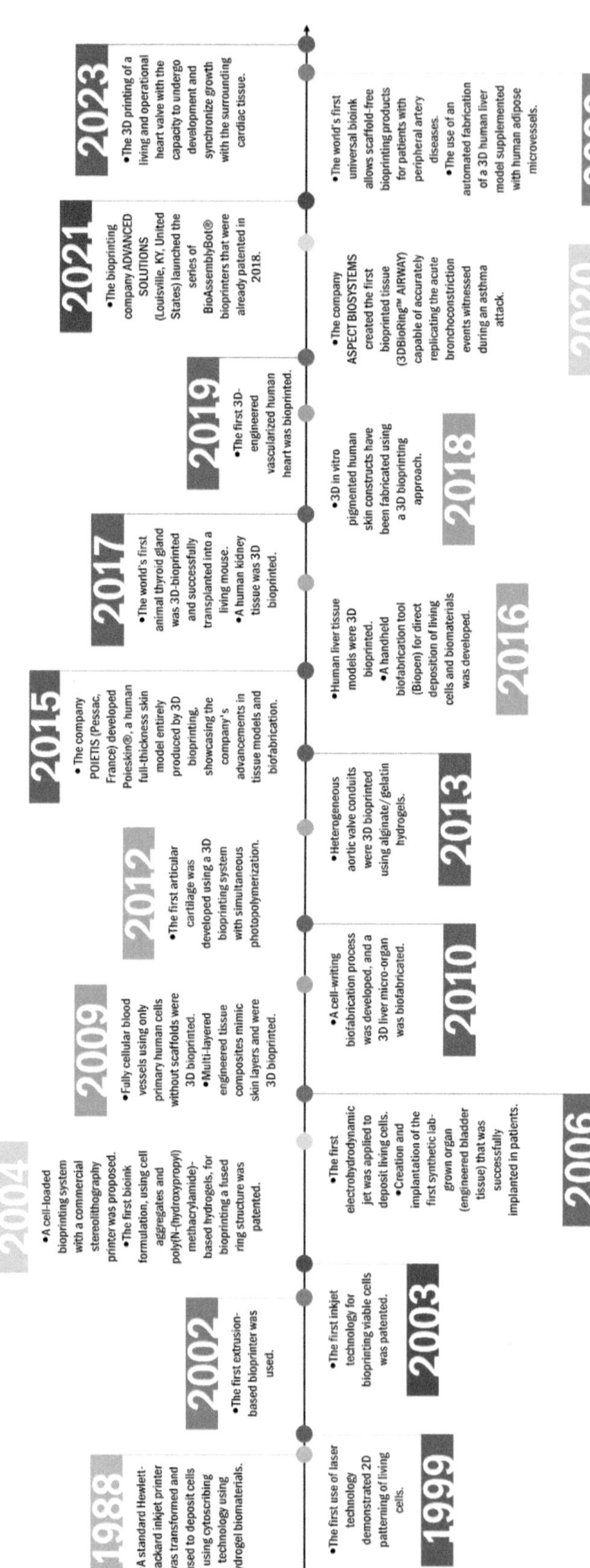

Fig. 4 A brief timeline of different key events in the bioprinting evolution.

bioprinting methods such as extrusion-based, droplet-based, laser-assisted, and vat polymerization-based bioprinting. Other than these pioneering bioprinters, several other companies (not cited hereinafter) use value add-ons to provide more affordable and accessible 3D bioprinters. These advancements highlight the significant contributions of these bioprinting technologies to the fields of tissue engineering and regenerative medicine, paving the way for innovative applications and breakthroughs in the creation of complex biological structures. Information regarding the described 3D bioprinter companies is provided in Table 2.

4.1 ADVANCED SOLUTIONS

In 2019, the company ADVANCED SOLUTIONS (Louisville, KY, United States) introduced the BioBot Basic bioprinter. It is the world's first polar coordinate-based bioprinter. It is a small yet powerful entry-level bioprinter designed for researchers and academics. The bioprinter uses extrusion bioprinting technology (Cambron, 2020). The BioBot Basic bioprinter's accomplishments in 3D bioprinting extend beyond organ-specific constructs to include foundational technologies such as microscaffolds and bioinks (Aleman et al., 2021; Dikici et al., 2020; Rousselle et al., 2022). Since then, the company has made significant advancements in the field of bioprinting with the BioAssemblyBot® bioprinter. It utilizes a six-axis bioprinter featuring a robotic arm for the precise deposition of various materials in 3D space, facilitating the process of multi-material bioprinting. Moreover, this bioprinter has played a crucial role in various cutting-edge research projects, demonstrating its versatility and impact in the fields of tissue engineering and regenerative medicine (Moss et al., 2022). Some notable achievements include the contour skin printing platform, developed in 2018, which utilized the BioAssemblyBot® for contoured skin printing. In 2019, a "heart attack patch" using the BioAssemblyBot® had been created, demonstrating its potential in tissue engineering and regenerative medicine. In the same year, the company ADVANCED SOLUTIONS was awarded a patent for a vascularized *in-vitro* perfusion module, showcasing the technology's innovation created by 3D bioprinting (Golway and Hoying, 2019). In 2021, the company launched its BioAssemblyBot® series of bioprinters. BioAssemblyBot® 200, a versatile four-axis robotic 3D bioprinter, and BioAssemblyBot® 500, a six-axis biosafety cabinet bioprinter, are expanding their product offerings. The company is also planning a coordinated project with NASA for 2024, further demonstrating its commitment to innovation and collaboration.

4.2 CLUSTER TECHNOLOGY

The company CLUSTER TECHNOLOGY (Osaka, Japan), presented the DeskViewer™, operating on the principle of piezo-electronic inkjet printing. This system features four injectors with varying nozzle sizes, enabling the loading and printing of diverse cell types or protein solutions. Additionally, it provides flexibility, as the volume and diameter of the drops from the nozzle can be modified and adapted as needed (Fatimi et al., 2022). The company has achieved a significant milestone in the realm of 3D bioprinting by successfully creating human liver tissue chips (Matsusaki et al., 2013). This accomplishment represents a breakthrough in the field of organ-on-a-chip technology, offering a novel and advanced platform for studying human liver function in a controlled and physiologically relevant environment.

4.3 GESIM

The company GESIM (Radeberg, Germany) developed the BioScaffolder® bioprinter for versatile bioprinting applications. This system enables the bioprinting of diverse hard and soft biopolymers, whether with or without cells. It specializes in designing and bioprinting porous and multi-biomaterial structures tailored for tissue engineering (Fatimi et al., 2022). The BioScaffolder® employs advanced techniques such as sequential bioprinting, coaxial extrusion, and nanoliter pipetting (Klüver et al., 2022). The company's achievements in 3D bioprinting extend across multiple medical domains, including pelvic floor dysfunction, dentistry, cardiology, and oncology (Gaetani et al., 2012; Jiang et al., 2017; Jiang et al., 2020; Paul et al., 2019; Thattaruparambil Raveendran et al., 2019).

4.4 ENVISIONTEC

In the year 2000, the company ENVISIONTEC (Dearborn, MI, United States), a prominent player in the global 3D printing industry, pioneered the creation of the inaugural commercial extrusion-based 3D Bioplotter® bioprinter. This bioprinter, originally conceived by Mulhapt's group at the University of Freiburg, was subsequently brought to the commercial market through ENVISIONTEC's efforts (Pereira et al., 2018). The 3D Bioplotter® is a versatile rapid prototyping tool used for processing a variety of biomaterials for computer-aided tissue engineering. It is capable of processing a wide range of biomaterials, including hydrogels, soft polymers, and bioceramics (Fatimi et al., 2022). The system is designed to create 3D scaffolds with a defined outer form and an open inner structure, making them suitable for applications in bone regeneration, cell and organ printing, cartilage and skin production, and other tissue engineering fields (Chang et al., 2014; Jain et al., 2020; Wang et al., 2016; Yu et al., 2019; Zhou et al., 2020).

4.5 REGENHU

In 2009, the company REGENHU (Villaz-St-Pierre, Switzerland) launched its first instrument for bioprinting. The Biofactory®, which is an eight-printhead bioprinter in a biosafety enclosure, is designed to support various bioprinting modalities, encompassing both extrusion- and droplet-based techniques. This system facilitates the utilization of a diverse array of biomaterials, such as photocrosslinkable hydrogels, proteins, and high-viscosity biomaterials (Fatimi et al., 2022). Additionally, Biofactory® is an integrated system housed within a laminar flow hood, ensuring a sterile environment with precise control over temperature, humidity, and gas composition. On the other hand, the second bioprinter developed, 3D Discovery® Evolution, offers the capability to handle both macro and nano dimensions within a single instrument. It has the ability to generate tissue architectures that closely resemble those found in nature. With a diverse range of 11 printhead technologies integrated into a single instrument, this system allows for versatile applications (Fatimi et al., 2022). Furthermore, users have the flexibility to modify and adapt the configuration and specifications according to their requirements. The company's achievements in 3D bioprinting encompass a broad spectrum of tissues, ranging from cartilage and bone to cardiac and skin-related constructs (Bucciarelli et al., 2022; Horváth et al., 2015; Ng et al., 2018; Ng et al., 2016; Noor et al., 2019; Peiffer et al., 2020; Schwab et al., 2020; Somasekharan et al., 2020; Tan and Yeong, 2015). This versatility positions them at the forefront of regenerative medicine, with the potential to revolutionize medical interventions across multiple specialties.

4.6 ORGANOVO

In 2009, the company ORGANOVO (San Diego, CA, United States) introduced the NovoGen MMX™ bioprinter, a multi-material bioprinter relying on extrusion technology. The NovoGen MMX™ is a bioprinter capable of creating biological tissues such as liver, kidneys, intestines, skin, pancreas, and more. It includes two printheads, one for extracting cells and the other for hydrogels, scaffolds, or soft biomaterials (Choudhury et al., 2018a). This technology has been used in various studies to print structures composed of different types of cells and biomaterials, demonstrating its potential in tissue engineering and regenerative medicine (Fatimi et al., 2022). The company has made significant strides in the field of 3D bioprinting, achieving success in the fabrication of various complex biological structures. Notably, they have successfully produced kidney, tissue-engineered muscle, liver, and human intestinal tissue. (Bour et al., 2020; Lawlor et al., 2020; Madden et al., 2018; Norona et al., 2019). Although ORGANOVO no longer actively promotes this bioprinter, it continues to supply it primarily to pharmaceutical companies for applications such as drug screening (Thazhathukunnel et al., 2015).

4.7 ALLEVI

The company ALLEVI (Philadelphia, PA, United States) offered the Allevi bioprinter, which employs LED photocuring utilizing blue and UV light (Fatimi et al., 2022). This system facilitates working with various biomaterials. More recently, the Allevi 3 bioprinter was introduced. It is a pneumatic extrusion-based bioprinter that features a three-extruder system, allowing quick printing of multi-cell tissues and creating complex structures. With the option for photocuring in visible or UV light, the Allevi 3 supports a wide range of bioinks and biomaterials. Furthermore, the heated print bed offers temperature control, accommodating various material viscosities. The company's accomplishments extend to orthopedic applications through the 3D bioprinting of bone tissue, a crucial development for bone grafts and replacements (Roopavath et al., 2019; Sjöholm et al., 2020). In addition to these achievements, the company has engineered a liver model and cell-laden hydrogels, as well as different veterinary dosage forms (Ji et al., 2019; Mazzocchi et al., 2019; Moses et al., 2020).

4.8 ASPECT BIOSYSTEMS

The company ASPECT BIOSYSTEMS (Vancouver, BC, Canada) developed the RX1™ bioprinter powered by the Lab-on-a-Printer™ microfluidic technology (Beyer et al., 2014). The patented platform is a brand-new way of bioprinting, designed specifically to biofabricate physiologically complex and heterogeneous human tissues in a personalized manner for various applications in the life sciences. Moreover, this innovative technology enables the bioprinting of tissues with high cell densities, ensuring both high viability and a preserved phenotype. The RX1™ achieves this by utilizing low-viscosity biomaterials in its manufacturing process (Bsoul et al., 2016). Like ORGANOVO, the company ASPECT BIOSYSTEM exclusively offers its bioprinters through partnership programs. The company partners with both academic and industry specialists to create an array of intricate 3D tissue models representing various diseases, including neural, kidney, and liver toxicity, cardiotoxicity, and 3D cancer models (Abelseth et al., 2019; Addario et al., 2020; Dickman et al., 2020; Lee et al., 2019b; Sharma et al., 2020).

Besides introducing the RX1™ bioprinter, ASPECT BIOSYSTEMS has made significant strides in the creation and validation of bioprinted tissues for preclinical drug testing and transplantation. A noteworthy achievement includes the development of the 3DBioRing™ AIRWAY, the inaugural bioprinted tissue capable of faithfully reproducing acute bronchoconstriction events observed during an asthma attack. This breakthrough marks a substantial success and signifies a revolutionary advancement in the realm of biomedical research (Dickman et al., 2020).

4.9 INVENTIA LIFE SCIENCE

The company INVENTIA LIFE SCIENCE (Alexandria, Australia) developed RASTRUM™ bioprinter (Fatimi et al., 2022). This bioprinter has been built for 3D cell biology, accelerating drug discovery and biomedical research. It is based on drop-on-demand technology that facilitates the deposition of nanoliter droplets containing cells and matrix components, enabling the construction of 3D cell models in this manner (Mahmodi et al., 2021). The company has made significant strides in the field of 3D bioprinting, achieving success in the fabrication of various complex biological structures. Notably, they have successfully produced scaffolds for drug screening assays on cancer cells and drug testing platforms for breast cancer, a breakthrough with implications for multicellular models for drug discovery. Furthermore, the company has demonstrated the capability to 3D bioprint multicellular spheroids and liver models (Bock et al., 2023; Engel et al., 2022; Jung et al., 2022; Sullivan et al., 2023; Utama et al., 2020; Westhaus et al., 2023).

4.10 POIETIS

The NGB-R™ is a 4D bioprinting platform developed by the company POIETIS (Pessac, France) that is characterized by high precision and resolution. It features embedded in-line monitoring systems that can control the quality of each bioprinted layer, enabling the manufacture of controlled 3D cell structures and reproducible tissue models. The NGB-R™ bioprinter is a multimodal bioprinting system that combines laser-assisted, micro-valve, and extrusion bioprinting, offering true versatility in bioprinting from cells to spheroids and providing the possibility to work with a wide range of biomaterials and hydrogels (Aleman et al., 2021). The NGB-R™ is the first commercially available instrument to boast laser-assisted bioprinting, allowing for the deposition of microdroplets of cell bioink with a precision of a few microns . The company POIETIS has also developed Poieskin®, a full-thickness human skin model entirely produced by 3D bioprinting, showcasing the company's advancements in tissue models and biofabrication (Cadau et al., 2017).

4.11 REVOTEK

In 2015, the company REVOTEK (Sichuan, China) introduced the 3D blood vessel bioprinter. This bioprinter is based on scaffold-free bioprinting and relies on proprietary biosphere technology, making it particularly well-suited for crafting scaffold-free vascular structures. The company achieved a groundbreaking milestone by successfully 3D printing living, functional blood vessels using stem cells in a Rhesus monkey. The bioink used for the bioprinting process was made from stem cells derived from the fat tissue of monkeys in a microenvironment of growth factors and nutrients that can stimulate the cells to grow into the types of cells needed to form a functioning blood vessel. Furthermore, they successfully integrated these artificial vessels with the existing cells in the monkey's body (Kang and Zuo, 2016).

4.12 REGEMAT 3D

The company REGEMAT 3D (Granada, Spain) developed the Bio V1 bioprinter. It is optimized for osteochondral tissues and can be used in other applications as well. It features exchangeable printheads, allowing for a wide range of applications. More recently, the company introduced the REG4LIFE bioprinter. REGEMAT 3D's bioprinting systems have undergone optimization and validation for the precise printing of various tissue types such as cartilage, skin, bone, and cardiac tissue (Antich et al., 2020; Jiménez et al., 2017; Oberdiek et al., 2021; Zafeiris et al., 2021). Additionally, with the modular and exchangeable printing heads technology, these systems are designed to seamlessly operate with a diverse range of biomaterials, including, among others, collagen, nanocellulose, and thermoplastics.

4.13 CELLINK

The company CELLINK (Gothenburg, Sweden) introduced the Inkredible+™ bioprinter, which is a pneumatic-based extrusion system. This bioprinter allows 3D bioprinting with different cell types and bioinks in the same structure, and it supports a broad spectrum of biomaterials, including those that may exhibit high viscosity at room temperature. The dual heated printheads enable the printing of a wide variety of biomaterials, and the built-in UV crosslinking system allows for quick and easy bioprinting of living tissues. Furthermore, the company CELLINK developed a second bioprinter model. The BIO X™ is a 3D bioprinter that seamlessly integrates three distinct printheads. Operating on the extrusion principle, it has the capability to design structures using various cell types, such as endothelial cells, stem cells, or fibroblasts. Additionally, the BIO X™ is equipped with a germicidal UV light system, enabling the sterilization of the printing environment through light. In a more recent development, CELLINK unveiled the BIO X6™ bioprinter. This advanced system is equipped with six printheads, allowing the creation of multimaterial constructs

Table 2   Information concerning companies of 3D bioprinters.

Company (Headsquar)	Foundation	Fields	Products	Bioprinters	Bioprinted tissues or organs	References
ADVANCED SOLUTIONS (Louisville, KY, United States)	1987	3D bioprinting; Human microvessels; Tissue constructs.	Bioprinters and software; Bioprinting supplies; Biomaterials and bioinks; Incubators and perfusion systems.	BioBot Basic®	Microscaffolds for cell culture; Bioinks for tissue engineering of functional constructs; Human skin model.	(Rousselle *et al.*, 2022) (Aleman *et al.*, 2021) (Dikici *et al.*, 2020)
				BioAssemblyBot®	3D human liver model.	(Moss *et al.*, 2022)
CLUSTER TECHNOLOGY (Osaka, Japan)	1991	Nano-micromachining; Resin composite material technology; Chemical engineering; Electronic component.	Composite materials; 3D printers; Software; Micro droplet ejection devices; Inkjet heads.	DeskViewer™	Human liver tissue chips.	(Matsusaki *et al.*, 2013)
GESIM (Radeberg, Germany)	1995	Microarray technology; 3D bioprinting.	Instrumentation and microfluidics for microarrays; 3D bioprinters.	BioScaffolder®	Pelvic floor muscles; Periodontal tissue; Cardiac tissue; Multicellular tumor spheroids.	(Thattaruparambil Raveendran *et al.*, 2019) (Gaetani *et al.*, 2012) (Paul *et al.*, 2019) (Jiang *et al.*, 2020) (Jiang *et al.*, 2017)
ENVISIONTEC (Dearborn, MI, United States)	2002	3D printing; Printing materials.	Bioprinters; Biomaterial inks.	3D Bioplotter®	Blood vessels; Adipose tissue; Tracheal graft; Tooth tissue; Adipose tissue.	(Jain *et al.*, 2020) (Chang *et al.*, 2014) (Zhou *et al.*, 2020) (Wang *et al.*, 2016) (Yu *et al.*, 2019)
REGENHU (Villaz-St-Pierre, Switzerland)	2007	3D bioprinting; Human skin printing; Personalized medicine; Cellular drug discovery models.	Bioprinters; Bioprinting management software; Human cellular models; Human skin.	3D Discovery® Evolution	Cartilage tissue constructs; Engineered biological tissues; Constructs for bone regeneration; Cardiac patches.	(Somasekharan *et al.*, 2020) (Schwab *et al.*, 2020) (Peiffer *et al.*, 2020) (Bucciarelli *et al.*, 2022) (Noor *et al.*, 2019)
				Biofactory®	Skin; Air-blood tissue barrier; Skin tissue regeneration; 3D tubular construct.	(Ng *et al.*, 2018) (Ng *et al.*, 2016) (Horváth *et al.*, 2015) (Tan & Yeong, 2015)
				R-GEN series	No data	N/A

Contd.

Table 2 *Contd.*

Company (Headsquar)	Foundation	Fields	Products	Bioprinters	Bioprinted tissues or organs	References
ORGANOVO (San Diego, CA, United States)	2007	Bioprinted tissues; 3D bioprinting; Cell 3D models; Disease models.	Bioprinters; Bioprinted human tissues.	NovoGen MMX™	Kidney; Tissue-engineered muscle; Liver; Human intestinal tissue.	(Bour *et al.*, 2020) (Lawlor *et al.*, 2020) (Madden *et al.*, 2018) (Norona *et al.*, 2019)
ALLEVI (Philadelphia, PA, United States)	2013	3D bioprinting.	Bioprinters; Software; Biomaterial inks.	Allevi	Veterinary dosage forms; Bone graft; Osteochondral constructs; Cell-laden hydrogels; Liver model.	(Moses *et al.*, 2020) (Sjöholm *et al.*, 2020) (Roopavath *et al.*, 2019) (Ji *et al.*, 2019) (Mazzocchi *et al.*, 2019)
ASPECT BIOSYSTEMS (Vancouver, BC, Canada)	2013	3D bioprinting; Disease models; Therapeutics Bioprinted tissues; Tissue Engineering.	Bioprinters; Bioprinted tissues.	RX1™	Engineered neural tissues; Brain tissue; Renal tissue; 3D contractile smooth muscle tissues; Neural tissues.	(Sharma *et al.*, 2020) (Lee *et al.*, 2019b) (Addario *et al.*, 2020) (Dickman *et al.*, 2020) (Abelseth *et al.*, 2019)
INVENTIA LIFE SCIENCE (Alexandria, Australia)	2013	3D bioprinting; 3D biological constructs; 3D cell models; Drug discovery.	Bioprinters; 3D cell culture platforms; Hydrogels.	RASTRUM™	Scaffolds for drug screening assay on cancer cells; Multicellular spheroids; Multicellular models for drug discovery; Drug testing platforms for breast cancer; Liver models.	(Engel *et al.*, 2022) (Utama *et al.*, 2020) (Jung *et al.*, 2022) (Sullivan *et al.*, 2023) (Bock *et al.*, 2023) (Westhaus *et al.*, 2023)
POIETIS (Pessac, France)	2014	3D/4D bioprinting.	3D bioprinters; Bioprinted full thickness human skin model.	NGB-R™	Skin model; Functional mesenchymal stem cells patterns.	(Cadau *et al.*, 2017) (Pages *et al.*, 2015)
REVOTEK (Chengdu, China)	2014	Bioprinted organs; 3D bioprinting; Regenerative medicine; Medical imaging.	Bioprinters; Bioinks; 3D imaging software.	T-Series™	3D bioprinted blood vessels and implantation in rhesus monkeys.	(Kang & Zuo, 2016)

Contd.

Table 2 *Contd.*

Company (Headsquar)	Foundation	Fields	Products	Bioprinters	Bioprinted tissues or organs	References
REGEMAT 3D (Granada, Spain)	2015	Bioprinting systems; Regenerative medicine; Cell Therapies; Tissue engineering.	3D bioprinters; Software; Bioreactors; Biomaterials.	Bio V1	Bone tissue; Articular cartilage constructs.	(Antich *et al.*, 2020) (Zafeiris *et al.*, 2021) (Jiménez *et al.*, 2017)
				REG4LIFE	Bone substitute scaffolds.	(Oberdiek *et al.*, 2021)
CELLINK (Gothenburg, Sweden)	2016	Bioprocessing; Drug discovery; Molecular biology; 3D Bioprinting; Tissue Engineering.	Bioprinters; Software; Bioreactors; Bioinks and biomaterials; Tissue engineering kits; Cells and media.	Inkredible+™	Cartilage and skin tissue; Vascularized soft tissues; Skin constructs.	(Thayer *et al.*, 2018) (Shie *et al.*, 2020) (Lee *et al.*, 2020)
				BIO X™	Engineered neural tissues; Skin constructs; Wound dressing; Bone tissue; Autologous fat grafts.	(Ngo *et al.*, 2020) (Shie *et al.*, 2020) (Ramesh *et al.*, 2020) (Naseri *et al.*, 2020) (Oskarsdotter *et al.*, 2023)
				BIO X6™	Tissue-engineered heart valves.	(Jafari *et al.*, 2023)

using a combination of crosslinking modalities. Furthermore, this capability enables the fabrication of more intricate structures and the development of physiologically relevant models. The company's achievements in 3D bioprinting span a diverse range of tissues and organs, from cartilage and skin to neural tissues, bones, and heart valves (Jafari et al., 2023; Lee et al., 2020; Naseri et al., 2020; Ngo et al., 2020; Oskarsdotter et al., 2023; Ramesh et al., 2020; Shie et al., 2020; Thayer et al., 2018). These advancements collectively represent a groundbreaking contribution to regenerative medicine, potentially revolutionizing transplantation, personalized medicine, and therapeutic interventions across various medical disciplines.

5.   Future Challenges and Opportunities

Despite its potential, there are remaining challenges to be overcome in 3D bioprinting. One of the main challenges is finding suitable printing materials with excellent printability, biocompatibility, and desired mechanical properties (Mao et al., 2020). Another challenge is vascularization, which is crucial for constructing biomimetic structures like lung tissue (Barreiro Carpio et al., 2021). Additionally, future challenges in 3D bioprinting include preserving microscale and submicroscale resolution while enabling high-throughput and volumetric construct fabrication, as well as breaking the resolution limits, optimizing bioink composition, and developing new printing strategies to improve the technology's capabilities (Zandrini et al., 2023). Finally, 3D bioprinting technologies present a regulatory challenge due to the inclusion of living cells in the fabrication process. Traditional regulatory frameworks are designed for mass-manufactured therapies, posing complexities for the regulation of bespoke 3D bioprinted solutions (Mladenovska et al., 2023).

As the technology advances, it is expected to have a significant impact on regenerative medicine, drug screening, and personalized tissue engineering (Kačarević et al., 2018). 3D bioprinting, amid its challenges, offers transformative opportunities across various domains. One of its most promising prospects lies in personalized medicine, where the technology enables the creation of customized tissues and organs tailored to individual patient needs (Lam et al., 2023). This potential revolutionizes medical treatments, offering more effective and targeted solutions. In the realm of drug testing and development, bioprinted tissues provide a sophisticated platform for more accurate assessments, reducing reliance on animal testing and expediting the drug development process (Gao et al., 2021). The field of tissue engineering and regenerative medicine is significantly advanced by 3D bioprinting, offering solutions for organ transplantation and the repair of damaged tissues. Advancements in materials science further enhance the technology's capabilities, with ongoing research yielding novel biomaterials that improve biocompatibility and overall performance (Saini et al., 2021). The collaborative nature of 3D bioprinting, involving biologists, engineers, materials scientists, and clinicians, presents an opportunity for interdisciplinary innovation (Gu et al., 2020). Education and training in the medical field are transformed, allowing surgeons to hone their skills through practice on 3D-printed models before engaging in complex procedures. Moreover, the technology holds promise for space exploration, where on-demand organ and tissue fabrication could prove vital for the health and well-being of astronauts on long-duration space missions (Majumder and Ghosh, 2023). As 3D bioprinting continues to advance, its myriad opportunities promise to reshape healthcare, pharmaceuticals, education, and even space exploration, offering a glimpse into a future where precision medicine and regenerative therapies become commonplace (Ramadan and Zourob, 2021).

Conclusions and Remarks

The history of 3D bioprinting is a captivating journey marked by significant technological milestones and groundbreaking achievements. Over the years, researchers and companies have tirelessly pushed the boundaries of science and engineering to revolutionize the field of regenerative medicine. Several key conclusions and remarks can be drawn from the history of 3D bioprinting:

- *Evolution of technology:* The history of 3D bioprinting reflects a rapid evolution of technology. From its humble beginnings as a concept to the present-day capability of creating complex human tissues and organs, the technological advancements have been remarkable. The refinement of bioprinting techniques, materials, and precision has played a pivotal role in the field's progress.
- *Diverse applications:* The achievements in 3D bioprinting have led to diverse applications across various medical disciplines. The ability to print tissues such as cartilage, bone, skin, and even complex organs like the heart demonstrates the versatility of this technology. These achievements have profound implications for transplantation, personalized medicine, and therapeutic interventions.
- *Organ-on-a-chip technology:* The development of human tissue chips, such as the human liver tissue chip, represents a significant stride in creating more accurate models for drug testing and disease research. Organ-on-a-chip technology allows for the simulation of physiological conditions, enabling more reliable and predictive outcomes in drug development.
- *Bioinks and scaffolds:* The refinement of bioinks and the creation of micro scaffolds for cell culture showcase the importance of the materials used in bioprinting. Tailoring bioinks and scaffolds for specific tissues and applications enhances the precision and functionality of bioprinted constructs, contributing to the success of tissue engineering endeavors.
- *Challenges and future prospects:* Despite the remarkable achievements, challenges persist, including the need for vascularization in larger constructs, ensuring long-term viability, and addressing ethical considerations. Looking ahead, ongoing research aims to overcome these challenges, and the future of 3D bioprinting holds promise for more complex, functional tissues and organs.
- *Interdisciplinary collaboration:* The history of 3D bioprinting underscores the importance of interdisciplinary collaboration between experts in biology, materials science, engineering, and medicine. This collaborative effort has been essential in advancing the field and tackling complex challenges from various angles.

In conclusion, the history of 3D bioprinting is a testament to human ingenuity and the relentless pursuit of innovative solutions to pressing medical challenges. As the field continues to progress, the potential for transformative impact on healthcare and medical research remains high, opening doors to new possibilities in regenerative medicine and beyond.

References

Abelseth, E., Abelseth, L., De la Vega, L., Beyer, S.T. and Wadsworth, S.J. et al. (2019). 3D Printing of Neural Tissues Derived from Human Induced Pluripotent Stem Cells Using a Fibrin-Based Bioink. *ACS Biomaterials Science & Engineering, 5*(1), 234–243. doi: 10.1021/acsbiomaterials.8b01235.

Addario, G., Djudjaj, S., Farè, S., Boor, P. and Moroni, L. et al. (2020). Microfluidic bioprinting towards a renal in vitro model. *Bioprinting, 20*, e00108. doi: 10.1016/j.bprint.2020.e00108.

Agarwal, S., Saha, S., Balla, V.K., Pal, A. and Barui, A. et al. (2020). Current Developments in 3D Bioprinting for Tissue and Organ Regeneration–A Review. *Frontiers in Mechanical Engineering, 6.* doi: 10.3389/fmech.2020.589171.

Aleman, J., Sivakumar, H., DePalma, T., Zhou, Y. and Mazzocchi, A. et al. (2021). Engineering a thixotropic and biochemically tunable hyaluronan and collagen bioink for biofabrication of multiple tissue construct types. *bioRxiv,* 2021.2009.2001.458584. doi: 10.1101/2021.09.01.458584.

Antich, C., de Vicente, J., Jiménez, G., Chocarro, C. and Carrillo, E. et al. (2020). Bio-inspired hydrogel composed of hyaluronic acid and alginate as a potential bioink for 3D bioprinting of articular cartilage engineering constructs. *Acta Biomater, 106*, 114–123. doi: 10.1016/j.actbio.2020.01.046.

Atala, A., Bauer, S.B., Soker, S., Yoo, J.J. and Retik, A.B. et al. (2006). Tissue-engineered autologous bladders for patients needing cystoplasty. *The Lancet, 367*(9518), 1241–1246. doi: 10.1016/s0140-6736(06)68438-9.

Barreiro Carpio, M., Dabaghi, M., Ungureanu, J., Kolb, M. R. and Hirota, J.A. et al. (2021). 3D Bioprinting Strategies, Challenges, and Opportunities to Model the Lung Tissue Microenvironment and Its Function. *Frontiers in Bioengineering and Biotechnology, 9.* doi: 10.3389/fbioe.2021.773511.

Beyer, S.T., Walus, K., Mohamed, T. and Bsoul, A.A.M. (2014). Canada. Patent Application: CA2915737A1.

Bock, N., Forouz, F., Hipwood, L., Clegg, J. and Jeffery, P. et al. (2023). GelMA, Click-Chemistry Gelatin and Bioprinted Polyethylene Glycol-Based Hydrogels as 3D Ex Vivo Drug Testing Platforms for Patient-Derived Breast Cancer Organoids. *Pharmaceutics, 15*(1), 261.

Boland, T., Wilson, W.C. and Xu, T. (2006). United States. Granted Patent: US7051654B2.

Bour, R.K., Sharma, P.R., Turner, J.S., Hess, W.E. and Mintz, E.L. et al. (2020). Bioprinting on sheet-based scaffolds applied to the creation of implantable tissue-engineered constructs with potentially diverse clinical applications: Tissue-Engineered Muscle Repair (TEMR) as a representative testbed. *Connective Tissue Research, 61*(2), 216–228. doi: 10.1080/03008207.2019.1679800.

Bsoul, A., Pan, S., Cretu, E., Stoeber, B. and Walus, K. et al. (2016). Design, microfabrication, and characterization of a moulded PDMS/SU-8 inkjet dispenser for a Lab-on-a-Printer platform technology with disposable microfluidic chip. *Lab on a Chip, 16*(17), 3351–3361. doi: 10.1039/c6lc00636a.

Bucciarelli, A., Petretta, M., Grigolo, B., Gambari, L. and Bossi, A.M. et al. (2022). Methacrylated Silk Fibroin Additive Manufacturing of Shape Memory Constructs with Possible Application in Bone Regeneration. *Gels, 8*(12), 833. doi: 10.3390/gels8120833.

Bulanova, E.A., Koudan, E.V., Degosserie, J., Heymans, C. and Pereira, F.D.A.S. et al., (2017). Bioprinting of a functional vascularized mouse thyroid gland construct. *Biofabrication, 9*(3), 034105. doi: 10.1088/1758-5090/aa7fdd.

Cadau, S., Rival, D., Valerie, A., Chavan, M. and Fayol, D. et al. (2017). New bioprinted skin, cosmetic *in vitro* model. *Journal of Cosmetic Science, 68*(1), 85–90. doi: pubmed.ncbi.nlm.nih.gov/29465388.

Cambron, S. D. (2020). United States. Granted Patent: US10875243B2.

Chang, J.W., Park, S.A., Park, J.-K., Choi, J.W. and Kim, Y.-S. et al. (2014). Tissue-Engineered Tracheal Reconstruction Using Three-Dimensionally Printed Artificial Tracheal Graft: Preliminary Report. *Artif Organs, 38*(6), E95-E105. doi: 10.1111/aor.12310.

Chang, R., Emami, K., Wu, H. and Sun, W. (2010). Biofabrication of a three-dimensional liver micro-organ as an in vitro drug metabolism model. *Biofabrication, 2*(4), 045004. doi: 10.1088/1758-5082/2/4/045004.

Choudhury, D., Anand, S. and Naing, M.W. (2018a). The Arrival of Commercial Bioprinters - Towards 3D Bioprinting Revolution! *International Journal of Bioprinting, 4*(2), 1–20. doi: 10.18063/ijb.v4i2.139.

Choudhury, D., Tun, H.W., Wang, T. and Naing, M.W. (2018b). Organ-Derived Decellularized Extracellular Matrix: A Game Changer for Bioink Manufacturing? *Trends in Biotechnology, 36*(8), 787–805. doi: 10.1016/j.tibtech.2018.03.003.

Colosi, C., Shin, S.R., Manoharan, V., Massa, S. and Costantini, M. et al. (2016). Microfluidic Bioprinting of Heterogeneous 3D Tissue Constructs Using Low-Viscosity Bioink. *Advanced Materials, 28*(4), 677–684. doi: 10.1002/adma.201503310.

Cui, X., Breitenkamp, K., Finn, M.G., Lotz, M. and D'Lima, D.D. et al. (2012). Direct Human Cartilage Repair Using Three-Dimensional Bioprinting Technology. *Tissue Engineering Part A, 18*(11-12), 1304–1312. doi: 10.1089/ten.tea.2011.0543.

Dhariwala, B., Hunt, E. and Boland, T. (2004). Rapid Prototyping of Tissue-Engineering Constructs, Using Photopolymerizable Hydrogels and Stereolithography. *Tissue Engineering, 10*(9-10), 1316–1322. doi: 10.1089/ten.2004.10.1316.

Dickman, C.T.D., Russo, V., Thain, K., Pan, S. and Beyer, S.T. et al. (2020). Functional characterization of 3D contractile smooth muscle tissues generated using a unique microfluidic 3D bioprinting technology. *The FASEB Journal, 34*(1), 1652-1664. doi: 10.1096/fj.20190106 Dikici, S., Claeyssens, F., & MacNeil, S. (2020). Bioengineering Vascular Networks to Study Angiogenesis and Vascularization of Physiologically Relevant Tissue Models in Vitro. *ACS Biomaterials Science & Engineering, 6*(6), 3513–3528. doi: 10.1021/acsbiomaterials.0c00191.

Duan, B., Hockaday, L.A., Kang, K.H. and Butcher, J.T. (2013). 3D Bioprinting of heterogeneous aortic valve conduits with alginate/gelatin hydrogels. *Journal of Biomedical Materials Research Part A, 101A*(5), 1255–1264. doi: 10.1002/jbm.a.34420.

Duchi, S., Onofrillo, C., O'Connell, C.D., Blanchard, R. and Augustine, C. et al. (2017). Handheld Co-Axial Bioprinting: Application to *in situ* surgical cartilage repair. *Scientific Reports, 7*(1), 5837. doi: 10.1038/s41598-017-05699-x.

Engel, M., Belfiore, L., Aghaei, B. and Sutija, M. (2022). Enabling high throughput drug discovery in 3D cell cultures through a novel bioprinting workflow. *SLAS Technology, 27*(1), 32–38. doi: 10.1016/j.slast.2021.10.002.

Fatimi, A., Okoro, O.V., Podstawczyk, D., Siminska-Stanny, J. and Shavandi, A. et al. (2022). Natural hydrogel-based bio-Inks for 3D bioprinting in tissue engineering: A review. *Gels, 8*(3), 179. doi: 10.3390/gels8030179.

Forgacs, G., Jakab, K., Neagu, A. and Mironov, V. (2012). United States. Granted Patent: US8241905B2.

Foty, R.A., Pfleger, C.M., Forgacs, G. and Steinberg, M.S. (1996). Surface tensions of embryonic tissues predict their mutual envelopment behavior. *Development, 122*(5), 1611–1620. doi: pubmed.ncbi.nlm.nih.gov/8625847.

Gaetani, R., Doevendans, P.A., Metz, C.H. G., Alblas, J. and Messina, E. et al. (2012). Cardiac tissue engineering using tissue printing technology and human cardiac progenitor cells. *Biomaterials, 33*(6), 1782-1790. doi: 10.1016/j.biomaterials.2011.11.003.

Gao, G., Ahn, M., Cho, W.-W., Kim, B.-S. and Cho, D.-W et al. (2021). 3D Printing of Pharmaceutical Application: Drug Screening and Drug Delivery. *Pharmaceutics, 13*(9), 1373.

Gao, Q., He, Y., Fu, J.-z., Liu, A. and Ma, L. et al. (2015). Coaxial nozzle-assisted 3D bioprinting with built-in microchannels for nutrients delivery. *Biomaterials, 61*, 203–215. doi: 10.1016/j.biomaterials.2015.05.031.

Golway, M., Palmer, J.C., Eli, J.K., Bartlett, J.D. and Collins, E.H et al. (2018). United States. Granted Patent: US9910935B2.

Golway, M.W. and Hoying, J.B. (2019). United States. Granted Patent: US10392595B2.

Gu, Z., Fu, J., Lin, H. and He, Y. (2020). Development of 3D bioprinting: From printing methods to biomedical applications. *Asian Journal of Pharmaceutical Sciences, 15*(5), 529–557. doi: 10.1016/j.ajps.2019.11.003.

Horváth, L., Umehara, Y., Jud, C., Blank, F. and Petri-Fink, A. et al. (2015). Engineering an in vitro air-blood barrier by 3D bioprinting. *Sci Rep, 5*(1), 7974. doi: 10.1038/srep07974.

Hull, C.W. (1986). United States. Granted Patent: US4575330A.

Ilic, D. and Liovic, M. (2022). Industry updates from the field of stem cell research and regenerative medicine in February 2022. *Regenerative Medicine, 17*(6), 327–336. doi: 10.2217/rme-2022-0046.

Jafari, A., Vahid Niknezhad, S., Kaviani, M., Saleh, W. and Wong, N. et al. (2023). Formulation and Evaluation of PVA/Gelatin/Carrageenan Inks for 3D Printing and Development of Tissue-Engineered Heart Valves. *Advanced Functional Materials, n/a*(n/a), 2305188. doi: 10.1002/adfm.202305188.

Jain, S., Yassin, M.A., Fuoco, T., Liu, H. and Mohamed-Ahmed, S. et al. (2020). Engineering 3D degradable, pliable scaffolds toward adipose tissue regeneration; optimized printability, simulations and surface modification. *Journal of Tissue Engineering, 11*, 2041731420954316. doi: 10.1177/2041731420954316.

Jansen, J., Thompson, J.M., Dugan, M.J., Nolan, P. and Wiemann, M.C. et al (2002). Peripheral Blood Progenitor Cell Transplantation. *Therapeutic Apheresis, 6*(1), 5-14. doi: 10.1046/j.1526-0968.2002.00392.x.

Jayasinghe, S.N., Qureshi, A.N. and Eagles, P.A.M. (2006). Electrohydrodynamic Jet Processing: An Advanced Electric-Field-Driven Jetting Phenomenon for Processing Living Cells. *Small, 2*(2), 216–219. doi: 10.1002/smll.200500291.

Ji, S., Almeida, E. and Guvendiren, M. (2019). 3D bioprinting of complex channels within cell-laden hydrogels. *Acta Biomater, 95*, 214–224. doi: 10.1016/j.actbio.2019.02.038.

Jiang, T., Munguia-Lopez, J.G., Flores-Torres, S., Grant, J. and Vijayakumar, S. et al. (2017). Directing the Self-assembly of Tumour Spheroids by Bioprinting Cellular Heterogeneous Models within Alginate/Gelatin Hydrogels. *Sci Rep, 7*(1), 4575. doi: 10.1038/s41598-017-04691-9.

Jiang, T., Munguia-Lopez, J.G., Gu, K., Bavoux, M.M. and Flores-Torres, S. et al., (2020). Engineering bioprintable alginate/gelatin composite hydrogels with tunable mechanical and cell adhesive properties to modulate tumor spheroid growth kinetics. *Biofabrication, 12*(1), 015024. doi: 10.1088/1758-5090/ab3a5c.

Jiménez, G., Antich, C., Marchal, J., Baena, J. and Sabata, R. et al. (2017). Design of 3D bioprinted articular cartilage of MSCs-loaded for osteochondral injuries. *Cytotherapy, 19*(5, Supplement), S27-S28. doi: 10.1016/j.jcyt.2017.02.056.

Jung, M., Skhinas, J.N., Du, E.Y., Tolentino, M.A.K. and Utama, R.H. et al. (2022). A high-throughput 3D bioprinted cancer cell migration and invasion model with versatile and broad biological applicability. *Biomaterials Science, 10*(20), 5876-5887. doi: 10.1039/d2bm00651k.

Kačarević, Ž.P., Rider, P.M., Alkildani, S., Retnasingh, S. and Smeets, R. et al. (2018). An Introduction to 3D Bioprinting: Possibilities, Challenges and Future Aspects. *Materials, 11*(11), 2199. doi: 10.3390/ma11112199.

Kang, H.-W., Lee, S.J., Ko, I.K., Kengla, C. and Yoo, J.J. et al. (2016). A 3D bioprinting system to produce human-scale tissue constructs with structural integrity. *Nat Biotechnol, 34*(3), 312–319. doi: 10.1038/nbt.3413.

Kang, Y. and Zuo, X. (2016). China. Patent Application: CN106039419A.

King, S.M., Higgins, J.W., Nino, C.R., Smith, T.R. and Paffenroth, E.H. et al. (2017). 3D Proximal Tubule Tissues Recapitulate Key Aspects of Renal Physiology to Enable Nephrotoxicity Testing. *Frontiers in Physiology, 8*(123). doi: 10.3389/fphys.2017.00123.

Klebe, R.J. (1988). Cytoscribing: A method for micropositioning cells and the construction of two- and three-dimensional synthetic tissues. *Experimental Cell Research, 179*(2), 362–373. doi: 10.1016/0014-4827(88)90275-3.

Klüver, E., Baltzer, M., Langer, A. and Meyer, M. (2022). Additive Manufacturing with Thermoplastic Collagen. *Polymers, 14*(5), 974.

Koch, L., Deiwick, A., Schlie, S., Michael, S. and Gruene, M. et al. (2012). Skin tissue generation by laser cell printing. *Biotechnology and Bioengineering, 109*(7), 1855–1863. doi: 10.1002/bit.24455.

Lam, E.H.Y., Yu, F., Zhu, S. and Wang, Z. et al. (2023). 3D Bioprinting for Next-Generation Personalized Medicine. *International Journal of Molecular Sciences, 24*(7), 6357.

Landers, R., Hübner, U., Schmelzeisen, R. and Mülhaupt, R. (2002). Rapid prototyping of scaffolds derived from thermoreversible hydrogels and tailored for applications in tissue engineering. *Biomaterials, 23*(23), 4437–4447. doi: 10.1016/S0142-9612(02)00139-4.

Lawlor, K.T., Vanslambrouck, J.M., Higgins, J.W., Chambon, A. and Bishard, K. et al. (2020). Cellular extrusion bioprinting improves kidney organoid reproducibility and conformation. *Nature Materials, 20*(2), 260–271. doi: 10.1038/s41563-020-00853-9.

Lee, A., Hudson, A.R., Shiwarski, D.J., Tashman, J.W. and Hinton, T.J. et al. (2019a). 3D bioprinting of collagen to rebuild components of the human heart. *Science, 365*(6452), 482–487. doi: 10.1126/science.aav9051.

Lee, C., Abelseth, E., de la Vega, L. and Willerth, S.M. (2019b). Bioprinting a novel glioblastoma tumor model using a fibrin-based bioink for drug screening. *Materials Today Chemistry, 12*, 78–84. doi: 10.1016/j.mtchem.2018.12.005.

Lee, S., Sani, E.S., Spencer, A.R., Guan, Y. and Weiss, A.S. et al. (2020). Human-Recombinant-Elastin-Based Bioinks for 3D Bioprinting of Vascularized Soft Tissues. *Advanced Materials, 32*(45), 2003915. doi: 10.1002/adma.202003915.

Lee, W., Debasitis, J.C., Lee, V.K., Lee, J.-H. and Fischer, K. et al. (2009). Multi-layered culture of human skin fibroblasts and keratinocytes through three-dimensional freeform fabrication. *Biomaterials, 30*(8), 1587–1595. doi: 10.1016/j.biomaterials.2008.12.009.

Levato, R., Webb, W.R., Otto, I.A., Mensinga, A. and Zhang, Y. et al. (2017). The bio in the ink: cartilage regeneration with bioprintable hydrogels and articular cartilage-derived progenitor cells. *Acta Biomater, 61*, 41–53. doi: 10.1016/j.actbio.2017.08.005.

Li, J., Chen, M., Fan, X. and Zhou, H. (2016). Recent advances in bioprinting techniques: approaches, applications and future prospects. *Journal of Translational Medicine, 14*(1), 271. doi: 10.1186/s12967-016-1028-0.

Madden, L.R., Nguyen, T.V., Garcia-Mojica, S., Shah, V. and Le, A.V. et al. (2018). Bioprinted 3D Primary Human Intestinal Tissues Model Aspects of Native Physiology and ADME/Tox Functions. *iScience, 2*, 156–167. doi: 10.1016/j.isci.2018.03.015.

Madiedo-Podvrsan, S., Belaïdi, J.-P., Desbouis, S., Simonetti, L. and Ben-Khalifa, Y. et al., (2021). Utilization of patterned bioprinting for heterogeneous and physiologically representative reconstructed epidermal skin models. *Sci Rep, 11*(1), 6217. doi: 10.1038/s41598-021-85553-3.

Mahmodi, H., Piloni, A., Utama, R.H. and Kabakova, I. (2021). Mechanical mapping of bioprinted hydrogel models by brillouin microscopy. *Bioprinting, 23*, e00151. doi: 10.1016/j.bprint.2021.e00151.

Majumder, N. and Ghosh, S. (2023). 3D biofabrication and space: A 'far-fetched dream' or a 'forthcoming reality'? *Biotechnology Advances, 69*, 108273. doi: 10.1016/j.biotechadv.2023.108273.

Mandrycky, C., Wang, Z., Kim, K. and Kim, D.-H. (2016). 3D bioprinting for engineering complex tissues. *Biotechnology Advances, 34*(4), 422–434. doi: 10.1016/j.biotechadv.2015.12.011.

Mao, H., Yang, L., Zhu, H., Wu, L. and Ji, P et al. (2020). Recent advances and challenges in materials for 3D bioprinting. *Progress in Natural Science: Materials International, 30*(5), 618–634. doi: 10.1016/j.pnsc.2020.09.015.

Matsusaki, M., Sakaue, K., Kadowaki, K. and Akashi, M. (2013). Three-Dimensional Human Tissue Chips Fabricated by Rapid and Automatic Inkjet Cell Printing. *Adv Healthc Mater, 2*(4), 534–539. doi: 10.1002/adhm.201200299.

Mazzocchi, A., Devarasetty, M., Huntwork, R., Soker, S. and Skardal, A. et al. (2019). Optimization of collagen type I-hyaluronan hybrid bioink for 3D bioprinted liver microenvironments. *Biofabrication, 11*(1), 015003. doi: 10.1088/1758-5090/aae543.

Mladenovska, T., Choong, P.F., Wallace, G.G. and O'Connell, C.D. (2023). The regulatory challenge of 3D bioprinting. *Regenerative Medicine, 18*(8), 659–674. doi: 10.2217/rme-2022-0194.

Mohebi, M.M. and Evans, J.R.G. (2002). A Drop-on-Demand Ink-Jet Printer for Combinatorial Libraries and Functionally Graded Ceramics. *Journal of Combinatorial Chemistry, 4*(4), 267–274. doi: 10.1021/cc010075e.

Moses, J.C., Saha, T. and Mandal, B.B. (2020). Chondroprotective and osteogenic effects of silk-based bioinks in developing 3D bioprinted osteochondral interface. *Bioprinting, 17*, e00067. doi: 10.1016/j.bprint.2019.e00067.

Moss, S.M., Schilp, J., Yaakov, M., Cook, M. and Schuschke, E. et al. (2022). Point-of-use, automated fabrication of a 3D human liver model supplemented with human adipose microvessels. *SLAS Discovery, 27*(6), 358–368. doi: 10.1016/j.slasd.2022.06.003.

Naseri, E., Cartmell, C., Saab, M., Kerr, R.G. and Ahmadi, A. et al. (2020). Development of 3D Printed Drug-Eluting Scaffolds for Preventing Piercing Infection. *Pharmaceutics, 12*(9), 901. doi: 10.3390/pharmaceutics12090901.

Ng, W.L., Qi, J.T.Z., Yeong, W.Y. and Naing, M.W. (2018). Proof-of-concept: 3D bioprinting of pigmented human skin constructs. *Biofabrication, 10*(2), 025005. doi: 10.1088/1758-5090/aa9e1e.

Ng, W.L., Yeong, W.Y. and Naing, M.W. (2016). Polyelectrolyte gelatin-chitosan hydrogel optimized for 3D bioprinting in skin tissue engineering. *International Journal of Bioprinting, 2*(1), 10. doi: 10.18063/ijb.2016.01.009.

Ngo, T.B., Spearman, B.S., Hlavac, N. and Schmidt, C.E. (2020). Three-Dimensional Bioprinted Hyaluronic Acid Hydrogel Test Beds for Assessing Neural Cell Responses to Competitive Growth Stimuli. *ACS Biomaterials Science & Engineering, 6*(12), 6819–6830. doi: 10.1021/acsbiomaterials.0c00940.

Nguyen, D.G., Funk, J., Robbins, J.B., Crogan-Grundy, C. and Presnell, S.C. et al., (2016). Bioprinted 3D Primary Liver Tissues Allow Assessment of Organ-Level Response to Clinical Drug Induced Toxicity In Vitro. *PLoS One, 11*(7), e0158674. doi: 10.1371/journal.pone.0158674.

Noor, N., Shapira, A., Edri, R. and Gal, I., Wertheim, L. et al. (2019). 3D Printing of Personalized Thick and Perfusable Cardiac Patches and Hearts. *Advanced Science, 6*(11), 1900344. doi: 10.1002/advs.201900344.

Norona, L.M., Nguyen, D.G., Gerber, D.A., Presnell, S.C. and Mosedale, M. et al. (2019). Bioprinted liver provides early insight into the role of Kupffer cells in TGF-β1 and methotrexate-induced fibrogenesis. *PLoS One, 14*(1), e0208958. doi: 10.1371/journal.pone.0208958.

Norotte, C., Marga, F.S., Niklason, L.E. and Forgacs, G. (2009). Scaffold-free vascular tissue engineering using bioprinting. *Biomaterials, 30*(30), 5910–5917. doi: 10.1016/j.biomaterials.2009.06.034.

O'Connell, C.D., Di Bella, C., Thompson, F., Augustine, C. and Beirne, S. et al. (2016). Development of the Biopen: a handheld device for surgical printing of adipose stem cells at a chondral wound site. *Biofabrication, 8*(1), 015019. doi: 10.1088/1758-5090/8/1/015019.

Oberdiek, F., Vargas, C.I., Rider, P., Batinic, M. and Görke, O. et al. (2021). Ex Vivo and In Vivo Analyses of Novel 3D-Printed Bone Substitute Scaffolds Incorporating Biphasic Calcium Phosphate Granules for Bone Regeneration. *International Journal of Molecular Sciences, 22*(7), 3588. doi: 10.3390/ijms22073588.

Odde, D.J. and Renn, M.J. (1999). Laser-guided direct writing for applications in biotechnology. *Trends in Biotechnology, 17*(10), 385–389. doi: 10.1016/s0167-7799(99)01355-4.

Oskarsdotter, K., Nordgård, C.T., Apelgren, P., Säljö, K. and Solbu, A.A. et al. (2023). Injectable In Situ Crosslinking Hydrogel for Autologous Fat Grafting. *Gels, 9*(10), 813.

Pages, E., Rémy, M., Keriquel, V., Correa, M.M. and Guillotin, B. et al. (2015). Creation of highly defined mesenchymal stem cell patterns in three dimensions by laser-assisted bioprinting. *Journal of Nanotechnology in Engineering and Medicine, 6*(2), 021006. doi: 10.1115/1.4031217.

Paul, K., Darzi, S., McPhee, G., Del Borgo, M.P. and Werkmeister, J.A. et al. (2019). 3D bioprinted endometrial stem cells on melt electrospun poly ε-caprolactone mesh for pelvic floor application promote anti-inflammatory responses in mice. *Acta Biomater, 97*, 162–176. doi: 10.1016/j.actbio.2019.08.003.

Peiffer, Q.C., de Ruijter, M., van Duijn, J., Crottet, D. and Dominic, E. et al. (2020). Melt electrowriting onto anatomically relevant biodegradable substrates: Resurfacing a diarthrodial joint. *Materials & design, 195*, 109025–109025. doi: 10.1016/j.matdes.2020.109025.

Pereira, F.D. A.S., Parfenov, V., Khesuani, Y.D., Ovsianikov, A. and Mironov, V. et al. (2018). Commercial 3D Bioprinters. In A. Ovsianikov, J. Yoo and V. Mironov (Eds.), *3D Printing and Biofabrication* (pp. 535–549). Cham: Springer International Publishing.

Ramadan, Q. and Zourob, M. (2021). 3D Bioprinting at the Frontier of Regenerative Medicine, Pharmaceutical, and Food Industries. *Frontiers in Medical Technology, 2*. doi: 10.3389/fmedt.2020.607648.

Ramesh, S., Kovelakuntla, V., Meyer, A.S. and Rivero, I.V. (2020). Three-dimensional printing of stimuli-responsive hydrogel with antibacterial activity. *Bioprinting*, e00106. doi: 10.1016/j.bprint.2020.e00106.

Reeser, K. and Doiron, A.L. (2019). Three-Dimensional Printing on a Rotating Cylindrical Mandrel: A Review of Additive-Lathe 3D Printing Technology. *3D Printing and Additive Manufacturing, 6*(6), 293–307. doi: 10.1089/3dp.2019.0058.

Roopavath, U.K., Soni, R., Mahanta, U., Deshpande, A.S. and Rath, S.N. et al. (2019). 3D printable SiO2 nanoparticle ink for patient specific bone regeneration. *RSC Advances, 9*(41), 23832–23842. doi: 10.1039/c9ra03641e.

Rousselle, A., Ferrandon, A., Mathieu, E., Godet, J. and Ball, V. et al. (2022). Enhancing cell survival in 3D printing of organoids using innovative bioinks loaded with pre-cellularized porous microscaffolds. *Bioprinting, 28*, e00247. doi: 10.1016/j.bprint.2022.e00247.

Saini, G., Segaran, N., Mayer, J.L., Saini, A. and Albadawi, H. et al. (2021). Applications of 3D Bioprinting in Tissue Engineering and Regenerative Medicine. *Journal of Clinical Medicine, 10*(21), 4966.

Schwab, A., Hélary, C., Richards, R.G., Alini, M. and Eglin, D. et al. (2020). Tissue mimetic hyaluronan bioink containing collagen fibers with controlled orientation modulating cell migration and alignment. *Materials Today Bio, 7*, 100058. doi: 10.1016/j.mtbio.2020.100058.

Sharma, R., Smits, I.P.M., De La Vega, L., Lee, C. and Willerth, S.M. et al. (2020). 3D Bioprinting Pluripotent Stem Cell Derived Neural Tissues Using a Novel Fibrin Bioink Containing Drug Releasing Microspheres. *Frontiers in Bioengineering and Biotechnology, 8*(57), 1–12. doi: 10.3389/fbioe.2020.00057.

Shie, M.-Y., Lee, J.-J., Ho, C.-C., Yen, S.-Y. and Ng, H.Y. et al. (2020). Effects of gelatin methacrylate bio-ink concentration on mechano-physical properties and human dermal fibroblast behavior. *Polymers, 12*(9), 1930. doi: 10.3390/polym12091930.

Sjöholm, E., Mathiyalagan, R., Rajan Prakash, D., Lindfors, L. and Wang, Q. et al. (2020). 3D-Printed Veterinary Dosage Forms—A Comparative Study of Three Semi-Solid Extrusion 3D Printers. *Pharmaceutics, 12*(12), 1239. doi: 10.3390/pharmaceutics12121239.

Skardal, A., Mack, D., Kapetanovic, E., Atala, A. and Jackson, J.D. et al. (2012). Bioprinted Amniotic Fluid-Derived Stem Cells Accelerate Healing of Large Skin Wounds. *STEM CELLS Translational Medicine, 1*(11), 792–802. doi: 10.5966/sctm.2012-0088.

Somasekharan, T.L., Kasoju, N., Raju, R. and Bhatt, A. (2020). Formulation and Characterization of Alginate Dialdehyde, Gelatin, and Platelet-Rich Plasma-Based Bioink for Bioprinting Applications. *Bioengineering, 7*(3), 108. doi: 10.3390/bioengineering7030108.

Sullivan, M. A., Lane, S., Volkerling, A., Engel, M. and Werry, E.L. et al. (2023). Three-dimensional bioprinting of stem cell-derived central nervous system cells enables astrocyte growth, vasculogenesis, and enhances neural differentiation/function. *Biotechnology and Bioengineering, 120*(10), 3079–3091. doi: 10.1002/bit.28470.

Tan, B., Gan, S., Wang, X., Liu, W. and Li, X. et al. (2021). Applications of 3D bioprinting in tissue engineering: advantages, deficiencies, improvements, and future perspectives. *Journal of Materials Chemistry B, 9*(27), 5385–5413. doi: 10.1039/d1tb00172h.

Tan, E.Y.S. and Yeong, W.Y. (2015). Concentric bioprinting of alginate-based tubular constructs using multi-nozzle extrusion-based technique. *International Journal of Bioprinting, 1*(1), 8. doi: 10.18063/ijb.2015.01.003.

Thattaruparambil Raveendran, N., Vaquette, C., Meinert, C., Samuel Ipe, D. and Ivanovski, S. et al. (2019). Optimization of 3D bioprinting of periodontal ligament cells. *Dental Materials, 35*(12), 1683–1694. doi: 10.1016/j.dental.2019.08.114.

Thayer, P.S., Orrhult, L.S. and Martínez, H. (2018). Bioprinting of Cartilage and Skin Tissue Analogs Utilizing a Novel Passive Mixing Unit Technique for Bioink Precellularization. *JoVE*(131), e56372. doi: 10.3791/56372.

Thazhathukunnel, T., Chow, A. and Amirfar, V.A. (2015). Is 3D printing the future of health care? *Pharmacy Today, 21*(6), 56.

Thorpe, D., Belcher, S. and Nicholson, J. (2020). United States. Patent Application: US20200130277A1.

Tripathi, S., Mandal, S.S., Bauri, S. and Maiti, P. (2023). 3D bioprinting and its innovative approach for biomedical applications. *MedComm, 4*(1), e194. doi: 10.1002/mco2.194.

Utama, R.H., Atapattu, L., O'Mahony, A.P., Fife, C.M. and Baek, J. et al. (2020). A 3D Bioprinter Specifically Designed for the High-Throughput Production of Matrix-Embedded Multicellular Spheroids. *iScience, 23*(10). doi: 10.1016/j.isci.2020.101621.

Vanaei, S., Parizi, M.S., Salemizadehparizi, F. and Vanaei, H.R. (2021). An Overview on Materials and Techniques in 3D Bioprinting Toward Biomedical Application. *Engineered Regeneration, 2*, 1–18. doi: 10.1016/j.engreg.2020.12.001.

Wang, X.-F., Song, Y., Liu, Y.-S., Sun, Y.-c. and Wang, Y.-g et al. (2016). Osteogenic differentiation of three-dimensional bioprinted constructs consisting of human adipose-derived stem cells in vitro and in vivo. *PLoS One, 11*(6), e0157214. doi: 10.1371/journal.pone.0157214.

Westhaus, A., Cabanes-Creus, M., Dilworth, K.L., Zhu, E. and Salas Gómez, D. et al. (2023). Assessment of Pre-Clinical Liver Models Based on Their Ability to Predict the Liver-Tropism of Adeno-Associated Virus Vectors. *Human Gene Therapy, 34*(7-8), 273–288. doi: 10.1089/hum.2022.188.

Wilson Jr., W.C. and Boland, T. (2003). Cell and organ printing 1: Protein and cell printers. *The Anatomical Record Part A: Discoveries in Molecular, Cellular, and Evolutionary Biology, 272A*(2), 491–496. doi: 10.1002/ar.a.10057.

Yu, C., Zhu, W., Sun, B., Mei, D. and Gou, M. et al. (2018). Modulating physical, chemical, and biological properties in 3D printing for tissue engineering applications. *Applied Physics Reviews, 5*(4). doi: 10.1063/1.5050245.

Yu, H., Zhang, X., Song, W., Pan, T. and Wang, H. et al. (2019). Effects of 3-dimensional Bioprinting Alginate/Gelatin Hydrogel Scaffold Extract on Proliferation and Differentiation of Human Dental Pulp Stem Cells. *Journal of Endodontics, 45*(6), 706–715. doi: 10.1016/j.joen.2019.03.004.

Zafeiris, K., Brasinika, D., Karatza, A., Koumoulos, E. and Karoussis, I.K. et al. (2021). Additive manufacturing of hydroxyapatite–chitosan–genipin composite scaffolds for bone tissue engineering applications. *Materials Science and Engineering: C, 119*, 111639. doi: 10.1016/j.msec.2020.111639.

Zandrini, T., Florczak, S., Levato, R. and Ovsianikov, A. (2023). Breaking the resolution limits of 3D bioprinting: future opportunities and present challenges. *Trends in Biotechnology, 41*(5), 604–614. doi: 10.1016/j.tibtech.2022.10.009.

Zhang, Y., Li, G., Wang, J., Zhou, F. and Ren, X. et al. (2023). Small Joint Organoids 3D Bioprinting: Construction Strategy and Application. *Small*, 2302506. doi: 10.1002/smll.202302506.

Zhou, X., Nowicki, M., Sun, H., Hann, S.Y., Cui, H., Esworthy, T., Lee, J.D., Plesniak, M. and Zhang, L.G. (2020). 3D Bioprinting-Tunable Small-Diameter Blood Vessels with Biomimetic Biphasic Cell Layers. *ACS Applied Materials & Interfaces, 12*(41), 45904–45915. doi: 10.1021/acsami.0c14871.

Overview of 3D Bioprinting Technology

Harshada M. Adhyapak,[1] *Santosh L. Gaonkar*[1*]
and *Namratha B.*[2]

1. Introduction

3D printing can transform any physical object, previously represented geometrically, into a tangible entity through the gradual integration of materials. In recent times, there has been a notable upsurge in the utilization of 3D printing technology. It was Charles Hull who initially introduced and made commercially available the concept of 3D printing in 1980. Presently, 3D printing finds its predominant application in the creation of prosthetic heart pumps, jewelery lines, 3D printed corneas, PGA rocket engines, the Amsterdam steel bridge, and other items closely associated with the food and aviation industries. CAD (computer-aided design) drawings serve as the foundation for the direct layer-by-layer fabrication of three-dimensional (3D) structures using 3D printing technology. The innovative and adaptable nature of 3D printing technology has established it as a significant advancement in the field of technology (Shahrubudin et al., 2019).

Currently, the materials that can be fabricated through the utilization of 3D printing technology encompass an array of substances such as metals, ceramics, materials based on graphene, and traditional thermoplastics. The advent of 3D printing technology has the potential to incite revolutions within industries and prompt alterations in manufacturing practices. The incorporation of 3D printing technology into manufacturing processes is anticipated to yield cost savings and expedite production timelines. Furthermore, consumer demands are poised to exert a more substantial influence on the realm of production. Customers are afforded greater authority in determining the specifications of the final product and can request customization accordingly. In parallel, the proximity of 3D printing technology facilities to customers will facilitate enhanced responsiveness and adaptability in manufacturing processes, thereby improving quality control measures. It is noteworthy that at present, 3D printing has become a prevalent and widespread practice worldwide (Kačarević et al.,

---

[1] Department of Chemistry, Manipal Institute of Technology, Manipal Academy of Higher Education, Manipal, India
[2] Department of Chemistry, The Yenepoya Institute of Arts, Science, Commerce and Management, Mangaluru, India.
* Corresponding author: sl.gaonkar@manipal.edu

2018). The domains of agriculture, healthcare, the automotive industry, and the aerospace industry are among those that are increasingly employing 3D printing technology for the purpose of mass customization and production of open-source designs. The utilization of 3D printing technology in the manufacturing sector comes with several disadvantages. To illustrate, the adoption of 3D printing technology will diminish the necessity for labor in manufacturing, thereby inevitably exerting a substantial influence on the economies of nations that heavily depend on low-skilled occupations (Ozbolat, 2017).

2. The Evolution of 3D Bioprinting

The historical account of 3D bioprinting is an engrossing odyssey that interweaves advancements in technology, healthcare, and biomaterials. The notion of technology of 3D bioprinting can be traced back to the 1980s, when additive manufacturing techniques were devised, enabling the gradual deposition of materials to fabricate three-dimensional objects. Though these initial methodologies were predominantly employed for constructing rudimentary prototypes and models, it became evident that similar principles could be applied to the realm of medicine (Thayer et al., 2020). The main origins of three-dimensional bioprinting can be traced back to the early 2000s. when researchers initiated an investigation into the concept of printing biological tissues and structures. A significant milestone in this field occurred in the mid-2000s with the groundbreaking work conducted by Dr. Gabor Forgacs and his team at the University of Missouri. They achieved the printing of living cells using an inkjet-like method, wherein droplets containing cells suspended in bioink were deposited onto a substrate to form rudimentary tissue structures. This pivotal work established the fundamental basis for the field and generated widespread interest in the potential applications of 3D bioprinting in regenerative medicine (Sigaux et al., 2019).

In the subsequent years, researchers have delved deeper into refining bioprinting techniques and expanding the range of biomaterials that can be printed. A crucial focus during this process has been the development of bioinks, which are materials compatible with living cells. Various natural and synthetic polymers, hydrogels, and components of the extracellular matrix have been thoroughly investigated as potential bioinks. The objective of these explorations is to create a supportive environment for cell growth and tissue development (Kačarević et al., 2018).

Advancements in the realm of imaging technologies, particularly magnetic resonance imaging (MRI) along with computed tomography (CT), have also played a vital role in the advancement of 3D bioprinting. These cutting-edge technologies have facilitated the precise delineation of patient-specific anatomical structures, thereby enabling the fabrication of individualized and tailored tissue constructs (Valeria and Charalampos, 2018). As the discipline has progressed, researchers have successfully showcased the bioprinting of increasingly intricate tissues and organs. Notably, in 2013, scientists at Heriot-Watt University in Scotland achieved the remarkable feat of bioprinting a miniature liver utilizing human cells. Subsequent milestones encompassed the bioprinting of cardiac tissue, blood vessels, and even fully functional miniature organs. Organovo, a pioneering bioprinting enterprise established in 2007, emerged as one of the frontrunners in the commercialization of technology of 3D bioprinting for the purposes of pharmaceutical testing and drug development (Arslan-Yildiz et al., 2016).

The subsequent years witnessed a notable upsurge in collaborative endeavors across disciplines such as engineering, biology, materials science, and medical expertise, aimed at surmounting the obstacles associated with bioprinting. Scholars directed their efforts towards ameliorating the vascularization of printed tissues, enhancing the survival of cells, and progressing the incorporation of diverse cell types within intricate structures (Choudhury et al., 2018).

In the 2020s, the realm of three dimensional bioprinting attained a level of maturation wherein it transitioned from experimental showcases to pragmatic applications. Bioprinted tissues were increasingly utilized for drug testing, disease modeling, and, on certain occasions, transplantation research. The technology persisted in advancing, tackling concerns pertaining to scalability, standardization, and regulatory considerations (Murphy and Atala, 2014).

3. Cornerstones of 3D Bioprinting Technology

The future of regenerative medicine along with biomedical research is being influenced by the emergence of new trends in 3D bioprinting technology. A significant trend in this field involves the development of vascularized tissues, which addresses a crucial challenge in the bioprinting process. To overcome this challenge, researchers are exploring innovative methods, such as integrating endothelial cells and sacrificial materials, to create intricate vascular networks within the bioprinted constructs. This advancement holds great potential for producing larger and more metabolically active tissues by ensuring a sufficient supply of nutrients and effective waste removal. Another noteworthy trend in 3D bioprinting is the shift towards high-throughput techniques for drug screening applications (Jessop et al., 2017). As technological progress continues, the capacity to simultaneously or rapidly produce multiple tissue models through printing enhances the efficacy of drug testing procedures, thereby permitting a more comprehensive screening of pharmaceutical compounds. Moreover, the integration of bioprinting with other cutting-edge technologies, like artificial intelligence and machine learning, is gaining momentum. Such technologies contribute to the optimization of bioprinting parameters, resulting in enhanced precision, velocity, and predictive modeling of tissue development. The investigation of innovative bioink formulations, encompassing the utilization of sophisticated biomaterials and extracellular matrix components, is nurturing the generation of more biomimetic and functional tissues (Zhou et al., 2021).

Furthermore, there is a growing inclination towards collaborative interdisciplinary research, whereby experts from the areas of biology, engineering, along with materials science collaborate to surmount challenges and stimulate innovation in the realm of 3D bioprinting. These emerging trends collectively foreshadow a future wherein bioprinting technologies continue to progress, thereby unveiling novel possibilities for personalized medicine, tissue engineering, and transformative applications in healthcare (Vanaei et al., 2020).

4. Bioprinting Techniques

3D bioprinting comprises various methodologies, each possessing its array of benefits and implementations (Figure 1). The trio of primary techniques within the realm of 3D bioprinting encompass inkjet-based bioprinting, extrusion-based bioprinting, and laser-based bioprinting (Li et al., 2016).

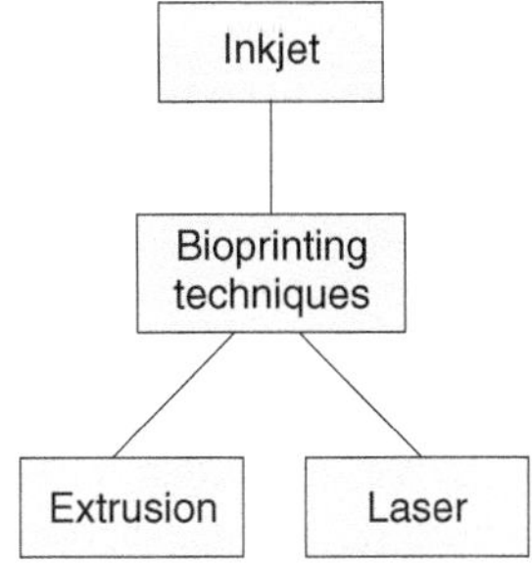

Fig. 1 Types of bioprinting techniques

4.1 Inkjet-Based Bioprinting

Principle: Analogous to the conventional inkjet printing methodology, this approach encompasses the expulsion of droplets of biological ink from a printing apparatus onto a substrate in a regulated design.

Advantages: Noteworthy rapidity in the printing process, capability to attain elevated precision, and appropriateness for the replication of intricate cellular configurations.

Applications: Employed in scenarios where meticulousness and celerity are of paramount importance, such as fabricating tissue models for pharmaceutical experimentation (Sina et al., 2019).

4.2   Extrusion-Based Bioprinting

The employed methodology entails the utilization of a pneumatic or mechanical extrusion system for the purpose of propelling or retracting bioink through a nozzle. This process facilitates the deposition of the bioink layer by layer, thereby resulting in the formation of the intended structure.

Advantages: This approach possesses the capability to accommodate a diverse range of bioinks exhibiting varying viscosities. Consequently, it permits the integration of different cell types and biomaterials.

Applications: The aforementioned technique is particularly well-suited for the printing of intricate and expansive tissues and organs, such as cartilage or blood vessels (Ibrahim and Monika, 2016).

4.3   Laser-Based Bioprinting

Principle: The utilization of a laser for precise focusing on a donor slide containing material leads to the generation of pressure, which in turn propels the bioink onto a receiving substrate in a designated pattern.

Advantages: This technique provides excellent resolution and precision, making it ideal for printing complex structures and delicate tissues.

Applications: It finds utility in scenarios that necessitate high resolution, such as the creation of intricate tissue models and the construction of biological structures on a micro-scale.

These methodologies are often categorized based on their respective printing mechanisms; however, variations and hybrid approaches continue to emerge, signifying the dynamic nature of 3D bioprinting technology. Researchers remain actively engaged in exploring enhancements and innovations to augment printing speed, cell viability, resolution, and the assortment of printable biomaterials. The selection of a specific bioprinting technique is contingent upon the specific requirements of the intended application, including factors such as the type of tissue or organ being printed, the desired level of resolution, and the mechanical properties of the resulting construct (Allen et al., 2022).

5.   Bioinks

Bioinks play a crucial role in 3D bioprinting technology, serving as the substance used to place living cells, biomaterials, and other bioactive agents layer by layer to construct 3D structures. These structures can vary from basic tissue models to intricate organs, providing a basis for a wide range of applications like tissue engineering, regenerative medicine, and drug testing. Bioinks must satisfy specific requirements to ensure that they are compatible with living organisms, capable of being printed, and able to support the viability and functionality of cells (Guvendiren, 2019). The development of bioinks is an area of active investigation, with ongoing efforts directed towards enhancing their printability, stability, and biological performance. Progress in bioink technology contributes to the precision and adaptability of 3D bioprinting, bringing us closer to achieving functional and implantable tissues and organs for therapeutic purposes (Selcan et al., 2018).

6.   Types of Bioinks

6.1   Hydrogels

Hydrogels are widely favored as bioinks because of their aqueous composition and resemblance to the ECM (extracellular matrix) in living tissues. Alginate, agarose, gelatin, and hyaluronic acid are common hydrogel materials. These materials provide a supportive milieu for cellular proliferation and allow for the sequential deposition of cells during the printing process. Hydrogels play a pivotal and multifaceted role in three dimensional bioprinting technology, serving as the fundamental building blocks of bioink formulations. These polymer networks, which are cross-linked and water-based, possess a significant water content and display viscoelastic characteristics, rendering them highly compatible with the intricate nature of living cells (Ramiah et al., 2020). In the realm of three-dimensional bioprinting, hydrogels serve as bio-inks that enclose living cells, providing a printable and biocompatible medium for the most precise deposition of cells, layer by layer. The malleable physical and chemical attributes of hydrogels enable researchers to customize them to imitate the specific traits of target tissues, such as rigidity, permeability, and decay rates. The aqueous composition of hydrogels closely resembles the natural extracellular matrix, fostering an environment conducive to cellular proliferation, differentiation, and nutrient transport (Fatimi et al., 2022).

Additionally, hydrogels possess the potential to be altered in order to include bioactive compounds, like growth factors, which augment their capability to govern cellular actions and impact the advancement of tissues. On the whole, the distinctive characteristics of hydrogels render them essential in the process of 3D bio fabrication, permitting the creation of intricate, biomimetic structures that have applications in the domain of regenerative medicine, tissue engineering and the progression of personalized healthcare (Janitha and Ambalangodage, 2020).

6.2 Extracellular Matrix (ECM) Components

Bioinks frequently include ECM (extracellular matrix) components to replicate the natural conditions of tissues. Collagen, fibrin, and laminin are some of the examples of ECM proteins that are utilized to augment cell attachment, migration, and differentiation. The ECM, which plays a crucial role in 3D bioprinting technology, functions as a biomimetic scaffold that closely imitates the microenvironment of living tissues. Within the realm of 3D bioprinting, the ECM serves as a foundational element that is integrated into bioinks. This intricate network of proteins, polysaccharides, and glycoproteins not only provides structural support, but also exerts an influence on cellular behaviors like migration, adhesion,proliferation, and differentiation (Abaci and Guvendiren, 2020).

The inclusion of ECM constituents in bioinks enhances the bioactive properties of printed structures, thereby facilitating the generation of functional tissues. Collagen, fibrin, and laminin are commonly employed ECM components in the realm of 3D bioprinting due to their compatibility with diverse cell types and their ability to foster a tissue-specific milieu. The role of ECM extends beyond mere structural support, as it significantly contributes to the overall functionality and integrity of bioprinted tissues. Through the integration of ECM within the bioink formulations, 3D bioprinting endeavors to emulate the natural signals that govern cellular behavior, thereby promoting the development of intricate, biomimetic tissues with most potential applications in regenerative medicine, tissue engineering, and particularly the advancement of tailored medical therapies (Dzobo et al., 2019).

6.3 Synthetic Polymers

Synthetic polymers have a vital role in 3D bioprinting technology, as they provide the most precise manipulation of material properties and functionalities that are necessary for the creation of personalized bioinks. These polymers, such as polyethylene glycol (PEG), polycaprolactone (PCL), and poly lactic-co-glycolic acid (PLGA), offer adaptability to bioink formulations by enabling customization of mechanical strength, rates of degradation, and compatibility with the living organism (Khoeini et al., 2021). Synthetic polymers possess various advantages, such as customizable stiffness and mechanical properties that are essential for imitating specific characteristics of tissues. Their ability to degrade can be finely adjusted, allowing for the controlled release of bioactive molecules or the gradual modification of printed tissues after implantation. Moreover, synthetic polymers act as a framework or structural support within the bioink, assisting in the precise deposition of cells and facilitating tissue organization during the process of bioprinting (Sonu et al., 2021).

In addition to providing stability to the printed structure, these polymers also offer the flexibility to incorporate other biomaterials, growth factors, or cells to create bioinks tailored to meet the specific requirements of diverse organs and tissues. The inclusion of synthetic polymers in bioinks expands the possibilities of three dimensional bioprinting, enabling the creation of intricate polymers with a wide range of applications, including tissue regeneration, organ engineering, drug delivery systems, and the advanced medical therapeutics (Parak et al., 2019).

6.4 Cellulose-Based Materials

Various materials derived from cellulose are playing a vital role in advancing the field of three dimensional bioprinting technology. These materials possess unique characteristics that contribute to the development of bioinks with improved properties for tissue engineering along with regenerative medicine. One such material, nitrocellulose, which is derived from cellulose nanofibers, is particularly noteworthy due to its biocompatibility, high surface area, and impressive mechanical strength. These properties make nanocellulose an excellent candidate for serving as a three-dimensional scaffold in bioinks, providing a supportive structure for the precise deposition of living cells during the bioprinting process (Afrinal et al., 2022). Furthermore, cellulose-based materials have adjustable properties, allowing researchers to customize bioinks to mimic the specific requirements of different tissues. For example, the surface chemistry and porosity of cellulose-based materials can be modified to create bioinks that closely resemble the natural microenvironment of target tissues. The sustainability of cellulose, sourced from renewable plant-based origins, aligns with the increasing focus on eco-friendly practices in bioprinting. Cellulose-based bioinks show promise in promoting cell adhesion, proliferation, and differentiation, thereby facilitating the development of functional tissues. As researchers continue to explore the potential of cellulose-based materials, their versatility and biocompatibility make them valuable components in the pursuit of fabricating intricate and biomimetic structures using 3D bioprinting techniques (Wan et al., 2022).

6.5 Bioceramics

The development of 3D bioprinting technology is greatly aided by bioceramics, especially in the areas of tissue engineering and regenerative medicine. Hydroxyapatite, which is a type of bioceramic, is a prominent choice due to its composition that closely resembles the mineral component found in natural bone. The incorporation of bioceramics into the bioinks used in 3D bioprinting serves to enhance the structural and mechanical properties of the printed constructs which makes them highly suitable for applications in the engineering of bone tissue (Salah et al., 2022). The inclusion of bioceramics in the bio-inks provides a scaffold that possesses high compressive strength, mimicking the stiffness of natural bone and contributing to the overall stability of the printed structure. Additionally, bioceramics offer a biomimetic microenvironment that facilitates the proliferation,adhesion, and differentiation of cells, which are vital processes for the successful regeneration of bone tissue. This integration of bioceramics into bioinks is particularly advantageous in the fabrication of bone substitutes and implants, where the objective is to create constructs that not only provide structural support to the surrounding tissues but also actively participate in the regeneration process. The usage of bioceramics in 3D bioprinting highlights its potential to revolutionize orthopedic treatments by offering customized solutions for bone defects, fractures, and personalized implants that align with the intricate anatomy along with mechanical properties of native bone tissue (Guvendiren, 2019).

6.6 Decellularized Extracellular Matrix (dECM)

This whole process entails the utilization of natural tissues that have undergone decellularization to extract cellular components, thereby leaving behind the extracellular matrix (ECM). The dECM (decellularized ECM) can be transformed into a bio-ink, which creates a tissue-specific microenvironment for the introduction of seeded cells. Using a meticulous decellularization procedure, the dECM retains the intricate structure of the ECM while eliminating cellular components. This acellular matrix serves as a fundamental bioink, functioning as a natural scaffold that facilitates the precise deposition of living cells during the bioprinting process. The bioactive molecules present within the dECM, including growth factors and signaling proteins, actively contribute to the regulation of cellular behavior, exerting influence over processes such as migration,adhesion and differentiation (Claire et al., 2019). Moreover, the utilization of dECM enables the replication of tissue-specific microenvironments, fostering the development of functional tissues that closely resemble their native counterparts. The immunomodulatory properties of dECM further mitigate the risk of immune responses when bioprinted tissues are transplanted. Additionally, the proteins contained within the dECM confer mechanical strength and stability to the printed constructs, which is of utmost importance in applications involving load-bearing tissues. On the whole, the incorporation of dECM in 3D bioprinting not only enhances the biomimicry of bioprinted tissues, but also contributes to their structural integrity, functionality, and potential for successful integration into host tissues (Dzobo et al., 2019).

7. Combination Bioinks

Researchers are presently engaged in the exploration of hybrid or combination bioinks that integrate multiple substances, each with a designated purpose. To illustrate, a bioink might encompass a hydrogel to support cellular growth, synthetic polymers to ensure structural integrity, and growth factors to enhance cellular behavior. The utilization of combination inks constitutes a remarkable advancement in 3D bioprinting technology, as it provides a versatile method to fabricate bioinks that harness the advantageous attributes of multiple materials. These inks, frequently composed of a fusion of natural and synthetic polymers, hydrogels, and other biomaterials, allow researchers to capitalize on the complementary characteristics of each constituent (James and Mulgaonkar, 2022). The utilization of various materials affords the opportunity to finely adjust the physical, mechanical, and biochemical attributes, thus catering to the diverse demands of distinct tissues and organs. To illustrate, a composite ink can incorporate a hydrogel to ensure biocompatibility, a synthetic polymer for structural reinforcement, and specific growth factors to direct cellular behavior. This strategy enhances the overall printability, cell viability, and tissue-specific functionality of the bioink. The capacity to fabricate bioinks with customized and synergistic properties renders combination inks a valuable asset in 3D bioprinting, broadening the range of various applications in tissue engineering, regenerative medicine along with the creation of more intricate and biomimetic constructs for advanced medical interventions (Ahasan and Bashir, 2019)

8. Applications

The convergence of biology, materials science along with computer-aided design has resulted in the emergence of 3D bioprinting, which holds great potential for advancing medical research, and personalized medicine, and ultimately improving patient care (Aathma et al., 2021). This revolutionary technique opens up new possibilities for creating functional tissues and organs that are tailored to meet the particular needs of individual patients. In doing so, it addresses the persistent challenges of organ shortages and compatibility issues in transplantation. As we delve deeper into the field of 3D bioprinting, its potential applications extend beyond regenerative medicine to encompass drug discovery, disease modeling, and the development of biofabricated implants. The remarkable ability to accurately recreate intricate biological structures has significant implications, providing unprecedented opportunities to explore and manipulate the complex interactions between cells, signaling pathways, and microenvironments. This journey represents the fusion of technology and biology, marking the dawn of a new era where the boundaries of what is achievable continue to expand, reshaping the landscape of medicine and deepening our understanding of life itself (Figure 2).

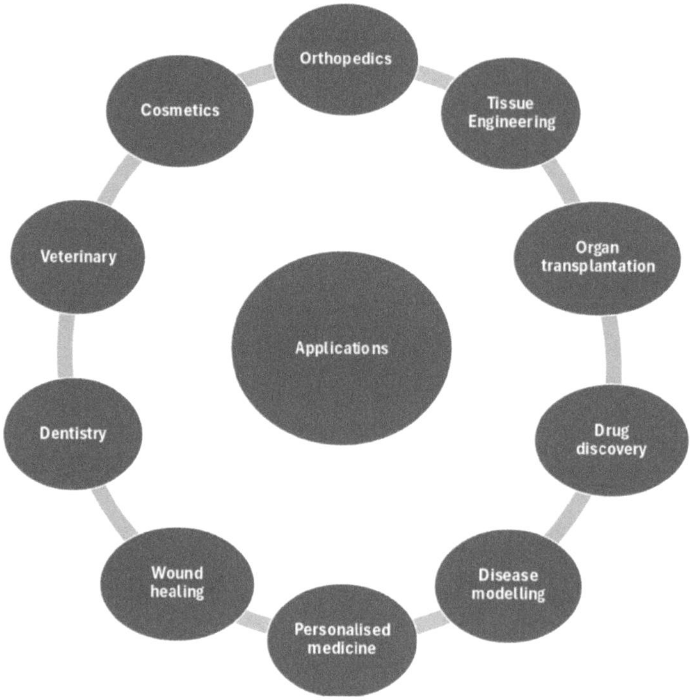

Fig. 2   Applications of 3D Bioprinting Technology

8.1   *Tissue Engineering*

The multifaceted applications of three dimensional bioprinting in the field of tissue engineering have opened up a new realm of possibilities for the generation and regeneration of biological tissues. One particularly significant application involves the precise construction of intricate tissue scaffolds. Through the utilization of 3D bioprinters, it is now possible to deposit bioinks that consist of a various combination of living cells, growth factors, and biomaterials with an exceptional level of spatial accuracy. This level of precision permits the recreation of complex tissue architectures. The ability to achieve such complexity is vital in the engineering of tissues that possess mechanical properties and structural intricacies that closely resemble those of native tissues. Additionally, 3D bioprinting plays an important role in the development of vascularized constructs, a challenge that has long plagued tissue engineering. By providing a network for the delivery of nutrients along with oxygen, this technology enables the sustenance of larger and more complex tissues. (Zhang and Zhang, 2015). Another notable application lies in the generation of functional organoids and in vitro tissue models. These constructs, produced through 3D printing, serve as accurate representations of human tissues, enabling scientists to investigate diseases, assess drug reactions, and acquire insights into tissue development and functionality within a controlled setting. These models are particularly valuable in the field of personalized medicine, as they allow for the precise evaluation of drug effectiveness and toxicity, surpassing the capabilities of traditional two-dimensional cell cultures (Matai et al., 2020).

Furthermore, 3D bioprinting plays a pivotal role in advancing regenerative medicine by offering a platform for the production of transplantable tissues and organs. This technology facilitates the step-by-step assembly of tissues with precise cellular compositions, thereby fostering the creation of implantable constructs that can seamlessly integrate with the recipient organism. Consequently, this has the potential to address the scarcity of donor organs and mitigate the risk of immune rejection by utilizing the patient's own cells during the printing process (Sanjairaj et al., 2018). In conjunction with these applications, 3D bioprinting plays a crucial role in the fabrication of biocompatible implants for the purpose of repairing and replacing tissues. From bone grafts to cartilage implants, 3D bioprinting enables the personalization of implants according to the anatomical and physiological requirements of individual patients, thereby enhancing the integration and functionality of these implants (Gu et al., 2018).

8.2 Organ Transplantation

Currently, 3D bioprinting technology is on the verge of revolutionizing the field of organ transplantation, presenting a wide range of applications that tackle crucial challenges related to the scarcity of donor organs and compatibility issues. One pivotal application entails the potential of bioprinting complete organs with intricate architectures employing a patient's own cells. This personalized approach not only mitigates the risk of immune rejection but also obviates the necessity for immunosuppressive medications, which frequently accompany traditional transplant procedures (Gilbert et al., 2018). The capability to accurately deposit bioinks containing diverse cell types, growth factors along with biomaterials layer by layer enables the production of functional and vascularized organs, surmounting the limitations of conventional transplantation techniques. Moreover, 3D bioprinting permits the fabrication of organ scaffolds, providing a blueprint for cell growth and tissue regeneration. These scaffolds can be infused with patient-specific cells, fostering the advancement of fully operational organs externally. This application holds the potential of substantially reducing transplant waiting times and augmenting the pool of accessible organs (Cui et al., 2016).

Moreover, the utilization of 3D bioprinting plays an important role in the area of tissue engineering, specifically in the creation of tissue patches or grafts for the purpose of organ repair. Through the development of personalized constructs that accurately replicate the microenvironment of specific organs, bioprinting facilitates the transplantation of functional tissue segments, thereby contributing to the regeneration of damaged organs. This approach proves to be particularly pertinent in addressing situations where there is a compromise in partial organ function, offering a targeted and minimally invasive alternative to the conventional method of whole organ transplantation (Li et al., 2016).

8.3 Drug Discovery and Testing

The applications of three-dimensional bioprinting in pharmaceutical research are extensive and hold significant potential for advancement. One prominent application lies in the creation of physiologically relevant tissue models and organoids that accurately reproduce the microenvironments of human organs (Satpathy et al., 2018).

Researchers have the ability to utilize 3D bioprinting in order to fabricate intricate three-dimensional structures consisting of diverse cell types, extracellular matrices, and biochemical stimuli, thus emulating the intricate nature of human tissues. These sophisticated models provide a detailed representation of in vivo conditions in contrast to conventional two-dimensional cell cultures, thereby establishing a foundation for investigating drug responses with greater accuracy. By incorporating cells specific to individual patients, 3D bioprinted tissues allow for personalized drug testing, enabling researchers to evaluate how individuals may react to specific treatments and ultimately contribute to the advancement of precision medicine (Peng et al., 2017). Furthermore, the utilization of three-dimensional bioprinting serves to facilitate the establishment of disease models, thereby granting researchers the opportunity to investigate the mechanisms of a very wide range of diseases within a controlled and repeatable setting. These said models play an important role in comprehending the progression of diseases and identifying potential targets for pharmaceutical intervention. For example, the creation of cancer spheroids or organoids through the means of 3D bioprinting permits a more precise examination of tumor behavior and the response to anticancer medications in comparison to conventional models, ultimately enhancing the efficacy of drug discovery endeavors (Ma et al., 2018).

Within the realm of drug delivery research, the implementation of 3D bioprinting technology allows for the fabrication of drug-eluting implants and tissue-engineered constructs, which can be further utilized for the sustained release of therapeutic agents. This innovation ensures the meticulous regulation of drugs' spatial distribution within the printed structures, thereby optimizing strategies for drug delivery and ultimately enhancing the efficacy of therapeutic outcomes (Gao et al., 2021).

8.4   Disease Modeling

3D bioprinting facilitates the generation of intricate disease models, providing researchers with the opportunity to investigate diseases in a regulated setting. This is particularly advantageous when it comes to comprehending intricate diseases such as cancer and neurological disorders. A notable application involves the production of highly authentic and physiologically significant tissue models using 3D bioprinting methods. By accurately depositing bioinks that consist of a combination of cells, biomaterials, and growth factors, researchers have the ability to construct three-dimensional structures that closely resemble the microarchitecture along with the cellular composition of specific tissues impacted by diseases. This further allows for the creation of organoids or tissue constructs which are disease-specific, thereby replicating the complexity of in vivo environments and presenting a superior alternative to conventional two-dimensional cell cultures (Memic et al., 2017).

3D bioprinted disease models hold significant value in the examination of intricate diseases such as cancer, neurodegenerative disorders, and cardiovascular conditions. To illustrate, in the realm of cancer research, 3D bioprinted tumor models effectively capture the diversity and interplay between cancer cells, stromal cells, and the extracellular matrix, thus presenting a more precise depiction of tumor behavior and reaction towards treatments. In the field of neurodegenerative disease modeling, three-dimensional bioprinting facilitates the replication of brain-like structures, enabling researchers to explore the progression of ailments like Alzheimer's and Parkinson's in a more authentic context (Amanda et al., 2023).

8.5   Personalized Medicine

The utilization of this technology permits the development of tissues and organs that are specifically designed for individual patients, thereby creating the way for the field of personalized medicine. This encompasses the construction of implants, prosthetics, and other medical devices that are customized to fit the unique anatomical and physiological characteristics of each patient. One significant application of this technology involves the creation of patient-specific tissues and organs which can be used for transplantation. By employing bioinks that consist of a patient's own cells, the process of 3D bioprinting facilitates the production of tailor-made implants that effectively minimize the risk of rejection along with enhancing the overall success rate of transplant procedures (Germain et al., 2022).

In the realm of pharmaceutical advancement, the application of 3D bioprinting expedites the creation of tissue models that are cultivated outside of the body and can imitate the intricate nuances of an individual's response to treatment. This enables a more precise evaluation of drug efficacy and the formulation of tailored treatment plans. Furthermore, this technology assumes a pivotal role in the realm of disease replication, as it empowers researchers to fabricate three-dimensional structures that accurately mimic the distinct characteristics of an individual's ailment. This facilitates a deeper comprehension of the mechanisms that drive disease and the development of treatments that target these specific attributes. In general, the integration of 3D bioprinting into the practice of personalized medicine is revolutionizing the field by customizing therapeutic interventions to align with the specific genetic, anatomical, and physiological attributes of each patient, thus inaugurating a novel era of meticulousness and efficacy in the domain of healthcare (Lam et al., 2023).

8.6 Dental Applications

One noteworthy application pertains to the production of personalized dental implants and prosthetics. By utilizing the technique of 3D bioprinting, dental experts can fabricate highly accurate copies of a patient's oral structures, encompassing both teeth and gums. This allows for the creation of tailor-made implants that seamlessly integrate with the patient's existing dentition, thereby not only enhancing the aesthetic outcome but also elevating the functionality and comfort of dental prosthetics. Furthermore, the utilization of 3D bioprinting facilitates the generation of bioactive frameworks for tissue engineering in the realm of dental regenerative medicine (Mohd et al., 2023). The implementation of this technology enables the reconstruction of damaged oral tissues, such as periodontal ligaments or alveolar bone, thereby stimulating the regeneration of a patient's natural dental structures. Moreover, 3D bioprinting additionally contributes to the development of precise and patient-specific models for pre-surgical planning and dental education. This offers practitioners the opportunity to visualize intricate anatomical structures and simulate procedures prior to actual interventions. All in all, the utilization of 3D bioprinting in the field of dentistry is propelling the advancement of precision, customization, and regenerative capacity within dental treatments, signifying a momentous evolution in the practice of oral healthcare (Ramaiah et al., 2020).

8.7 Bioprinted Skin for Wound Healing

3D bioprinting is utilized in the production of synthetic skin for wound healing. These biofabricated skin structures can be employed further in the treatment of burn victims and individuals with chronic wounds, presenting a more efficient and personalized solution. Through the utilization of 3D bioprinting, scientists can accurately deposit layers of bioinks that contain living cells, growth factors, and biomaterials to construct three-dimensional structures that closely mimic the intricate architecture of natural skin. This facilitates the creation of skin grafts that are specific to each patient, possessing customized thickness, elasticity, and pigmentation, thus ensuring optimal integration and functional restoration upon transplantation. The bioprinted skin not only acts as a physical barrier, but also stimulates cellular regeneration and tissue repair, thereby expediting the process of wound healing (Guvendiren, 2019). Additionally, 3D bioprinting allows for the inclusion of various types of cells that include keratinocytes, fibroblasts, and endothelial cells, thereby replicating the complex cellular interactions that are crucial for skin functionality. This contributes to the development of bioprinted skin that is vascularized and innervated, promoting an enhanced blood supply and the integration of nerves in the regenerated tissue. Additionally, this technology enables the direct incorporation of antimicrobial agents or therapeutic substances into the printed constructs, addressing the issue of infection control and creating a favorable environment for healing. Furthermore, this technology also finds application in the field of drug testing, as 3D bioprinted skin models provide an opportunity for evaluating the effectiveness of topical treatments and wound care products, thereby reducing the necessity for animal testing (Jessop et al., 2017).

8.8 Orthopedics

3D bioprinting technology is increasingly emerging as a transformative force in the field of orthopedics, presenting innovative possibilities for the treatment of musculoskeletal conditions. A crucial application of this technology involves the production of tailored implants and scaffolds for the regeneration of bones and cartilages. 3D bioprinting paves the way for the creation of intricate structures by employing bioinks that encompass living cells, growth factors, and biomaterials. This facilitates the development of personalized implants that conform to the patient's anatomical specifications. Such an individualized approach enhances the integration of the implant, diminishes the likelihood of rejection, and improves overall treatment outcomes (Stanco et al., 2020). Likewise, 3D bioprinting empowers the production of intricate models that aid in surgical planning. This enables orthopedic surgeons to visualize and rehearse procedures on replicas that accurately replicate the patient's specific conditions prior to actual interventions. Additionally, this technology plays a vital role in the fabrication of artificial joints and ligaments, offering alternatives to joint replacement surgeries. By emulating the biomechanics and structure of natural tissues, 3D bioprinting in orthopedics holds immense potential in advancing regenerative therapies, enhancing patient mobility, and addressing the distinctive challenges associated with musculoskeletal disorders (Koçak et al., 2021).

8.9 Cosmetic and Aesthetic Procedures

3D bioprinting can be employed in the context of cosmetic and aesthetic procedures, to generate customized tissues, such as ear cartilage or soft tissue implants. By doing so, the precision and natural appearance of cosmetic interventions can be enhanced. A key area where this technology can be applied is in the creation of biofabricated tissues for reconstructive surgery or augmentation procedures. Through the precise deposition of bioinks that contain patient-specific cells and biomaterials, 3D bioprinting enables the fabrication of customized implants that seamlessly integrate with existing tissues. This approach minimizes the risk of rejection and enhances aesthetic outcomes (Vijayavenkataraman et al., 2016). The value of this technology is particularly evident in procedures like breast reconstruction or facial contouring, where achieving natural proportions and textures is of utmost importance. Moreover, 3D bioprinting contributes to the advancement of skin substitutes and dermal fillers, offering alternatives for tissue regeneration and wrinkle reduction. The ability to recreate intricate tissue structures and mimic the natural aging process makes 3D bioprinting a most promising tool for the progression of cosmetic and aesthetic procedures. Consequently, it provides safer and more tailored interventions that align with individual preferences and anatomical variations (Pu et al., 2023)

8.10 Veterinary Medicine

The utilization of this technology extends to the field of veterinary medicine, where it serves to produce implants, prosthetics, and tissues for animals, ultimately enhancing their general health and state of being. A noteworthy application of this technology involves the production of personalized implants and prosthetics that are tailored to the distinctive anatomies of individual animals, thus effectively addressing congenital abnormalities or injuries with a high level of precision (Gu et al., 2020). Within the realm of regenerative medicine, the implementation of 3D bioprinting facilitates the creation of tissue scaffolds, which in turn promote the regeneration of damaged tissues such as bones and cartilages in companion animals or livestock. This capability holds significant value, particularly when it comes to addressing musculoskeletal injuries or degenerative conditions associated with aging. Furthermore, 3D bioprinting plays a crucial role in advancing more ethically sound practices for drug testing, as it generates in vitro models that accurately replicate the physiological characteristics of specific animal organs. This innovative approach diminishes the reliance on traditional methods of animal testing. In the field of veterinary surgery, this technology assists in preoperative planning by enabling the creation of patient-specific models based on medical imaging data. This, in turn, enables veterinarians to visualize complex anatomical structures and simulate surgical procedures. All in all, 3D bioprinting harbors the potential to revolutionize veterinary medicine by providing tailored solutions that enhance diagnostic precision, treatment outcomes, and the overall well-being of animals (Tan et al., 2021).

9. The Plus Side of 3D bioprinting

3D bioprinting technology presents a plethora of advantages that possess the capacity to revolutionize the realm of regenerative medicine and biomedical research. One notable advantage rests in its capability to fabricate highly intricate and personalized biological constructs with meticulousness and intricacy, thereby enabling the reproduction of anatomically precise tissues and organs. This degree of personalization is vital in surmounting the obstacles faced in organ transplantation, as 3D bioprinting facilitates the generation of tissues tailored to the particular requirements and genetic composition of individual patients. The technology facilitates the integration of diverse cell types, biomaterials, and signaling molecules into a singular printed structure, emulating the innate intricacy of living tissues. Furthermore, 3D bioprinting permits the spatial arrangement of distinct cell types within a construct, fostering tissue functionality and the potential for interactions among multiple cells (Dongxu et al., 2022).

Another notable benefit lies in the capacity for high-throughput screening in the realm of drug discovery along with its development. Tissue models created through the process of 3D bioprinting possess the ability to serve as more physiologically relevant platforms for drug testing, yielding a closer approximation to human tissues when compared to traditional 2D cell cultures. Consequently, this not only amplifies the precision of preclinical trials but also diminishes dependence on animal models. Moreover, 3D bioprinting contributes to advancements in the field of disease modeling by granting researchers the capability to replicate pathological conditions and analyze disease progression within a controlled laboratory environment. Furthermore, this technology plays a crucial role in personalized medicine by enabling the generation of patient-specific tissues for drug testing and transplantation. Such an individualized approach exhibits the potential to enhance treatment outcomes while minimizing the likelihood of immune rejection. Additionally, 3D bioprinting contributes to the development of tissue engineering strategies, which in turn facilitate the repair and regeneration of impaired tissues and organs (Mazzocchi et al., 2019). The versatility of this technology can extend to the creation of implantable devices, including bioprinted scaffolds that offer support for tissue growth and integration within the human body. Despite the vast possibilities that 3D bioprinting presents, certain challenges related to scalability, vascularization, and long-term functionality remain. Nevertheless, the advantages of 3D bioprinting underscore its potential to revolutionize medical research, patient care, and the future landscape of regenerative medicine (Kačarević et al., 2018).

10. Hindrances

While 3D bioprinting technology holds great promise in the field of medicine and healthcare, it is not without its drawbacks and ethical considerations. One notable disadvantage pertains to the intricate nature and associated challenges of printing functional and vascularized organs. The replication of human tissues, including the intricate networks of blood vessels, proves to be a complex task with current bioprinting techniques. This limitation impedes the ability to create fully functioning organs, which in turn affects the efficacy of transplants and potentially restricts the range of treatable conditions (Chameettachal et al., 2019). Furthermore, a significant drawback lies in the long-term safety and effectiveness of 3D bioprinted organs. It is imperative that the biological and biomechanical properties of printed tissues closely resemble those of natural tissues in order to avoid potential rejection or adverse reactions in recipients. Achieving such a high level of precision necessitates extensive research and validation, and concerns persist regarding unforeseen complications that may arise over time (Gilbert et al., 2018).

The ethical implications surrounding 3D bioprinting also encompass issues such as the possibility for the misuse and commodification of human tissues. There is a risk that the technology could be exploited for purposes other than therapeutic use, raising concerns about the creation of organs for non-essential purposes or even for financial gain. Striking a balance between promoting innovation and preventing unethical practices necessitates thoughtful consideration and the establishment of robust regulatory frameworks (Patuzzo et al., 2018).

Furthermore, the financial burden linked with the utilization of 3D bioprinting technology represents a noteworthy drawback. The machinery, components, and specialized knowledge necessary for bioprinting are currently high-priced, which presents difficulties in terms of widespread acceptance and availability. This situation gives rise to apprehensions regarding the potential exacerbation of disparities in healthcare, as solely individuals with financial resources would be able to avail themselves of these advanced medical interventions (Jovic et al., 2020).

11. Challenges

While 3D bioprinting presents significant potential, its widespread adoption and application are impeded by various obstacles (Figure 3). One primary impediment stems from the intricate nature of replicating the complex microarchitectures found in natural tissues. Overcoming this challenge necessitates achieving the requisite level of precision and intricacy in the printing process to replicate the hierarchical organization observed in living tissues, which remains a formidable hurdle. Furthermore, ensuring the viability of cells throughout the bioprinting process represents another critical challenge. Effectively balancing printing speed, temperature, and the selection of bioink materials is crucial to optimize the prevention of cellular damage and the preservation of the functionality of the printed tissues.

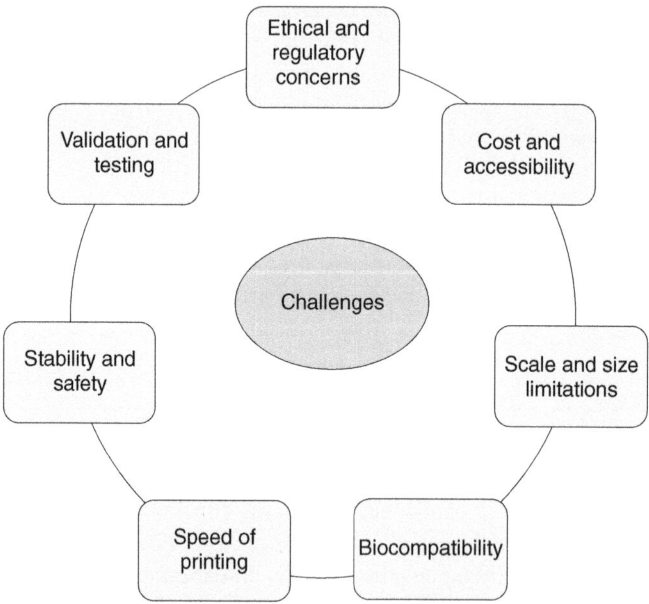

Fig. 3 The challenges associated with 3D bioprinting technology

The integration of blood vessels into bioprinted constructs is crucial for the viability of larger and metabolically active tissues, thus making vascularization a significant obstacle. The clinical relevance of bioprinted structures can be limited by the absence of a functional vascular network, which affects their thickness and complexity. Additionally, selecting suitable biomaterials for bioink formulations that replicate the mechanical along with biochemical properties of native tissues remains a persistent challenge. Critical considerations include ensuring biocompatibility, avoiding immune responses, and promoting long-term stability. The scalability of the bioprinting process is another notable challenge, particularly when aiming to produce tissues or organs of clinically relevant sizes. Innovative solutions are required to scale up such bioprinting processes without compromising the integrity and functionality of the printed constructs. The advancement of 3D bioprinting is also hindered by regulatory hurdles and ethical considerations (Agarwal et al., 2020)

The necessity for standardized protocols, safety assessments, and regulatory frameworks for bioprinted products adds complexity to their translation from the laboratory to clinical applications. Additionally, ethical concerns related to the acquisition of cells, specifically stem cells, and the potential for bioprinting to generate intricate biological entities raise ethical inquiries that necessitate attention. Despite these challenges, ongoing research and technological advancements persistently push the boundaries of 3D bioprinting, providing glimpses of a future wherein the technology can surmount these obstacles and deliver transformative resolutions in the field of regenerative medicine along with tissue engineering (Stanco et al., 2020).

12.   Ethics Associated with 3D Printed Organs

The ethical considerations surrounding the utilization of 3D printed organs give rise to a multitude of intricate deliberations that intersect with various domains of medicine, technology, and society. One noteworthy ethical concern centers around the fair and just distribution of this groundbreaking technology. As the advancement and accessibility of 3D printing of organs progress, inquiries emerge regarding the means to guarantee that all individuals, irrespective of their socioeconomic standing, can derive benefits from these life-preserving breakthroughs. The issues of equitable allocation and affordability necessitate careful navigation in order to avoid exacerbating existing disparities in healthcare provision (Patuzzo et al., 2018). Another ethical aspect involves the potential commodification of organs. Employing 3D printing technology introduces the possibility that organs might be treated as marketable commodities, thereby prompting apprehensions regarding the commercialization of human anatomical components. Striking a harmonious equilibrium between fostering innovation and safeguarding against exploitative practices is of paramount importance to upholding the ethical standards governing organ transplantation (Kirillova et al., 2020).

In addition, the ethical considerations surrounding the long-term safety and effectiveness of 3D printed organs are of utmost importance. To ensure that these bioprinted organs meet rigorous standards of quality and safety prior to being implanted in human bodies, it is imperative that thorough testing and regulation are in place. The research and development process should be guided by ethical frameworks that prioritize transparency, informed consent, and the well-being of patients. Furthermore, in the realm of 3D printed organs, concerns regarding privacy arise. Given that this technology relies on detailed patient-specific data, safeguarding individuals' privacy becomes a matter of great significance. The ethical implementation of 3D printed organs necessitates robust data protection measures and the acquisition of informed consent for the utilization of personal medical information (Gilbert et al., 2018).

13.   The Emerging Technologies

The future of regenerative medicine and biomedical research is being shaped by the emergence of new developments in 3D bioprinting technology. One noteworthy development pertains to the creation of vascularized tissues, which addresses a crucial challenge in the areas of bioprinting. To form intricate vascular networks within bioprinted constructs, researchers are exploring innovative methods, such as the incorporation of endothelial cells and sacrificial materials. This advancement shows promise in the production of larger and more metabolically active tissues by ensuring sufficient nutrient supply and efficient waste removal. Additionally, there is a notable shift towards the utilization of high-throughput bioprinting for drug screening purposes (Gilbert et al., 2018). As technology progresses, the capacity to print numerous tissue models concurrently or in quick succession enhances the efficacy of drug testing procedures, thereby enabling more comprehensive screening of pharmaceutical compounds. Furthermore, the incorporation of bioprinting with other cutting-edge technologies like artificial intelligence and machine learning, is gaining momentum. These technologies can contribute to the refinement of bioprinting parameters, resulting in improved precision, speed, and predictive modeling of tissue development. The investigation into novel bioink formulations, including the utilization of sophisticated biomaterials and extracellular matrix components, is fostering the production of more biomimetic and functional tissues. Additionally, the inclination towards collaborative interdisciplinary research is growing, with experts from the fields of biological sciences, engineering, and materials science working together to overcome obstacles and stimulate innovation in 3D bioprinting. These emerging trends collectively signify a future in which bioprinting technologies continue to progress, unlocking new possibilities for personalized medicine, tissue engineering, and transformative applications in healthcare (Chameettachal et al., 2019).

14.   Safety of 3D Bio Printed Medical Products

The preservation of the well-being of 3D bioprinted medical products is a matter of utmost importance in the advancement and utilization of this innovative technology. A primary concern revolves around the compatibility of the materials employed in the printing process with living organisms. It is of vital significance that the biomaterials chosen for bioprinting closely replicate the characteristics of human tissues to minimize the possibility of rejection or undesirable reactions upon implantation. Thorough testing and validation procedures are indispensable to ensure the safety and effectiveness of these materials, addressing concerns associated with their toxicity, capacity to provoke an immune response, and long-term durability (Patuzzo et al., 2018). The intricate complexity of the human anatomy presents an additional challenge in terms of safety in the realm of three-dimensional bioprinting. The accurate reproduction of intricate tissue structures, including vascular networks, is pivotal for the proper functioning of bioprinted organs. Insufficient blood supply can give rise to complications such as tissue death and impaired organ function. Researchers are actively engaged in the refinement of bioprinting techniques to tackle this challenge, with a particular emphasis on the creation of vascularized tissues that closely resemble the natural circulatory system (Gilbert et al., 2018). In addition to the considerations surrounding materials and structures, the sterility of the bioprinting process is of utmost importance to prevent infections and guarantee the safety of patients. The risk of introducing contaminants during the printing or post-printing phases must be minimized through rigorous quality control measures and adherence to sterile manufacturing practices. Any compromise in terms of sterility could expose individuals receiving 3D bioprinted medical products, particularly in the context of organ transplants, to serious health hazards.

Long-term surveillance is a crucial element of 3D bioprinting. It is imperative to conduct comprehensive studies following the implantation of bioprinted organs in order to evaluate their endurance and functionality over extended durations. This necessitates the continuous assessment of potential complications, such as immune reactions, tissue degradation, and unforeseen physiological responses. Given the progressive nature of bioprinting technology, continuous monitoring is necessary to identify and address any unanticipated safety concerns that may arise as the technology advances. Furthermore, ethical considerations encompass the safety of 3D bioprinted medical products. It is essential to engage in transparent and thorough communication with patients, providing them with comprehensive information about potential risks, benefits, and uncertainties, in order to obtain informed consent. Robust regulatory frameworks and ethical guidelines must be established to govern the development, testing, and deployment of 3D bioprinted products, ensuring that ethical standards are upheld throughout the entire process (Gilbert et al., 2018; Patuzzo et al., 2018).

15.   Future Prospects

The future potentials of 3D bioprinting technology bring about immense promise and are on the verge of transforming various aspects of medicine and biomedical research. One of the most notable potentials resides in the progress of personalized medicine. As the technology develops further, the capacity to fabricate tissues and organs that are specifically tailored for individual patients, for the purpose of transplantation or drug testing, could pave the way for a new era of customized medical treatments. This personalized approach holds the capacity to enhance treatment outcomes, mitigate the risk of rejection in transplantation, and augment the effectiveness of pharmaceutical interventions. Furthermore, 3D bioprinting can be expected to play a crucial role in addressing the worldwide crisis of organs' scarcity, by offering a viable solution for their fabrication of according to the existing demand. The possibility of bioprinting complete organs, such as kidneys or hearts, could alleviate the current limitations faced in organ transplantation and provide life-saving alternatives to patients who are on waiting lists. Additionally, the technology is projected to have the utmost significant impact on the field of regenerative medicine, as it enables the repair and replacement of damaged or degenerated tissues.

Advancements in the techniques used for bioprinting and bioink formulations can create functional tissues that seamlessly integrate with the host. This could provide new therapeutic options for individuals who have injuries, congenital defects, or degenerative conditions. In the areas of drug development, the ability of 3D bioprinting to produce tissue models that accurately mimic physiological conditions could improve the reliability of preclinical trials, reducing the reliance on animal models and speeding up the drug discovery process. As the technology continues to progress, the incorporation of other innovative technologies like artificial intelligence and advanced imaging techniques could further increase the precision and efficiency of bioprinting processes. Nevertheless, some challenges need to be addressed to fully unlock the transformative potential of 3D bioprinting. These challenges include vascularization, scalability, and ensuring long-term functionality. Despite these obstacles, the ongoing advancements in research and development indicate a future where 3D bioprinting becomes a widely adopted medical technology. This technology has the potential to offer groundbreaking solutions for personalized healthcare, organ transplantation, and regenerative medicine on a global scale (Arslan-Yildiz et al., 2016)

Conclusion

The technology of 3D bioprinting represents a radical and transformative force that intersects the fields of biology, engineering, and medicine. This convergence has resulted in a significant reshaping of the landscape within tissue engineering and regenerative medicine. This comprehensive examination serves to underscore the foundational principles that underpin 3D bioprinting, while also shedding light on its various applications in the realms of organ transplantation, disease modelling, and tissue repair. Although the potential of this technology is immense, there are obstacles that must be overcome, such as the development of functional bioinks and the achievement of vascularization within printed tissues. These challenges require collaborative and concerted efforts in order to advance the field in the future. However, despite these hurdles, it is important to recognize the significance of ongoing research and collaboration, as they hold the promise of personalized medicine and the potential to revolutionize therapies and drug discovery. As 3D bioprinting continues to progress, its transformative impact will continue to unfold, offering a glimpse into a future where the boundaries of tissue engineering are continuously surpassed, thus paving the way for groundbreaking medical applications.

References

Abaci, A. and Guvendiren, M. (2020) Designing Decellularized Extracellular Matrix-Based Bioinks for 3D Bioprinting. *Advanced Healthcare Materials*, 9(24), c2000734. doi:10.1002/adhm.202000734.

Afrinal, F., Khaswar, S., Yessie, W.S., Jaydee, C., Daniel, P., Bhushan, M., John, F. and Farah, F. (2022) 3D printed cellulose based product applications. *Materials Chemistry Frontiers*, 6, 254–279. doi:10.1039/D1QM00390A.

Ahasan, H. and Bashir, K. (2019) Development of clay based novel hybrid bio-ink for 3D bio-printing process. *Journal of Manufacturing Processes*, 38, 76–87. doi:10.1016/j.jmapro.2018.12.034.

Agarwal, S., Saha, S., Balla, V.K., Aniruddha, P., Ananya, B. and Bodhak, S. (2020) Current developments in 3D bioprinting for tissue and organ regeneration-a review. *Frontiers in Mechanical Engineering*, 6, 589171. doi:10.3389/fmech.2020.589171.

Allen, Z., Anuradha, S. and Swaminathan, S. (2022) Design considerations of bioinks for laser bioprinting technique towards tissue regenerative applications. *Bioprinting*, 27, e00205. doi:10.1016/j.bprint.2022.e00205.

Amanda, C. J., Sonali, S. Sydney, S. Victor, A.S., Julie, W., Zachary, L., Ryan, F., Leili, R. and Stephanie, M.W. (2023) 3D bioprinting for organ and organoid models and disease modelling. *Expert Opinion on Drug Discovery*, 18 (9), 1043–1059. doi:10.1080/17460441.2023.2234280.

Arslan-Yildiz, A., El Assal, R., Chen, P., Guven, S., Inci, F. and Demirci, U. (2016) Towards artificial tissue models: Past, present, and future of 3D bioprinting. *Biofabrication*, 8(1), 014103. doi:10.1088/1758-5090/8/1/014103.

Aathma, M.B., Kausalya, N.M., Bhagesh, B.H., Anarghya, H., Keerthana, K., Aparajita, S., Carol F.L., Keshav, D.V.S., Dharshini, G., Dhivya, D.S., Selinda, M., Shweta, C., Sree, R.R.D.K., Bobby, P. and Nirmal, M. (2021) An insight on advances and applications of 3d bioprinting: A review. *Bioprinting*, 24, e00176. doi:10.1016/j. bprint.2021.e00176.

Chameettachal, S., Yeleswarapu, S., Sasikumar, S., Shukla, P., Hibare, P., Bera, A.K., Bojedla, S.S.R. and Pati, F. (2019) 3D Bioprinting: Recent Trends and Challenges. *Journal of the Indian Institute of Science*, 99, 375–403. doi:10.1007/s41745-019-00113-z.

Choudhury, D., Anand, S. and Naing, M.W. (2018) The arrival of commercial bioprinters - Towards 3D bioprinting revolution! *International Journal of Bioprinting*, 4(2), 139. doi: 10.18063/IJB.v4i2.139.

Claire, Y., Xuanyi, M., Wei, Z., Pengrui, W., Kathleen, L.M., Jacob, S., Anna, K., Alexandria, H. and Shaochen, C. (2019) Scanningless and continuous 3D bioprinting of human tissues with decellularized extracellular matrix. *Biomaterials*, 194, 1–13. doi:10.1016/j.biomaterials.2018.12.009.

Cui, H., Nowicki, M., Fisher, J.P. and Zhang, L.G. (2016). 3D Bioprinting for Organ Regeneration. *Advanced Healthcare Materials*, 6(1), 1601118.doi:10.1002/adhm.201601118.

Dongxu, K., Changmei, N. and Xi, Y. (2022) Evolution of 3D bioprinting-from the perspectives of bioprinting companies, Bioprinting, 25, e00193. doi10.1016/j.bprint.2022.e00193.

Dzobo, K., Motaung, K.S.C.M. and Adesida, A. (2019) Recent trends in decellularized extracellular matrix bioinks for 3D printing: An updated review. *International Journal of Molecular Sciences*, 20 (18), 4628. doi:10.3390/ijms20184628.

Fatimi, A., Okoro, O.V., Podstawczyk, D., Siminska-Stanny, J. and Shavandi, A. (2022) Natural Hydrogel-Based Bio-Inks for 3D Bioprinting in Tissue Engineering: A Review. *Gels* 8(3), 179. doi:10.3390/gels8030179.

Gao, G., Ahn, M., Cho, W., Kim, B.S. and Cho, D.W. (2021) 3D Printing of Pharmaceutical Application: Drug Screening and Drug Delivery. *Pharmaceutics*, 13(9), 1373. doi:10.3390/pharmaceutics13091373.

Germain, N., Dhayer, M., Dekiouk, S. and Marchetti, P. (2022) Current Advances in 3D Bioprinting for Cancer Modeling and Personalized Medicine. *International Journal of Molecular Sciences*, 23(7), 3432. doi:10.3390/ijms2307343.

Gilbert, F., O'Connell, C.D., Mladenovska, T. and Dodds, S. (2018) Print Me an Organ? Ethical and Regulatory Issues Emerging from 3D Bioprinting in Medicine. *Science and Engineering Ethics*, 24(1), 73–91. doi:10.1007/s11948-017-9874-6.

Gu, B.K., Choi, D.J., Park, S.J., Kim, Y.J. and Kim, C.H. (2018) 3D Bioprinting Technologies for Tissue Engineering Applications. *Advances in Experimental Medicine and Biology*,1078, 15–28. doi:10.1007/978-981-13-0950-2_2.

Gu, Z., Fu, J., Lin, H. and He, Y. (2020) Development of 3D bioprinting: From printing methods to biomedical applications. *Asian Journal of Pharmaceutical Sciences*, 15 (5), 529–557. doi:10.1016/j.ajps.2019.11.003.

Guvendiren, M. (2019) *3D Bioprinting in Medicine: Technologies, Bioinks, and Applications*, United States: Springer International Publishing. 209 doi:10.1007/978-3-030-23906-0.

Ibrahim, T.O. and Monika, H. (2016) Current advances and future perspectives in extrusion-based bioprinting. *Biomaterials* 76, 321-343. doi:10.1016/j.biomaterials.2015.10.076.

James, S. and Mulgaonkar, S. (2022) Study on parameter optimization of 3D bioprinting of hybrid bio-inks. *The International Journal of Advanced Manufacturing Technology*, 119, 7063–7074. doi:10.1007/s00170-021-08561-7.

Janitha, M.U. and Ambalangodage, C.J. (2020) Hydrogel-based 3D bioprinting: A comprehensive review on cell-laden hydrogels, bioink formulations, and future perspectives. *Applied Materials Today*, 18, 100479. doi:10.1016/j. apmt.2019.100479.

Jessop, Z.M., Al-Sabah, A., Gardiner, M.D., Combellack, E., Hawkins, K. and Whitaker, I.S. (2017) 3D bioprinting for reconstructive surgery: Principles, applications and challenges. *Journal of Plastic, Reconstructive and Aesthetic Surgery*, 70(9), 1155–1170. doi:10.1016/j.bjps.2017.06.001.

Jovic, T.H., Combellack, E.J., Jessop, Z.M. and Whitaker, I.S. (2020) 3D Bioprinting and the Future of Surgery. *Frontiers in Surgery*, 27(7), 609836. doi: 10.3389/fsurg.2020.609836.

Kačarević, Ž.P., Rider, P.M., Alkildani, S., Retnasingh, S., Smeets, R., Jung, O., Ivanišević, Z., Barbeck, M. and Barbeck, M. (2018) An introduction to 3D bioprinting: Possibilities, challenges and future aspects. *Materials*, 11(11), 2199. doi:10.3390/ma11112199.

Khoeini, R., Nosrati, H., Akbarzadeh, A., Eftekhari, A., Kavetskyy, T., Khalilov, R., Ahmadian, E., Nasibova, A., Datta, P., Roshangar, L., Dante, C.D., Soodabeh, D., Magali, C. and Ibrahim, T.O. (2021) Natural and Synthetic Bioinks for 3D Bioprinting. *Advanced NanoBiomed Research*, 1(8). doi:10.1002/anbr.202000097.

Koçak, E., Yıldız, A. and Acartürk, F. (2021) Three dimensional bioprinting technology: Applications in pharmaceutical and biomedical area. *Colloids and Surfaces B: Biointerfaces*, 197, 111396. doi:10.1016/j.colsurfb.2020.111396.

Kirillova, A., Bushev, S., Abubakirov, A. and Sukikh, G. (2020) Bioethical and Legal Issues in 3D Bioprinting. *International Journal of Bioprinting* 6(3), 272. doi: 10.18063/ijb.v6i3.272.

Lam, E.H.Y., Yu, F., Zhu, S. and Wang, Z. (2023) 3D Bioprinting for Next-Generation Personalized Medicine. *International Journal of Molecular Sciences*, 24(7), 6357. doi:org/10.3390/ijms24076357.

Li, J., Chen, M., Fan, X. and Zhou, H. (2016) Recent advances in bioprinting techniques: Approaches, applications and future prospects. *Journal of Translational Medicine*, 14(1). doi:10.1186/s12967-016-1028-0.

Ma, X., Liu, J., Zhu, W., Tang, M., Lawrence, N., Yu, C., Gou, M. and Chen, S. (2018) 3D bioprinting of functional tissue models for personalized drug screening and in vitro disease modeling. *Advanced Drug Delivery Reviews*, 132, 235–251. doi:10.1016/j.addr.2018.06.011.

Matai, I., Kaur, G., Seyedsalehi, A., McClinton, A. and Laurencin, C.T. (2020) Progress in 3D bioprinting technology for tissue/organ regenerative engineering. *Biomaterials*, 226, 119536. doi:10.1016/j.biomaterials.2019.119536.

Memic, A., Ali, N., Bahram, M., Julio, A.V.C., Musab, A., Alireza, D., Mohsen, A. and Mehdi, N. (2017) Bioprinting technologies for disease modeling. Biotechnology Letters, 39 (9), 1279–1290. doi:10.1007/s10529-017-2360-z.

Mohd, N., Razali, M., Fauzi, M.B. and Abu, K.N.H. (2023) In Vitro and In Vivo Biological Assessments of 3D-Bioprinted Scaffolds for Dental Applications. *International Journal of Molecular Sciences*, 24(16), 12881. doi:10.3390/ijms241612881.

Murphy, S. and Atala, A. (2014) 3D bioprinting of tissues and organs. *Nature Biotechnology,* 32, 773–785. doi:10.1038/nbt.2958.

Ozbolat, I.T. (2017) *3D Bioprinting: Fundamentals, Principles and Applications.* London, United Kingdom: Academic Press, 1–337.

Parak, A., Pradeep, P., du Toit, L.C., Kumar, P., Choonara, Y.E. and Pillay, V. (2019) Functionalizing bioinks for 3D bioprinting applications. *Drug Discovery Today*, 24 (1), 198–205. doi:10.1016/j.drudis.2018.09.012.

Patuzzo, S., Goracci, G., Gasperini, L. and Ciliberti, R. (2018) 3D Bioprinting Technology: Scientific Aspects and Ethical Issues. *Science and Engineering Ethics,* 24(2), 335–348. doi: 10.1007/s11948-017-9918-y.

Peng, W., Datta, P., Ayan, B., Ozbolat, V., Sosnoski, D. and Ozbolat, I.T. (2017) 3D bioprinting for drug discovery and development in pharmaceutics. *Acta Biomaterialia,* 15(57), 26–46. doi:10.1016/j.actbio.2017.05.025.

Pu, Y., Yıkun, Ju., Yue, Hu., Xiaoyan, X., Bairong, F. and Lanjie Lei (2023) Emerging 3D bioprinting applications in plastic surgery. Biomaterials Research, 27 (1), doi: 10.1186/s40824-022-00338-7.

Ramiah, P., du Toit, L.C., Choonara, Y.E., Kondiah, P.P.D. and Pillay, V. (2020) Hydrogel-Based Bioinks for 3D Bioprinting in Tissue Regeneration. *Frontiers in Materials*, 7. doi:10.3389/fmats.2020.00076.

Salah, M., Naini, F.B. and Tayebi, L. (2022) 3D Printing and Bioprinting of Biomaterials and Bioceramic Scaffolds: Clinical Outcomes and Implications in Bone Tissue Engineering and Maxillofacial Reconstructive Surgery. In: Choi, A.H., Ben-Nissan, B. (eds) *Innovative Bioceramics in Translational Medicine II.* Vol 18. Singapore: Springer. doi:10.1007/978-981-16-7439-6_2.

Sanjairaj, V., Wei-Cheng, Y., Wen, F.L., Chi-Hwa, W., Jerry, Y.H.F. (2018) 3D bioprinting of tissues and organs for regenerative medicine. *Advanced Drug Delivery Reviews*, 132, 296–332. doi:10.1016/j.addr.2018.07.004.

Satpathy, A., Datta, P., Wu, Y., Ayan, B., Bayram, E. and Ozbolat, I.T. (2018) Developments with 3D bioprinting for novel drug discovery. *Expert Opinion on Drug Discovery*, 13 (12), 1115–1129. doi:10.1080/17460441.2018.1542427.

Selcan, P.G., Ilyas, I., Yu, S.Z., Ali, K. and Mehmet, R.D. (2018) Bioinks for 3D bioprinting: an overview. *Biomaterial Sciences*, 6, 915–946. doi: 10.1039/C7BM00765E.

Shahrubudin, N., Lee, T.C. and Ramlan, R. (2019) An overview on 3D printing technology: Technological, materials, and applications. *Procedia Manufacturing*, 35, 1286–1296. doi:10.1016/j.promfg.2019.06.089.

Sigaux, N., Pourchet, L., Breton, P., Brosset, S., Louvrier, A. and Marquette, C.A. (2019) 3D Bioprinting: principles, fantasies and prospects. *Journal of Stomatology, Oral and Maxillofacial Surgery*, 120 (2) 128–132. doi:10.1016/j.jormas.2018.12.014.

Sina, A.M., Saeid, M. and Roger, J.N. (2019) Inkjet dispensing technologies: recent advances for novel drug discovery. *Expert Opinion on Drug Discovery,* 14(2), 101–113. doi: 10.1080/17460441.2019.1567489.

Sonu, K., Abhimanyu, T. and Sabu, T. (2021) 3D Bioprinting of Nature-Inspired Hydrogel Inks Based on Synthetic Polymers. *ACS Applied Polymer Materials,* 3 (8) 3685–3701. doi: 10.1021/acsapm.1c00567.

Stanco, D., Urbán, P,. Tirendi, S., Ciardelli, G. and Barrero, J. (2020) 3D bioprinting for orthopaedic applications: Current advances, challenges and regulatory considerations. *Bioprinting,* 20, e00103. doi:10.1016/j.bprint.2020.e00103.

Tan, B., Gan, S., Wang, X., Liu, W. and Li, X. (2021) Applications of 3D bioprinting in tissue engineering: advantages, deficiencies, improvements, and future perspectives. *Journal of Materials Chemistry B,* 5385–5413. doi:10.1039/d1tb00172h.

Thayer, P., Martinez, H. and Gatenholm, E. (2020) History and Trends of 3D Bioprinting. *3D Bioprinting Principles and Protocols,* UK: Humana Press Inc., 3–18. doi:10.1007/978-1-0716-0520-2_1.

Valeria, F. and Charalampos, T. (2018) Recent advances on the development of phantoms using 3D printing for imaging with CT, MRI, PET, SPECT, and ultrasound. *Medical Physics,* 45 (9), e740-e760. doi:10.1002/mp.13058.

Vanaei, S., Parizi, M.S., Vanaei, S., Salemizadehparizi, F. and Vanaei, H.R. (2021) An Overview on Materials and Techniques in 3D Bioprinting Toward Biomedical Application. *Engineered Regeneration,* 2, 1–18. doi:10.1016/j.engreg.2020.12.001.

Vijayavenkataraman, S., Lu W.F. and Fuh, J.Y.H. (2016) 3D bioprinting of skin: a state-of-the-art review on modelling, materials, and processes. *Biofabrication,* 8 (3), 032001. doi: 10.1088/1758-5090/8/3/032001.

Wan, J.W.N.L., Sajab, M.S., Mohamed, A.P. and Kaco, H. (2022) Recent Advances in 3D Bioprinting: A Review of Cellulose-Based Biomaterials Ink. *Polymers,* 14(11), 2260. doi:10.3390/polym14112260.

Zhang, X. and Zhang, Y. (2015) Tissue Engineering Applications of Three-Dimensional Bioprinting. *Cell Biochemistry and Biophysics,* 72(3), 777–782. doi:10.1007/s12013-015-0531-x.

Zhou, J., Tian, Z., Tian, Q., Peng, L., Li, K., Luo, X., Wang, D., Yang, Z., Jiang, S., Sui, X., Huang, J., Liu, S., Hao, L., Tang, P., Yao, Q. and Guo, Q. (2021) 3D bioprinting of a biomimetic meniscal scaffold for application in tissue engineering. *Bioactive Materials,* 6 (6), 1711-1726. doi: 10.1016/j.bioactmat.2020.11.027.

Strategies in 3D Bioprinting

Ashis Kumar Bera,[1] *Anwesha Ghosh,*[1] *Amit Ghosh,*[2]
Lubna Zeenat,[2] *MD Abdullah,*[1] *Mansi Dixit,*[1]
and *Falguni Pati*[1,2]*

1. Introduction

Most of the preclinical research and current understanding of physiology and pathology comes from 2D/3D cell culture systems and animal models. Although a 2D or 3D cell culture simplifies experiments and produces faster results, its use in clinical research and translational medicine is limited due to a lack of tissue-level architecture (Cukierman et al., 2002; Rimann & Graf-Hausner, 2012; Duval et al., 2017). Tissue architecture, cell-cell and cell-matrix interactions, and biophysical signals from the 3D niche are all important aspects of the system that are overlooked in reductionist 2D and even 3D cell cultures. However, in the animal model, species-level genetic and behavioral alterations are not always as predictive as they are in clinical contexts. Additionally, ethical concerns and regulations force tissue engineering for an alternative approach (Jackson & Thomas, 2017; Yamada & Cukierman, 2007). Thus, 3D tissue models that more closely resemble the tissue-level architectural organization of human biology are desired for these applications.

Tissue engineering and regenerative medicine have made rapid advances in the development of multifunctional, three-dimensional (3D) tissue constructs, as well as innovative treatment techniques for tissue regeneration or organ replacement (Murphy & Atala, 2014; Kang et al., 2016; Mandrycky et al., 2016; Mikos et al., 2006). Biofabrication offers a potential method for developing complex 3D biological constructs capable of reproducing the functional organization of human tissues while allowing for physiologically realistic cell interactions (Pati et al., 2014). Although the 3D printing technology is commonly used to reproducibly make products with complicated geometry and architecture in home, design, arts, and science, the potential of its translation in tissue engineering came to the attention of the community not long ago (Murphy et al., 2014). Bioprinting falls under the broad flagship category of additive manufacturing. It is a multidisciplinary approach based on material science, mechanics, biology, medicine, and engineering, contributing equally to

---

[1] Department of Biomedical Engineering, Indian Institute of Technology Hyderabad, Kandi, India.
[2] Centre for Interdisciplinary programs, Indian Institute of Technology Hyderabad, Kandi, India.
* Corresponding author: falguni@bme.iith.ac.in

creating a tissue analogue like in vivo. In 3D bioprinting, biomaterials, including embedded cells, known as "bioink," are deposited on the collecting substrate layer by layer in the required patterns defined by the printer. Such techniques are enabled by extraordinary accuracy in bioink dispensing by robotics, allowing for the reproducible production of biological structures with minimum aberrations in shape, architecture, and, eventually, function. The entire bioprinting process is automated, with no human operators needed for high-throughput tissue development for in vitro tissue models or translational purposes. Traditionally, the three essential components of TE (cells, biomaterials, and growth factors) are mixed to create a construct that may be implanted immediately or matured in vitro before transplantation (Groll et al., 2014). Here, we discuss the various aspects of bioprinting technology, paying special attention to the various strategies employed in biofabrication for reconstructing 3D tissue structure. Furthermore, we also discuss the current approaches and their limitations. The new developments and future prospects of this technology are also emphasized.

2.   General Consideration of Bioprinting

The bioprinting process workflow generally begins with data acquisition using magnetic resonance imaging (MRI), computed tomography (CT), optical coherence tomography (OCT), and photoacoustic tomography (PAT) images of the diseased tissue or organ to be constructed (Jorgensen et al., 2020; Zhang et al., 2018) (Figure 1. step 1). These medical imaging data sets contain fundamental details about the volumetric shape of tissues and organs, but microstructure and even cellular information cannot be obtained using these approaches (Figure 1. step 2). Advanced microscopy (fluorescent, confocal, or two-photon) may reveal further information at the cellular level; however, the structures that may be photographed are often restricted in size, and primary tissue must be sacrificed (Albanna et al., 2018). This data can be readily imported into a computer to construct the entire structure by computer-aided design or mathematical modeling, figuring out how closely to imitate the topographical features to match them in vivo equivalents. Currently, MRI or CT data sets are mainly utilized to create the overall volume, while information regarding the infill is often designed using open-source or proprietary bioprinted software (Figure 1. step 3). This is still a limiting factor for more innovative bioprinting procedures, therefore the entire power of the technology has yet to be unveiled.

The process is then followed by selecting biomaterials and cells that can support the encapsulated cells while having physical and chemical properties appropriate for a specific set of bioprinting procedures. Biomaterials, like the ECM in native tissue, play a significant role in cell attachment, proliferation, tissue maturation, and functioning (Figure 1. step 4). Depending on the target tissue, where mechanical strength is the principal attribute, such as bone tissue, materials must analyze its degradation profile over time to regenerate (Freed et al., 1994). Functionalization of biomaterials (e.g., fibronectin, laminin, and R.G.D.) (Liu et al., 2012; Hoffman, 2012) can also be achieved by providing the synthetic materials used in bioprinting with the appropriate physical properties. Besides materials, encapsulated cells comprised as a critical component of the bioink. Depending on the target tissue structures, cells can be dispersed in the bioink as single cells or aggregated as a spheroid (Bhise et al., 2016). While single cell dispersion provides for greater flexibility in producing scaffolds with high precision, spheroid may be employed for larger scaffolds with high cell density (Figure 1. step 5). After considering bioink, the printing process must be chosen based on the bioink and the target scaffold in order to better imitate hierarchical architecture similar to real tissue (Figure 1. step 6). There is a broad range of fabrication systems accessible today, but each process has limitations, and no approach is considered superior to another. Here, we focus on the three most relevant fabrication techniques for fabricating hydrogel-based materials suitable for 3D bioprinting: laser-induced forward transfer, inkjet bioprinting, and extrusion-based bioprinting. These techniques are described in detail and compared to each other in the following section.

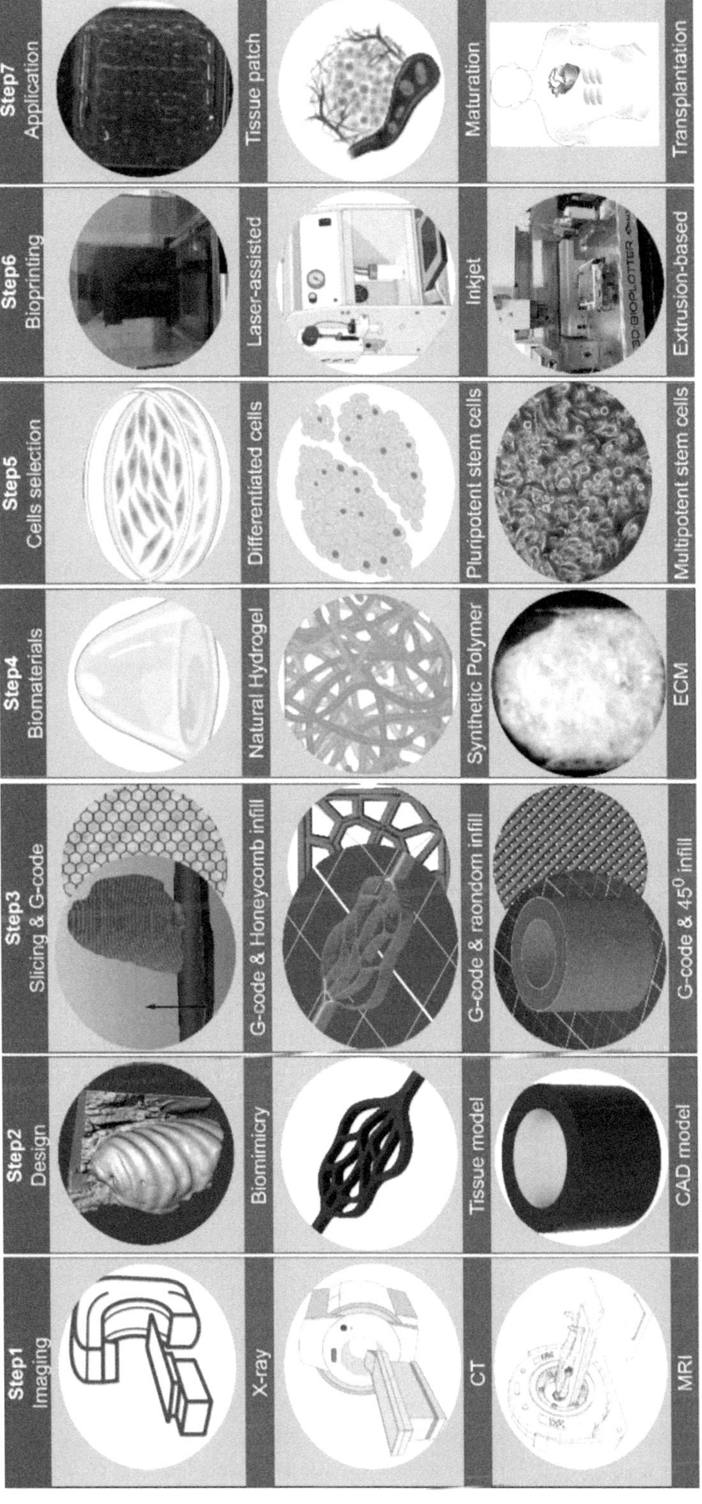

Fig. 1　Schematic representation of different steps of 3D bioprinting strategies.

3. Laser-induced Forward Transfer

Laser-assisted bioprinting (LaBP) also known as Laser-induced forward transfer (LIFT) techniques, include three main components: a pulsed laser, a donor slide, and a receiving substrate. The movement of the donor and substrate layer can be adjusted to build both 2D and 3D structures. Modified LIFT comprises two versions: matrix-assisted pulsed laser evaporation direct writing (MAPLE-DW) and absorbing film-assisted laser-induced forward transfer (AFA-LIFT). The two techniques differ in the setup of the donor-layer used, MAPLE-DW constitutes two different layers: a supporting laser-transparent layer and a laser absorbing layer. While AFA-LIFT has three different layers; in addition to laser-transparent supporting layers and laser-absorbing layers, there is a deposition layer. The laser-absorbing layer is metal coated (100 nm), and on absorbing the laser it fosters the evaporation of the coating, which in turn builds a high-pressure bubble propelling the material to the surface and eventually assisting in the final deposition. The receiving layer on the other hand is coated with hydrogel (20–40 μm) that cushions the impact for cell deposition and prevents drying of the material (Jungst et al., 2016). The resolution of LIFT techniques is quite high and is mainly dependent on the energy and the duration of the laser pulse, the thickness of the deposited material and its properties (Duocastella et al., 2008). LaBP has been used to develop a proof-of-concept for the fabrication of a 3D-cornea using functional biomaterials and human stem cells (Sorkio et al., 2018). Further LaBP along with GelMA as a supporting material has been used to develop arrays of spheroids with high printing speed and high cell viability (Hakobyan et al., 2020). Bone and cartilage engineering have been performed using LaBP to reinforce tricalcium silicate-based bioink and generate electrospun injectable nanofibers ensuring biocompatibility and a mechanically robust environment (Li et al., 2023).

4. Inkjet Bioprinting

Inkjet bioprinting is one of the initial bioprinting approaches known as table-top bioprinting (Winston C.R., Winston C.R., 1962; Steven I. Zoltan S.H., 1972). Early studies have shown that inkjet-based bioprinting offers distinct benefits over extrusion bioprinting in terms of contactless, speed, high resolution, and precise control over the deposition droplets. It is a precise and repeatable technique used to deposit cells and biomaterials in droplet form, enabling a variety of patterns for diverse applications (Freed et al., 1994). The combination of cells, biomaterials, and bioactive chemicals known as bioinks is one of the key elements of inkjet-based bioprinting. Based on the type of driving force employed, inkjet bioprinting is majorly divided into three types: thermal, electrostatic, and piezoelectric inkjet bioprinting (Figure 2) (Li et al., 2018). The different types of Inkjet bioprinters available for biomedical applications are low cost, easy to operate, possess a fast fabrication speed, high resolution, and high throughput droplet generation. The print resolution for inkjet bioprinting lies between 10 to 50 μm. In various applications, it is shown that the bioink viscosity is not more than 10 mPa-s. It is also shown that the cell viability after printing is greater than 85% (Zhou et al., 2019).

4.1 *Thermal Inkjet Bioprinting*

The mechanism of thermal inkjet-bioprinting starts by heating the thermal actuator inside the cartridge near the nozzle head, which generates small sized air bubbles to eject the bioink into droplet form on the print bed (Figure 2A). At first, a quick electric pulse is supplied to the thermal actuator, which suddenly raises the temperature close to 300°C. After that, the heated actuator evaporates the bioink, creating an air bubble that drives the bioink outside in droplet form (Cui et al., 2009).

4.2 *Electrostatic Inkjet Bioprinting*

Droplets are generated by changing the fluid volume inside the bioink loaded cartridge (Figure 2B). The increase in voltage between the electrode and the pressure plate raises the chamber volume, activating the bioink flow from the nozzle head in a droplet fashion. The deflected pressure plate returns to its normal form when the charge is turned off. The increased pressure then forces the droplets out (Kamisuki et al., 1998). Because of its electrostatic-driven power, electrostatic printing is inexpensive; nevertheless, its tiny orifices frequently clog.

4.3 Piezoelectric Inkjet Bioprinting

The name suggests that this type of bioprinting is accelerated by piezoelectric force (Figure 2C). An actuator is attached at the bottom of the extrusion head, where altered voltage is applied to change the shape of the present actuator. After that, the fluid chamber volume is changed, leading to pressure difference, and then, gradually, bioink droplets come out from the nozzle head, incapacitating the surface tension. According to published reports, printheads may be classified into four categories in piezoelectric printing: shear mode printhead, push mode printhead, bend mode printhead, and squeeze mode nozzle printhead (Li et al., 2018).

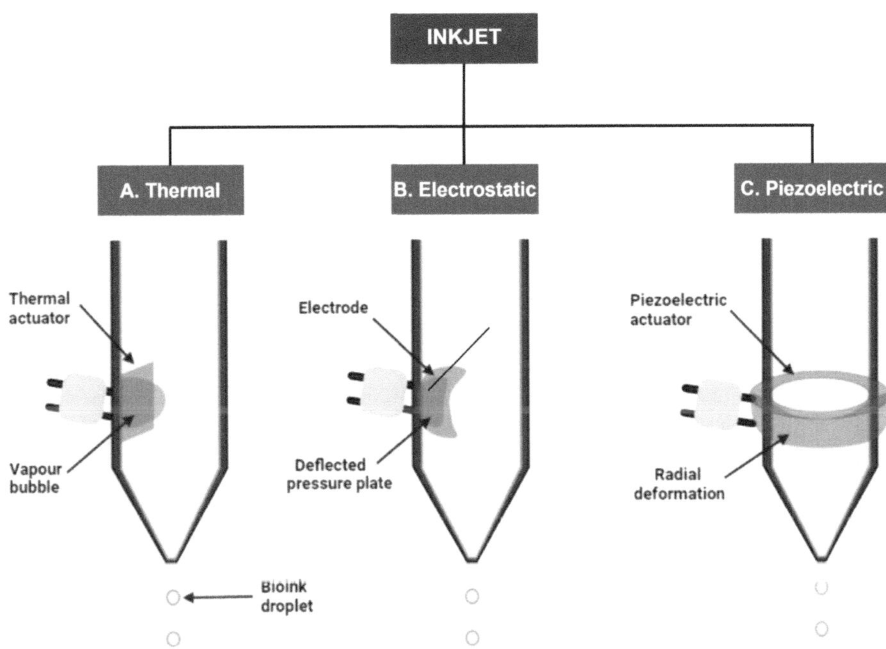

Fig. 2 Different types of inkjet bioprinting strategies. Schematic diagrams of different mechanisms of inkjet bioprinting. (A) Thermal inkjet bioprinting, (B) Electrostatic inkjet bioprinting, (C) Piezoelectric inkjet bioprinting.

4.4 Biomaterials for Inkjet Bioprinting

Currently available biomaterials for inkjet bioprinting include natural polymers, like Collagen 1, Alginate, Gelatin, Hyaluronic acid, silk, and Chitosan, whereas synthetic polymers include polyethylene glycol (PEG), Polycaprolactone (PCL), Polylactic Acid (PCL), and Poly (lactic-co-glycolic acid) (PLGA). The range of applications includes biomedical engineering of different tissues, regenerative medicine, drug delivery systems, and drug formulation (Li et al., 2018; Zhou, et al., 2019). Among the different biomaterials used in inkjet bioprinting, hydrogels made up of hydrophilic polymers have many advantages that make them a suitable material for inkjet bioprinting. Hydrogel viscosity can be controlled when printing different 3D structures with a unique property of rapid water absorption and swelling when embedded in a modulation solution for 3D tissue constructs (Chai et al., 2017). After printing, it can be crosslinked physically, chemically, or thermally to retain the shape without degradation. It is suggested that crosslinking of the hydrogel during printing can lead to channel clogging; therefore, crosslinking should occur after printing. It also maintains the shape fidelity after printing and allows the transfer of nutrients and dissolved oxygen to the cells. The ECM mimicking hydrogels have important components of the natural ECM that enhance better cell attachment, proliferation, migration, and transdifferentiation into different lineages with suitable biomolecular cues. ECM hydrogels also preserve the tissue microenvironment for cellular growth, providing native-like growth conditions for the biological construct (Kyle et al., 2017).

4.5 Biomedical Application of Inkjet Bioprinting

Inkjet 3D scaffolds play a significant role in tissue and organ regeneration. Three essential components of a well-built 3D scaffold are mechanical strength, cytocompatibility, and structural integrity. As discussed above, cytocompatibility of inkjet bioprinting has been shown to come up with the standards for tissue engineering and regenerative medicine. Along with biological functional scaffold fabrication in various applications in the field of biomedical engineering (Kuma et al., 2021), inkjet bioprinting has a profound application in pharmaceutical drug formulation, drug-loaded vesicle formulation, drug coating, biomaterial patterning, cell-free scaffold fabrication, and drug screening (Li et al., 2020).

Many processes and considerations must be made throughout the formulation process to optimize a drug's pharmacological, physical, and chemical qualities. Conventional drug formulation methods are based on the crystal formation of drug solutions that take several days. Advancing these preparation strategies, inkjet printing has been used to speed up the process with higher accuracy and purity. The formation of very small volume (5-20 pL) droplets enhances rapid evaporation and crystallization (Buanz et al., 2013). Similarly, for drug-loaded vesicle formulation, tablets of various sizes and shapes have been produced by inkjet bioprinting, allowing for the manipulation of dosage and adjustment of the drug release profile. Next is the ability to coat drugs in various biomedical transplantable stents, including highly and weakly soluble ones, demonstrated using inkjet bioprinting technology. Due to its ability to print at high resolution in the micrometer range, inkjet bioprinting is a desirable patterning approach for metal particles and polymers (Tekin et al., 2008). Additionally, three-dimensional matrices or constructs that may imitate the extracellular milieu and offer a platform for tissue regeneration and cell proliferation are called cell-free scaffold fabrications. Instead of seeding scaffolds with living cells as is typically done in traditional tissue engineering, cell-free scaffolds concentrate on providing structural support and signals for the recruitment of endogenous cells and the development of tissues. Regenerative medicine and tissue healing are only two of the biological uses for these scaffolds. Drug screening refers to checking the various parameters of a drug to ensure an effective treatment strategy of its appropriate dose in a very short time and a controlled manner. New drugs are being screened by Inkjet bioprinting, which is becoming increasingly popular in drug screening because its drop-on-demand technique allows for the production of ink droplets with a varied and adjustable volume range (from pL to L), ensuring the uniformity of drug chemical responses (Daly et al., 2015).

5. Extrusion-based Bioprinting

Extrusion bioprinting is most widely used due to its scalability, practicality, affordability, and potential to print clinical-scale tissue. Extrusion bioprinting was first introduced in 2002. Cell-based ink is extruded like thread or filament using mechanical and pneumatic pressure. In extrusion bioprinting, two or more printing heads are attached that are capable of extruding bioink composed of a single and different combination of materials, growth factors, and cells by exerting continuous pressure that helps in the dispersion of the bioink thread through a small-scale nozzle. The cartridge is fixed during printing, and the arms move in different directions, but the movement depends on the printer's design and model. Extrusion bioprinting has an edge over other bioprinting approaches in terms of print speed; pressure with high viscous bioink reduces harsh conditions, shear stress, and shock on the cells, which helps to improve cellular viability.

Extrusion bioprinting has numerous advantages. The significant advantage of this method is scalability, which is the potential to print patient-specific constructs that mimic biological tissue, which is very difficult with the help of other bioprinting methods. Printing with high cell concentration and high viscosity (600 kPa s) nearly equal to native tissue is another advantage. The disadvantage of this approach is the lowest resolution (~100 µm) of all the existing bioprinting techniques, Hydrogel deformation, and potential nozzle clogging. The applicability of extrusion bioprinting is also tuned with multi-material and coaxial techniques. It is suitable to 3D bio print different biological constructs, including liver, kidney, blood vessels, tracheal graft, adipose tissue, and other engineered tissue. Pneumatic extrusion printing may be the best method for using specific polymers, such as Gelatin, silk fibroin, polyethylene glycol, GelMA, and other hosts of self-gelling/entangling inks because they possess shear thinning. Fabricating hollow filaments with tiny channels and concentric multilayered round biological structures is ideally suited for the coaxial nozzle approach. Additionally, the devices are easily adjustable to the properties of newly created materials by simply modifying the extrusion nozzle dimensions. They are also readily accessible commercially.

Table 1   Comparison of different 3D bioprinting techniques

Technique	Features	Advantages	Disadvantages	Cost and Effect on cells	References
Laser-assisted 3D bioprinting	A laser pulse is propelled onto a ribbon containing bioinks, the latter are extruded	High viscosity bioinks and high-cell density can be easily handled with high precision and resolution.	Expensive and time taking process.	High. Cell viability is >95%	(Murphy et al., 2014)
Inkjet bioprinting	Bioink is expelled in the form of droplets by piezoelectric, thermal or electromagnetic forces.	Inexpensive with high speed, fast.	Droplet size and placement are still a challenge. High viscosity bioinks also pose difficulty in being inkjetted.	Low. Cell viability is >85%	(Murphy, et al., 2014)
Extrusion	The ink moves through a nozzle either on the application of pneumatic or mechanical force or a screw-based system.	High viscosity bioinks and high cell density can be printed	Cells may be affected due to shear forces applied inside the nozzle.	Medium. Cell viability is low ~40%	(Murphy et al., 2014) (Pati et al., 2014)

6. Consideration for Bioink Development

Cells reside in a complex dynamic microenvironment referred to as extracellular matrix (Hu et al., 2022). The ECM is a heterotypic mixture of various biophysical and biochemical cues and this composition varies according to tissue type and function. Tissue engineering comes into play to develop biomimetic materials that can serve as a realistic cellular microenvironment (Zhang et al., 2021). Ideally the developed biomaterial should not only act as a support scaffold but also provides the niche specific cues required for cellular growth proliferation differentiation. These preceding events eventually affect the cellular signaling pathway required for proper functioning of the particular tissue. With the advancement in fields of tissue engineering and regenerative medicines in the early 90s, researchers around the globe recognized that the 2D cell culture technique fails to mimic the in vitro cellular response (Duval et al., 2017). In order to surpass the primary limitation, emerging studies have encapsulated specific cells within the biomimetic hydrogels to recreate the bulk cellular microenvironment for more effective development of engineered functional tissue. These 3D polymeric systems mostly involve natural polymers, synthetic polymers, hybrid hydrogels like different polymeric blends or nanocomposite hydrogels. Further these polymeric hydrogels are often mixed with different growth factors, bioactive molecules and functionalized peptides to provide the suitable environment required for proper cellular activity (Nicolas et al., 2020). The 2D tissue culture plate oversimplifies the native microenvironment. In 2D systems, cells are adhered to each other and to the substratum in one direction and the cells can migrate freely without any physical constraints while in 3D systems, the cells get adhered from all directions, thereby creating the apical-basal polarity and the required junctions to hold the cells together to prevent paracellular diffusion (Del et al., 2019). Eventually, all these events correspond to native like cellular functions.

However, cells in vivo are not just trapped in a specific 3D extracellular matrix but their microenvironment varies dynamically with time or in response to physical stimuli like stress. Therefore, the evolution of 3D cell encapsulated polymeric hydrogels with time and in response to some physical stimuli provides the concept of mimicking the 4D cellular macroenvironment. The bioink developed for bioprinting must be biocompatible for implantation of the printed construct within the biological system. The main factors that should be considered are for preventing any immune reaction in response to the printed tissue implantation and secured integration of the printed construct at its specific physiological location without creating any chaos in vivo; generally biocompatibility of a bioink is studied by incorporation of specific cell types within the hydrogel (Gungor-Ozkerim et al., 2018) and the material is studied for cell growth proliferation differentiation and expression. Approximately 80-90% of cell viability with good expression or specific markers after seven days of in vivo cell culture qualifies the bioink to be biocompatible with the natural ECM where the cell resides. It is mainly composed of glycosaminoglycans, proteins, collagen, fibronectin, laminin, and elastin. Collagen (Hölzl et al., 2016) is the most common and abundant protein for all tissues in mammals although the type and distribution of collagen fibrils vary in a time specific manner but it is the main contributor that provides the tissue with the required tensile strength to withstand the maximum strain level natural biomaterials like derivatives of collagen gelatin decellularized extracellular matrix are commonly used as bioink for 3D printing (Schwab et al., 2020). These natural biomaterials can be cross-linked to form water soluble hydrogels which have added advantages for being used as cellular nations as they are structurally similar to native ECM with easy handling and tunable mechanical properties. Additionally, cells in vivo require certain biochemical cues that assist cells to develop second cell surface fibronectin or are immobilized with various functional groups and specified peptide sequences that directly interact with cells and affect the cellular behavior (Bachmann et al., 2019; Yamada et al., 2019).

6.1   *Porosity Degradability and Mechanical Strength*

The second important parameter for choosing a suitable biomaterial as bioink is the presence of sustainable interstitial space force within the polymeric network. The porosity of the hydrogel scaffold depends on concentration or density of the polymer as well as the degree of cross linking of the scaffold (Foudazi et al., 2023). The presence of pores allows diffusion of nutrients from culture media for cell survival and prevents hypoxia of the cells residing in the inner core of the hydrogel network. The hydrogel also provides available space in a physically confined macro environment for homogeneous distribution of media within the polymeric network. Implantation of a porous construct allows local angiogenesis to take place which is an important determinant for vascularized tissue constructs however increased pore sizes or increased pore densities decreases the stiffness of the hydrogel scaffold which can negatively affect the cell growth by affecting the ECM secretion and regeneration of the functionalized tissue to take place. Therefore a macroscale porosity affects the microarchitecture of the cell environment and control of the intricate porosity which is the guiding factor towards development of a functionalized engineered tissue construct (Baur et al., 2023; Annabi et al., 2010).

6.2   Mechanical Stiffness

Native tissue has a mechanical property ranging from kilopascals to megapascals depending upon the physiological location and its specific function (Luo et al., 2022). An engineered tissue construct needs restoration of its mechanical strength in addition to its biological functionalities (Zhang et al., 2018). The mechanical stiffness of the native tissue is largely due to the intrinsic pattern of an organization of collagen fibrils. In a specified architecture 3D organ printing often fails to attain such high mechanical stiffness. 3D organ printing often fails to attain the hierarchical organization of the fibrillar network. This is due to the rigorous procedure for bioink preparation which involves unfolding of the collagen fibril and refolding of the fibrillar network by different crosslinking procedures and biodegradation . The choice of the bioink for bioprinting must be biodegradable for regeneration of the target tissue to take place; the degradation of the construct should be homogeneous in nature and the rate of degradation of the bioprinted tissue should be keep pace with the regeneration of the new tissue. A bioink which has a good biodegradation rate but is not so biocompatible can lead to improper secretion of extracellular matrix and therefore suboptimal development of the target tissue; natural biomaterials are mainly biodegradable and the degradation is mainly through the action of various enzymes. A lot of synthetic polymers are also biodegradable in nature where the mechanism of degradation is mainly through chemical deterioration or hydrogelation of the functional groups like ether, ester or amide bonds. However some polyesters or poly acids or polyamides have a hydrolysable backbone. Rapid degradation of such polymers results in significant loss of mechanical strength in the first place and also an accumulation of glycolic acid that can generate an intense inflammatory response (Raghuwanshi et al., 2019). Natural polymers are often blended with synthetic. To enhance its mechanical stiffness there are four tensile strength hardness creep failures. Some of the parameters need to be considered by choosing a bioink for 3D bioprinting of specific tissue stiffness. The stiffness of different biological tissue is diverse and this diversity is not only attributed to tissue complexity and function but also to other factors like hydration age and strength of the native tissue (Simionescu et al., 2014).

7.   3D Bioprinting: Modeling and Computational Simulation

The fluidic part of the 3D bioprinting process is bioink, which contains cells and material, so cells can be expensive, and during the experiment, trial and error are tedious and time-consuming. Blending modeling and simulation works as a catalyst to decrease this trial and error and speeds up the process. The rheological properties of bioink are crucial for cellular viability and maintaining the construct's shape fidelity and structural integrity. Computational simulation is a potential tool to predict the outcome virtually with a wide range of bioink viscoelastic properties, nozzle geometry, and applied pressure. In addition, the computational simulation accurately correlates the amount of shear stress exerted on cells, the applied pressure, and the nozzle geometry, ultimately determining the survivability of cells. Bioink modeling was done using the Herschel Bulkley model to understand the fluid flow inside the printing head. Emmermacher et al. accurately showed how pressure drops on the printing head, and shear parameters varied at the outlet with the help of analytical calculations and validation with CFD and numerical simulation (Emmermacher et al., 2020). The simulation also predicts the difference that arises in printed tissue during printing because of the conical or cylindrical nozzle in terms of shear parameters and cell alignment. The model enables us to measure the mechanical properties of hydrogel to estimate the flow rate of cell-laden hydrogel by changing the density of cells.

A simulation of the material flow in bioprinting techniques is needed to understand the relationships between needle shape, printing settings, material properties, and mechanical forces during extrusion. Predicting the extruded strand's form or the mechanical force exerted on the cells can be helpful. The printing process may be optimized through computational simulations, and novel bioink formulations can be developed with minimal experimentation. Paxton et al. developed a mathematical model to theoretically understand the pressure-driven, shear-thinning extrusion of bioink through a nozzle in a 3D bioprinter (Paxton et al., 2017). The model predicts the variation of shear stress and residence time for cells at the inner part of the nozzle and the effect of different parameters on cytocompatibility.

7.1   Consideration of Process Parameters and Printing Outcomes: Experimental and Theoretical Approach

In the biomedical sciences, TE and RM are fascinating domains. The principal objective is to create implantable tissue constructs to replace, restore, and promote the regeneration of the damaged organ. Bioink must possess some desired characteristics, such as favorable viscoelasticity, faster in situ gelation, and better resolution during bioprinting. Hence, it reduces the post-maturation time, ultimately reducing the hostile physical and immunological effects on cells. So, for a better and optimum construct, bioink and its related parameters play a vital role but also depend on the bioprinting technique. For instance, the viscosity of bioink may help in the faster maturation of biological constructs.

To overcome these challenges during the bioprinting and maintaining cellular viability, an optimum shear thinning property is necessary to mitigate the effect of higher shear stress on cells. In shear thinning fluid, when the pressure is applied for extrusion, its viscosity decreases, and bioink quickly passes through the nozzle. The clinical functionality of 3D bioprinted tissue constructs is established based on the retention of cell functions like cell viability, cell proliferation, differentiation, maturation, and immunological functionality, and printing fidelity like construct size, resolution, and stability of complex shape. All these characters have relied on multiple process parameters and geometrical features of bioprinting, including nozzle shape, diameter, applied pressure, flow rate, print speed, and rheological nature of bioink.

In 3D bioprinting, layer by layer, the disposition of cell-laden ink and multilayers construct and try to mimic the native biological tissue. Still, during this process, multiple parameters are involved due to many technical challenges related to the motility and viability of living cells. These challenges are overcome by incorporating computational simulations to analyze the effect of process parameters. Digitally, this helps print viable constructs with optimum functionality. Cell viability is compromised on the substrate in noncontact bioprinting techniques such as laser-assisted bioprinting (LaBP). Hydrogels with shear-thinning properties are very suitable for addressing the issue since they lower viscosity when shear stress is applied at a high rate. Exposure to laser energy without any quartz-based laser absorbing layer harms cellular viability and causes genetic damage. According to theoretical calculations, introducing a laser photo absorption medium minimizes UV exposure and provides the cells less than 0. 1% of the incident UV rays. An earlier study shows that nearly 95% cell viability can be achieved by using low-frequency visible light-based lasers with a breast cancer cell line.

7.2   Rheological Behavior of Bioink

Printing fidelity and cell functionality strongly depend on the rheological properties of bioink. Printability is directly impacted by several important rheological characteristics, including viscosity, shear stress, viscoelasticity, bioink flow, and shear rate. Computational Fluid Dynamics (CFD) is a popular tool for determining flow dynamics in simple and complex designs. In particular, CFD can compute inner parameters like pressure, velocity, and shear stress of microfluidics that are difficult to detect experimentally. It is commonly known that shear stress, in particular, and inner nozzle pressures significantly affect the survival of cells. Thus, the viability of cells decreases with increasing shear stress. For instance, it was found by Blaeser et al. that cells subjected to low shear stress (<5 kPa) exhibit high cellular viability (up to 96%). In contrast, cells subjected to high shear stress (>10 kPa) exhibit dropped cellular viability (91% and 76%, respectively).

The internal resistance to flow in 3D bioprinting is called viscosity, while extrusion bioprinting may print materials with a broad range of viscosities. Shear-thinning fluid is ideal for improving functioning and preventing nozzle clogging in bioprinting. A low-viscosity bioink print minimizes nozzle clogging and is less likely to distort during printing. However, printing with a highly viscous bioink makes it difficult to extrude and requires considerable pressure, which can harm encapsulated cells. For bioprinting, non-Newtonian shear thinning fluids make the best bioink because they reduce shear stress on cells, maximize shape retention, and reduce nozzle clogging. Rheology needs to be performed to determine the viscoelastic region and the key strain/stress points before bioprinting. The viscoelastic region where the sample's uniform frequency load progressively increases could be identified using the amplitude sweep test.

In hydrogel-based bioinks, the flow properties of hydrogels describe how they respond to shear stresses, highlighting the interaction between shear stress (or viscosity) and shear rate. This flow behavior is usually classed as Newtonian or non-Newtonian.

7.3 Applied Pressure and Nozzle Geometry

The applied pressure is the bioink's force for its extrusion from the nozzle. During the bioprinting process, the bioink extruded from the nozzle cells undergoes shear stress and deformation, affecting the cells' viability, so this effect is strongly related to applied pressure and nozzle geometry. The applied force is also involved in maintaining the flow rate (Bera et al., 2022). The existing study suggests that nozzle geometry is essential and imparts cell shear stress. Conical nozzle geometry has higher maximum wall stress than cylindrical nozzle, influencing cell viability in the bio-printed construct. The nozzle diameter and type have direct effects on cell viability. A smaller nozzle diameter leads to a higher velocity gradient, higher shear stress, and, consequently, higher cell damage.

7.4 Viscosity Modification and Bioink Screening

The viscosity of bioink is influenced by several factors, including solvents, temperature, molecular weight, and biological additives like growth factors. There are numerous ways to adjust the viscosity for better printing. GelMA viscosity is increased by strontium nanoparticles (1. 5 mg/mL), which also exhibit improved shape retention. While encasing, chitosan enhanced its osteogenic capacity and promoted the growth of cells while CNFs (cellulose nanofibers) enhanced rheological features. The best possible substitutes to increase the shear thinning ability of bioink and improve shape retention in post-printing are nanoparticles or nano-fibrillated cellulose.

7.5 Print Speed

In 3D bioprinting, print speed refers to the rate at which the printer head moves along the x, y, and z axes to deposit the cell-laden hydrogel and prints the 3D structure layer-by-layer. Synchronization of print speed and bioink flow are determining factors for better cellular viability and mechanical properties of the filament; when the applied pressure increases, the flow rate of the bioink increases, requiring an increase in printing speed . If the flow rate of the bioink is lower than the print speed, it may have a discontinuous filament or low-grade mechanical and structural integrity. The ink spreads laterally to provide broader printed lines if the print speed exceeds the ink's velocity (Bera et al., 2022).

8.   Cell Source, Selection, and Consideration to Preserve Cell Viability

For inkjet bioprinting, various important factors (Figure 3) need to be considered for the preparation of the bioink is to attain higher cell viability after bioprinting. Bioink, which mainly contains polymer material and cells together, makes it an important consideration to thrive in the application of biofabrication of different kinds of tissues. In this expression, the source of cells is an important factor. Basically, there are various cell sources for inkjet-based bioprinting. Primary cells are isolated from tissues by enzymatic digestion methods that, after printing, mimic the physiological microenvironment, but one major limitation of the primary cell line is its difficult process of isolation and viability. On the other hand, immortal cell lines are easy to obtain and frequently used in bioprinting, but in terms of native tissue microenvironment, it does not mimic completely; also, with time in 2D culture, immortal cell lines are genetically altered, which may not be suitable for different applications. Cells from embryos like embryonic stem cells, induced pluripotent stem cells, mesenchymal stem cells, and other pluripotent or multipotent stem cells can develop into a variety of cell types, making them useful for applications in inkjet bioprinting for various tissue engineering applications (West-Livingston et al., 2020).

Depending on the cell type origin, epithelial cells are top seeded on bioprinted constructs for attachment growth and proliferation, whereas mesothelial cells are encapsulated inside the hydrogel and bioprinted to grow. For the development of vascularization in bioprinted constructs, endothelial cells are used, and for increasing the complexity, more immune cells (like macrophages, monocytes and neutrophils) are incorporated (Ghosh et al., 2023). The viability and functionality of cells before printing depend on the availability of oxygen, nutrients, pH level, physiological temperature, and growth factors, whereas post-printing viability depends on shear stress generated during bioprinting. Therefore, it is important to carefully choose the printing parameters (such as nozzle size and printing speed) to minimize shear stress and maintain cell integrity. Developing bio inks with appropriate rheological characteristics to enable droplet extrusion via the printing nozzle requires careful consideration of viscosity, shear-thinning behavior, and gelation kinetics (Mota et al., 2020).

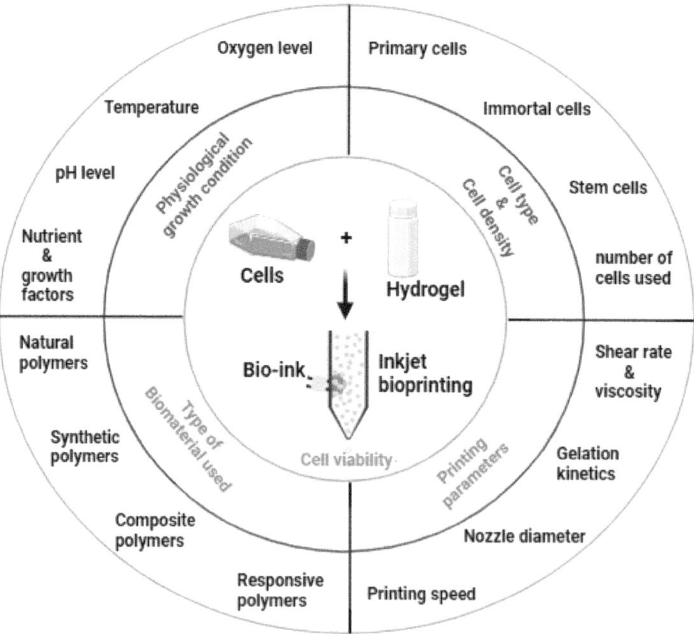

Fig. 3   Schematics represent the different factors considered for better cell viability in inkjet bioprinting.

Besides all these, initial cell density and print resolution are the most important factors in obtaining maximum cell viability during printing to replicate intricate tissue architectures precisely.

9.   4D Bioprinting

The term came into existence in 2013 and soon it was used in actuation, soft robotics and other fields including bioprinting. 4D bioprinting encompasses the use of stimuli-responsive materials that demonstrate a change in shape and functionality over time. It also refers to 3D bioprinted constructs that can be transformed (cell maturation) with respect to time (Yang et al., 2019).

9.1   Stimuli-responsive Materials

9.1.1   Thermo-responsive materials

Thermo-responsive materials that exhibit excellent printability and processibility such as collagen, gelatin, PEG (poly ethylene glycol), PNIPAM (poly(N-isopropylacrylamide)), PNVCL (poly(N-vinylcaprolactam)), poly(ε-caprolactone) dimethacrylate, PU (polyurethane) are used to achieve shape morphing effects (64–66). Thermo-responsive polymers with a glass transition temperature greater than 58°C cannot be used as bioinks for 4D bioprinting as cell survival will be compromised (Zafar, 2019). Scaffolds designed from acrylated epoxidized soybean oil (AESO), Gel/Chit-H+ hydrogel are sensitive to temperature, therefore, undergo shape transformation and sol-gel transition and thus assist in 4D bioprinting (Miao et al., 2016; Wen et al., 2020). Smart valves printed with alginate/PNIPAM have been designed to close upon hot water exposure and to open when exposed to cold water. Thermo-responsive Pluronic F-127 has been known for healing skin burns in combination with a coordination complex of zinc and metformin. Sol-gel transition is also exhibited by thermosensitive hydroxypropyl chitin (HPCT), N-acetylglucosamine (NAG) and carboxymethyl chitosan (CMCS)-based hydrogel; the latter has been employed for the treatment of diabetes using cell engineering.

9.1.2   Magneto-responsive materials

Hydrogels stimulated by magnetic fields are momentous candidates for bioprinting. Magneto-responsive materials with additives such as para and ferromagnetic nanoparticles. Nanoparticles can serve in DDS (drug delivery systems) (Javaid and Haleem, 2019). For instance, hydrogel of agar/PEG infused with Fe_3O_4 has been used to treat traumatized soft tissues (Ulbrich et al., 2016). PDMS poly(dimethylsiloxane) reinforced with Fe-based NPs (nanoparticles) have been bioprinted to fabricate anisotropic scaffolds (Zhu et al., 2018), PEGDA (Polyethylene glycol diacrylate) infused with Fe_3O_4 NPs have been bioprinted for use in biomedical applications (Kuhnt et al., 2022).

9.1.3   Moisture-responsive materials

Shape-morphing materials that operate on swelling and deswelling mechanisms find use in actuating and soft-robotics (Maraveas et al., 2022). PEGDA, silk fibroin, cellulose, microcrystalline cellulose (MCC) modified with stearoyl moieties undergo shape charge upon desorption and sorption (Zhang et al., 2015). For instance, water and ethanol vapor-based stimuli have been used to cause reversible actuation of silk fibroin films (Ganesan et al., 2022).

9.1.4   pH-responsive materials

Many functional groups in response to environmental pH changes, respond by gaining or losing protons and in turn cause shape morphing of the biomaterial (Kalva et al., 2021). Biomaterials such as collagen, gelatin, chitosan, alginate, hyaluronic acid and synthetic materials such as PAA (poly(acrylic acid)), PHIS (poly(histidine)), PASP (poly (aspartic acid)) are sensitive to pH and thus their properties and shape can be altered by it (Lai et al., 2021; Chowdhury et al., 2021; Hussain et al., 2021).

9.1.5 *Biologically responsive materials*

These materials respond to biological molecules, enzymes, glucose (El-Husseiny et al., 2022). The change in peptide sequences and biomolecules alter the material properties and thus cause shape-morphing effects (Wan et al., 2020). A 4D printed construct with fibrin deposition and calcification has been developed using enzymatic stimuli of thrombin and alkaline phosphatase Devillard et al., 2018).

9.1.6 *Multi-responsive materials*

Many synthesized materials can demonstrate response to more than one stimulus. For example, graphene incorporated in PNIPAM is dual responsive, metallopolymers show the triple shape morphing effect (TSME) (Meure et al., 2022) with two temporary shapes. PEAK (poly (aryl ether ketone)) with grafted carboxylic acid pyridine (Yang et al., 2022) and poly (D, L-lactide-co-trimethylene carbonate) (PLMC)/poly (trimethylene carbonate) (PTMC)/Fe3O4 (Wan et al., 2022) (also exhibit TSME.

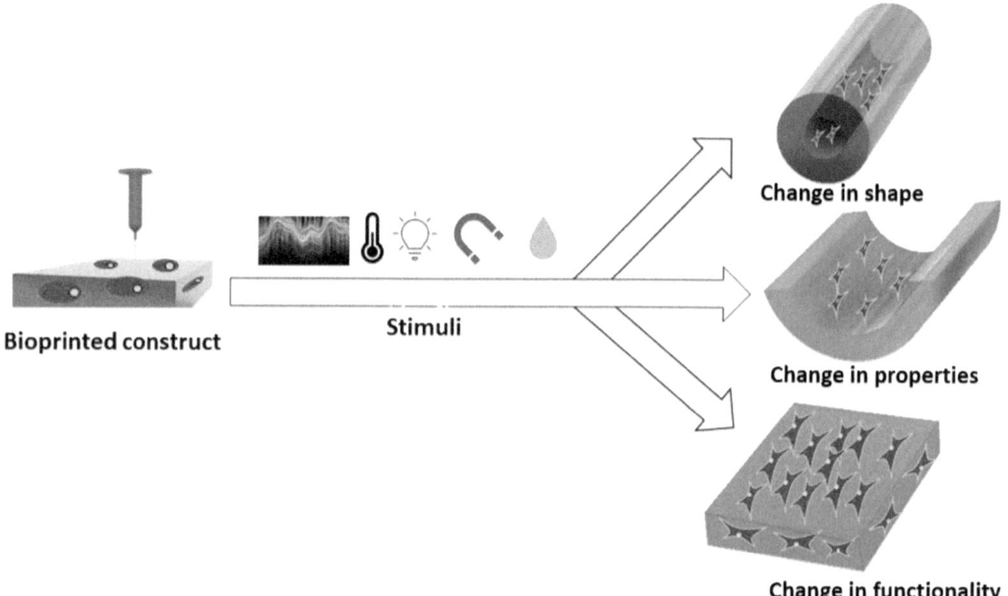

Fig. 4   The figure represents the dynamic changes (such as change in shape, property and function) exhibited by a 3D bioprinted construct upon application of various stimuli (such as water, temperature, magnetic field, light).

10. Validation and Strategies to Achieve Functional Organs

Validation is the process of making something legally approved and acceptable. Achieving functional organs via bioprinting is a complex and multidisciplinary process that requires a blend of scientific knowledge, medical approaches, and tissue engineering. It focuses on cell maturation and angiogenesis, two crucial tissue engineering and regenerative medicine components (Jorgensen et al., 2019). The intricate journey emphasizes pivotal components like cell maturation, angiogenesis, and remodeling (Kong et al., 2023).

Cell maturation validation entails ensuring that the chosen cell types undergo appropriate differentiation to acquire the characteristics of mature, functional cells. This is frequently preceded by a careful selection of cell sources, focusing on cells capable of differentiating into the specific cell types required for the target organ (Gaebel et al., 2011). Cell maturation strategies include optimizing culture conditions, growth factors, and signaling pathways to guide cells through developmental stages. Mimicking the natural microenvironment of organs with tailored biomaterials and scaffolds is critical for cell maturation (Jorgensen et al., 2019; Yeo et al., 2023). Validation efforts include evaluating mature marker expression, functionality, and the ability of cells to perform organ-specific tasks.

Angiogenesis, or the formation of new blood vessels, is required for the engineered organ to have a functional vascular network. This may include assessing the potency and functionality of the vascular network, as well as ensuring adequate perfusion for nutrient and oxygen delivery to cells (Wolf et al., 2012). Angiogenesis strategies include incorporating endothelial cells into engineered tissue, using growth factors to stimulate vessel formation, and developing biomaterials that promote vascular ingrowth. It is critical to mimic the intricate vascular architecture of the target organ (Zhu et al., 2021). Cell maturation and angiogenesis strategies intertwine in a coordinated approach. Mature cells in a well-vascularized environment are critical for the proper functioning of engineered organs (Tomasina et al., 2019). To achieve a balanced and functional outcome, scientists often fine-tune these strategies iteratively, adjusting the balance between cell types, optimizing culture conditions, and refining vascularization approaches (Xu et al., 2018). Here, we have discussed some of the strategies and validation approaches.

10.1 Biomaterial Selection

The choice of biomaterials in bioprinting is a critical success factor, as they serve as the bioink for constructing intricate organ structures. These biomaterials serve multiple functions, requiring biocompatible properties, providing structural support, and mimicking the native extracellular matrix (ECM) of the target organ. Biocompatibility ensures that the materials used do not cause adverse reactions when introduced into living tissues, promoting compatibility with the biological environment. Structural support is critical for preserving the integrity and shape of the 3D-printed organ, and biomaterials such as polycaprolactone (PCL) excel in this role due to their robust mechanical properties (Dixit et al., 2023). Furthermore, exploring various hydrogels, bioinks, and scaffold materials results in the mimicry of the native ECM. Natural materials, such as gelatin derived from collagen, closely replicate the composition of the ECM, providing a favorable environment for cellular activities. Interdisciplinary efforts of researchers include precisely exploring optimal biomaterial combinations tailored to each organ, demonstrating the intricate balance required for bioprinting success. This emphasizes the importance of biomaterials in shaping the future of bioprinting for regenerative medicine and organ transplantation, as evidenced by ongoing studies and advancements in the field (Murphy et al., 2014).

10.2 Vascularization and Perfusion

Ensuring an adequate blood supply is of the utmost importance in organ bioprinting because it is essential to the survival and functionality of the engineered tissues. The difficulty is replicating the intricate vascular networks that allow r nutrient and oxygen exchange and efficient waste removal in natural organs (Murphy et al., 2023). One approach involves creating microchannels within the bioprinted structure to mimic the small blood vessels that permeate natural tissues. These microchannels serve as conduits for circulating vital fluids, promoting the vital processes of nutrient delivery and waste elimination. Another avenue of study is the incorporation of pre-formed blood vessels into the bioprinted organ, leveraging existing vascular structures to improve perfusion (Poldervaart et al., 2014). Achieving proper vascularization is essential for sustaining the metabolic needs of cells and supporting the maturation and functionality of the bioprinted tissue (Kolesky, 2014).

10.3 Biologically Functional and Matured Organs

Bioprinted organs must mature and develop proper biological functions. Mimicking the natural maturation process involves creating conducive microenvironments, promoting cell-cell interactions, and providing appropriate biochemical cues (Poldervaart et al., 2014). It involves using growth factors, biomimetic environments, and dynamic culture systems (Groll et al., 2016). Bioprinted organs must undergo maturation to develop proper biological functions. This involves creating conducive microenvironments, cell-cell interactions, and providing biochemical cues using growth factors, biomimetic environments, and dynamic culture systems. The process of bioprinting organs represents a groundbreaking leap in the field of regenerative medicine, offering the potential to create functional replacement organs for transplantation. However, the successful bioprinting of organs goes beyond the initial fabrication stage. An essential subsequent step is the maturation of bioprinted tissues, a complex and dynamic process that aims to cultivate a microenvironment conducive to developing proper biological functions.

Maturation involves arranging various factors to mimic the intricate conditions found in natural organ development. One key aspect is the creation of microenvironments within the bioprinted structures. These microenvironments are critical in providing the necessary cues for cells to differentiate, organize, and mature into specific functional tissues. Facilitating cell-cell interactions is another crucial element of the maturation process. Cells within an organ do not function in isolation; instead, they engage in intricate communication networks that influence their behavior and functionality (Li et al., 2021). In the context of bioprinting, promoting cell-cell interactions involves ensuring that the printed cells are arranged to mirror the natural organization of tissues. This spatial arrangement encourages the development of cellular connections and communication, contributing to the overall maturation of the bioprinted organ. Providing biochemical cues is fundamental to steering the differentiation and maturation of bioprinted tissues. Growth factors, signaling molecules, and other biochemical components are introduced into the bioprinted structures to simulate the natural biochemical environment of developing organs (Pereira et al., 2021). This mimicking of native cues helps guide cells through their maturation pathways, ensuring they acquire the specific functions characteristic of the intended organ.

Biomimetic environments and dynamic culture systems are employed to enhance the maturation process. Biomimetic environments replicate the natural conditions of the target organ, including factors such as temperature, pH, and mechanical forces (Luo et al., 2018). Dynamic culture systems involve exposing the bioprinted tissues to controlled and variable conditions, such as fluid flow or mechanical stretching, to enhance their development and maturation further (Luo et al., 2019). In essence, the maturation of bioprinted organs is a sophisticated and intricately orchestrated process. It involves the integration of multiple parameters, including microenvironmental conditions, cell-cell interactions, and biochemical signaling, all aimed at guiding the bioprinted tissues toward functional maturity (Masri et al., 2022). This approach holds great promise for advancing the field of regenerative medicine, bringing us closer to the realization of fully functional, bioprinted organs for transplantation and therapeutic applications.

The maturation of bioprinted organs is critical in creating functional and viable tissues. This intricate process is analogous to the natural development of organs in the human body and involves several key aspects aimed at achieving proper biological functions. Creating conducive microenvironments is a fundamental step in the maturation of bioprinted organs. These microenvironments are carefully engineered to mimic the intricate conditions found in native tissues (Figure 5) (Luo et al., 2019).

10.4 Immunomodulation

The immune response is a significant challenge in organ transplantation. Bioprinted organs should ideally be designed to minimize immune rejection. Strategies include using patient-specific cells,

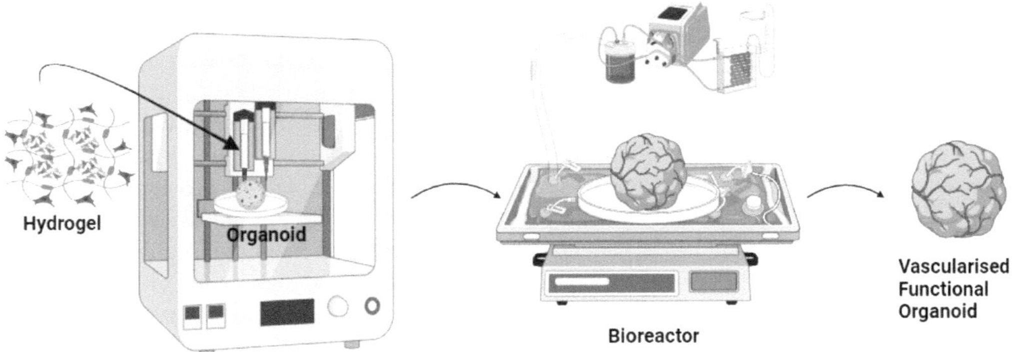

Fig. 5 Schematic representation of 3D bioprinting and tissue maturation process.

incorporating immunomodulatory factors, and developing techniques to avoid immune recognition (Elalouf, 2021). Immunomodulation signifies the premeditated manipulation of the immune system to guide macrophages toward a phenotype that nurtures tissue regeneration. The design of 3D-printed constructs plays a pivotal role in this process. Cautiously selected materials, often biocompatible polymers or hydrogels, form the structural foundation, creating an environment conducive to cellular interactions. These constructs may incorporate bioactive molecules, such as growth factors and cytokines, strategically released over time through controlled delivery systems. By mimicking the architecture and composition of native tissue, 3D bioprinting allows for the precise engineering of microenvironments, guiding macrophages toward states essential for successful tissue regeneration (Dutta et al., 2023).

10. 5 Biomechanical Considerations

Organs have unique biomechanical properties that contribute to their function. Bioprinting must consider these mechanical aspects, such as tissue stiffness, elasticity, strength, and flexibility. Mimicking the native biomechanics is crucial for the long-term success of the bioprinted organ (Chae et al., 2023). A key component is scaffold stiffness, designed to mimic the degrees of stiffness found in various body tissues. This makes sense because biomechanical cues have a significant effect on cellular behavior. To direct cell fate and promote tissue development in a way that closely resembles physiological processes, the stiffness of the scaffold should match that of the original tissue (Bera & Pati, 2023; Krishna & Sankar, 2023). The interconnected voids within the scaffold structure are represented by porosity, which becomes another crucial aspect. The porosity features of native tissues are unique and necessary for critical processes like cell migration, oxygen exchange, and nutrition diffusion (Khajehmohammadi et al., 2023). The bioprinting process is carefully optimized to fabricate a scaffold that hits a balance, providing enough porosity to support cell viability and fostering an environment favorable to tissue integration. The mechanical characteristics of the bioprinted hydrogel are crucial; these include tensile strength, elasticity, and compressive strength. It is essential to match these mechanical properties of the intended tissue (Ma et al., 2018). Furthermore, the mechanical integrity of the construct is crucial for its longevity in preserving structural stability and resistance to physiological forces. Cell signaling and tissue development are regulated by biomechanical cues that are finely woven into the bioprinted scaffold. Scaffold stiffness, porosity, and mechanical properties must thus harmoniously converge (Parak et al., 2019). A comprehensive approach ensures that the bioprinted structures function as real microenvironments, offering the necessary cues for appropriate cell behavior and spatial organization and ultimately helping fully realize tissue regeneration.

Conclusion and Outlook

Additive manufacturing, often known as 3D bioprinting in the medical industry, has rapidly evolved into a very active field of study and is already being used to fabricate medical implants. Fabricating soft tissue analogues for translational applications requires additional improvement for future consideration. One of the advantages of 3D bioprinting is its ability to manufacture encapsulated cells and materials with tissue-level hierarchical architecture via a computer-controlled automated robotic hand dispensing system. However, clinically relevant bioprinted constructions must exhibit functioning and effectiveness while also possessing biomechanical properties that closely resemble their target tissue equivalents. Depending on the size of the target tissue and its design, biomaterials and bioprinting processes need to choose a better mimic native tissue. Three main types of bioprinting processes suited for hydrogel-based 3D bioprinting: LIFT, inkjet printing, and extrusion-based printing have been covered. While each technique has advantages and limitations, extrusion-based dispensing is the only method capable of producing therapeutically relevant constructs, in spite of a lower resolution than LIFT or inkjet printing. With our discussion of material preparation and rheological profiles of non-Newtonian flow and other related flow phenomena, we created the primary criteria to be considered while developing novel bioinks. The bioink should exhibit shear thinning behavior, a high damping factor ratio, and shear recovery properties for extrusion-based bioprinting. During extrusion, the cell-encapsulated materials experience a tremendous amount of shear stress, which can be detrimental to the cell viability; the shear stress can be optimized by the bioink flow ratio, nozzle diameter, or print speed. For better optimization of flow behavior and cellular impact, mathematical modeling may be used to optimize printing process parameters, as well as for time-consuming and experimental error. Although bioprinting techniques enable the fabrication of complex architecture similar to native tissue, the overhang region is a fundamental restriction for all existing bioprinting procedures. To create a hanging geometry, the bioprinted constructs can be further modified using procedures known as 4D bioprinting. Stimulus-sensitive materials created using standard 3D bioprinting procedures allow particular stimuli to fold into the required stable architecture that holds the whole framework. Finally, all bioprinted constructs must mature in vitro before being used as a drug screening model, transplantation via dynamic flow, or immunomodulation.

References

Albanna M., Binder K.W., Murphy S.V., Kim J., Qasem S.A. et al. In Situ Bioprinting of Autologous Skin Cells Accelerates Wound Healing of Extensive Excisional Full-Thickness Wounds. Sci Rep. 2019 Feb; 9(1): 1856.

Annabi N., Nichol J.W., Zhong X., Ji C., Koshy S., Khademhosseini A., et al. Controlling the Porosity and Microarchitecture of Hydrogels for Tissue Engineering. Tissue Eng Part B Rev. 2010 Aug; 16(4): 371.

Bachmann M., Kukkurainen S., Hytönen V.P., Wehrle-Haller B. Cell adhesion by integrins. Physiol Rev. 2019 Jul; 99(4): 1655–99.

Baur E., Hirsch M., Amstad E.. Porous 3D Printable Hydrogels. Adv Mater Technol. 2023 May; 8(9): 2201763.

Bera A.K., Pati F. 3D Bioprinting of Skin Tissue Model. In: Pant A.B., Dwivedi A., Ray R.S., Tripathi A., Upadhyay A.K., Poojan S., editors. Skin 3-D Models and Cosmetics Toxicity [Internet]. Singapore: Springer Nature Singapore; 2023. p. 83–104. Available from: https://doi. org/10. 1007/978-981-99-2804-0_5

Bera A.K., Sriya Y., Pati F., Formulation of Dermal Tissue Matrix Bioink by a Facile Decellularization Method and Process Optimization for 3D Bioprinting toward Translation Research. Macromol Biosci. 2022 Aug 1; 22(8).

Bhise N.S., Manoharan V., Massa S., Tamayol A., Ghaderi M., Miscuglio M., et al. A liver-on-a-chip platform with bioprinted hepatic spheroids. Biofabrication. 2016 Jan; 8(1): 14101.

Blaeser A., Duarte Campos D.F., Puster U., Richtering W., Stevens M.M., Fischer H. Controlling Shear Stress in 3D Bioprinting is a Key Factor to Balance Printing Resolution and Stem Cell Integrity. Adv Healthc Mater. 2016 Feb; 5(3): 326–33.

Buanz A.B.M., Telford R., Scowen I.J., Gaisford S. Rapid preparation of pharmaceutical co-crystals with thermal inkjet printing. CrystEngComm. 2013; 15(6): 1031–5.

Chae S., Ha D.H., Lee H. 3D bioprinting strategy for engineering vascularized tissue models. Int J bioprinting. 2023; 9(5): 748.

Chai Q., Jiao Y., Yu X. Hydrogels for Biomedical Applications: Their Characteristics and the Mechanisms behind Them. Gels (Basel, Switzerland). 2017 Jan; 3(1).

Chowdhury J., Anirudh P.V., Karunakaran C., Rajmohan V., Mathew A.T., Koziol K., et al. 4D Printing of Smart Polymer Nanocomposites: Integrating Graphene and Acrylate Based Shape Memory Polymers. Polymers (Basel). 2021 Oct; 13(21).

Cui X., Boland T. Human microvasculature fabrication using thermal inkjet printing technology. Biomaterials. 2009 Oct; 30(31): 6221–7.

Cukierman E., Pankov R., Yamada K.M., Cell interactions with three-dimensional matrices. Curr Opin Cell Biol. 2002 Oct; 14(5): 633–9.

Daly R., Harrington T.S., Martin G.D., Hutchings I.M., Inkjet printing for pharmaceutics - A review of research and manufacturing. Int J Pharm. 2015 Oct; 494(2): 554–67.

Del Bakhshayesh A.R., Asadi N., Alihemmati A., Tayefi Nasrabadi H., Montaseri A., Davaran S., et al. An overview of advanced biocompatible and biomimetic materials for creation of replacement structures in the musculoskeletal systems: Focusing on cartilage tissue engineering. J Biol Eng. 2019; 13(1): 1–21.

Devillard C.D., Mandon C.A., Lambert S.A., Blum L.J., Marquette C.A. Bioinspired Multi-Activities 4D. Printing Objects: A New Approach Toward Complex Tissue Engineering. Biotechnol J. 2018 Dec; 13(12): e1800098.

Dixit M., Singh N., Das P., Datta P. Bioprinting in Pharmaceuticals. In: Banerjee S., editor. Additive Manufacturing in Pharmaceuticals [Internet]. Singapore: Springer Nature Singapore; 2023. p. 293–325. Available from: https://doi. org/10. 1007/978-981-99-2404-2_9

Duocastella M., Fernández-Pradas J.M., Serra P., Morenza J.L. Jet formation in the laser forward transfer of liquids. Appl Phys A Mater Sci Process. 2008; 93(2): 453–6.

Dutta S.D., Patil T.V., Ganguly K., Randhawa A., Lim K.T. Unraveling the potential of 3D bioprinted immunomodulatory materials for regulating macrophage polarization: State-of-the-art in bone and associated tissue regeneration. Bioact Mater [Internet]. 2023; 28: 284–310. Available from: https://www. sciencedirect. com/science/article/pii/S2452199X23001664

Duval K., Grover H., Han L.H., Mou Y., Pegoraro A.F. et al. Modeling Physiological Events in 2D vs. 3D Cell Culture. Physiology (Bethesda). 2017 Jul; 32(4): 266–77.

Elalouf A. Immune response against the biomaterials used in 3D bioprinting of organs. Transpl Immunol. 2021 Dec; 69: 101446.

El-Husseiny H.M., Mady E.A., Hamabe L., Abugomaa A., Shimada K, Yoshida T., et al. Smart/stimuli-responsive hydrogels: Cutting-edge platforms for tissue engineering and other biomedical applications. Mater Today Bio [Internet]. 2022; 13:100186. Available from: https://www. sciencedirect. com/science/article/pii/S2590006421000946

Emmermacher J., Spura D., Cziommer J., Kilian D., Wollborn T., Fritsching U., et al. Engineering considerations on extrusion-based bioprinting: interactions of material behavior, mechanical forces and cells in the printing needle. Biofabrication. 2020 Mar; 12(2): 25022.

Foudazi R., Zowada R., Manas-Zloczower I., Feke D.L. Porous Hydrogels: Present Challenges and Future Opportunities. Langmuir. 2023 Feb; 39(6): 2092–111.

Freed, L.E., Vunjak-Novakovic, G., Biron, R.J., Eagles, D.B., Lesnoy, D.C., Barlow, S.K., Langer R. Biodegradable Polymer Scaffold for Tissue Engineering. Nat Biotechnol [Internet]. 1994; 12: 689–93. Available from: papers3://publication/uuid/2AF9C0E1-DBF9-49E3-8E4F-171D8C9E801B

Gaebel R., Ma N., Liu J., Guan J., Koch L., Klopsch C., et al. Patterning human stem cells and endothelial cells with laser printing for cardiac regeneration. Biomaterials. 2011 Dec; 32(35): 9218–30.

Ganesan M., Kumar R., Satapathy D.K. Bidirectional Actuation of Silk Fibroin Films: Role of Water and Alcohol Vapors. Langmuir. 2022 May; 38(19): 6066–75.

Ghosh A., Ghosh S., Pati F., Duraiswamy S., Complexity in in-vitro tumor microenvironment reconstruction for drug screening and personalized medicine. Bioprinting [Internet]. 2023; 36:e00316. Available from: https://www. sciencedirect. com/science/article/pii/S2405886623000593

Groll J., Boland T., Blunk T., Burdick J.A., Cho D.W. et al. Biofabrication: reappraising the definition of an evolving field. Biofabrication. 2016 Jan; 8(1): 13001.

Gudapati H., Dey M., Ozbolat I. A comprehensive review on droplet-based bioprinting: Past, present and future. Biomaterials. 2016 Sep; 102: 20–42.

Gungor-Ozkerim P.S., Inci I., Zhang Y.S., Khademhosseini A., Dokmeci M.R. Bioinks for 3D bioprinting: an overview. Biomater Sci. 2018 May; 6(5): 915.

Hakobyan D., Médina C., Dusserre N., Stachowicz M.L., Handschin C., Fricain J.C., et al. Laser-assisted 3D bioprinting of exocrine pancreas spheroid models for cancer initiation study. Biofabrication. 2020 Apr; 12(3): 35001.

Hoffman A.S. Hydrogels for biomedical applications. Adv Drug Deliv Rev [Internet]. 2012; 64: 18–23. Available from: https://www. sciencedirect. com/science/article/pii/S0169409X12002700

Hölzl K., Lin S., Tytgat L., Van Vlierberghe S., Gu L., Ovsianikov A. Bioink properties before, during and after 3D bioprinting. Biofabrication. 2016 Sep; 8(3).

Hu M., Ling Z., Ren X. Extracellular matrix dynamics: tracking in biological systems and their implications. J Biol Eng [Internet]. 2022; 16(1): 1–13. Available from: https://doi. org/10. 1186/s13036-022-00292-x

Hussain K., Aslam Z., Ullah S., Shah M.R. Synthesis of pH responsive, photocrosslinked gelatin-based hydrogel system for control release of ceftriaxone. Chem Phys Lipids. 2021 Aug; 238:105101.

Imamura Y., Mukohara T., Shimono Y., Funakoshi Y., Chayahara N., Toyoda M., et al. Comparison of 2D and 3D-culture models as drug-testing platforms in breast cancer. Oncol Rep. 2015 Apr; 33(4): 1837–43.

Jackson S.J., Thomas G.J. Human tissue models in cancer research: looking beyond the mouse. Vol. 10, Disease models & mechanisms. England; 2017. p. 939–42.

Javaid M., Haleem A. 4D printing applications in medical field: A brief review. Clin Epidemiol Glob Heal [Internet]. 2019; 7(3): 317–21. Available from: https://www. sciencedirect. com/science/article/pii/S2213398418302082

Jorgensen A.M., Yoo J.J., Atala A. Solid Organ Bioprinting: Strategies to Achieve Organ Function. Chem Rev. 2020 Oct; 120(19): 11093–127.

Jungst T., Smolan W., Schacht K., Scheibel T., Groll J. Strategies and Molecular Design Criteria for 3D Printable Hydrogels. Chem Rev. 2016; 116(3): 1496–539.

Kalva N., Uthaman S., Lee S.J., Lim Y.J., Augustine R., Huh K.M., et al. Degradable pH-responsive polymer prodrug micelles with aggregation-induced emission for cellular imaging and cancer therapy. React Funct Polym [Internet]. 2021; 166(February):104966. Available from: https://doi. org/10. 1016/j. reactfunctpolym. 2021. 104966

Kamisuki S., Hagata T., Tezuka C., Nose Y., Fujii M., Atobe M. A low power, small, electrostatically-driven commercial inkjet head. In: Proceedings MEMS 98 IEEE Eleventh Annual International Workshop on Micro Electro Mechanical Systems An Investigation of Micro Structures, Sensors, Actuators, Machines and Systems (Cat No98CH36176. 1998. p. 63–8.

Kang H.W., Lee S.J., Ko I.K., Kengla C., Yoo J.J. et al. A 3D bioprinting system to produce human-scale tissue constructs with structural integrity. Nat Biotechnol. 2016 Mar; 34(3): 312–9.

Khajehmohammadi M., Azizi Tafti R., Nikukar H. Effect of porosity on mechanical and biological properties of bioprinted scaffolds. J Biomed Mater Res A. 2023 Feb; 111(2): 245–60.

Kolesky D.B., Truby R.L., Gladman A.S., Busbee T.A., Homan K.A., Lewis J.A. 3D bioprinting of vascularized, heterogeneous cell-laden tissue constructs. Adv Mater. 2014 May; 26(19): 3124–30.

Kong Z., Wang X. Bioprinting Technologies and Bioinks for Vascular Model Establishment. Int J Mol Sci. 2023 Jan; 24(1).

Krishna D.V., Sankar M.R. Extrusion based bioprinting of alginate based multicomponent hydrogels for tissue regeneration applications: State of the art. Mater Today Commun [Internet]. 2023; Available from: https://api. semanticscholar. org/CorpusID:257194976

Krstic M., Rogic Miladinovic Z., Barudzija T., Mladenovic A., Suljovrujic E. Stimuli-responsive copolymeric hydrogels based on oligo(ethylene glycol) dimethacrylate for biomedical applications: An optimisation study of pH and thermoresponsive behaviour. React Funct Polym [Internet]. 2022; 170: 105140. Available from: https://www. sciencedirect. com/science/article/pii/S1381514821003321

Kuhnt T., Camarero-Espinosa S., Takhsha Ghahfarokhi M., Arreguín M., Cabassi R., Albertini F., et al. 4D Printed Shape Morphing Biocompatible Materials Based on Anisotropic Ferromagnetic Nanoparticles. Adv Funct Mater. 2022; 32(50): 1–11.

Kumar P., Ebbens S., Zhao X. Inkjet printing of mammalian cells – Theory and applications. Bioprinting [Internet]. 2021; 23:e00157. Available from: https://www. sciencedirect. com/science/article/pii/S2405886621000300

Kyle S., Jessop Z.M., Al-Sabah A., Whitaker I.S. 'Printability' of Candidate Biomaterials for Extrusion Based 3D Printing: State-of-the-Art. Adv Healthc Mater. 2017; 6(16): 1–16.

Lai J., Ye X., Liu J., Wang C., Li J., Wang X., et al. 4D printing of highly printable and shape morphing hydrogels composed of alginate and methylcellulose. Mater Des [Internet]. 2021; 205:109699. Available from: https:// www. sciencedirect. com/science/article/pii/S0264127521002513

Li J., Liu Y., Zhang Y., Yao B., Enhejirigala, Li Z., et al. Biophysical and Biochemical Cues of Biomaterials Guide Mesenchymal Stem Cell Behaviors. Front cell Dev Biol. 2021; 9:640388.

Li W., Liu Z., Tang F., Jiang H., Zhou Z., Hao X., et al. Application of 3D Bioprinting in Liver Diseases. Micromachines. 2023; 14(8): 1–19.

Li X, Chen J., Liu B., Wang X., Ren D., Xu T. Inkjet Printing for Biofabrication. In: Ovsianikov A., Yoo J., Mironov V., editors. 3D Printing and Biofabrication [Internet]. Cham: Springer International Publishing; 2018. p. 283–301. Available from: https://doi. org/10. 1007/978-3-319-45444-3_26

Li X., Liu B., Pei B., Chen J., Zhou D., Peng J., et al. Inkjet Bioprinting of Biomaterials. Chem Rev. 2020; 120(19): 10793–833.

Liu W., Thomopoulos S., Xia Y. Electrospun nanofibers for regenerative medicine. Adv Healthc Mater. 2012; 1(1): 10–25.

Luo T., Tan B., Zhu L., Wang Y., Liao J. A Review on the Design of Hydrogels With Different Stiffness and Their Effects on Tissue Repair. Front Bioeng Biotechnol. 2022 Jan; 10: 817391.

Luo Y., Lin X., Huang P. 3D Bioprinting of Artificial Tissues: Construction of Biomimetic Microstructures. Macromol Biosci. 2018 Jun; 18(6):e1800034.

Luo Y., Wei X., Huang P. 3D bioprinting of hydrogel-based biomimetic microenvironments. J Biomed Mater Res B Appl Biomater. 2019 Jul; 107(5): 1695–705.

Ma X., Yu C., Wang P., Xu W., Wan X., Lai C.S.E., et al. Rapid 3D bioprinting of decellularized extracellular matrix with regionally varied mechanical properties and biomimetic microarchitecture. Biomaterials. 2018 Dec; 185: 310–21.

Mandrycky C., Wang Z., Kim K., Kim D.H. 3D bioprinting for engineering complex tissues. Biotechnol Adv. 2016; 34(4): 422–34.

Maraveas C., Bayer I.S., Bartzanas T. 4D printing: Perspectives for the production of sustainable plastics for agriculture. Biotechnol Adv. 2022; 54:107785.

Masri S., Zawani M., Zulkiflee I., Salleh A., Fadilah N.I.M., Maarof M., et al. Cellular Interaction of Human Skin Cells towards Natural Bioink via 3D-Bioprinting Technologies for Chronic Wound: A Comprehensive Review. Int J Mol Sci. 2022 Jan; 23(1).

Meurer J., Bätz T., Hniopek J., Jäger M., Zechel S., Schmitt M., et al. Synthesis and Characterization of Metallopolymer Networks featuring Triple Shape-Memory Ability Based on Different Reversible Metal Complexes. Polymers (Basel). 2022; 14(9).

Miao S., Zhu W., Castro N.J., Nowicki M., Zhou X., Cui H., et al. 4D printing smart biomedical scaffolds with novel soybean oil epoxidized acrylate. Sci Rep [Internet]. 2016; 6(March): 1–10. Available from: http://dx. doi. org/10. 1038/srep27226

Mikos A.G., Herring S.W., Ochareon P., Elisseeff J., Lu H.H. et al. Engineering complex tissues. Tissue Eng. 2006 Dec; 12(12): 3307–39.

Mohammadalizadeh Z., Bahremandi-Toloue E., Karbasi S. Recent advances in modification strategies of pre- and post-electrospinning of nanofiber scaffolds in tissue engineering. React Funct Polym [Internet]. 2022; 172:105202. Available from: https://www. sciencedirect. com/science/article/pii/S138151482200044X

Mota C., Camarero-Espinosa S., Baker M.B., Wieringa P., Moroni L. Bioprinting: From Tissue and Organ Development to in Vitro Models. Chem Rev. 2020; 120(19): 10547–607.

Murphy A.R., Allenby M.C. In vitro microvascular engineering approaches and strategies for interstitial tissue integration. Acta Biomater. 2023 Nov; 171: 114–30.

Murphy S.V., Atala A. 3D bioprinting of tissues and organs. Nat Biotechnol. 2014 Aug; 32(8): 773–85.

Naficy S., Gately R., Gorkin R., Xin H., Spinks G.M. 4D Printing of Reversible Shape Morphing Hydrogel Structures. Macromol Mater Eng. 2017; 302(1): 1–9.

Nicolas J., Magli S., Rabbachin L., Sampaolesi S., Nicotra F., Russo L. 3D Extracellular Matrix Mimics: Fundamental Concepts and Role of Materials Chemistry to Influence Stem Cell Fate. Biomacromolecules. 2020 Jun; 21(6): 1968–94.

Parak A., Pradeep P., du Toit L.C., Kumar P., Choonara Y.E., Pillay V. Functionalizing bioinks for 3D bioprinting applications. Drug Discov Today. 2019 Jan; 24(1): 198–205.

Pati F., Jang J., Ha D.H., Won Kim S., Rhie J.W. et al. Printing three-dimensional tissue analogues with decellularized extracellular matrix bioink. Nat Commun. 2014 Jun 2; 5.

Paxton N., Smolan W., Böck T., Melchels F., Groll J., Jungst T. Proposal to assess printability of bioinks for extrusion-based bioprinting and evaluation of rheological properties governing bioprintability. Biofabrication. 2017 Nov; 9(4): 44107.

Pereira R.F., Lourenço B.N., Bártolo P.J., Granja P.L. Bioprinting a Multifunctional Bioink to Engineer Clickable 3D Cellular Niches with Tunable Matrix Microenvironmental Cues. Adv Healthc Mater. 2021 Jan; 10(2):e2001176.

Poldervaart M.T., Gremmels H., van Deventer K., Fledderus J.O., Oner F.C., Verhaar M.C., et al. Prolonged presence of VEGF promotes vascularization in 3D bioprinted scaffolds with defined architecture. J Control release Off J Control Release Soc. 2014 Jun; 184: 58–66.

Raghuwanshi V.S., Garnier G., Characterisation of hydrogels: Linking the nano to the microscale. Adv Colloid Interface Sci. 2019 Dec; 274.

Rimann M., Graf-Hausner U. Synthetic 3D multicellular systems for drug development. Curr Opin Biotechnol. 2012 Oct; 23(5): 803–9.

Schwab A., Levato R., D'Este M., Piluso S., Eglin D., Malda J. Printability and Shape Fidelity of Bioinks in 3D Bioprinting. Chem Rev. 2020 Oct; 120(19): 11028–55.

Simionescu B.C., Ivanov D. Natural and Synthetic Polymers for Designing Composite Materials. In: Antoniac IV, editor. Handbook of Bioceramics and Biocomposites [Internet]. Cham: Springer International Publishing; 2014. p. 1–54. Available from: https://doi. org/10. 1007/978-3-319-09230-0_11-1

Sorkio A., Koch L., Koivusalo L., Deiwick A., Miettinen S., Chichkov B., et al. Human stem cell based corneal tissue mimicking structures using laser-assisted 3D bioprinting and functional bioinks. Biomaterials [Internet]. 2018; 171: 57–71. Available from: https://www. sciencedirect. com/science/article/pii/S0142961218302898

Steven I., Zoltan S.H., Pulsed Droplet Ejecting System. United State Pat [Internet]. 1972; 2(19): 1–29. Available from: https://patentimages. storage. googleapis. com/30/f4/62/e9b75605352fb0/US10679987. pdf

Tekin E., Smith P.J., Schubert U.S. Inkjet printing as a deposition and patterning tool for polymers and inorganic particles. Soft Matter. 2008; 4(4): 703–13.

Tomasina C., Bodet T., Mota C., Moroni L., Camarero-Espinosa S. Bioprinting Vasculature: Materials, Cells and Emergent Techniques. Mater (Basel, Switzerland). 2019 Aug; 12(17).

Ulbrich K., Holá K., Šubr V., Bakandritsos A., Tuček J., Zbořil R. Targeted Drug Delivery with Polymers and Magnetic Nanoparticles: Covalent and Noncovalent Approaches, Release Control, and Clinical Studies. Chem Rev. 2016 May; 116(9): 5338–431.

Wan X., He Y., Liu Y., Leng J. 4D printing of multiple shape memory polymer and nanocomposites with biocompatible, programmable and selectively actuated properties. Addit Manuf. 2022; 53(December 2021).

Wan Z., Zhang P., Liu Y., Lv L., Zhou Y. Four-dimensional bioprinting: Current developments and applications in bone tissue engineering. Acta Biomater [Internet]. 2020; 101: 26–42. Available from: https://www. sciencedirect. com/science/article/pii/S1742706119307172

Wen H., Li J., Payne G.F., Feng Q., Liang M., Chen J., et al. Hierarchical patterning via dynamic sacrificial printing of stimuli-responsive hydrogels. Biofabrication. 2020 Apr; 12(3):35007.

West-Livingston L.N., Park J., Lee S.J., Atala A., Yoo J.J. The Role of the Microenvironment in Controlling the Fate of Bioprinted Stem Cells. Chem Rev. 2020 Oct; 120(19):11056–92.

Winston C.R., Winston C.R. United State patent. 1962;

Wolf M.T., Daly K.A., Reing J.E., Badylak S.F. Biologic scaffold composed of skeletal muscle extracellular matrix. Biomaterials. 2012 Apr; 33(10): 2916–25.

Xu Y., Hu Y., Liu C., Yao H., Liu B., Mi S. A Novel Strategy for Creating Tissue-Engineered Biomimetic Blood Vessels Using 3D Bioprinting Technology. Mater (Basel, Switzerland). 2018 Sep; 11(9).

Yamada, K.M. and Cukierman, E. (2007). Modeling tissue morphogenesis and cancer in 3D. Cell, 130(4): 601–610.

Yamada Y., Onda T., Wada Y., Hamada K., Kikkawa Y., Nomizu M. Structure-Activity Relationships of RGD-Containing Peptides in Integrin αvβ5-Mediated Cell Adhesion. ACS Omega. 2023 Feb; 8(5): 4687–93.

Yang G.H., Yeo M., Koo Y.W., Kim G.H. 4D Bioprinting: Technological Advances in Biofabrication. Macromol Biosci. 2019 May; 19(5): e1800441.

Yang S., He Y., Leng J. Zwitterionic Poly(aryl ether ketone) with Water-Actuated, Reshaping-Reconfiguration Ability and Triple Shape Memory Effect. ACS Appl Polym Mater. 2022; 4(6): 4286–97.

Yeo M., Sarkar A., Singh Y.P., Derman I.D., Datta P., Ozbolat I.T. Synergistic coupling between 3D bioprinting and vascularization strategies. Biofabrication. 2023 Nov; 16(1).

Zafar M.Q., Zhao H. 4D Printing: Future Insight in Additive Manufacturing. Met Mater Int [Internet]. 2019; 26: 564–85. Available from: https://api. semanticscholar. org/CorpusID:202641174

Zhang K., Geissler A., Standhardt M., Mehlhase S., Gallei M., Chen L., et al. Moisture-responsive films of cellulose stearoyl esters showing reversible shape transitions. Sci Rep. 2015; 5: 1–13.

Zhang W., Liu Y., Zhang H. Extracellular matrix: an important regulator of cell functions and skeletal muscle development. Cell Biosci. 2021 Dec; 11(1).

Zhang X.N., Wang Y.J., Sun S., Hou L., Wu P., Wu Z.L., et al. A Tough and Stiff Hydrogel with Tunable Water Content and Mechanical Properties Based on the Synergistic Effect of Hydrogen Bonding and Hydrophobic Interaction. Macromolecules. 2018 Oct; 51(20): 8136–46.

Zhang Y.S., Oklu R., Dokmeci M.R., Khademhosseini A. Three-Dimensional Bioprinting Strategies for Tissue Engineering. Cold Spring Harb Perspect Med. 2018 Feb; 8(2).

Zhou D., Chen J., Liu B., Zhang X., Li X., Xu T. Bioinks for jet-based bioprinting. Bioprinting [Internet]. 2019; 16:e00060. Available from: https://www. sciencedirect. com/science/article/pii/S2405886619300260

Zhu J., Wang Y., Zhong L., Pan F., Wang J. Advances in tissue engineering of vasculature through three-dimensional bioprinting. Dev Dyn an Off Publ Am Assoc Anat. 2021 Dec; 250(12): 1717–38.

Zhu M., Li W., Dong X., Yuan X., Midgley A.C., Chang H., et al. In vivo engineered extracellular matrix scaffolds with instructive niches for oriented tissue regeneration. Nat Commun. 2019 Dec 1; 10(1).

Zhu P., Yang W., Wang R., Gao S., Li B., Li Q. 4D Printing of Complex Structures with a Fast Response Time to Magnetic Stimulus. ACS Appl Mater Interfaces. 2018; 10(42): 36435–42.

Recent Advances in 3D Bioprinting

Laura Mendoza Cerezo,[1] *Alfonso Carlos Marcos Romero,*[1]
Antonio Macías García,[2] *Juan Pablo Carrasco Amador,*[1]
Jesús Manuel Rodríguez Rego[1*]

1. Introduction

3D printing, also called additive manufacturing, is a process that creates three-dimensional objects from a digital file by depositing successive layers of material, such as plastic, metal or resin, until the complete object is formed. The first patent application for a 3D printer was filed in 1981 by Hideo Kodama, a researcher at the Nagoya Municipal Institute of Industrial Research in Nagoya, Japan (Kodama, 1981). Although the idea was innovative, Kodama's project was terminated due to a lack of funding and little interest in the scientific community, as its potential applications were not fully understood. In the 1980s, three French engineers, Alain Le Méhauté, Olivier de Witte and Jean-Claude André, revisited the possibility of creating a 3D printer, basing their idea on the technology of solidifying photosensitive resins using UV light (Yanar et al., 2020). Their project, submitted to the French National Centre for Scientific Research (CNRS), was also not well received due to a lack of apparent application areas and a shortage of funds for its development. Finally, in 1983, Chuck Hull, co-founder of 3D Systems, revolutionized the world with the invention of stereolithography, considered the first 3D printing technology. It uses a laser to solidify layers of photosensitive resin, shaping three-dimensional objects from a digital design. Five years later, Scott Crump, founder of Stratasys, took 3D printing a step further with the creation of fused deposition technology (Groth et al., 2014). This method, one of the most popular today, uses a filament of thermoplastic material that is melted and extruded layer by layer to create objects with precision.

3D printing has revolutionised the way in which objects are designed, manufactured and prototyped in a wide range of sectors. This technology, which has experienced exponential growth in the last decade, opens up a world of possibilities in a variety of fields, including medicine (Li

[1] Department of Graphic Expression, University of Extremadura, Spain.
[2] Department of Mechanical, Energy and Materials Engineering. School of Industrial Engineering. University of Extremadura. Avenida de Elvas, Badajoz. Spain.
* Corresponding author: jesusrodriguezrego@unex.es

et al., 2015). Thus, the evolution of 3D printing has led to a breakthrough in the development of new medical devices and custom-made prostheses, through the computational processing and design of the desired part and its subsequent generation by additive manufacturing. The fabrication of biologically inert tissue constructs has employed a variety of 3D printing techniques, replacing non-medical materials with medically suitable ones, such as metals, polymers, ceramics and hydrogels (Kalaskar, 2022), each depending on the specific application. For the moulding of these materials, the technologies currently used are material extrusion, powder bed fusion, binder jetting, and vat photopolymerization (Ozbolat, 2017).

Despite the recognised contribution of 3D printing to the solution of various medical problems, it has numerous limitations such as the lack of precision in the placement of cells for the colonisation of the construct, the low cell density that it supports as these can only be placed on the surface of the grown scaffold and the absence of vascular networks necessary for the generation of oxygenated and viable thick tissues (Bioprinting Toward Organ Fabrication: Challenges and Future Trends: Online, 2017). Thus, while the early days of 3D printing in medicine have been successful in creating anatomical models and customised prostheses, over time technologies have evolved towards bioprinting, which seeks to create functional three-dimensional biological structures using living cells, biomaterials and biomolecules, with precise control over porosity and internal architecture, and making it possible to manufacture structures with customised mechanical and structural properties. In addition, 3D bioprinting offers the possibility of incorporating drug molecules or proteins to enhance cellular response and create personalised, multifunctional structures. These features open up a world of possibilities for tissue regeneration by providing an optimal cellular environment that guides and facilitates the repair process. Bioprinting technologies are at an early stage of development but have the potential to revolutionize medicine and medical research, improving the lives of millions of people and changing the way medicine will be practised in the future. They fall into three main categories: extrusion bioprinting, laser bioprinting and droplet bioprinting, each with characteristics that make them more suitable for different functions.

To understand the different bioprinting technologies, it is crucial to understand the technologies used in medicine that laid the foundations for their development: FDM (Fused Deposition Modeling) 3D printing and SLA (Stereolithography) 3D printing. These two techniques, although different in their operation, share the same fundamental principle: additive manufacturing. This is done by adding material layer by layer, as if building the object from the bottom up (Kafle et al., 2021), making it an appropriate manufacturing technique for rapid prototyping in various fields of engineering and biomedicine (Ngo et al., 2018).

The 3D printing process begins with the digitization of the structure to be reproduced three-dimensionally, either by developing it with CAD programmes, digital sculpture programmes or digitization of pre-existing objects using 3D scanners, or even computerised tomography. The file extension obtained must be converted to standard tessellation language (*.stl*) file, where, in the case of CAD files, the continuous geometry of the file is converted to small triangles (Wong and Hernandez, 2012). Finally, the new file obtained is exported to a model cutting software able to create a toolpath for the 3D printer, indicating the instructions to be followed, and consequently generating a file processable by the printer (*gcode*).

2.   FDM 3D Printing

2.1   *Elements of an FDM 3D Printer*

FDM 3D printing is one of the most popular and accessible 3D printing technologies, and is based on layer-by-layer fused material deposition to create three-dimensional objects from a digital file (Dong et al., 2012). A FDM 3D printer consists of the following parts:

- **Extruder:**   This is the component that melts the filament and deposits it on the printing platform. It is composed of a motor, a gear, and a nozzle.
- **Nozzle:**   This is the part of the extruder that extrudes the molten filament. Its diameter determines the resolution of the print and can vary from 0.1 mm to 1.2 mm, depending on the desired application.
- **Printing bed:**   This is the surface on which the molten material is deposited. It can be heated or not heated, to ensure the adhesion of the first printed layer, depending on the material used.
- **X-axis motor:**   This is the motor that allows the movement of the extruder on the X-axis.
- **Y-axis motor:**   This s the motor that allows the movement of the extruder on the Y-axis.
- **Z-axis motor:**   This is the motor that allows the movement of the extruder on the Z-axis. The set of motors of the three axes (X, Y and Z) allows the free movement of the extruder in the three axes of space.
- **Base:**   This is the structure that supports the entire printer.
- **Software:**   This is the program that controls the printer and converts the 3D file into instructions for the machine.

2.2 Printing Process

During the 3D printing process, specialized software included in the printer takes an STL (digital 3D model) file and prepares it for printing. This process involves splitting the model into layers and orienting it correctly on the printing platform. The filament of the chosen thermoplastic material is then heated and extruded through a thin nozzle, depositing the molten material layer by layer on the platform, which is at a specific temperature. The nozzle and platform are moved precisely on the X, Y and Z axes, following the instructions of the software, to create the three-dimensional shape of the original model. This way, 3D parts can be created directly from a digital design with high accuracy (Acierno and Patti, 2023).

2.3 Types of Materials

Most FDM printers available in the market have a maximum operating temperature of around 300°C. This limits the use of the machine to materials with relatively low melting points, excluding those with exceptionally high melting points. Among the most used materials in FDM are the thermoplastic polymers ABS and PLA, due to their printing properties and suitable melting point. There are alternatives such as polyamide (PA), polycarbonate (PC), polymethylmethylacrylate (PMMA), polyethylene (PE) and polypropylene (PP), each with their own specific characteristics and applications. The choice of the appropriate material will depend on the properties and characteristics desired for the final part to be printed (Mohan et al., 2017). In medicine, the materials used are polycaprolactone (PCL), polylactic acid (PLA) and polyurethane (PU) (Tetsuka and Shin, 2020).

3. SLA 3D Printing

3.1 Elements of a SLA 3D Printer

Stereolithography or SLA 3D printing is one of the most precise and highest resolution 3D printing technologies. It is a technique based on photopolymerization, producing the selective solidification of a photosensitive resin. It uses a mobile photon source to propagate a chain polymerisation process that results in the photo-crosslinking of the pre-existing macromolecules in the material used (Bagher and Jin, 2019).

A SLA 3D printer consists of the following parts:

- **Laser:**   This component emits a beam of ultraviolet light to solidify the resin.
- **Galvanometer:**   This is a system that controls the movement of the laser in the XY plane.
- **Resin tank:**   This is the container in which the photosensitive resin is placed.

- **Printing platform:**   This is the surface on which the solidified resin is deposited, which may be movable or fixed.
- **Z-axis:**   This is the axis that controls the movement of the printing platform in the vertical direction.
- **Base:**   This is the structure that supports the entire printer.
- **Software:**   This is the program that controls the printer and converts the 3D file into instructions for the machine.

3.2   Printing Process

SLA 3D printing works like drawing a three-dimensional object with light. A computer-controlled laser projects a pattern onto a photosensitive resin surface. The light solidifies the resin where it hits, creating a layer of the object. The process is repeated layer by layer until the object is complete (Melchels et al., 2010). The first layer of the 3D print is adhered to the support platform by solidifying it with the laser. Then, the platform is lowered a little and more liquid resin is applied on top of the previous layer. A new light pattern is exposed on the resin, solidifying a second layer that adheres to the first. The depth of solidification is greater than the height of the platform's descent, ensuring a strong bond between the two layers. This process is repeated layer by layer until the 3D object is complete (Melchels et al., 2010).

3.3   Types of Materials

In SLA 3D printing, resins are used, mainly polyesters (FPP, PLA, PCL, PCL, PCL/PEG/Chitosan), polycarbonates (PTMC, PTMC/Gelatin, Trimethylolpropane Carbonate) or polyethers (PEG, PEG/ Chitosan, PEO/PEG, Poly tetrahydrofuran ether). Generally, the photosensitive resin used in SLA 3D printing is based on cationic photopolymerization or hybrid photopolymerization, during which the wavelength of the laser beam used is 355 nm (Quan et al., 2020). At this wavelength, both radical and cationic photopolymerization could be performed, which is an advantage, as the resins for cationic photopolymerization are smaller and the price of the initiator is high, as well as having a long induction period for photopolymerization, so hybrid photosensitive resins are often adopted (Quan et al., 2020), widening the range of possibilities. Both in medicine and in the field of tissue engineering research, biocompatible resins are used, of which a considerable range is available (Guttridge et al., 2022).

3.4   Bioprinting Technologies

Although 3D printing technology is being widely used in medicine to produce customised prostheses or bioabsorbable scaffolds, the material used to generate three-dimensional structures does not have the capacity to generate new tissues from the patient's cells, requiring the development of other technologies suitable for the deposition of material with the capacity to encapsulate cells inside. Following the same operating model as conventional 3D printers, bioprinting is a technology that uses biocompatible materials that can be loaded with cells, producing the least possible damage to the cells before, during and after the bioprinting process.

3.5   Requirements for the Ideal Bioprinter

A bioprinter capable of generating a biomimetic structure with the highest possible accuracy and maintainence of the appropriate properties for the survival of the reproduced tissue must meet the following requirements (Xu, 2014):

- **High resolution:**   To achieve the creation of functional tissues, the bioprinter needs millimetre precision to properly reproduce their structure, including the microvasculature, canals and other microscopic structures that are essential for the correct proliferation of cells.

- **High throughput:** An ideal bioprinter will be able to print tissue in a reasonable time, compatible with tissue survival needs and clinical application.
- **Ability to dispense multiple materials simultaneously:** Since most tissue constructs are not composed of a single cell type, the ideal bioprinter should be able to simultaneously dispense multiple bioinks with different biochemical and mechanical properties to create more complex structures.
- **Biocompatibility:** Bioprinter materials and components that are in contact with cells or bioinks must be biocompatible to ensure cell survival.
- **Cell viability:** Through precise control of temperature, pressure, and light exposure, the bioprinter must ensure the best possible conditions during the printing process for the cells, minimising their stress.
- **Process repeatability:** The generation of consistent and reliably reproducible structures is essential for the manufacture of fabrics with predictable characteristics and to ensure the quality of the final product.
- **Control of bioink dispensability:** The bioprinter must allow precise control of the bioink properties by adjusting the temperature, applied pressure (in case of extrusion bioprinting) and printing speed, ensuring the formation of suitable structures with the desired properties.

3.6   Extrusion Bioprinters

These types of bioprinters are the most widely used due to their simplicity of use and their ability to generate larger three-dimensional structures. They work, like conventional FDM 3D printers, by depositing successive layers of materials, in this case using biomaterials such as hydrogels through the forces exerted by pneumatic pressure or mechanical tools (piston or screw) (Yu, 2020). The process begins with loading the biomaterial into a cartridge or syringe, which is placed into an extrusion device, which controls the flow of the biomaterial through the nozzle. The nozzle moves precisely over a printing platform and deposits the biomaterial layer by layer to create the desired structure, while controlling the temperature to ensure that neither the biomaterial nor the cells are damaged during the printing process. Simultaneously, the bioprinting platform can be heated to maintain an optimal temperature. Some bioprinter models also incorporate a humidification system to prevent the biomaterial from drying out during the printing process.

The bioprinter control software allows the adjustment of print parameters such as print speed, pressure applied to the bioink and nozzle temperature to suit the material being printed.

There are currently 3 types of extrusion bioprinters:

- **Pneumatic:** These use compressed air to push the biomaterial through the nozzle. This technology has a lower printing precision.
- **Piston-driven:** These use a piston to push the biomaterial through the nozzle. A constant volumetric flow rate is maintained and controlled directly by the syringe piston, so the average exit velocity does not depend on the rheological properties of the material but only on the geometry of the system (Chiesa, 2020).
- **Screw-driven:** These use a rotating screw to push the biomaterial through the nozzle. This technology is more accurate than pneumatic bioprinting, but also has greater cell damage (Ning, 2020).

Advantages

It can extrude cell-loaded bioink into continuous strands that allow the design of a biomimetic structure on a large scale due to its fast printing speed (Online, 2024). In addition, extrusion technology allows the use of a wide selection of biomaterials, including synthetic polymers, cell-loaded hydrogels, cell aggregates and microcarriers, as it enables the use of a wide range of biomaterial viscosities (Unagolla and Jayasuriya, 2020).

Disadvantages

The resolution of bioprinted parts is relatively low, and due to shear damage to the cells as they pass through the nozzle during the extrusion process, cell viability is often poor (Koch et al., 2020).

3.7 Conventional Extrusion Bioprinters

Some of the extrusion bioprinters currently on the market and their characteristics are described below:

- **BIOX from Cellink:**   This is a user-friendly pneumatic extrusion bioprinter with a resolution of up to 1 μm. It has Clean Chamber Technology, which prevents contamination of the prints made, and a UV LED light curing system of 365, 405, 485 and 520 nm. It can print different materials thanks to the interchangeable heads that adapt to each of them, with a maximum of 3 different printheads. It includes an automatic calibration system.
- **GeSiM BS5.3/CB from GeSiM:**   This includes a gradient mixing system of thermoplastic biopolymers to create structures with customized properties. In addition, it is integrated into a clean bench to ensure a sterile printing environment, and decentralized units optimize space and heat dissipation. It offers automatic nozzle alignment for greater precision, and also includes printing beds for SBS well plates. Its Nanoliter pipetting module enables precise deposition of cells and proteins during printing, offering resource savings, and its on-board washing system simplifies liquid handling.
- **TISSUE SCRIBE by 3D Cultures:**   This is a compact bioprinter that stands out for its versatility and ease of use. It has a single nozzle capable of printing a wide range of materials, including, among others, gelatin, gelatin-MA, alginate, chitosan, collagen, silicone rubber, PDMS, pluronic, meeting various research needs. The 3 available models adapt to different syringes (1 mL, 3 mL and 10 mL), while the interchangeable nozzles allow greater flexibility by having the ability to push and retract the material, facilitating the printing of complex structures, even with thick materials. The secondary platform for calibration and changing the physical zero-point Z simplifies the printing process and allows the use of tips of different lengths.
- **BIO V1 from REGEMAT:**   This is a highly customisable extrusion bioprinter, with several heads prepared for different materials and a resolution of 150 μm in the XY axes and 0. 4 μm in the Z axis. It also has modules for light curing of materials using UV, infrared and blue light, and allows the extrusion of materials from $-20°C$ to $100°C$. It includes two interchangeable beds and can be cooled or heated.
- **Allevi 3 by Allevi3D:**   This is a multi-material bioprinter with an automatic calibration system that includes an integrated camera to allow real-time monitoring of the printing process. It is equipped with visible light for light-curing materials.
- **LulzBot Bio Printer by LulzBot 3D Printers:**   This is a bioprinter that uses FRESH (Freeform Reversible Embedding of Suspended Hydrogels) technology, which allows the bioprinter to bioprint materials on a thermo-reversible viscous gel that can be subsequently liquefied by temperature, thus avoiding the generation of substrates.

3.8 Extrusion Bioprinters with Higher Degrees of Freedom of Movement

The versatility of a bioprinter is defined by the number of movements its nozzle can perform. These movements, known as degrees of freedom, can be linear (displacements on the X, Y and Z axes) or angular (turns on the same X, Y and Z axes) . The more degrees of freedom a bioprinter has, the more complex and precise the printing of 3D structures will be. Thus, a bioprinter with 6 degrees of freedom can move the nozzle in any direction in space, as if it were drawing in the air, while one with only 3 degrees of freedom can only move the nozzle in a straight line along the X, Y and Z axes, as if it were drawing a line on a table.

- **Advanced Solutions BioAssemblyBot500 (BAB500):** This is a six-axis robotic arm bioprinter housed in a Class II, Type A biosafety cabinet to ensure a sterile sample environment. It features integrated environmental control and up to ten interchangeable heads or "hands" that allow different ways to control pressure, temperature, or UV exposure. It features machine vision and artificial intelligence, and a print speed of up to 200 µl/min and a resolution of 5µm.

3.9 *Extrusion Bioprinters Enabling Bioprinting of Cellular Aggregates*

These bioprinters allow biomaterials to be deposited with high precision, which is essential for creating 3D structures of the desired shape and size. This is especially important for the bioprinting of cell aggregates, as these structures are small and complex.

- **FABION2 from 3D Bioprinting Solutions:** This enables the creation of complex tissue structures using tissue spheroids and a variety of hydrogels. Its screw-like print head facilitates the precise injection of spheroids and high cell density printing. In addition, the process enables the synthesis of extracellular matrix proteins within the spheroids, resulting in highly viable and functional tissue constructs. With a laser positioning system that offers a precision of 5µm, the bioprinter can create more complex structures.

3.10 *Extrusion Bioprinters Supporting other Bioprinting Modalities*

This category of bioprinters can combine other types of bioprinting with extrusion, providing greater flexibility in bioprinting and choice of bioinks.

- **REGENHU R-GEN 100:** This supports up to five printing tools and combines jetting, contact dispensing and electro-writing technologies with multiple auxiliary process options for simple or complex constructions. It can bioprint thermo-responsive polymers (collagen, elastin, poloxamer, biopolymers), thermoplastics (polycaprolactone, PLA, poly(lactic-coglycolic acid), polyurethane), ceramics and metals (hydroxyapatite, calcium phosphates, magnesium, silver), photoreticulable bioinks (functionalized PEG, GelMA, HAMA, light-curable silicones) and other commonly used biomaterials (alginate, cellulose, hyaluronic acid, silk fibroin, gellan gum, chitosan, peptide gels, decellularized ECM, graphene, carbon nanotubes).
- **EnvisionTEC 3D-Bioplotter from EnvisionTEC:** This has up to five print heads, an accuracy of up to 1 µm, and features the ability to include a turntable to enable the printing of cylindrical structures, including a 365 nm UV curing head. It achieved the first FDA-approved 3D printed regenerative bone graft substitute product.
- **Fluicell Biopixlar:** This is a bioprinter with microfluidic technology to accurately deposit cells on the printing surface, promoting intercellular communication and ensuring high cell viability. In addition, it does not require bioink, eliminating the risks of toxicity and variability associated with this material. It has the ability to produce a wide variety of 3D structures, from simple cell arrays to complex organoids. It includes a gamepad-style controller to control the deposition of each cell and can generate the desired print patterns.

4. Inkjet-based Bioprinters

With its origins in the publishing industry for printing text and images, the development of inkjet technology extended its applications from two-dimensional (2D) to three-dimensional (3D) (Li et al., 2020) so that its application can now be seen in research fields such as polymer moulding or tissue engineering. Inkjet bioprinting involves the assembly of biologically relevant materials with a predesigned pattern to achieve desired biological functions. These materials range from generic biomaterials without cellular components (polymers or pharmaceuticals) to functional biomaterials (growth factors, proteins and DNA) and cells (Li et al., 2020). Thus, this technology works by depositing small droplets of bioink on a substrate to create three-dimensional structures, with the associated advantage of avoiding contact with other elements. It physically manipulates a bioink solution to generate droplets on a receiving substrate by harnessing gravity, atmospheric pressure and the fluid mechanics of the bioink solution (Gudapati et al., 2017).

Advantages

It exhibits higher cell viability and deposition precision than in extrusion bioprinting.

Disadvantages

Cell death is induced by processes such as increased temperature or frequency. Electrostatic inkjet bioprinting, thermal inkjet bioprinting and piezoelectric inkjet bioprinting are prone to clogging. The resolution of microvalve bioprinters is lower than that of thermal and piezoelectric bioprinters.

4.1   Continuous Inkjet Bioprinting

Continuous inkjet printing is based on a constant flow of ink which, under controlled pressure, is transformed into a liquid column. This column breaks up into individual droplets due to the Plateau-Rayleigh instability of the fluid, which then passes through charging plates that give them an electrical charge. The charged droplets are then directed through deflection plates which, by modulating the electric field, precisely control the location of each droplet on the printing substrate. If a droplet is not required for the current print, it is deflected and reintroduced into the ink circulation system to minimize material waste (Li et al., 2020). This method presents some challenges for bioprinting, as it is a complex system with a risk of ink contamination during the recirculation process, which also needs to keep ejecting ink at all times to avoid clogging (Iwanaga et al., 2015). Therefore, it is not a technology commonly used in bioprinting.

4.2   Drop-on-demand Inkjet Bioprinting

In continuous inkjet printing a constant flow is produced which is divided into small packages (droplets) with the same volume, but a lower surface area. Due to Plateau-Rayleigh instability, in drop-on-demand inkjet bioprinting droplets are produced only when the ejection signal is reached, allowing greater precision, and do not need to be pre-loaded, resulting in higher efficiency of the bioprinting process (Li et al., 2020). In addition, the ink circulation process is eliminated, making the process simpler. This type of bioprinting deposits the bioink droplets onto the substrate in a precise and controlled process. The printer nozzle is manually positioned at the desired location and, using a carefully calibrated pressure pulse with a frequency generally between 1 and 20 KHz, creates resonance in the chamber behind the nozzle, ejecting a drop of the bioink. In the absence of the pressure pulse, the surface tension in the nozzle holds the liquid in place, and the static pressure in the nozzle can be controlled to ensure a stable meniscus, ensuring more accurate droplet deposition (Derby, 2010).

There are four methods of generating the pressure pulse to induce droplet generation, off which piezoelectric inkjet bioprinting and microvalve inkjet bioprinting have been the preferred technologies for the manufacture of commercial bioprinters currently available on the market:

4.3   Thermal Inkjet Bioprinting

Thermal inkjet bioprinting uses a small thin-film thermal actuator located in the fluid chamber. By applying an electric current to the heater, the temperature of the fluid in direct contact is raised above its boiling point to between 250-350°C, creating a small vapour bubble (Cui et al., 2012a). Although the applied temperature is extremely high compared to the cell survival temperature, as the application time is very short, the total temperature of the liquid will only increase by 4-10°C above the ambient temperature (Cui et al., 2012). When the current is interrupted, heat transfer causes the bubble to collapse rapidly, generating an expansion and contraction process that provides the pressure impulse needed to accurately eject a drop of bioink. It has been speculated that the heat supplied during the bioprinting process for droplet generation may be producing a self-initiated temporal reprogramming induced by the tension generated by the small droplets surrounding the cells, due to rapid stretching and compression of the cell membranes in a fraction of a second. This sudden variation in tension can send signals to the cell nucleus that induce the expression of the most primitive or original genes, triggering dedifferentiation (Morales, 2023).

4.4   Piezoelectric Inkjet Bioprinting

Piezoelectric actuators are a type of device that can transform electrical energy into mechanical energy by means of the piezoelectric effect, attributed to an asymmetric centre of a material's crystal structure or molecular chain, which induces spontaneous polarisation or polarisation under an applied force. Thus, electrical input energy is transferred into outputs of force, displacement or motion efficiently and accurately (Gao et al., 2020).

In piezo inkjet bioprinting, the pressure pulse is generated by a direct mechanical drive via a piezo actuator. In other words, a voltage pulse applied to the piezo actuator generates a deformation in the wall of the chamber where the bioink is located. This deformation produces an abrupt change in the volume of the chamber, which drives the ejection of a droplet with precision. In this way, the optimization of piezo inkjet bioprinting is achieved by fine-tuning the actuation mode of the piezo elements and the characteristics of the applied voltage pulse. While inkjet bioprinting may result in the death of some cells, the percentage of cells affected is relatively low, as cell viability in this process is usually above 85%, often exceeding that of extrusion printing.

- **BioScaffolder Analytic 3D Bioprinter:**   This is a modular, multi-head 3D bioprinting system that employs temperature-controlled piezoelectric micropipetting technology, enabling high-throughput prints at very low volumes, from pico to nanoliter scale. With up to four independent Z-axes, it can print a wide variety of materials, including pasty materials. It includes a fused electrospinning printing option and a high-temperature piston extruder for high-viscosity polymers.
- **FUJIFILM Dimatix DMP-2850:**   This is a fluid materials printer that uses a disposable piezoelectric inkjet cartridge with the ability to optimize the characteristics of droplets as they are ejected from the nozzle. It includes a microelectromechanical systems (MEMS) -based cartridge-type printhead that allows researchers to fill it with their own study fluids.

5.   Electrostatic Inkjet Bioprinting

In electrostatic inkjet bioprinting, droplets are generated by electrostatic manipulation of the fluid chamber volume. The printer applies an electrical charge between the pressure plate and the electrode, causing a curvature in the pressure plate and creates a force that increases the volume of the chamber, which causes the ink in the reservoir to flow into the chamber. When the charge is deactivated, the pressure plate returns to its original shape, the volume inside the chamber is reduced and droplets are ejected by the increased pressure (Zhou et al., 2019). The driving force depends on the coulomb force between the charges.

This type of bioprinting stands out for its energy efficiency by using little electrical energy and its gentle handling of the bioink. Unlike other methods, it does not generate heat during droplet formation, which protects cell integrity. In addition, the low printing frequency (around 2 kHz) minimizes the possibility of cell damage from sonication, a concern present in other techniques operating at higher frequencies (15-25 kHz). However, the size of the nozzle in this method has two limitations: it is relatively fixed and susceptible to clogging.

5.1   Microvalve Inkjet Bioprinting

The microvalve inkjet bioprinting system consists of a three-axis mobile robotic platform, different microvalve print heads and an individual gas regulation system for each print head that provides the necessary pneumatic pressure and valve opening time control (Long Ng et al., 2017).

The bioink is stored in a pressurised fluid chamber, and its flow is controlled by the microvalves, which consist of a solenoid coil and a plunger that act as a magnet and a miniature piston. When a voltage pulse is applied to the coil, a magnetic field is generated which pushes the plunger upwards, unlocking the orifice. This opens the door, releasing a drop of bioink with millimetre precision when the back pressure is high enough to overcome the surface tension in the orifice. The back pressure inside the fluid chamber, together with the opening time of the microvalve, determines the size and velocity of the droplet. Meanwhile, the movement of the nozzle guides the droplet to its final destination on a substrate. During bioprinting, parameters such as pneumatic pressure, nozzle geometry, cell concentration and bioink constituents determine droplet volume and cell viability (Faulkner-Jones, 2015).

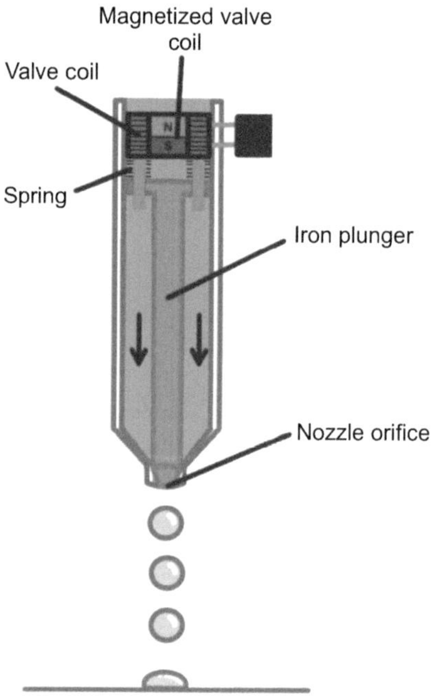

Fig. 1   Microvalve inkjet bioprinting

- **Black Drop Biodrucker Gmbh from The Bioprinting Company:**   This is a bioprinter with a rapid exchange system for bioink cartridges, optimized for non-contact, on-demand bioprinting of cell-loaded bioinks, with an adapter that allows micro-extrusion of highly viscous materials. Using a shear stress control system, it achieves higher levels of post-print cell viability than other printing modalities.
- **Inventia's RASTRUM:**   This is a microvalve-based 3D bioprinter that combines drop-on-demand technology with modifiable synthetic matrix systems. It has several independent nozzles that allow the simultaneous deposition of up to 8 different fluids, being able to deposit up to 1,000 drops per second on the surface of the plate with its 2-axis linear motion control system.

5.2 *Electro-hydrodynamic Inkjet Bioprinting*

Electrohydrodynamic inkjet bioprinting uses electrostatic forces to induce the movement of bioink, generates droplets, stretching them until they break and consequently depositing them on a substrate, obtaining a high-resolution 2D pattern (Online, 2024) and creating three-dimensional structures with millimetre precision. In electrohydrodynamic systems, a solution is passed through a positively charged metal needle, reacting to the charge, and generating repulsive Coulombic forces on its surface, causing the meniscus at the tip of the needle to deform into a Taylor cone, the conical ink meniscus in the nozzle orifice that forms when pressure is applied to the solution in the chamber. If the voltage is high enough, the electrostatic repulsion at the surface can overcome the surface tension at the apex of the liquid cone, causing it to disintegrate due to the Plateau-Rayleigh instability of the fluid and creates a jet of droplets. Thus, by adjusting the electric field strength, both a continuous droplet jet and on-demand droplet dispensing can be obtained, although unlike drop-on-demand inkjet bioprinting, electrohydrodynamic inkjet printing cannot print a single droplet at a time.

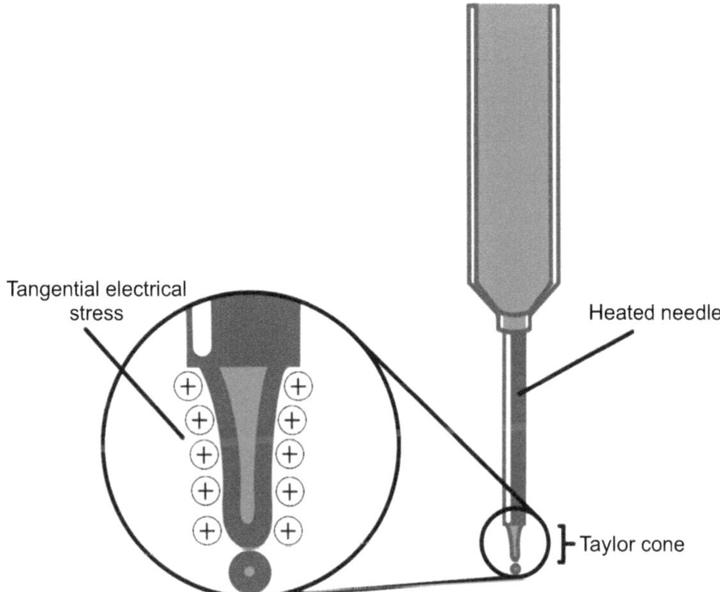

Fig. 2 Electrohydrodynamic inkjet bioprinting

- **CHIMERA from Ourobionics:** This is an advanced biofabrication platform enabling 4D bioprinting through electric field manipulation technology and microfluidic gradient bioprinting. It includes biofabrication technologies with module upgrades, such as electrohydrodynamic cell jetting, 3D bioelectropulverisation, microfluidic gradient bioprinting, cell electrospinning/ fusion and cell electrospinning.

5.3 *Bioprinting Based on Vat Polymerization*

The application of polymerization-based 3D printing to tissue engineering and regenerative medicine in a vat emerges as a novel technique to overcome some of the problems existing with current techniques. In this process, a light source, either ultraviolet or visible, selectively solidifies a photosensitive liquid resin layer by layer inside a vat, where it is transformed into a pre-designed three-dimensional structure. The photosensitive liquid resin together with the cells and growth factors form the bioink. This technology enables the fabrication of complex structures with high resolution and precision, ideal for the creation of customised structures, tissues and organs for medical applications.

Advantages

It does not require extrusion through a nozzle (no shear stresses on the cells) and is faster (limits exposure time to non-physiological conditions) and more accurate; additionally, it allows the generation of more complex structures due to its high resolution.

Disadvantages

It induces cell damage during bioprinting when UV light is used. Hence, filling the vat requires more biomaterial, cells and biomolecules than needed for structure generation.

6.   Stereolithography-based Bioprinters (SLA)

SLA bioprinting, similar to SLA fabrication in 3D printing, creates 3D tissue structures layer-by-layer by converting a 3D model into a series of overlapping 2D images, each representing a cross-section of the model in a specific plane. This method of image processing similar to biomedical imaging devices, such as MRI or CT scans, allows its use in combination with these technologies, and can process simple geometries and complex tissue structures, facilitating the generation of models for biomedical studies and the recreation of tissues for transplantation (Online, 2024). In this type of bioprinting, the biomaterials used as bioink must be photosensitive, so that, after irradiation with the appropriate light source, the cross-linking process takes place. It is therefore concluded that the key element in the resolution and precision of the structures bioprinted with this technology is the light source, since its characteristics determine the properties of the scaffold generated. There are two types of SLA bioprinting:

- **Monophotonic method:** In this method the photoinitiator generates free radicals after absorbing a high-energy photon. SLA 3D bioprinting systems based on visible and UV light use this method of photopolymerization.
- **Multiphoton or two-photon method:** In this method the photoinitiator in the excited transition state generates free radicals after sequentially absorbing multiple low-energy photons (Li and Fourkas, 2007). Two-photon bioprinting systems using infrared light as an illumination source are based on this method.

The bioprinting process begins by mixing the biocompatible photosensitive polymer with the cells to be used to generate the three-dimensional tissue to create the bioink. The bioink is then added to the vat of the SLA bioprinter and the manufacturing platform is irradiated with the light source above the vat point by point, following the determined pattern, to generate a solidified layer. Inside the vat, a platform descends to a defined height after the solidification of the first layer and cross-links the second layer. This process is repeated layer by layer until the entire structure is cross-linked.

During the bioprinting process, cell damage occurs due to the light source used, usually UV light. UV light is known to induce DNA damage in mammalian cells, causing bipyrimidine photoproducts and photo-oxidation damage (Outaleb and Kadmiri, 2020). Therefore, bioprinting processes based on visible light-induced SLA have been developed, achieving a decrease in cell damage.

- **TissueRay™ 3D Bioprinter from Tissuelabs:** This is a 3D bioprinter that uses digital mask stereolithography (MSLA) technology to create complex structures from biomaterials. It works with a light system based on a high-resolution (4K) LCD screen that projects patterns layer by layer, solidifying the liquid biomaterial with ultraviolet light. It is used to fabricate microfluidic devices, organs-on-chip, cellular structures and medical implants.
- **CELLINK's Quantum X bio:** This is an immersion laser lithography (DiLL)-enabled 3D microfabrication system that enables printing on a variety of substrates, including microfluidic systems for organs or lab-on-a-chip applications. It enables printing on microfluidic systems, including custom microfluidic channels and commercial microfluidic chips. It also enables printing of high structures and the use of custom resins.

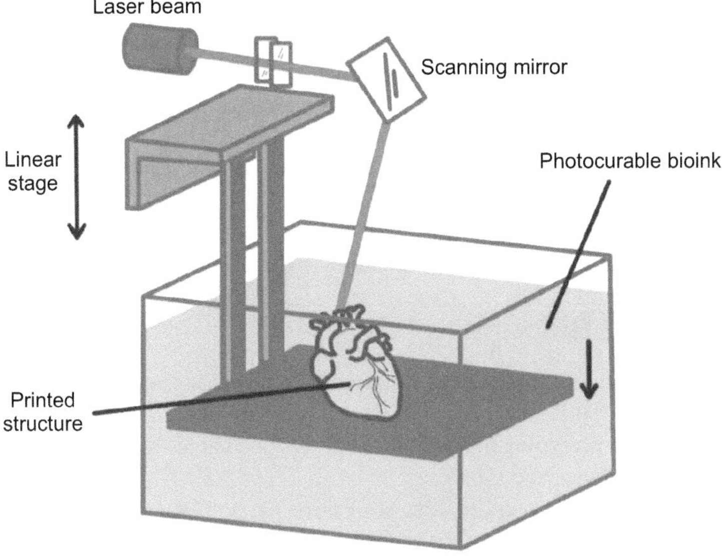

Fig. 3   Stereolithography-based bioprinters (SLA)

6.1   *Light Processing-based Bioprinters (DLP)*

This bioprinting method uses a very similar procedure to SLA bioprinting to generate three-dimensional structures, except that instead of irradiating the photosensitive bioink dot by dot with the light source to generate each layer with the set pattern, it uses a projector to project the light and photocure the image of the layer in a single pass (Deng et al., 2019). In contrast to SLA bioprinting, the projector is located under the flask, so that as the manufacturing platform is irradiated and solidifies the first layer, the platform rises to solidify successive layers. This is a method with complex printing capability and high structure generation speed, although, due to the resolution requirements of the digital light mirrors and the size of the project area, the printable area is reduced compared to that of SLA technology (Zheng et al., 2020). As in the case of SLA bioprinting, the light source used can also be visible light to reduce cell damage during the bioprinting process (Online, 2024).

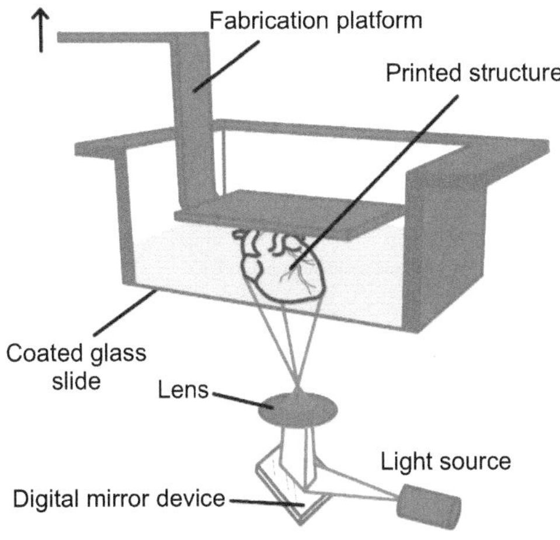

Fig. 4   Light processing based bioprinters (DLP)

- **CELLINK's BIONOVA X:**   This is a high-resolution 3D bioprinter that uses digital light processing (DLP) technology to print 3D living cellular structures directly into multiwell plates. It enables lateral and vertical multi-material printing, enabling multiple stiffness of bioprinted structures, and uses a 405 nm light source (visible light) to minimise cell damage during bioprinting.
- **LUMEN X™ Gen 3 from CELLINK:**   This is a DLP bioprinter that uses visible light to generate three-dimensional structures. The manufacturing platform is autoclavable, so the sterility of the process is not compromised. It allows the material stiffness to be adjusted and biomechanical gradients to be created according to the needs of the tissue.

7. Laser-assisted Bioprinters (LAB)

Laser technologies are breaking new ground in tissue engineering and regenerative medicine, as they enable the precise organisation of biomaterials into well-defined three-dimensional structures through high-resolution prototyping methods. This precision enables the creation of highly complex and functional artificial tissues and organs.

Laser-assisted bioprinters generally consist of three parts: a donor slide (or ribbon) composed of a transparent glass layer, a thin layer of laser-absorbing metal and a thin layer of bioink, a pulsed laser beam and a receiver slide facing the ribbon (Kačarević, 2018). The tape is itself composed of three parts:

- A support that does not absorb the laser, composed of materials such as glass or quartz.
- A thin metal film that absorbs the laser by coating the substrate, composed of materials such as gold or titanium.
- A thin layer of organic compounds prepared within a liquid phase, such as culture medium or collagen, disposed on the surface of the metal.

The LAB technique works by creating a small cavitation-like bubble within the bioink when the metal film underneath the hydrogel is vaporised by a laser pulse. This bubble expands and then contracts, generating a jet that propels a droplet of the bioink from the tape to the substrate, as if a shot were fired (Keriquel, 2017).

This technology stands out for its picolitre-level resolution, which means it can control cell density and three-dimensional spatial organisation with unmatched precision, even at the single-cell level, a significant advance in tissue engineering.

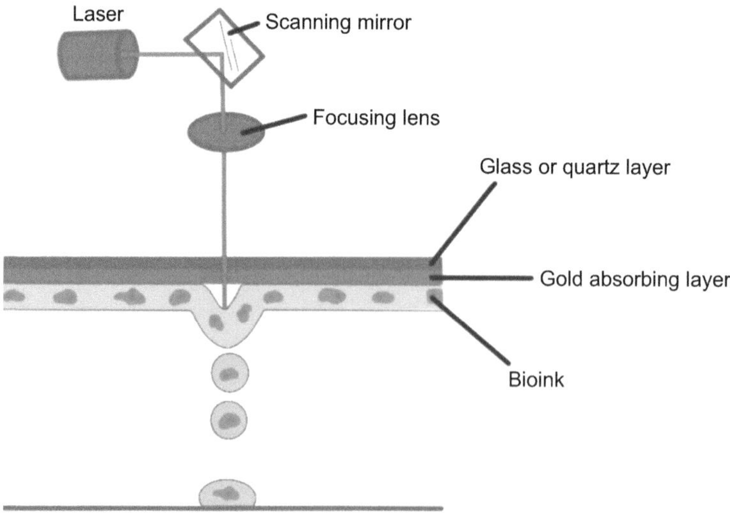

Fig. 5   Laser-assisted bioprinters (LAB)

Advantages

It can deposit material with high precision and print resolution, allowing isolation of cells or aggregates of cells with a high concentration. The absence of contact with other materials prevents contamination and blockages.

Disadvantages

It is an expensive process with low scalability. Its productivity is lower than other bioprinting techniques due to the limited variety of biomaterials that can be transferred in each laser pulse.

- **Poietis' NGB-R Bioprinter:** This is a multimodal 4D bioprinting system that combines laser-assisted, microvalve-assisted and extrusion-assisted bioprinting, enabling bioprinting from cells to spheroids, and enabling the use of a wide range of biomaterials and hydrogels. It has a six-axis robotic arm that can print to an accuracy of 10 µm, and includes an integrated microscope that enables online monitoring of cell printing.

8.   Challenges and Future Prospects

Over the past decade, bioprinting has emerged as a revolutionary technology with the potential to transform regenerative medicine, tissue engineering and pharmacology. As we move towards a future where bioprinting is increasingly likely to be used routinely in medicine and research, the evolution of various bioprinting technologies plays a crucial role in reliably recreating tissues to make this a reality. Thus, despite current advances in bioprinting technologies, there several challenges remain and future perspectives that need to be addressed to maximise their clinical and commercial potential, such as the need to develop more bioactive and biodegradable biomaterials, improving post printing cell viability and functionality, increasing the production scale and speed, and validating the safety and efficacy of printed tissues in large-scale clinical trials. All this requires the constant evolution of bioprinting technologies to adapt to new discoveries and achieving the ability to perfectly recreate something as complex as the structure of living tissue.

Achieving this goal requires the collaboration of experts in diverse areas such as cell biology, tissue engineering, material science, robotics, bioinformatics and regenerative medicine, leveraging the diversity of knowledge and skills to address technical and scientific challenges, identifying innovative solutions and ensuring the viability and functionality of printed tissues.

In addition, it is essential to advance in the standardisation of bioprinting processes and technologies and to establish clear regulations to ensure the quality and safety of bioprinted products. Furthermore, the integration of bioprinting with other emerging technologies, such as artificial intelligence and personalised medicine, will open up new opportunities for innovation and improved clinical outcomes.

References

A. Bagheri and J. Jin, 'Photopolymerization in 3D Printing', *ACS Appl. Polym. Mater.*, vol. 1, no. 4, pp. 593–611, Apr. 2019, doi: 10.1021/acsapm.8b00165.

A. Faulkner-Jones, 'Bioprinting of human pluripotent stem cells and their directed differentiation into hepatocyte-like cells for the generation of mini-livers in 3D', *Biofabrication*, vol. 7, no. 4, p. 044102, Oct. 2015, doi: 10.1088/1758-5090/7/4/044102.

A. Kafle, E. Luis, R. Silwal, H.M. Pan, P.L. Shrestha et al. '3D/4D Printing of Polymers: Fused Deposition Modelling (FDM), Selective Laser Sintering (SLS), and Stereolithography (SLA)', *Polymers*, vol. 13, no. 18, Art. no. 18, Jan. 2021, doi: 10.3390/polym13183101.

A. Outaleb and N.E. Kadmiri, 'Effects of UV radiation on DNA: Review', *J. Anal. Sci. Appl. Biotechnol.*, vol. 2, no. 2, Art. no. 2, Dec. 2020, doi: 10.48402/IMIST.PRSM/jasab-v2i2.24095.

'Bioprinting Toward Organ Fabrication: Challenges and Future Trends | IEEE Journals & Magazine | IEEE Xplore'. Accessed: Feb. 27, 2024. [Online]. Available: https://ieeexplore.ieee.org/abstract/document/6423824

B. Derby, 'Inkjet Printing of Functional and Structural Materials: Fluid Property Requirements, Feature Stability, and Resolution', *Annu. Rev. Mater. Res.*, vol. 40, no. 1, pp. 395–414, 2010, doi: 10.1146/annurev-matsci-070909-104502.

C. Dong, M. Petrovic and I.J. Davies, 'Applications of 3D printing in medicine: A review', *Ann. 3D Print. Med.*, vol. 14, p. 100149, May 2024, doi: 10.1016/j.stlm.2024.100149.

C. Groth, N.D. Kravitz, P.E. Jones, J.W. Graham and W.R. Redmond et al. 'Three-dimensional printing technology', *J. Clin. Orthod. JCO*, vol. 48, no. 8, pp. 475–485, Aug. 2014.

C. Guttridge, A. Shannon, A. O'Sullivan, K.J. O'Sullivan and L.W. O'Sullivan et al. 'Biocompatible 3D printing resins for medical applications: A review of marketed intended use, biocompatibility certification, and post-processing guidance', *Ann. 3D Print. Med.*, vol. 5, p. 100044, Mar. 2022, doi: 10.1016/j.stlm.2021.100044.

'3D Printed Tissue Models: Present and Future | ACS Biomaterials Science & Engineering'. Accessed: Feb. 28, 2024. [Online]. Available: https://pubs.acs.org/doi/full/10.1021/acsbiomaterials.6b00129?casa_token=osokhuh9XpsAAAAA%3AWEmNK0Ba2Lj63kv5mpgXQmYH40uFifkDFRq_a1Zifi6x5BuX3YY2TcWg7VJC0wOWMyEQ45cac2Ysjw

D. Acierno and A. Patti, 'Fused Deposition Modelling (FDM) of Thermoplastic-Based Filaments: Process and Rheological Properties—An Overview', *Materials*, vol. 16, no. 24, Art. no. 24, Jan. 2023, doi: 10.3390/ma16247664.

D.M. Kalaskar, *3D Printing in Medicine*. in Woodhead Publishing Series in Biomaterials. Elsevier Science, 2022. [Online]. Available: https://books.google.es/books?id=fTi0zgEACAAJ

D. Zhou, J. Chen, B. Liu, X. Zhang, X. Li et al., 'Bioinks for jet-based bioprinting', *Bioprinting*, vol. 16, p. e00060, Dec. 2019, doi: 10.1016/j.bprint.2019.e00060.

"Electrohydrodynamic jet printed conducting polymer for enhanced chemiresistive gas sensors - Journal of Materials Chemistry C (RSC Publishing) DOI:10.1039/D0TC05719C'. Accessed: Mar. 02, 2024. [Online]. Available: https://pubs.rsc.org/en/content/articlehtml/2021/tc/d0tc05719c

F. Koch, K. Tröndle, G. Finkenzeller, R. Zengerle, S. Zimmermann et al., 'Generic method of printing window adjustment for extrusion-based 3D-bioprinting to maintain high viability of mesenchymal stem cells in an alginate-gelatin hydrogel', *Bioprinting*, vol. 20, p. e00094, Dec. 2020, doi: 10.1016/j.bprint.2020.e00094.

F.P.W. Melchels, J. Feijen and D.W. Grijpma, 'A review on stereolithography and its applications in biomedical engineering', *Biomaterials*, vol. 31, no. 24, pp. 6121–6130, Aug. 2010, doi: 10.1016/j.biomaterials.2010.04.050.

H. Gudapati, M. Dey and I. Ozbolat, 'A comprehensive review on droplet-based bioprinting: Past, present and future', *Biomaterials*, vol. 102, pp. 20–42, Sep. 2016, doi: 10.1016/j.biomaterials.2016.06.012.

H. Kodama, 'Automatic method for fabricating a three-dimensional plastic model with photo-hardening polymer', *Rev. Sci. Instrum.*, vol. 52, no. 11, pp. 1770–1773, Nov. 1981, doi: 10.1063/1.1136492.

H. Quan, T. Zhang, H. Xu, S. Luo, J. Nie et al., 'Photo-curing 3D printing technique and its challenges', *Bioact. Mater.*, vol. 5, no. 1, pp. 110–115, Mar. 2020, doi: 10.1016/j.bioactmat.2019.12.003.

H. Tetsuka and S.R. Shin, 'Materials and technical innovations in 3D printing in biomedical applications', *J. Mater. Chem. B*, vol. 8, no. 15, pp. 2930–2950, Apr. 2020, doi: 10.1039/D0TB00034E.

I. Chiesa., 'Modeling the Three-Dimensional Bioprinting Process of β-Sheet Self-Assembling Peptide Hydrogel Scaffolds', *Front. Med. Technol.*, vol. 2, 2020, Accessed: Feb. 28, 2024. [Online]. Available: https://www.frontiersin.org/articles/10.3389/fmedt.2020.571626

I.T. Ozbolat, K.K. Moncal and H. Gudapati, 'Evaluation of bioprinter technologies', *Addit. Manuf.*, vol. 13, pp. 179–200, Jan. 2017, doi: 10.1016/j.addma.2016.10.003.

J.M. Unagolla and A.C. Jayasuriya, 'Hydrogel-based 3D bioprinting: A comprehensive review on cell-laden hydrogels, bioink formulations, and future perspectives', *Appl. Mater. Today*, vol. 18, p. 100479, Mar. 2020, doi: 10.1016/j.apmt.2019.100479.

J. Yu, 'Current Advances in 3D Bioprinting Technology and Its Applications for Tissue Engineering', *Polymers*, vol. 12, no. 12, Art. no. 12, Dec. 2020, doi: 10.3390/polym12122958.

K.V. Wong and A. Hernandez, 'A Review of Additive Manufacturing', *Int. Sch. Res. Not.*, vol. 2012, p. e208760, Aug. 2012, doi: 10.5402/2012/208760.

L.Li and J.T. Fourkas, 'Multiphoton polymerization', *Mater. Today*, vol. 10, no. 6, pp. 30–37, Jun. 2007, doi: 10.1016/S1369-7021(07)70130-X.

L. Ning, 'Process-induced cell damage: pneumatic versus screw-driven bioprinting', *Biofabrication*, vol. 12, no. 2, p. 025011, Feb. 2020, doi: 10.1088/1758-5090/ab5f53.

N. Mohan, P. Senthil, S. Vinodh and N. Jayanth, 'A review on composite materials and process parameters optimisation for the fused deposition modelling process', *Virtual Phys. Prototyp.*, vol. 12, no. 1, pp. 47–59, Jan. 2017, doi: 10.1080/17452759.2016.1274490.

N. Yanar, P. Kallem, M. Son, H. Park, S. Kang et al., 'A New era of water treatment technologies: 3D printing for membranes', *J. Ind. Eng. Chem.*, vol. 91, pp. 1–14, Nov. 2020, doi: 10.1016/j.jiec.2020.07.043.

P. A. Morales, 'Thermal inkjet bioprinting drastically alters cell phenotype', *Biofabrication*, vol. 15, no. 3, p. 031001, May 2023, doi: 10.1088/1758-5090/acd3b3.

S. Deng, J. Wu, M.D. Dickey, Q. Zhao and T. Xie et al. 'Rapid Open-Air Digital Light 3D Printing of Thermoplastic Polymer', *Adv. Mater.*, vol. 31, no. 39, 2019, doi: 10.1002/adma.201903970.

S. Iwanaga, K. Arai and M. Nakamura, 'Inkjet Bioprinting', in *Essentials of 3D Biofabrication and Translation*, A. Atala and J.J. Yoo, Eds., Boston: Academic Press, 2015, pp. 61–79. doi: 10.1016/B978-0-12-800972-7.00004-9.

Stereolithography 3D Bioprinting | Springer Nature Experiments. Accessed: Mar. 03, 2024. [Online]. Available: https://experiments.springernature.com/articles/10.1007/978-1-0716-0520-2_6

T.D. Ngo, A. Kashani, G. Imbalzano, K.T.Q. Nguyen and D. Hui et al. 'Additive manufacturing (3D printing): A review of materials, methods, applications and challenges', *Compos. Part B Eng.*, vol. 143, pp. 172–196, Jun. 2018, doi: 10.1016/j.compositesb.2018.02.012.

T. Xu, 'Principles of Bioprinting Technology', in *Regenerative Medicine Applications in Organ Transplantation*, G. Orlando, J. Lerut, S. Soker and R.J. Stratta, Eds., Boston: Academic Press, 2014, pp. 67–79. doi: 10.1016/B978-0-12-398523-1.00006-9.

'Volumetric Bioprinting of Complex Living-Tissue Constructs within Seconds - Bernal - 2019 - Advanced Materials - Wiley Online Library'. Accessed: Mar. 03, 2024. [Online]. Available: https://onlinelibrary.wiley.com/doi/full/10.1002/adma.201904209

V. Keriquel, 'In situ printing of mesenchymal stromal cells, by laser-assisted bioprinting, for in vivo bone regeneration applications', *Sci. Rep.*, vol. 7, Dec. 2017, doi: 10.1038/s41598-017-01914-x.

W. Long Ng, J. Min Lee, W. Yee Yeong and M.W. Naing, 'Microvalve-based bioprinting – process, bio-inks and applications', *Biomater. Sci.*, vol. 5, no. 4, pp. 632–647, 2017, doi: 10.1039/C6BM00861E.

X. Cui, K. Breitenkamp, M.G. Finn, M. Lotz and D.D. D'Lima et al. 'Direct Human Cartilage Repair Using Three-Dimensional Bioprinting Technology', *Tissue Eng. Part A*, vol. 18, no. 11–12, pp. 1304–1312, Jun. 2012, doi: 10.1089/ten.tea.2011.0543.

X. Cui, T. Boland, D.D. D'Lima and M.K. Lotz, 'Thermal Inkjet Printing in Tissue Engineering and Regenerative Medicine', *Recent Pat. Drug Deliv. Formul.*, vol. 6, no. 2, pp. 149–155, 2012a.

X. Gao., 'Piezoelectric Actuators and Motors: Materials, Designs, and Applications', *Adv. Mater. Technol.*, vol. 5, no. 1, p. 1900716, 2020, doi: 10.1002/admt.201900716.

X. Li, 'Inkjet Bioprinting of Biomaterials', *Chem. Rev.*, vol. 120, no. 19, pp. 10793–10833, Oct. 2020, doi: 10.1021/acs.chemrev.0c00008.

Y. Li, D. Li, B. Lu, D. Gao and J. Zhou et al. 'Current status of additive manufacturing for tissue engineering scaffold', *Rapid Prototyp. J.*, vol. 21, no. 6, pp. 747–762, Jan. 2015, doi: 10.1108/RPJ-03-2014-0029.

Ž.P. Kačarević, 'An Introduction to 3D Bioprinting: Possibilities, Challenges and Future Aspects', *Materials*, vol. 11, no. 11, Art. no. 11, Nov. 2018, doi: 10.3390/ma11112199.

Z. Zheng, D. Eglin, M. Alini, R. Richards, L. Qin et al., 'Visible Light-Induced 3D Bioprinting Technologies and Corresponding Bioink Materials for Tissue Engineering: A Review', *Engineering*, vol. 7, Sep. 2020, doi: 10.1016/j.eng.2020.05.021.

5

Futuristic Application of 3D Bioprinted Organs

Rashmi Ramakrishnan[1]* and *Haneen Moustafa*[1]

1. Introduction

Three-dimensional (3D) bioprinting is a computer-assisted technology that involves the rapid printing of functional materials and their supporting components in a layer-by-layer manner on a substrate to create complex living tissues and organs having the desired 3D cellular architecture and functions. The most significant difference between 3D printing and 3D bioprinting appears in the type of materials used to fabricate the final construct. Traditional 3D printing utilizes non-biological materials such as plastics, metals, alloys, ceramics, polymer resins, rubber or composite materials to create 3D objects, having potential applications across a wide range of industries, including manufacturing, prototypes, customized parts and many more. In contrast, 3D bioprinting involves additional complexities and technical challenges, of employing living cell types, biomaterials, growth and differentiation factors that are biocompatible and conducive to cell growth, which can enable the creation of tissue-like structures or entire organs with biological functionality, such as vasculature, cellular organization, and tissue-specific properties. Navigating these intricacies necessitates the fusion of technologies spanning engineering, biomaterial science, cell biology, physics, and medicine. 3D bioprinting finds widespread applications in biomedicine including, but not limited to, tissue engineering, microphysiological systems, drug screening, disease modelling, precision medicine and biomedical devices (Dey and Ozbolat, 2020; Murphy and Atala, 2014).

2. 3D Bioprinting Strategies

The three central approaches to 3D bioprinting are biomimicry, autonomous self-assembly, and mini tissue building blocks. Combinations of these are expected to be a requirement for printing a complex 3D biological structure with multiple functional, structural, and mechanical characteristics. A typical bioprinting process can be generally divided into three phases: 1) pre-processing, which includes imaging and digital 3D design, and material/cell selection. Raw imaging data acquired from imaging

---

[1] CÚRAM, Science Foundation Ireland Research Centre for Medical Devices, University of Galway, Galway, Ireland.
* Corresponding author: rashmi.ramakrishnan@universityofgalway.ie; roshrashmi@gmail.com

modalities like X-rays, CT-scans, ultrasounds, or MRI scans are processed using tomographic reconstruction to produce 2D cross-sectional images. 3D models are then generated via computer-aided design and computer-aided manufacturing (CAD-CAM) tools and mathematical modeling techniques. The material selection and cell source are specific to the tissue/organ. The biomaterials/bioinks can be natural, synthetic, or composite polymers as well as decellularized ECMs. Cells may be stem/primary cells-allogeneic or autologous sources or cell lines. 2) *processing/bioprinting* - This involves processing by automated deposition of cells and/or biomaterials of interest and 3) *post-processing*. In post-processing, the printed construct is either transplanted *in vivo directly or* after a period of *in vitro* maturity or is reserved for *in vitro* testing (Murphy and Atala, 2014).Figure 1 illustrates this process.

The main technologies used for deposition and patterning of biological materials are inkjet, extrusion, laser-assisted and stereolithography based bioprinting. Understanding the advantages and limitations is crucial for selecting the most suitable technique based on the specific requirements of tissue engineering projects, considering factors such as the resolution, speed, bioink material and cell viability.

2.1 Inkjet-based Bioprinting

Inkjet 3D bioprinting, a non-contact technique, known as drop-on-demand printers expels bioink droplets onto a substrate by thermal or acoustic (piezoelectric or electrostatic) forces, enabling high-speed printing and integration of multiple printing heads for concentration gradients in heterogeneous tissue structures. Thermal inkjet bioprinting uses electric heating generation of vapor bubbles to force droplets out. The piezoelectric actuator triggers piezoelectric crystals through high-frequency electrical energy or electrostatic forces to break the liquid into droplets. The benefits include high print speed (10,000 droplets/s), low cost, cell viability (>85% with cell densities of 10^6 cells/ml), compatibility with many biological materials and wide availability. However, the risk of exposing cells and materials to thermal and mechanical stress, low droplet directionality, uneven droplet size, easy clogging of the nozzle, limited ink viscosity, and unreliable cell encapsulation pose major limitations for usage in 3D bioprinting. Inkjet-based bioprinting is commonly used to fabricate skin, cartilage, bone, liver and blood vessels.

2.2 Extrusion Based Bioprinting

3D extrusion bioprinting dispenses bioinks through a nozzle by using either air pressure (pneumatic) or mechanical methods (piston or screw), allowing the creation of large-scale constructs with high structural integrity. Microextrusion 3D bioprinting excels in printing high-viscosity bioinks, achieving high cell densities and scaffold-free structures, ease of operation; however, it faces limitations in resolution and imposes high shear stress on cells. It can use cell densities of 10^8 cells/ml and has a survival rate in the range of 40-85%. Increasing print resolution (5-200 μm) and speed (10-50 μm/s) is a challenge in microextrusion bioprinting technology. It is commonly used to fabricate aortic valves, skin, branched vascular trees, nerves, muscle, and *in vitro* pharmacokinetic and tumor models.

2.3 Laser-assisted Bioprinting

Laser-assisted bioprinting (LAB) utilizes focused laser pulses to achieve high precision, resolution and shape fidelity, making it suitable for micropatterned structures. LAB is compatible with a range of viscosities (1–300 mPa/s) with speed up to 1,600 mm/s with cell densities of 10^8 cells/ml and cell viability of 85-95%. LAB does not use a nozzle, therefore, there are no clogging concerns. However, the cytotoxicity of photocrosslinkers, UV light sources, cost, and the long printing process are few drawbacks. It is commonly used to fabricate bone, cartilage, blood vessels, skin and adipose tissue.

2.4 Stereolithography

Stereolithography-based bioprinting uses UV light or a laser to cross-link polymers, offering high resolution (200 nm - 6 µm) without clogging during the printing process. The technique utilizes light-sensitive hydrogels that are deposited in a layer-by-layer fashion to form a 3D structure. The speed of this method is very fast (about 40,000 mm/s) with cell densities of $>10^6$ cells/ml and viability of more than 90%. However, long-term exposure of cells to intense UV radiation can affect their cell viability. Commonly used to fabricate bone, nerve, liver, cardiac, blood vessels, cartilage, cornea, etc (Dey and Ozbolat, 2020; Z. Gu et al., 2020; Murphy and Atala, 2014; Reddy et al., 2023).

3.   4D bioprinting-The Fourth Dimension of Bioprinting

Fourth-dimensional (4D) bioprinting has emerged in recent years, which adds the additional dimension of time within the printed 3D scaffolds. During the 4D bioprinting process, an external stimulus like physical, chemical, and biological stimuli are exposed to the printed construct, causing a change in shape or functionality. Contrary to static fabrication technologies such as 3D printing, electrospinning, and salt leaching, stimuli-responsive materials used in 4D printing possess programmable attributes, allowing for controlled deformations and functional changes, as well as unique features such as the ability to self-fold, twist, and swell, resulting in complex constructs. One of the potential uses of 4D bioprinting with stimuli-responsive biomaterials is the development of implantable medical devices that can adapt to changes in the body over time while also self-assembling and self-healing. The biomaterial inks used in 4D bioprinting applications typically combine traditional bioprinting biomaterials with stimuli-responsive biomaterials. Among these, shape-memory biomaterials, a subset of stimuli-responsive biomaterials, exhibit programmable properties enabling controlled deformation of printed structures. Shape memory polymers (SMPs) and shape memory hydrogels (SMHs) are prominent examples, with SMPs reverting to their original form upon exposure to stimuli such as pH, redox, temperature, enzyme, and mechanical force, or some readily available and easily-controlled external stimuli such as light, ultrasound, electric, and magnetic. On the other hand SMHs excel in cell encapsulation for 4D bioprinting. Biological stimuli can be glucose, enzymes, and other biomolecules. A select few stimuli-responsive biomaterials are detailed in Table 1. 4D bioprinting is a s promising approach to fabricate functional constructs for tissue regeneration applications. Nonetheless, hurdles hinder its clinical adoption; many current stimuli-responsive biomaterials lack bioactivity, only facilitating basic shape alterations. Moreover, they often lose structural integrity with repeated deformations and may necessitate harsh chemicals to induce transformations, posing risks in clinical scenarios (Agarwal et al., 2021; Faber et al., 2023). Future research should focus on enhancing stimuli-responsive biomaterials to address these limitations.

4.   Futuristic Applications of 3D Bioprinted Organs

4.1 3D Bioprinting in Tissue Engineering and Regenerative Medicine

3D bioprinting provides an innovative approach to address tissue engineering and regenerative medicine limitations, available with the current approaches. The objective of tissue engineering and regenerative medicine is to mimic native tissue through the creation of functional tissue constructs to address damage sustained by repair. In the traditional tissue engineering approach, cells are seeded onto a porous and mechanically stable scaffold, for cell proliferation and tissue formation. This approach is advantageous in terms of achieving optimal structural support with suitable degradation kinetics; cellular microenvironment modulation; ease in exchange of nutrients and waste, to and from cells within the scaffold. However, these methods have demonstrated limitations in their success when used *in vivo*, both logistically and economically, as they are randomized in nature with non-uniform pore distribution, limited cell density, viability, reproducibility, absence

Table 1　Different stimuli-responsive biomaterials for 4D printing applications

Stimulus Type	Examples of Stimuli-responsive Biomaterials	Advantages	Applications	Limitations	Reference
Temperature	n-isopropylacrylamide polymers (pNIPAM)	Non-invasive	Biomedical applications; Bone, muscle, and cardiovascular tissue engineering; Drug delivery applications; Cell sheet engineering	Cells cultivated with these thermo-responsive polymers are themselves also sensitive towards changes in the environmental temperature; low temperatures induce a cold stress and impair metabolic activity, and extremely high temperatures affect cell viability as well	(Agarwal et al., 2021; Bril et al., 2022; Faber et al., 2023; Tamay et al., 2019; Wells et al., 2019, 2019; W. Zhou et al., 2020)
	Poly(n-cyclopropylacrylamide) (PNCPAm)				
	Poly(n-vinylcaprolactam)				
	Polyurethane				
	Polycaprolactones				
	Pluronics				
	Poloxamers				
	Elastin-like polypeptides				
	Chitosan				
pH	Chitosan	Solubility, Degradability; Swelling; Surface activity. and self-assembly; Non-invasive	Biomedical applications; Wound dressings; Drug and gene delivery; Controlled release of drugs and other therapeutic molecules	Cells can be sensitive to changes in pH; pH-sensitive systems may be activated during implantation or administration, making these systems susceptible to off-target delivery.	
	Poly(acrylamide)				
	Poly(lactic-co-glycolic acid) (PLGA)				
	PLA-poly(ethyleneimine)				
	N-carboxyethyl chitosan/ dibezaldehyde-terminated PEG				
	β-cyclodextrin-modified Alginate; diethylenetriamine-modified Alginate				

Contd.

Table 1 *Contd.*

Stimulus Type	Examples of Stimuli-responsive Biomaterials	Advantages	Applications	Limitations	Reference
Magnetic field	Superparamagnetic iron oxide nanoparticles Eg: γ- iron oxide (Fe_2O_3) nanoparticles	Superparamagnetic properties; Non-invasive; Useful with heat-labile bonds or Thermosensitive materials	Biomedical applications; Bone tissue remodelling; Soft robotic and surgical applications; Bone/Cartilage Tissue engineering; Drug delivery system	Magnetic NPs smaller than 50 nm are able to cross biological membranes and adversely affect the function of the tissues by inducing inflammation, generating reactive oxygen Species, impeding DNA function, and driving cells to apoptosis	
	pNIPAM-co-acrylic acid				
	Polypropylene fumarate with Fe_2O_3 nanoparticles				
	Polydimethylsiloxane and Fe particles (PDMS/Fe)				
	PCL/Fe-doped hydroxyapatite (HAP)				
	Magnetic hydrogel composed of HEMA, EGDMA, and SMA				
	Bioactive glass/PCL scaffold embedded with magnetic Fe_3O_4 nanoparticles				
	Tetramethylazanium hydroxide				
Electric field	Gelatin methacryloyl (GelMA)	Electric-field induced cell alignment; Swelling properties; Non-invasiveness; Enhance cellular uptake of drugs or nanoparticles; Ease of use; Inexpensive	Tissue regeneration of muscle; Helps in osteogenic differentiation; Biosensors; Blood vessels and nerve tissue regeneration	Need to place electrodes in the polymer matrix, limiting use to topical or subdermal implants	
	Polyaniline				
	Polypyrrole				
	Polythiophene				
	Ethylene vinyl acetate				
	Polyethylene				
	Pluronic F127				

Contd.

Table 1   *Contd.*

Stimulus Type	Examples of Stimuli-responsive Biomaterials	Advantages	Applications	Limitations	Reference
Light (UV, visible, NIR, and lasers of various wavelength)	Urethane diacrylate and linear semicrystalline polymer	Non-invasive; Drug release in light-responsive biomaterials	Biomedical applications; Soft robotics; Cardiac/ Nervous tissue engineering; Cell culture platforms	Poor tissue penetration; Damaging effects on healthy tissues depending on penetration depth, diameter of the light beam, exposure duration or the light intensity	
	GelMA and PEGDA				
	Graphene nanohybrid				
	Incorporation of azobenzene, spiropyran, or dithienylethene moiety, or photocleavable crosslinkers, like o-nitrobenzyl esters- based polymers				
	pNIPAM functionalized with spirobenzopyran				
Ultrasound	PLA-b-PEG	Non-invasive	Bioimaging in medicine	Limitations in penetration depth; Limitation in methods to deliver the materials to targeted tissues before stimulation	
	Melamine-embedded Poly(vinyl alcohol)				
	Chitosan / Alginate				
	Poly(methacrylic acid) (PMAA)				
	Poly(2-oxazoline) micelles				
Enzymes	Poly(styrenyl ether trehalose	Enzymatic crosslinking; Enzyme-responsive degradation; Non-invasive; Smart delivery systems; Biological and metabolic roles; Selectivity; Less-toxic;	Biomedical applications; 3D screening platforms; Tissue engineering	Release of the drug before reaching the intended target	
	PEG				
	Polydimethylsiloxane,				
	Polyethylenimine				
	PEGylated alkynylated peptide dendrimer				
	MMP-sensitive HA				

of vascular and neural networks and do not allow for customized options. 3D bioprinting marks a groundbreaking advancement in both bioengineering and the biomedical field, offering the ability to fabricate patient-specific autologous organs and tissues, diminishing the risk of activation of the immune system. Bioprinting can develop complex organ/tissue structures with precise positioning and architectural control like shape, pore geometry, and interconnectivity, mimicking human physiology with high reproducibility and repeatability. Co-printing multiple types of cells composed of various materials can be used to achieve structural and biochemical complexity of living tissue/ organs in a heterocellular microenvironment (Agarwal et al., 2021; Z. Gu et al., 2020; Tripathi et al., 2023). 3D bioprinting has been widely used in various application areas and few applications are listed in Table 2.

4.2   3D Bioprinting Organs for Transplantation

Organ failure, stemming from factors such as aging, illnesses, accidents, and congenital defects, presents a significant medical hurdle. Organ manufacturing utilising cutting-edge 3D-printing technology has emerged as a growing area of research aimed at the transition of engineered solid organs to the clinic, addressing the shortage of organ donors and mitigating the risk of immune rejection and waiting time. While flat, tubular, and hollow non-tubular engineered organs have already been implanted in patients, in vitro formation of a fully functional solid organ at a translatable scale has not yet been achieved. Major challenges in organ bioprinting include complexity and unpredictability of the 3D organ printing process, including issues such as biomaterial selection, biocompatibility, biodegradability, cell source, cell types, cell viability, interconnectivity, tissue vascularization, innervations, shape fidelity, scale-up, and restoration of complex functionality of the printed tissue. The achievement of this milestone heavily relies on comprehending the mechanisms involved in embryonic organogenesis. However, further research is essential to overcome the technical, biological, regulatory and ethical challenges related with 3D bioprinting for its widespread clinical implementation (Jorgensen et al., 2020; Reddy et al., 2023; Y. Wu et al., 2023). The Food and Drug Administration (FDA) regulates 3D printed organs in the USA. Health Canada (HC) has issued preliminary recommendations to assist medical device manufacturers in formulating regulations for bioprinting in Canada. In Europe, the European Medical Devices Directive, the Active Implantable Medical Devices Directive, and the In-vitro Diagnostic Medical Devices Directive of the European Union (EU) govern the regulation of 3D printing health technology. Implantable devices, including 3D organs, are classified as high-risk and necessitate an independent design dossier review (Jorgensen et al., 2020; Panja et al., 2022). Major milestones in the development of 3D bioprinting technology in the area of tissue engineering and organ bioprinting are illustrated in Figure 1 and 2.

Scientists have printed living organs like the heart, liver, kidney, lungs, bone, cornea and skin. Few advancements in the area of tissue engineering and organ printing are listed in Table 2. Atala and his colleagues developed the first lab-grown or engineered bladder for successful transplantation in humans, implanted in patients in 1999. Researchers created a functional experimental solid organ, a miniature kidney that secretes urine. Engineered functional, experimental solid organs (penile tissues and livers) using a strategy to recycle donor organs, with promising applications to other solid organs, such as the kidney and pancreas were developed. Researchers successfully implanted engineered vaginas into four girls with rare genetic defects in 2005 (Adamowicz et al., 2017; Jorgensen et al., 2020). Patient-specific ear-shaped cartilage were implanted by utilizing expanded microtia chondrocytes in conjunction with a biodegradable scaffold (G. Zhou et al., 2018). Scientists have utilized a patient's own cells and biological materials to produce the world's first 3D vascularized engineered heart through printing technology (Noor et al., 2019). Multilayered vascularized 3D-printed skin graft designed for implantation (Baltazar et al., 2020). Researchers bioprinted a functional prototype of a pancreas, achieving stable blood flow in pigs (Klak et al., 2023). Scientists reported engineered uterus that can sustain pregnancy and live delivery pre-clinically (Magalhaes et al., 2020).

Table 2   3D Bioprinting for different tissue engineering application

Target Organ	Bioink	Printing Type	Cell Types	Study Period	Significant Result	Reference
Skin	Fibrinogen/ Collagen	Inkjet	Fibroblasts; Keratinocytes	8 weeks	Novel proof-of-concept validation of a mobile skin bioprinting system that provides rapid on-site management of extensive wounds.	(Albanna et al., 2019)
	Alginate/ Gelatin/ Cellulose/ Fibrinogen	Extrusion	Primary dermal keratinocytes (HDKs) and fibroblasts (HDFs)	21 days	Epidermal-dermal functional construct.	(Ramakrishnan et al., 2022)
	Collagen/ Matriderm	Laser-assisted	NIH/3T3 fibroblasts; HaCaT keratinocytes	11 days	Some blood vessels were found to be arising from the wound bed.	(Michael et al., 2013)
	Gelatin/ Alginate/ Fibrinogen/ Laminin	Extrusion	HDFs; HaCaT	21 days	Histological evaluation showed thinner epidermal thickness which could be improved by means of prolonging the culture duration and optimizing the medium components.	(J. Liu et al., 2022)
	Plasma derived-Fibrin	Extrusion	HDFs; HDKs	3 weeks (21 days)	Bioprinted skin displayed well-developed stratum corneum and basal membrane, offering a cost-effective method for developing normal human skin suitable for clinical and commercial use.	(Cubo et al., 2016)
	Polyvinylpyrrolidone (PVP)/ Collagen	Inkjet	HDFs	10 days	The combination of electrospun nanofibrous matrices and 3D bioprinted constructs	(Ng et al., 2018)
	GelMA/ Polyethylene oxide (PEO)	Hand-held Extrusion	NIH/3T3	7 days	A portable handheld extrusion bioprinter was developed for *in situ* wound dressing.	(Ying et al., 2020)
Cardiac	Alginate/PEGDA-Fibrinogen (PF)	Extrusion	iPSC- derived cardiomyocytes (CMs), HUVECs	14 days	Bioprinted ECs exhibit regeneration ability by restoring blood flow through revascularization.	(Maiullari et al., 2018)
	Gelatin/mTgase cross-linking	Extrusion	hBone marrow derived-MSCs; Necnatal rat CMs	21 days	Generated stable cell aligning microchannels.	(Tijore et al., 2018)
	GelMA/ Cardiac dECM	Extrusion	Human cardiac progenitor cells (hCPCs); rat-CFBs	14 days	Patches were retained on rat hearts and showed vascularization over 14 days *in vivo*.	(Bejleri et al., 2018)

Contd.

Table 2 *Contd.*

Target Organ	Bioink	Printing Type	Cell Types	Study Period	Significant Result	Reference
	Collagen	Extrusion (FRESH)	iPSC-derived CMs	7 days	Cardiac ventricles printed with human cardiomyocytes showed synchronized contractions, directional action potential propagation, and wall thickening up to 14% during peak systole.	(A. Lee et al., 2019)
	GelMA/ Fibronectin	Extrusion	Cardiac myocytes, Fibroblasts	7 days	Cell survival increased with incorporation of adhesion molecules and lowering of GelMA concentration.	(Koti et al., 2019)
	PCL/ hdECM	Extrusion	hCPCs, hMSCs	28 days	This 3D pre-vascularized stem cell patch effectively delivered the stem cells via the epicardial delivery route	(Jang et al., 2017)
	Prepolyglycerol sebacate/ Polypyrrole/ TEMPO oxidized nanocellulose (pre-PGS-PPy: TOCNF)	Extrusion	H9c2 cells	4 days	Multifunctional cardiac patches for long-term drug release therapies after Myocardial Infarction	(Ajdary et al., 2020)
Cornea	Collagen/ Alginate	Extrusion	Corneal keratocytes	7 days	Showed survival of keratocytes with cell viability at days 1 and 7 with post-printing >90% and 83%, respectively.	(Isaacson et al., 2018)
	PEG-PCL fibers reinforced GelMa	Extrusion	Rat- limbal stromal stem cells (LSSCs)	7 days	The result demonstrated that fiber hydrogel and serum-free media synergize to provide an optimal environment for the maintenance of keratocyte phenotype and the regeneration of damaged corneal stroma.	(Kong et al., 2020)
	Alginate/ Gelatin	DLP/ Extrusion	Human corneal epithelial cell (HCEC) line	--	Geometry-controllable corneal substitutes with possibility of producing substitutes for other cornea-like shell structures with different scale and geometry features, such as the glomerulus, atrium, and oophoron, more biological evaluation required.	(B. Zhang et al., 2019)

Contd.

Table 2 *Contd.*

Target Organ	Bioink	Printing Type	Cell Types	Study Period	Significant Result	Reference
	rh-Laminin/ Collagen	Laser-assisted	Human ESC-derived limbal epithelial stem cells (hESC-LESC), hADMSCs	7 days	First study to demonstrate the feasibility of 3D laser-assisted bioprinting for corneal applications using human stem cells and successful fabrication of layered 3D bioprinted tissues mimicking the structure of the native corneal tissue..	(Sorkio et al., 2018)
	PVA/ Chitosan	Extrusion	hADMSCs	7 days	Preliminary biostability studies showed that composite constructs were compatible with hASCs even after 30 days of degradation, showing potential for these cells to be differentiated to the stroma layer in future.	(Ulag et al., 2020)
	GelMA/ PEGDA	DLP	Rabbit corneal epithelial cells (rCECs), rADMSCs	28 days	Bi-layer cells-laden corneal scaffold is applied in a rabbit keratoplasty model. The post-operative outcome reveals efficient sealing of corneal defects, re-epithelialization and stromal regeneration.	(He et al., 2022)
	HA-based dopamine with hydrazone crosslinking	Extrusion	hADMSCs and hADMSC-derived corneal stromal keratocytes, hPSCs- derived neurons	21 days	Human stem cell derived corneal stromal model with innervation.	(Mörö et al., 2022)
Bone	PEG/PLGA	Extrusion	Bone marrow-derived MSCs	15 days	PEG/PLGA bioprinted scaffolds address challenges associated with post-fabrication cell seeding and biomolecule deposition by patterning biological contents within structures to achieve optimal structure	(Sawkins et al., 2015)
	PEG/GelMA	Inkjet	hMSCs	21 days	Scaffolds demonstrated an improvement of mechanical properties and osteogenic and chondrogenic differentiation.	(Gao et al., 2015)
	Collagen/nano- HAP	Laser-assisted	MSCs, D1 cell line	42 days	*In situ* printing of mesenchymal stromal cells, associated with collagen and nano-HAP, in order to favor bone regeneration, in a calvarial defect model in mice	(L. Li et al., 2017)

Contd.

Table 2   *Contd.*

Target Organ	Bioink	Printing Type	Cell Types	Study Period	Significant Result	Reference
	PCL/ RGD-γ-irradiated Alginate/ nano-HA	Extrusion/ FDM	Bone marrow-derived MSCs	14 days	Gene activated MSC-laden constructs were then implanted subcutaneously, directly post fabrication, and were found to support superior levels of vascularization and mineralization compared to cell-free controls.	(Cunniffe et al., 2017)
	PCL with resveratrol & strontium ranelate	Extrusion	MSCs, monocyte-derived osteoclasts, ECs	21 days	Bone scaffolds containing the small dual molecules had combinational advantages in enhancing angiogenesis and inhibiting osteoclast activities, and they synergistically promoted MSC osteogenic differentiation in critical-sized rat mandibular bone defect models .	(W. Zhang et al., 2020)
	Octacalcium phosphate (OCP)/ GelMA	SLA	HUVECs spheroids, Mouse multipotent mesenchymal C3H10T1/2 cells	14 days	Osteoblastic differentiation and formation of the capillary-like structures	(Anada et al., 2019)
	GelMA biofunctionalized with bone particles (BPs)	Extrusion	Cells in BPs	28 days	This study demonstrates the feasibility of bioprinted viable BPs and may have some potential for patient-specific chairside clinical translation.	(Ratheesh et al., 2020)
Cartilage	Fibrinogen/ Gelatin/ HA/ Glycerol	Extrusion	Human bone marrow stem/ stromal cells (hBMSCs), HUVECs	14 days	3D bioprinting of prevascularized implants for the repair of critically sized bone defects	(Nulty et al., 2021)
	HA/ Allyl-functionalized poly(glycidol)/ PCL	Extrusion	Human & Equine MSCs	21 days	Embedded hMSCs showed good cell survival for at least 21 days in culture	(Stichler et al., 2017)
	PCL/ dECM	Extrusion	Human inferior turbinate-tissue derived MSCs (hTMSCs), hADMSCs, rat Myoblast cells (L6)	14 days	Chondrogenic differentiation of cells within the construct, with greater expression of SOX9 and type II collagen	(Pati et al., 2014)

Contd.

Table 2 *Contd.*

Target Organ	Bioink	Printing Type	Cell Types	Study Period	Significant Result	Reference
	Nanofibrillated cellulose/alginate (Nasal cartilage)	Extrusion	Human bone MSCs and human nasal chondrocytes	60 days	Subcutaneous implantation in nude mice	(Apelgren et al., 2017)
	Collagen/ nano-HAP	Laser-Assisted	MSCs	2 months	LAB can be used for the *in situ* printing of MSCs in bioink, in order to favor bone regeneration, in a calvarial defect model in mice	(Keriquel et al., 2017)
Meniscus	ColMA/ Collagen/ Chondroitin sulfate methacrylate	Extrusion	Human bone marrow MSC	4 weeks	Cells were present up to 4 weeks post printing	(Klarmann et al., 2023)
	Nanofibrillated cellulose/ Alginate	Inkjet	Human nasoseptal chondrocytes (hNC)	7 days	Short term study showing bioink characterization and cell viability preliminary studies.	(Markstedt et al., 2015)
	Alginate/ PLA nanofibers	Extrusion	hADMSCs	8 weeks (56 days)	Human medial knee meniscus digitally modeled using magnetic resonance images was bioprinted and evaluated over 8 weeks *in vitro*	(Narayanan et al., 2016)
	Alginate/ Gelatin/ Carboxymethylated cellulose nanocrystal	Extrusion	Human knee articular chondrocytes (NHAC-kn)	28 days	The formulated bioink is printable, stable under cell culture conditions, biocompatible, and able to maintain the native phenotype of chondrocytes	(Semba et al., 2023)
	GelMA/ Meniscal ECM/ PCL	Dual-nozzle + multi temperature printing system	Meniscal fibrocartilage chondrocytes	8 weeks (56 days)	Cell viability, mechanics, biodegradation and tissue formation *in vivo* were performed to ensure that the scaffold had sufficient feasibility and functionality	(Jian et al., 2021)
	Meniscal dECM	Extrusion	Porcine-derived fibrochondrocytes	5 days	Development of decellularized meniscus ECM-derived inks with rheological properties for printability, enabling the fabrication of mechanically functional meniscal tissue equivalents. Further *in vivo* studies are required.	(B. Wang et al., 2023)

Contd.

Table 2 *Contd.*

Target Organ	Bioink	Printing Type	Cell Types	Study Period	Significant Result	Reference
	PCL/ Meniscus ECM functionalized with kartogenin (KGN)-loaded PLGA microspheres (PCL/ MECM-KGN μS)	FDM	Synovium-derived MSCs	21 days	Synergistic effect of the MECM and sustained release of KGN can endow the PCL/MECM-KGN μS scaffolds with excellent cell vitality preservation and chondrogenic activity.	(H. Li et al., 2021)
	PLA with Carbohydrate	Extrusion	hMSC	28 days	*In vivo* stability and biocompatibility showed improved behaviour of the construct with angiogenic activity.	(Gupta et al., 2020)
Trachea	PCL/ Alginate	Extrusion	Rabbit nasal epithelial cells, Rabbit auricular chondrocytes	12 months (1 yr)	Artificial trachea was effective in the regeneration of respiratory epithelium, but not in cartilage regeneration.	(J.H. Park et al., 2019)
	PCL/ Fibrin	Extrusion	MSCs	8 weeks (56 days)	Successful integration of the implanted 3D printed tracheal grafts with the adjacent trachea	(Chang et al., 2014)
	PCL/ Collagen / HA	Extrusion	MSCs	2 weeks (14 days)	First study of its kind to fabricate bioprinted tracheal constructs with separate cartilage and smooth muscle regions	(Ke et al., 2019)
	Silk fibroin methacrylate	DLP;4D Bioprinting	Rabbit auricular chondrocytes, Rabbit nasal turbinate stem cells	8 weeks (56 days)	Trachea scaffold implantation in a partial resection rabbit model	(S. H. Kim et al., 2020)
	PCL/ Atelocollagen	Extrusion	Human nasal chondrocytes and human nasal turbinate stem cells	8 weeks (56 days)	3D bioprinting of a trachea-mimetic cellular construct of a clinically relevant size	(J. H. Park et al., 2021)
Esophagus	PCL	Extrusion	Rabbit MSCs	3 weeks (21 days)	Repairs partial esophageal defects; but doesn't allow circumferential reconstruction.	(S. Y. Park et al., 2016)
	Poly(L-lactide-co-ε-caprolactone)	Extrusion	A10 cells (myoblasts), L929, hMSCs	7 days	Overall design limited by the rotating mandrel	(Tan et al., 2015)

Contd.

Table 2 *Contd.*

Target Organ	Bioink	Printing Type	Cell Types	Study Period	Significant Result	Reference
	PLGA porous microspheres/ Agarose/ Collagen	Extrusion	L929, Rat2 cells (fibroblasts), A10 (smooth muscle), C2C12 cells (myoblasts), TR146 cells (ECs), hMSCs	14 days	High risk of collapse of a longer construct	(Tan et al., 2016)
Intestine	PEGDA/ Acrylic acid	SLA	Caco-2	3 weeks (21 days)	Developed intestinal structure including crypt/villus architecture with photopolymerizable hydrogel.	(Creff et al., 2019)
	GelMA/ PEGDA/ LAP	SLA	Caco-2,NIH/3T3	21 days	The resulting model shows a cellular distribution and co-localization for both epithelial and stromal compartments resembling native tissue.	(Torras et al., 2023)
	Novogel	Extrusion	Intestinal myofibroblast, Intestinal epithelial cells (hIECs), Caco-2	21 days	GI toxicity of the model. The 3D intestinal tissue demonstrates a polarized epithelium with tight junctions and specialized epithelial cell types and expresses functional and inducible CYP450 enzymes.	(Madden et al., 2018)
	GelMA/ PEGDA/ LAP & tartrazine	SLA	Caco-2, HT29-MTX, Human intestinal fibroblasts (HIF)	21 days	3D bioprinted model of the intestinal mucosa with improved physiological features: villus-like architecture and stromal compartment for evaluating drug permeability.	(Macedo et al., 2023)
Blood vessels	GelMA/ HA/ Glycerol/ Fibrinogen	Extrusion	HUVECs, Smooth muscle cells (SMCs)	7 days	A bionic vascular vessel with dual layers was fabricated successfully, and kept good viability and functionality.	(Jin et al., 2022)
	Alginate/ GelMA/ PEGTA	Extrusion	HUVECs, MSC	21 days	Bioink formulation may also have significant potential in engineering large-scale vascularized tissue constructs towards applications in organ transplantation and repair.	(Jia et al., 2016)
	Gelatin/mTG, Pluronic F127	SLA	HUVECs	72 h	Approach for constructing integrated vasculature for tissue engineering.	(Y. Liu et al., 2019)
	Polydopamine-coated calcium silicate/ PCL	Extrusion	Wharton's jelly MSCs, HUVECs	14 days	Approach may be effective for building deep bone structures with complex vascular networks	(Chen et al., 2018)

Contd.

Table 2   *Contd.*

Target Organ	Bioink	Printing Type	Cell Types	Study Period	Significant Result	Reference
Liver	Pluronic 127/ Alginate	Extrusion	Human hepatoma cell line, HepG2/C3A	7 days	Study findings demonstrate high viability and liver-specific metabolic activity, as assessed by synthesis of urea, albumin, and expression levels of the detoxifying CYP1A2 enzyme of cells embedded in the 3D hydrogel system, useful for investigating drug-induced hepatotoxicity.	(Gori et al., 2020)
	GelMA/ dECM	DLP	Hepatocytes hiHep cells	5 days	Liver dECM was found to not only improve the printability but also the hiHep cell viability of GelMA-based bioinks	(Mao et al., 2020)
	NovoGel 2.0	Extrusion	Hepatocytes, HSCs, ECs	4 weeks (28 days)	A bioprinted liver model to model liver injury leading to fibrosis	(H. Lee & Cho, 2016)
	Alginate/ Plasma/ Methyl-cellulose/ Fibrin/ Collagen	Extrusion	HepG2 cells, HUVECs, NHDFs	14 days	Core-shell bioprinting was shown to be a valuable tool to study cell-cell interactions and to develop complex tissue-like models.	(Taymour et al., 2022)
	Galactosylated alginate	Inkjet	Primary mouse hepatocytes	2 days	The fabricated GA-gel was able to successfully promote adhesion of hepatocytes.	(Arai et al., 2017)
Kidney	Kidney dECM/ Gelatin/ HA/ Glycerol	Extrusion	Primary kidney cells	2 weeks (14 days)	Exhibit the structural and functional characteristics of the native renal tissue	(Ali et al., 2019)
	Fibrinogen/ Gelatin	Inkjet	PTEC-TERT1 cells	2 months (56 days)	Construction of a bioprinting method for creating 3D human renal proximal tubules *in vitro*	(Homan et al., 2016)
	Bacterial nanocellulose/ Alginate	Extrusion	HUVECs	14 days	Developing an interconnected microchannels macro porosity and vascular like lumen structure in the kidney	(Sämfors et al., 2019)
	Polyethylene vinyl acetate (PEVA)	Extrusion	HK-2s, Caco-2s, and GEs cells	--	3D bioprinted *in vitro* secondary hyperoxaluria model by mimicking intestinal-oxalate-malabsorption-related kidney stone disease	(Yoon et al., 2022)
Urethra	PCL/ PLCL/ Fibrin/ Gelatin/ HA	Inkjet	Urothelial cells (UCs), SMCs	7 days	Active proliferation and expression of specific biomarkers	(K. Zhang et al., 2017)

Contd.

Table 2 *Contd.*

Target Organ	Bioink	Printing Type	Cell Types	Study Period	Significant Result	Reference
	GelMA/ Alginate/ eight-arm PEG acrylate (PEGOA)	Extrusion	Bladder urothelial cells, SMCs	2 weeks (14 days)	Printed urethra mimics the histology of the native urethra	(Pi et al., 2018)
	PLGA/PCL/Triethyl citrate (TEC)	Extrusion	Mouse fibroblast cells; L929	7 days	Mimic the natural urethral tissue in mechanical properties and cell bioactivity	(Xu et al., 2020)
	Collagen-carbodiimide crosslinking	Extrusion	SCaBER cells	3 days	Construction of a new type I collagen-based tubular scaffold is presented that possesses intrinsic radial elasticity	(Versteegden et al., 2017)
Nerves	Alginate/ Agarose/ Carboxymethyl-chitosan	Extrusion	Cortical human neural stem cell	11 days	Formation of synaptic contacts, establishment of networks, and spontaneous activity of differentiated neurons	(Q. Gu et al., 2016)
	Fibrinogen/ HA	Extrusion	Schwann cells	7 days	Schwann cells exhibited high viability immediately after printing and maintained proliferation over time. Schwann cells and DRG neurons aligned parallel to the 3D printed strands.	(England et al., 2017)
	GelMA/ PEGDA	Extrusion	BMSC	21 days	Embedded BMSCs in the inner layer significantly enhanced PC12 cell proliferation and neurite outgrowth, indicating accelerated nerve regeneration potential. GelMA/PEGDA combination improved mechanical strength while retaining biocompatibility.	(J. Liu et al., 2021)
	Gelatin/ Alginate	Extrusion	Schwann cells	4 weeks	Schwann cells maintained high viability and exhibited improved functionality, including increased expression of neurotrophic factors (NGF, BDNF, GDNF, PDGF), when cultured in 3D bioprinted scaffolds compared to traditional 2D culture methods.	(Z. Wu et al., 2020)

Contd.

Table 2   *Contd.*

Target Organ	Bioink	Printing Type	Cell Types	Study Period	Significant Result	Reference
Adipose	Agarose/ GelMA	Extrusion	ADMSCs/ ADSCs spheroids	14 days	Taking advantage of the self-assembling ability of spheroids and the controlled arrangement of bioprinting technologies, mature adipose tissue can be regenerated.	(Colle et al., 2020a)
	Nanocellulose/ Alginate/HA	Extrusion	Mouse MSC cell line C3H10T1/2	14 days	Alginate in the hydrogel may restrict the mobility of encapsulated hADSCs, impairing the differentiation potential of the cells.	(Henriksson et al., 2017)
	HAMA/ GelMA/ PEG-4A	Extrusion	HWA	19 days	3D HAMA/GelMA hydrogel facilitated spontaneous adipogenic differentiation of white progenitor cells without exogenous induction.	(Qi et al., 2018)
	Agarose/ GelMA	Extrusion	ADMSCs/ ADSCs spheroids	14 days	Taking advantage of the self-assembling ability of spheroids and the controlled arrangement of bioprinting technologies, mature adipose tissue can be regenerated.	(Colle et al., 2020b)

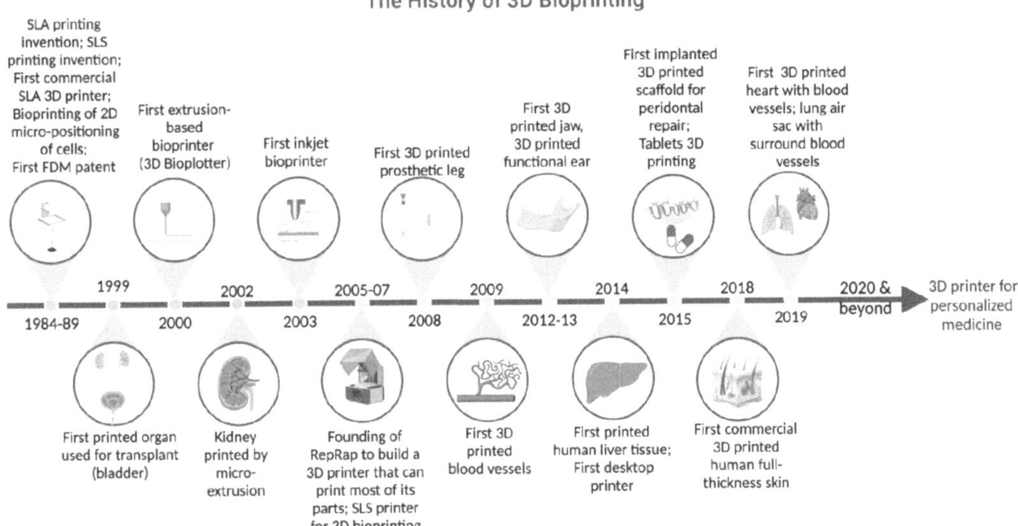

Fig. 1 Major milestones in the development of 3D bioprinting technology in tissue engineering and organ printing; created in Biorender.com.

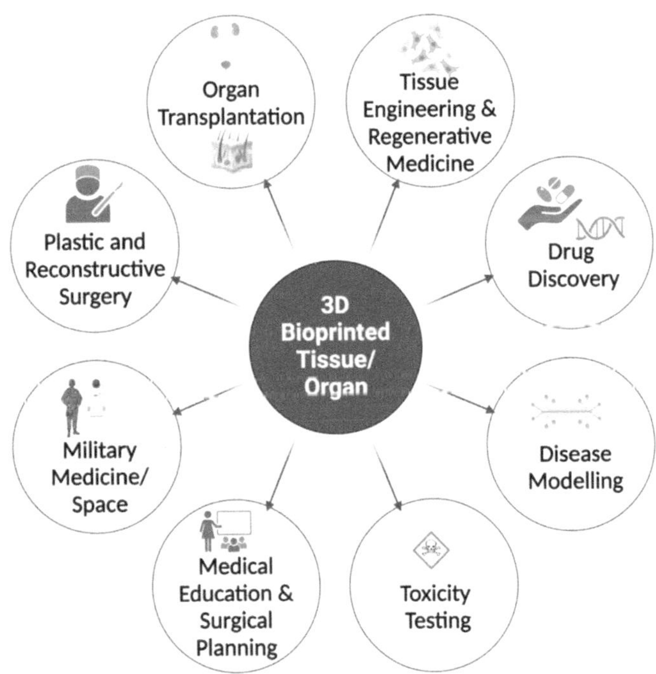

Fig. 2 Illustration of various application of 3D bioprinted tissues or organs in biomedical research; illustration made using Biorender.com

In situ bioprinting or intraoperative bioprinting is a promising application of 3D bioprinting to pattern de novo tissue directly onto the desired location in the body, which would minimize the gap between implant-host interfaces such as chronic wounds in the skin or bone defect. With the help of medical imaging, the topology of printed tissue can be designed to fit into the wound/defects. This allows for precise deposition of diverse cellular structures, hydrogels, and soluble factors within the affected areas. Vascularization presents a significant obstacle, especially in situ bioprinting.

Solutions such as incorporating oxygen-generating biomaterials or oxygen-filled microparticles into the bioink, or implementing sacrificial porous structures within the bioprinted tissue using meshed filaments, can address this challenge. There are few reports in this domain (Pagan et al., 2023; Pazhouhnia et al., 2022). Scientists report proof-of-concept validation of a mobile skin bioprinting system that provides rapid on-site management of extensive wounds. The same group also reports a mobile full-thickness skin bioprinting system, which can be used as a bedside option as well (Albanna et al., 2019).

4.3 3D Bioprinting in Plastic and Reconstructive Surgery

3D bioprinting technology allows the design of individualized grafts for each patient's custom needs, resulting in a higher degree of precision, fit, aesthetics, biocompatibility and lower immunogenicity. Few applications of 3D printing/bioprinting include skin flaps, rhinoplasty, hand printing, breast implants, prosthesis, bone, cartilage, nerve, and others. Few bioprinted studies are listed in Table 2. Farrell et al. reported a custom-made hand model with a replica of the bone using PLA and joint structures covered with several layers of silicone to simulate skin coverage (Farrell et al., 2020). Li et al. used 3D scanning and *in situ* bioprinting technologies to regenerate cartilage and bone defects (L. Li et al., 2017). 3D printing is widely used for craniomaxillofacial surgeries in mandible, midface, orbit, frontal sinus, cranial vault reconstructions. Researchers are investigating the use of patient-specific cells to create customized skin grafts that correspond to the individual's unique skin characteristics, improving wound healing and scar reduction outcomes. Researchers have 3D printed vascularized and perfusable skin graft using human keratinocytes, fibroblasts, pericytes, and endothelial cells, which might overcome the limitations of graft survival observed in a vascular skin substitute (Baltazar et al., 2020). Researchers have used 3D printed breast implants for in patients with breast ptosis: 2-stage reconstruction (Tomita et al., 2017). Several clinical trials are on-going in this area, anticipating successful commercialisations.

4.4 3D Bioprinting of Microfluidics and Organ-on-a-Chip Systems

The current focus within the translational medical research community is shifting towards emphasizing complex human factors and conditions, rather than solely relying on animal-based *in vivo* models and cell-based *in vitro* models. When comparing 2D and 3D models, there are significant differences, especially in terms of proteins, biomarkers, gene expression, drug response, resistance, cell morphology, cell growth and migration. Animal models have interspecial differences in physiology and metabolism compared to humans and does not allow comprehensive prediction of physiological reactions, drug-induced toxicity, potential side effects, and treatment efficiency and is limited by ethical controversies. Human cell-derived organoids, a 3D dimensional cellular complex with a certain spatial structure generated by cells differentiated from stem cells cultured *in vitro,* is a promising option for drug screening, personalized medicine, and disease modelling. Through the use of 3D printing technology, researchers address limitations in precise cell positioning, thus mimicking natural tissue structures (Leung et al., 2022; Tabatabaei Rezaei et al., 2023).

Advancements in microfluidics, tissue engineering, and cell biology have contributed to the development of microengineered organ-on-a-chip platforms. Organs-on-a-chip are systems containing engineered or natural miniature tissues grown inside microfluidic chips, designed to recapitulate key functional aspects of organs' and tissues' microenvironments and functions within a microscale culture. All organ-on-a-chip platforms have three critical and defining characteristics: The 3D nature for tissue culture, integration of multiple cell types (such as parenchymal, stromal, vascular and immune cells); and modelling of biomechanical forces relevant to the tissue being modelled (such as stretch forces for lung tissues or haemodynamic shear forces for vascular tissues) (Low et al., 2021). Organ-on-a-chip can be single organ-on-a-chip system, which allows evaluation of the response of a specific organ to a compound or mixture of compounds and multi organs-on-a-chip system also known as body-on-a-chip or human-on-a-chip system, which studies the systemic interactions between organs. There is no perfect standard material, as different materials have their advantages and disadvantages. The most commonly used materials for fabrication of microfluidic devices are silicone rubber, such as poly(dimethylsiloxane) (PDMS), glass, and thermoplastics such as PS, poly(methyl methacrylate) (PMMA), polycarbonate (PC) or cyclic olefin copolymer (Leung et al., 2022). Creating functional tissues within the organ-on-a-chip system uses two approaches. In a top-down or organotypic approach, a primary tissue for example, an organ slice from a biopsy or engineered tissue such as a preformed organoid is incorporated into the system, whereas in a bottom-up approach, isolated cells from primary, immortalized lines or stem cell-derived sources are cultured inside a microfluidic environment, which supports the remodelling of the cells into a functional neo-tissue (Y. Wang et al., 2023). The challenges include biomaterial selection, cell sourcing, universal culture medium, platform design, linking multiple platforms, regulations and commercialization (Low et al., 2021). Figure 3 gives an illustration of different organ-on-a-chip platforms and various applications are explained below.

4.5 Organs-on-a-Chip for Drug Discovery

Drug development and screening can be costly, time-consuming, involving high-risk procedures that necessitate preclinical validation and clinical trial evaluation before market release. This selection process involves screening the drug for toxicity, metabolism, biological activity, pharmacological efficacy and medicinal value. Despite this thorough and lengthy process, which typically spans 12-15 years for drug approval, approximately 50% of drug failures are attributed to unpredictable toxicity and inefficacy. Ma et al. employed digital light processing to produce liver lobule structures, creating a 3D printed hexagonal anatomical feature comprising both parenchymal and non-parenchymal tissue components. This intricate structure demonstrated enhanced morphological organization, higher liver-specific gene expression levels, and increased secretion of metabolic products compared to both 2D monolayer culture and a 3D model with only hepatic progenitor cells. The system's projection optics enabled the generation of light patterns at micrometer-level resolution, facilitating the rapid biofabrication of the liver lobule hydrogel construct within seconds with minimal UV exposure (Ma et al., 2021). Miller et al. used SLA to create biomimetic 3D structures with a focus on vascularized systems. The purpose of this research was to improve the authenticity of microfluidic vascular implants and valves, resulting in more accurate organ-on-a-chip models for lung, liver, and cardiac microsystems. Scientists have developed a highly functional human-derived body-on-a-chip platform that integrates multiple human cell derived tissues with a common blood supply system for drug toxicity testing and personalized medicine. The purpose of this research was to improve the authenticity of microfluidic vascular implants and valves, resulting in more accurate organ-on-a-chip models for lung, liver, and cardiac microsystems (Jodat et al., 2018; Low et al., 2021; Tabatabaei Rezaei et al., 2023; Vunjak-Novakovic et al., 2021; Y. Wang et al., 2023). Researchers developed first engineered miniature 3D human brains/organoids resembling the normal human blood brain barrier (Scientists have successfully created kidney organoids from urine cells (F et al., 2019).

4.6 Disease Modelling on a Chip

The use of various human organoids, spheroid organ-on-a-chip systems, such as the brain and lungs, has proven to be a valuable tool for investigating infectious diseases, genetic disorders, and cancer. They enable studies of systemic disease in the human setting for diseases that currently have minimal alternative models available, including cancer metastasis, inflammation, fibrosis, aging, asthma, vascular abnormalities, neural disorders, myopathies, kidney disorders, gut health and infections. Lee et al. also developed a multi-layer 3D liver fibrosis-on-a-chip system that incorporates hepatocytes, activated stellate cells, and endothelial cells. This disease model showed liver fibrosis characteristics such as collagen buildup, cell death, and decreased liver function (Ingber, 2022; Jodat et al., 2018; Kanabekova et al., 2022; Leung et al., 2022).

4.7 Cancer Models on a Chip

The combination of spheroid culture and microfluidic platform may be a successful strategy in the organ-on-a-chip systems to simulate the *in vivo* tumor microenvironment modelling in terms of angiogenesis, tumor growth, intravasation, extravasation and metastasis for studying cancer models as well as drug screening of anticancer candidates. The option of patient-derived tumours-on-chips for screening chemotherapeutics enables treatment comparison and optimization towards using this technology for precision medicine. Several tumour-on-a-chip models include neural glioblastoma, renal cell carcinoma, lung, pancreatic, colorectal, ovarian, prostate and cervical cancer (Low et al., 2021). Patient-derived pancreatic ductal epithelial cells were used to create a pancreas-on-a-chip to understand the cystic fibrosis transmembrane conductance regulator protein and its role in insulin secretion (Shik Mun et al., 2019). Reid et al. used 3D bioprinting to create tumoroid arrays for studying the tumorigenesis and microenvironmental redirection of breast cancer cells. A lung cancer-on-a-chip equipped with a pH sensor, a trans-epithelial/trans-endothelial electrical resistance (TEER) impedance sensor and a fluorescence microscope was developed for real-time monitoring of cellular responses to different concentrations of the anticancer drugs, doxorubicin, and docetaxel (Leung et al., 2022).

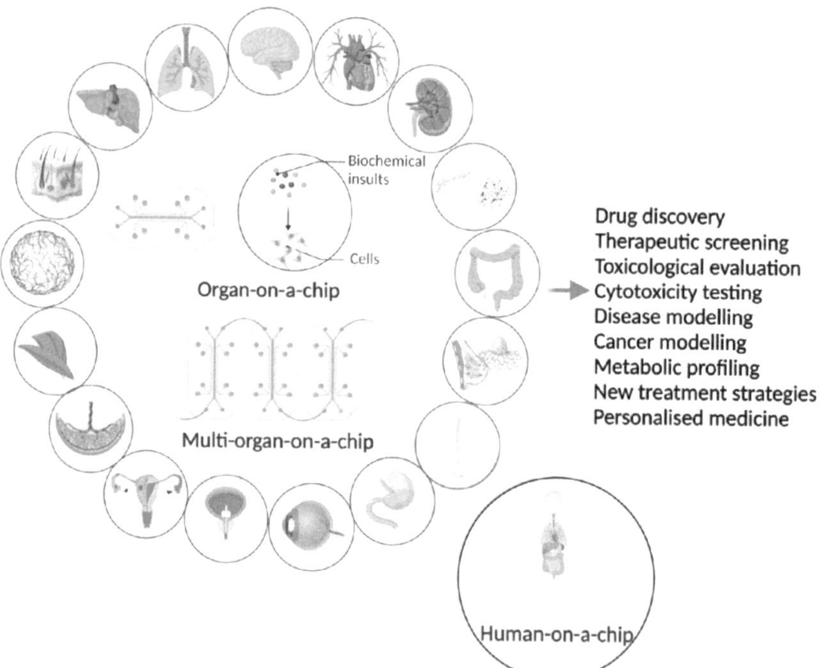

Fig. 3   Organ-on-a-chip and disease-on-a-chip platforms for studying human physiology and pathophysiology for various therapeutic applications; Illustration created with BioRender.com.

4.8 Organs-on-a-Chip for Toxicological Assessment

Organ-on-a-chip models for liver, heart, kidney, skin, lung, intestine, vasculature and brain are traditionally targeted for toxicity studies. This enables the study of complex organ to organ interactions for pharmacokinetic/pharmacodynamic modelling, absorption, distribution, metabolism and excretion (ADME) profiling, quantitative systems pharmacology and other computational modelling (Low et al., 2021). Physiome-on-a-chip created interconnected microphysiological systems involving 10 organs for quantitative biology and pharmacology studies (Edington et al., 2018). Whereas, developmental toxicological vulnerabilities have been assessed with the use of placenta-on-a-chip models that can recapitulate the ability of compounds to cross or affect the maternal-fetal barrier. 3D placental barrier-on-a-chip microdevices were studied as an *in vitro* model of transporter-mediated drug efflux in the human placental barrier using trophoblasts and placental endothelial cells (Blundell et al., 2018). 3D placental barrier-on-a-chip microdevices with BeWo trophoblast cells and HUVECs were explored in evaluating complicated placental responses to NPs exposure *in vitro* (Yin et al., 2019).

4.9   Organs-on-a-Chip for Biological Evaluation of Medical Devices

One of the main prerequisites to quality of a biomaterial/medical device for clinical use is the biocompatibility evaluation at the cellular and tissue levels. ISO 10993 Biological Evaluation of Medical Devices Parts provides a framework for studying biological evaluation of medical devices. According to the standard, an assessment for biological effects from the exposure of a medical device or material to the human body can include testing such as process genotoxicity, carcinogenicity and reproductive toxicity (ISO 10993-3:2014), hemocompatibility (ISO 10993-4:2017), *in vitro* cytotoxicity (ISO 10993-5:2009), local effects after implantation (ISO 10993-6:2016), skin sensitization (ISO 10993-10:2021), systemic toxicity (ISO 10993-11:2017), Toxicokinetic study (ISO 10993-16:2017),and irritation (ISO 10993-23:2021). Conventional test methods have many disadvantages in anticipating the results of clinical scenarios and have variability in results among labs (Gruber and Nickel, 2023). In a physiological setting characterized by heterocellular nature, assessing biocompatibility with a single cell type is inadequate. The cell population used for the evaluation should be tailored according to the specific application and target organ. Primary cells are more representative of tissues compared to cell lines, increasing the physiological relevance of data. Organ-on-a-chips are useful *in vitro* models bridging the gap between conventional cell cultures and animal models or human subjects. Single or multiple-organ-on-a-chip models enable multi-parametric read-outs of organ functions via endpoint measurements using cantilevers, integrated electrodes, sensors and high throughput studies, offering insights into the integrated biology of both humans and animals (Leung et al., 2022; Vunjak-Novakovic et al., 2021).

4.10   3D Bioprinting in Military Medicine

3D printing is a game-changer to help print parts for battlefield repairs and surgical instruments and biomaterials on demand. To combat veterans with severe head injuries, customized 3D printed cranial implants are used to restore damaged skulls to their original shape and density. Scientists have improved upon the 3D bioprinting technique to develop engineered skeletal muscle as a potential therapy for replacing diseased or damaged muscle tissue. Scientists have developed mobile 3D printers for *in situ* bioprinting of skin cells on burn wounds for on-site management, which can help injured service members to recover from war wounds. Another interesting method involves harvesting cells from a soldier with burn injuries to facilitate the printing of a bandage with biomaterial, thereby accelerating the healing process (Albanna et al., 2019; J. H. Kim et al., 2018; Pazhouhnia et al., 2022; Varkey et al., 2019).

4.11   3D Bioprinting in Space

Bioprinting in microgravity has the potential to produce food and medicine on demand in future space missions. Microgravity settings can be advantageous for bioprinting complex structures and tissues that are difficult to manufacture under earth's gravity due to lack of certain structural support. In 2014, NASA launched usage of 3D printers using fused deposition modeling to the

International Space Station (ISS) to explore the potential of additive manufacturing for in-space applications and demonstrate the capability to manufacture parts and tools in orbit. The 3D printing in zero-G investigations, demonstrated 3D printing with inorganic materials such as plastic in microgravity. Researchers were able to print cardiac tissues using the ISS's 3D BioFabrication Facility (Tabury et al., 2023). Scientists performed the first successful bioprinting of a human knee meniscus with MSCs in orbit using the ISS's 3D BioFabrication Facility. Protein-based artificial retina manufacturing developed and validated space-based manufacturing methods for artificial retinas. A study from ESA (European Space Agency) and the German Space Agency, demonstrated the function of a prototype for a portable handheld bioprinter, Bioprint FirstAid that creates a patch from a patient's own skin cells for customized bandages that could accelerate healing on future missions to the Moon and Mars (Van Ombergen et al., 2023; Warth et al., 2023).

4.12 3D Bioprinting in Medical Education and Surgical Training

3D printed models have increasingly gained popularity by offering realistic and customizable models of human anatomy and pathology for educating medical students, nurses, young residents, and junior surgeons. The 3D printed models enable educators to create intricate simulations of complex anatomical challenges that may be difficult to convey through traditional educational methods, allowing students to analyze and strategize interventions. By utilizing medical imaging data, 3D bioprinting can produce patient-specific anatomical models that replicate individual variations in anatomy and pathology. This enables trainees to practice surgical procedures on models that closely resemble the patient's anatomy, improving pre-operative planning. Bioprinted models can simulate surgical scenarios, allowing trainees to practice procedures in a risk-free environment before operating on patients This enhances surgical skills, improves proficiency, and reduces the learning curve associated with complex surgeries. Bioprinting technology fosters innovation in medical education and surgical training by enabling the development of novel teaching tools, simulation platforms, and surgical techniques. It facilitates research into tissue engineering, regenerative medicine, and personalized healthcare (Meyer-Szary et al., 2022; Ye et al., 2020).

5. Challenges and Prospects

3D bioprinting has achieved the creation of multiple human-scale tissues with functionality nearing the transplantation threshold. However, further enhancements are necessary to progress in areas such as functional organ bioprinting for transplantation. The major challenges in 3D bioprinting organs include: (i) *Biomaterial selection*- biomaterials for 3D bioprinting must be biocompatible, biodegradable, immune-compatible, scalable and sterilizable with desired functional, mechanical, and printing characteristics; utilizing decellularized tissue-specific extracellular matrix (ECM) scaffolds as printable material holds significant promise for organ printing, (ii) *Cell source*- deeper understanding of the heterogeneous cell populations and their physiology within tissues is necessary; researchers can select appropriate cell sources tailored to the specific requirements and objectives of 3D bioprinting applications; maintaining cell viability and functionality during both the bioprinting process and post-printing stages is crucial for ensuring the optimal performance of printed tissues without triggering immune responses when implanted into the body, (iii) *Complexity and heterogeneity*-achieving the complexity and heterogeneity found in natural tissues, including different cell types, extracellular matrix compositions, and organization, to mimic native tissue structure and function accurately, (iv) *Vascularization and innervation*-replicating the intricate network of blood vessels within printed tissues to provide necessary nutrients and oxygen and remove waste efficiently and innervations are essential for the long-term survival of the tissue and integration of the organ to the host, (v) *Maturation* of the printed construct before transplantation *in vivo* or for *in vitro* testing, (vi) *Bioprinter technology*-improving the resolution and precision of bioprinting techniques to accurately recreate tissue microarchitecture and achieve finer details, is crucial for tissue functionality and integration; combining bioprinter technologies can be a strategy to overcome technical challenges, (vii) *Scalability and commercialisation-* developing bioprinting methods that are scalable, cost-effective for producing larger tissues and organs efficiently while, maintaining high printing speeds to minimize cell damage and maintain viability; automated robotic technologies that incorporate each of the components of the biofabrication production line may be promising, (viii) *Ethical considerations-*ethical considerations while using human samples pertaining to confidentiality of donors and getting informed consent of donors is important, ix) *Regulatory approval-* navigating regulatory frameworks to ensure that bioprinted tissues and organs meet safety and efficacy standards for clinical use, which involves addressing concerns related to long-term performance, quality control, and ethical considerations. Addressing these challenges requires interdisciplinary collaboration among researchers from fields such as biology, engineering, materials science, and medicine, along with advancements in technology and innovative approaches in bioprinting methodologies. Indeed, the establishment of good practices and approved standard protocols, patient-derived specific models and less complex scalable models could guarantee the usage of 3D bioprinted platforms as a keystone to close the gap between the pre-clinical and clinical studies.

References

Adamowicz, J., Pokrywczynska, M., Van Breda, S.V., Kloskowski, T. and Drewa, T et al. (2017). Concise Review: Tissue Engineering of Urinary Bladder; We Still Have a Long Way to Go? *STEM CELLS Translational Medicine, 6*(11), 2033–2043. https://doi.org/10.1002/sctm.17-0101

Agarwal, T., Hann, S.Y., Chiesa, I., Cui, H., Celikkin, N et al. (2021). 4D printing in biomedical applications: Emerging trends and technologies. *Journal of Materials Chemistry B, 9*(37), 7608–7632. https://doi.org/10.1039/D1TB01335A

Ajdary, R., Ezazi, N.Z., Correia, A., Kemell, M., Huan, S. et al. (2020). Multifunctional 3D-Printed Patches for Long-Term Drug Release Therapies after Myocardial Infarction. *Advanced Functional Materials, 30*(34), 2003440. https://doi.org/10.1002/adfm.202003440

Albanna, M., Binder, K.W., Murphy, S.V., Kim, J., Qasem, S.A. et al. (2019). In Situ Bioprinting of Autologous Skin Cells Accelerates Wound Healing of Extensive Excisional Full-Thickness Wounds. *Scientific Reports, 9*(1), 1856. https://doi.org/10.1038/s41598-018-38366-w

Ali, M., Pr, A.K., Yoo, J.J., Zahran, F., Atala, A. et al. (2019). A Photo-Crosslinkable Kidney ECM-Derived Bioink Accelerates Renal Tissue Formation. *Advanced Healthcare Materials, 8*(7), 1800992. https://doi.org/10.1002/adhm.201800992

Anada, T., Pan, C.-C., Stahl, A.M., Mori, S., Fukuda, J. et al. (2019). Vascularized Bone-Mimetic Hydrogel Constructs by 3D Bioprinting to Promote Osteogenesis and Angiogenesis. *International Journal of Molecular Sciences, 20*(5), 1096. https://doi.org/10.3390/ijms20051096

Apelgren, P., Amoroso, M., Lindahl, A., Brantsing, C., Rotter, N. et al. (2017). Chondrocytes and stem cells in 3D-bioprinted structures create human cartilage in vivo. *PloS One, 12*(12), e0189428. https://doi.org/10.1371/journal.pone.0189428

Arai, K., Yoshida, T., Okabe, M., Goto, M., Mir, T.A. et al. (2017). Fabrication of 3D-culture platform with sandwich architecture for preserving liver-specific functions of hepatocytes using 3D bioprinter. *Journal of Biomedical Materials Research Part A, 105*(6), 1583–1592. https://doi.org/10.1002/jbm.a.35905

Baltazar, T., Merola, J., Catarino, C., Xie, C.B., Kirkiles-Smith, N.C. et al. (2020). Three Dimensional Bioprinting of a Vascularized and Perfusable Skin Graft Using Human Keratinocytes, Fibroblasts, Pericytes, and Endothelial Cells. *Tissue Engineering. Part A, 26*(5–6), 227–238. https://doi.org/10.1089/ten.TEA.2019.0201

Bejleri, D., Streeter, B.W., Nachlas, A.L.Y., Brown, M.E., Gaetani, R. et al. (2018). A Bioprinted Cardiac Patch Composed of Cardiac-Specific Extracellular Matrix and Progenitor Cells for Heart Repair. *Advanced Healthcare Materials, 7*(23), 1800672. https://doi.org/10.1002/adhm.201800672

Blundell, C., Yi, Y.-S., Ma, L., Tess, E.R., Farrell, M.J. et al. (2018). Placental Drug Transport-on-a-Chip: A Microengineered In Vitro Model of Transporter-Mediated Drug Efflux in the Human Placental Barrier. *Advanced Healthcare Materials, 7*(2), 1700786. https://doi.org/10.1002/adhm.201700786

Bril, M., Fredrich, S. and Kurniawan, N.A. (2022). Stimuli-responsive materials: A smart way to study dynamic cell responses. *Smart Materials in Medicine, 3*, 257–273. https://doi.org/10.1016/j.smaim.2022.01.010

Chang, J.W., Park, S.A., Park, J.-K., Choi, J.W., Kim, Y.-S. et al. (2014). Tissue-Engineered Tracheal Reconstruction Using Three-Dimensionally Printed Artificial Tracheal Graft: Preliminary Report. *Artificial Organs, 38*(6), E95–E105. https://doi.org/10.1111/aor.12310

Chen, Y.-W., Shen, Y.-F., Ho, C.-C., Yu, J., Wu, Y.-H. A. et al. (2018). Osteogenic and angiogenic potentials of the cell-laden hydrogel/mussel-inspired calcium silicate complex hierarchical porous scaffold fabricated by 3D bioprinting. *Materials Science and Engineering: C, 91*, 679–687. https://doi.org/10.1016/j.msec.2018.06.005

Colle, J., Blondeel, P., De Bruyne, A., Bochar, S., Tytgat, L. et al. (2020a). Bioprinting predifferentiated adipose-derived mesenchymal stem cell spheroids with methacrylated gelatin ink for adipose tissue engineering. *Journal of Materials Science. Materials in Medicine, 31*(4), 36. https://doi.org/10.1007/s10856-020-06374-w

Colle, J., Blondeel, P., De Bruyne, A., Bochar, S., Tytgat, L. et al. (2020b). Bioprinting predifferentiated adipose-derived mesenchymal stem cell spheroids with methacrylated gelatin ink for adipose tissue engineering. *Journal of Materials Science: Materials in Medicine, 31*(4), 36. https://doi.org/10.1007/s10856-020-06374-w

Creff, J., Courson, R., Mangeat, T., Foncy, J., Souleille, S. et al. (2019). Fabrication of 3D scaffolds reproducing intestinal epithelium topography by high-resolution 3D stereolithography. *Biomaterials, 221*, 119404. https://doi.org/10.1016/j.biomaterials.2019.119404

Cubo, N., Garcia, M., Del Cañizo, J.F., Velasco, D. and Jorcano, J.L. et al. (2016). 3D bioprinting of functional human skin: Production and in vivo analysis. *Biofabrication, 9*(1), 015006. https://doi.org/10.1088/1758-5090/9/1/015006

Cunniffe, G.M., Gonzalez-Fernandez, T., Daly, A., Sathy, B.N., Jeon, O. et al. (2017). * Three-Dimensional Bioprinting of Polycaprolactone Reinforced Gene Activated Bioinks for Bone Tissue Engineering. *Tissue Engineering. Part A, 23*(17–18), 891–900. https://doi.org/10.1089/ten.tea.2016.0498

Dey, M. and Ozbolat, I.T. (2020). 3D bioprinting of cells, tissues and organs. *Scientific Reports, 10*(1), 14023. https://doi.org/10.1038/s41598-020-70086-y

Edington, C.D., Chen, W.L.K., Geishecker, E., Kassis, T., Soenksen, L.R. et al. (2018). Interconnected Microphysiological Systems for Quantitative Biology and Pharmacology Studies. *Scientific Reports, 8*(1), 4530. https://doi.org/10.1038/s41598-018-22749-0

England, S., Rajaram, A., Schreyer, D.J. and Chen, X. (2017). Bioprinted fibrin-factor XIII-hyaluronate hydrogel scaffolds with encapsulated Schwann cells and their *in vitro* characterization for use in nerve regeneration. *Bioprinting, 5*, 1–9. https://doi.org/10.1016/j.bprint.2016.12.001

F, S., Mb, R., T, M., A, R., C, A., J, J., L, G., M, V., A, V., M, V et al. (2019). Tubuloids derived from human adult kidney and urine for personalized disease modeling. *Nature Biotechnology, 37*(3). https://doi.org/10.1038/s41587-019-0048-8

Faber, L., Yau, A. and Chen, Y. (2023). Translational biomaterials of four-dimensional bioprinting for tissue regeneration. *Biofabrication, 16*(1), 012001. https://doi.org/10.1088/1758-5090/acfdd0

Farrell, D.A., Miller, T.J., Chambers, J.R., Joseph, V.A. and McClellan, W.T. et al. (2020). Three-Dimensionally-Printed Hand Surgical Simulator for Resident Training. *Plastic and Reconstructive Surgery, 146*(5), 1100–1102. https://doi.org/10.1097/PRS.0000000000007025

Gao, G., Schilling, A.F., Hubbell, K., Yonezawa, T., Truong, D. et al. (2015). Improved properties of bone and cartilage tissue from 3D inkjet-bioprinted human mesenchymal stem cells by simultaneous deposition and photocrosslinking in PEG-GelMA. *Biotechnology Letters, 37*(11), 2349–2355. https://doi.org/10.1007/s10529-015-1921-2

Gori, M., Giannitelli, S.M., Torre, M., Mozetic, P., Abbruzzese, F. et al. (2020). Biofabrication of Hepatic Constructs by 3D Bioprinting of a Cell-Laden Thermogel: An Effective Tool to Assess Drug-Induced Hepatotoxic Response. *Advanced Healthcare Materials, 9*(21), 2001163. https://doi.org/10.1002/adhm.202001163

Gruber, S. and Nickel, A. (2023). Toxic or not toxic? The specifications of the standard ISO 10993-5 are not explicit enough to yield comparable results in the cytotoxicity assessment of an identical medical device. *Frontiers in Medical Technology, 5*, 1195529. https://doi.org/10.3389/fmedt.2023.1195529

Gu, Q., Tomaskovic-Crook, E., Lozano, R., Chen, Y., Kapsa, R.M. et al. (2016). Functional 3D Neural Mini-Tissues from Printed Gel-Based Bioink and Human Neural Stem Cells. *Advanced Healthcare Materials, 5*(12), 1429–1438. https://doi.org/10.1002/adhm.201600095

Gu, Z., Fu, J., Lin, H. and He, Y. (2020). Development of 3D bioprinting: From printing methods to biomedical applications. *Asian Journal of Pharmaceutical Sciences, 15*(5), 529–557. https://doi.org/10.1016/j.ajps.2019.11.003

Gupta, S., Sharma, A., Vasantha Kumar, J., Sharma, V., Gupta, P.K. et al. (2020). Meniscal tissue engineering *via* 3D printed PLA monolith with carbohydrate based self-healing interpenetrating network hydrogel. *International Journal of Biological Macromolecules, 162*, 1358–1371. https://doi.org/10.1016/j.ijbiomac.2020.07.238

He, B., Wang, J., Xie, M., Xu, M., Zhang, Y. et al. (2022). 3D printed biomimetic epithelium/stroma bilayer hydrogel implant for corneal regeneration. *Bioactive Materials, 17*, 234–247. https://doi.org/10.1016/j.bioactmat.2022.01.034

Henriksson, I., Gatenholm, P. and Hägg, D.A. (2017). Increased lipid accumulation and adipogenic gene expression of adipocytes in 3D bioprinted nanocellulose scaffolds. *Biofabrication, 9*(1), 015022. https://doi.org/10.1088/1758-5090/aa5c1c

Homan, K.A., Kolesky, D.B., Skylar-Scott, M.A., Herrmann, J., Obuobi, H. et al. (2016). Bioprinting of 3D Convoluted Renal Proximal Tubules on Perfusable Chips. *Scientific Reports, 6*, 34845. https://doi.org/10.1038/srep34845

Ingber, D.E. (2022). Human organs-on-chips for disease modelling, drug development and personalized medicine. *Nature Reviews Genetics, 23*(8), 467–491. https://doi.org/10.1038/s41576-022-00466-9

Isaacson, A., Swioklo, S. and Connon, C.J. (2018). 3D bioprinting of a corneal stroma equivalent. *Experimental Eye Research, 173*, 188–193. https://doi.org/10.1016/j.exer.2018.05.010

Jang, J., Park, H.-J., Kim, S.-W., Kim, H., Park, J.Y. et al.. (2017). 3D printed complex tissue construct using stem cell-laden decellularized extracellular matrix bioinks for cardiac repair. *Biomaterials, 112*, 264–274. https://doi.org/10.1016/j.biomaterials.2016.10.026

Jia, W., Gungor-Ozkerim, P.S., Zhang, Y.S., Yue, K., Zhu, K. et al. (2016). Direct 3D bioprinting of perfusable vascular constructs using a blend bioink. *Biomaterials, 106*, 58–68. https://doi.org/10.1016/j.biomaterials.2016.07.038

Jian, Z., Zhuang, T., Qinyu, T., Liqing, P., Kun, L. et al. (2021). 3D bioprinting of a biomimetic meniscal scaffold for application in tissue engineering. *Bioactive Materials, 6*(6), 1711–1726. https://doi.org/10.1016/j.bioactmat.2020.11.027

Jin, Q., Jin, G., Ju, J., Xu, L., Tang, L. et al. (2022). Bioprinting small-diameter vascular vessel with endothelium and smooth muscle by the approach of two-step crosslinking process. *Biotechnology and Bioengineering, 119*(6), 1673–1684. https://doi.org/10.1002/bit.28075

Jodat, Y.A., Kang, M.G., Kiaee, K., Kim, G.J., Martinez, A.F.H. et al. (2018). Human-Derived Organ-on-a-Chip for Personalized Drug Development. *Current Pharmaceutical Design, 24*(45), 5471–5486. https://doi.org/10.2174/1381612825666190308150055

Jorgensen, A.M., Yoo, J.J. and Atala, A. (2020). Solid Organ Bioprinting: Strategies to Achieve Organ Function. *Chemical Reviews, 120*(19), 11093–11127. https://doi.org/10.1021/acs.chemrev.0c00145

Kanabekova, P., Kadyrova, A. and Kulsharova, G. (2022). Microfluidic Organ-on-a-Chip Devices for Liver Disease Modeling In Vitro. *Micromachines, 13*(3), 428. https://doi.org/10.3390/mi13030428

Ke, D., Yi, H., Est-Witte, S., George, S., Kengla, C. et al. (2019). Bioprinted trachea constructs with patient-matched design, mechanical and biological properties. *Biofabrication, 12*(1), 015022. https://doi.org/10.1088/1758-5090/ab5354

Keriquel, V., Oliveira, H., Rémy, M., Ziane, S., Delmond, S. et al. (2017). In situ printing of mesenchymal stromal cells, by laser-assisted bioprinting, for in vivo bone regeneration applications. *Scientific Reports, 7*, 1778. https://doi.org/10.1038/s41598-017-01914-x

Kim, J.H., Seol, Y.-J., Ko, I.K., Kang, H.-W., Lee, Y.K. et al. (2018). 3D Bioprinted Human Skeletal Muscle Constructs for Muscle Function Restoration. *Scientific Reports, 8*(1), 12307. https://doi.org/10.1038/s41598-018-29968-5

Kim, S.H., Seo, Y.B., Yeon, Y.K., Lee, Y.J., Park, H.S. et al. (2020). 4D-bioprinted silk hydrogels for tissue engineering. *Biomaterials, 260*, 120281. https://doi.org/10.1016/j.biomaterials.2020.120281

Klak, M., Wszoła, M., Berman, A., Filip, A., Kosowska, A. et al. (2023). Bioprinted 3D Bionic Scaffolds with Pancreatic Islets as a New Therapy for Type 1 Diabetes-Analysis of the Results of Preclinical Studies on a Mouse Model. *Journal of Functional Biomaterials, 14*(7), 371. https://doi.org/10.3390/jfb14070371

Klarmann, G.J., Piroli, M.E., Loverde, J.R., Nelson, A.F., Li, Z et al. (2023). 3D printing a universal knee meniscus using a custom collagen ink. *Bioprinting, 31*, e00272. https://doi.org/10.1016/j.bprint.2023.e00272

Kong, B., Chen, Y., Liu, R., Liu, X., Liu, C. et al. (2020). Fiber reinforced GelMA hydrogel to induce the regeneration of corneal stroma. *Nature Communications, 11*(1), 1435. https://doi.org/10.1038/s41467-020-14887-9

Koti, P., Muselimyan, N., Mirdamadi, E., Asfour, H. and Sarvazyan, N.A. et al. (2019). Use of GelMA for 3D printing of cardiac myocytes and fibroblasts. *Journal of 3D Printing in Medicine, 3*(1), 11–22. https://doi.org/10.2217/3dp-2018-0017

Lee, A., Hudson, A.R., Shiwarski, D.J., Tashman, J.W., Hinton, T.J. et al. (2019). 3D bioprinting of collagen to rebuild components of the human heart. *Science, 365*(6452), 482–487. https://doi.org/10.1126/science.aav9051

Lee, H. and Cho, D.-W. (2016). One-step fabrication of an organ-on-a-chip with spatial heterogeneity using a 3D bioprinting technology. *Lab on a Chip, 16*(14), 2618–2625. https://doi.org/10.1039/C6LC00450D

Leung, C.M., de Haan, P., Ronaldson-Bouchard, K., Kim, G.-A., Ko, J. et al. (2022). A guide to the organ-on-a-chip. *Nature Reviews Methods Primers, 2*(1), 1–29. https://doi.org/10.1038/s43586-022-00118-6

Li, H., Liao, Z., Yang, Z., Gao, C., Fu, L. et al. (2021). 3D Printed Poly(ε-Caprolactone)/Meniscus Extracellular Matrix Composite Scaffold Functionalized With Kartogenin-Releasing PLGA Microspheres for Meniscus Tissue Engineering. *Frontiers in Bioengineering and Biotechnology, 9*. https://doi.org/10.3389/fbioe.2021.662381

Li, L., Yu, F., Shi, J., Shen, S., Teng, H. et al. (2017). In situ repair of bone and cartilage defects using 3D scanning and 3D printing. *Scientific Reports, 7*(1), 9416. https://doi.org/10.1038/s41598-017-10060-3

Liu, J., Zhang, B., Li, L., Yin, J. and Fu, J et al. (2021). Additive-lathe 3D bioprinting of bilayered nerve conduits incorporated with supportive cells. *Bioactive Materials, 6*(1), 219–229. https://doi.org/10.1016/j.bioactmat.2020.08.010

Liu, J., Zhou, Z., Zhang, M., Song, F., Feng, C. et al. (2022). Simple and robust 3D bioprinting of full-thickness human skin tissue. *Bioengineered, 13*(4), 10090–10100. https://doi.org/10.1080/21655979.2022.2063651

Liu, Y., Zhang, Y., Jiang, W., Peng, Y., Luo, J. and Xie, S. et al., (2019). A Novel Biodegradable Multilayered Bioengineered Vascular Construct with a Curved Structure and Multi-Branches. *Micromachines, 10*(4), Article 4. https://doi.org/10.3390/mi10040275

Low, L.A., Mummery, C., Berridge, B.R., Austin, C.P. and Tagle, D.A. et al. (2021). Organs-on-chips: Into the next decade. *Nature Reviews. Drug Discovery, 20*(5), 345–361. https://doi.org/10.1038/s41573-020-0079-3

Ma, C., Peng, Y., Li, H. and Chen, W. (2021). Organ-on-a-Chip: A new paradigm for drug development. *Trends in Pharmacological Sciences, 42*(2), 119–133. https://doi.org/10.1016/j.tips.2020.11.009

Macedo, M.H., Torras, N., García-Díaz, M., Barrias, C., Sarmento, B. et al. (2023). The shape of our gut: Dissecting its impact on drug absorption in a 3D bioprinted intestinal model. *Biomaterials Advances, 153*, 213564. https://doi.org/10.1016/j.bioadv.2023.213564

Madden, L.R., Nguyen, T.V., Garcia-Mojica, S., Shah, V., Le, A.V. et al. (2018). Bioprinted 3D Primary Human Intestinal Tissues Model Aspects of Native Physiology and ADME/Tox Functions. *iScience, 2*, 156–167. https://doi.org/10.1016/j.isci.2018.03.015

Magalhaes, R.S., Williams, J.K., Yoo, K.W., Yoo, J.J. and Atala, A. et al. (2020). A tissue-engineered uterus supports live births in rabbits. *Nature Biotechnology, 38*(11), 1280–1287. https://doi.org/10.1038/s41587-020-0547-7

Maiullari, F., Costantini, M., Milan, M., Pace, V., Chirivì, M. et al. (2018). A multi-cellular 3D bioprinting approach for vascularized heart tissue engineering based on HUVECs and iPSC-derived cardiomyocytes. *Scientific Reports, 8*(1), 13532. https://doi.org/10.1038/s41598-018-31848-x

Mao, Q., Wang, Y., Li, Y., Juengpanich, S., Li, W., Chen, M. et al. (2020). Fabrication of liver microtissue with liver decellularized extracellular matrix (dECM) bioink by digital light processing (DLP) bioprinting. *Materials Science and Engineering: C, 109*, 110625. https://doi.org/10.1016/j.msec.2020.110625

Markstedt, K., Mantas, A., Tournier, I., Martínez Ávila, H., Hägg, D. et al. (2015). 3D Bioprinting Human Chondrocytes with Nanocellulose–Alginate Bioink for Cartilage Tissue Engineering Applications. *Biomacromolecules, 16*(5), 1489–1496. https://doi.org/10.1021/acs.biomac.5b00188

Meyer-Szary, J., Luis, M.S., Mikulski, S., Patel, A., Schulz, F. et al. (2022). The Role of 3D Printing in Planning Complex Medical Procedures and Training of Medical Professionals-Cross-Sectional Multispecialty Review. *International Journal of Environmental Research and Public Health, 19*(6), 3331. https://doi.org/10.3390/ijerph19063331

Michael, S., Sorg, H., Peck, C.-T., Koch, L., Deiwick, A. et al. (2013). Tissue Engineered Skin Substitutes Created by Laser-Assisted Bioprinting Form Skin-Like Structures in the Dorsal Skin Fold Chamber in Mice. *PLoS ONE, 8*(3), e57741. https://doi.org/10.1371/journal.pone.0057741

Mörö, A., Samanta, S., Honkamäki, L., Rangasami, V.K., Puistola, P. et al. (2022). Hyaluronic acid based next generation bioink for 3D bioprinting of human stem cell derived corneal stromal model with innervation. *Biofabrication, 15*(1), 015020. https://doi.org/10.1088/1758-5090/acab34

Murphy, S.V. and Atala, A. (2014). 3D bioprinting of tissues and organs. *Nature Biotechnology, 32*(8), 773–785. https://doi.org/10.1038/nbt.2958

Narayanan, L.K., Huebner, P., Fisher, M.B., Spang, J.T., Starly, B. et al. (2016). 3D-Bioprinting of Polylactic Acid (PLA) Nanofiber–Alginate Hydrogel Bioink Containing Human Adipose-Derived Stem Cells. *ACS Biomaterials Science & Engineering, 2*(10), 1732–1742. https://doi.org/10.1021/acsbiomaterials.6b00196

Ng, W.L., Goh, M.H., Yeong, W.Y. and Naing, M.W. (2018). Applying macromolecular crowding to 3D bioprinting: Fabrication of 3D hierarchical porous collagen-based hydrogel constructs. *Biomaterials Science, 6*(3), 562–574. https://doi.org/10.1039/C7BM01015J

Noor, N., Shapira, A., Edri, R., Gal, I., Wertheim, L. et al. (2019). 3D Printing of Personalized Thick and Perfusable Cardiac Patches and Hearts. *Advanced Science (Weinheim, Baden-Wurttemberg, Germany), 6*(11), 1900344. https://doi.org/10.1002/advs.201900344

Nulty, J., Freeman, F.E., Browe, D.C., Burdis, R., Ahern, D.P. et al. (2021). 3D bioprinting of prevascularised implants for the repair of critically-sized bone defects. *Acta Biomaterialia, 126*, 154–169. https://doi.org/10.1016/j.actbio.2021.03.003

Pagan, E., Stefanek, E., Seyfoori, A., Razzaghi, M., Chehri, B. et al. (2023). A handheld bioprinter for multi-material printing of complex constructs. *Biofabrication, 15*(3), 035012. https://doi.org/10.1088/1758-5090/acc42c

Panja, N., Maji, S., Choudhuri, S., Ali, K.A. and Hossain, C.M. et al. (2022). 3D Bioprinting of Human Hollow Organs. *AAPS PharmSciTech, 23*(5), 139. https://doi.org/10.1208/s12249-022-02279-9

Park, J.H., Ahn, M., Park, S.H., Kim, H., Bae, M. et al. (2021). 3D bioprinting of a trachea-mimetic cellular construct of a clinically relevant size. *Biomaterials*, *279*, 121246. https://doi.org/10.1016/j.biomaterials.2021.121246

Park, J.-H., Yoon, J.-K., Lee, J.B., Shin, Y.M., Lee, K.-W. et al. (2019). Experimental Tracheal Replacement Using 3-dimensional Bioprinted Artificial Trachea with Autologous Epithelial Cells and Chondrocytes. *Scientific Reports*, *9*(1), 2103. https://doi.org/10.1038/s41598-019-38565-z

Park, S.Y., Choi, J.W., Park, J.-K., Song, E.H., Park, S.A. et al. (2016). Tissue-engineered artificial oesophagus patch using three-dimensionally printed polycaprolactone with mesenchymal stem cells: A preliminary report. *Interactive CardioVascular and Thoracic Surgery*, *22*(6), 712–717. https://doi.org/10.1093/icvts/ivw048

Pati, F., Jang, J., Ha, D.-H., Won Kim, S., Rhie, J.-W. et al. (2014). Printing three-dimensional tissue analogues with decellularized extracellular matrix bioink. *Nature Communications*, *5*(1), 3935. https://doi.org/10.1038/ncomms4935

Pazhouhnia, Z., Beheshtizadeh, N., Namini, M.S. and Lotfibakhshaiesh, N. (2022). Portable hand-held bioprinters promote in situ tissue regeneration. *Bioengineering & Translational Medicine*, *7*(3), e10307. https://doi.org/10.1002/btm2.10307

Pi, Q., Maharjan, S., Yan, X., Liu, X., Singh, B. et al. (2018). Digitally Tunable Microfluidic Bioprinting of Multilayered Cannular Tissues. *Advanced Materials (Deerfield Beach, Fla.)*, *30*(43), e1706913. https://doi.org/10.1002/adma.201706913

Qi, D., Wu, S., Kuss, M.A., Shi, W., Chung, S. et al. (2018). Mechanically robust cryogels with injectability and bioprinting supportability for adipose tissue engineering. *Acta Biomaterialia*, *74*, 131–142. https://doi.org/10.1016/j.actbio.2018.05.044

Ramakrishnan, R., Kasoju, N., Raju, R., Geevarghese, R., Gauthaman, A. et al. (2022). Exploring the Potential of Alginate-Gelatin-Diethylaminoethyl Cellulose-Fibrinogen based Bioink for 3D Bioprinting of Skin Tissue Constructs. *Carbohydrate Polymer Technologies and Applications*, *3*, 100184. https://doi.org/10.1016/j.carpta.2022.100184

Ratheesh, G., Vaquette, C. and Xiao, Y. (2020). Patient-Specific Bone Particles Bioprinting for Bone Tissue Engineering. *Advanced Healthcare Materials*, *9*(23), 2001323. https://doi.org/10.1002/adhm.202001323

Reddy, V.S., Ramasubramanian, B., Telrandhe, V.M. and Ramakrishna, S. (2023). Contemporary standpoint and future of 3D bioprinting in tissue/organs printing. *Current Opinion in Biomedical Engineering*, *27*, 100461. https://doi.org/10.1016/j.cobme.2023.100461

Sämfors, S., Karlsson, K., Sundberg, J., Markstedt, K. and Gatenholm, P. et al. (2019). Biofabrication of bacterial nanocellulose scaffolds with complex vascular structure. *Biofabrication*, *11*(4), 045010. https://doi.org/10.1088/1758-5090/ab2b4f

Sawkins, M.J., Mistry, P., Brown, B.N., Shakesheff, K.M., Bonassar, L.J. et al. (2015). Cell and protein compatible 3D bioprinting of mechanically strong constructs for bone repair. *Biofabrication*, *7*(3), 035004. https://doi.org/10.1088/1758-5090/7/3/035004

Semba, J.A., Mieloch, A.A., Tomaszewska, E., Cywoniuk, P. and Rybka, J.D. et al. (2023). Formulation and evaluation of a bioink composed of alginate, gelatin, and nanocellulose for meniscal tissue engineering. *International Journal of Bioprinting*, *9*(1), 621. https://doi.org/10.18063/ijb.v9i1.621

Shik Mun, K., Arora, K., Huang, Y., Yang, F., Yarlagadda, S. et al. (2019). Patient-derived pancreas-on-a-chip to model cystic fibrosis-related disorders. *Nature Communications*, *10*(1), 3124. https://doi.org/10.1038/s41467-019-11178-w

Sorkio, A., Koch, L., Koivusalo, L., Deiwick, A., Miettinen, S. et al. (2018). Human stem cell based corneal tissue mimicking structures using laser-assisted 3D bioprinting and functional bioinks. *Biomaterials*, *171*, 57–71. https://doi.org/10.1016/j.biomaterials.2018.04.034

Stichler, S., Böck, T., Paxton, N., Bertlein, S., Levato, R. et al. (2017). Double printing of hyaluronic acid/poly(glycidol) hybrid hydrogels with poly(ε-caprolactone) for MSC chondrogenesis. *Biofabrication*, *9*(4), 044108. https://doi.org/10.1088/1758-5090/aa8cb7

Tabatabaei Rezaei, N., Kumar, H., Liu, H., Lee, S.S., Park, S.S. et al. (2023). Recent Advances in Organ-on-Chips Integrated with Bioprinting Technologies for Drug Screening. *Advanced Healthcare Materials*, *12*(20), e2203172. https://doi.org/10.1002/adhm.202203172

Tabury, K., Rehnberg, E., Baselet, B., Baatout, S. and Moroni, L. et al. (2023). Bioprinting of Cardiac Tissue in Space: Where Are We? *Advanced Healthcare Materials*, *12*(23), 2203338. https://doi.org/10.1002/adhm.202203338

Tamay, D.G., Dursun Usal, T., Alagoz, A.S., Yucel, D., Hasirci, N. et al. (2019). 3D and 4D Printing of Polymers for Tissue Engineering Applications. *Frontiers in Bioengineering and Biotechnology*, *7*, 164. https://doi.org/10.3389/fbioe.2019.00164

Tan, Y.J., Leong, K.F., An, J., Chian, K.S., Tan, X. et al. (2015). Fabrication and *in vitro* analysis of tubular scaffolds by melt-drawing for esophageal tissue engineering. *Materials Letters*, *159*, 424–427. https://doi.org/10.1016/j.matlet.2015.07.061

Tan, Y.J., Tan, X., Yeong, W.Y. and Tor, S.B. (2016). Hybrid microscaffold-based 3D bioprinting of multi-cellular constructs with high compressive strength: A new biofabrication strategy. *Scientific Reports, 6*(1), 39140. https://doi.org/10.1038/srep39140

Taymour, R., Chicaiza-Cabezas, N.A., Gelinsky, M. and Lode, A. (2022). Core–shell bioprinting of vascularized in vitro liver sinusoid models. *Biofabrication, 14*(4), 045019. https://doi.org/10.1088/1758-5090/ac9019

Tijore, A., Irvine, S.A., Sarig, U., Mhaisalkar, P., Baisane, V. et al. (2018). Contact guidance for cardiac tissue engineering using 3D bioprinted gelatin patterned hydrogel. *Biofabrication, 10*(2), 025003. https://doi.org/10.1088/1758-5090/aaa15d

Tomita, K., Yano, K., Taminato, M., Nomori, M. and Hosokawa, K. et al. (2017). DIEP Flap Breast Reconstruction in Patients with Breast Ptosis: 2-Stage Reconstruction Using 3-Dimensional Surface Imaging and a Printed Mold. *Plastic and Reconstructive Surgery. Global Open, 5*(10), e1511. https://doi.org/10.1097/GOX.0000000000001511

Torras, N., Zabalo, J., Abril, E., Carré, A., García-Díaz, M. et al. (2023). A bioprinted 3D gut model with crypt-villus structures to mimic the intestinal epithelial-stromal microenvironment. *Biomaterials Advances, 153*, 213534. https://doi.org/10.1016/j.bioadv.2023.213534

Tripathi, S., Mandal, S.S., Bauri, S. and Maiti, P. (2023). 3D bioprinting and its innovative approach for biomedical applications. *MedComm, 4*(1), e194. https://doi.org/10.1002/mco2.194

Ulag, S., Ilhan, E., Sahin, A., Karademir Yilmaz, B., kalaskar, D.M. et al. (2020). 3D printed artificial cornea for corneal stromal transplantation. *European Polymer Journal, 133*, 109744. https://doi.org/10.1016/j.eurpolymj.2020.109744

Van Ombergen, A., Chalupa-Gantner, F., Chansoria, P., Colosimo, B.M., Costantini, M. et al., (2023). 3D Bioprinting in Microgravity: Opportunities, Challenges, and Possible Applications in Space. *Advanced Healthcare Materials, 12*(23), 2300443. https://doi.org/10.1002/adhm.202300443

Varkey, M., Visscher, D.O., van Zuijlen, P.P.M., Atala, A. and Yoo, J.J. et al. (2019). Skin bioprinting: The future of burn wound reconstruction? *Burns & Trauma, 7*, 4. https://doi.org/10.1186/s41038-019-0142-7

Versteegden, L.R., van Kampen, K.A., Janke, H.P., Tiemessen, D.M., Hoogenkamp, H.R. et al. (2017). Tubular collagen scaffolds with radial elasticity for hollow organ regeneration. *Acta Biomaterialia, 52*, 1–8. https://doi.org/10.1016/j.actbio.2017.02.005

Vunjak-Novakovic, G., Ronaldson-Bouchard, K. and Radisic, M. (2021). Organs-on-a-chip models for biological research. *Cell, 184*(18), 4597–4611. https://doi.org/10.1016/j.cell.2021.08.005

Wang, B., Barceló, X., Von Euw, S. and Kelly, D.J. (2023). 3D printing of mechanically functional meniscal tissue equivalents using high concentration extracellular matrix inks. *Materials Today Bio, 20*, 100624. https://doi.org/10.1016/j.mtbio.2023.100624

Wang, Y., Gao, Y., Pan, Y., Zhou, D., Liu, Y. et al. (2023). Emerging trends in organ-on-a-chip systems for drug screening. *Acta Pharmaceutica Sinica. B, 13*(6), 2483–2509. https://doi.org/10.1016/j.apsb.2023.02.006

Warth, N., Berg, M., Schumacher, L., Boehme, M., Windisch, J. et al. (2023). Bioprint FirstAid: A handheld bioprinter for first aid utilization on space exploration missions. *Acta Astronautica, 215*. https://doi.org/10.1016/j.actaastro.2023.11.033

Wells, C.M., Harris, M., Choi, L., Murali, V.P., Guerra, F.D. et al. (2019). Stimuli-Responsive Drug Release from Smart Polymers. *Journal of Functional Biomaterials, 10*(3), 34. https://doi.org/10.3390/jfb10030034

Wu, Y., Qin, M. and Yang, X. (2023). Organ bioprinting: Progress, challenges and outlook. *Journal of Materials Chemistry B, 11*(43), 10263–10287. https://doi.org/10.1039/D3TB01630G

Wu, Z., Li, Q., Xie, S., Shan, X. and Cai, Z. et al. (2020). In vitro and in vivo biocompatibility evaluation of a 3D bioprinted gelatin-sodium alginate/rat Schwann-cell scaffold. *Materials Science and Engineering: C, 109*, 110530. https://doi.org/10.1016/j.msec.2019.110530

Xu, Y., Meng, Q., Jin, X., Liu, F. and Yu, J. et al. (2020). Biodegradable Scaffolds for Urethra Tissue Engineering Based on 3D Printing. *ACS Applied Bio Materials, 3*(4), 2007–2016. https://doi.org/10.1021/acsabm.9b01151

Ye, Z., Dun, A., Jiang, H., Nie, C., Zhao, S. et al. (2020). The role of 3D printed models in the teaching of human anatomy: A systematic review and meta-analysis. *BMC Medical Education, 20*(1), 335. https://doi.org/10.1186/s12909-020-02242-x

Yin, F., Zhu, Y., Zhang, M., Yu, H., Chen, W. et al. (2019). A 3D human placenta-on-a-chip model to probe nanoparticle exposure at the placental barrier. *Toxicology in Vitro: An International Journal Published in Association with BIBRA, 54*, 105–113. https://doi.org/10.1016/j.tiv.2018.08.014

Ying, G., Manríquez, J., Wu, D., Zhang, J., Jiang, N. et al. (2020). An open-source handheld extruder loaded with pore-forming bioink for in situ wound dressing. *Materials Today. Bio, 8*, 100074. https://doi.org/10.1016/j.mtbio.2020.100074

Yoon, J., Singh, N.K., Jang, J. and Cho, D.-W. (2022). 3D bioprinted in vitro secondary hyperoxaluria model by mimicking intestinal-oxalate-malabsorption-related kidney stone disease. *Applied Physics Reviews*, 9(4), 041408. https://doi.org/10.1063/5.0087345

Zhang, B., Xue, Q., Hu, H., Yu, M., Gao, L. et al. (2019). Integrated 3D bioprinting-based geometry-control strategy for fabricating corneal substitutes. *Journal of Zhejiang University. Science. B*, 20(12), 945–959. https://doi.org/10.1631/jzus.B1900190

Zhang, K., Fu, Q., Yoo, J., Chen, X., Chandra, P. et al. (2017). 3D bioprinting of urethra with PCL/PLCL blend and dual autologous cells in fibrin hydrogel: An in vitro evaluation of biomimetic mechanical property and cell growth environment. *Acta Biomaterialia*, 50, 154–164. https://doi.org/10.1016/j.actbio.2016.12.008

Zhang, W., Shi, W., Wu, S., Kuss, M., Jiang, X. et al. (2020). 3D printed composite scaffolds with dual small molecule delivery for mandibular bone regeneration. *Biofabrication*, 12(3), 035020. https://doi.org/10.1088/1758-5090/ab906e

Zhou, G., Jiang, H., Yin, Z., Liu, Y., Zhang, Q. et al. (2018). In Vitro Regeneration of Patient-specific Ear-shaped Cartilage and Its First Clinical Application for Auricular Reconstruction. *EBioMedicine*, 28, 287–302. https://doi.org/10.1016/j.ebiom.2018.01.011

Zhou, W., Qiao, Z., Nazarzadeh Zare, E., Huang, J., Zheng, X. et al. (2020). 4D-Printed Dynamic Materials in Biomedical Applications: Chemistry, Challenges, and Their Future Perspectives in the Clinical Sector. *Journal of Medicinal Chemistry*, 63(15), 8003–8024. https://doi.org/10.1021/acs.jmedchem.9b02115

Ethics Associated with 3D-Printed Organs

Manjoosha RY,[1] Greeshma N,[1] Ashtami J,[2] Mohanan PV[2] and Renu John[1]*

1. Introduction

Regenerative medicine is a broad field of science, which aims to "replace or regenerate human cells, tissue, or organs to restore or establish normal human function" (Mason and Dunnill, 2008). Tissue engineering is one of the pillars of regenerative medicine. Research in this area has shown promise in bridging the gap between the need for transplants and the lack of available organs. 3D bioprinting, an innovative tissue engineering technology, is a complex process involving several stages, such as model reconstruction of the organ, choosing biomaterials, and deciding the combination of multiple cell types, followed by processing using appropriate printing technologies (Place et al., 2009). Examples of 3D printed organs employed for transplantation include 3D bioprinted bone, tissue-engineered skin, and liver organoids (de Kanter et al., 2023).

Three-dimensional printing is possible through technologies such as additive manufacturing, rapid prototyping, and solid free-form manufacturing. Typically, 3D bioprinting involves automatic layer-by-layer deposition of "bioinks", which are made of live cells, polymeric hydrogels, and other bioactive substances (such as growth factors) (Lei and Wang, 2016). The 3D printed biological constructs are made of multiple cells/tissues as well as acellular constructions, along with smart surface features that can influence cellular activity. Biocompatible and biodegradable polymers commonly employed in bioprinting include synthetic polymers such as poly (lactic-co-glycolic acid) or polyurethane, and natural polymers such as gelatin, alginate, collagen, and hyaluronic acid (Song et al., 2021).

Based on the working principle and mechanism of action, additive manufacturing techniques for bioprinting 3D organs are classified into several categories. Inkjet-based printing is one of the

[1] Department of Biomedical Engineering, Indian Institute of Technology Hyderabad, Sangareddy, Telangana.
[2] Division of Toxicology, Biomedical Technology Wing, Sree Chitra Tirunal Institute of Medical Science and Technology, Thiruvananthapuram, Kerala.
* Corresponding author: renujohn@bme.iith.ac.in

commonly used techniques, wherein layers of droplets are deposited in a non-contact mode, usually in a drop-on-demand manner via acoustic, piezoelectric, or thermal inkjet nozzles (Boland et al., 2006). Extrusion-based bioprinting is another common technique, which incorporates an automatic robotic system and a fluid dispensing system. The deposition of bioink is precise and continuous, based on the programmed CAD model, through single or multiple nozzles which are usually controlled by a pressure-driven system (Ozbolat and Hospodiuk, 2016). Stereolithography (SLA) techniques are the most mature, and widely used 3D bioprinting techniques in industry that can print large-size models (Quan et al., 2020). In this technique, a CAD model initiates the deposition of photosensitive material on the surface, while in parallel, a concentrated laser beam induces cross-linking of selective photosensitive materials point by point. Each layer is thus printed sequentially until the 3D construct is completely fabricated (Magalhães et al., 2020; Song et al., 2021).

The organ bioprinting process is typically divided into three stages: pre-processing, bioprinting, and post-processing. The pre-processing stage involves two major steps: the preparation of the bioink, and creating the organ model. Bioink preparation mainly involves *in vitro* cell culture, to either form cell suspensions (in hydrogels or other thermoresponsive polymers) or to grow aggregates of specific sizes. The organ models are designed by acquiring high-resolution images of the target organ. Consequently, the acquired images are processed to prepare the CAD design and bioprinting process blueprints. In the bioprinting stage, one of the above-mentioned fabrication modalities is used to print the organ. Thereafter during the post-processing stage, the printed cells undergo maturation to form the target tissues. This process is ideally executed in an incubator or a bioreactor, after which the organs are set for implantation (Datta et al., 2018; Patuzzo et al., 2017).

As 3D bioprinting technology is evolving, with claims of being a new paradigm in medicine, the plausible ethical and moral implications related to the development and translation of this technology need to be analyzed critically (Trommelmans et al., 2009a). The objective should be to get a wider perspective on the entire tissue engineering process, including the translation from preclinical to clinical stage, for successful transplantation and future evaluations, instead of concentrating on the isolated steps of the 3D bioprinting process. In this chapter, the key ethical considerations for research and the successful translation of 3D bioprinted organs are summarized. Certain guidelines that can be employed by all the stakeholders – the scientists, clinicians, engineers, businessmen, lawmakers, and the general public, are also discussed so that appropriate measures and actions can be taken at a much earlier stage.

2. Benefits of 3D Bioprinted Organs

2.1 Personalization

The first and foremost advantage of the use of 3D-printed organs is the possibility of customization or personalization of the product. This technology can help in developing tissues and organs that can be tailored to fit various individual patient needs. In case a patient's own cells are used, the compatibility is significantly improved, and the risk of transplant rejection is reduced. Also, it is more ethical as the use of donor or animal tissues is avoidable. Additionally, customization includes preclinical drug delivery studies and personalized drugs suiting the genetic makeup of the 3D printed organ. This allows for effective drug response, thus aiding in fast recovery with milder complications (Kloc and Ghobrial, 2014).

2.2 Organ Donors can be Replaced

It was reported that 154,324 patients were registered for organ transplantation in the U.S. in 2009 (Aslanyan, 2016). Most of the patients kept waiting and hoping for an organ, while 8,863 of them couldn't survive, and only 18% of the patients got the organ they registered for. Additionally, successful transplantation involves receiving a healthy organ while managing tissue rejections and combating infections (Jiménez Oliver, 2023). Further, there are certain organs that cannot come from living donors. The 3D bioprinted organs could, thus, reduce the reliance on organ donations. Also, the waiting times due to shortage of organ donors are vastly reduced, thus giving every patient an equal second chance, thereby enhancing the quality of life. This could also end the illegal trade and sale of human organs (Scheper-Hughes, 2000).

2.3 Risk of Rejection is Reduced

To minimize the risk of organ rejection, several immunosuppressive drugs with a high dose are to be taken by the patient to suppress the body's natural immune response. Several of these drugs are non-specific, and can be toxic to other parts of the body, as well (Shin, 2022). Further, reduction in the body's immune response can increase the chances of other infections. 3D printed organs can be thoroughly tested for the drug delivery pathways and immune response using organ-on-chip platforms in the preclinical phase, thereby reducing the risk of rejection.

2.4 Precision of 3D Printed Organs

3D bioprinting allows for the creation of complex architectures, complete with intricate vasculatures and membranes for gas and nutrient exchange. Also, use of specific biomaterials can improve the biocompatibility and biodegradability of the organ (wherever required), while preserving its shape and functionality (Agarwal et al., 2020). Furthermore, 3D printed tissues and organs have the potential to solve certain issues related to congenital defects. For example, congenital tracheomalacia and tracheal stenosis are common amongst prematurely born babies (Shopova et al., 2023). While surgical treatments have certain limitations, 3D printed parts have shown great promise in the preclinical and clinical trials (Frejo and Grande, 2019). Apart from these, several other benefits include the possibility of performing disease modeling and drug testing studies on the 3D printed organs using organ-on-chip models. Gender differences associated with transplantations can also be circumvented. For example, there have been reports of differences in kidney anatomy and function in different genders (van Daal et al., 2020). In addition, the risk of infection, the action of immunosuppressive agents, and ultimately, rejection rates are also gender-dependent. All these issues can be overcome by the use of 3D printed organs.

On the whole, 3D printed organs have the potential to revolutionize healthcare, by offering personalized and regenerative solutions for organ failure. However, it is essential to consider overcoming the ethical, moral, and regulatory challenges, before 3D printed organs are available for commercial use.

3. Ethical Considerations

Though hugely promising, 3D printed organs raise several ethical issues, regarding clinical research, to translation to the patients, in addition to the impact on society at large. These issues have to be assessed systematically as the technology develops as the research is transitioning from the preclinical to the clinical stage.

3.1 Tissue Selection and Handling

The choice of the cell or tissue source is one of the critical issues requiring ethical debate, especially with the use of embryonic stem cells (ESCs) and animal-derived tissue components. In the case of ESCs, there exist several short-term *in vivo* studies that have been successful. However, certain long-term studies have indicated that these cells may lead to tumors and malignant cancers (Herberts and Kwa, 2011). Another discussion is around the question of whether an embryo should be recognized as a human life. This is because embryos are often derived from living or aborted foetuses or from embryoblasts usually left over from IVF procedures (Welin, 2014). With animal-derived tissue, the question is whether appending animal material to humans necessarily "dehumanizes" an individual. The same ethical argument exists with transplanted organs as well. Ultimately, the use of bioprinted organs should be decided based on whether the intermingling between animal and human tissues affects human reasoning and moral capacities (Patuzzo et al., 2017). Induced pluripotent stem (iPS) cells, developed as an alternative to ESCs, could be considered as an ethical substitute if the conditions of complete pluripotency without the risk of damaging mutations are met (Power and Rasko, 2011). Alternately, use of patient-specific cells to develop customized bioprinted organs can be considered as an option, to avoid the ethical issues associated with cell sources.

Ethical issues around tissue collection include invasiveness of the extraction procedure, donor confidentiality, and consent and storage conditions of the collected tissue. It is expected that the tissues collected from the donor cause minimum harm or pain to the donor (Oerlemans et al., 2010). Safeguarding the privacy and confidentiality of the donor data and medical records requires discussion around whether the process is to be made completely anonymous, or if certain data is to be kept original to return the clinical findings (Otto et al., 2016; Vijayavenkataraman et al., 2016).

3.2   Risk and Safety

Despite the potential of bioprinted organs, there are several risks and safety issues to be thoroughly assessed. The use of living cells poses threats of mutagenesis, immunogenicity, and tumorigenicity to the recipient (Kirillova et al., 2020). The bioactive components in the printed organ-or scaffold material may introduce pathogens or other contaminants, or may introduce cytotoxic byproducts (Gilbert, Viaña, et al., 2018). The implant's dynamic interactions within the human body environment are unpredictable, and in most cases, the implantation process is irreversible (Kashi and Saha, 2009; Trommelmans et al., 2009a). For example, treatments involving autologous cells may be ethically clear, however, there have been reports of patients developing lesions in the kidneys after undergoing stem cell therapy (Thirabanjasak et al., 2010).

Though it is challenging to perform risk-benefit analysis, the safety and efficacy of the technology are to be thoroughly evaluated through *in vitro* and *in vivo* preclinical trials. In the case of clinical trials, several recommendations have been suggested by several groups for the appropriate design and execution of the trials. Randomized control trials are to be performed wherever possible, whereas it is unacceptable to perform first-in-human trials on healthy or stable patients (Trommelmans et al., 2009a). Long-term follow-ups, with registries are also required to collect long-term data of the clinical trial participants, which can assist in tracing adverse events and monitoring successful regeneration (Hildebrandt, 2020; Jacques and Suuronen, 2020).

3.3   Consent Conditions

Informed consent is an important precondition for every phase of 3D printed organ development and its clinical applications. This starts from the tissue donors and their families' consent regarding privacy, equitable access, long-term use, and storage. In addition, the consent should be voluntary and should not be coerced or pressured (Musmade et al., 2013). There are several conditions while obtaining consent. There are particular challenges when the patient is in an emergency situation and lacks decisional capacity (Kirillova et al., 2020). The patients' desperation for a cure or the uncertainty regarding the possible complications from the trial may affect the validity of the consent (Trommelmans et al., 2008b).

It is, therefore, essential for medical professionals to maintain transparency, carefully explain and provide all the relevant information. The information presented should include the source of tissues and other components of the implant, the probable risks and benefits associated, alternative treatment options, and a complete disclosure of interests (Baker et al., 2016; Trommelmans et al., 2008a). Additionally, the information must be presented in a language that the patient understands, and supported by the provision of consultation with a medical professional, along with necessary educational material (Taylor et al., 2014; Vijayavenkataraman et al., 2016).

3.4 Ownership and Commodification

Another ethical question often asked is in the donated tissue or engineered organ ownership claim context. The ownership can be claimed either by the tissue donor, the parties that were involved in making the organ, or the patient who received the organ/implant. In addition, there is the issue of intellectual property rights over the engineered organ – whether the product can be patented, and if it is, whether the rights belong to the patient, researcher or the product maker (Sekar et al., 2021). It has been argued that patenting would foster innovation and prevent product misuse while maintaining quality (de Kanter et al., 2023; Vermeulen et al., 2017). However, access to scientific benefits may become unequal and inaccessible, and patenting may also hinder open research (Lavoie, 2011). It has been argued that patients retain the right to autonomy over their organs and their bodies (Harbaugh, 2015). Nevertheless, from a scientific perspective, it has been debated that there should be provisions to conceal the steps involved in the bioprinting process. There have been suggestions to adopt a "portfolio approach", which can provide means of incentivizing the company's innovation while providing accessible and approachable healthcare (Li et al, 2014; Varkey and Atala, 2015).

3.5 Sociocultural Considerations

There are several ethical dilemmas while discussing the societal impact and cultural concerns of the usage of bioprinted organs. These include issues regarding organ access and justice, the use of organs for enhancement and longevity, impacts on healthcare markets, biosecurity, and preservation of human morals and values. Firstly, it is expected that the high costs associated with bioprinting organs and the requirement of expertise, machinery, and a trained workforce can affect the accessibility of these organs (Datta et al., 2023). Also, there is a question of who should be held accountable, in case something goes wrong (Allon et al., 2017). Additionally, some scientists argue that the tissue-engineered products may also improve human longevity, with claims of "reverse aging". Such treatments can raise questions regarding the normalization of reckless lifestyles, support for organ donation, and also whether such treatments for cosmetic or physical enhancements should be considered normal (Oerlemans, van Hoek, et al., 2013; Rhodes, 2013). These issues can, in turn, escalate already existing socioeconomic disparities. Therefore, it is essential that equal access to these implants and treatments is ensured, and regulations put in place for benefit-sharing and accountability.

While these bioprinted organs can provide alternatives for several ethically controversial practices, they also raise several issues regarding trade practices. For example, though bioprinted organs can help in ending illegal organ trade, there is a possibility of the generation of new black markets for tissue-engineered organs, which in turn have to be tightly regulated (Singh et al., 2020; Welin, 2014). Furthermore, with the increasing accessibility of these implants, concerns have been raised regarding unregulated use, which can lead to bioterrorism as well (Gilbert, O'Connell, et al., 2018). Though bioprinted organs can be considered more natural than mechanical implants, the "naturalness" of the product is often debated. One perception to be consider is whether the product is on par with an organ transplant from a donor (Vijayavenkataraman et al., 2016). On the other hand, in certain cultures and religions, there are moral concerns regarding issues such as the source of tissues used for bioprinting the organs, or the use of these implants. For example, the use of porcine tissues is unacceptable in some cultures and the use of any animal-derived components might be unacceptable for others (Datta et al., 2023; Oerlemans et al., 2010). It is, therefore, essential to consider other sources such as autologous or plant-based sources to circumvent these ethical concerns (Contessi Negrini et al., 2020).

4. Way Forward

With advances in technology, 3D printing in particular, different stakeholders should actively engage to formulate a focused Ethical, Legal, and Social Aspects (ELSA) framework for the development and use of 3D printed organs. Equal representation from different stakeholders, which include scientists, researchers, clinicians, engineers, businessmen, lawmakers, and the general public, is required to facilitate the translation of this technology to clinical use. Government intervention, in terms of policies and regulatory frameworks, should be assessed and evaluated at the early stages of the development of this technology. Particularly, considering the disparities among different cultures, religions, and regions, there is a need for agreement among scientists from these diverse communities and nations on a common code of conduct (Chan, 2018). The first requirement is an appropriate classification of bioprinted organs – whether it is to be classified as a drug, biologic, a medical device or a 'combination product'. This is important because each type of product has a different review and approval procedure, and ultimately the purpose of the review process is to check the safety and efficacy of the implant (Smith, 2006). It is also necessary to establish proper guidelines for collection procedures and storage of donor tissues, as well as for ownership rights in the case of biobanking (Master et al., 2020; Trommelmans et al., 2009b). An additional requirement is to set uniform frameworks for the maintenance of cell culture standards, the use of quality biomaterials, and manufacturing practices, in general (Oerlemans, Feitz, et al., 2013).

Responsible conduct is imperative from various outlets, including the scientists, researchers and clinicians involved, in addition to media personnel. Particularly, print media can have the ability to influence patients' understanding of health issues and educate them. Concerns have been raised in certain cases where the published content created biases, promoted stereotypes, or inflated the hopes and expectations of the patients which affected the patient's consent to undergo treatments (Young et al., 2008). Scientific reports and mass media publications must be critically evaluated, so that the reports are not misleading or exaggerated while setting realistic expectations (Gilbert, Viaña, et al., 2018). In addition, consent should be taken after providing comprehensive information using appropriate tools and providing adequate examples regarding the risks and benefits, to aid in good understanding and decision-making (Falagas et al., 2009). Scientists and clinicians should be adequately trained to gain the necessary expertise, in addition to understanding the ethical implications of the use of these bioprinted organs. It has also been reported that clinicians have less confidence in industry-sponsored clinical trials, and prefer government-funded trials to avoid ethical and moral issues (de Vries et al., 2008). Especially, during the commercialization of the products, the potential conflicts of interest must be dealt with, by providing complete interest disclosure, or by maintaining independent oversight mechanisms (Lu et al., 2015; Taylor et al., 2014). Another regulatory discussion involves the question of whether licensing of the products is required, to prevent the risk of falling into the wrong hands (Vijayavenkataraman et al., 2016). Finally, discussion is also required regarding liabilities such as long-term maintenance, assurance of product quality, and the parties accountable in case of complications (Hutchison and Sparrow, 2016; Nicholson, 2013).

Public involvement is an essential part of the development of the ELSA framework for the smooth clinical translation of bioprinted organs. On the one hand, it is imperative for scientists to engage with the public to provide reliable and accurate information and counter misinformation to empower people to make informed decisions. On the other hand, the patients and the public must also critically question the researchers on the assumptions and implications of the use of these products. Finally, as members of society, everyone is responsible for actively engaging in conversations surrounding the use of these bioprinted organs. Vijayaraghavan et al. (2016) have several recommendations for establishing an all-encompassing regulatory framework with a special focus on 3D printed organ technology. These recommendations include involving local and global experts, policy, and lawmakers to set up regulatory panels while discussing and debating on the risks, benefits, and economic considerations of implementing and accepting this technology. A proper ethics framework has to be established, considering all the ethical challenges discussed above, while also consulting with legal experts to acquire clarity on IP rights and patents. Also, strict guidelines are required for licensing, auditing, and usage of the products.

Conclusions

3D bioprinting technology has the therapeutic potential to print tissues and organs, presenting innovative healthcare solutions that can provide large-scale public health benefits. However, the ethical implications accompanying the use of this technology are complex and multifaceted, requiring thorough debate and discussion by ethicists, scientists, engineers, businessmen, and lawmakers. All innovators and stakeholders have a moral obligation to provide comprehensive risk-benefit information to the patients and the public. Governments and national and international regulatory bodies play a significant role in formulating strategies for processes such as the classification of these products, approval guidelines, licensing and patenting rules. The long-term objective should be to frame stringent policies and regulatory frameworks to monitor the successful translation of this technology for public welfare.

References

Agarwal, S., Saha, S., Balla, V.K., Pal, A., Barui, A. et al. (2020). Current Developments in 3D Bioprinting for Tissue and Organ Regeneration–A Review. *Frontiers in Mechanical Engineering, 6.* https://doi.org/10.3389/fmech.2020.589171

Allon, I., Ben-Yehudah, A., Dekel, R., Solbakk, J.-H., Weltring, K.-M. et al. (2017). Ethical issues in nanomedicine: Tempest in a teapot? *Medicine, Health Care and Philosophy, 20*(1), 3–11. https://doi.org/10.1007/s11019-016-9720-7

Aslanyan, L. (2016). *Advantages of 3D Bioprinting: What the Future Holds.* Izumi International. https://info.izumiinternational.com/advantages-of-bioprinting

Baker, H.B., McQuilling, J.P. and King, N.M.P. (2016). Ethical considerations in tissue engineering research: Case studies in translation. *Methods, 99,* 135–144. https://doi.org/10.1016/j.ymeth.2015.08.010

Boland, T., Xu, T., Damon, B. and Cui, X. (2006). Application of inkjet printing to tissue engineering. *Biotechnology Journal, 1*(9), 910–917. https://doi.org/10.1002/biot.200600081

Chan, S. (2018). Research Translation and Emerging Health Technologies: Synthetic Biology and Beyond. *Health Care Analysis, 26*(4), 310–325. https://doi.org/10.1007/s10728-016-0334-2

Contessi Negrini, N., Toffoletto, N., Farè, S. and Altomare, L. (2020). Plant Tissues as 3D Natural Scaffolds for Adipose, Bone and Tendon Tissue Regeneration. *Frontiers in Bioengineering and Biotechnology, 8.* https://doi.org/10.3389/fbioe.2020.00723

Datta, P., Barui, A., Wu, Y., Ozbolat, V., Moncal, K.K. et al (2018). Essential steps in bioprinting: From pre- to post-bioprinting. *Biotechnology Advances, 36*(5), 1481–1504. https://doi.org/10.1016/j.biotechadv.2018.06.003

Datta, P., Cabrera, L.Y. and Ozbolat, I.T. (2023). Ethical challenges with 3D bioprinted tissues and organs. *Trends in Biotechnology, 41*(1), 6–9. https://doi.org/10.1016/j.tibtech.2022.08.012

de Kanter, A.-F.J., Jongsma, K.R., Verhaar, M.C. and Bredenoord, A.L. (2023). The Ethical Implications of Tissue Engineering for Regenerative Purposes: A Systematic Review. *Tissue Engineering Part B: Reviews, 29*(2), 167–187. https://doi.org/10.1089/ten.teb.2022.0033

de Vries, R.B.M., Oerlemans, A., Trommelmans, L., Dierickx, K. and Gordijn, B. et al. (2008). Ethical Aspects of Tissue Engineering: A Review. *Tissue Engineering Part B: Reviews, 14*(4), 367–375. https://doi.org/10.1089/ten.teb.2008.0199

Falagas, M.E., Korbila, I.P., Giannopoulou, K.P., Kondilis, B.K. and Peppas, G. et al. (2009). Informed consent: how much and what do patients understand? *The American Journal of Surgery, 198*(3), 420–435. https://doi.org/10.1016/j.amjsurg.2009.02.010

Frejo, L. and Grande, D.A. (2019). 3D-bioprinted tracheal reconstruction: an overview. *Bioelectronic Medicine, 5*(1), 15. https://doi.org/10.1186/s42234-019-0031-1

Gilbert, F., O'Connell, C.D., Mladenovska, T. and Dodds, S. (2018). Print Me an Organ? Ethical and Regulatory Issues Emerging from 3D Bioprinting in Medicine. *Science and Engineering Ethics, 24*(1), 73–91. https://doi.org/10.1007/s11948-017-9874-6

Gilbert, F., Viaña, J.N.M., O'Connell, C.D. and Dodds, S. (2018). Enthusiastic portrayal of 3D bioprinting in the media: Ethical side effects. *Bioethics, 32*(2), 94–102. https://doi.org/10.1111/bioe.12414

Harbaugh, J.T. (2015). Do You Own Your 3D Bioprinted Body? *American Journal of Law & Medicine, 41*(1), 167–189. https://doi.org/10.1177/0098858815591512

Herberts, C.A. and Kwa, M.S. (2011). *Risk factors in the development of stem cell therapy.* https://doi.org/10.1186/1479-5876-9-29

Hildebrandt, M. (2020). Horses for courses: an approach to the qualification of clinical trial sites and investigators in ATMPs. *Drug Discovery Today*, *25*(2), 265–268. https://doi.org/10.1016/j.drudis.2019.10.003

Hutchison, K. and Sparrow, R. (2016). What Pacemakers Can Teach Us about the Ethics of Maintaining Artificial Organs. *Hastings Center Report*, *46*(6), 14–24. https://doi.org/10.1002/hast.644

Jacques, E. and Suuronen, E.J. (2020). The Progression of Regenerative Medicine and its Impact on Therapy Translation. *Clinical and Translational Science*, *13*(3), 440–450. https://doi.org/10.1111/cts.12736

Jiménez Oliver, K. (2023). Overview of Organ Donation. *Mexican Journal of Medical Research ICSA*, *11*(21), 55–63. https://doi.org/10.29057/mjmr.v11i21.10007

Kashi, A. and Saha, S. (2009). Ethics in Biomaterials Research. *Journal of Long-Term Effects of Medical Implants*, *19*(1), 19–30. https://doi.org/10.1615/JLongTermEffMedImplants.v19.i1.30

Kirillova, A., Bushev, S., Abubakirov, A. and Sukikh, G. (2020). Bioethical and Legal Issues in 3D Bioprinting. *International Journal of Bioprinting*, *6*(3), 272. https://doi.org/10.18063/ijb.v6i3.272

Kloc, M. and Ghobrial, R. (2014). Chronic allograft rejection: A significant hurdle to transplant success. *Burns and Trauma*, *2*(1), 3. https://doi.org/10.4103/2321-3868.121646

Lavoie, M. (2011). The Role of Social Scientists in Accelerating Innovation in Regenerative Medicine. *Review of Policy Research*, *28*(6), 613–630. https://doi.org/10.1111/j.1541-1338.2011.00525.x

Lei, M. and Wang, X. (2016). Biodegradable polymers and stem cells for bioprinting. *Molecules*, *21*(5), 1–14. https://doi.org/10.3390/molecules21050539

Li, P.H. (2014). 3D Bioprinting Technologies: Patents, Innovation and Access. *Law, Innovation and Technology*, *6*(2), 282–304. https://doi.org/10.5235/17579961.6.2.282

Lu, L., Arbit, H.M., Herrick, J.L., Segovis, S.G., Maran, A. et al. (2015). Tissue Engineered Constructs: Perspectives on Clinical Translation. *Annals of Biomedical Engineering*, *43*(3), 796–804. https://doi.org/10.1007/s10439-015-1280-0

Magalhães, L.S.S.M., Santos, F.E.P., Elias, C. de M.V., Afewerki, S., Sousa, G.F. et al. (2020). Printing 3D Hydrogel Structures Employing Low-Cost Stereolithography Technology. *Journal of Functional Biomaterials*, *11*(1), 12. https://doi.org/10.3390/jfb11010012

Mason, C. and Dunnill, P. (2008). A brief definition of regenerative medicine. *Regenerative Medicine*, *3*(1), 1–5. https://doi.org/10.2217/17460751.3.1.1

Master, Z., Crowley, A.P., Smith, C., Wigle, D., Terzic, A. et al. (2020). Stem cell preservation for regenerative therapies: ethical and governance considerations for the health care sector. *Npj Regenerative Medicine*, *5*(1), 23. https://doi.org/10.1038/s41536-020-00108-w

Musmade, P., Nijhawan, L., Udupa, N., Bairy, K., Bhat, K. et al. (2013). Informed consent: Issues and challenges. *Journal of Advanced Pharmaceutical Technology & Research*, *4*(3), 134. https://doi.org/10.4103/2231-4040.116779

Nicholson, J. (2013). Reflections on the Ethics of Biomaterials Science. *The New Bioethics*, *19*(1), 54–63. https://doi.org/10.1179/2050287713Z.00000000021

Oerlemans, A.J.M., Feitz, W.F.J., van Leeuwen, E. and Dekkers, W.J.M. (2013). Regenerative Urology Clinical Trials: An Ethical Assessment of Road Blocks and Solutions. *Tissue Engineering Part B: Reviews*, *19*(1), 41–47. https://doi.org/10.1089/ten.teb.2012.0136

Oerlemans, A.J.M., Rodrigues, C.H.C.M.L., Verkerk, M.A., van den Berg, P.P. and Dekkers, W.J.M. et al. (2010). Ethical Aspects of Soft Tissue Engineering for Congenital Birth Defects in Children—What Do Experts in the Field Say? *Tissue Engineering Part B: Reviews*, *16*(4), 397–403. https://doi.org/10.1089/ten.teb.2009.0666

Oerlemans, A.J.M., van Hoek, M.E.C., van Leeuwen, E., van der Burg, S. and Dekkers, W.J.M. et al (2013). Towards a Richer Debate on Tissue Engineering: A Consideration on the Basis of NEST-Ethics. *Science and Engineering Ethics*, *19*(3), 963–981. https://doi.org/10.1007/s11948-012-9419-y

Otto, I.A., Breugem, C.C., Malda, J. and Bredenoord, A.L. (2016). Ethical considerations in the translation of regenerative biofabrication technologies into clinic and society. *Biofabrication*, *8*(4), 042001. https://doi.org/10.1088/1758-5090/8/4/042001

Ozbolat, I.T. and Hospodiuk, M. (2016). Current advances and future perspectives in extrusion-based bioprinting. *Biomaterials*, *76*, 321–343. https://doi.org/10.1016/j.biomaterials.2015.10.076

Patuzzo, S., Goracci, G., Gasperini, L. and Ciliberti, R. (2017). 3D Bioprinting Technology: Scientific Aspects and Ethical Issues. *Science and Engineering Ethics*, *24*, 335–348. https://doi.org/10.1007/s11948-017-9918-y

Place, E.S., Evans, N.D. and Stevens, M.M. (2009). Complexity in biomaterials for tissue engineering. *Nature Materials*, *8*(6), 457–470. https://doi.org/10.1038/nmat2441

Power, C. and Rasko, J.E.J. (2011). Will Cell Reprogramming Resolve the Embryonic Stem Cell Controversy? A Narrative Review. *Annals of Internal Medicine*, *155*(2), 114. https://doi.org/10.7326/0003-4819-155-2-201107190-00007

Quan, H., Zhang, T., Xu, H., Luo, S., Nie, J. et al. (2020). Photo-curing 3D printing technique and its challenges. *Bioactive Materials, 5*(1), 110–115. https://doi.org/10.1016/j.bioactmat.2019.12.003

Rhodes, R. (2013). Bioethics: Looking Forward and Looking Back. *The American Journal of Bioethics, 13*(1), 13–16. https://doi.org/10.1080/15265161.2013.747318

Scheper-Hughes, N. (2000). The Global Traffic in Human Organs. *Current Anthropology, 41*(2), 191–224. https://doi.org/10.1086/300123

Sekar, M.P., Budharaju, H., Zennifer, A., Sethuraman, S., Vermeulen, N. et al., (2021). Current standards and ethical landscape of engineered tissues—3D bioprinting perspective. *Journal of Tissue Engineering, 12*, 204173142110276. https://doi.org/10.1177/20417314211027677

Shin, A. (2022). *The History, Current Status, Benefits, and Challenges of 3D Printed Organs.* http://arxiv.org/abs/2207.13212

Shopova, D., Yaneva, A., Bakova, D., Mihaylova, A., Kasnakova, P. et al. (2023). (Bio) printing in Personalized Medicine—Opportunities and Potential Benefits. *Bioengineering, 10*(3), 287. https://doi.org/10.3390/bioengineering10030287

Singh, S., Choudhury, D., Yu, F., Mironov, V. and Naing, M.W. et al. (2020). In situ bioprinting – Bioprinting from benchside to bedside? *Acta Biomaterialia, 101*, 14–25. https://doi.org/10.1016/j.actbio.2019.08.045

Smith, D.S. (2006). The Government's role in advancing regenerative medicine and tissue engineering – science, safety, and ethics. *Periodontology 2000, 41*(1), 16–29. https://doi.org/10.1111/j.1600-0757.2006.00177.x

Song, D., Xu, Y., Liu, S., Wen, L. and Wang, X. et al. (2021). Progress of 3D Bioprinting in Organ Manufacturing. *Polymers, 13*(18), 3178. https://doi.org/10.3390/polym13183178

Taylor, D.A., Caplan, A.L. and Macchiarini, P. (2014). Ethics of bioengineering organs and tissues. *Expert Opinion on Biological Therapy, 14*(7), 879–882. https://doi.org/10.1517/14712598.2014.915308

Thirabanjasak, D., Tantiwongse, K. and Thorner, P.S. (2010). Angiomyeloproliferative Lesions Following Autologous Stem Cell Therapy. *Journal of the American Society of Nephrology, 21*(7), 1218–1222. https://doi.org/10.1681/ASN.2009111156

Trommelmans, L., Selling, J. and Dierickx, K. (2008a). Ethical reflections on clinical trials with human tissue engineered products. *Journal of Medical Ethics, 34*(9), e1–e1. https://doi.org/10.1136/jme.2007.022913

Trommelmans, L., Selling, J. and Dierickx, K. (2008b). Informing participants in clinical trials withex vivo human tissue-engineered products: what to tell and how to tell it? *Journal of Tissue Engineering and Regenerative Medicine, 2*(4), 236–241. https://doi.org/10.1002/term.82

Trommelmans, L., Selling, J. and Dierickx, K. (2009a). Is tissue engineering a new paradigm in medicine? Consequences for the ethical evaluation of tissue engineering research. *Medicine, Health Care and Philosophy, 12*(4), 459–467. https://doi.org/10.1007/s11019-009-9192-0

Trommelmans, L., Selling, J. and Dierickx, K. (2009b). The importance of the values attached to cells for a good informed consent procedure in cell donation for tissue engineering purposes. *Cell and Tissue Banking, 10*(4), 293–299. https://doi.org/10.1007/s10561-009-9123-6

van Daal, M., Muntinga, M.E., Steffens, S., Halsema, A. and Verdonk, P. et al. (2020). Sex and Gender Bias in Kidney Transplantation: 3D Bioprinting as a Challenge to Personalized Medicine. *Women's Health Reports, 1*(1), 218–223. https://doi.org/10.1089/whr.2020.0047

Varkey, M. and Atala, A. (2015). Organ bioprinting: a closer look at ethics and policies. *Wake Forest JL & Pol'y, 5*, 275.

Vermeulen, N., Haddow, G., Seymour, T., Faulkner-Jones, A. and Shu, W. et al. (2017). 3D bioprint me: a socioethical view of bioprinting human organs and tissues. *Journal of Medical Ethics, 43*(9), 618–624. https://doi.org/10.1136/medethics-2015-103347

Vijayavenkataraman, S., Lu, W.F. and Fuh, J.Y.H. (2016). 3D bioprinting – An Ethical, Legal and Social Aspects (ELSA) framework. *Bioprinting, 1–2*, 11–21. https://doi.org/10.1016/j.bprint.2016.08.001

Welin, S. (2014). Ethical Issues in Tissue Engineering. In *Tissue Engineering* (pp. 809–838). Elsevier. https://doi.org/10.1016/B978-0-12-420145-3.00023-7

Young, M.E., Norman, G.R. and Humphreys, K.R. (2008). Medicine in the Popular Press: The Influence of the Media on Perceptions of Disease. *PLoS ONE, 3*(10), e3552. https://doi.org/10.1371/journal.pone.0003552

Challenges in 3D-Bioprinting Techniques

Elif Ilhan,[1*] *Dilruba Baykara,*[1,2] *Beyza Topcu*[1,3]
and *Oguzhan Gunduz*[1,2]

1. Introduction

Biomedical engineering has used three-dimensional (3D) printing as a potent production platform more and more in the last twenty years. Tissue engineering has great potential with 3D printing since it may offer a reliable and quick method of assembling functional tissue *in vitro* (D. J. Richards et al., 2013). All these components can be assembled efficiently with 3D printing by utilizing biomaterials, printing techniques, and cell delivery strategies. While early approaches involved printing intricate scaffolds and then seeding cells, more recent approaches aim to reduce the number of stages and provide both cells and structure simultaneously using scaffold-free or scaffold-based designs (Kim et al., 1998; Miller et al., 2012). By layer-by-layer positioning of materials, biomolecules, or even living cells in the products, such technologies considerably enhance our ability to create a variety of complex and personalized biomedical goods accurately, effectively, inexpensively, and with high reproducibility. Even though 3D printing has made remarkable strides in biomedical engineering, additional work remains to be done to create new and significantly better biomedical goods using this technology. Specifically, there are numerous obstacles in the way of 3D printing materials, techniques, and applications that need to be overcome before millions of patients may access innovative and high-quality products (Lai et al., 2021).

Depending on the basic working principles for fabricating tissue structures three major methods are applied mostly: extrusion, droplet, and laser-based bioprinting (Ilhan et al., 2021). The most widely used bioprinting method is extrusion-based, primarily because it can create more complex 3D structures. The fluid dispensing system and robotic system for bioprinting are combined to create the extrusion-based bioprinting process. The deposition system uses computer control to disperse biological printing. The outcome is the exact deposition of enclosed cells inside the

---

[1] Center for Nanotechnology & Biomaterials Application and Research (NBUAM), Marmara University, Turkey.
[2] Department of Metallurgical and Materials Engineering, Faculty of Technology, Marmara University, Istanbul, Turkey.
[3] Department of Bioengineering, Faculty of Engineering, Marmara University, Istanbul, Turkey
[*] Corresponding author: eliffguven@gmail.com

required three-dimensional structures in the form of cylindrical filaments (Ozbolat and Hospodiuk, 2016). The utilization of high pressures and small-diameter nozzles in extrusion-based bioprinting is associated with reduced cell viability due to process-induced stress, with potential risks such as nozzle clogging and compromised structural integrity, along with drawbacks of lower resolution and accuracy (Dababneh and Ozbolat, 2014; Tanzeglock et al., 2009). Bioprinters employing laser technology are alternatively referred to as laser-assisted printers and laser-direct printers. Laser-assisted printers offer high print resolution through factors like laser power, exposure time, laser spot size, and light wavelength. However, they are hindered by drawbacks such as slow speed, high costs, and material limitations for 3D printing applications. Additionally, the complexities of reaction kinetics and curing treatments contribute to their intricacy (Bedir et al., 2020). Inkjet bioprinting represents an economical method wherein bio-inks can be effectively dispersed in a controlled manner, contributing to its cost-effectiveness. Inkjet bioprinting faces limitations such as a restricted viscosity range and prolonged printing times, which constrain bioink composition; additionally, the technique used by the actuator, particularly in thermal modes, can adversely affect cell viability (Velasco et al., 2018; Zheng et al., 2011).

Natural and synthetic polymers are particularly suitable materials for 3D printing applications (Ilhan et al., 2020). Natural materials offer diverse properties for 3D printing, serving as promising advanced materials with stability, cell adhesion, and biocompatibility. These materials can be processed into bio-inks for 3D bioprinting, particularly in constructing composite scaffolds vital for fields like tissue engineering and regenerative medicine. Despite these advantages, there are limitations to address, including the need for improvements in the biocompatibility and mechanical properties of certain natural materials, enhancements in bio-inks, and accelerated development of advanced bioprinters (Su et al., 2022). Synthetic biopolymers, in general, exhibit commendable formability characteristics, yet are frequently associated with diminished biocompatibility, posing challenges in their integration within biological systems. Potential disadvantages of 3D bioprinting may include biocompatibility issues, limitations in their ability to support cell growth, and difficulty in resembling biological tissue (Schuurman et al., 2013). Despite the promising features of 3D bioprinting technology, there are still difficulties, such as the inability to facilitate vascularization, insufficient cell sources, challenges in maintaining cell viability during bioprinting, and inadequate biomimicry. In addition to biological, material-related and printer-related challenges, management challenges are among the most common parameters . The still high costs of 3D bioprinters, the lack of standards, regulation, automation and customization problems, along with logistics issues are seen as difficulties in disseminating 3D bioprinters (Shahrubudin et al., 2020).

In this chapter, we take a thorough look at the challenges faced by 3D bioprinting, as depicted in figure 1, pointing out its weaknesses and places where it needs improvement. The information is presented in detail and organized under different headings for better clarity.

2. Technical Challenges of 3D Bioprinting

2.1 *Challenges in Materials*

The materials used in the health sector have been constantly changing and developing for centuries. The procurement and production of materials used for treatment purposes has always been a problem in the transition between ages. This problem still exists today in different forms and dimensions. Tissue engineering studies using biomaterials offer innovative and promising approaches to solve these problems. The fact that these biomaterials are natural, and synthetic is of great importance in terms of diversity. However, synthesis, production and procurement of biomaterials have their difficulties in terms of cost and time. The technological and economic biodiversity of the country you live in can be given as an example. Biodiversity in the ecosystem, which varies between continents and even between regions, is a perspective that should be evaluated in the development

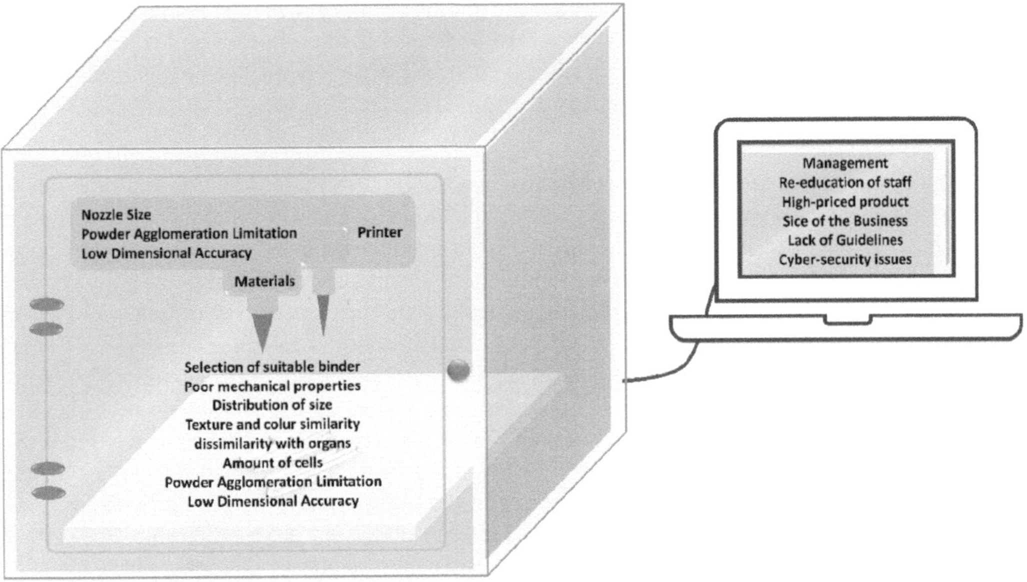

Fig. 1   Challenges of 3D bioprinting

of the infrastructure of biomedical applications that continue to progress. For example, in a 3D bioprinting study, when deducting the supply of devices, consumables and biomaterials required, for a classical 3D bioprinting study if the necessary materials come from an overseas region, they must arrive intact. Additionally, in case of an insufficient supply of materials and devices, the process of biomaterial synthesis and scaffold production may be disrupted and halted.

2.1.1   Solutions

In 3D bioprinting techniques, the printability of biomaterials and bio-inks together with their biological properties is a fundamental issue at the centre of the challenges in 3D bioprinting (Gillispie et al., 2023). For each 3D bioprinting technique, different parameters need to be considered in the use of biomaterials that are evaluated specifically for each bioprinting technique. When these parameters are evaluated with a deductive approach; viscosity, rheology, surface tension, mechanical strength, toxicity, cytotoxicity, degradation, and swelling behaviour of these solutions should be considered in order to provide optimum conditions for bioinks based on biomaterials (Cai et al., 2022). In this regard, when these features are elaborated respectively;

- Viscosity is modelled by the Mark-Houwink Sakurada equation (η = k.MA).
  (k and are constants, M is the molecular weight)

Based on the above equation, the viscosity of the solutions varies according to the M of the materials. Besides, ambient temperature, homogeneous distribution, percentage of biomaterial in the solution and solvent preference also affect the solution viscosity (Robb and Lennox, 2011; Sin and Tueen, 2019). In short, viscosity, which is the resistance of liquids or solutions to flow, is one of the factors that directly affect the behaviour of the solution prepared during 3D printing by moving inversely proportional to the flow rate. The viscosity rate may vary according to the preferred extrusion technique and region. When it is very high, it becomes difficult for the solution to reach the needle tip, maintain a continuous flow (shear rate), and accelerate according to the speed parameter in G-Codes, For these reasons, the prepared solutions may dry up and remain at the needle tip; they may even clog the needle tip (Zhang et al., 2020). Extra time is spent to make the blocked needle tip usable again or a new needle is required. This leads to a loss of time and cost. Additionally, increased pressure values or flow rates in the devices used to reach the needle tip and maintain a continuous flow can lead to mechanical and physical damage to the devices. Moreover, high pressure values can cause the nanofibre caps or filaments to be thicker and wider than they should be. In such cases, although the desired pore size and density cannot be obtained, a filled scaffold can be printed (Gunduz et al., 2018).

- **Rheology**

Rheology is a science that describes and analyzes the process of deformation and flow rate of materials under certain stresses (Darvell, 2018; Summerscales and Grove, 2014). Analyzing the flow behaviour of materials provides an advantage in making decisions according to application areas and using appropriate materials. By examining the behaviours of bio-inks through tests such as Dynamic strain sweep test, Interval-thixotropic-tests, amplitude sweep test, evaluation of shear-thinning; viscosity vs shear strain rate, shear stress etc, shear strain rates are compared. Through these comparisons, we obtain more detailed data about the printability of pure or composite bioinks. In this way, it is possible to determine the phase transitions and permanent deformation range of bio-inks under certain tension forces. For example, the suitability of bioinks with linear viscoelastic range (LVR) is determined according to additive manufacturing (AM) techniques and the extent to which biomaterials affect viscosity and shear rate in the use of composite bioinks is determined. At the same time, detailed information can be obtained about the degradation and recovery of printed scaffolds under certain pressures by hysteresis loop analysis. In short, while rheology analyses enable the evaluation of parameters such as temperature and pressure range required for optimum printability of bio-inks it also allows interpretation of cell viability, mechanical strength and bioactive behaviour.

- **Surface Tension**

Surface tension is the energy required for each unit area (cm^2) increase of liquids and the resistance to this increase and external forces (Owais et al., 2017).

$$\gamma = -\rho g \left(h + \frac{r}{3} \right)$$

The surface tension, formalised above, is affected by the density (ρ), the acceleration due to gravity (m/s^2), the amount of capillary rise (h) and the radius of the capillary (Brindha et al., 2016). According to these units, the information and approaches we will obtain about the optimization processes of the solutions are evolving. In this case, surface tension and density, which are directly proportional to the surface tension according to the equation, can be counted among the issues experienced during printing. In classical AM applications, electrospray or electrospinning techniques prevent the formation of stable and continuous results. Especially in electrospinning, the surface tension and viscosity of the solution are important parameters to be optimized (Guo et al., 2022.). This is because in solutions with high surface tension, the formation of unstable beads and the production of a stable nanofibre may not occur (Li et al., 2021). To avoid this problem, the surface tension should be reduced and optimized along with the optimization of the viscosity during nanofiber fabrication (Ayati et al., 2022). Especially in high molecular weight polymers or high concentration solutions, high surface tension is a highly likely issue, and in these cases, the use of Tween 80, a non-ionic surfactant at certain concentrations, decreases the surface tension (γ) of the solution and allows a more stable, and successful electrospun operation (Wu et al., 2023).

- **Mechanical Strength**

The layer-by-layer printing principle of 3D bioprinting approaches, which have been developing for the last three decades, enables more controlled and regular printing with bio-inks. Bioinks containing sensitive organisms and molecules such as living cells, biomolecules, proteins, bioactive agents, and growth factors (VEGF, EGF, FGF, etc.), are supported by biomaterials and used to produce mechanically stronger scaffolds to prevent existing problems. In particular, it is necessary to produce layered and porous scaffolds in which living cells and biomolecules are evenly distributed. In printing trials without equal distribution, imbalance and failure are experienced in the adhesion and proliferation rates of cells. Layer-by-layer printing studies adjust the thickness balance and size of the filaments forming each layer of the scaffolds. In addition to these parameters that can be adjusted with the device parameters, elastic modulus, compressive strength, maximum strain, flexural modulus, fatigue, and tensile strength analyses and evaluations of the biomaterials used should be performed. If the viscosity of the bio-inks used in the designs to provide the required mechanical strength is higher, it may be necessary to use a slower shear rate. In this case, according to the scale and design of the scaffold produced, the printing time required is prolonged. The prolonged process is a major disadvantage for bio-inks, which are susceptible to contamination and degradation. At the same time, it is possible that high porosity and optimum pore size ratio cannot be obtained as a result of the thicker and tougher structure of the scaffolds designed for printing. As a result, the physical and morphological structures of the scaffold designs are very important for their resistance to the desired compression and tension stress, vascularization , angiogenesis and cell proliferation in tissue engineering studies in general.

- **Swelling and degradation**

Swelling and degradation tests are two forms of analysis that concern both physical structure and chemical structure (Venkata Krishna and Ravi Sankar, 2023; W. Wu, 2020). We have mentioned the mechanical strength of the scaffolds prepared with 3D bioprinting techniques according to the production forms. The development of proliferation, vascularization and angiogenesis, which gain a success percentage according to mechanical strength; swelling and degradation behaviour are significantly affected. When a classical swelling test is considered, the pore sizes of the scaffold, which can change according to the swelling behaviour of the scaffold, can lead to changes in the initially targeted scaffold design. When the degradation test is approached with the same logic, considering that the treatment period of a classic wound is between 4-6 weeks; the structure must be stable throughout the process (Wallace et al., 2023). At this point, especially the insufficient strength of water-soluble biomaterials is among the problems experienced in 3D bioprinting studies. However, the use of chemical, physical or enzymatic cross-linking methods can prevent this problem (Ghavaminejad et al., 2020). However, the viscosity, which is directly proportional to the degree of crosslinking as well as the crosslinking technique applied, may cause disruptions in the printing process (Belyadi et al., 2019). Especially during interactive 3D bioprinting of crosslinker-loaded bioinks in extrusion-based printers, blockages may occur at the needle tip due to the changing chemical structure.

2.1.2 *Natural Polymers*

Natural biomaterials are polymers of protein, polysaccharide or glycosaminoglycan origin. The use of these polymers in living tissue such as keratin, collagen, silk, gelatin, cellulose, alginate, chitosan and hyaluronic acid in bioinks increases intercellular interaction, adhesion, proliferation and biocompatibility. These materials with low cytotoxicity and toxicity should be used as composites (Chakrapani et al., 2022; Pradhan et al., 2020; Sionkowska et al., 2020; Varanko et al., 2020). This is because they have some disadvantages.

Keratin refers to the whole intermediate filament-forming proteins found in vertebrate epithelium and corneous tissues (Aramwit, 2016). Keratins, which are divided into alpha-keratins and beta-keratins according to their preferred sources for the extraction procedure, are extracted by different methods such as ionic liquids, alkaline extraction, reduction oxidation, microwave irradiation or steam explosion. When the characteristic behaviours of the extracted keratins are analyzed , they stand out with their high biocompatibility and biodegradation, high polarity, and high chemical reactivity properties.

Type I Collagen which constitutes about 90% of the protein mass in mammalian connective tissues, forms the basis of these bioinks due to its self-organizing properties into fibrils. However, a major challenge is the low mechanical properties of collagen bioinks, especially at low concentrations. To address this, researchers explore two main approaches: These are using supportive hydrogels like gelatin slurry to improve printability, albeit with concerns about gelatin diffusion, and increasing the storage modulus of collagen bioinks to enhance printability for direct extrusion bioprinting.

Silk, a common protein polymer, is produced by a variety of insects such as spiders, silkworms and bees, each with different characteristics. Silks, which differ according to their species and variety, have unique primary sequences, structural features and fibroin compositions for each silk variety (Gupta et al., 2020). Additionally, properties such as biocompatibility, low degradation rate, low immunogenicity, and good mechanical strength, like those of silk fibroin (SF) are particularly attractive for soft tissue engineering applications such as cartilage, ligaments, and skin (Institute of Electrical and Electronics Engineers et al., 2019). However, regulation of viscosity, poor cross-linking and the risk of cytotoxicity from chemical residues due to cross-linking of SF make bioprinting and in vivo applications difficult (Rodriguez et al., 2017).

Gelatin, sourced from natural collagen, is a water-soluble protein renowned for its numerous advantageous characteristics (Hong et al., 2019). Gelatin based scaffolds exhibit high biocompatibility, bioactivity, suitable biodegradability, and non-immunogenicity. These attributes render gelatin based hydrogels, and scaffolds ideal candidates for use as extracellular matrices across diverse biomedical applications (He et al., 2020). Hence, it is among the polymers frequently preferred in bioprinting techniques such as extrusion-based 3D printing, but its direct effect on ambient temperature makes the bioprinting process difficult (Li et al., 2018). Therefore, depending on the type of device used or the scaffold design, optimum conditions (37°C) can be achieved by heating the device head and/or device table and working under low pressure forces (Leucht et al., 2020).

Cellulose, a widely available natural polymer, is commonly used in scaffolds for its high biocompatibility and rigidity due to hydrogen bond crosslinking (Lin et al., 2023). Cellulose, which is classified in different groups, can be mainly grouped as cellulose nanofibrils (CNFs), cellulose nanocrystals (CNCs), and bacterial nanocellulose (BNC) (Wang et al., 2020).

Alginate polymer, a linear polysaccharide composed of guluronic and mannuronic acids, usually obtained from the cell walls of brown algae is considered to be a low-cost marine material. It has various desirable properties such as non-toxic, biodegradable and non-immunogenic (K.Y. Lee and Mooney, 2012) (Abka-khajouei et al., 2022) In addition to these properties, there are approaches that the proportional distribution of acids in its chemical structure affects an optimum bioprinting and mechanical strength (Gorroñogoitia et al., 2022).

Chitosan, obtained by deacetylation of chitin, is found in crustaceans, insects or in the exoskeletons of fungi (Szymańska and Winnicka, 2015). Chitosan polymer, which can be synthesised with high and low molecular weights, can cause failures in scaffold designs due to its low mechanical strength and gelation rate. Nonadhesive, biocompatible, and enzymatically degradable **hyaluronic acid (HA)** which is a naturally occurring polysaccharide found in connective tissues. It is composed of D-glucuronic acid and N-acetyl-D-glucosamine units (Guvendiren et al., 2012). Thanks to vital roles in cellular functions like attachment, proliferation, and migration properties HA is utilized in cartilage and neural tissue engineering, as well as drug delivery systems due to its ability to support tissue growth and provide controlled release of therapeutic agents (Sundararaghavan and Burdick, 2011). But HA based bioinks have limitations in bioprinting due to their weak post-printing shape stability which is insufficient (Noh et al., 2019).

2.1.3 Synthetic Polymers

Synthetic polymers used in both hard and soft tissue applications highlight their ability to tune functional properties and rheological behaviour through various methods such as monomer selection, architectural control and post-polymerisation functionalization (S. Kumar, 2021). But synthetic polymers are generally incompatible with direct cell incorporation due to the printing process conditions and properties such as high melting point, solubility in organic solvents, and challenges in encapsulating cells (Chen et al., 2023). Due to these limitations and the lack of biological cues found in the natural extracellular matrix (ECM), which are crucial for stimulating cellular proliferation and differentiation as well as providing sites for cellular recognition, synthetic polymers account for only 10% of bioprinting systems (Raees et al., 2023). The polymers studied to improve the mechanical properties of the scaffolds designed in this direction are added to the bio-ink after they are made suitable for cell viability with different conditions and techniques (Schaefer et al., 2023).

Additionally, the integrity of 3D printed objects is jeopardized by bacterial contamination in biomaterials, polymeric materials, and viable cells utilized in grafts and transplants. This issue needs to be resolved immediately. It is essential to comprehend how 3D topography and extracellular matrix (ECM) interact to facilitate biofilm growth on 3D printed materials. According to research, preventing the production of biofilms might be the answer. It is suggested that using bioinks or ink-substrates with possible antibacterial effects is a workable way to lessen the danger and infection related to implantation (Muthukrishnan, 2021).

3. Challenges of Production Method in 3D Printing

In 3D printing, computer-designed models are transformed into physical objects by converting them into a series of coordinates that can be read by a printer. This data is then used to create successive layers generated by laser optics or ink-based print heads, and a computer-controlled platform moves accordingly. In this process, the objects are produced layer by layer. There are several established 3D printing technologies for modern polymers, including light-based printing processes, extrusion-based processes and inkjet printing (thermal or piezoelectric) (Jiang et al., 2020). In this section, the 3D printing processes and the challenges that arise during printing are examined and summarised in detail.

3.1 Extrusion Printing

3D Extrusion printing is a widely used technique in tissue engineering and regenerative medicine. It is used to create structures or scaffolds that contain cells (Naghieh and Chen, 2021). In this printing technique, where pneumatic and mechanical forces are responsible for the ejection of the material, the material is deposited in continuous strips by different mechanisms, as shown in figure 2. An extrusion bioprinter usually consists of three main units: a container (e.g. a syringe) that holds biomaterials, a dispensing head that ejects the biomaterial, and a pick-up stage where the bioink is collected. The print resolution can be influenced by the settings for these three units and the printing process. Numerous studies in this context have shown that the width and height of the printed strands can be influenced by the height of the nozzle, the nozzle diameter, the speed of the dispensing head and the flow rate of the extruded bioink (Malekpour and Chen, 2022). With this printing technique, the application of the correct pressure, the use of the correct nozzle, the correct speed of movement of the print head and the amount of material dispensed is decisive for the printing process (Ravoor et al., 2023). While the printing dynamics, such as extrusion pressure, nozzle size and printing speed, are closely linked, the rheological nature of the inks influences the resolution of the printed structure. The combined design of optimized ink rheology and printing dynamics plays an important role in creating defect-free 3D printed structures (Malekpour and Chen, 2022). In the extrusion bioprinting technique, living cells are incorporated into the hydrogel, which enables the printing of 3D structures. The printability of the designed structure is important as it can affect the accuracy of the scaffolds printed using this technique and therefore the performance of the cells (Naghieh and Chen, 2021). Therefore, there is a balance between printability and cell viability in this technique (Hou et al., 2023). This method also has important limitations.

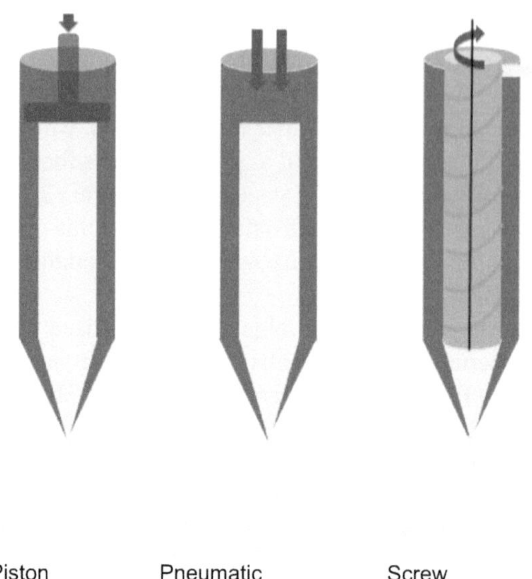

Fig. 2   Schematic Representation of Extrusion printing

3.1.1 Shear stress

The bioink used in extrusion printing systems is passed under pressure through a nozzle of known size. Depending on different velocity gradients, the bioink flows through the nozzle. It was found that extrusion bioprinting increases the shear stress in the region around the nozzle. As a result, the cells in the region near the wall move more slowly, which leads to the deformation of the cells. In this system, in which the nozzle diameter and viscosity also play a role, shear stress is identified as the main cause of cell death (Lepowsky et al., 2018).

Mechanotransduction refers to the ability of living tissues to respond locally to mechanical forces and physical microenvironments. This process involves an important mechanism that regulates biological responses such as cell growth, differentiation, shape change and cell death.

The most common model assumes conformational changes that start at cell surface proteins leading to signal transduction in the cytoplasm. Extracellular proteins such as integrins, focal adhesins and fates are initiators of force transmission. Mechanical stress redirects these proteins to cytoskeletal proteins (actin, myosin IIs and actin). Factors involved in mechanotransduction include calcium and ion channels, mechanosensitive ion channels that open fibronectin, and G protein-coupled receptors. The signal propagates from the cytoskeleton to the nucleus, resulting in a variety of biological responses ranging from cell deformation to cell growth and differentiation (Boularaoui et al., 2020).

3.1.2 Nozzle Geometry

Another parameter that influences cell viability and pressure sensitivity is the nozzle geometry. Studies have shown that conical and cylindrical nozzle geometries influence cell viability and cell damage. Conical needles have the advantage of low air pressure and less cell damage (Billiet et al., 2014). Therefore, nozzle geometry is important for reducing cell damage and successful printing in extrusion-based bioprinting.

3.2 Inkjet Printing

In this method, also known as droplet printing, the bioink is sprayed from the spray nozzle in the device as droplets in a volume range of nanoliters to picoliters (Kumar et al., 2021). Combined with precise computer control, this technology enables the rapid printing of high-resolution materials down to 50 µm by spraying a large number of droplets onto the substrate. A computer is used to print the designed model (Xie et al., 2020a). The computer sends an electrical signal to move the nozzle, which sprays the bioink and the substrate to which the material is applied. The drop-by-drop application of the bioink influences the exact resolution of the printed model. The two most important parameters that affect print quality are droplet size reduction and print speed control (Lee et al., 2015). To optimize droplet size, parameters such as nozzle diameter, material viscosity, printing mechanism and substrate wettability need to be fine-tuned (Caviezel et al., 2008) As shown in Figure 3, inkjet printing is divided into thermal and piezoelectric printing. This distinction is based on the operating principle and the spraying mode. The heating device plays an important role in the thermal inkjet printer. This device surrounds the inkjet device. When the signal is received, it heats up quickly and causes spraying to take place. In the piezoelectric inkjet printing method, which is more widely researched today, the place where the fluid material flows is coated with piezoelectric material. The piezoelectric printing nozzle undergoes mechanical deformation in response to the electric field. With the signal sent, the piezoelectric material contracts and the fluid material used for printing is ejected from the nozzle (Kumar et al., 2021). There are some challenges with these methods.

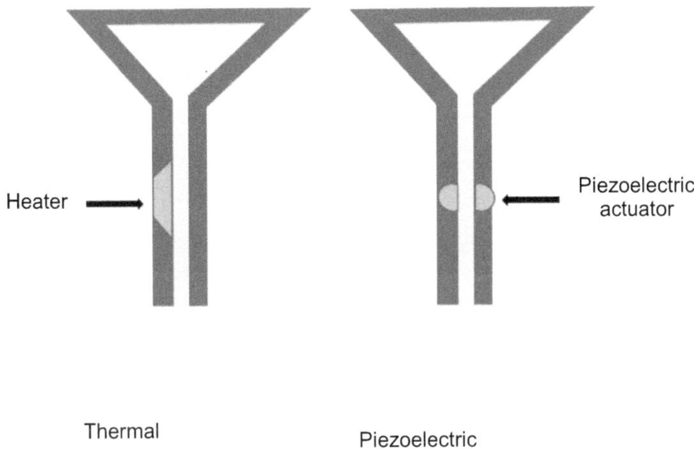

Fig. 3   Schematic Representation of Inkjet Printing

3.2.1   Mechanical Interaction

The risks of possible clogging of the nozzles or a high cell density, which leads to the cells being exposed to thermal and mechanical stresses, are the greatest challenges of this printing technique. Biomass with a low polymer concentration has a low cell density. An increase in polymer concentration or cell density can lead to clogging of the nozzles (Xie et al., 2020a). An alternative way to increase the print resolution of low-viscosity bioinks is therefore the use of crosslinkers. These materials can be crosslinked with pH, chemicals or ultraviolet light after spray deposition. However, crosslinkers can have negative effects on the cells during bioprinting. The chemicals used for chemical modification can produce toxic products for the cells (Azizi Machekposhti et al., 2019). The correlation between extrusion pressure, duration of mechanical shear and cell density should be defined and optimized accordingly to avoid negative effects on cell stability (Adhikari et al., 2021).

3.3   Light-based 3D Printing

Selective laser melting (SLM), selective laser sintering (SLS), DLP printing, and laser-assisted printing are examples of light-based 3D printing. When the basic working principle is compared,

DLP and laser-assisted printing methods are based on photopolymerization reactions, while SLM and SLS printing techniques apply the melting of the powdered material at high temperatures generated by the laser (Zhang et al., 2020). The SLA printing technique uses UV light to solidify the photopolymer layer and initiate the polymerization chain reaction. The components of the technique are shown in figure 4. After the solidification of the layer, the platform is lowered vertically to allow the uncured liquid resin to spread over the top of the layer. The top layer is polymerized until the designed 3D structure is formed (Xie et al., 2020a). A resin tank, beam-curable polymer resin, laser source, XY scanning mirror, and a moving table are the main components required for SLA (Stereolithography) printing (Fisher et al., 2002). With a fundamentally similar operating principle, digital light processing (DLP) printing uses ultraviolet (UV) light (or visible light) from a digital projector to project the image of the pattern simultaneously across the resin. The higher resolution of the designed structure depends on some parameters. The curing time, layer thickness, amount of photopolymer, and photoinitiator are important parameters. Selective laser melting (SLM) is a fusion process based on the selective laser sintering (SLS) printing technique of fusing fine powder grains arranged regularly on a platform. In the SLS printing technique, laser energy is used. In the SLS technique, electron beams are used. These beams are used to scan models controlled by CAD data files. The powder particles are heated and as a result, neighbouring powders fuse by molecular diffusion to form a layer. To produce the next layer, the platform is lowered and new powder grains are fused. The production of the 3D structure is completed. Heat treatment methods can be preferred for unbonded powder particles to reach a certain density after removal (Xie et al., 2020a). While these techniques have advantages such as high resolution and fast printing, they also have some disadvantages.

3.3.1   Cost Challenge

Light-based bioprinters are an expensive production technology for tissue engineering studies. The large quantities of bioinks required for the device and the lack of information on parameter tuning have led to significant limitations in the adoption of this technology (Pérez-Cortez et al., 2023). In terms of cost, the resin used in SLA is more expensive than the tools used in other printing techniques (Mehdiyev and Felhő, 2023). Light-curable biomaterials have price limitations. Most commercially available light-based resins require a large amount of material depending on the design of the resin container. Synthesizing these high-volume bioinks for a single production run is time-consuming, labour-intensive, and expensive. It is important to design the resin containers in a way that reduces material consumption. In addition, some processes may need to be applied after printing. These processes include steps to remove excess resin and improve it (Pérez-Cortez et al., 2023).

3.3.2   Photoinitiator

One of the challenges of laser bioprinting is that it leads to lower cell viability (Bishop et al., 2017). The photopolymerization process is triggered by the free radicals in the structure of the photoinitiator, which is decomposed by UV light or visible light. When bioprinting in the presence of the cell, the free radicals of the photoinitiator are likely to react with components present in the cell membrane or within the cell. This can lead to the formation of reactive oxygen species (ROS). As a result, cell damage may occur. The exposure time of cells to photoinitiators is an important parameter. It plays an important role in the encapsulation of cells by photopolymerization (Xu et al., 2015).

4.   Challenge of Functional in Vitro Models

While half a million patients worldwide are waiting for an organ transplant, it has been determined that there are more than 100,00 people on the waiting list for organ transplants in the United States. It is a serious problem that people die every day because they cannot get a vital organ (Parihar et al., 2022; Zhang, 2022). For decades, doctors, biologists and bioengineers have been

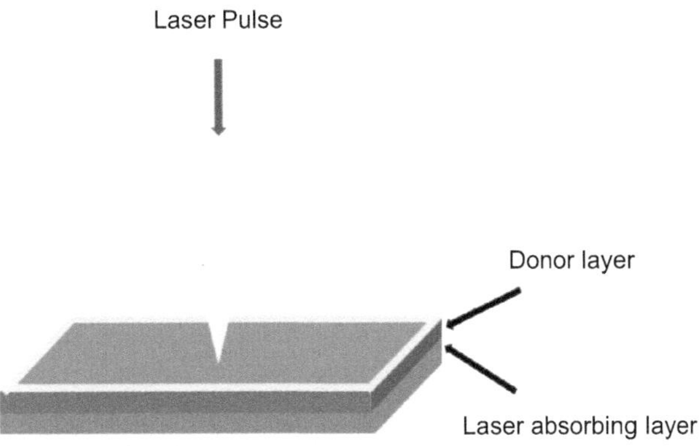

Fig. 4   Schematic Representation of Light-based Printing

trying to mimic the complex processes that take place in healthy and diseased tissue by recreating the human body *in vitro* (Bassi et al., 2021). Bioprinting technology, developed to overcome these problems, aims to overcome all limitations through the controlled combination and precise accumulation of cells and biomaterials to create natural tissue-like tissues and organs. Bioprinting is an emerging alternative technology to tissue and organ engineering. This technology, which has a multidisciplinary infrastructure, is developing rapidly (Zhang, 2022). This is a challenging and exciting process. Studies have been conducted to develop in vitro models for various applications. These include studies such as 2D cell culture-based monolayer, multilayer or co-culture models, 3D organoids, 3D-printed and organ systems on a chip. When these systems are evaluated, they have advantages and disadvantages (Kutlehria and Sachdeva, 2021). The challenges of bioprinting technology include many areas such as biocompatibility, vascularization, cell viability and function, reproducibility and standardization, and cost. In this section, more detailed information will be given about these difficulties.

4.1 Bioink

The bioink developed for successful printing of the targeted tissue or organ must be a supporting material, both biochemically and physically, for the cell to survive and differentiate. Biochemically, chemokines, adhesion factors, signalling proteins and growth factors are important for the survival of the cell, as well as physically, in terms of the mechanical and structural properties of the extracellular matrix. Tissue-appropriate selected bioinks have important roles such as serving as temporary substitutes for tissue functions, organizing tissue regeneration, and directing integration within the host tissue (Cui et al., 2017). Biocompatibility is one of the basic features to minimize the possibility of encountering host rejection of the organ to be produced with the bioprinting technique and to prevent complications or rejection. Bioinks, also defined as cell-encapsulated biomaterials, currently have limitations in the development of compatible formulations for cell printing. Solvents used in materials to be used for bioprinting, high temperatures and viscosity of the materials may cause difficulties in printing (Wragg et al., 2019). In the printing technique that requires high viscosity, the shear force that increases with the high pressure applied during the extrusion process is a factor that negatively affects cell viability (Yang et al., 2020).

Cell behaviour in mechanotransduction may be negative, and as a result, stem cells may be directed to undesirable lineages. In addition, cross-linking should be applied to the structure produced after printing. However, cross-linking made by chemical, thermal or enzymatic means has the risk of cytotoxicity and DNA damage. For example, the effects of UV light used as a photopolymerization agent on DNA need to be investigated for a long time (Fedorovich et al., 2009). Synthetic materials are obtained using non-biological sources and chemical production techniques.

The excellent mechanical properties of these materials are polymers used in 3D printing technology. The most commonly used synthetic polymers include poly (lactic acid) (PLA), poly(glycolic acid) (PGA), polylactic-co-glycolic acid (PLGA), polyurethane (PU), and polycaprolactone (PCL). Polycaprolactone (PCL) polymer, which is easy to shape for printing, has a significant limitation in encapsulating cells. Synthetic polymers, which are relatively biologically inert, present challenges in easily incorporating them for 3D printing because the use of heat, organic solvents and toxic activators for printing affects the activity and growth of cells (Liu and Wang, 2020).

Natural materials have become interesting materials in 3D printing technology due to their advantages such as biocompatibility, biodegradability, increasing cell adhesion, and improving self-organisation of cells. Various studies have been conducted on the use of natural materials such as hyaluronic acid, chitosan, gelatin, and collagen. The relatively limited options of natural materials cannot meet the increasing demand due to limitations such as low mechanical properties and precise production control (Ma et al., 2024a). Further research is also needed on the risk of inflammation and infection of these natural polymers. There is a need for toxicity studies on the by-products of the breakdown of materials produced from non-human organisms such as alginate and gelatine, which enter the bloodstream and are cleared by the kidneys and liver (Jovic et al., 2020). To solve this problem, it is important to develop combinations that meet biomechanical requirements. However, different formulations need to be developed for each printing technology. Because it is not possible for every formulation to be suitable for all printing techniques (Cui et al., 2017; Hölzl et al., 2016)

4.2 Cell Sourcing

The selection of cells for 3D bioprinting of tissues or organs was critical for their application in future clinical applications. 3D printed tissues and organs that represent native tissue consist of multiple cell types with specific biological functions in addition to primary functional cell types. These cells include various cell types that provide the necessary environment for the functional development and maintenance of primary cells and play a role in supportive and structural functions (Cui et al., 2017). The aim is to design a structure that aims to realistically mimic the physiological properties of cells and maintain their normal functions in the in vivo environment. The use of primary cells in 3D printing by isolating cells from the patient to reduce negative immune reactions has the potential to lead to significant advances in this field. In addition to the difficulty of isolating primary cells, they also have life-limiting effects (Xie et al., 2020b; Xie et al., 2020a). In addition, the presence of genetic diseases, accessibility of certain cell types and ethical aspects are other challenges. They are sensitive to parameters such as temperature and pressure changes during 3D printing. This may cause cell death. In addition, the life span of these cells is limited. Replication potential decreases with each pass and may cause difficulty. Ethical rules are the biggest limitation for cells derived from human tissues. Approval from ethics committees may be required to obtain these cells. Also, limited human experiments are among the issues that remain unclear regarding the behaviour of autology cells.

Stem cells represent a renewable cell source for regenerative medicine due to their ability to differentiate into other cell types. In addition to the advantages of using them, there are also some limitations. These limitations include the potential risk of tumour formation in undifferentiated pluripotent stem cells, the risks of genetic and epigenetic abnormalities, and the complex and time-consuming process of induced pluripotent stem cells (iPSCs) (Ma et al., 2024b). The risk of teratoma formation as a result of the use of these cells and the potential strengthening of maligenesis still affect the scientific world as a concern. In one study, Japanese researchers decided to stop the experiment on humans using induced pluripotent stem cells as a result of genomic mutation (Jovic et al., 2020).

In addition, as stem cells undergo differentiation, there is a risk of decreased proliferation capacity. As a result of complete differentiation, their ability to divide is lost. In order to overcome this difficulty and to keep the proliferation ability of the cells constant, differentiation into progenitor cells should be ensured (Ma et al., 2024b).

4.3　Vascularization

Vasculogenesis is a process of de novo blood vessel formation in embryos, which involves interactions between vascular and endothelial progenitor cells and growth factors (Mir et al., 2023). This formation saw the presence of vascularized tissues supporting tissue-specific functions throughout the body, comprising a variety of vessels ranging from millimeter-sized, small diameter vessels to micron-sized capillary networks (D. Richards et al., 2016). These vascularized tissues support tissue function by facilitating oxygen and nutrient delivery, waste removal, and immune cell circulation (Jafarkhani et al., 2019). Thanks to this perfusion, a continuous cycle is formed in the human body, which ensures adequate nutrition of the tissues. Therefore, vascularisation and angiogenesis formation are necessary for the existence of healthy tissues. However, in tissue engineering studies, the desired treatment and implant application for each damaged tissue cannot give a successful result (Masson-Meyers and Tayebi, 2021). This major problem is more common in areas with extensive tissue damage. In large implant or scaffold applications, the rate of angiogenesis formation may remain low. Hypoxia that may occur at this point causes apoptosis and tissue loss in the target area. For these reasons, scaffold designs are specially designed with 3D printing techniques to ensure adequate vascularisation and angiogenesis. These techniques include; written moulding strategy, coaxial extrusion strategy, sacrificial material strategy, lithography-based printing strategy, and inkjet printing strategy (H. Lee et al., 2021). It is important that the preferred materials in the application of the mentioned techniques are angiogenic biomaterials. At this stage, surface chemistry, surface topography, hardness, degradation, porosity and biocompatibility of the materials gain importance. If examples of studies are given, studies using natural biomaterials are generally seen. Biomaterials such as collogen, silk fibroin, alginate, chitosan, hylonic acid, fibrin and GelMA are being studied.

4.4　The limits of Biomimicry

Biomimicry (Biomimetics) draws inspiration from nature to develop new materials and technologies, particularly focusing on biomolecules and their supramolecular organization. Despite the challenges posed by nature's efficiency in creating biomimetic materials, the text explores various building blocks used in bottom-up arrangements, including organosilanes, carbon allotropes, dendrimers, carbohydrates, nucleic acids, amino acids, and lipids. It also highlights common approaches to producing synthetic biomimetic materials, emphasizing the importance of building blocks and their supramolecular arrangement in the process (Moldoveanu and David, 2022; Moreira et al., 2015). Biomimicry, which is based on imitating nature, tries to impose the structures in question on the structural and physiological structures in nature. For example; cellular, porous structures in nature, such as beehive wooden cellular structures, honeycombs, and spongy bone, can lead to ECM designs. These structures offer extraordinary properties that can be adapted and diversified through design, making them valuable for a variety of applications. In AM, these structures are known as lattice structures; they are extensively examined and used in terms of properties such as compatibility, energy absorption, impact absorption, acoustic absorption, vibration, insulation explosion protection, heat insulation and thermal control (Chaturvedi et al., 2022; Du Plessis et al., 2020). However, sometimes there may not be sufficient results regarding the printability of the designs discussed because the success rate of optimum scaffold production varies as a result of the printability of complex structures found in nature through AM technologies and the sensitivity of bioinks s and devices.

5.　Challenges in Management

5.1　Cost-effectiveness

Effective scaling and commercialization of bio-printed tissues pose significant challenges, especially in light of complex aspects related to tissue design, cell source, and production logistics inherent in contemporary methodologies. Importantly, these approaches often necessitate a high level of customization to adapt to the unique needs of individual patients, thus presenting significant barriers to cost-effectiveness. As businesses consider investments in this emerging field, a smart strategy requires exploring ways to alleviate the financial burdens inherent in personalized materials and designs. A feasible approach in the short term involves the development of general or universal scaffolds. This involves creating basic structures that can be adapted to various organs and offer a potentially more cost-effective alternative to proprietary solutions. Additionally, an exploration of components designed to streamline and save money on the manufacturing process is emerging as a promising avenue for companies navigating the complex landscape of personalized 3D printed tissue replacements.

Utilizing acellular scaffolds and populating them with the patient's own cells is a viable and effective alternative strategy. This methodology not only has the potential to improve costs but also serves to reduce the risks associated with allogeneic rejection. While the adoption of a customized tissue engineering paradigm like 3D bioprinting may require significant initial expenses, a critical consideration lies in judiciously balancing these costs against the possibility of prolonged and costly lifelong interventions such as dialysis or surgical treatment. When conducting a cost-effectiveness analysis for personalized tissue engineering, it becomes clear that a one-time intervention, while initially costly, can be more financially advantageous than ongoing non-therapeutic treatments that a patient may require throughout their lifetime. This realization highlights the importance of carefully considering the economic environment in which short-term investments can yield long-term benefits and potentially transform the treatment landscape for conditions that require innovative and sustainable medical interventions (Murphy et al., 2020).

In the field of 3D printing, the manufacturing procedure requires the successive layering of material to form an object on a defined bed or platform. However, this bed/platform exhibits limited dimensions and thus imposes restrictions on the size of printable objects. The resulting limitations lead to challenges in scalability, which is a major issue in the field of AM. This limitation arises from the natural dimensions of the bed/platform and is particularly noticeable when encountering objects of significant size that exceed the spatial boundaries of the construction platform. A traditional approach in such cases involves reducing the object through scaling. However, this fit-for-purpose solution falls short when dealing with printing different sets of parts with different dimensions. In such scenarios, directly applying scaling to fit bed dimensions would be impractical. Instead, a comprehensive re-engineering of the entire platform for object printing is required, thus adding a significant layer of complexity to the production process. A critical understanding that the size constraint is intricately intertwined with the design features of the 3D printing apparatus and associated cost considerations are warranted. The dimensions of the bed/platform not only determine upper thresholds of printable object sizes but also impose important considerations on the scalability of the printing process. Consequently, the complexities associated with size constraints contribute significantly to broader discourses on the optimization of 3D printing systems and require a nuanced investigation of design principles and cost implications to advance progressive developments in this field (Malik et al., 2022; Thomas-Seale et al., 2018).

5.2 *Standardization*

The field of 3D bioprinting technology lacks standardized protocols for the technology itself and its related components, such as bioprinting materials, bioinks, cell sources, and general bioprinting processes. While there are already recommendations for 3D printer manufacturers and standards for AM terminology as outlined in ISO/DIS 17296-1, there is still a great need to develop manufacturing guidelines tailored to the intricate field of bioprinting and to further standardize the process (Food and Drug Administration, 2017).

There is currently a lack of established standards for the materials used in bioprinting, which is causing delays in product creation. However, the introduction of standardized materials and manufacturing processes could speed up the translation of bioprinted structures into clinical applications. This would also allow producers to streamline their procedures for particular structures or products and reduce the sources needed to develop base materials and technical processes. It's not just materials that need standardization, but also cell culture media and bioinks. Systems of quality control that can detect issues throughout the production process are also important for ensuring the safety, effectiveness, and reproducibility of printed products. Developing a comprehensive standards framework for 3D bioprinting is critical. This framework should cover materials, processes, and quality control parameters. By doing so, it can increase the efficiency of product development, reduce costs, and accelerate the translation of bioprinting technologies into clinical applications. This will ultimately improve the landscape of regenerative medicine (Hunsberger et al., 2017).

5.3 *Automation and Personalization*

Automated design processes can be integrated into personalized manufacturing to identify regulatory mechanisms that are crucial in achieving consistent and predictable results. However, when it comes to personalized designs, the artistic aspect often overshadows engineering principles due to the complex nature of anatomical designs. Fortunately, advancements in 3D imaging and modelling software now allow for computational processes that incorporate explicit design parameters. This advancement enables the automation and tailoring of personalized construct creation that seamlessly adapts to the patient's unique anatomical configuration and injury requirements (Kengla et al., 2017).

Advanced 3D imaging and modelling software allows the creation of customized structures based on specific design parameters. This software enables the creation of printed structures based on 3D models obtained with medical imaging technologies. These structures are based on the principle of placement of determined scanning architecture, material properties and cell types in specific regions. Integration of these computational processes not only ensures accuracy but also streamlines the manufacturing process and increases repeatability. An indepth understanding of fundamental biological processes such as biomaterial self-assembly, tissue healing processes, and harmonious assembly of printed structures is important in determining design criteria. This information plays an important role in the clinical applications and regulatory processes of personalized printed structures. It also encourages harmonious progress of technological developments and regulatory requirements. In many respects, bioprinting embodies a paradigm reminiscent of 4D printing, marked by the dynamic rearrangement of cells and gradual degradation of scaffold materials post-implantation. The complexities inherent in these complex 4D prints require a solid research foundation to comprehensively predict their results (Tibbits, 2012). Accordingly, building a repository of knowledge through systematic research efforts becomes indispensable for navigating the complex interplay of biological, engineering, and regulatory dimensions inherent in the evolving field of bioprinting. The synergy of rigorous research initiatives and technological advances holds the promise of ushering in an era where personalized bioprinting is not only an innovative concept but also a clinically sound and regulatory reality.

5.4 *Regulation*

The integration of 3D bioprinted tissues and organs into clinical practice is poised to revolutionize healthcare; however, it faces formidable regulatory challenges. Despite the multitude of manufacturing methodologies, the Food and Drug Administration (FDA) presently evaluates 3D printed medical devices and conventionally manufactured products through a uniform regulatory framework. A notable legislative development in this area is the 21st Century Cures Act, which defines regencrative medicine treatments as meeting the definition of 'regenerative medicine therapy'. Cell treatments, human cell and tissue products, therapeutic tissue engineering products, combination products utilizing these therapeutic approaches, and gene therapies that result in long-term alterations to cells or tissues fall under this category. To shape the course of 3D bioprinting in healthcare, FDA proactively disseminated thorough advice tailored for 3D printer manufacturers (Food and Drug Administration, 2017). However, the regulatory landscape becomes complex when considering functional 3D bioprinted structures that host living cells and bioactive materials. First, the fundamental difference between these constructs from conventional clinical products stems from the complex mechanisms at play and long-term repercussions in the human host that have not yet been elucidated. Secondly, the versatile nature of tissue structures poses a regulatory dilemma, since mechanisms of action rely on a large number of active ingredients, making compliance with a standardized definition of strength difficult. Thirdly, the fabrication and product characterization of these structures pose significant complexity; seemingly inconspicuous changes in the manufacturing process can cause profound and unpredictable changes in the properties of the product. Consequently, a convincing and clear regulatory pathway is essential to stay away from the emergence of burdensome and unnecessary regulatory pathways. Regulatory frameworks must rigorously explain how current legal framework and policy governing traditional device manufacturing apply to non-traditional organizations, such as medical institutions and academic institutions, that engage in the creation of 3D printed personalized devices.

Positively, current guidance and regulatory frameworks put forward by the FDA and other domestic regulatory agencies demonstrate awareness of these multifaceted issues. Furthermore, confluence of production processes in technology and increasing emphasis on standardization and codification of optimal procedures for the creation and manufacture of printed structures offer ways in which some inherent regulatory challenges can be effectively alleviated. The combination of evolving regulatory frameworks and technological advances holds promise for the seamless integration of 3D bioprinting into mainstream healthcare and heralds a paradigm shift in therapeutic interventions (Murphy et al., 2020).

5.5 Logistics

The logistical challenges inherent in the transportation of products containing living cells and tissues are compounded by their inherent environmental and time-sensitive nature. This complexity is particularly pronounced when contemplating the manufacturing of patient-specific tissues or organs. Patient-care facilities are unlikely to possess 3D printing capabilities or the requisite infrastructure for the clinical-grade production of cells and materials, thereby necessitating a sophisticated logistical chain to bridge these gaps. Present cold storage shipping protocols, conceived decades ago, fall short of meeting the precision and performance standards requisite for the transportation of living biological products. To address this deficiency, the conceptualization and implementation of a novel shipping system are imperative. Such a system should be meticulously designed to ensure the requisite stability, effective communication, data collection, and documented compliance, taking into account the intricacies associated with the transfer of medical data essential for the design of fabricated tissues or organs.

Given the scarcity of facilities equipped with the requisite expertise, technology, and resources for the production of tissues and organs for transplantation, a centralized logistical model may prove indispensable, at least in the initial phases of implementation. This could entail the strategic establishment of several major facilities capable of undertaking comprehensive biofabrication processes. In such a scenario, patient-derived cells and materials would be transported to these centralized biofabrication facilities, where the manufacturing process would take place. Subsequently, the biofabricated organs would undergo systematic shipping protocols for their return to the patient. The blueprint for the shipping logistics could draw inspiration from established practices within traditional organ procurement and transplantation programs. Such programs have historically prioritized the development of optimal systems and practices for organ procurement, multi-site coordination, preservation, and transportation. Adapting and augmenting these practices to align with the unique demands of shipping living biological products would be integral to the successful establishment of an efficient and reliable logistical framework for the burgeoning field of biofabrication. Additionally, this approach may also necessitate the strategic distribution of major biofabrication facilities, mirroring the geographical considerations inherent in organ-procurement programs, to maximize efficiency and minimize transportation-related challenges.

6. Conclusion and Future Perspectives

In the past decade, bioprinting has evolved from basic cell dispensing to creating intricate structures like alveolar models and heart-like tissues. Despite the daunting goal of constructing entire organs cell-by-cell, its achievement could revolutionize medicine (Kang et al., 2016; Lee et al., 2019). Future bioprinting endeavours should prioritize addressing key challenges to advance the field, beyond hardware development and commercialization. Creating a whole organ, layer by layer, from cells to proteins, using a machine, is a significant undertaking. If successful, it could revolutionize both medicine and engineering. Hence, it is crucial to approach all the mentioned challenges with a deep understanding of the actual complexities involved in addressing them. Subsequent research efforts should prioritize identifying the essential challenges that will genuinely advance the field, rather than pursuing tangential directions. Recent years have seen a surge in bioprinting hardware development, with costs ranging from a few thousand to several hundred thousand. Biologists express concerns that high-cost systems may not adequately address crucial challenges in tissue reconstruction, while engineers highlight the precision in biomaterial dispensing offered by the hardware, underscoring the need for a shared responsibility between the two disciplines. A balanced approach calls for engineering tools focused on biological challenges rather than solely on speed and cost. Prioritizing functional properties over high-resolution biomaterial dispensing, this approach aims to identify barriers to bioprinting complex tissues. Achieving the goal of bioprinting ideal organs for human implantation requires a well-balanced collaboration between engineering and biology. To sum up, while numerous obstacles lie ahead, the promising future of bioprinting is justified, and the rapid progress in recent advancements suggests a positive outlook.

References

Abka-khajouei, R., Tounsi, L., Shahabi, N., Patel, A.K., Abdelkafi, S. et al. (2022). Structures, Properties and Applications of Alginates. In *Marine Drugs* (Vol. 20, Issue 6). MDPI. https://doi.org/10.3390/md20060364

Adhikari, J., Roy, A., Das, A., Ghosh, M., Thomas, S. et al. (2021). Effects of Processing Parameters of 3D Bioprinting on the Cellular Activity of Bioinks. In *Macromolecular Bioscience* (Vol. 21, Issue 1). https://doi.org/10.1002/mabi.202000179

Aramwit, P. (2016). Introduction to biomaterials for wound healing. *Wound Healing Biomaterials*, 2, 3–38. https://doi.org/10.1016/B978-1-78242-456-7.00001-5

Azizi Machekposhti, S., Mohaved, S. and Narayan, R.J. (2019). Inkjet dispensing technologies: recent advances for novel drug discovery. In *Expert Opinion on Drug Discovery* (Vol. 14, Issue 2). https://doi.org/10.1080/17460441.2019.1567489

Bedir, T., Ulag, S., Ustundag, C.B. and Gunduz, O. (2020). 3D bioprinting applications in neural tissue engineering for spinal cord injury repair. In *Materials Science and Engineering C*. https://doi.org/10.1016/j.msec.2020.110741

Belyadi, H., Fathi, E. and Belyadi, F. (2019). Hydraulic fracturing chemical selection and design. *Hydraulic Fracturing in Unconventional Reservoirs*, 107–120. https://doi.org/10.1016/B978-0-12-817665-8.00008-4

Billiet, T., Gevaert, E., De Schryver, T., Cornelissen, M. and Dubruel, P. et al. (2014). The 3D printing of gelatin methacrylamide cell-laden tissue-engineered constructs with high cell viability. *Biomaterials*, *35*(1). https://doi.org/10.1016/j.biomaterials.2013.09.078

Boularaoui, S., Al Hussein, G., Khan, K.A., Christoforou, N. and Stefanini, C. et al. (2020). An overview of extrusion-based bioprinting with a focus on induced shear stress and its effect on cell viability. In *Bioprinting* (Vol. 20). https://doi.org/10.1016/j.bprint.2020.e00093

Brindha, J., Privita Edwina, R.G., Rajesh, P.K. and Rani, P. (2016). *Influence of rheological properties of protein bio-inks on printability: a simulation and validation study*. 3, 3285–3295. www.sciencedirect.comwww.materialstoday.com/proceedings

Cai, Y., Chang, S.Y., Gan, S.W., Ma, S., Feng Lu, W. et al. (2022). Nanocomposite bioinks for 3D bioprinting. *Acta Biomaterialia*, *151*, 45–69. https://doi.org/10.1016/j.actbio.2022.08.014

Caviezel, D., Narayanan, C. and Lakehal, D. (2008). Adherence and bouncing of liquid droplets impacting on dry surfaces. *Microfluidics and Nanofluidics, 5*(4). https://doi.org/10.1007/s10404-007-0248-2

Chakrapani, G., Zare, M. and Ramakrishna, S. (2022). *Biomaterials from the value-added food wastes.* https://doi.org/10.1016/j.biteb.2022.101181

Chaturvedi, I., Jandyal, A., Wazir, I., Raina, A., Irfan, M. et al. (2022). *Biomimetics and 3D printing-Opportunities for design applications.* https://doi.org/10.1016/j.sintl.2022.100191

Chen, X.B., Fazel Anvari-Yazdi, A., Duan, X., Zimmerling, A., Gharraei, R. et al. (2023). Biomaterials / bioinks and extrusion bioprinting. In *Bioactive Materials* (Vol. 28, pp. 511–536). KeAi Communications Co. https://doi.org/10.1016/j.bioactmat.2023.06.006

Cui, H., Nowicki, M., Fisher, J.P. and Zhang, L.G. (2017). 3D Bioprinting for Organ Regeneration. In *Advanced Healthcare Materials* (Vol. 6, Issue 1). https://doi.org/10.1002/adhm.201601118

Dababneh, A.B. and Ozbolat, I.T. (2014). Bioprinting Technology: A Current State-of-the-Art Review. *Journal of Manufacturing Science and Engineering, Transactions of the ASME.* https://doi.org/10.1115/1.4028512

Darvell, B.W. (2018). Rheology. *Materials Science for Dentistry, 92–120.* https://doi.org/10.1016/B978-0-08-101035-8.50004-3

Du Plessis, A., Babafemi, A.J., Chandra Paul, S., Panda, B., Tran, J.P. et al. . (2020). *Biomimicry for 3D concrete printing: A review and perspective.* https://doi.org/10.1016/j.addma.2020.101823

Fedorovich, N.E., Oudshoorn, M.H., van Geemen, D., Hennink, W.E., Alblas, J. e al. (2009). The effect of photopolymerization on stem cells embedded in hydrogels. *Biomaterials, 30*(3). https://doi.org/10.1016/j.biomaterials.2008.09.037

Fisher, J.P., Dean, D. and Mikos, A.G. (2002). Photocrosslinking characteristics and mechanical properties of diethyl fumarate/poly(propylene fumarate) biomaterials. *Biomaterials, 23*(22), 4333–4343. https://doi.org/10.1016/S0142-9612(02)00178-3

Food and Drug Administration. (2017). Technical Considerations for Additive Manufactured Medical Devices:Guidance for Industry and Food and Drug Administration Staff Document. In *Center for Devices and Radiological Health.*

Ghavaminejad, A., Ashammakhi, N., Wu, X.Y., Khademhosseini, A. and Khademhosseini, Ali et al. (2020). *Crosslinking Strategies for Three-Dimensional Bioprinting of Polymeric Hydrogels.* https://doi.org/10.1002/smll.202002931

Gillispie, G.J., Copus, J., Uzun-Per, M., Yoo, J.J., Atala, A. et al. (2023). *The correlation between rheological properties and extrusion-based printability in bioink artifact quantification.* https://doi.org/10.1016/j.matdes.2023.112237

Gorroñogoitia, I., Urtaza, U., Zubiarrain-Laserna, A., Alonso-Varona, A. and Zaldua, A.M. et al. (2022). A Study of the Printability of Alginate-Based Bioinks by 3D Bioprinting for Articular Cartilage Tissue Engineering. *Polymers, 14*(2). https://doi.org/10.3390/polym14020354

Guo, Y., Wang, X., Shen, Y., Dong, K., Shen, L. et al. (2022). *Research progress, models and simulation of electrospinning technology: a review.* https://doi.org/10.1007/s10853-021-06575-w

Gupta, S., Alrabaiah, | Hussam, Christophe, M., Mohammad Rahimi-Gorj et al (2020). *Evaluation of silk-based bioink during pre and post 3D bioprinting: A review.* https://doi.org/10.1002/jbm.b.34699

Guvendiren, M., Purcell, B. and Burdick, J.A. (2012). Photopolymerizable Systems. *Polymer Science: A Comprehensive Reference: Volume 1-10, 1–10,* 413–438. https://doi.org/10.1016/B978-0-444-53349-4.00227-2

He, H., Li, D., Lin, Z., Peng, L., Yang, J. et al. (2020). Temperature-programmable and enzymatically solidifiable gelatin-based bioinks enable facile extrusion bioprinting. *Biofabrication, 12*(4), 045003. https://doi.org/10.1088/1758-5090/AB9906

Hölzl, K., Lin, S., Tytgat, L., Van Vlierberghe, S., Gu, L. et al. (2016). Bioink properties before, during and after 3D bioprinting. In *Biofabrication* (Vol. 8, Issue 3). https://doi.org/10.1088/1758-5090/8/3/032002

Hong, S., Kim, J.S., Jung, B., Won, C. and Hwang, C. et al. (2019). Coaxial bioprinting of cell-laden vascular constructs using a gelatin-tyramine bioink. *Biomaterials Science, 7*(11), 4578–4587. https://doi.org/10.1039/c8bm00618k

Hou, Y.C., Cui, X., Qin, Z., Su, C., Zhang, G. et al. (2023). Three-dimensional bioprinting of artificial blood vessel: Process, bioinks and challenges. *International Journal of Bioprinting, 9*(4). https://doi.org/10.18063/ijb.740

Hunsberger, J.G., Goel, S., Allickson, J. and Atala, A. (2017). Five Critical Areas that Combat High Costs and Prolonged Development Times for Regenerative Medicine Manufacturing. *Current Stem Cell Reports, 3*(2), 77–82. https://doi.org/10.1007/s40778-017-0083-7

Ilhan, E., Ozerol, E. A., Alpdagtas, S., Sengor, M., Ustundag, C.B. et al (2021). *Biofunctional Inks for 3D Printing in Skin Tissue Engineering.* 229–259. https://doi.org/10.1007/978-981-16-4667-6_7

Ilhan, E., Ulag, S., Sahin, A., Yilmaz, B.K., Ekren, N. et al. (2020). Fabrication of tissue-engineered tympanic membrane patches using 3D-Printing technology. *Journal of the Mechanical Behavior of Biomedical Materials, 114*(November 2020), 104219. https://doi.org/10.1016/j.jmbbm.2020.104219

Institute of Electrical and Electronics Engineers, IEEE Thailand Section, & Thai Biomedical Engineering Association. (2019). *BMEiCON-2019 : the 12th Biomedical Engineering International Conference : November 19-22, 2019, Ubon Ratchathani, Thailand and Pakse, Laos.*

Jafarkhani, M., Salehi, Z., Aidun, A. and Shokrgozar, M.A. (2019). *Bioprinting in Vascularization Strategies.* https://doi.org/10.29252/ibj.23.1.9

Jiang, Z., Diggle, B., Tan, M.L., Viktorova, J., Bennett, C.W. et al. (2020). Extrusion 3D Printing of Polymeric Materials with Advanced Properties. In *Advanced Science* (Vol. 7, Issue 17). John Wiley and Sons Inc. https://doi.org/10.1002/advs.202001379

Jovic, T.H., Combellack, E.J., Jessop, Z.M. and Whitaker, I.S. (2020). 3D Bioprinting and the Future of Surgery. In *Frontiers in Surgery* (Vol. 7). https://doi.org/10.3389/fsurg.2020.609836

Kang, H.-W., Lee, S.J., Ko, I.K., Kengla, C., Yoo, J.J. et al. (2016). A 3D bioprinting system to produce human-scale tissue constructs with structural integrity. *Nature Biotechnology, 34*(3), 312–319. https://doi.org/10.1038/nbt.3413

Kengla, C., Renteria, E., Wivell, C., Atala, A., Yoo, J.J. et al. (2017). Clinically Relevant Bioprinting Workflow and Imaging Process for Tissue Construct Design and Validation. *3D Printing and Additive Manufacturing, 4*(4), 239–247. https://doi.org/10.1089/3dp.2017.0075

Kim, S.S., Utsunomiya, H., Koski, J.A., Wu, B.M., Cima, M.J. et al (1998). Survival and Function of Hepatocytes on a Novel Three-Dimensional Synthetic Biodegradable Polymer Scaffold With an Intrinsic Network of Channels. *Annals of Surgery, 228*(1).

Kumar, P., Ebbens, S. and Zhao, X. (2021). Inkjet printing of mammalian cells – Theory and applications. In *Bioprinting* (Vol. 23). https://doi.org/10.1016/j.bprint.2021.e00157

Kumar, S. (2021). Synthetic polymer-derived single-network inks/bioinks for extrusion-based 3D printing towards bioapplications. *Cite This: Mater. Adv, 2,* 6928. https://doi.org/10.1039/d1ma00525a

Kutlehria, S. and Sachdeva, M.S. (2021). Role of In Vitro Models for Development of Ophthalmic Delivery Systems. In *Critical reviews in therapeutic drug carrier systems* (Vol. 38, Issue 3). https://doi.org/10.1615/CritRevTherDrugCarrierSyst.2021035222

Lai, J., Wang, C. and Wang, M. (2021). 3D printing in biomedical engineering: Processes, materials, and applications. *Applied Physics Reviews, 8*(2), 21322. https://doi.org/10.1063/5.0024177

Lee, A., Hudson, A.R., Shiwarski, D.J., Tashman, J.W., Hinton, T.J. et al. (2019). 3D bioprinting of collagen to rebuild components of the human heart. *Science (New York, N.Y.), 365*(6452), 482–487. https://doi.org/10.1126/science.aav9051

Lee, H., Jang, T.S., Han, G., Kim, H.W. and Jung, H. Do. et al. (2021). Freeform 3D printing of vascularized tissues: Challenges and strategies. *Journal of Tissue Engineering, 12,* 1–34. https://doi.org/10.1177/20417314211057236

Lee, K.Y. and Mooney, D.J. (2012). Alginate: properties and biomedical applications. *Progress in Polymer Science, 37*(1), 106. https://doi.org/10.1016/J.PROGPOLYMSCI.2011.06.003

Lee, V.K., Dias, A., Ozturk, M.S., Chen, K., Tricomi, B. et al. (2015). 3D bioprinting and 3D imaging for stem cell engineering. In *Bioprinting in Regenerative Medicine.* https://doi.org/10.1007/978-3-319-21386-6_2

Lepowsky, E., Muradoglu, M. and Tasoglu, S. (2018). Towards preserving post-printing cell viability and improving the resolution: Past, present, and future of 3D bioprinting theory. In *Bioprinting* (Vol. 11). https://doi.org/10.1016/j.bprint.2018.e00034

Leucht, A., Volz, A.-C., Rogal, J., Borchers, K. and Kluger, P.J. et al. (2020). *Advanced gelatin-based vascularization bioinks for extrusion-based bioprinting of vascularized bone equivalents.* https://doi.org/10.1038/s41598-020-62166-w

Li, Y., Zhu, J., Cheng, H., Li, G., Cho, H. et al. (2021). Developments of Advanced Electrospinning Techniques: A Critical Review. In *Advanced Materials Technologies* (Vol. 6, Issue 11). John Wiley and Sons Inc. https://doi.org/10.1002/admt.202100410

Li, Z., Huang, S., Liu, Y., Yao, B., Hu, T. et al. (2018). *Tuning Alginate-Gelatin Bioink Properties by Varying Solvent and Their Impact on Stem Cell Behavior.* https://doi.org/10.1038/s41598-018-26407-3

Lin, L., Jiang, S., Yang, J., Qiu, J., Jiao, X. et al. (2023). Application of 3D-bioprinted nanocellulose and cellulose derivative-based bio-inks in bone and cartilage tissue engineering. *International Journal of Bioprinting, 9.* https://doi.org/10.18063/ijb.v9i1.637

Liu, F. and Wang, X. (2020). Synthetic polymers for organ 3D printing. In *Polymers* (Vol. 12, Issue 8). https://doi.org/10.3390/polym12081765

Ma, Y., Deng, B., He, R. and Huang, P. (2024a). Advancements of 3D bioprinting in regenerative medicine: Exploring cell sources for organ fabrication. *Heliyon, 10*(3), e24593. https://doi.org/10.1016/j.heliyon.2024.e24593

Ma, Y., Deng, B., He, R. and Huang, P. (2024b). Advancements of 3D bioprinting in regenerative medicine: Exploring cell sources for organ fabrication. *Heliyon, 10*(3), e24593. https://doi.org/10.1016/j.heliyon.2024.e24593

Malekpour, A. and Chen, X. (2022). Printability and Cell Viability in Extrusion-Based Bioprinting from Experimental, Computational, and Machine Learning Views. In *Journal of Functional Biomaterials* (Vol. 13, Issue 2). https://doi.org/10.3390/jfb13020040

Malik, A., Ul Haq, M.I., Raina, A. and Gupta, K. (2022). 3D printing towards implementing Industry 4.0: sustainability aspects, barriers and challenges. *Industrial Robot, 49*(3), 491–511. https://doi.org/10.1108/IR-10-2021-0247

Masson-Meyers, D.S. and Tayebi, L. (2021). Vascularization strategies in tissue engineering approaches for soft tissue repair. *Journal of Tissue Engineering and Regenerative Medicine, 15*(9), 747. https://doi.org/10.1002/TERM.3225

Miller, J.S., Stevens, K.R., Yang, M.T., Baker, B.M., Nguyen, D.-H.T et al. (2012). Rapid casting of patterned vascular networks for perfusable engineered three-dimensional tissues. *Nature Materials, 11*(9), 768–774. https://doi.org/10.1038/nmat3357

Mir, A., Lee, E., Shih, W., Koljaka, S., Wang, A. et al. (2023). 3D Bioprinting for Vascularization. In *Bioengineering* (Vol. 10, Issue 5). MDPI. https://doi.org/10.3390/bioengineering10050606

Moldoveanu, S. and David, V. (2022). Affinity, immunoaffinity, and aptamer type HPLC. *Essentials in Modern HPLC Separations*, 559–569. https://doi.org/10.1016/B978-0-323-91177-1.00008-9

Moreira, F., Guerreiro, J., Brandão, L. and Sales, M.G. (2015). Synthesis of molecular biomimetics. In *Biomimetic Technologies: Principles and Applications* (pp. 3–31). https://doi.org/10.1016/B978-0-08-100249-0.00001-X

Murphy, S.V, De Coppi, P. and Atala, A. (2020). Opportunities and challenges of translational 3D bioprinting. *Nature Biomedical Engineering, 4*(4), 370–380. https://doi.org/10.1038/s41551-019-0471-7

Muthukrishnan, L. (2021). *Imminent antimicrobial bioink deploying cellulose, alginate, EPS and synthetic polymers for 3D bioprinting of tissue constructs*. https://doi.org/10.1016/j.carbpol.2021.117774

Naghieh, S. and Chen, X. (2021). Printability—A key issue in extrusion-based bioprinting. In *Journal of Pharmaceutical Analysis* (Vol. 11, Issue 5). https://doi.org/10.1016/j.jpha.2021.02.001

Noh, I., Kim, N., Tran, H.N., Lee, J. and Lee, C. et al. (2019). 3D printable hyaluronic acid-based hydrogel for its potential application as a bioink in tissue engineering. *Biomaterials Research, 23*(1). https://doi.org/10.1186/s40824-018-0152-8

Owais, A., Khaled, M. and Yilbas, B.S. (2017). *3.9 Hydrophobicity and Surface Finish*. https://doi.org/10.1016/b978-0-12-803581-8.09172-4

Ozbolat, I.T. and Hospodiuk, M. (2016). Current advances and future perspectives in extrusion-based bioprinting. In *Biomaterials*. https://doi.org/10.1016/j.biomaterials.2015.10.076

Parihar, A., Pandita, V., Kumar, A., Parihar, D.S., Puranik, N. et al. (2022). 3D Printing: Advancement in Biogenerative Engineering to Combat Shortage of Organs and Bioapplicable Materials. In *Regenerative Engineering and Translational Medicine* (Vol. 8, Issue 2). https://doi.org/10.1007/s40883-021-00219-w

Pérez-Cortez, J.E., Sánchez-Rodríguez, V.H., Gallegos-Martínez, S., Chuck-Hernández, C., Rodriguez, C.A. et al. (2023). Low-Cost Light-Based GelMA 3D Bioprinting via Retrofitting: Manufacturability Test and Cell Culture Assessment. *Micromachines, 14*(1). https://doi.org/10.3390/mi14010055

Pradhan, S., Brooks, A.K. and Yadavalli, V.K. (2020). *Nature-derived materials for the fabrication of functional biodevices*. https://doi.org/10.1016/j.mtbio.2020.100065

Raees, S., Ullah, F., Javed, F., Akil, H.M., Jadoon Khan, M. et al. (2023). Classification, processing, and applications of bioink and 3D bioprinting: A detailed review. In *International Journal of Biological Macromolecules* (Vol. 232). Elsevier B.V. https://doi.org/10.1016/j.ijbiomac.2023.123476

Ravoor, J., Elsen, S.R., Thangavel, M., Arumugam, D. and Karuppan, D. et al. (2023). Development of hybrid multi-head, multi-material paste and ink extrusion type 3D printer for biomedical applications. *Journal of Asian Ceramic Societies, 11*(4). https://doi.org/10.1080/21870764.2023.2247210

Richards, D.J., Tan, Y., Jia, J., Yao, H. and Mei, Y. et al. (2013). 3D Printing for Tissue Engineering. *Israel Journal of Chemistry, 53*(9–10), 805–814. https://doi.org/https://doi.org/10.1002/ijch.201300086

Richards, D., Jia, J., Yost, M., Markwald, R. and Mei, Y. et al. (2016). 3D Bioprinting for Vascularized Tissue Fabrication. *Annals of Biomedical Engineering 2016 45:1, 45*(1), 132–147. https://doi.org/10.1007/S10439-016-1653-Z

Robb, B. and Lennox, B. (2011). The electrospinning process, conditions and control. *Electrospinning for Tissue Regeneration*, 51–66. https://doi.org/10.1533/9780857092915.1.51

Rodriguez, M.J., Brown, J., Giordano, J., Lin, S.J., Omenetto, F.G. et al. (2017). Silk based bioinks for soft tissue reconstruction using 3-dimensional (3D) printing with in vitro and in vivo assessments. *Biomaterials, 117*, 105–115. https://doi.org/10.1016/j.biomaterials.2016.11.046

Schaefer, N., Andrade Mier, M.S., Sonnleitner, D., Murenu, N., Ng, X.J. et al. (2023). Rheological and Biological Impact of Printable PCL-Fibers as Reinforcing Fillers in Cell-Laden Spider-Silk Bio-Inks. *Small Methods*, 7(10). https://doi.org/10.1002/smtd.202201717

Schuurman, W., Levett, P.A., Pot, M.W., van Weeren, P.R., Dhert, W.J.A. et al. (2013). Gelatin-methacrylamide hydrogels as potential biomaterials for fabrication of tissue-engineered cartilage constructs. *Macromolecular Bioscience*, 13(5), 551–561. https://doi.org/10.1002/mabi.201200471

Shahaboddin Ayati, S., Karevan, M., Stefanek, E., Bhia, M. and Akbari, M. et al. (2022). *Nanofibers Fabrication by Blown-Centrifugal Spinning*. https://doi.org/10.1002/mame.202100368

Shahrubudin, N., Koshy, P., Alipal, J., Kadir, M.H.A. and Lee, T.C. et al. (2020). Challenges of 3D printing technology for manufacturing biomedical products: A case study of Malaysian manufacturing firms. *Heliyon*, 6(4), e03734. https://doi.org/https://doi.org/10.1016/j.heliyon.2020.e03734

Sin, L.T. and Tueen, B.S. (2019). Rheological Properties of Poly (Lactic Acid). *Polylactic Acid*, 203–225. https://doi.org/10.1016/B978-0-12-814472-5.00006-6

Sionkowska, A., Gadomska, M., Musiał, K. and Piatek, J. (2020). Hyaluronic Acid as a Component of Natural Polymer Blends for Biomedical Applications: A Review. *Molecules*, 25(18). https://doi.org/10.3390/MOLECULES25184035

Su, C., Chen, Y., Tian, S., Lu, C. and Lv, Q. et al. (2022). Natural Materials for 3D Printing and Their Applications. *Gels*, 8(11). https://doi.org/10.3390/gels8110748

Summerscales, J. and Grove, S. (2014). Manufacturing methods for natural fibre composites. *Natural Fibre Composites: Materials, Processes and Applications*, 176–215. https://doi.org/10.1533/9780857099228.2.176

Sundararaghavan, H.G. and Burdick, J.A. (2011). Cell Encapsulation. *Comprehensive Biomaterials*, 5, 115–130. https://doi.org/10.1016/B978-0-08-055294-1.00163-X

Szymańska, E. and Winnicka, K. (2015). Marine drugs Stability of Chitosan-A Challenge for Pharmaceutical and Biomedical Applications. *Mar. Drugs*, 13, 1819–1846. https://doi.org/10.3390/md13041819

Tanzeglock, T., Soos, M., Stephanopoulos, G. and Morbidelli, M. (2009). Induction of mammalian cell death by simple shear and extensional flows. *Biotechnology and Bioengineering*. https://doi.org/10.1002/bit.22405

Thomas-Seale, L.E.J., Kirkman-Brown, J.C., Attallah, M.M., Espino, D.M. and Shepherd, D.E.T. et al. (2018). The barriers to the progression of additive manufacture: Perspectives from UK industry. *International Journal of Production Economics*, 198, 104–118. https://doi.org/https://doi.org/10.1016/j.ijpe.2018.02.003

Tibbits, S. (2012). Design to Self-Assembly. *Architectural Design*, 82(2), 68–73. https://doi.org/https://doi.org/10.1002/ad.1381

Varanko, A., Saha, S. and Chilkoti, A. (2020). *Recent trends in protein and peptide-based biomaterials for advanced drug delivery*. https://doi.org/10.1016/j.addr.2020.08.008

Velasco, D., Quílez, C., Garcia, M., del Cañizo, J.F. and Jorcano, J.L. et al. (2018). 3D human skin bioprinting: a view from the bio side. *Journal of 3D Printing in Medicine*. https://doi.org/10.2217/3dp-2018-0008

Venkata Krishna, D. and Ravi Sankar, M. (2023). Persuasive factors on the bioink printability and cell viability in the extrusion-based 3D bioprinting for tissue regeneration applications. *Engineered Regeneration*, 4, 396–410. https://doi.org/10.1016/j.engreg.2023.07.002

Wallace, H.A., Basehore, B.M. and Zito, P.M. (2023). Wound Healing Phases. *StatPearls*. https://www.ncbi.nlm.nih.gov/books/NBK470443/

Wang, X., Wang, Q. and Xu, C. (2020). *Nanocellulose-Based Inks for 3D Bioprinting: Key Aspects in Research Development and Challenging Perspectives in Applications-A Mini Review*. https://doi.org/10.3390/bioengineering7020040

Wragg, N.M., Burke, L. and Wilson, S.L. (2019). A critical review of current progress in 3D kidney biomanufacturing: Advances, challenges, and recommendations. In *Renal Replacement Therapy* (Vol. 5, Issue 1). https://doi.org/10.1186/s41100-019-0218-7

Wu, C., Wang, H. and Cao, J. (2023). Tween-80 improves single/coaxial electrospinning of three-layered bioartificial blood vessel. *Journal of Materials Science: Materials in Medicine*, 34(1), 1–15. https://doi.org/10.1007/S10856-022-06707-X/FIGURES/14

Wu, W. (2020). Study on 3D printing technology and mechanical properties of a nano-enhanced composite hydrogel bio-ink. *Micro & Nano Letters*. https://doi.org/10.1049/mnl.2019.0712

Xie, Z., Gao, M., Lobo, A.O. and Webster, T.J. (2020a). 3D bioprinting in tissue engineering for medical applications: The classic and the hybrid. In *Polymers* (Vol. 12, Issue 8). https://doi.org/10.3390/POLYM12081717

Xie, Z., Gao, M., Lobo, A.O. and Webster, T.J. (2020b). 3D bioprinting in tissue engineering for medical applications: The classic and the hybrid. In *Polymers* (Vol. 12, Issue 8). MDPI AG. https://doi.org/10.3390/POLYM12081717

Xu, L., Sheybani, N., Yeudall, W.A. and Yang, H. (2015). The effect of photoinitiators on intracellular AKT signaling pathway in tissue engineering application. *Biomaterials Science*, 3(2). https://doi.org/10.1039/c4bm00245h

Yang, Q., Gao, B. and Xu, F. (2020). Recent Advances in 4D Bioprinting. In *Biotechnology Journal* (Vol. 15, Issue 1). https://doi.org/10.1002/biot.201900086

Zhang, J., Hu, Q., Wang, S., Tao, J. and Gou, M. et al. (2020). Digital light processing based three-dimensional printing for medical applications. *International Journal of Bioprinting*, 6(1), 12–27. https://doi.org/10.18063/ijb.v6i1.242

Zhang, S., Li, G., Man, J., Zhang, S., Li, J et al. (2020). *Fabrication of Microspheres from High-Viscosity Bioink Using a Novel Microfluidic-Based 3D Bioprinting Nozzle.* https://doi.org/10.3390/mi11070681

Zhang, W. (2022). Recent Progress in Bioprinting: From Bioink Design to Applications. In *Bioengineering* (Vol. 9, Issue 12). https://doi.org/10.3390/bioengineering9120785

Zheng, Q., Lu, J., Chen, H., Huang, L., Cai, J. et al. (2011). Application of inkjet printing technique for biological material delivery and antimicrobial assays. *Analytical Biochemistry*, *410*(2), 171–176. https://doi.org/https://doi.org/10.1016/j.ab.2010.10.024

Advantages and Disadvantages of 3D Bioprinting

Rashmi Ramakrishnan[1] and Abhirami Dinesan[2]*

1. Introduction

Three dimensional (3D) bioprinting is an advanced technology that has emerged from the existing additive manufacturing technique 3D printing. The custom fabricating technique of 3D printing has the potential to drastically upend the global consumer market and spark a manufacturing revolution. Over the past decades, 3D bioprinting has been extensively used for the fabrication of a wide range of tissues/organs. This not only lays the groundwork for the ultimate goal of organ replacement, but also serves as a valuable *in vitro* model for exploring pharmacokinetics, drug screening and related search endeavours. The origins of 3D printing date back to the 1980's, with a significant milestone occurring when Charles Hull patented the first commercial 3D printing technology in 1984. This pivotal moment marked the inception of 3D printing and laid the foundation for the development of 3D bioprinting. Bioprinting made its debut in 1988, when Robert J Klebe utilized an inkjet printer to print cells, further expanding the possibilities of this technology. In 1999, Odde and Renn pioneered the use of laser-assisted bioprinting for living cells, aiming to create models with intricate anatomical structures (Gu et al., 2020).

There are various approaches to 3D bioprinting, comprising biomimicry, autonomous self-assembly and mini-tissue building blocks. In 2001, there was a significant advancement in medical technology, where Atala and his team 3D printed bladder-shaped scaffolds and subsequently infused it with human cells for tissue engineering purposes. Functional bladders, cultivated through the bioprinting of tissue derived from a patient's own cells, have already been successfully transplanted into the human body, marking a significant achievement in the field (Atala, 2011). In 2003, Boland et al revolutionized bioprinting with a modified office inkjet printer, which later served as the basis for all modern bioprinters. In 2004, Gabor Forgacs pioneered the first printer using living cells without

[1]   CÚRAM, Science Foundation Ireland Research Centre for Medical Devices, University of Galway, Galway, Ireland.
[2]   Amrita School of Nanosciences and Molecular Medicine, Amrita Institute of Medical Sciences and Research Centre, Amrita Vishwa Vidyapeetham, Ernakulam, India.
*   Corresponding author: rashmi.ramakrishnan@universityofgalway.ie; roshrashmi@gmail.com

the need for cell scaffolding (Kachouie et al., 2010). In 2006, the initial instance of printing involving the encapsulation of cells within hydrogels occurred, where liver cells were bioprinted to create an *in vitro* model utilized for pharmacokinetic investigations (Chang et al., 2006). In 2009, Norotte et al. employed bioprinting techniques to engineer vascular tissue devoid of scaffolds (Norotte et al, 2009). In 2012, Skardal and colleagues experimented with *in situ* bioprinting on mouse models (Skardal et al., 2012). In 2019 Noor et al. developed the first perfusable scale-down 3D printed heart. Ramasamy et al. synthesized an artificial skin using an extrusion-based 3D bioprinter (Ramasamy et al., 2021). Researchers are continually exploring the potential of bioprinting to fabricate other functional organs, expanding the scope of possibilities.

2. Workflow of 3D Bioprinting

3D bioprinting entails the precise layering of biomaterials to construct intricate, living structures. In essence, the procedure can be summarized through three fundamental stages: pre-bioprinting, bioprinting and post-bioprinting. The initial stage, known as the preparatory or pre-bioprinting phase is the designing of anatomically accurate 3D models. Raw imaging data from medical imaging modalities like X-ray, computed tomography (CT) and magnetic resonance imaging (MRI) can be processed using tomographic reconstruction to produce 2D cross-sectional images which can be converted into 3D models via computer graphics software such as computer-aided design and computer-aided manufacturing (CAD-CAM) and mathematical modelling techniques. Additionally, the preparatory phase encompasses the critical selection of biomaterials, bioinks, cell types, extracellular matrix (ECM) proteins and bioactive molecules for use in the subsequent steps. Common biomaterials used are synthetic, natural or composite polymers as well as decellularized ECM. Cell sources may be allogeneic or autologous stem cells, primary cells or cell lines depending on the field of application. Through the application of CAD, the internal and external features of the scaffold architecture, including aspects like porosity and pore sizes, can be integrated into the 3D model of the tissue defect (Kačarević et al., 2018). This crucial stage ensures the accurate translation of the anatomical details from medical imaging into the digital model, contributing to the success of 3D bioprinting.

Moving on to the processing or bioprinting phase, it involves the actual printing of tissues using additive manufacturing techniques. The utilization of machine learning algorithms plays a crucial role in enhancing various parameters during the printing process. This includes optimizing the quality of the process and the printed parts, as well as predicting potential anomalies. Bioinks, which are liquid mixtures encompassing cells, matrix materials, and nutrients, are loaded into a printer cartridge and then precisely deposited. Since different cell types naturally compose every tissue in the body, the technologies used for 3D bioprinting such as inkjet, microextrusion or laser-assisted printers, must ensure the stability and viability of cells throughout the manufacturing process as well. This step is crucial for translating the designed 3D models into tangible biological constructs through the bioprinter (Shin et al., 2022).

The final stage is referred to as post-processing/bioprinting. Here, the printed tissues may require a period of maturation in a bioreactor before transplantation, where the printed tissues undergo structural development and functional maturation, which assess the quality of printed results in various bioprinting procedures. Alternatively the 3D tissue may be used for *in vitro* applications. Validation of potential maturity factors through experimentation is vital for advancing tissue maturation and preserving tissue properties. Frequent challenges encountered during the post-printing phase include discrepancies between the envisioned printed results and the actual outcomes concerning design and cell proliferation (Zhao et al., 2021). Figure 1 explains the technical details in each phase of bioprinting.

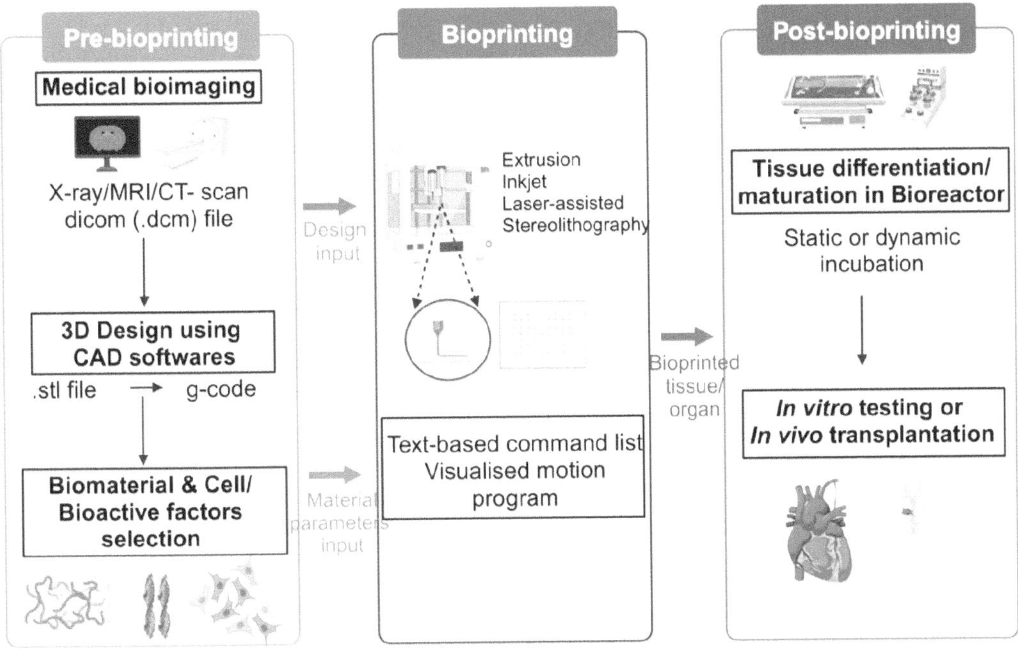

Fig. 1 Bioprinting process comprises pre-bioprinting, bioprinting and post-bioprinting stages which will result in creation of 3D bioprinted organ/tissue for *in vitro* testing or *in vivo* implantation. Here, data from the medical bioimaging input/acquisition is used to generate the 3D CAD model, where a visualized motion program is generated, and instructions to print the construct are transmitted to the computer using a text-based command to print the design. Abbreviations: MRI, magnetic resonance imaging; CT, computed tomography; DICOM, digital imaging and communications in medicine; CAD, computer-aided design; STL, STereoLithography File Format; g-code, geometric Code (Illustration created with BioRender.com).

3. Types of 3D Bioprinting

3.1 *Extrusion-based Bioprinting*

Extrusion-based bioprinting is the most common method which incorporates semi-solid extrusion (SSE) or fused deposition modelling (FDM) and has found extensive applications across diverse biomedical fields. Extrusion-based bioprinting extrudes bioink (typically from a syringe) via a nozzle using mechanical or pneumatic forces to generate continuous microfilaments, which are then deposited on the receiving substrate and stacked into desired shapes. Extrusion-based bioprinters commonly feature multiple print heads, enabling the simultaneous deposition of various materials within a single construct. This functionality empowers researchers to fabricate constructs that exhibit regional variations in biomaterials, cell types, cell densities, and signalling molecules, facilitating the creation of complex and heterogeneous tissue models. The common extrusion-based bioprinting can be classified into pneumatic, piston and screw-driven. A pneumatic-driven extrusion system utilizes compressed air to realize liquid dispensing. Mechanical driven liquid dispensing systems such as piston-driven are suitable for extrusion of high viscosity biomaterials whereas screw-driven extrusions provide more volumetric control. However, screw-driven systems might damage the cells loaded in the bioink (Gu et al., 2020).

3.2 *Inkjet-based Bioprinting*

Inkjet based bioprinting represents a non-contact approach that relies on the expulsion of liquid droplets onto a substrate. This method is notably cost-effective and exhibits compatibility with living materials. It can be subdivided into continuous inkjet (CIJ) printing and drop-on-demand (DOD) inkjet printing. DOD can be divided as thermal, piezoelectric and electrostatic, based on the difference in droplet motivation mechanisms. Thermal inkjet bioprinting uses controllable impulsive voltage to heat the thermal actuator (e.g., film resistor) to a high temperature (typically 200-300°C), inducing the formation of an expanded bubble that exerts pressure to propel the ink through a narrow nozzle onto the substrates. Following ejection, the bioink in the nozzle is supplied by thermal actuator cooling and nozzle capillary siphoning. Despite the high temperatures capable of denaturing hydrogel material, the heating duration is sufficiently brief to have no negative influence on the stability of biocomponents. (Boland et al., 2006). Thermal inkjet bioprinting is widely used in various kinds of biologics including protein and cells. Piezoelectric technology operates by utilizing transient pressure exerted by a piezoelectric actuator to generate drops. Unlike thermal technology, the piezoelectric approach does not rely on heat, eliminating the risk of orifice clogging. This non-thermal characteristic ensures that droplets maintain their directionality, exhibiting a consistent and uniform size. The absence of heat in the piezoelectric method not only contributes to preventing clogging issues but also expands its applicability to temperature-sensitive materials. Similarly, electrostatic inkjet bioprinting exploits instantaneous volume increase to achieve ejection, by which an impulse voltage is applied to a platen and a motor, leading to a bend on platen for extrusion of bioink (Gu et al., 2020).

3.3   *Laser-assisted Bioprinting*

Laser-assisted bioprinting (LAB) utilizes laser pulses to precisely deposit biomaterials, cells and other bioinks to build 3D tissue constructs layer by layer. This method typically comprises three components, a pulsed laser source, a ribbon coated with liquid biological substances deposited on a metal film and a recipient substrate. The laser beam is directed at the ribbon, causing the liquid biological substance to evaporate. The laser pulse creates a high-pressure bubble that injects the bioink droplet from a donor slide onto the acceptor substrate. This allows precise control over the amount and pattern of deposition. The receiving substrate incorporates a biopolymer or cell culture medium to maintain cellular adhesion and sustained growth post the transfer of cells from the ribbon. LAB can achieve very high resolution on the order of single cells. The laser spot size and biomaterial properties determine the minimum printable feature size, typically 10-100 μm which enables construction of intricate and heterogeneous tissues. LAB is notable for having mild conditions that maintain high cell viability after printing. The short laser pulses minimize damage and the lack of nozzlesprevents shear stress. A wide range of cells like stem cells, endothelial cells, etc and organoids can be printed with this technique (Yu et al., 2020).

3.4   *Stereolithography*

Stereolithography (SLA), particularly utilizing photocuring-based bioprinting, is a bioprinting technique that harnesses the photopolymerization properties of photosensitive polymers under precisely controlled lighting to create intricate 3D structures. According to different light scanning modes, photocuring-based bioprinting can further be classified into SLA, and digital light processing (DLP). SLA bioprinting constructs 3D tissue structures by layering materials incrementally. To achieve this, the intended 3D model is transformed into a series of sliced 2D images. Each image represents a cross-section of the solid 3D model at a specific plane from the top, thus serving as the input for the SLA 3D bioprinting procedure. In SLA bioprinting, a liquid resin containing photopolymerizable molecules is exposed to a specific pattern of light, usually from a laser or projector. The light triggers polymerization, causing the resin to solidify layer by layer, ultimately forming the desired 3D object. The quality of printed parts is frequently influenced by the properties of the light source, impacting resolution and accuracy. Additionally, adjusting illumination conditions can fine-tune the mechanical properties of the scaffold. In SLA bioprinting, biomaterials

Table 1   Different types of 3D Bioprinting methods and their properties

Parameters	Different types of 3D Printing				References
	Extrusion	*Inkjet*	*Laser-assisted*	*Stereolithography*	
Printing process	Serial line by line	Serial drop by drop	Serial drop by drop	Parallel & Continuous (projection-based)	(Agarwal et al., 2020) (Gu et al., 2020) (Reddy et al, 2023)
Actuator	Pneumatic pressure/ Mechanical pressure/ (piston or screw) Electromagnetic driver	Piezoelectric pulse/ Thermal induced pulse/ Acoustic actuator/ Pneumatic actuator	Laser induced pulse	Laser-based curing- UV and visible light projection	
Printing Speed / Accuracy	Low-medium 10-50 µm/s	Medium-High (up to 10 000 droplets/s)	Moderate-High 200-1600 mm/s	High	
Resolution	Medium (100 µm)	High (50 µm)	High (50 µm)	High (200 nm - 6 µm)	
Dispensing mechanism	Screw/ Pneumatic/ Piston	Thermal/Piezoelectric/ Electrostatic	Laser-assisted	Photo-polymerization of photo initiators	
Supported Viscosity	30 to 6×10^7 mPa/s	Less than 0.1 Pa/s	1-300 mPa/s	No limitation	
Vertical Printing Quality	Good	Poor	Medium	Good	
Gelation Methods	Chemical/Photo- crosslinking/Temperature/	Chemical/ Photo-crosslinking	Chemical/ Photo-crosslinking	Photo-crosslinking	
Cell Viability	40-80%	>85%	85-95%	>85%	
Cell Density	Medium (10^8 cells/ml)	Low (10^6 cells/ml)	High (>10^8 cells/ml)	Medium (>10^6 cells/ml)	
Fabrication Time	Short	Medium	High	Medium	
Structural and Mechanical integrity	High	Low	Low	High	
Scalability	Yes	Yes	Limited	Yes	
Material Choice	Thermo/Photo-sensitive	Thermo/pH/Photo-sensitive	Photosensitive	Photosensitive	
Cost	Low-Medium	Low	High	Medium	
Ease of Operation	Easy	Difficult	Medium	Easy	

Contd.

Table 1 *Contd.*

Parameters	Different types of 3D Printing				References
	Extrusion	Inkjet	Laser-assisted	Stereolithography	
Example of Biomaterials used	GelMA; Alginate; PLA fibers; Collagen; Hyaluronic acid; Gelatin; Fibrin; PU	Collagen; Alginate; Fibrin; Poly (ethylene glycol) dimethacrylate (PEGDMA)	Collagen; Alginate; nano-Hydroxyapatite (nHA); Matrigel	PEGDA; GelMA	
Application/ Target Tissues	Skin; Vascular; Cartilage; Bone; Liver; Muscle/Tendon; Brain; Cardiac; Nerve	Skin; Vascular; Cartilage; Bone; Lung	Vascular; Skin; Bone; Cartilage; Adipose; Nerve	Skin; Vascular; Bone; Cartilage; Spinal cord	
Advantages	Printability of high cell density and highly viscous bioinks; Low cost	Low cost; Flexible printing; High cell viability; High resolution; High throughput non-contact printing	Non-contact, nozzle-free printing; High precision and resolution; High cell density and viability	High cell viability; High variety of printable bioinks; High resolution of bioprinting; Low printing time	
Limitations	Cell damage due to mechanical stress generated during printing; Lower resolution; Clogging nozzles	Lack of precision in droplet placement and size; Nozzle clogging; Risk of exposing cells to mechanical and thermal stress; Possibility of cell agglomeration and sedimentation; Limited printable materials (liquid only)	Time-consuming; Slow printing speed; Low flow rate caused by fast gelation; Low scalability and comparatively high costs	Potential cytotoxicity caused by the laser system under UV light; Lengthy post-processing; Crosslinking requires transparent and photosensitive bioink limiting choice of additives and cell density	

need to be capable of photo-crosslinking. SLA enables high-resolution printing and precise control over the shape and structure of the printed tissue or organ models, making it a valuable technique in tissue engineering and regenerative medicine research (Crook, 2020). The precision to construct intricate designs with superior detail has made SLA bioprinting appealing for diverse applications, spanning from the creation of implantable scaffolds to the development of advanced tissue models on microfluidic chips.

There are already many companies in medical bioprinting and few are: EnvsionTEC (Germany), RegenHu (Switzerland), Poetis (France), Organovo (USA), Sciperio/nScript (USA), Cellink (Sweden/USA), Allevi (formerly BioBots, USA), BioDevices (USA), 3Dynamics systems (USA), Advanced Solutions (USA), Aspect Biosystems (Canada), REGEMAT3D (Spain), Rokit (South Korea), 3D Bioprinting Solutions (Russia), Regenovo (China), BIO3D (Singapore) (Kirillova et al, 2020).

4.   Bioinks for 3D Bioprinting

Bioinks are specialized biomaterials designed for loading into 3D printers to construct intricate tissue-like structures, typically containing living cells, and possibly bioactive components suspended in a biocompatible matrix, which provides support and structure for the cells to grow and differentiate. Bioinks can be scaffold-based and scaffold-free. The scaffold-based bioinks consist of cells and supporting structures like hydrogels, microcarriers, or decellularized ECM. The second type is scaffold-free, where no biomaterials serve as cell carriers; instead, only cell aggregates are directly printed. Bioinks can be composed of either natural biomaterials, synthetic biomaterials independently, or a blend of both, forming hybrid biomaterials. The composition of bioink can vary depending on the specific application and the type of tissue being printed, along with cells such as stem cells, differentiated cells, or even cell lines. An ideal bioink material should possess several key attributes, including the ability to be easily printed, high mechanical strength, shape fidelity and stability, resistance to dissolution in cell culture media, appropriate biodegradability for tissue regeneration, non-toxic and non-immunogenic properties, with the capacity to facilitate cell adhesion and their phenotypic functions. Furthermore, these materials should be readily manufacturable, cost-effective, and commercially accessible (Gungor-Ozkerim et al., 2018). Tables 2 and 3 provide an explanation of the various bioinks and cell types used for 3D bioprinting.

5.   Applications of 3D Bioprinting

3D bioprinting is attracting increasing attention with its ability to fabricate geometrically complex constructs for prototypes, multi-material parts, medical devices, and engineered tissues and holds tremendous potential across many more applications. Here are a few major applications for 3D bioprinting, with an emphasis on biomedical healthcare:

5.1   3D Bioprinting in Tissue Engineering and Organ Transplantation

One of the primary applications of 3D bioprinting is in tissue engineering, where it can be used to fabricate tissue constructs for regenerative medicine. In recent times, there has been a significant surge in the scarcity of organs for transplant recipients worldwide. This has led to an urgent demand within the healthcare sector for artificial alternatives. Organ printing is the 3D construction of functional cellular tissue that can replace organs made by additive biofabrication with computational technology. Researchers are working towards bioprinting complex organs like the liver, kidney, heart, bladder, trachea, esophagus, and pancreas, which could help alleviate the shortage of donor organs. The 3D bioprinted urinary bladder was made to replace a patient's defective bladder and continues to function after 14 years (Anthony Atala et al., 2006). In 2014, a British surgeon successfully implanted a 3D printed pelvis for a man who lost half his pelvis to bone cancer. Another group in Southampton used 3D printing technology to replace a patient's hip which was crushed in a car accident. The first 3D printed skull transplant has taken place in the Netherlands. In 2019, researchers at the Human Genome and Stem Cell Research Institute in Brazil, achieved a significant milestone by successfully bioprinting a miniature liver. In 2022, a woman received a custom-printed ear created from her own harvested cells. In 2023, scientists produced replicas of full-thickness human skin to help regenerate skin for severe wounds. The 3D-printed skin could benefit burn victims, reconstructive surgery, and patients with chronic wounds, such as diabetic ulcers (Jorgensen et al., 2023) (Gungor-Ozkerim et al., 2018) (Gu et al., 2022). Table 3 explains a few examples of 3D bioprinting systems in tissue engineering and regenerative applications.

5.2   3D Bioprinting for Microfluidics and Organ-On-a-Chip Platforms

Organs-on-a-chips are systems containing engineered or natural miniature tissues grown inside microfluidic chips. By integrating innovations in tissue engineering and microfabrication, organ-on-a-chip have emerged as a cutting-edge experimental platform for simulating human physiology including the interstitial flow, blood/airflow, diffusion, breathing motions, peristalsis-like motion, concentration gradient of molecules, cardiac contractility, and electrophysiology to study human pathophysiology and assess the impact of therapeutic interventions within the body. This microfluidic form of microphysiological system comes in various sizes and shapes, but they all contain hollow channels comprising intricate networks of hair-thin microchannels lined by living cells and tissues cultured under dynamic fluid flow. These channels serve to direct and manage minuscule volumes of solution, ranging from picoliters to milliliters. By culturing various cells such as the brain, lung, heart, blood vessel, and skin on these microfluidic chips, the physiological and mechanical properties of tissues were simulated. This enables efficient and precise screening through the dynamic environment within the microfluidic chip, unlike the static environment of the existing plastic-based cell culture. It can be a single-organ-on-a-chip system offering a high degree of biological authenticity, allowing evaluation of the response of a specific organ to a compound/ mixture of compounds or multi-organ- or body- or human-on-a-chip systems which can provide a framework to examine the potential interaction of one organ with at least one other, principally through the exchange of metabolites or soluble signalling molecules (Leung et al., 2022). There is no perfect standard material for fabrication of organ-on-a-chip systems, thermoplastics and poly(dimethylsiloxane) (PDMS) are widely used. Other materials include glass, silicon, paper, resins or combinations of these materials.

Various human organ-on-a-chip systems have been employed to replicate intricate diseases and rare genetic disorders, to study hosts-microbiomes interactions, to simulate inter-organ physiology, and to mimic human clinical reactions to drug toxicity, cancer metastasis (cancer-on-a-chip), inflammation, radiation, toxins, and infectious agents. Collecting readouts from these devices can be done by *in situ*, offline or end-point measurements. *In situ* measurements are carried out while operating a recirculating organ-on-a-chip system enabling near real-time monitoring of cell states and functionality. This can be are done using integrated electrodes to measure various electromechanical signals like transepithelial electrical resistance (TEER), cantilevers for cell/tissue contractility, integrated biochemical sensors for measurement of various soluble analytes, such as secreted proteins (immunosensors), dissolved oxygen or can be coupled to an optical set-up for live-cell imaging. Offline readouts from sampling recirculating mediums can be used to evaluate soluble biomarkers using assay kits or liquid chromatography/mass spectrometry (LC/MS). End point measurements can be used to study transcriptome and proteome level analysis by expression of specific biomarkers using immunohistochemical and/or cytochemical techniques next-generation sequencing (Leung et al., 2022).

In 2004, the initial publication on utilizing microfluidic technology to model organs and systemic-level functions in human physiology and disease research marked a significant milestone. Subsequently, the groundbreaking breathing lung device, also known as the lung-on-a-chip, was developed in 2010. This landmark achievement sparked the progression of biologically inspired

Table 2   Properties of commonly used biopolymers for bioink development in 3D bioprinting

Bioink / Natural Biomaterials	Crosslinking Mechanism	Bioprinting Application — Bioink	Target	Bioprinting	Advantages	Disadvantages	References
Collagen (Natural component of ECM)	Temperature/ Photo-crosslinking- UV/ Chemical-Glutaraldehyde, Carbodiimide, Genipin, Vitamin Riboflavin, Tannic acid	Collagen	Skin	Droplet	Biocompatible; Contains native cell adhesion ligands; Modifiable	Mechanical instability; Slow gelation rate; Fast degradation rate	(Turnbull et al., 2018- NOT FOUND IN REFS)
		Collagen/GelMA	Skin	Extrusion			
		Matrigel/Collagen I/ Laminin/Collagen IV	Cornea	Laser			
		Collagen/nano-Hydroxyapatite	Bone	Laser			
Hyaluronic acid (HA) (Non-sulfated glycosaminoglycan distributed widely throughout connective, epithelial, and neural tissues)	Photo-crosslinking/ Chemical-Glutaraldehyde/ Carbodiimide divinyl sulfone	HA with dopamine and carbohydrazide modification (HA-DA-CDH)	Cornea	Extrusion	Rapid gelation; Cell proliferation promoter; Easy to modify; Viscoelastic and hygroscopic properties	Rapid degradation and low mechanical strength; Need chemical modification to regulate the rheology	(Gaetani et al., 2015; Di Bella et al., 2018; Keriquel et al., 2010; Li et al., 2023)
		HA/Gelatin	Cardiac	Inkjet			
		Nano-HA	Bone	Laser			
		HA/GelMA	Cartilage	Extrusion			
		Glycidal methacrylate-HA (GM-HA)	Liver	Droplet			
		Laminin/HA	Cornea	Laser			
		HA/GelMA	Bone	Extrusion			
Fibrin (Insoluble protein formed during blood clotting)	Enzymatic/ Ionic	Fibrin	Skin	Extrusion	Cytocompatibility; Cell binding sites for attachment, proliferation; Low immunogenicity; Easily purified from blood providing autologous source; Superior elasticity	Mechanical instability; Low shear thinning; Fast degradation	(Skardal et al., 2012)
		Fibrin/Gelatin, Glycerol/ HA	Cardiac	Extrusion			
		Fibrinogen/ Collagen	Skin	Inkjet			
		Collagen/Gelatin/ Fibrinogen/Alginate	Cardiac	Extrusion			

Table 2 *Contd.*

Bioink / Natural Biomaterials	Crosslinking Mechanism	Bioprinting Application — Bioink	Target	Bioprinting	Advantages	Disadvantages	References
Gelatin (Protein derived from partial hydrolysis of collagen)	Thermal/ Chemical-Glutaraldehyde, Transglutaminase, Horseradish peroxidase (HRP)- H_2O_2, Carbodiimide, Genipin	Gelatin/ Alginate	Liver	Extrusion	Biocompatible; Water solubility; Thermally reversible; Non-immunogenicity; Thermoresponsive sol-gel transition behaviour; Cell-friendly binding domains; Ease of chemical modification	Low shape fidelity and rigidity; Low viscosity	(Lam et al., 2019)
		GelMA)/ Methylacrylated HA (HAMA)	Cartilage	SLA			
		Gelatin/ PEG	Liver	DLP			
		Fibronectin/ Gelatin	Cardiac	Laser			
Alginate (Naturally-derived biopolymer from brown algae)	Ionic	Alginate/ Gelatin	Skin	Extrusion	Biocompatibility; Low toxicity; Low price; Rapid gelation; Suitable for cell encapsulation; Ease of crosslinking using divalent cations	Covalent crosslinking required for strength; Lack cell adhesion site; Highly hydrophilic and biodegradable	(Milazzo et al., 2019)
		Alginate/ PLGA	Skin	Extrusion			
		Alginate/ Gelatin/ Fibrinogen	Liver	Extrusion			
		Alginate/ ColMA	Cornea	Extrusion			
		Alginate/ Nanocellulose/ Collagen	Cornea	Extrusion			
Chitosan (Cationic polysaccharide produced by partial deacetylation of chitin obtained from the outer skeleton of shellfish or from fungal fermentation	pH/Chemical -Genipin/ Glutaraldehyde	Chitosan	Skin	Extrusion	Biocompatibility; Antibacterial properties; Mucoadhesive and homeostatic features	Mechanical instability; Poor solubility; Slow gelation rate; Lack of cell-binding domains	(Ulag et al., 2020; Maturavongsadit et al., 2021)
		Chitosan/ Gelatin	Skin	Extrusion			
		Chitosan/ PVA	Cornea	Extrusion			
		Alginate/ Gelatin/ Carboxymethyl chitosan	Bone	Extrusion			
		Chitosan/ β-glycerophosphate/ Hydroxyethyl cellulose/ Cellulose nanocrystals	Bone	Extrusion			

Contd.

Table 2 *Contd.*

Bioink / Natural Biomaterials	Crosslinking Mechanism	Bioprinting Application — Bioink	Target	Bioprinting	Advantages	Disadvantages	References
Silk (Protein isolated from *Bombyx mori*)	Enzymatic/Thermal/pH Sonication/ Chemical- HRP-H_2O_2	Silk fibroin-glycidyl methacrylate	Bone	DLP	Non-toxic; Gradual degradation; Low immunogenicity; High viscosity and shear thinning; Cost effective	Inducement of nozzle clogging; Lack of cell biding for cell adherence; Limited cell growth and function	(Ni et al., 2023)
		Silk fibroin (SF)/ hydroxypropyl methylcellulose	Cartilage	Extrusion			
		SF/ Decellularized liver matrix/ Gelatin	Liver	Extrusion			
		SF/ Gelatin/ human placenta ECM	Soft tissue constructs	Extrusion			
		SF/ Collagen	Cartilage	Extrusion			
Cellulose (Polysaccharide isolated from plants, many forms of algae and the oomycetes)	Ionic (Ca2+)	Alginate sulfate/ Nanocellulose	Cartilage	Extrusion	High mechanical properties and shape fidelity; Non-toxic	Non-biodegradation *in vivo*; Low cell adhesion	(Müller et al.,2017; Ramakrishnan et al., 2022; Li et al., 2023)
		Alginate/ Gelatin/ Diethylaminoethyl cellulose/ Fibrinogen	Skin	Extrusion			
		Nanofibrillated cellulose (NFC)/ Alginate/ nanofibrillated cellulose (NFC)/ HA	Cartilage	Inkjet			
		Alginate/ Methyl-cellulose	Liver	Extrusion			
		Alginate/ Nanocellulose	Cardiac	Extrusion			
Agarose (Polysaccharide extracted from seaweed)	Thermal/Chemical/Ionic	Collagen/ Agar	Cornea	Drop-on-demand	High mechanical strength when cross-linked; Low price; Non/low-toxic	Poor cell adhesion; Low cell adhesion and spreading; Brittle; Fairly slow degradation	(López-Marcial et al., 2018)
		Collagen/ Agarose/ Alginate	Cartilage	Extrusion			
		n,o-Carboxymethyl chitosan/ Agarose	Nerve	Extrusion			

Contd.

Table 2 *Contd.*

Bioink — Natural Biomaterials	Crosslinking Mechanism	Bioprinting Application — Bioink	Target	Bioprinting	Advantages	Disadvantages	References
Decellularized ECM (Isolated ECM from inhabiting native cell comprising different components such as collagen, GAGs, chondroitin sulphate,HA, elastin, etc)	Thermal/Chemical	Liver decellularized ECM (dECM)	Liver	Droplet	Biocompatibility; Retains the natural microenvironmental Promotes cell growth and differentiation; Printability; Thermoresponsive nature	Low viscosity; Complicated process of decellularization and costly; Requires complete decellularization and sterilization of dECM	(T.-Y. Lu et al., 2013; J. Jang et al., 2017;Li et al., 2023)
		Liver dECM/ GelMA	Liver	Extrusion			
		Gelatin-RGD/ Amniotic membrane dECM	Cornea	Extrusion			
		Cornea-derived dECM	Cornea	Extrusion			
		GelMA/ dECM	Liver	Droplet			
Hydroxyapatitite (Naturally-occurring mineral form of calcium apatite found in teeth and bones)	Methanol	PEGDMA/ Bioactive glass (BG)/ Hydroxyapatite	Bone	Inkjet	Good shape fidelity and produce porous	Low printability; Limited tissue specificity; Low cell adhesion	(Bogala, 2022)
		Nano-hydroxyapatite	Bone	Laser-assisted			
		Alginate/ Nano-hydroxyapatite	Bone	Laser-assisted			
		Alginate/ PVA/ Hydroxyapatite	Bone	Extrusion			
		PCL/ PEG/ Hydroxyapatite	Bone	Extrusion			
Matrigel (ECM proteins derived from the Engelbreth-Holm-Swarm mouse sarcoma)	Thermal	Alginate/ Gelatin/ Matrigel	Lung	Extrusion	Promotes vascularization; Imparts high cell survival rates; Good shape fidelity	Batch-to-batch variability; Undefined composition; Poorly organized architecture	(Flores- Torres et al., 2021)
		Alginate/ Methylcellulose/ Matrigel/ Fibrin	Liver	Extrusion			
		Matrigel	Ovary	Inkjet			

Contd.

Table 2 *Contd.*

Bioink / Natural Biomaterials	Crosslinking Mechanism	Bioprinting Application			Advantages	Disadvantages	References
		Bioink	Target	Bioprinting			
Synthetic Biomaterials Polyethylene Glyccl (PEG)	Thermoplastic/ Thermal/ Photo-crosslinking/Chemical -Genipin	Silk fibroin/ PEG	Skin	Droplet	Good shape fidelity and rigidity; Biocompatibility, Non-immunogenicity; widely used sacrificial bio-ink	Hydrophobicity; Long degradation time; Lack of cell adhesion site	(Maiullari et al., 2018; Cui et al., 2012)
		PEG/ Chitosan	Skin	Extrusion			
		PEG monoacrylate-Fibrinogen/ Alginate	Cardiac	Extrusion			
		Silk fibroin/ PEG	Cartilage	SLA			
		PEGDMA	Cartilage	Inkjet			
		Gelatin/ PEG	Liver	Extrusion			
Polylactic Acid (PLA)/ Poly(lactic-co-glycolic acid) (PLGA)	Thermoplastic Thermal/ Photo-crosslinking/ Chemical-Genipin	PLA/ Chitosan/ HA	Dermis	Extrusion	FDA approved; Good shape fidelity and rigidity; Biodegradable; Biocompatible	Hydrophobicity; Long degradation time; Lack of cell adhesion site	(H. Wang et al., 2023)
		PLA/ Hydroxyapatite	Bone	Extrusion			
		Hydroxyapaptite/ PLGA-RGD functionalised	Bone	Extrusion			
		PLGA with Gly-Phe-Hyp-Gly-Arg	Bone	FDM			
		PLGA/ Calcium Sulfate	Bone	FDM			
Polycaprolactone (PCL)	Thermoplastic Thermal/ Photo-crosslinking/Chemical - Genipin	PCL/ Collagen	Epidermis/ dermis	Inkjet	FDA approved; Good shape fidelity and rigidity; Low melting point and high stability	Hydrophobicity; Long degradation time; Lack of cell adhesion site; Unsuitable for cell encapsulation	(H. Wang et al., 2023)
		PCL/ Alginate	Cartilage	Extrusion			
		PCL/ Alginate	Cartilage	Inkjet			
		Collagen/ PCL	Liver	Extrusion			
		Gelatin/ Collagen/ PCL	Liver	Extrusion			
		GelMA/ PEG-PCL fibers	Cornea	Extrusion			

Contd.

Table 2 *Contd.*

Bioink / Natural Biomaterials	Crosslinking Mechanism	Bioprinting Application			Advantages	Disadvantages	References
		Bioink	Target	Bioprinting			
Poly(vinyl alcohol) (PVA)	Glutaraldehyde/ Chemical-Genipin	Alginate/ Hydroxyapatite/ PVA	Bone	Extrusion	Biodegradable; Biocompatible; thermostable; Water-soluble; Excellent adhesive properties; Transparency	Low cell affinity; Hydrophilicity causes uncontrolled swelling	(H. Wang et al., 2023)
		PVA/ Gelatin/ Carrageenan	Cardiac-heart valve	Extrusion			
		PVA	Tablets	FDM			
		PVA functionalised with cis-5-norbornene-endo-2, 3-dicarboxylic anhydride (PVA-Nb / solubilized decellularized cartilage ECM	Cartilage	Extrusion			
Pluronic	Thermo-responsive/ Photo-polymerization/ Ionic	Pluronic F127/ GelMA	Blood vessels	Extrusion	Sacrificial material; Stimuli-responsive properties	Unsuitable for long-term structural support; Poor mechanical strength; Poor cell adhesion	(Gopinathan & Noh, 2018)
		dECM/ Pluronic F127	Blood vessels	Extrusion			
		Pluronic F127/ HA	Nerve	Extrusion			
		Pluronic F127/ Alginate	Bone	Extrusion			

Table 3 Bioprinted Constructs for different tissue engineering applications

Area of Application	Bioprinting Type	Bioink Composition	Cell types	Bioprinter	Significant Result	Reference
Skin	Extrusion	Fibrin/ Gelatin/ Glycerol/ HA	Human keratinocytes (HDKs), fibroblasts (HDFs), dark-melanocytes, microvascular endothelial cells (ECs) (HMVECs), follicle papillae cells and pre-adipocytes (HPAs)	Integrated tissue and organ printer (ITOP)	Human tissue derived multicellular full thickness bioprinted skin facilitated human-like skin architecture *in vivo* with lesser scar formation	(Jorgensen et al., 2023) (Ramakrishnan et al., 2022)
	Droplet	PVA/ Collagen	HDFs	Biofactory, RegenHU Switzerland	A novel printing method with a controlled number of droplets with layer deposition	(Ng et al., 2018)
	Extrusion	Alginate/ Gelatin/ Diethylaminoethyl cellulose/ Fibrinogen	HDFs, HDKs	3D Discovery Bioprinter, RegenHu Switzerland	Long term culture of 4 weeks with epidermal-dermal functionality	(Ramakrishnan et al., 2022)
	Extrusion	Recombinant human type III collagen/ GelMA	HaCaT, HDFs	Biomaker 2, SunP Biotech	Enhanced wound healing and hair follicle development on *in vivo* rat model	(Yang et al., 2022)
	Extrusion	PGA/ Collagen/ Fibronectin	HDKs, HECs, HDFs	BioX, Cellink, Sweden	Human-tissue derived bioprinted skin	(Baltazar et al., 2023)
	Extrusion	Gelatin/ Collagen I/ Elastin/Fibrinogen/ Laminin, and Entactin	HDKs, HDFs	3D Discovery Bioprinter, RegenHu Switzerland	Four primary layers of the epidermis were developed with tight junction barriers	(Derr et al., 2019)
	Extrusion	Methylcellulose/ Alginate with gallium-crosslinking	HDFs	Allevi 2, USA	Antibacterial property	(Rastin et al., 2021)
	Hand-held extrusion / robotic arm methods	Fibrin/ HA	hMSCs	Microfluidic print held made using 3D Systems, USA	Handheld bioprinter for wound-conformal delivery of skin precursor sheets	(Cheng et al., 2020)

Contd.

Table 3 *Contd.*

Area of Application	Bioprinting Type	Bioink Composition	Cell types	Bioprinter	Significant Result	Reference
Cardiac	Extrusion	Omentum-derived dECM/ Gelatin	iPSCs-derived cardiomyocytes and ECs	3D Discovery Bioprinter, RegenHu Switzerland	Vacsularised and perfusable cardiac equivalent matching the immunological, cellular, biochemical, and anatomical characteristics	(Noor et al., 2019)
	Extrusion (Coaxial)	Alginate/ PEG-monoacrylate-Fibrinogen	HUVECs, iPSC-derived cardiomyocytes, Fibroblasts	--	Engineered cardiac tissue with host's vasculature	(Maiullari et al., 2018)
	SLA	Collagen	rMSCs	EnvisionTEC 3D-Bioplotter, Germany	Remodeling capacity with increasing elastin, vimentin, alpha SMA, and CD31 throughout the 12 weeks	(Maxson et al., 2019)
	Inkjet	HA/ Gelatin	Human cardiac-derived progenitor cells (hCMPCs)	Bioscaffolder, Germany	Translational approach to enhance hCMPC delivery	(Gaetani et al., 2015)
	Extrusion	Alginate/ Gelatin	Vascularised spheroid with human cardiac fibroblasts (CFs), human coronary artery ECs (HCAECs) and iPSC-derived cardiomyocytes	BioX, Cellink, USA	Epicardial transplantation in myocardial infarction model following permanent left anterior descending artery ligation	(Roche et al., 2023)
	Extrusion	Laminin-521	Patient-derived cardiomyocytes	Inkredible+, CellInk, USA	Cardiac tissue model	(Wolfe et al., 2023)
	Extrusion	GelMA/ Alginate with gold nanorods	Neonatal rat cardiomyocytes	NovoGen MMX Bioprinter, Organovo, USA	Gold nanorods improved the electrical propagation between cardiac cells and promoted their Functionality	(Zhu et al., 2017)
Pancreas	Extrusion	Pectin/ Alginate/ Pluronic F127	MIN6 cells, THP1-reporter cell line	Biobots, USA	The structure supports the survival of cells and has the capability of immune regulation	(Hu et al., 2021)
	Extrusion	Alginate/ Methylcellulose	Pancreatic cells	BioScaffolder 3.1, GeSiM mbH, Germany	The islets could produce insulin and glucagon in the structure	(Duin et al., 2019)

Contd.

Table 3   *Contd.*

Area of Application	Bioprinting Type	Bioink Composition	Cell types	Bioprinter	Significant Result	Reference
	DLP	HAMA/ Pancreatic dECM	Primary islets	China	Pancreatic islet organoids	(D. Wang et al., 2023)
	Extrusion	PANC-1- Plasma/ Alginate/ Methylcellulose	PANC-1	Inkredible 3D printer Cellink, Sweden	Pancreatic tumour modelling	(Banda Sánchez et al., 2023)
	Extrusion	Pancreatic dECM/ GelMA/ HAMA with lithium phenyl-2,4,6-trimethyl-benzoyl phosphinate (LAP) photoinitiator	Pancreatic islet cells	BioX, Cellink, Sweden	Transplantation of porcine pancreatic islets in the form of 3D bionic scaffolds into NOD-SCID mice without induced diabetes	(Klak et al., 2023)
	Extrusion	Pancreatic dECM/ Fibrinogen/ Alginate	hMSCs/HUVECs	3D-Bioplotter, EnvisionTEC, Germany	Vascularised pancreatic grafts	(Idaszek et al., 2021)
Cornea	DLP/ Extrusion-	Alginate/ Gelatin	Human Corneal epithelial cell line		Geometry-controllable corneal substitutes	(B. Zhang et al., 2019)
	Extrusion	GelMA	Human corneal keratocytes	Bioscaffolder, SYS-ENG, Germany	3D printed HK seeded corneal stroma with synthesis of the specific collagens and proteoglycan by the seeded keratocytes	(Kilic Bektas & Hasirci, 2020)
	Extrusion	Gelatin/ Arg-Gly-Asp; RGD)/ commercial lyophilized bovine amniotic membrane (AM)	Human corneal ECs	Edison Invivo, ROKIT, Korea	3D bioprinted R5- hCEC-laden AM endothelial grafts in a descemetorhexis-induced corneal endothelial decompensation model in rabbits	(H. Kim et al., 2019)
	SLA/ Extrusion	Alginate/ Gelatin/ Collagen	Acellular	SLA- Formlabs, USA/ Extrusion -Bio X, Cellink,USA	High throughput/rapid printing on large scale	(Kutlehria et al., 2020)

organ-on-a-chip devices, shaping the advancements seen in organ-on-a-chip technology today (Deng et al., 2023). Y.S. Zhang et al. developed a human thrombosis-on-a-chip using a 3D printing method in 2016, combined with micro-molding by incorporating GelMA hydrogel bioink mixed with fibroblasts. Endothelialized micro-channels were injected with a mixture of human blood to replicate clot formation. This biomimetic model allows for advanced *in vitro* studies targeting thrombosis and related variations, surpassing existing comparable research (Zhang et al., 2016). In 2019, H. Lee and colleagues developed a liver-on-a-chip platform featuring a biliary system, achieved through the integration of various liver cell types and ECMs within a custom microfluidic chip using a nozzle-based 3D bioprinting method (H. Lee et al., 2019).

Table 4   Human organs-on-a-chip platforms for disease/cancer modelling, drug development and personalized medicine.

System	Model type	Cell Types	Features	References
Respiratory / Lung-on-a-chip	Lung	Calu-3 cells	3D-printed molds to manufacture a chip model with an open well design and with lower and upper layers to mimic the human lung	(Shrestha et al., 2019)
	Influenza A virus infection- SARS-CoV-2	Human brain microvascular endothelial cells (ECs) (HBMVECs), Human lung alveolar type 2 (hAT2), Human pulmonary alveolar epithelial cells (HPAEpiCs,) Human pulmonary microvascular ECs (HPMECs), Human bronchial/tracheal epithelial cell (NHBEs)	Confirmation of change in airway cell morphology after the virus infection in 3D. Confirmation of virus entry and cytokine changes according to drug treatment concentration	(Si et al., 2021)
	Cystic fibrosis (2-Channel;PDMS)	HPMECs	Hyperinflammation in cystic fibrosis	(Plebani et al., 2022)
Kidney-on-a-chip	Renal transport, Nephrotoxicity (3-Channel; Plastic)	Proximal tubule epithelial (CiPTEC-OAT1) cells	Proximal tubule model for nephrotoxicity and drug interaction studies	(Vormann et al., 2021)
	Filtration barrier (2-Channel; PDMS)	hiPS-cell-derived podocytes	Human glomerular function with mature human podocytes may facilitate drug development and personalized-medicine applications	(Musah et al., 2017)
	Lowe Syndrome and Dent II Disease Tubulopathy (2-Channel; Plastic)	Human proximal tubule cell line HK-2	Replication of clinical phenotype	(Naik et al., 2021)

Contd.

Table 4 *Contd.*

System	Model type	Cell Types	Features	References
Gut/Intestine-on-a-chip	Intestinal inflammation	Human colorectal carcinoma-derived (Caco-2) intestinal epithelial cells, human capillary ECs or human lymphatic microvascular ECs	Model to study villus injury with compromised intestinal barrier function	(H. J. Kim, et al., 2016)
	Inflammatory bowel disease (2-Channel;PDMS)	Organoid-derived intestinal epithelial cells, human colon crypt-derived epithelial and primary microvascular ECs (HIMECs)	Recapitulated the effects of proinflammatory cytokines in the intestinal epithelial barrier in inflammation-associated injury to investigate leaky gut in human beings.	(Apostolou et al., 2021)
	Bacterial infection, microbiome (2-Channel;PDMS)	Patient-derived organoids primary human colon epithelial cells, HIMECs	Species-specific sensitivity to Escherichia coli infection	(Tovaglieri et al., 2019)
	SARS-CoV-2 virus infection (2-Channel;PDMS)	Human large intestine HIMECs, epithelial cells, HUVECs	Human preclinical model for studying coronavirus related pathology as well as for testing of potential anti-viral or anti-inflammatory therapeutics.	(Bein et al., 2021)
Liver-on-a-chip	Hepatitis B Virus infection	Hepatocytes (HepG2-NTCP|), PHH, 3T3-J2, Kupffer cell (KC), Huh 7, human hepatocytes	Fabrication of a system to confirm long-term HBV infection in 3D using patient-derived PHH; Analysis of immune response according to HBV infection; Confirmation of changes in immune factor expression with Kupffer cells	(Ortega-Prieto et al., 2018)
	Hepatitis B Virus infection (1-Channel;Plastic)	HepG2/NTCP cells, HepaRG cells, PHH HepDE19 cells, NIH/3T3, J2 cells, KC	Platform to study innate immune and cytokine responses after viral infection-associated injury	(Ortega-Prieto et al., 2018)
	Steatosis (1-Channel;Plastic)	Hepatocytes, microvascular cardiac ECs, HepG2/C3A	Drug toxicity	(Ehrlich et al., 2018)
	Drug-induced liver injury (2-Channel;PDMS)	Hepatocytes, liver sinusoidal ECs (LSECs), KC, stellate cells	Human and cross species drug toxicities	(K.-J. Jang et al., 2019)
Brain-on-a-chip	Parkinson disease (2-Channel;PDMS)	Neuron, microglial, astrocyte, pericytes	α-Synuclein pathology in a human brain-chip to assess blood-brain barrier disruption	(Pediaditakis et al., 2021)
	Fungal meningitis of *Cryptococcus neoformans* (3-Channel;PDMS)	Human neural stem cells, brain microvascular ECs and brain vascular pericytes	Fungal invasion of blood brain barrier	(J. Kim et al., 2021)

Contd.

Table 4   *Contd.*

System	Model type	Cell Types	Features	References
Eye-on-a-chip	Retinopathy (2-Channel;PDMS)	Retinal pigmented epithelial, 7 retinal (iPS org)	Microphysiological model of the human retina integrating more than seven different essential retinal cell types derived from hiPSCs used for studying underlying pathology of retinal diseases and drug toxicity	(Achberger et al., 2019)
	Corneal barrier function	Human CEpCs	Capable of simulating tear volume, tear flow, shear, friction, air exposure and blinking associated tear movement	(Bennetet al., 2018)
	Corneal barrier function	HCE-T cells	Spatiotemporal determination of metabolite activities	(Abdalkader et al,2021)
Heart-on-a-chip	Heart contractility, cardiotoxicity (3D printed PDMS + plastic)	iPSCs- derived Cardiomyocytes	Endothelialized-myocardium-on-a-chip platform for cardiovascular toxicity evaluation	(Y. S. Zhang,, et al., 2016)
	Cardiotoxicity	iPSCs- derived Cardiomyocytes	Cardiac model for drug discovery and screening	(Miller et al., 2021)
Uterus-on-a-chip	Endometrial remodelling (5-Channel;PDMS)	Stromal and endometrial cells	Menstrual cycle-dependent endometrial differentiation	(Ahn et al., 2021)
	Endometrial remodelling (2-Channel;PDMS)	HUVECs, stromal and endometrial cells	Uterine contraception, drug efficacy	(Gnecco et al., 2017)
Placenta-on-a-chip	Placental barrier (2-Channel;PDMS)	Trophoblast	Drug transport	(Blundell et al., 2018)
Cartilage-on-a-chip	Osteoarthritis (2-Channel;PDMS)	Synovial fibroblast, chondrocytes	Monocyte extravasation, drug efficacy in the articular joint	(Mondadori et al., 2021)
Skin-on-a-chip	Skin irritation (2-Channel;Plastic)	Keratinocytes	Drug and chemical toxicity	(Y. S. Zhang et al., 2016)
Pancreas-on-a-chip	Diabetes mellitus (1-Channel;Plastic)	Pancreatic islets	Glucose-sensitive insulin secretion	(Glieberman et al., 2019)
Cancer-on-a-chip	Breast cancer (3-Channel;PDMS)	Human dermal lymphatic ECs, MDA-MB-231, BT474, and A549	Breast cancer lymphangiogenesis	(Cho et al., 2021)
	Breast cancer (2-Channel;ECM gel)	Human mammary epithelial cell line (MCF10A), Human dermal microvascular ECs, HEK-293T cells	Mutation-induced cancer progression, angiogenesis	(Kutys et al., 2020)

Contd.

Table 5 *Contd.*

System	Model type	Cell Types	Features	References
	Lung (Non-small-cell lung cancer) (2-Channel;PDMS)	H1975 human NSCLC adenocarcinoma cells, primary lung alveolar or small airway epithelial cells	Site-dependent cancer growth	(Hassell et al., 2017)
	Colorectal cancer (3-Channel;PDMS)	ECs, fibroblasts, HCT116 cancer cells	Microphysiological system platform for the study of colorectal cancer drug efficacy	(Hachey et al., 2021)
	Lung cancer	Human NSCLC, A549, human fetal lung fibroblast (HFL1) cell lines, HUVECs	Model to investigate the role of the stromal cells in lung tumorigenesis and chemotherapy	(S. W. Lee et al., 2018)
	Pancreatic Ductal Adenocarcinoma	Human dermal fibroblasts, HUVECs, human pancreatic ductal adenocarcinoma (hPDAC) cells from patient derived organoids	3D model with perfused vascular network, to accurately recapitulate a dynamic tumor microenvironment for drug screening.	(Lai et al., 2020)
	Colorectal cancer	Endothelial colony-forming cell-derived ECs (ECFC-EC), normal lung fibroblasts (NHLF), and colorectal cancer cells (HCT116 and SW480)	Microphysiological system (MPS) platform for the study of colorectal cancer pathological and pharmacological studies.	(Hachey et al., 2021)
	Liver cancer	HepG2	Platform for the study of liver cancer pathological and pharmacological studies.	(S. Lu et al., 2018)

5.3 3D Bioprinting in Drug Discovery and Development

Bioprinted tissues provide physiologically relevant models for drug screening and toxicity testing. Since the majority of drug toxicity tests and assays are conducted using conventional 2D monolayer *in vitro* culture systems that do not replicate the natural 3D tissue microenvironment, and many studies that pass preclinical trials ultimately fail in clinical trials. The primary cause for the failure rate is the lack of biomimetic physiologically relevant 3D *in vitro* models for testing drug toxicity. The bioprinted tissues have the potential to serve as *in vitro* models for drug testing, enabling the assessment of drug toxicity. This approach can yield results comparable to future *in vivo* testing, ultimately mitigating the high attrition rate and associated research expenses. There are several liver-on-a-chip platforms, with both parenchymal and non-parenchymal cells to recapitulate normal and disease mechanisms. Table 4 lists few examples. These serve as an *in vitro* model for drug metabolism to evaluate drug pharmacodynamic and pharmacokinetic profiling, alongside other organs involved in drug absorption, distribution and excretion connected in a recirculating circuit for drug screening and development (Leung et al., 2022).

5.4 3D Bioprinting in Disease Modelling for Studying Infectious Diseases

Lack of adequate experimental models has impeded the understanding of infection pathogenesis and the development of effective medications. While conventional *in vitro* human cell culture platforms, such as monolayer cultures of immortalized human cell lines, offer cost-effective and convenient screening for experimental targets, they fall short in capturing the complex and dynamic responses of human organs. Consequently, models that accurately replicate human-pathogen interactions remain elusive. Animal models have contributed to vaccine and treatment research for infectious diseases; however, their inability to fully mimic human-pathogen interactions and ethical issues, compromises the reliability of experimental outcomes. There is also increasing pressure from society and governments to find alternatives to animal testing. Bioprinting technology facilitates the creation of *in vitro* disease models that closely mimic various disease pathologies, aiding in studying disease progression, identifying new therapeutic targets, and devising personalized treatment strategies. Despite this advancement, the utilization of sophisticated *in vitro* tissue models in infectious disease research is still in its infancy, resulting in limited success with 3D bioprinting-based approaches. In recent years, microfluidic organs-on-a-chip have emerged as promising tools for modeling infectious diseases (Shi et al, 2019). A few examples are provided in Table 4.

5.5   3D Bioprinting in Recapitulating 3D Tumor Microenvironment for Cancer Modelling

The approval of anticancer therapeutic strategies continues to face delays due to the absence of models capable of accurately replicating *in vivo* cancer physiology. Conventional *in vitro* models lack the ability to mimic the organ and tissue structures, fluid flows, and mechanical stimuli found in human body compartments. Conversely, *in vivo* animal models struggle to recreate the characteristic human tumor microenvironment necessary for studying cancer behavior and progression. The tumor microenvironment is a dynamic and intricate setting comprising various stromal cells, including fibroblasts, endothelial cells, lymphatic vascular networks, pericytes, and immune cells from both adaptive and innate immunity (such as T and B lymphocytes, tumor-associated macrophages, and natural killer cells) and ECM components. These will foster a bi-directional and complex communication network with tumor cells to regulate numerous cellular processes and activation of several pathways, ultimately promoting tumor cell proliferation, invasion, plasticity and metastasis. In such a scenario, great efforts are focused on developing advanced culture models to recapacitate the key *in vivo* tumour microenvironment interactions, such as organ-on-a-chip (specifically, cancer-on-a-chip), which can be used to understand the underlying molecular pathways, and identify new targeted therapeutic strategies. Figure 2 illustrates cancer-on-a-chip system and few examples of such models are listed in Table 4.

Organ- and cancer-on-a-chip research might be used as a keystone to bridge the gap between pre-clinical and clinical investigations if best practices, approved standard protocols, patient-derived specific models, and less complex scalable models were established. Emulate (USA), Mimetas, (Netherlands), Elvesys (France), AxoSim,(USA), TaraBiosystems (USA), Nortis Bio (USA), BioIVT (USA), AlveoliX (Switzerland), TissUse, (Germany) BiomimX (Italy) are few companies developing organ-on-a-chip models.

5.6   3D Bioprinting for Animal-free Meat

According to the Food and Agriculture Organization (FAO) of the United Nations, global meat demand is projected to triple or quadruple by 2050, reaching 455 million metric tons. Cultured meat is considered to be a viable alternative to conventional flesh to satisfy the increasing human demand for meat and for addressing health and sustainability concerns such as the mass killing of livestock, animal welfare issues, by-product waste, and diseases associated with meat consumption. 3D Food Printing (3DFP) is a promising avenue to produce cultured meat that closely resembles animal flesh meat and for large scale production. Selective laser sintering, binder jetting, inkjet printing, stereolithography, extrusion printing, are employed for 3D printing meat. 3D printing meat utilizes materials that are derived from *in vitro* cell culture (muscle cells), meat by-products/ wastes,

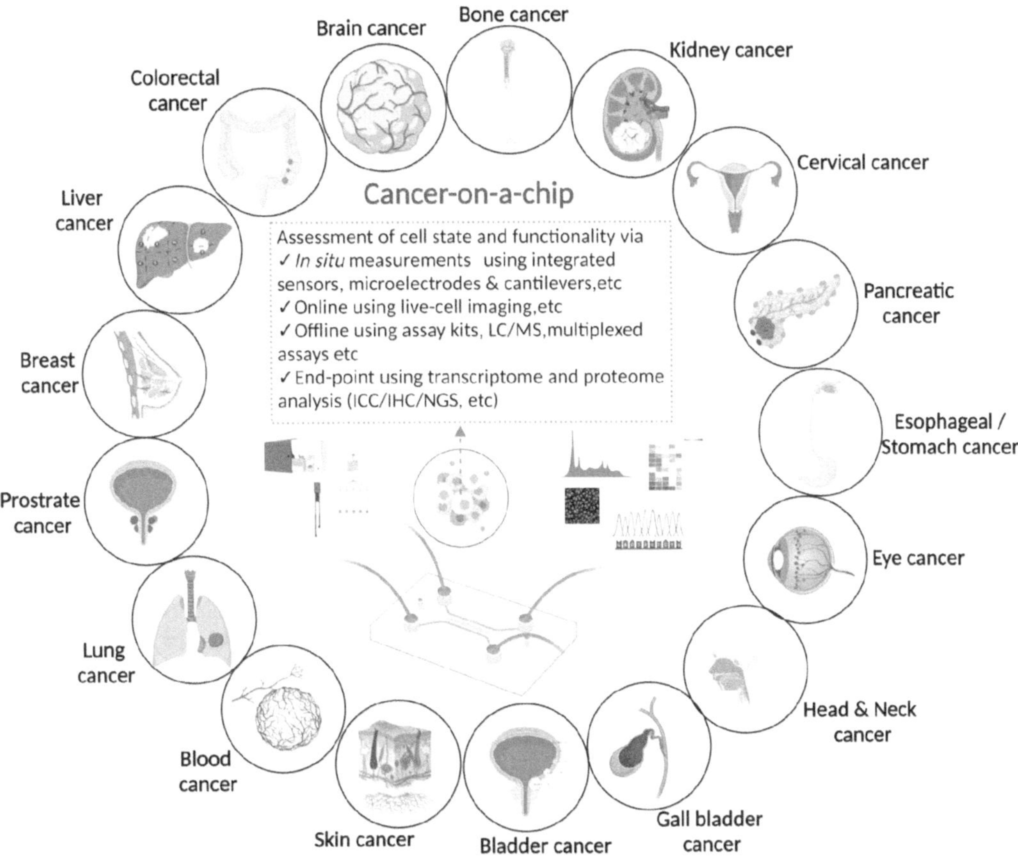

Fig. 2 Cancer-on-a-chip platforms recapitulating the tumor microenvironment to study cancer pathophysiology. Abbreviations: LC/MS, liquid chromatography/mass spectrometry; IHC, immunohistochemical/or ICC, immunocytochemical techniques; NGS, next-generation sequencing; Illustration created with Biorender.com.

insects, and plant-based materials like starch, pea protein, beetroot, chickpeas, coconut fat, algae proteins. Strict regulations to ensure food safety at all links and improvement of nutritional health and flavor/sensory properties of the 3D printed meat needs to be taken care of. Mosa Meat, known for producing the world's first lab-grown burger under Dr. Mark Post, and Singapore's Shiok Meats remain at the forefront (Guo et al., 2023), (Tibrewal et al., 2023). In 2021, the Singapore Food Agency (SFA) made history by becoming the first regulatory authority worldwide to approve the commercialization of a cultured meat product, after it was considered safe for consumption. Kang et al. developed a tendon-gel integrated bioprinting technology for the first time to fabricate whole cut steak-like meat (Kang et al., 2021). Steaks were created by printing a soft meat paste mixture that mimics the nutritional properties and taste of traditional beefsteaks (Tibrewal et al., 2023). Aleph Farms Ltd. and Israel Institute of Technology have demonstrated the viability of producing cultured meat using 3D printing technology in space (K. Handral et al, 2022). Jeong et al reported steak-like cultured meat with the proper mixture of fat and muscle using DLP bioprinting (Jeong et al., 2022). In 2023, FDA accepted GOOD Meat's cultivated chicken as safe.

5.7   3D Bioprinting in Veterinary Medicine

Although the main driving force behind innovation in 3D bioprinting has been utility in human medicine, recent efforts investigating its veterinary application have begun to emerge. 3D bioprinting has been utilized to create bone, cardiovascular, cartilage, corneal and neural constructs in animal species (Jamieson et al., 2021). 3D printed customized implants and prosthetics for animals can be tailored to fit individual patients' anatomy, leading to improved outcomes in procedures such as orthopedic surgeries or dental implants. Bioprinted tissues and scaffolds hold promise for regenerative medicine in veterinary care like bioprinted cartilage or bone constructs which can be used to repair musculoskeletal injuries in animals, offering a potential alternative to traditional treatments. Bioprinted tissue models can serve as valuable tools for drug testing and disease modeling in veterinary medicine. Bioprinted anatomical models are more attractive than cadavers and other ready-made organ models, for surgical training in veterinary medicine, allowing veterinary students to practice surgical procedures in a controlled environment before operating on live animals. Bioprinting holds potential for aiding conservation efforts for endangered species. Bioprinting techniques could be used to create tissue samples or even organs from preserved cells, helping to preserve genetic diversity and prevent extinction. However, technological limitations as well as ethical and regulatory challenges have impeded clinical acceptance.

6.   Advantages of 3D Bioprinting

3D printing has made significant inroads into various industries, including healthcare, biomedical, dental, aerospace, manufacturing and many more. The global 3D bioprinting industry is experiencing rapid growth, with projections indicating an expansion from $18.3 billion in 2022 to over $83 billion by 2029. The advantages of the 3D bioprinting industry are manifold. 3D bioprinting presents a transformative approach to healthcare, with the potential to revolutionize organ transplantation, regenerative medicine, and medical research. Some of the benefits include:

(1) **Rapid prototyping of complex structures**   Unlike traditional machining methods, 3D bioprinting enables the creation of complex structures to produce intricate designs and geometries with precise control that are challenging or impossible to achieve using conventional manufacturing processes, often requiring assemblies of multiple components. This innovative technology allows for the precise layering of bioink, containing living cells and supportive biomaterials, to construct intricate three-dimensional designs and also allows for quick modification of a design before mass production. This capability allows for the replication of intricate tissue architectures found in natural organs, enhancing their functionality.

(2) **Allows for automation, minimizing human errors**   This automation ensures consistent and accurate placement of biological materials, reducing the risk of human error in manual handling. Automation in 3D bioprinting enables the establishment of standardized processes and protocols, reducing variability and errors caused by human factors such as individual technique or judgment. These algorithms can identify potential issues such as nozzle clogging, material inconsistency, or structural deformities during printing and take corrective actions autonomously, reducing the need for manual intervention and minimizing the risk of errors going unnoticed.

(3) **Replacement of organ donors**   3D bioprinting may enable the fabrication of fully functional artificial organs for transplantation, eliminating the need for donor organs altogether and solving the organ shortage crisis. This could significantly alleviate the shortage of donor organs and save countless lives.

(4) **Prevention of immune rejection**   By using a patient's own cells or compatible materials, the risk of organ rejection is minimized, leading to better patient outcomes and reducing the need for immunosuppressive drugs.

(5) **Human-relevant models and disease modelling for high throughput screening**   3D bioprinting allows researchers to recreate complex disease states *in vitro* by engineering tissues and organs with specific pathophysiological features. These disease models can be used to study disease mechanisms, test potential therapeutics, and high-throughput screening of drugs and compound drug toxicity in a human-relevant context, while addressing ethical concerns,

reducing costs, and accelerating the pace of biomedical research and drug development. This will also allow to monitor treatment and drug effects closely.

(6) Replacement of animal testing   Traditional animal testing often lacks direct relevance to human physiology and can produce misleading results. By bioprinting human tissues and organs using human cells, researchers can develop more accurate models that better mimic human biology, offering a more reliable alternative to animal testing.

(7) Replacement of human volunteers for drug testing   Bioprinted tissues offer a versatile platform for assessing the safety of pharmaceutical compounds and potential drug candidates. Researchers can use these models to evaluate drug-induced toxicity, identify adverse effects, and optimize drug formulations before advancing to clinical trials, thereby minimizing the risks associated with human exposure to potentially harmful substances.

(8) Sustainability through waste reduction   3D printing technology has greater precision by using only the necessary amount of material, lesser energy and need for space than the traditional methods, making the process more cost-effective and sustainable.

7.   Challenges in 3D Bioprinting

Researchers continue to explore innovative solutions, including improved bioink formulations, advanced printing techniques, and enhanced post-printing maturation processes, to overcome the current challenges and enhance the overall efficacy of bioprinted constructs. Few of the challenges are:

(1) Inconsistencies in structural integrity   Engineering tissue complexity, post-print tissue maturation and maintenance, standardized and scalable manufacture are a challenge. The mechanical properties of bioprinted constructs, such as stiffness and tensile strength, may vary and often fall short of mimicking the native tissue. Achieving the right balance between mechanical support and biocompatibility remains a substantial hurdle.

(2) Limited material selection and compatibility   The choice of biomaterials for the bioinks plays a crucial role in determining the mechanical properties of the printed constructs. Finding materials that are both printable and capable of replicating the mechanical characteristics of diverse tissues remains a complex task.

(3) Cell viability and functionality   During the bioprinting process, cells may experience shear stress, mechanical forces, temperature variations, and other environmental changes that can affect their viability and functionality and lead to improper function of the implanted tissue. Maintaining high cell viability and ensuring that the printed cells retain their desired functions post-printing is a persistent challenge. Bioprinting requires sources of cells that are readily available, easy to expand in culture, nonimmunogenic and that can reproduce all the functions of the tissue or organ system. Potentially, combinations of various mature and/or multipotent cell sources can be applied to efficiently reproduce the cell phenotypes needed for specific tissues. A well characterized and reproducible source of cells, along with a greater understanding of the heterogeneous cell types present in the tissues, is required.

(4) Absence of vasculature   Most bioprinted tissues still lack some functional elements, such as vasculature, lymphatics, and multiple supporting cell types. Vasculature is essential for the long-term viability of any bioprinted tissue construct.

(5) Lack of innervations   Innervations help to integrate the tissue with host neurovascular networks, resulting in accelerated functional tissue regeneration and long-term survival.

(6) Tissue maturation   There are no guidelines for assembly and maturation of tissues after 3D bioprinting. Tissue maturation conditions are one of the key factors to obtain physiologically relevant implantable organs.

(7) Regulatory challenges   Lack of guidelines for standardised testing and ensuring safety are delaying development and commercialization.

(8) Clinical translation and Commercialization   There are many hurdles when it comes to clinical translation of bioprinting tissues and organs. The well-known challenges are the source of cells, biomaterial selection, scalable manufacturing technologies, long-term storage and transportation of these constructs without adverse effects on structural integrity, cell viability and function. Integration of quality control measures and standardized protocols for cell sourcing, bioprinting, and preservation and collaboration with regulatory agencies is essential to ensure reproducibility and safety in clinical applications.

(9) Ethical & Legal considerations   Confidentiality, informed consent for donation, material modification, and storage, as well as future use, including those for commercial and research purposes, should be upheld when using donor tissues or cells for 3D bioprinting. In clinical trials involving 3D bioprinted platforms, attempting reverse implantation could potentially exacerbate harm to patients. Legal regulations encompass various intellectual property rights, such as patents, copyrights, design rights, and trademarks, among others. Establishing regulations that address these issues is crucial (Murphy & Atala, 2014), (Bliley et al, 2022), (Vijayavenkataraman, 2023) (Kirillova et al., 2020) (H. Zhang & Wu, 2023).

8. Perspectives

Overcoming these challenges is essential to realize the full potential of bioprinting technology in clinical settings and to advance the field of regenerative medicine towards the development of functional, implantable tissues and organs for patients in need. Further development of standardized clinical-grade 3D bioprinters and biocompatible bioinks, patient-derived specific models along with the establishment of GMP-compliant cell manufacturing centers allied to medical facilities, will indeed play a crucial role in enabling wider adoption of 3D bioprinting technology in clinical practice. The field of 3D bioprinting holds immense potential for future growth and innovation within the broader realm of additive manufacturing technologies and impact across diverse applications in healthcare, research, and beyond.

References

Abdalkader, R., Chaleckis, R., Wheelock, C.E. and Kamei, K. (2021). Spatiotemporal determination of metabolite activities in the corneal epithelium on a chip. *Experimental Eye Research, 209,* 108646.

Achberger, K., Probst, C., Haderspeck, J., Bolz, S., Rogal, J. et al., (2019). Merging organoid and organ-on-a-chip technology to generate complex multi-layer tissue models in a human retina-on-a-chip platform. *ELife, 8,* e46188.

Agarwal, S., Saha, S., Balla, V.K., Pal, A., Barui, A. et al. (2020). Current Developments in 3D Bioprinting for Tissue and Organ Regeneration–A Review. *Frontiers in Mechanical Engineering, 6,* 589171.

Ahn, J., Yoon, M.-J., Hong, S.-H., Cha, H., Lee, D. et al. (2021). Three-dimensional microengineered vascularised endometrium-on-a-chip. *Human Reproduction, 36*(10), 2720–2731.

Apostolou, A., Panchakshari, R.A., Banerjee, A., Manatakis, D.V., Paraskevopoulou, M.D. et al. (2021). A Novel Microphysiological Colon Platform to Decipher Mechanisms Driving Human Intestinal Permeability. *Cellular and Molecular Gastroenterology and Hepatology, 12*(5), 1719–1741.

Atala, A. (2011). Tissue engineering of human bladder. *British Medical Bulletin, 97*(1), 81–104.

Atala, Anthony, Bauer, S.B., Soker, S., Yoo, J.J. and Retik, A.B. et al. (2006). Tissue-engineered autologous bladders for patients needing cystoplasty. *The Lancet, 367*(9518), 1241–1246.

Baltazar, T., Jiang, B., Moncayo, A., Merola, J., Albanna, M.Z. et al. (2023). 3D bioprinting of an implantable xeno-free vascularized human skin graft. *Bioengineering & Translational Medicine, 8*(1), e10324.

Banda Sánchez, C., Cubo Mateo, N., Saldaña, L., Valdivieso, A., Earl, J. et al. (2023). Selection and Optimization of a Bioink Based on PANC-1-Plasma/Alginate/Methylcellulose for Pancreatic Tumour Modelling. *Polymers, 15*(15), 3196.

Bein, A., Kim, S., Goyal, G., Cao, W., Fadel, C. et al. (2021). Enteric Coronavirus Infection and Treatment Modeled With an Immunocompetent Human Intestine-On-A-Chip. *Frontiers in Pharmacology, 12,* 718484.

Bennet, D., Estlack, Z., Reid, T. and Kim, J. (2018). A microengineered human corneal epithelium-on-a-chip for eye drops mass transport evaluation. *Lab on a Chip, 18*(11), 1539–1551.

Bliley, J.M., Shiwarski, D.J. and Feinberg, A.W. (2022). 3D-bioprinted human tissue and the path toward clinical translation. *Science Translational Medicine*, *14*(666), eabo7047.

Blundell, C., Yi, Y., Ma, L., Tess, E.R., Farrell, M.J. et al. (2018). Placental Drug Transport-on-a-Chip: A Microengineered In Vitro Model of Transporter-Mediated Drug Efflux in the Human Placental Barrier. *Advanced Healthcare Materials*, *7*(2), 1700786.

Bogala, M.R. (2022). Three-dimensional (3D) printing of hydroxyapatite-based scaffolds: A review. *Bioprinting*, *28*, e00244.

Boland, T., Xu, T., Damon, B. and Cui, X. (2006). Application of inkjet printing to tissue engineering. *Biotechnology Journal*, *1*(9), 910–917.

Chang, R., Starly, B., Sun, W., Culbertson, C., Holtorf, H. et al. (2006). Freeform Bioprinting of Liver Encapsulated in Alginate Hydrogels Tissue Constructs for Pharmacokinetic Study. The University of Texas at Austin. Retrieved January 31, 2024, from https://repositories.lib.utexas.edu/handle/2152/80104

Cheng, R.Y., Eylert, G., Gariepy, J.-M., He, S., Ahmad, H. et al. (2020). Handheld instrument for wound-conformal delivery of skin precursor sheets improves healing in full-thickness burns. *Biofabrication*, *12*(2), 025002.

Cho, Y., Na, K., Jun, Y., Won, J., Yang, J.H. et al. (2021). Three-Dimensional In Vitro Lymphangiogenesis Model in Tumor Microenvironment. *Frontiers in Bioengineering and Biotechnology*, *9*, 697657.

Crook, J.M. (Ed.). (2020). *3D Bioprinting: Principles and Protocols*. Methods in Molecular Biology (Vol. 2140). New York, NY: Springer US. Retrieved February 4, 2024, from https://link.springer.com/10.1007/978-1-0716-0520-2

Cui, X., Breitenkamp, K., Finn, M.G., Lotz, M. and D'Lima, D.D. et al. (2012). Direct Human Cartilage Repair Using Three-Dimensional Bioprinting Technology. *Tissue Engineering Part A*, *18*(11–12), 1304–1312.

Deng, S., Li, C., Cao, J., Cui, Z., Du, J. et al. (2023). Organ-on-a-chip meets artificial intelligence in drug evaluation. *Theranostics*, *13*(13), 4526–4558.

Derr, K., Zou, J., Luo, K., Song, M.J., Sittampalam, G.S. et al. (2019). Fully Three-Dimensional Bioprinted Skin Equivalent Constructs with Validated Morphology and Barrier Function. *Tissue Engineering Part C: Methods*, *25*(6), 334–343.

Di Bella, C., Duchi, S., O'Connell, C.D., Blanchard, R., Augustine, C., (2018). *In situ* handheld three-dimensional bioprinting for cartilage regeneration. *Journal of Tissue Engineering and Regenerative Medicine*, *12*(3), 611–621.

Duin, S., Schütz, K., Ahlfeld, T., Lehmann, S., Lode, A. et al. (2019). 3D Bioprinting of Functional Islets of Langerhans in an Alginate/Methylcellulose Hydrogel Blend. *Advanced Healthcare Materials*, *8*(7), 1801631.

Ehrlich, A., Tsytkin-Kirschenzweig, S., Ioannidis, K., Ayyash, M., Riu, A. et al. (2018). Microphysiological flux balance platform unravels the dynamics of drug induced steatosis. *Lab on a Chip*, *18*(17), 2510–2522.

Flores-Torres, S., Peza-Chavez, O., Kuasne, H., Munguia-Lopez, J.G., Kort-Mascort, J., Ferri, L., Jiang, T., et al. (2021). Alginate gelatin–Matrigel hydrogels enable the development and multigenerational passaging of patient-derived 3D bioprinted cancer spheroid models. *Biofabrication*, *13*(2), 025001.

Gaetani, R., Feyen, D.A.M., Verhage, V., Slaats, R., Messina, E. et al. (2015). Epicardial application of cardiac progenitor cells in a 3D-printed gelatin/hyaluronic acid patch preserves cardiac function after myocardial infarction. *Biomaterials*, *61*, 339–348.

Glieberman, A.L., Pope, B.D., Zimmerman, J.F., Liu, Q., Ferrier, J.P et al. (2019). Synchronized stimulation and continuous insulin sensing in a microfluidic human Islet on a Chip designed for scalable manufacturing. *Lab on a Chip*, *19*(18), 2993–3010.

Gnecco, J.S., Pensabene, V., Li, D.J., Ding, T., Hui, E.E et al. (2017). Compartmentalized Culture of Perivascular Stroma and Endothelial Cells in a Microfluidic Model of the Human Endometrium. *Annals of Biomedical Engineering*, *45*(7), 1758–1769.

Gopinathan, J. and Noh, I. (2018). Recent trends in bioinks for 3D printing. *Biomaterials Research*, *22*(1), 11.

Gu, Z., Fu, J., Lin, H. and He, Y. (2020). Development of 3D bioprinting: From printing methods to biomedical applications. *Asian Journal of Pharmaceutical Sciences*, *15*(5), 529–557.

Gungor-Ozkerim, P.S., Inci, I., Zhang, Y. S., Khademhosseini, A. and Dokmeci, M.R. et al. (2018). Bioinks for 3D bioprinting: An overview. *Biomaterials Science*, *6*(5), 915–946.

Guo, X., Wang, D., He, B., Hu, L. and Jiang, G. et al. (2023). 3D Bioprinting of Cultured Meat: A Promising Avenue of Meat Production. *Food and Bioprocess Technology*. Retrieved March 12, 2024, from https://link.springer.com/10.1007/s11947-023-03195-x

Hachey, S.J., Movsesyan, S., Nguyen, Q.H., Burton-Sojo, G., Tankazyan, A. et al. (2021). An *in vitro* vascularized micro-tumor model of human colorectal cancer recapitulates *in vivo* responses to standard-of-care therapy. *Lab on a Chip*, *21*(7), 1333–1351.

Hassell, B.A., Goyal, G., Lee, E., Sontheimer-Phelps, A., Levy, O. et al. (2017). Human Organ Chip Models Recapitulate Orthotopic Lung Cancer Growth, Therapeutic Responses, and Tumor Dormancy In Vitro. *Cell Reports*, *21*(2), 508–516.

Hu, S., Martinez-Garcia, F.D., Moeun, B.N., Burgess, J.K., Harmsen, M.C., Hoesli, C. et al. (2021). An immune regulatory 3D-printed alginate-pectin construct for immunoisolation of insulin producing β-cells. *Materials Science and Engineering: C*, *123*, 112009.

Idaszek, J., Volpi, M., Paradiso, A., Nguyen Quoc, M., Górecka, Ż. et al. (2021). Alginate-based tissue-specific bioinks for multi-material 3D-bioprinting of pancreatic islets and blood vessels: A step towards vascularized pancreas grafts. *Bioprinting*, *24*, e00163.

Jamieson, C., Keenan, P., Kirkwood, D., Oji, S., Webster, C. et al. (2021). A Review of Recent Advances in 3D Bioprinting With an Eye on Future Regenerative Therapies in Veterinary Medicine. *Frontiers in Veterinary Science*, *7*, 584193.

Jang, J., Park, H.-J., Kim, S.-W., Kim, H., Park, J.Y. et al. (2017). 3D printed complex tissue construct using stem cell-laden decellularized extracellular matrix bioinks for cardiac repair. *Biomaterials*, *112*, 264–274.

Jang, K.-J., Otieno, M.A., Ronxhi, J., Lim, H.-K., Ewart, L. et al. (2019). Reproducing human and cross-species drug toxicities using a Liver-Chip. *Science Translational Medicine*, *11*(517), eaax5516.

Jeong, D., Seo, J. W., Lee, H., Jung, W.K., Park, Y.H. et al. (2022). Efficient Myogenic/Adipogenic Transdifferentiation of Bovine Fibroblasts in a 3D Bioprinting System for Steak-Type Cultured Meat Production. *Advanced Science*, *9*(31), 2202877.

Jorgensen, A.M., Gorkun, A., Mahajan, N., Willson, K., Clouse, C. et al. (2023). Multicellular bioprinted skin facilitates human-like skin architecture in vivo. *Science Translational Medicine*, *15*(716), eadf7547.

K. Handral, H., Hua Tay, S., Wan Chan, W. and Choudhury, D. (2022). 3D Printing of cultured meat products. *Critical Reviews in Food Science and Nutrition*, *62*(1), 272–281.

Kačarević, Ž., Rider, P., Alkildani, S., Retnasingh, S., Smeets, R. et al. (2018). An Introduction to 3D Bioprinting: Possibilities, Challenges and Future Aspects. *Materials*, *11*(11), 2199.

Kachouie, N.N., Du, Y., Bae, H., Khabiry, M., Ahari, A.F. et al. (2010). Directed assembly of cell-laden hydrogels for engineering functional tissues. *Organogenesis*, *6*(4), 234–244.

Kang, D.-H., Louis, F., Liu, H., Shimoda, H., Nishiyama, Y. et al. (2021). Engineered whole cut meat-like tissue by the assembly of cell fibers using tendon-gel integrated bioprinting. *Nature Communications*, *12*(1), 5059.

Keriquel, V., Guillemot, F., Arnault, I., Guillotin, B., Miraux, S. et al. (2010). *In vivo* bioprinting for computer- and robotic-assisted medical intervention: Preliminary study in mice. *Biofabrication*, *2*(1), 014101.

Kilic Bektas, C. and Hasirci, V. (2020). Cell loaded 3D bioprinted GelMA hydrogels for corneal stroma engineering. *Biomaterials Science*, *8*(1), 438–449.

Kim, B.S., Gao, G., Kim, J.Y. and Cho, D. (2019). 3D Cell Printing of Perfusable Vascularized Human Skin Equivalent Composed of Epidermis, Dermis, and Hypodermis for Better Structural Recapitulation of Native Skin. *Advanced Healthcare Materials*, *8*(7), 1801019.

Kim, H.J., Li, H., Collins, J.J. and Ingber, D.E. (2016). Contributions of microbiome and mechanical deformation to intestinal bacterial overgrowth and inflammation in a human gut-on-a-chip. *Proceedings of the National Academy of Sciences*, *113*(1). Retrieved March 12, 2024, from https://pnas.org/doi/full/10.1073/pnas.1522193112

Kim, H., Jang, J., Park, J., Lee, K.-P., Lee, S. et al. (2019). Shear-induced alignment of collagen fibrils using 3D cell printing for corneal stroma tissue engineering. *Biofabrication*, *11*(3), 035017.

Kim, J., Lee, K.-T., Lee, J.S., Shin, J., Cui, B. et al. (2021). Fungal brain infection modelled in a human-neurovascular-unit-on-a-chip with a functional blood–brain barrier. *Nature Biomedical Engineering*, *5*(8), 830–846.

Kirillova, A., Bushev, S., Abubakirov, A. and Sukikh, G. (2020). Bioethical and Legal Issues in 3D Bioprinting. *International Journal of Bioprinting*, *6*(3), 272.

Klak, M., Wszoła, M., Berman, A., Filip, A., Kosowska, A. et al. (2023). Bioprinted 3D Bionic Scaffolds with Pancreatic Islets as a New Therapy for Type 1 Diabetes—Analysis of the Results of Preclinical Studies on a Mouse Model. *Journal of Functional Biomaterials*, *14*(7), 371.

Kutlehria, S., Dinh, T.C., Bagde, A., Patel, N., Gebeyehu, A. (2020). High-throughput 3D bioprinting of corneal stromal equivalents. *Journal of Biomedical Materials Research Part B: Applied Biomaterials*, *108*(7), 2981–2994.

Kutys, M.L., Polacheck, W.J., Welch, M.K., Gagnon, K.A., Koorman, T. et al. (2020). Uncovering mutation-specific morphogenic phenotypes and paracrine-mediated vessel dysfunction in a biomimetic vascularized mammary duct platform. *Nature Communications*, *11*(1), 3377.

Lai, B.F.L., Lu, R.X.Z., Hu, Y., Davenport Huyer, L., Dou. et al. (2020). Recapitulating Pancreatic Tumor Microenvironment through Synergistic Use of Patient Organoids and Organ-on-a-Chip Vasculature. *Advanced Functional Materials*, *30*(48), 2000545.

Lam, T., Dehne, T., Krüger, J.P., Hondke, S., Endres, M. et al. (2019). Photopolymerizable gelatin and hyaluronic acid for stereolithographic 3D bioprinting of tissue-engineered cartilage. *Journal of Biomedical Materials Research Part B: Applied Biomaterials, 107*(8), 2649–2657.

Lee, H., Chae, S., Kim, J.Y., Han, W., Kim, J. et al. (2019). Cell-printed 3D liver-on-a-chip possessing a liver microenvironment and biliary system. *Biofabrication, 11*(2), 025001.

Lee, S.W., Kwak, H.S., Kang, M.-H., Park, Y.-Y et al. (2018). Fibroblast-associated tumour microenvironment induces vascular structure-networked tumouroid. *Scientific Reports, 8*(1), 2365.

Leung, C.M., De Haan, P., Ronaldson-Bouchard, K., Kim, G.-A., Ko, J. et al. (2022). A guide to the organ-on-a-chip. *Nature Reviews Methods Primers, 2*(1), 33.

Li, W., Liu, Z., Tang, F., Jiang, H., Zhou, Z. et al. (2023). Application of 3D Bioprinting in Liver Diseases. *Micromachines, 14*(8), 1648.

López-Marcial, G.R., Zeng, A.Y., Osuna, C., Dennis, J., García, J. M et al. (2018). Agarose-Based Hydrogels as Suitable Bioprinting Materials for Tissue Engineering. *ACS Biomaterials Science & Engineering, 4*(10), 3610–3616.

Lu, S., Cuzzucoli, F., Jiang, J., Liang, L.-G., Wang, Y. et al. (2018). Development of a biomimetic liver tumor-on-a-chip model based on decellularized liver matrix for toxicity testing. *Lab on a Chip, 18*(22), 3379–3392.

Lu, T.-Y., Lin, B., Kim, J., Sullivan, M., Tobita, K. et al. (2013). Repopulation of decellularized mouse heart with human induced pluripotent stem cell-derived cardiovascular progenitor cells. *Nature Communications, 4*(1), 2307.

Maiullari, F., Costantini, M., Milan, M., Pace, V., Chirivì, M. et al. (2018). A multi-cellular 3D bioprinting approach for vascularized heart tissue engineering based on HUVECs and iPSC-derived cardiomyocytes. *Scientific Reports, 8*(1), 13532.

Maturavongsadit, P., Narayanan, L.K., Chansoria, P., Shirwaiker, R. and Benhabbour, S.R. et al. (2021). Cell-Laden Nanocellulose/Chitosan-Based Bioinks for 3D Bioprinting and Enhanced Osteogenic Cell Differentiation. *ACS Applied Bio Materials, 4*(3), 2342–2353.

Maxson, E.L., Young, M.D., Noble, C., Go, J.L., Heidari, B. et al. (2019). In vivo remodeling of a 3D-Bioprinted tissue engineered heart valve scaffold. *Bioprinting, 16*, e00059.

Miller, K.L., Xiang, Y., Yu, C., Pustelnik, J., Wu, J. et al. (2021). Rapid 3D BioPrinting of a human iPSC-derived cardiac micro-tissue for high-throughput drug testing. *Organs-on-a-Chip, 3*, 100007.

Mondadori, C., Palombella, S., Salehi, S., Talò, G., Visone, R. et al. (2021). Recapitulating monocyte extravasation to the synovium in an organotypic microfluidic model of the articular joint. *Biofabrication, 13*(4), 045001.

Müller, M., Öztürk, E., Arlov, Ø., Gatenholm, P. and Zenobi-Wong, M. et al. (2017). Alginate Sulfate–Nanocellulose Bioinks for Cartilage Bioprinting Applications. *Annals of Biomedical Engineering, 45*(1), 210–223.

Murphy, S.V. and Atala, A. (2014). 3D bioprinting of tissues and organs. *Nature Biotechnology, 32*(8), 773–785.

Musah, S., Mammoto, A., Ferrante, T.C., Jeanty, S.S.F., Hirano-Kobayashi, M. et al. (2017). Mature induced-pluripotent-stem-cell-derived human podocytes reconstitute kidney glomerular-capillary-wall function on a chip. *Nature Biomedical Engineering, 1*(5), 0069.

Naik, S., Wood, A.R., Ongenaert, M., Saidiyan, P., Elstak, E.D. et al. (2021). A 3D Renal Proximal Tubule on Chip Model Phenocopies Lowe Syndrome and Dent II Disease Tubulopathy. *International Journal of Molecular Sciences, 22*(10), 5361.

Ng, W.L., Goh, M.H., Yeong, W.Y. and Naing, M.W. (2018). Applying macromolecular crowding to 3D bioprinting: Fabrication of 3D hierarchical porous collagen-based hydrogel constructs. *Biomaterials Science, 6*(3), 562–574.

Ni, T., Liu, M., Zhang, Y., Cao, Y. and Pei, R. (2020). 3D Bioprinting of Bone Marrow Mesenchymal Stem Cell-Laden Silk Fibroin Double Network Scaffolds for Cartilage Tissue Repair. *Bioconjugate Chemistry, 31*(8), 1938–1947.

Noor, N., Shapira, A., Edri, R., Gal, I., Wertheim, L (2019). 3D Printing of Personalized Thick and Perfusable Cardiac Patches and Hearts. *Advanced Science, 6*(11), 1900344.

Norotte, C., Marga, F.S., Niklason, L.E. and Forgacs, G. (2009). Scaffold-free vascular tissue engineering using bioprinting. *Biomaterials, 30*(30), 5910–5917.

Ortega-Prieto, A.M., Skelton, J.K., Wai, S.N., Large, E., Lussignol, M. et al. (2018). 3D microfluidic liver cultures as a physiological preclinical tool for hepatitis B virus infection. *Nature Communications, 9*(1), 682.

Pediaditakis, I., Kodella, K.R., Manatakis, D.V., Le, C.Y., Hinojosa, C.D et al. (2021). Modeling alpha-synuclein pathology in a human brain-chip to assess blood-brain barrier disruption. *Nature Communications, 12*(1), 5907.

Plebani, R., Potla, R., Soong, M., Bai, H., Izadifar, Z. et al. (2022). Modeling pulmonary cystic fibrosis in a human lung airway-on-a-chip. *Journal of Cystic Fibrosis, 21*(4), 606–615.

Ramakrishnan, R., Kasoju, N., Raju, R., Geevarghese, R., Gauthaman, A. et al. (2022). Exploring the Potential of Alginate-Gelatin-Diethylaminoethyl Cellulose-Fibrinogen based Bioink for 3D Bioprinting of Skin Tissue Constructs. *Carbohydrate Polymer Technologies and Applications*, 3, 100184.

Ramasamy, S., Davoodi, P., Vijayavenkataraman, S., Teoh, J.H., Thamizhchelvan, A.M. et al. (2021). Optimized construction of a full thickness human skin equivalent using 3D bioprinting and a PCL/collagen dermal scaffold. *Bioprinting*, 21, e00123.

Rastin, H., Ramezanpour, M., Hassan, K., Mazinani, A., Tung, T.T. et al. (2021). 3D bioprinting of a cell-laden antibacterial polysaccharide hydrogel composite. *Carbohydrate Polymers*, 264, 117989.

Reddy, V.S., Ramasubramanian, B., Telrandhe, V.M. and Ramakrishna, S. (2023). Contemporary standpoint and future of 3D bioprinting in tissue/organs printing. *Current Opinion in Biomedical Engineering*, 27, 100461.

Roche, C.D., Lin, H., Huang, Y., De Bock, C.E., Beck, D. et al. (2023). 3D bioprinted alginate-gelatin hydrogel patches containing cardiac spheroids recover heart function in a mouse model of myocardial infarction. *Bioprinting*, 30, e00263.

Shi, D., Mi, G., Wang, M. and Webster, T.J. (2019). In vitro and ex vivo systems at the forefront of infection modeling and drug discovery. *Biomaterials*, 198, 228–249.

Shin, J., Lee, Y., Li, Z., Hu, J., Park, S.S. et al. (2022). Optimized 3D Bioprinting Technology Based on Machine Learning: A Review of Recent Trends and Advances. *Micromachines*, 13(3), 363.

Shrestha, J., Ghadiri, M., Shanmugavel, M., Razavi Bazaz, S., Vasilescu, S. et al. (2019). A rapidly prototyped lung-on-a-chip model using 3D-printed molds. *Organs-on-a-Chip*, 1, 100001.

Si, L., Bai, H., Rodas, M., Cao, W., Oh, C.Y., Jiang, A. et al. (2021). A human-airway-on-a-chip for the rapid identification of candidate antiviral therapeutics and prophylactics. *Nature Biomedical Engineering*, 5(8), 815–829.

Skardal, A., Mack, D., Kapetanovic, E., Atala, A., Jackson, J.D. et al. (2012). Bioprinted Amniotic Fluid-Derived Stem Cells Accelerate Healing of Large Skin Wounds. *Stem Cells Translational Medicine*, 1(11), 792–802.

Tibrewal, K., Dandekar, P. and Jain, R. (2023). Extrusion-based sustainable 3D bioprinting of meat & its analogues: A review. *Bioprinting*, 29, e00256.

Tovaglieri, A., Sontheimer-Phelps, A., Geirnaert, A., Prantil-Baun, R., Camacho, D.M. et al. (2019). Species-specific enhancement of enterohemorrhagic E. coli pathogenesis mediated by microbiome metabolites. *Microbiome*, 7(1), 43.

Ulag, S., Ilhan, E., Sahin, A., Karademir Yilmaz, B., Kalaskar, D.M. et al. (2020). 3D printed artificial cornea for corneal stromal transplantation. *European Polymer Journal*, 133, 109744.

Vijayavenkataraman, S. (2023). 3D bioprinting: Challenges in commercialization and clinical translation. *Journal of 3D Printing in Medicine*, 7(2), 3DP8.

Vormann, M.K., Vriend, J., Lanz, H.L., Gijzen, L., Van Den Heuvel, A., et al. (2021). Implementation of a Human Renal Proximal Tubule on a Chip for Nephrotoxicity and Drug Interaction Studies. *Journal of Pharmaceutical Sciences*, 110(4), 1601–1614.

Wang, D., Guo, Y., Zhu, J., Liu, F., Xue, Y. et al. (2023). Hyaluronic acid methacrylate/pancreatic extracellular matrix as a potential 3D printing bioink for constructing islet organoids. *Acta Biomaterialia*, 165, 86–101.

Wang, H., Bi, S., Shi, B., Ma, J., Lv, X. et al. (2023). Recent Advances in Engineering Bioinks for 3D Bioprinting. *Advanced Engineering Materials*, 25(19), 2300648.

Wolfe, J.T., He, W., Kim, M.-S., Liang, H.-L., Shradhanjali, A. et al. (2023). 3D-bioprinting of patient-derived cardiac tissue models for studying congenital heart disease. *Frontiers in Cardiovascular Medicine*, 10, 1162731.

Yang, Y., Xu, R., Wang, C., Guo, Y., Sun, W. et al. (2022). Recombinant Human Collagen-Based Bioinks for the 3D Bioprinting of Full-thickness Human Skin Equivalent. *International Journal of Bioprinting*, 8(4), 611.

Yu, J., Park, S.A., Kim, W.D., Ha, T., Xin, Y.-Z. (2020). Current Advances in 3D Bioprinting Technology and Its Applications for Tissue Engineering. *Polymers*, 12(12), 2958.

Zhang, B., Xue, Q., Hu, H., Yu, M., Gao, L. et al. (2019). Integrated 3D bioprinting-based geometry-control strategy for fabricating corneal substitutes. *Journal of Zhejiang University-SCIENCE B*, 20(12), 945–959.

Zhang, H. and Wu, C. (2023). 3D printing of biomaterials for vascularized and innervated tissue regeneration. *International Journal of Bioprinting*, 9(3), 706.

Zhang, Y.S., Arneri, A., Bersini, S., Shin, S.-R., Zhu, K. et al. (2016). Bioprinting 3D microfibrous scaffolds for engineering endothelialized myocardium and heart-on-a-chip. *Biomaterials*, 110, 45–59.

Zhang, Y.S., Davoudi, F., Walch, P., Manbachi, A., Luo, X. et al. (2016). Bioprinted thrombosis-on-a-chip. *Lab on a Chip*, 16(21), 4097–4105.

Zhao, H., Xu, J., Zhang, E., Qi, R., Huang, Y. et al. (2021). 3D Bioprinting of Polythiophene Materials for Promoting Stem Cell Proliferation in a Nutritionally Deficient Environment. *ACS Applied Materials & Interfaces*, 13(22), 25759–25770.

Zhu, K., Shin, S.R., Van Kempen, T., Li, Y., Ponraj, V., et al. (2017). Gold Nanocomposite Bioink for Printing 3D Cardiac Constructs. *Advanced Functional Materials*, 27(12), 1605352.

Materials for 3D Bioprinting

Humira Assad[1] and *Ashish Kumar*[2*]

1. Introduction

In recent years, the intersection of advanced technology and biomedical research has led to the emergence of 3D BP as a groundbreaking field within medical science (Assad et al., 2023). This innovative approach combines principles of additive manufacturing with biological sciences, enabling the precise fabrication of intricate three-dimensional structures with profound implications for regenerative medicine (RM) and beyond (Sachdev, 2022). By leveraging a diverse array of biomaterials, cells, and bioactive factors, 3D BP holds the potential to revolutionize how we approach challenges in healthcare, offering new avenues for tissue regeneration, DD, and personalized medicine (Ankita, 2022). Central to the success of 3D BP is the selection and optimization of materials used in the process. The materials employed in 3D BP must possess a unique set of characteristics to facilitate cell growth, differentiation, and tissue maturation. Ideally, these materials should be biocompatible, providing a supportive environment for cell attachment, proliferation, and function (Piras, 2017; Zhang, 2022). They should also be bioresorbable, allowing for the gradual degradation of the scaffold as new tissue forms, thereby minimizing the risk of inflammation or rejection. Additionally, materials must exhibit appropriate mechanical properties to mimic the mechanical cues present in native tissues, ensuring structural integrity and functionality (Kačarević, 2018; Bartolo, 2022).

Natural polymers, like collagen, alginate, and gelatin, have garnered significant attention as key components in BP materials owing to their biocompatibility and resemblance to the extracellular matrix (ECM) found in living tissues (Liu, 2018). These polymers offer a biomimetic environment for cell adhesion, migration, and differentiation, promoting tissue regeneration and integration upon implantation. Furthermore, their tunable properties allow for the customization of mechanical strength, degradation rate, and bioactivity, making them versatile candidates for a wide range of applications (Park, 2017). Synthetic polymers, including polyurethane (PU), polyethylene glycol (PEG), and poly (lactic-co-glycolic acid) (PLGA), offer additional advantages in terms of mechanical

[1] Department of Chemistry, School of Chemical Engineering and Physical Sciences, Lovely Professional University, India.
[2] Nalanda College of Engineering, Bihar Engineering University, Science, Technology and Technical Education Department, Government of Bihar, Bihar, India.
* Corresponding author: drashishchemlpu@gmail.com

strength, stability, and process ability. These materials can be precisely engineered to achieve desired characteristics like pore size, porosity, and degradation kinetics, making them suitable for the synthesis of intricate tissue scaffolds with controlled construction and functionality (Liu and Wang, 2020). However, their synthetic nature may raise concerns regarding biocompatibility and immunogenicity, necessitating thorough biocompatibility testing and optimization (Wang, 2019; R.G and A.P, 2023). In addition to polymers, hydrogels have arisen as guaranteeing resources for 3D BP applications owing to their high water content, biocompatibility, and capability to encapsulate cells and bioactive molecules (Unagolla, 2020; Abdollahiyan, 2020). Hydrogels offer a supportive matrix for cell encapsulation and proliferation while maintaining a hydrated microenvironment conducive to cell survival and function. Moreover, their shear-thinning behavior and rapid gelation kinetics enable precise deposition and patterning of cells and biomaterials, facilitating the fabrication of complex tissue constructs with spatial control over cell distribution and organization (Abbadessa, 2016; Rajabi, 2021; Maniglia, 2020).

The field of 3D BP has seen significant advancements in material design, fabrication techniques, and biomedical applications. Researchers are exploring innovative strategies to enhance the functionality and bioactivity of bioprinted tissues, such as incorporating bioactive molecules, cell-laden microspheres, and stimuli-responsive materials. Moreover, the integration of advanced imaging techniques, computational modeling, and bioprinter technologies is enabling the development of patient-specific tissue constructs with tailored properties and functionalities (Assad, 2023). Despite these exciting developments, several challenges remain to be addressed in the field of 3D BP, including achieving vascularization, scaling up production, and ensuring long-term functionality and integration of bioprinted tissues. Additionally, regulatory and ethical considerations surrounding the use of bioprinted tissues for clinical applications require careful scrutiny and standardization to ensure safety and efficacy. In this chapter, we aim to provide a comprehensive overview of the current state-of-the-art in materials for 3D BP, highlighting recent advancements, challenges, and future prospects. By examining the properties, fabrication methods, and biomedical applications of BP materials, we seek to elucidate their pivotal role in advancing the field of medicine, ultimately paving the way for the development of functional, transplantable tissues and organs.

2. Criteria for Optimal 3D BP Materials

The range of materials available for 3D BP is growing as the field of material science advances. There are a number of things to carefully examine in order to select appropriate materials with the needed mechanical and functional properties and to ensure a successful printing process. We will now go into greater detail about the essential qualities of the best materials for 3D BP.

(a) *Printability:*   It refers to the capacity of materials to be accurately and efficiently deposited within a designated area within a defined timeframe (Kyle, 2017; Jain, 2019). The precision of the product's size and structure after 3D printing is causally linked to this performance. The demand for printability of materials will vary depending on the printing technology used. For instance, the viscosity of the substance can be severely limited when using inkjet BP. For the layered construction of intricate three-dimensional structures to occur, the material must be able to cross-link quickly. High viscosity materials can be utilized in micro-extrusion BP to preserve the original 3D shape after printing, and cross-linking can build the final stable structure after printing. As a result, the material must possess a certain cross-linking mechanism or shear thinning qualities. Many new materials are being reported for 3D BP at the moment, but ultimately these materials can only be used in a few straightforward printing processes, losing their usefulness.

(b) *Biocompatibility*:   The definition of biocompatibility has changed over time, from the original need for materials to coexist with tissues and organs and not have any negative local or systemic effects, to the more recent requirement that materials be able to positively interact with the host tissues and/or immune systems in order to achieve the goal of controlling the activity and function of host cells, tissues, and organs (Saroia, 2018; Williams, 2018). Currently, little limitations are placed on the biocompatibility of materials when using 3D BP to create medical models, rehabilitation tools, prostheses, surgical guides, and more. But when 3D BP is used to create scaffolds for tissue engineering (TE), implantable medical devices, and cell-filled tissue and organ substitutes, it is imperative that they have good biocompatibility. Materials science views the chemical composition, structural morphology, surface features, surface charge, and mechanical properties of the materials as the primary determinants of biocompatibility. Thus, the 3D BP materials can be altered in order to increase the biocompatibility through:

- Surface tampering which includes altering the charge strength of the surface, modifying the topology of the material, controlling the hydrophilicity and hydrophobicity of the outer layer, and covering it with bioactive molecules.
- Compositing or hybridizing various materials, such as merging the benefits of synthetic and natural materials to enhance the mechanical characteristics and biocompatibility of materials for 3D BP.
- Using the biomimicry principle to create materials that have a structure and function that are identical to or comparable to those that already exist *in vivo*.

(c) *Appropriate mechanical properties:*   When it comes to putting the printed structures' functions into practice, materials with a certain mechanical strength that can withstand external forces while maintaining their initial shape and structure are crucial. Selection and design of materials with varying mechanical properties (Lv, 2018) should be based on the actual application goals (Courtney, 2006; Kokubo, 2003). When constructing tissues and organs using 3D BP, it is crucial to select materials with suitable mechanical properties tailored to the diverse mechanical demands of the target tissues and organs. Additionally, sacrificial materials possessing robust mechanical qualities should be chosen to provide support during the printing process, especially for natural polymer materials with limited mechanical strength (Jang, 2017). After printing is finished, the support material must be simple to remove from the constructed objects. In the meantime, the support material itself or the products should not negatively affect the structure and other characteristics of the printed constructions after removal.

(d) *Biodegradability:*   3D BP materials should progressively break down in the body following implantation, as cells proliferate and ECM (Albayati, 2020) is produced (Nair, 2007; Martina, 2007). The rate of breakdown should coincide with the rate of generation of new tissue and the rate at which cells create ECM (Albayati, 2020) to replace implanted materials. Additionally, the breakdown products must be rapidly eliminated, easily metabolized, and non-toxic

(e) *Sterilization stability:*   An essential first step in the biological applications of biomaterials is sterilization (Qiu, 2017; Benson, 2002; Gil, 2014). Biomaterials are typically sterilized by physical or chemical methods, such as autoclaving, e-beam or gamma irradiation, heat/steam treatment, ethylene oxide treatment, ethanol incubation, and other methods that destroy all microbiological life. Every type of sterilization technique has a unique set of benefits and drawbacks as well as an appropriate range.

As a result, at least one type of sterilization technique must be compatible with the materials used in 3D BP. To put it another way, after being treated with the proper sterilization procedure, the materials must maintain their inherent properties or exhibit controlled performance degradation within an acceptable range.

3.   Common Materials in 3D Bioprinting

Metals, ceramics, and thermoplastics were the first materials to be deposited via 3D printing in non-biological applications. Organic solvents, higher processing temperatures, or cross-linking agents cannot be used while working with living cells or biomaterials (Ramadan, 2021). Thus, the focus continues to be on discovering biological materials that work well with printing processes and can meet the functional and mechanical requirements for tissue constructs (Arslan-Yildiz, 2021). The three most important characteristics of the biomaterials employed in 3D BP are printability, homogeneity in disintegration, and biocompatibility. Biomaterials are commonly characterized as organic or synthetic materials used in biological applications for the purpose of repairing or replacing any organ in the body (Assad, 2021). Based on their chemical composition, they are divided into four categories: composites, metals, polymers, and ceramics. Metals and composites have a high mechanical strength in addition to having a greater resistance to corrosion than other groups of materials (Assad, 2021; Assad et al, 2023; Assad, 2024). Polymers stand out from other materials because they are both biocompatible (BC) and biodegradable (Shim, 2017). Thermoplastic polymers are the most useful materials for 3D BP. However, they fall into two main categories for 3D BP: natural polymers and synthetic polymers (which are frequently separated from human or animal tissues). Furthermore, the word "bioink" is essential in the tissue and organ bioprinting sectors. Bioinks are made in a cellular matrix and contain both biomaterials and living cells. Compared to standard 3D printing materials, bioinks must have a print temperature lower than physiological temperatures and contain non toxic, bioactive ingredients (Gungor-Ozkerim, 2018). Because they contain materials that are suitable for them, bioinks employ both synthetic and natural polymers. Bioinks are being utilized to print a wide variety of materials, including ceramics, hydrogels, elastomers, and polymers, in 3D (O'Grady, 2019). This section discusses the benefits and limitations of certain materials for 3D BP.

3.1 Synthetic Polymers

High in strength and resistance, synthetic polymers (SP) are created artificially by humans in a laboratory with chemicals and the requisite conditions for their synthesis. The primary benefit of SP is in their easy modification due to their ability to tolerate variations in temperature and pH. Additionally, their enhanced resistance and mechanical strength allow them to be processed to meet specific requirements (Sachdeva, 2022). SP are ideal for 3D BP models because of their shallow gelation temperature, which is lower than that of natural polymers, which have a very high melting temperature. As a result, the created polymers are inert, difficult to break down, and have a high tensile strength. Below is a description of a few regularly used SP.

3.1.1 Polyurethane

A class of linearly segmented polymers known as PU are made up of organic (or hard segment) and oligodiol (or soft segment) units connected by carbamate (or urethane) linkages ($-NH-(C=O)-O-$). Because of their superior mechanical qualities and superior biocompatibility , polyurethanes (PUs), which can be either biodegradable or non-biodegradable have found extensive application in the biomedical field. Chemical composition determines the physicochemical and physiochemical characteristics of polymeric units (PUs), including their biodegradability, PH sensitivity, and thermos-sensitivity (Tsai, , 2015). For instance, ionic hydrophilic groups are frequently added to PU during its synthesis to convert it into an ionomer and cause it to disperse in water. The compositions of the soft segment oligodiols have a significant impact on the thermos- sensitivity of PU hydrogels (Hsiao, 2018). Acrylate groups are thermos-sensitive PUs that can be used for 3D printing of cells and tissues. They also function as an ultraviolet (UV) curing site. The majority of PUs that are currently in use are bioinert and non-biodegradable, therefore their uses in organ 3D printing are restricted. Our lab and others have recently made substantial use of biodegradable polymers (PUs) for 3D printing of bio-artificial organs because of their exceptional mechanical qualities, highly biocompatible materials, and adjustable chemical architectures. For center nerve repair, for instance, the aforementioned waterborne thermos-sensitive was printed at 37°C using the FDM process (Hsieh, 2015). After being 3D printed, neural stem cells (NSCs) with a cell density of 4×10^6 cells/ml demonstrated similar survivability and differentiation capacity when immersed in a waterborne PU hydrogel of the right stiffness. For the purpose of neuro regeneration, neural-like constructs made from human fibroblasts co-printed with FoxD3 plasmids in PU hydrogel may be used. Using Ho et al.'s waterborne thermos-responsive polymeric ultra-violet hydrogel as a "bioink," cells could be directly reprogrammed for customized cartilage tissue engineering (Ho, 2018).

The researchers also created a novel biodegradable elastomeric polymer (PU) and used it to 3D print supporting templates for cell migration, accommodation, growth, and proliferation. (Huang, 2013). This biodegradable elastomeric PU has been used in numerous biomedical applications over the last ten years, including hierarchical vascular/nerve networks, rabbit vein restoration overcoats, and conduits for peripheral nerve repair (Midha, 2019). Specifically, "a double-layer PU-collagen conduit with superior hydrophilicity, biocompatibilities, and mechanical qualities was 3D printed to serve as guides and bridges between the proximal and distal stumps for the repair of extensive peripheral nerve damage (Cui, 2009). Notably, a double-nozzle, low-temperature deposition 3D printer operating at $-20°C$ was used to produce a tubular PU-adipose stem cells (ASCs)/gelatin/ alginate/fibrinogen construct (He, 2011)". By including cryoprotectants in the hydrogels, such as dextran-40, glycerol, and DMSO, the ASCs were able to survive the freeze 3D printing stage. For over a month, cell activity was successfully maintained below $-80°C$. Cell viability in the hydrogels containing 5% DMSO after thawing was almost 80%, which was substantially higher than that of other methods of cell preservation. Because the cryo-protectants prevent ice crystals from forming during the freezing and thawing processes, there may be a lower chance of cell injury. Consequently, the cryo-protectant that uses 3D printing technology becomes a straightforward, easy, labor-saving, and practical technique for the preservation of bio-artificial organs in the future (Wang, 2010).

Moreover, our DIY double-nozzle low-temperature deposition 3D printer automatically produced a hybrid hierarchical PU-cell/hydrogel construct (Wang, 2013). The integrated biodegradable elastomeric PU with tunable biodegradation properties and good biocompatibility was composed of PCL and PEG. Pulsatile cultures of the 3D vascular templates with a principal axis were conducted in a bioreactor. Additional research has been done to develop neuronal and vascular networks in a complex bioartificial organ at the same time (Wang, 2013).

3.1.2 Polypropylene

Many uses for polypropylene (PP) have been developed, including as in prostheses and sutures. PP's molecular weight and dispersion, crystalline structure, and tactility are its defining characteristics. This inexpensive polymer has many qualities, including dimensional stability, flame resistance, transparency, and recyclability (RW, 1975; Zhang, 2022). Because it is lightweight and fatigue resistant, PP is used in low-strength applications. It is mostly used for packaging and storing and is semi-rigid (Gope, 2022). Because they are transparent and have good heat and impact resistance, they are utilized in syringes, inhalation systems, containers, caps, and closures. It is also utilized in the pharmaceutical, medical device, syringe, and diagnostics areas since it has reduced density, commendable chemical resistance, minimal toxicity, excellent electrical insulation, limited moisture absorption, decreased flammability, and an easy sterilization process (Zhang, 2019). Combining degradable and bioresorbable PP with hemp and coir fibers can result in joints and bone fixings with a high elongation property that help patients feel less discomfort (Pandiyaraj, 2016). Additionally, polypropylene has anti-thrombogenic properties that can be improved to support plasma protein adsorption, adhesion, and platelet activation, all of which are critical for biomedical applications. By employing the cold atmospheric pressure plasma (CAPP) aided polymerization process to add functional groups to the polymer's surface, the enhancement aims to improve blood compatibility (Lim, 2014).

Conventional sutures' biocompatibility raises serious concerns about immunological reactions, also known as hypersensitivity emerging from sutures, in which the sutures function as an antigen and initiate an immune response. It has been discovered that polypropylene is the ideal material to address biocompatibility concerns and offer a more effective treatment strategy. Immune incompatibility affects deep tissue and wound closure, causing discomfort to the dermal layer.

Any such incompatible cases should be consulted well in advance of undergoing a certain surgery since they can impact healthcare management and raise healthcare costs (Senarath-Yapa, 2014). For female pelvic floor dysfunction, tissue rejection and prosthetic mesh degradation persisted; the standard treatment involves employing synthetic grafts for pelvic reconstruction (Cheng, 2017). Because adipose-derived stem cells (ADSCs) have a high differentiation potential and the capacity to self-renew, employing polypropylene-based mesh integrated with ADSCs has found use in the therapy of dysfunction. This allows for the facilitation of TE (Winnacker, 2016; Gavrila, 2020). Although PP's poor mechanical qualities make it unsuitable for use in load-bearing applications, its remarkable fiber-forming qualities have allowed it to be used in the treatment of ventral incisional hernias and as a source of tetracycline for dental therapy. Chemically crosslinking PP for utilization in biomedical contexts is continuously being researched and developed. To obtain the required qualities and biocompatibility, there are a few possible approaches and considerations. One strategy that could be employed is the use of reactive molecules or functional groups that are capable of undergoing crosslinking reactions. For example, thiol-ene or thiol-epoxy procedures can be used to crosslink polypropylene chains by introducing thiol groups.

3.1.3   *Poly (lactic-co-glycolic acid)*

The FDA has approved PLGA, also known as linear aliphatic polyester is a synthetic copolymer of lactic acid and glycolic acid (Astete, 2006), (Liu, 2020). A popular copolymer having a composition of 75% lactic acid and 25% glycolic acid is known as PLGA 75:25. Due to the asymmetric carbon atom in the monomer lactic acid, it has two optical isomers: d (+) lactic acid and l (–) lactic acid (Gavrila, 2020). It is widely distributed as an intermediate or end product in the metabolism of carbohydrates in all living things, including humans, animals, plants, and microbes. In the meanwhile, small amounts of glycolic acid can be found in nature. By severing the ester connections inside its chains while wet, PLGA can be hydrolyzed. Either acidic monomers like lactic acid and glycolic acid or harmless salts like lactate (the salt form of lactic acid) and glycolate (the salt form of glycolic acid) are the end products of PLGA decomposition. Research has demonstrated that the amount of time needed for PLGA breakdown is correlated with the ratio of monomers, which is reflected in the molecular makeup. In comparison to lactide-predominant polymers, the amount of glycolide units increases with degrading time (Samadi, 2013).

Depending on its composition, PLGA can dissolve in a range of organic solvents. Polymers with higher glycolide content may require the use of fluorinated solvents, such as 1, 1, 1, 3, 3, 3-hexafluoroisopropanol, while those with higher lactide content dissolve in chlorinated solvents. The glass transition temperature of PLGA solutions typically lies between -40 and $-60°C$. We have created many low-temperature RP methods in the author's group to deposit synthetic PLGA solutions by themselves or in combination with other polymers. "Hybrid constructs with strong mechanical properties, tunable biodegradability, and acceptable in vivo biocompatibility , such as PLGA-gelatin, PLGA-collagen, PLGA/hydroxyapatite, PLGA/hydroxyapatite/phosphorylated chitosan etc., can be created by 3D printing different material systems together using double or multi nozzle 3D bioprinters (Li, 2019; Wang et al, 2017; Wang, 2017)". Large organ repair, regeneration, replacement, and restoration have all benefited greatly from the widespread usage of 3D printed constructs for bone, cartilage, nerve, and liver restoration. Simultaneously, the idea of neuralization and vascularization of large-scale 3D printed tissues has spread quickly throughout the globe (Marrella, 2018; Zhang, 2008).

3.1.4   *Polyethylene glycol*

PEG, sometimes referred to as poly(oxyethylene) or poly (ethylene oxide) (PEO), is a synthetic polyether with a linear and branching structure that is hydrophilic, biocompatible, and non-immunogenic. The FDA has authorized PEG in biomedicine as a promising option for cell encapsulation. Although PEG hydrogels are not biodegradable by nature, they can be made more biodegradable by adding segments that break down more quickly. The hydrolytical blocks that are most frequently utilized are PCL, PGA, and PLA (Jiang, 2008). The synthetic polymer that has been studied the most for soft tissue repair is undoubtedly PEG and its variants. Because PEG hydrogels lack cell-adhesive domains, they are unable to create the perfect environment for supporting tissue development and cell adhesion on their own. However, by using physical, ionic, or covalent crosslinking, the two hydroxyl groups of PEG-diol in the PEG molecules can be modified into different functional groups (such as acrylate, thiol, or carboxyl), which are useful for hydrogel production or conjugating with biomolecules (Shan, 2012). PEG is frequently chemically changed by adding acrylate groups to produce photopolymerizable PEGDA, which encapsulates cells fast. In extrusion-based 3D printing, PEGDA photopolymerized by UV light has been used to create scaffolds for TE with improved mechanical qualities. PEG hydrogels have recently seen the emergence of bioactive modification as a key tactic for controlling particular biological responses. To give cells an environment that mimics the ECM (M.R, 2020) , biomolecules such as growth factors, enzyme-sensitive peptides (ESPs), and cell-adhesive peptides (CAPs) have been used. Zhu evaluated the bioactive PEG hydrogels and their manufacturing methods in 2010 (Zhu, 2010). Villanueva et al. used PEG hydrogels incorporating Arg-Gly-Asp (RGD) to dynamically mechanically load cartilage BP in order to study the role of cell-matrix interactions. During mechanical stimulations, RGD-incorporated PEG hydrogels could enhance the chondrocyte phenotype and matrix production. This indicates that cell-matrix interactions play a crucial role in mediating cell activities through 3D printing (Villanueva, 2009). To optimize hybrid "bioinks" and bolster the mechanical properties of engineered hard tissues, researchers have combined PEG with GelMA. Employing inkjet-based printing techniques alongside CAPs, ESPs, and growth factors, researchers observed a notable augmentation in mesenchymal stem cell differentiation into cartilage and bone (Burmeister, 2018).

3.2 Natural Polymers

One can obtain naturally occurring polymers by a variety of physical, chemical, or biological techniques. Natural polymers are more tissue-friendly because they are compatible, able to withstand fluid, and easily soluble in a variety of solvents, including cell culture solutions and phosphate buffers. These characteristics allow it to be printed layer by layer, creating a model that, in a steady environment, will resemble a real organ (Bonandrini, 2014; Ozbolat, 2016). Among the most crucial attributes of these naturally derived polymers is their capacity to mimic cells or tissues, undergo proliferation, maturation, and differentiation, and synchronize with surrounding structures when provided with a controlled environment, including optimal temperature, sufficient hydration, and suitable growth medium (Derby, 2012; Toh, 2014; Hou, 2015). A significant disadvantage of natural polymers is that their activities are all significantly impacted by changes in the surrounding environment, such as temperature rises, dehydration, or the type of solvent in which they are dissolved. The following list includes several naturally occurring polymers that are frequently used: chitosan, collagen, alginate, and gelatin.

3.2.1 Chitosan

One well-known natural polymer used in TE is chitosan. It is a good choice for TE because of its inexpensive cost, biodegradability, antibacterial qualities, and biocompatibility. The exoskeletons of marine crustaceans, including lobsters, krill, prawns, and crabs, serve as the primary source of raw material for chitosan. It has a flexible structure, a lot of functional groups, and can be 3D printed into a variety of forms and sizes (Ding, 2021). Wu. employed chitosan hydrogel for directed cell growth in 2017 (Wu, 2017). Cheng et al. simultaneously synthesized a composite of chitosan and poly (ethylene glycol)-diacrylate/poly (caprolactone)-diacrylate for 3D printing using photopolymerization (Cheng, 2017). For bone TE, Lee et al. created scaffolds based on chitosan, gelatin, and hydroxyapatite (Lee, 2017). Elviri et al. employed chitosan scaffold to improve cell proliferation, while Morris et al. used chitosan and PEG diacrylate as bioink to print scaffolds using stereolithography (Mossesson, 2005; Elviri, 2017). Chitosan's poor strength restricts its application in TE, despite its many benefits (Bakshi, 2020). To address structural flaws, nano-sized materials were incorporated as fillers into chitosan and evenly dispersed throughout the entire matrix. Sadeghianmaryan et al. utilized 3D printing technology to impregnate sodium alginate and nano-hydroxyapatite (nHA) onto a printed chitosan scaffold, resulting in the creation of a chitosan/sodium alginate/nano-hydroxyapatite scaffold (Sadeghianmaryan, 2022). According to the compression test and the live/dead cell analysis, nHA improved cell survival and adhesion while also raising the scaffold's elastic modulus.

3.2.2 Gelatin

Gelatin, derived from the breakdown of collagen, is a naturally occurring protein that displays amphoteric behavior due to the presence of both alkaline and acidic amino acid functional groups (Lu, 2022). Mammalian gelatin has been employed as a biomaterial for regenerative purposes. Gelatin has low immunogenicity, is water soluble, non-cytotoxic, biocompatible, and stimulates cell adhesion. Owing to these features, gelatin hydrogel, also known as gelatin methacryloyl becomes a popular medium for DIW printing (GelMA). A novel method for printing cell-filled GelMA structures was proposed by Liu et al. (Liu, 2017). Lee et al. evaluated two varieties of GelMA for BP using cells (Lee, 2016). They stated that in the printed structures of A and B GelMA, cell survival reached up to 75%. Due to their high porosity and low stiffness, these components may be able to promote cell proliferation and survival. Gelatin derived from mammals has found application as a biomaterial with regenerative properties. Gelatin and its byproducts are extensively utilized in 3D bioprinting due to their favorable characteristics, including high biocompatibility, low immunogenicity, non-toxicity, water solubility, and ability to enhance cell adhesion (Park, 2017; Wang, 2013). The unique sol-gel transition in the gelatin combination appears at 28°C, which is also the melting temperature of the G hydrogel. Because of this, gelatin-based solutions' special thermal properties allow for the injection or extrusion of cells and/or bioactive materials using 3D BP plungers, and then the stacking of those materials at temperatures that are generally tolerated for the environment, between 1 and 28°C. In addition, hydrogels and solutions based on gelatin are employed both during and after 3D printing processes in order to maintain the structural integrity of the manufactured objects and to create niches within the prefabricated structures for cells and bioactive materials. These qualities have made gelatin hydrogel, such as GelMA, popular and widely used in DIW printing. However, there are two major disadvantages to natural gelatin-based hydrogels in the realm of 3D organ printing (Liu, 2018):

- Limited mechanical strength,
- Structural instability at physiological temperatures.

The physiological, cross-linked gel phases (or structures) are seen to degrade rapidly upon placing the printed, unit-filled 3D assemblies in culture conditions at around 37°C. The reason for this is that the inherent cross-linking between the gelatin molecules disorganizes at a melting point of 28°C, impairing the structural integrity of the three-dimensional (3D) forms. Stated differently, in a culture media, gelled gelatin-based structures dissolve instantaneously due to reversible, physical cross-linking linkages. In order to create a stable structure through 3D printing, gelatin structures must be reinforced even more (Rutz, 2015; Nagel, 2013).

3.2.3 Collagen

Over the past few decades, natural collagen has become a popular scaffold material for TE. It can greatly enhance osteoblasts, chondroblasts, and mesenchymal stem cells' adhesion, proliferation, and differentiation capacities on porous scaffolds (Nagel, 2013). In particular, cell seeding on the pore surface is facilitated by the collagen scaffold's pore size range of 50–150 μm. Collagen (Sachdeva, 2022) is thought to be able to bind to integrin receptors on the cell membrane and encourage cell adhesion and proliferation because it shares the same RGD peptide domains as gelatin. However, hydrogel potential (pH) and temperature can easily alter the characteristics of acid-soluble collagen solution, which complicates the process of 3D printing collagen solutions under ambient conditions. The reasoning behind this is that, when the solution reaches neutralization at 37°C, collagenases and metalloproteinase can rapidly degrade the collagen molecules into amino acids. Collagen molecules also have a tendency to congregate to create hydrogel. Collagen types I and II in particular have been widely used for 3D printed cartilage and bone healing scaffolds. The utilization of 3D printed scaffolds for tissue repair offers three distinct advantages. Firstly, unlike conventional TE porous scaffolds, most 3D printed scaffolds incorporate scaled-up passageways that facilitate the transport of nutrients, oxygen, and metabolites. Secondly, the gradient structural morphology and material composites of 3D printed scaffolds enable the realization of diverse functionalities. Lastly, biocompatible materials for hard/soft tissue/organ engineering can directly incorporate living cells. The articular cartilage, for instance, has a gradient cell density and a zonal ECM distribution extending from the articular surface to the calcified cartilage. One of the primary shortcomings of traditional tissue-engineered articular cartilage is its inability to replicate the mechanical and biological characteristics of individual zones of natural cartilage. In contrast, BP methods may produce precisely shaped constructions with precise cell distribution (Weadcock, 1996). The designed zonal cartilage created by BP collagen type II hydrogel constructions with a gradient chondrocyte density was the subject of a study by Ren et al. Collagen type II was found to be crucial in promoting chondrogenic differentiation and to be capable of preserving chondrocyte phenotypes in this investigation. The distribution of ECM within the 3D printed zonal cartilage exhibited a gradient pattern that correlated positively with chondrocyte density. To enhance biological effects, adjustments were made to the cell density and distribution pattern across various zonal areas during the bioprinting process (Ren, 2016). The limited applicability of pure collagen hydrogels as "bioinks" in 3D bioprinting of tissues and organs stems from their low viscosity and rapid degradation rate. To address this, blending collagen with other polymers like hyaluronic acid, fibrin, agarose, and alginate has become the preferred approach. This modification enhances viscosity, controls degradation rate, and improves printability, thus expanding the utility of collagen-based bioinks in bioprinting applications (Nagel, 2013).

3.2.4 Alginate

Brown algae provide the anionic polysaccharide known as alginate, sometimes referred to as algin. The word "alginate" can refer to any of the derivatives of alginic acid as well as the acid itself. It is typically used to describe the salts of alginic acid, which are made up of "β-d-mannuronic acid (M block) and α-l-glucuronic acid (G block) (Pawar, 2012; Eskens, 2020).

Alginate has shown special interest in wound healing, medication delivery, and RM because it dissolves in water and can be chemically crosslinked by divalent cations like barium (Ba^{2+}), strontium (Sr^{2+}), and calcium (Ca^{2+}) ions (Lee, 2012; Choi, 2017). The physiochemical characteristics of the alginate solution are intimately associated with the ratio of the M to G block. While a lower G/M ratio enhances flexibility, a greater G/M ratio gives polymeric structure and mechanical qualities stiffness (Stanton, 2015). Alginate and composite alginate hydrogels have been widely employed as cell-filled "bioinks" in certain 3D BP technologies due to their excellent chemical gelling ability, quick biodegradability, and superior biocompatibility (Axpe, 2016). (Several methods can be used to accomplish alginate-related 3D BP processes. These include pre-cross-linked alginate hydrogel coextruded with cells, coaxial nozzle-assisted crosslinking deposition with cross-linker spraying over the extruded cell-laden hydrogel, and cell-laden hydrogel bio-plotting in a plotting medium (cross-linker pool) (Ahn, 2012). In the field of tissue/organ 3D printing, each of these 3D BP processes has advantages and disadvantages. Two common occurrences in 3D BP with alginate are as follows. The first is that the low phase changing temperature (sol-gel transition point) and shear thinning characteristic of pure alginate solution make it difficult to print layer by layer into a high scale-up construct. Another frequent occurrence is that oxidation processes might adjust the sluggish biodegradation rate of alginate molecules (Wong, 2000). Organ 3D printing may benefit more from the oxidized alginate molecules with the right rate of degradation. Jia et al. concentrated on oxidizing alginate molecules in order to regulate the printability and degradability of alginate. Before printing, the oxidized alginate solutions might be optimized to produce precise lattice structures with improved accuracies (Jia, 2014). It is also possible to load human adipose-derived stem cells (hADSCs) into the oxidized alginate solutions. In their study, the alginate's concentration (conc.) and oxidation percentage (ox.) were compiled. The findings showed that whilst 5% ox.–15% conc. alginate was linked to an enhanced spreading cell phenotype that would promote osteogenesis, 0% ox.-8% conc. alginate produced a round cell shape that might be applicable to chondrogenesis. It was suggested that the best formulation of their "bioinks" for 3D BP be 5% ox.–15% conc. alginate.

Conclusion and Outlook

In the realm of 3D BP, the selection and engineering of suitable materials stand as the cornerstone for success. From synthetic to natural polymeric materials, each offers unique properties and functionalities crucial for fabricating intricate tissue structures. These materials provide a biomimetic microenvironment that supports cell adhesion, proliferation, and differentiation, laying the groundwork for applications in TE, RM, and DD. In this chapter, we have embarked on a comprehensive exploration of the materials crucial for advancing the field of 3D BP. Recognizing that the success of BP hinges on the selection of appropriate materials, we have delved into the criteria guiding this selection process. Moreover, we have scrutinized a diverse array of materials, spanning from natural to SP, each offering unique advantages and functionalities essential for fabricating complex tissue structures.

Looking ahead, the future of materials for 3D BP holds immense promise and potential for transformative advancements. Researchers are exploring novel biomaterials with enhanced biocompatibility, mechanical properties, and bio-functionalities to expand the capabilities of BP technology. Currently, the limited availability of biomaterials suitable for 3D bioprinting underscores the urgent need for further research in this area. Such endeavors hold promise for potentially saving the lives of numerous patients awaiting transplants. Furthermore, interdisciplinary collaborations between material scientists, biologists, engineers, and clinicians will drive innovation and accelerate the translation of 3D BP from bench to bedside. As the field progresses, we anticipate witnessing the fabrication of functional and implantable tissues and organs with unprecedented fidelity and physiological relevance. This progress will open new avenues for personalized medicine, organ transplantation, disease modeling, and drug screening, revolutionizing the landscape of healthcare and regenerative therapies. With ongoing research endeavors and technological innovations, 3D BP stands poised to realize its full potential as a transformative approach in RM and TE, shaping the future of healthcare for generations to come.

References

Abbadessa, A. *A synthetic thermosensitive hydrogel for cartilage bioprinting and its biofunctionalization with polysaccharides.* Biomacromolecules, 2016. 17(6): p. 2137–2147.

Abdollahiyan, P. *Hydrogel-based 3D bioprinting for bone and cartilage tissue engineering.* Biotechnology journal, 2020. 15(12): p. 2000095.

Ahn, S., et al., *Cells (MC3T3-E1)-laden alginate scaffolds fabricated by a modified solid-freeform fabrication process supplemented with an aerosol spraying.* Biomacromolecules, 2012. 13(9): p. 2997-3003.

Albayati, M.R., *Synthesis, crystal structure, Hirshfeld surface analysis and DFT calculations of 2-[(2, 3-dimethylphenyl) amino]-N'-[(E)-thiophen-2-ylmethylidene] benzohydrazide.* Journal of Molecular Structure, 2020. 1205: p. 127654.

Ankita IV, S., *A Review on Techniques and Biomaterials Used in 3D Bioprinting.* Cureus, 2022. 14(8).

Arslan-Yildiz, A., *Towards artificial tissue models: past, present, and future of 3D bioprinting.* Biofabrication, 2016. 8(1): p. 014103.

Assad, H. and A. Kumar, *Understanding functional group effect on corrosion inhibition efficiency of selected organic compounds.* Journal of Molecular Liquids, 2021. 344: p. 117755.

Assad, H., *A research combined experimental and computational approaches of succinylsulfathiazole hydrate as potent corrosion inhibitor for mild steel in acidic medium.* Journal of Molecular Liquids, 2023. 388: p. 122739.

Assad, H., *An overview of contemporary developments and the application of graphene-based materials in anticorrosive coatings.* Environmental science and pollution research, 2023: p. 1–20.

Assad, H., *Electrochemical and computational insights into the utilization of 2, 2-dithio bisbenzothiazole as a sustainable corrosion inhibitor for mild steel in low pH medium.* Environmental Research, 2024. 242: p. 117640.

Assad, H., A. Assad and A. Kumar, *Recent developments in 3D bio-printing and its biomedical applications.* Pharmaceutics, 2023. 15(1): p. 255.

Assad, H., I. Fatma and A. Kumar, *An overview of the application of graphene-based materials in anticorrosive coatings.* Materials Letters, 2023. 330: p. 133287.

Astete, C.E. and C.M. Sabliov, *Synthesis and characterization of PLGA nanoparticles.* Journal of biomaterials science, polymer edition, 2006. 17(3): p. 247–289.

Axpe, E. and M.L. Oyen, *Applications of alginate-based bioinks in 3D bioprinting.* International journal of molecular sciences, 2016. 17(12): p. 1976.

Bakshi, P.S., *Chitosan as an environment friendly biomaterial–a review on recent modifications and applications.* International journal of biological macromolecules, 2020. 150: p. 1072–1083.

Bartolo, P., *3D bioprinting: Materials, processes and applications.* CIRP Annals, 2022. 71(2): p. 577–597.

Benson, R.S., *Use of radiation in biomaterials science.* Nuclear Instruments and Methods in Physics Research Section B: Beam Interactions with Materials and Atoms, 2002. 191(1-4): p. 752–757.

Bonandrini, B., *Recellularization of well-preserved acellular kidney scaffold using embryonic stem cells.* Tissue Engineering Part A, 2014. 20(9-10): p. 1486–1498.

Burmeister, D.M., *Delivery of allogeneic adipose stem cells in polyethylene glycol-fibrin hydrogels as an adjunct to meshed autografts after sharp debridement of deep partial thickness burns.* Stem cells translational medicine, 2018. 7(4): p. 360–372.

Cheng, H., *Biocompatibility of polypropylene mesh scaffold with adipose-derived stem cells.* Experimental and Therapeutic Medicine, 2017. 13(6): p. 2922–2926.

Cheng, Y.-L. and F. Chen, *Preparation and characterization of photocured poly (ε-caprolactone) diacrylate/poly (ethylene glycol) diacrylate/chitosan for photopolymerization-type 3D printing tissue engineering scaffold application.* Materials Science and Engineering: C, 2017. 81: p. 66–73.

Choi, Y.-J., *3D cell printed tissue analogues: a new platform for theranostics.* Theranostics, 2017. 7(12): p. 3118.

Courtney, T., *Design and analysis of tissue engineering scaffolds that mimic soft tissue mechanical anisotropy.* Biomaterials, 2006. 27(19): p. 3631–3638.

Cui, T., *Rapid prototyping of a double-layer polyurethane–collagen conduit for peripheral nerve regeneration.* Tissue Engineering Part C: Methods, 2009. 15(1): p. 1–9.

Derby, B., *Printing and prototyping of tissues and scaffolds.* science, 2012. 338(6109): p. 921–926.

Ding, C., *Chitosan Wrapped Graphene/Polyurethane Composites with Improved Dielectric Properties for Capacitive Sensing.* Polymer Science, Series A, 2021. 63(5): p. 576–584.

Elviri, L., *Highly defined 3D printed chitosan scaffolds featuring improved cell growth.* Biomedical Materials, 2017. 12(4): p. 045009.

Eskens, O., G. Villani and S. Amin, *Rheological investigation of thermoresponsive alginate-methylcellulose gels for epidermal growth factor formulation.* Cosmetics, 2020. 8(1): p. 3.

Gavrila, D.E., *Advanced Polypropylene and Composites with Polypropylene with Applications in Modern Medicine*, in *Composite Materials.* 2020, IntechOpen London, UK.

Gil, E.S., *I mpact of Sterilization on the Enzymatic Degradation and Mechanical Properties of Silk Biomaterials.* Macromolecular Bioscience, 2014. 14(2): p. 257–269.

Gope, A.K., Y.-S. Liao and C.-F.J. Kuo, *Quality prediction and abnormal processing parameter identification in polypropylene fiber melt spinning using artificial intelligence machine learning and deep learning algorithms.* Polymers, 2022. 14(13): p. 2739.

Gungor-Ozkerim, P.S., *Bioinks for 3D bioprinting: an overview.* Biomaterials science, 2018. 6(5): p. 915–946.

He, K. and X. Wang, *Rapid prototyping of tubular polyurethane and cell/hydrogel constructs.* Journal of bioactive and compatible polymers, 2011. 26(4): p. 363–374.

Ho, L. and S.-h. Hsu, *Cell reprogramming by 3D bioprinting of human fibroblasts in polyurethane hydrogel for fabrication of neural-like constructs.* Acta biomaterialia, 2018. 70: p. 57–70.

Hou, R., *Natural polysaccharides promote chondrocyte adhesion and proliferation on magnetic nanoparticle/PVA composite hydrogels.* Colloids and Surfaces B: Biointerfaces, 2015. 132: p. 146–154.

Hsiao, S.-H. and S.-h. Hsu, *Synthesis and characterization of dual stimuli-sensitive biodegradable polyurethane soft hydrogels for 3D cell-laden bioprinting.* ACS applied materials & interfaces, 2018. 10(35): p. 29273–29287.

Hsieh, F.-Y. and S.-h. Hsu, *3D bioprinting: A new insight into the therapeutic strategy of neural tissue regeneration.* Organogenesis, 2015. 11(4): p. 153–158.

Huang, Y., K. He and X. Wang, *Rapid prototyping of a hybrid hierarchical polyurethane-cell/hydrogel construct for regenerative medicine.* Materials Science and Engineering: C, 2013. 33(6): p. 3220–3229.

Jain, S. *Printability and critical insight into polymer properties during direct-extrusion based 3D printing of medical grade polylactide and copolyesters.* Biomacromolecules, 2019. 21(2): p. 388–396.

Jang, J., *3D printed complex tissue construct using stem cell-laden decellularized ECM bioinks for cardiac repair.* Biomaterials, 2017. 112: p. 264–274.

Jia, J., *Engineering alginate as bioink for bioprinting.* Acta biomaterialia, 2014. 10(10): p. 4323–4331.

Jiang, Z., *Biodegradable and thermoreversible hydrogels of poly (ethylene glycol)-poly (ε-caprolactone-co-glycolide)-poly (ethylene glycol) aqueous solutions.* Journal of Biomedical Materials Research Part A: An Official Journal of The Society for Biomaterials, The Japanese Society for Biomaterials, and The Australian Society for Biomaterials and the Korean Society for Biomaterials, 2008. 87(1): p. 45–51.

Kačarević, Ž.P., *An introduction to 3D bioprinting: possibilities, challenges and future aspects.* Materials, 2018. 11(11): p. 2199.

Kokubo, T., H.-M. Kim and M. Kawashita, *Novel bioactive materials with different mechanical properties.* Biomaterials, 2003. 24(13): p. 2161–2175.

Kyle, S. , *Printability'of candidate biomaterials for extrusion based 3d printing: state-of-the-art. Adv Healthc Mater* 6 (16): 1700264. 2017.

Lee, B.H., *Synthesis and characterization of types A and B gelatin methacryloyl for bioink applications.* Materials, 2016. 9(10): p. 797.

Lee, C.-M., *Oxygen plasma treatment on 3D-printed chitosan/gelatin/hydroxyapatite scaffolds for bone tissue engineering.* Journal of nanoscience and nanotechnology, 2017. 17(4): p. 2747–2750.

Lee, K.Y. and D.J. Mooney, *Alginate: properties and biomedical applications.* Progress in polymer science, 2012. 37(1): p. 106–126.

Li, S., *Chitosans for tissue repair and organ three-dimensional (3D) bioprinting.* Micromachines, 2019. 10(11): p. 765.

Lim, V.F., *Recent studies of genetic dysfunction in pelvic organ prolapse: the role of collagen defects.* Australian and New Zealand Journal of Obstetrics and Gynaecology, 2014. 54(3): p. 198–205.

Liu, F. *Natural polymers for organ 3D bioprinting.* Polymers, 2018. 10(11): p. 1278.

Liu, F. and X. Wang, *Synthetic polymers for organ 3D printing.* Polymers, 2020. 12(8): p. 1765.

Liu, W., *Extrusion bioprinting of shear-thinning gelatin methacryloyl bioinks.* Advanced healthcare materials, 2017. 6(12): p. 1601451.

Lu, Y., *Application of gelatin in food packaging: A review.* Polymers, 2022. 14(3): p. 436.

Lv, S., *Designed biomaterials to mimic the mechanical properties of muscles.* Nature, 2010. 465(7294): p. 69–73.

Maniglia, B.C., *Preparation of cassava starch hydrogels for application in 3D printing using dry heating treatment (DHT): A prospective study on the effects of DHT and gelatinization conditions.* Food Research International, 2020. 128: p. 108803.

Marrella, A., *Engineering vascularized and innervated bone biomaterials for improved skeletal tissue regeneration.* Materials Today, 2018. 21(4): p. 362–376.

Martina, M. and D.W. Hutmacher, *Biodegradable polymers applied in tissue engineering research: a review.* Polymer International, 2007. 56(2): p. 145–157.

Midha, S *Advances in three-dimensional bioprinting of bone: progress and challenges.* Journal of tissue engineering and regenerative medicine, 2019. 13(6): p. 925–945.

Mosesson, M.W., *Fibrinogen and fibrin structure and functions.* Journal of thrombosis and haemostasis, 2005. 3(8): p. 1894–1904.

Nagel, T. and D.J. Kelly, *The composition of engineered cartilage at the time of implantation determines the likelihood of regenerating tissue with a normal collagen architecture.* Tissue Engineering Part A, 2013. 19(7-8): p. 824–833.

Nair, L.S. and C.T. Laurencin, *Biodegradable polymers as biomaterials.* Progress in polymer science, 2007. 32(8-9): p. 762–798.

O'Grady, B.J., *Spatiotemporal Control of Morphogen Delivery to Pattern Stem Cell Differentiation in Three-Dimensional Hydrogels.* Current protocols in stem cell biology, 2019. 51(1): p. e97.

Ozbolat, I.T. and M. Hospodiuk, *Current advances and future perspectives in extrusion-based bioprinting.* Biomaterials, 2016. 76: p. 321–343.

Pandiyaraj, K.N., *Tailoring the surface properties of polypropylene films through cold atmospheric pressure plasma (CAPP) assisted polymerization and immobilization of biomolecules for enhancement of anti-coagulation activity.* Applied Surface Science, 2016. 370: p. 545–556.

Park, J. *Cell-laden 3D bioprinting hydrogel matrix depending on different compositions for soft tissue engineering: Characterization and evaluation.* Materials Science and Engineering: C, 2017. 71: p. 678–684.

Pawar, S.N. and K.J. Edgar, *Alginate derivatization: A review of chemistry, properties and applications.* Biomaterials, 2012. 33(11): p. 3279–3305.

Piras, C.C., S. Fernández-Prieto and W.M. De Borggraeve, *Nanocellulosic materials as bioinks for 3D bioprinting.* Biomaterials science, 2017. 5(10): p. 1988–1992.

Qiu, Q.-Q., W.-Q. Sun and J. Connor, *4.12 Sterilization of Biomaterials of Synthetic and Biological Origin.* 2017.

Rajabi, M. *Chitosan hydrogels in 3D printing for biomedical applications.* Carbohydrate Polymers, 2021. 260: p. 117768.

Ramadan, Q. and M. Zourob, *3D bioprinting at the frontier of regenerative medicine, pharmaceutical, and food industries.* Frontiers in Medical Technology, 2021. 2: p. 607648.

Ren, X., *Engineering zonal cartilage through bioprinting collagen type II hydrogel constructs with biomimetic chondrocyte density gradient.* BMC musculoskeletal disorders, 2016. 17: p. 1–10.

RG, A.P., et al., *A review on the recent applications of synthetic biopolymers in 3D printing for biomedical applications.* Journal of Materials Science: Materials in Medicine, 2023. 34(12): p. 1–22.

Rutz, A.L., *A multi-material bioink method for 3D printing tunable, cell-compatible hydrogels.* Advanced materials (Deerfield Beach, Fla.), 2015. 27(9): p. 1607.

RW, P., *Human tissue reaction to sutures.* Ann Surg, 1975. 181: p. 144–150.

Sachdev IV, A., *A review on techniques and biomaterials used in 3D bioprinting.* Cureus, 2022. 14(8).

Sadeghianmaryan, A., *Fabrication of chitosan/alginate/hydroxyapatite hybrid scaffolds using 3D printing and impregnating techniques for potential cartilage regeneration.* International Journal of Biological Macromolecules, 2022. 204: p. 62–75.

Samadi, N., *The effect of lauryl capping group on protein release and degradation of poly (d, l-lactic-co-glycolic acid) particles.* Journal of controlled release, 2013. 172(2): p. 436–443.

Saroia, J., *A review on biocompatibility nature of hydrogels with 3D printing techniques, tissue engineering application and its future prospective.* Bio-Design and Manufacturing, 2018. 1: p. 265–279.

Senarath-Yapa, K., *Adipose-derived stem cells: a review of signaling networks governing cell fate and regenerative potential in the context of craniofacial and long bone skeletal repair.* International journal of molecular sciences, 2014. 15(6): p. 9314–9330.

Shan Wong, Y., *Engineered polymeric biomaterials for tissue engineering.* Current Tissue Engineering (Discontinued), 2012. 1(1): p. 41–53.

Shim, J.-H., *Effects of 3D-printed polycaprolactone/β-tricalcium phosphate membranes on guided bone regeneration.* International Journal of Molecular Sciences, 2017. 18(5): p. 899.

Stanton, M., J. Samitier and S. Sanchez, *Bioprinting of 3D hydrogels.* Lab on a Chip, 2015. 15(15): p. 3111–3115.

Teixeira-Costa, B.E. and C.T. Andrade, *Chitosan as a valuable biomolecule from seafood industry waste in the design of green food packaging.* Biomolecules, 2021. 11(11): p. 1599.

Toh, W.S. and X.J. Loh, *Advances in hydrogel delivery systems for tissue regeneration.* Materials Science and Engineering: C, 2014. 45: p. 690–697.

Tsai, Y.-C., *Synthesis of thermoresponsive amphiphilic polyurethane gel as a new cell printing material near body temperature.* ACS applied materials & interfaces, 2015. 7(50): p. 27613-27623.

Unagolla, J.M. and A.C. Jayasuriya, *Hydrogel-based 3D bioprinting: A comprehensive review on cell-laden hydrogels, bioink formulations, and future perspectives.* Applied materials today, 2020. 18: p. 100479.

Villanueva, I., C.A. Weigel and S.J. Bryant, *Cell–matrix interactions and dynamic mechanical loading influence chondrocyte gene expression and bioactivity in PEG-RGD hydrogels.* Acta biomaterialia, 2009. 5(8): p. 2832–2846.

Wang, X. and H. Xu, *Incorporation of DMSO and dextran-40 into a gelatin/alginate hydrogel for controlled assembled cell cryopreservation.* Cryobiology, 2010. 61(3): p. 345–351.

Wang, X., *3D printing of tissue/organ analogues for regenerative medicine*, in *Handbook of Intelligent Scaffolds for Tissue Engineering and Regenerative Medicine*. 2017, Jenny Stanford Publishing. p. 567–580.

Wang, X., *Advanced polymers for three-dimensional (3D) organ bioprinting.* Micromachines, 2019. 10(12): p. 814.

Wang, X., B.L. Rijff and G. Khang, *A building-block approach to 3D printing a multichannel, organ-regenerative scaffold.* Journal of tissue engineering and regenerative medicine, 2017. 11(5): p. 1403–1411.

Wang, X., K. He and W. Zhang, *Optimizing the fabrication processes for manufacturing a hybrid hierarchical polyurethane–cell/hydrogel construct.* Journal of Bioactive and Compatible Polymers, 2013. 28(4): p. 303–319.

Weadock, K.S., *Effect of physical crosslinking methods on collagen-fiber durability in proteolytic solutions.* Journal of Biomedical Materials Research: An Official Journal of The Society for Biomaterials and The Japanese Society for Biomaterials, 1996. 32(2): p. 221–226.

Williams, D.F., *On the mechanisms of biocompatibility.* Biomaterials, 2008. 29(20): p. 2941–2953.

Winnacker, M. and B. Rieger, *Poly (ester amide) s: recent insights into synthesis, stability and biomedical applications.* Polymer Chemistry, 2016. 7(46): p. 7039–7046.

Wong, T.Y., L.A. Preston and N.L. Schiller, *Alginate lyase: review of major sources and enzyme characteristics, structure-function analysis, biological roles, and applications.* Annual Reviews in Microbiology, 2000. 54(1): p. 289–340.

Wu, Q., *3D printing of microstructured and stretchable chitosan hydrogel for guided cell growth.* Advanced Biosystems, 2017. 1(6): p. 1700058.

Xavier, J.R., *Bioactive nanoengineered hydrogels for bone tissue engineering: a growth-factor-free approach.* ACS nano, 2015. 9(3): p. 3109–3118.

Zhang, C., *Synthesis and characterization of biodegradable elastomeric polyurethane scaffolds fabricated by the inkjet technique.* Biomaterials, 2008. 29(28): p. 3781–3791.

Zhang, L.-K., *Bone marrow stem cells combined with polycaprolactone-polylactic acid-polypropylene amine scaffolds for the treatment of acute liver failure.* Chemical Engineering Journal, 2019. 360: p. 1564–1576.

Zhang, P., *Investigation on the temperature control accuracy of a print head for extrusion 3D printing and its improved design.* Biomedicines, 2022. 10(6): p. 1233.

Zhang, W., W. Ye and Y. Yan, *Advances in photocrosslinkable materials for 3D bioprinting.* Advanced Engineering Materials, 2022. 24(1): p. 2100663.

Zhu, J., *Bioactive modification of poly (ethylene glycol) hydrogels for tissue engineering.* Biomaterials, 2010. 31(17): p. 4639–4656.

Bioinks for 3D Bioprinting

Priyanshu Shukla,[1] *Sourita Ghosh,*[1] *Soham Ghosh,*[1]
Saumya S K,[2] *Gaddam Kiranmai,*[1] *Aashwini Bhavsar,*[2]
Meenu T S[1] and *Falguni Pati*[1,2*]

1. Introduction

As the 21st century unfolded, increasing interest in repairing and fabricating functional tissues and organs has fueled the need for novel biofabrication approaches. Advancements in biomaterials and biotechnologies propelled three-dimensional (3D) bioprinting into a prominent position within biomedicine and tissue engineering, where conventional techniques fail to produce structures with the desired morphological, mechanical, anatomical, and biological properties. With the emergence of 3D bioprinting, precise heightened control has been provided to lay down the architecture of biofabricated 3D constructs. Its automated deposition process ensures a high degree of reproducibility. While still in its nascent stages, bioprinting's versatility accelerates its applications in tissue engineering, allowing for the fabrication of 3D tissue constructs with pre-programmed structures and geometries containing biomaterials and living cells, collectively referred to as bioink. The concept of 'bioink' has emerged as a promising solution to meet the complex requirements of biofabrication challenges. (Levato et al., 2017) Within the field of biofabrication, the term 'bioinks' may be defined as the composition of cell-encapsulating materials appropriate for processing by a biofabrication method. (Groll, n.d) (Moroni et al., 2016) Although not obligatory, biomaterials are not required when the bioink only comprises aggregated cells as cell spheroids or microtissues. Cells are an essential constituent of a bioink. Therefore, post-printing seeding cells on a 3D printed construct, formulated with polymers/hydrogel precursors such as thermoplastics that may include biological components but lack cells, can be classified as biomaterial inks but not bioinks. (Moroni et al., 2016) The bioink fabrication process demands meticulous attention to ensure optimal printing fidelity. This necessitates thorough consideration of rheological parameters like viscosity profile, shear-thinning or thickening behavior, and a strategy for post-printing gelation.

[1]   Department of Biomedical Engineering, Indian Institute of Technology Hyderabad, Kandi, India
[2]   Centre for Interdisciplinary Programs, Indian Institute of Technology Hyderabad, Kandi, India
*   Corresponding author: falguni@bme.iith.ac.in

Furthermore, safeguarding cell viability throughout the printing process, mitigating shear stress effects, and preserving post-printing bioactivity are essential for successful biofabrication. An ideal bioink is characterized by commendable biocompatibility, suitable mechanical properties, and optimal rheological behavior. (Chen et al et al., 2023). However, requirements of specific attributes within bioinks may differ based on the practical application being addressed. This chapter provides an indepth exploration of the diverse characteristics and properties of bioinks, encompassing recent trends in commercialization and presenting insights into the present scenario and future work in that direction.

2.   Crosslinking Strategies for Bioink

A crucial phase in the bioprinting workflow involves transforming a bioink into a sol-to-gel state commonly referred to as a crosslinked hydrogel. Crosslinking is a central process in 3D bioprinting and involves linking polymer chains through either physical methods, such as exposure to temperature, or chemical reactions, such as ion-mediated crosslinking, forming a stable hydrogel-based scaffold with an enmeshed, interconnected polymeric network. (GhavamiNejad et al., n.d) Various crosslinking methods are available, with thermal and ionic as physical crosslinking and photo and enzyme crosslinking as chemical crosslinking being commonly employed in bioprinting (Figure 1). Thermal crosslinking occurs in thermosensitive polymers, whereupon exposure to temperature variations induce crosslinking within polymer chains, leading to gelation in the 3D scaffold. Polymers like agarose, gelatin, and collagen naturally form hydrogels through thermal crosslinking, and some exhibit reversible crosslinking at critical temperatures. However, most natural polysaccharides and proteins can be transformed into thermally responsive hydrogels, typically exhibiting a sol-to-gel transition temperature below which the polymer chains undergo gelation.(Ward et al., n.d) Hydrogels formed through thermal crosslinking exhibit drawbacks, such as mechanical weakness and a longer gelation time than alternative methods.

Additionally, thermal crosslinking can lead to uncontrolled crosslinking, posing challenges in achieving desired material properties. Ionic crosslinking occurs when charged polymers are crosslinked with multivalent ions of opposite charge. This reversible process is commonly applied to hydrogels such as alginate and chitosan. Alginate, for instance, can be crosslinked by divalent metal ions, such as the addition of calcium (Ca^{2+}) ions, through spraying or bath-assisted printing, leading to rapid gelation of the solution. (Sardelli et al., n.d) In extrusion bioprinting, ionic crosslinking enables mild and instant gelation of the bioink as it comes out of the nozzle, offering better printability. However, drawbacks of ionic crosslinking include an uneven mechanical property due to uneven ion penetration within the printed construct, poor post-printing stability, as well as potential toxicity caused by ions affecting cell survival. (Demirtas et al., n.d). Despite these challenges, instant gelation under biomimetic conditions makes ionically crosslinked hydrogels an attractive candidate for 3D bioprinting applications. Chemical crosslinking is similar to ionic crosslinking, where the formation of a polymer network is initiated via covalent chemical bonds, mainly in the presence of crosslinking agents to obtain stable hydrogel constructs.

Photocrosslinking involves light-induced creation of a covalent bond between polymer chains, forming a crosslinked hydrogel construct. Photocurable polymers in the form of photosensitive hydrogels can be 3D printed and, upon exposure to laser or visible light, form stable 3D constructs. Some proteinaceous biopolymers, such as collagen, fibrin, and gelatin, with tyrosine residues, can undergo photocrosslinking in the presence of photoinitiators and a light source. For polymers that do not directly respond to light, the introduction of acrylate or methacrylate-based agents to polymer chains allows them to become photocurable. UV light is commonly used to crosslink these polymers. (Bertassoni et al., 2014). It is crucial to note that UV light may pose biological risks, potentially damaging encapsulated cells within the printed constructs and harming operators. Some widely used photocrosslinkable polymer bioprinting materials include gelatin-methacrylate (GelMA), (Bhise, n.d) (Zhu, n.d) silk fibroin-methacrylate (SFMA), (Hong, n.d) and hyaluronan-methacrylate (HAMA/MeHA). (Schuurmans et al., 2020). Enzyme crosslinking involves using enzymes to form covalent bonds between biopolymers. It is used during bioprinting due to the mild crosslinking mechanism and the overall process being biocompatible. Enzymes used during such crosslinking mechanisms like transglutaminase, (Zhou et al., n.d) tyrosinase (Ty), (Shi et al., 2018) and horseradish peroxidase (HRP) (Sakai et al., n.d) have been utilized for crosslinking hydrogels from materials such as gelatin, silk fibroin, and alginate. However, limitations include challenges in obtaining enzymes, resulting in hydrogels with limited mechanical properties and sensitivity to conditions like temperature and pH, impacting the crosslinking or bioprinting process. Despite these challenges, enzyme crosslinking remains a valuable approach in Bioprinting for its cell-friendly characteristics.

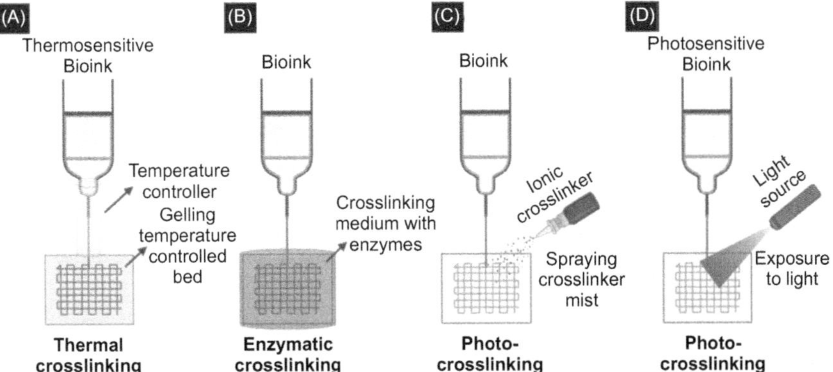

Fig. 1   Various crosslinking techniques for hydrogel scaffolds during 3D bioprinting. (A) Thermal crosslinking: adjusting the temperature during the crosslinking process - can be applied to thermoresponsive polymers that gel or denature at specific temperatures (e.g., agarose, gelatin); (B) Ionic Crosslinking: utilizes a spray delivery system to apply the crosslinking agent directly onto the hydrogel scaffold - can be advantageous for precise, localized crosslinking and rapid gelation; (C) Enzymatic Crosslinking: hydrogel scaffold is submerged in a liquid bath containing the crosslinker; (D) Photocrosslinking: utilizes ultraviolet (UV) light or other forms of electromagnetic radiation to trigger the crosslinking reaction - allows for rapid and spatially controlled crosslinking - ideal for precise patterning and fabrication.

3.   3D Bioprinting Modalities for Bioink

3.1   *Bioinks for Extrusion Printing*

Extrusion-based 3D bioprinting utilizes continuous pressure to extrude cylindrical bioink filaments through narrow nozzles, employing pneumatic, piston, or screw-driven mechanisms. This method allows for printing with inks with a range of viscosities with shear thinning behavior, making it suitable for various hydrogel polymer solutions encapsulating high cell densities. The technique is widely applied in biomanufacturing, producing large-scale 3D constructs with broad material applicability. However, challenges like hydrogel deformation in post-printed constructs, nozzle clogging with highly viscous biomaterial, and decreased cell viability due to shear forces exerted during printing persist. Extrusion-based 3D bioprinting remains prevalent in tissue engineering, driving advancements in regenerative medicine despite the associated limitations. (Morgan et al., n.d). Notably, research has explored innovative nozzle designs to mitigate hydrogel deformation and nozzle clogging issues, aiming to improve overall cell viability during printing. Furthermore, investigations into novel bioink formulations incorporate additives that improve the rheological properties of bioinks, thereby mitigating issues associated with filament width and enhancing overall printing resolution. These developments aim to achieve higher precision in the deposition of bioink filaments.

3.2 Bioinks for Inkjet Printing

Inkjet-based 3D bioprinting, developed in 1988, involves placing the bioink in a cartridge connected to the print head, and droplet generation is induced through either piezoelectric, thermal, or electrostatic effects, allowing for precise droplet size and deposition path control. The method demonstrates relatively high cell viability, around 90%, owing to the low viscosity of biomaterials used for bioink, minimizing the shear stress on cells. (Jayasinghe et al., n.d) Inkjet printing, with its cost-effective equipment resembling commercial printers, offers a lower cost for improving resolution than laser-based bioprinting. However, challenges with this printing technique include the unsuitability of high viscosity bioinks and using a bioink with high cell density and limited capacity for printing large-scale tissues. Recent research has emphasized the ongoing exploration of innovative bioink formulations compatible with inkjet printing technologies. These formulations enhance droplet stability, size uniformity, and printing fidelity. Studies have also delved into advancements in improving the actuation mechanisms responsible for droplet generation. (Gudapati et al., n.d) Piezoelectric, thermal, and electrostatic methods have been subject to optimization to address challenges related to bioink viscosity and improve printing speed without compromising cell viability. Additionally, researchers are investigating integrating microfluidic systems into inkjet printers for on-the-fly bioink modifications, enabling dynamic adjustments during the printing process.

3.3 Bioinks for Laser-Based Printing

Laser-assisted 3D bioprinting (LAB) applies pulsed lasers to induce physical response on the bioink deposition using direct writing as well as laser-induced phase transfer techniques. Without the need for nozzles, it avoids clogging issues and has broader applicability, accommodating bioinks with high viscous properties or bioinks laden with higher cell density. However, bioinks must adhere to the coating substrate and be viscoelastic for high-fidelity bioink deposition. Achieving a high resolution (~50μm) through precise optical devices ensures high cell viability due to the absence of shear stress during the printing process. Advancements in optical devices, including the integration of holographic patterning and dynamic focusing systems, contribute to achieving finer resolutions in laser-assisted bioprinting. However, the higher cost of lasers and complex control systems limits their practical applications, and there is a need to further understand the impact of lasers on cells. Recent studies have investigated laser source technologies, such as femtosecond lasers, that aim to improve the bioink's spatial precision and reduce collateral damage to encapsulated cells. Moreover, ongoing research into bioink formulations optimized for laser-induced printing has focused on achieving optimal viscosity and photopolymerization characteristics. (Guillotin, n.d)

4. Biomaterials in Bioink

Biomaterial solutions have been derived from natural sources or synthesized artificially with chemical modifications to polymers for bioink development for 3D bioprinting applications. Polymers are made up of long chains of organic biomolecules with the ability to retain high water content. Such polymers provide a hydrated environment to the encapsulated cells and are often referred to as hydrogels. These hydrogels support biological functions, including cell attachment, cell viability and proliferation, differentiation, and tissue regeneration. Based on the origin or the source of the polymer, they can be characterized either as natural or synthetic polymers. Natural polymers have the inherent property to support cell functionality, whereas synthetic polymers are biologically passive but demonstrate good mechanical properties. Synthetic polymers are composed of polymer chains that have been artificially created by synthesizing primary materials derived from fossil fuels such as coal, gas, or oil. The manipulation of properties such as the molecular weight of polymer chains and control over chemical reactions leading to macromolecule polymerization enables influencing and changing the rheological and mechanical properties in such lab-synthesized polymers. The ability to alter mechanical properties within synthetic polymers has led to the development of various 3D scaffolds created with cell-laden hydrogels that mimic the *in vivo* mechanical properties of native tissues. On the other hand, bioinks are typically not formulated directly with synthetic polymers due to their unsuitability for cell encapsulation. This is because organic solvents are often used in the synthesis of such polymers, and very specific printing conditions are required such as higher non-biocompatible temperatures for printing. Moreover, these materials often lack cell-adhesive ligands, limiting their ability to support cellular activities and restricting their direct use as bioinks. Instead, they should be used for biomaterial ink-based applications (Figure 2).

Consequently, synthetic polymers are frequently used as scaffold material or for printing to establish a 3D acellular construct with superior mechanical properties. Such printed frameworks are then used as supports to bioprint cell-laden hydrogels in the spaces left within the printed constructs, forming hybrid scaffolds; this approach is also called the hybrid bioprinting technique. In distinction, natural polymers are isolated from various natural sources such as flora, fauna, or even microorganisms. These polymers can be differentiated into three categories: firstly, polysaccharide-based natural polymers; secondly, protein polymers derived from the extracellular matrix (ECM); and thirdly, decellularized extracellular matrix (dECM) biomaterials.

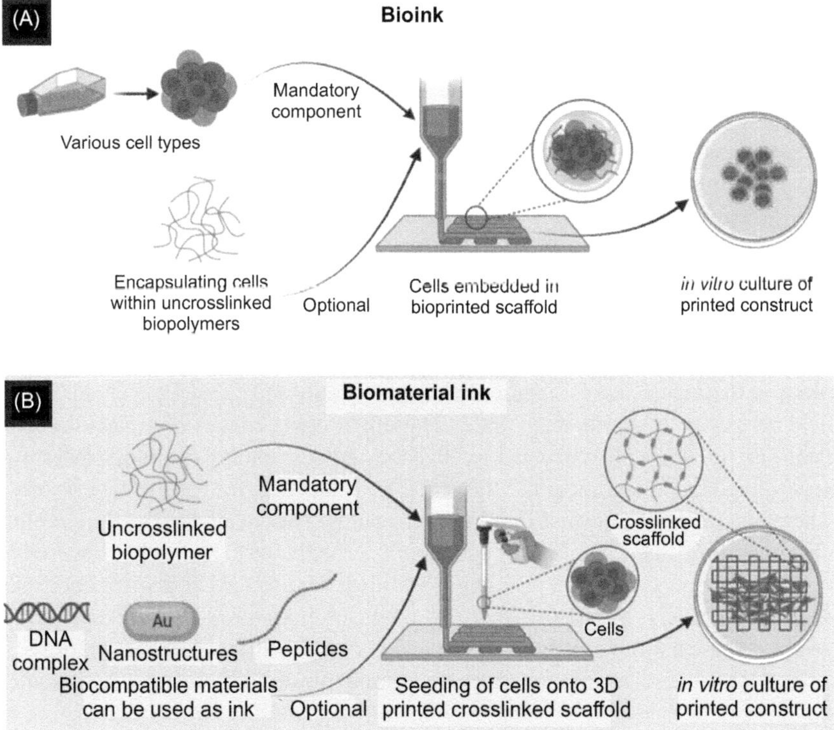

Fig. 2 The distinction between a cell-laden bioink and an acellular biomaterial ink is based on their structural composition and intended application. (A) In bioinks, cells are integral components of the printing formulation, and they may be incorporated through various strategies such as encapsulation into microcarriers, microgels, blended in the physical hydrogel, or hydrogel precursors. (B) Biomaterial inks inherently carry no cells within the ink formulation. Instead, cells are seeded in the second step onto the 3D printed construct, providing greater flexibility and overcoming biocompatibility limitations on the ink composition.

Alginate, chitosan, agarose, cellulose, carrageenan, dextran, and gellan gum are the most used carbohydrate-based natural biomaterials to prepare bioinks. Polysaccharides are ubiquitous, can be easily procured, and present with acceptable biocompatibility, immunological inertness, and simple gelation methods, which are favorable for cell-mediated printing. However, because of its inadequate capability to bind with cells due to the lack of cell-binding motifs, its modification or blending with other polymers is usually preferred, which can instead compromise the printing fidelity and stability of the gelated constructs.

Biomaterials sourced from the ECM, including collagen, gelatin, fibronectin, and hyaluronic acid, successfully emulate the cellular microenvironment, showcasing remarkable biocompatibility and biodegradability. However, their mechanical stability is comparatively limited, and the gelation process is often slow, necessitating further enhancements such as chemical modifications to augment their functionality. (He et al., 2023) Natural polymers derived from tissue-specific decellularized extracellular matrices (dECMs) possess distinct characteristics. As they are obtained directly from native tissues through the removal of cells, there is minimal immunogenicity. dECMs retain abundant natural ECM components, which include collagen, elastin, laminin, fibronectin, essential glycosaminoglycans (GAGs), along with the native components with 3D microarchitecture and microstructures of various types of organ-specific tissues. This unique composition provides an organ-specific tissue 3D microenvironment for the native cellular population, creating a conducive niche that encourages cellular functions such as population, aggregation, and ECM deposition, ultimately facilitating the generation of neo-tissues. Leveraging their biocompatible nature, tissue-specific dECMs have emerged as promising sources of bioinks for 3D bioprinting techniques and can be used to biofabricate various tissues and organs.

Bioinks derived from natural polymers, such as solubilized extracellular matrix (ECM) molecules, are typically characterized by unstable and weak bonding forces like hydrogen, ionic, and covalent bonds. Unlike native tissue, where ECM molecules are tightly assembled to form robust fibers, these bioinks exhibit lower mechanical strength and suboptimal printability due to low-viscosity hydrogels not holding 3D structures. Despite these disadvantages, the substantial benefits of natural polymers like ECM-based hydrogels, such as high similarity to native ECM components and microarchitectures, can offer a biomimetic microenvironment to encapsulated cells, which promotes cell adhesion, migration, cellular viability, and proliferation, as well as differentiation of encapsulated cells, therefore aiding tissue morphogenesis within bioprinted constructs.

4.1 Natural Bioinks

Naturally derived hydrogels possess inherent biocompatibility and can selectively direct cells toward physiological behaviors. (Catoria et al., 2022) These hydrogels consist of molecules recognized as physiological 'self' (Kaith et al., n.d) and for which they possess natural receptors, thereby prompting cell receptors to facilitate integration into the scaffold (Tang et al., n.d) and initiate essential cellular signaling and molecular mechanisms. The different printing parameters, such as printability, cellular density, biocompatibility, and rheological parameters, broadly vary due to the properties of natural polymers. Bioprinting processes and printing modalities, require further investigations and process optimization to biofabricate tissue constructs that can be mass-produced and scaled up. A usual approach to using these natural biomaterials when they have insufficient properties or are unsuitable for bioprinting technique, these biomaterials are homogenized with other biocompatible materials to create optimal bioinks.

4.1.1 Collagen-based bioink

Collagen is a hydrophilic protein that has structural and physicochemical properties similar to the structural components of the ECM present in the cells. (Akhmanova.n.d) (Li et al., n.d) Collagen has minimal antigenicity and excellent biocompatibility as it actively supports cellular attachment and biochemically regulates various cell functions, including metabolism, proliferation, adhesion, and migration. (Antoine et al., n.d) (Zhang et al., n.d) (Hesse et al., n.d) Collagen has been widely employed as a bioink in 3D printing applications (Murphy and Atala, 2014) to print corneal substitutes, (J.R. Jangamreddy et al., n.d) wound healing, (Zhang et al., n.d) bone, (Fan et al., n.d) and various tissue engineering approaches. (Sarrigiannidis, et al., n.d) (Dinescu et al., n.d) (Hu and Lo, n.d) Despite its usage in many biomedical applications, collagen bioink poses challenges in fabricating complex biocompatible scaffolds that closely mimic tissue *in vivo* structural architecture because of its poor printability. (Stepanovska et al., n.d) Gelatin methacrylate (GelMA) is a semisynthetic biopolymer with tunable chemical and physical characteristics that has been used for bioink formulations for various bioprinting applications. (Ghosh et al., n.d) (Rajabi et al., n.d) A study integrated the quick gelling property of GelMA with collagen's biocompatible and rheological properties to give the printed scaffold adequate mechanical properties. Drop-on-demand bioprinting technology was used to print this hybrid hydrogel to produce three-dimensional capillary-like structures utilizing HUVECs cocultured with hMSCs. (Tomasina et al., n.d)

Scaffolds were further created using the various collagen type I concentrations with Viscoll using an extrusion-based 3D bioprinting technique. (Osidak et al., n.d) This study assessed the printed scaffold's biocompatibility and mechanical properties. Another study described decellularized ECM (dECM) as a bioink for tissue bioprinting. (Pati et al., 2014) This study also showed the importance of tissue-specific dECM in providing several tissue-specific biochemical characteristics, including growth factors and cytokines, which operate as microenvironmental cues for tissue-specific differentiation. Another study evaluated the stability of the bioprinted structures with corneal stromal keratocytes (CSKs) encapsulated within a collagen type I bioink. After seven days of *in vitro* culture, the cellular proliferation, cell viability, and phenotypical morphology of the stromal cells in these 3D bioprinted models were evaluated. (Campos et al., 2019) The study's findings showed that corneal stromal tissue constructions with properties resembling those of native corneal stromal tissue could be successfully produced using their bioprinting technique. A study examined the bioprintability and rheological properties of collagen bioinks to culture primary chondrocyte cells for their application in cartilage tissue engineering by investigating the change in the mechanical strength of the bioprinted constructs before, during, and after the gelation (Beetov et al., n.d).

4.1.2   Gelatin

The acid and alkaline denaturation of collagen creates the biopolymer known as gelatin. (Andreazza et al., n.d) The gelatin solution is a thermosensitive and frequently used natural polymer for various biomedical and tissue engineering applications. There are multiple advantages of gelatin, such as its inherent biocompatibility, the biodegradable nature of the polymer, and its low antigenicity owing to the intrinsic Arg-Gly-Asp (RGD) residues present in gelatin backbone chains. (Jaipan et al., n.d) (Mushtaq et al., n.d) (Lukin et al., n.d) These properties make gelatin versatile for bioprinting applications. Wide ranges of concentrations of gelatin have been employed as a bioink material and as a composite with other biomaterials or with chemical modification for bioprinting applications. Gelatin-furfural bioink, hyaluronic acid (HA), and riboflavin as viscosity enhancers were crosslinked using visible light to build cell-laden bioprinted structures. The study examined the proliferation network formation and observed hetero cellular clustering and viability of mouse MSCs, C2C1 myoblasts, and STO fibroblast cells within the bioprinted monolayer and bilayer sheets. (Anilumar et al., n.d) A study assessed the cellular viability of human adipose-derived mesenchymal stromal cells (hASCs) in relation to bioactive glass employed in alginate-gelatin hydrogels in 3D bioprinted constructs. (Wei et al., n.d) Another study showed PCL and bioactive glass were used for solvent-based extrusion 3D bioprinting techniques to print various constructs. The fabricated scaffold's dimensions, physical characteristics, and dissolution were assessed over 28 days. The viability of hASCs was assessed after they were added to Alg-Gel composite hydrogel and bioprinted on the scaffolds. These findings highlighted the advantage of the solvent-based bioprinting technique for fabricating 3D scaffolds, showing initial cell viability exceeding 80% on the day of bioprinting but decreasing after a week of culture. (olan et al., n.d)

In another study, the gelatin-alginate hydrogel was used to bioprint an aortic valve canal containing cells designed from microcomputed tomography images. This program sliced imported STL files into layers and created fill and contour paths for each layer according to predetermined print parameters. They used an extrusion-based bioprinter to simultaneously bioprint encapsulated smooth muscle cells (SMCs) in the root portion of the bioprinted construct and interstitial leaflet cells within the leaflet portion according to the anatomical region. After printing, the bioprinted constructs had near-clinical dimensions close to anatomical conditions and were crosslinked in a $CaCl_2$ solution. They found that the optimum blend of gelatin and alginate was a critical factor influencing the print quality, allowing cellular proliferation and viability, expansion, and tissue maturation. (Duan et al., n.d). A study reported an alternative bioprinting method that combines polydimethylsiloxane (PDMS) ink, GelMA ink, and pluronic F127 fugitive ink to create vascularized 3D tissue structures based on the variations in thermally reversible gelation. Pluronic F127 fugitive-based hydrogel forms a liquid that flows at a cold temperature of 4°C, whereas GelMA-based bioink is a stiffer hydrogel ($G' > G''$) at 4°C, and these properties were used to generate hollow tubes. To promote endothelialization, endothelial cell suspension was injected, which created a 2D hierarchical bifurcating vascular network. They also printed multilayer tissue construct with two inks: a cell laden GelMA ink comprising human neonatal dermal fibroblasts (HNDFs) and Pluronic F127 ink. Pluronic was liquefied and removed from the hollow channels, and the endothelial cells were inserted in the hollow channels to generate vasculature in these three-dimensional constructs after the GelMA matrix had been crosslinked. This method aimed to reduce the time taken for bioprinting and create complex heterogeneous tissue structures with increased cell proliferation and viability for heterogeneous cell populations encapsulated within GelMA hydrogel. (Kolesy et al., 2014)

Gelatin's thermoresponsive properties allow users to tailor and be physically crosslinked during the bioprinting process via thermal gelation, leading to stable bioprinted constructs. A drawback to thermal crosslinking is that temperature-induced gelation is slow in the process, and bonds formed between polymer chains are weak and unstable. Gelatin-based hydrogels have been chemically modified to address this issue by adding photopolymerizable methacryloyl groups to gelatin backbone polymer chains. This allows for the formation of stronger bonds using photocrosslinking induced by UV light. A construct printed using GelMA is immediately photocrosslinked while the printing is going on or after the bioprinting process is done. (Gungor-ozkerim et al., n.d) GelMA is a very suitable bioink formulation for light-based bioprinting modalities because its crosslinking density can be tuned during the synthesis process or functionalization of gelatin by modulating methacryloyl group activation or by varying the duration or intensity of light used during photopolymerization, all the factors which ultimately alter the physiobiochemical properties of the bioprinted scaffold. Playing with photocrosslinking strategy, a study showcased a dual network hydrogel bioink formulation developed using methacrylated gelatin and modified hyaluronic acid for bioprinting applications. These scaffolds supported the cell survival post-printing and showcased good proliferation of mesenchymal stem cells, indicating their biocompatibility. This combination of the self-healing activity of the bioprinted strands with the modified HA and GelMA photo-crosslinking resulted in more stable tissue constructs with better mechanical properties. (Ding et al., n.d)

4.1.3 Fibrin

Fibrin, a fibrous protein originating from circulating soluble fibrinogen, constitutes a pivotal element in the coagulation cascade. (Gudapati et al., n.d) This bioink has established its application as a single-component bioink and in combination with thrombin–fibrinogen components to showcase its printability and effective usage in 3D bioprinting. (Melo et al., n.d) (Dell et al., n.d) A study done using extrusion-based 3D bioprinting replicated osteon-like patterns using endothelial cells and MSCs. Two-phase bioprinted scaffolds were shown to have enhanced neovascularization, and the strategy of incorporating fibrin-based bioink laden with multiple cell lines allowed the group to fabricate the bioprinted construct with osteogenic and vasculogenic functionalities. (Piard et al., n.d) In another study, concurrent bioprinting of polypropiolactone with fibrin bioink was used to mimic cortical bone properties. They observed optimal mechanical properties in the tissue constructs, with compression testing revealing a modulus similar to cortical bone. The embedding of HUVECs and hMSCs within fibrin hydrogels, followed by in vitro culturing, exhibited escalated expression of vascular markers. As seen in histological sections, subcutaneously implanting these bioprinted constructs in rats showed a significant rise in blood vessel count per unit area. Another study employed a composite bioink made up of a fibrin-gelatin complex for fabricating cardiac constructs containing cardiomyocytes and cardiac fibroblasts. (Tomoy, n.d) Their bioink formulation involved a series of steps-firstly, they employed furfuryl-gelatin visible-light crosslinking, and secondly, fibrinogen and calcium chloride chemical crosslinking was done on the bioink, which was followed by extrusion-based bioprinting of cell-laden constructs. This approach produced an extensively porous, well-networked construct demonstrating long-term stability and in vitro biocompatibility with cardiomyocytes, showcasing high troponin-1 cardiac marker expression. The bioink facilitated the coculturing of CMs and cardiac fibroblasts, which is pivotal for preserving cardiac wall physiology in vivo. A study highlighted the usage of fibrin bioink in 3D bioprinting to develop neural tissues that resemble a healthy brain. The hiPSC-derived neural progenitor cells encapsulated in fibrin hydrogel containing guggulsterone (anti-inflammatory) microspheres were printed layer-by-layer in dome-shaped structures. The viability of these constructs was assessed with neural marker expression associated with differentiation, specifically into dopaminergic neurons. (Anil Kumar et al., n.d)

4.1.4 Silk

Silkworm silk, characterized by its low-density structural protein with higher α-helix content and β-sheet content, exhibits robustness and is known to have a crystalline structure. A part of silk, the silk fibroin, is made up of 18 amino acids and forms a natural polymeric fibrin. (Schneider et al., n.d) Silk fibroin displays exceptional biodegradability, cellular compatibility, and mechanical strength. (Kim et al., n.d) (Lee et al., n.d) (Lee et al., n.d) Silk has been used extensively for tissue engineering applications and further has been applied for bioink formulation. (Egan et al., n.d) Huang et al. incorporated bacterial cellulose nanofibers (BCNFs) to boost the mechanical strength and refine the print resolution of silk fibroin/gelatin printed composite constructs. (Huang et al., n.d) Employing 3D printing and lyophilization, they fabricated hydrogel scaffolds based on silk fibroin, observing a substantial increase in tensile strength upon adding BCNFs. They introduced both large and fine pores into a pre-designed scaffold using 3D printing followed by lyophilization of the construct post printing. This method allowed fabrication of finer pores (~1–10 μm) to facilitate cell infiltration and larger sized pores (~300–600 μm) to safeguard thorough nutrient supply to cells within the printed constructs. Another study showcased 3D printing of a biomimetic meniscus 3D scaffold by applying a silk fibroin–gelatin-based bioink formulation. (Bandyopadhyay et al., n.d) The tissue engineered 3D printed scaffold displayed native tissue properties such as swelling index, mimetic mechanical strength, and biodegradability, ensuring *in vivo* like properties of the engineered scaffold. On top seeding of meniscal fibrochondrocytes on the biofabricated scaffolds, the cells maintained their morphology, showed good proliferation and viability and exhibited expression of total collagen and glycosaminoglycan markers.

4.1.5 Alginate

Alginate is a biopolymer that finds its primary sources in bacteria and marine algae, mainly isolated from brown algae. It has wide applications in tissue engineering, drug delivery, and various biological studies. It necessitates precise control over physical properties such as swelling index, mechanical strength, cellular attachment and proliferation, biodegradation, and positive interactions with bioactive molecules. (Sarker et al., n.d) Alginate has been extensively used as a single agent or in combination with other biomaterials as a bioink formulation. The earliest studies of alginate-based bioprinted constructs mimicked vasculature using various techniques, such as coaxial extrusion systems, (Falcone et al., n.d) droplet-based bioprinting, (Kotlarz et al., n.d) and laser-assisted bioprinting. (Yan et al., n.d) These constructs included heterogeneous tissue constructs incorporating multiple cell types. (Gudapati et al., n.d) A study demonstrated the fabrication of adipose tissue through 3D bioprinting by utilizing alginate and nanocellulose-based bioink to create grafts that exhibited substantial viability of graft *in vivo,* and neovascularization was observed for a culture period of 30 days. The alginate-based constructs maintained good printability, and the bioprinted grafts contained mature adipocytes and continuous vascular structures. Post-implantation, the bioprinted tissue displayed successful engraftment, with evident angiogenesis and vascularization within the graft. (Salio et al., n.d) In a different study, the preparation of alginate methacrylate systems and its rheological behavior before and after polymerization were explored for photocrosslinking-based 3D bioprinting. This research studied explored the impact of various properties of crosslinked alginate hydrogels on the grafting reaction time, revealing that prolonged grafting reaction times led to bioprinted constructs with less number of pores distributed homogeneously and less porosity, showing altered swelling, degradation, mechanical strength, and gelation time. (Mishbak et al., n.d) Additionally, a study focused on fabricating composite bioprinted scaffolds using alginate/carrageenan-based bioink via extrusion-based 3D bioprinting. The group studied suitable crosslinking concentrations, evaluated the rheological properties of the hydrogel-based bioink, and showed successful bioprinting using these hydrogels. The bioprinted scaffold demonstrated good cell viability and sufficient mechanical strength. (Stavarache et al., n.d)

4.2 *Synthetic Bioinks*

In 3D bioprinting, synthetic bioinks devoid of direct natural sourcing constitute a prevalent category among the bioink varieties. (Khoeini et al., n.d) Although natural bioinks have many material requirements, including enriched bioactive and biochemical components, they fail to maintain structural homogeneity and biomechanical properties. It leads to low mechanical properties, limited control, slow gelation, and challenges in the scalability of bioprinted constructs, and there might be potential immunogenic responses from animal-derived materials. Synthetic bioinks allow for the restoration of the limitations of natural bioinks. (Chimene et al., n.d). Bioinks produced synthetically offer distinctive advantages owing to their chemically defined constituents. These bioinks are characterized by enhanced and adjustable mechanical strength, precisely controlled biodegradability, and the capability for further chemical modifications. (Kumar, n.d) Biomaterials in synthetic bioinks allow for the introduction of crosslinking sites or biomimetic molecules, facilitating a consistency not commonly found in naturally derived polymers, which often exhibit variability from batch to batch. Examples of such synthetic polymers include PEG, poly(lactide-co-glycolide), and commonly used poly(caprolactone), referred to as PCL, and poly (l-lactic acid), known as PLA, as well as pluronic. (Chimene et al., n.d) However, only a subset of these polymers qualifies as genuine bioinks due to limitations in their ability to effectively encapsulate and integrate cells within the printed structure. Instead, they predominantly serve as supplementary biomaterials. Inkjet and extrusion printing methods stand out as popular strategies in bioprinting, primarily due to their capacity to fabricate constructs laden with cells within a physiologically relevant environment. These approaches offer a more conducive setting for cell survival during printing and proliferation in printed constructs. (Scribd, n.d)

4.2.1 *Polyethylene glycol (PEG)*

Poly (ethylene glycol) is one of the widely used synthetic polymers as bioink. This compound exhibits linear polyether characteristics and hydrophilic properties, allowing conjugation with various biomolecules such as proteins, liposomes, and enzymes. (Rutz et al., n.d) PEG is employed

Table 1   Summary of Synthetic bioinks

Biomaterial	Fabrication Method	Crosslinking	Tissue	Advantages	Disadvantages	References
PEG	Digital Light Processing (DLP) bioprinting	Photopolymerization	Cancer cell spheroid models	• Innovative bioink • Versatility in different cell culture models • High printing fidelity	• Biocompatibility with limited cell types • Complex and costly	(Kim et al., n.d)
	Extrusion based bioprinting	Covalent crosslinking	Dermal tissue	• Enhanced cell viability • Bioink with robust mechanical property	• Challenges in generalizing the bioink for other tissues • Low printing fidelity	(Rutz et al., n.d)
	Extrusion based bioprinting	Photopolymerization under UV radiation	Ear and nose	• Precise control over the PEG microsphere for better bioprinting of complex tissue. • Biocompatible with inculcating cell patterning.	• Limited mechanical strength • Issue with biodegradability. • Limited printing fidelity	(Xin et al., n.d)
	Inkjet-bioprinting	Photopolymerization	Bone and cartilage	• High speed and resolution • It has low cost compared with other tissue fabrication techniques. • It's a single step process • It has minimized print head clogging	• There is potential for cell damage • It has a limited range of suitable materials for bioprinting	(Gao et al., n.d)
PCL	Fused deposition modeling (FDM) and casting	Thermal crosslinking	Osteochondral tissue	• Variability in vertical pore distribution to mimic natural gradient of osteochondral tissue. • Achievement of cellular alignment. • Flexibility over tuning printing parameters. • Good mechanical strength	• The size limitation of the bioprinted construct. • -Require more bioink optimization for better attainment of tissue functionality and reproducibility.	(Nowicki i et al., n.d)
	Extrusion based bioprinting	Thermal crosslinking	Neural tissue construct	• Good conductive bioink • Potential neural regeneration	• Low printing fidelity • Limited biocompatibility.	(Vijayavenkataraman et al., n.d),

Contd.

Table 1 *Contd.*

Biomaterial	Fabrication Method	Crosslinking	Tissue	Advantages	Disadvantages	References
	Extrusion based bioprinting	Thermal crosslinking	Skin	• Biomimetic full-thickness skin construct • Enhanced biocompatibility • Precision and accuracy via 3D bioprinting	• Potential immune response • Low printing fidelity • Complexity in reproducibility	(Ramasamy et al., n.d)
	Extrusion based bioprinting	Thermal crosslinking	Urethra	• Urethral tissue equivalent • Enhanced mechanical properties • -Good printing fidelity	• Limited biocompatibility • Limited attainment of functionality	(Zhang et al., n.d)
PF-127	Pneumatic extrusion bioprinting	Cold method	Mesenchymal stem cells	• Printing optimization of hybrid hydrogel. • Good mechanical properties of the printed construct	• Scaffold collapse and corner drag in printed construct • Biomaterial ink without cells is a significant limitation as cells alter rheological properties	(Hibbert et al., n.d)
	Extrusion based bioprinting	Cold method	Sacrificial material for blood vessel generation	• Precise vascular architecture • Multilevel vasculature • Biocompatible scaffold	• Multistep complex process of fabrication • Issue maintaining functionality	(Xu et al., n.d)

as a bioink due to its several characteristics, including tunable mechanical properties, hydrophilicity, crosslinking versatility, controlled degradability, and reduced immunogenicity. The application of PEG in bioprinting is constrained due to toxic solvents during the synthesis process, reduced cellular recognition sites, limited biological cues, higher melting point issues, and intensity of photo-crosslinking parameters. (Khoeini et al., n.d) PEG demands modification to inculcate biocompatibility by adding cell adhesion components like RGD peptides. The PEG diol encompasses two hydroxyl end groups that possess the potential for conversion into various functional groups like carboxyl, methoxy, and thiol. Photopolymerization is the predominant approach for fabricating PEG hydrogels, offering enhanced temporal and spatial control during scaffold production. PEG-derived materials enable photo-crosslinking of hydrogels, contributing to superior mechanical stability post-bioprinting. (Xin et al., n.d)

PEG8NB was introduced as a novel direct light printing (DLP) resin and was formulated as a low-viscosity bioink, enabling the creation of precise hydrogels via a highly efficient thiol–norbornene photoclick reaction. The DLP-printed PEG8NB based hydrogels exhibited remarkable printability with high resolution printed scaffolds, with minimal photoinitiator concentrations and photoabsorbers. These hydrogels demonstrated versatility across several *in vitro* 2D models, facilitating development of endothelial networks in microfluidic channels and multicellular 3D spheroids. The investigation highlights the ability of PEG8NB as a responsive resin, propelling advancements in DLP bioprinting based applications. (Kim et al., n.d) The PEG crosslinking (PEGX) bioink was used to enhance the cell viability problem via covalent-based crosslinking. This covalent crosslinking approach enhanced the mechanical properties and significantly improved cell viability within the bioink matrix. (Rutz et al., n.d) PEG microgel bioink was utilized, demonstrating better efficacy in fabricating complex anatomically accurate 3D constructs of the ear and nose, that showed better stability devoid of secondary crosslinking. The hMSCs showed good proliferation in these 3D bioprinted constructs. (Xin et al., n.d) An acrylated PEG hydrogel was co-printed with the acrylated peptides via photopolymerization, which was used to bioprint human mesenchymal stem cells laden scaffolds to mimic bone and cartilage tissue and it was observed that cells showed good chondrogenic and osteogenic differentiation. (Gao et al., n.d) Photopolymerizable PEG based hydrogels serve as good biomaterials for tissue engineering purposes, especially tailored with bioactive peptides to recapitulate the characteristics of the natural extracellular matrix. These modified PEG and their derivatives contain degradable peptides, and their hydrogels are then susceptible to degradation by enzymes linked to cell migration. Incorporating functional groups like RGD residues into hydrogels that can be photopolymerized and are able to facilitate targeted cell adhesion, cell proliferation, and the production of extracellular matrix proteins within the hydrogel matrix. (Mann et al., n.d)

4.2.2 *Polycaprolactone (PCL)*

Polycaprolactone is classified as a semi-crystalline poly (alpha-hydroxy ester) with bioresorbable attributes. Its inherent high hydrophobicity and crystallinity contribute to its slow degradation rate. (Kumar et al., n.d) PCL displays a melting point of 63°C with a glass transition temperature of 60°C. PCL has good mechanical strength that is essential for structural support in bioprinting. It has excellent printing fidelity because of its thermoplastic nature as it melts around moderate temperatures and enables precise layer-by-layer printing of complex structures. (Hospodiuk et al., n.d) PCL-based biomaterials have been used with fused deposition modeling (FDM) and casting techniques to bioprint osteochondral tissue, as printed constructs show enhanced hMSC cell viability. (Nowicki et al., n.d) PCL was employed in neural tissue engineering with a chemical transformation into polypyrrole-b-polycaprolactone (PPy-b-PCL), conferring conductive properties. The bioprinted cell laden collagen/PPy-b-PCL construct showed good cellular viability. (Vijayavenkataraman et al., n.d) A full-thickness skin was biofabricated using extrusion-based 3D bioprinting using PCL/collagen scaffold with top-seeded keratinocytes (Ramasamy et al., n.d) The application of PCL/PLCL combined bioink to 3D bioprint urethra with a spiral scaffold design to mimic the native urethral microarchitecture. The urethral scaffold was laden with urothelial cells towards the inner layers and smooth muscle cells towards the outermost layer. (Zhang et al., n.d)

4.2.3 PF-127

Pluronic F-127 is a triblock co-polymer build-up of poly (propylene oxide) (PPO) and poly (ethylene oxide) (PEO). PF127 is a thermoresponsive polymer known for its amphiphilic nature, which has both hydrophilic and hydrophobic structures. Its unique property lies in its gel formation ability at specific temperatures and concentrations. (Hibbert et al., n.d) It undergoes sol-gel-transition in aqueous solutions and lower temperatures, forming a semi-solid gel that returns to its original liquid state once heated above gelation temperature. Several characteristics of PF-127 make it a suitable bioink, such as thermoresponsive gelation, injectability and printability, biocompatibility, tunable mechanical property, stability and support matrix, degradability, and sacrificial material. (Hibbert et al., n.d) A hybrid bioink with pluronic F-127 and alginate was used in a 3D bioprinting tissue construct where the printing parameters were optimized. (Hibbert et al., n.d) A new technique was developed using 3D bioprinting to create pre-vascularized constructs with vascular networks as seen in Figure 3. These cell-laden structures consisted of a decellularized extracellular matrix (dECM) with multilevel branched blood vessels. Herein, pluronic F127 was used as a sacrificial bioink to form the vasculature using a multi-nozzle 3D bioprinter. Pluronic was later removed, leaving hollow channels for attaching endothelial cells.

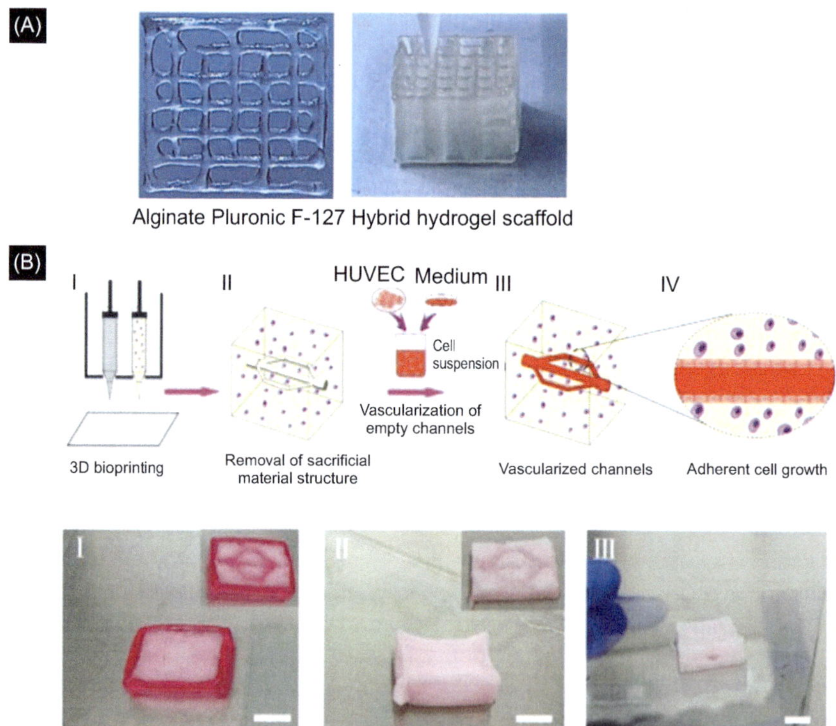

Fig. 3 Pluronic F-127 based bioinks for 3D bioprinting application (A) Pneumatic extrusion bioprinting via alginate-pluronic F-127 hybrid hydrogel. (Hibbert et al., n.d) (B) The 3D bioprinting of multichannel vasculature via pluronic F-127 sacrificial material. (Xu et al., n.d) (Reproduced with permission from)

4.3 Composite Bioinks

The absence of optimal bioink properties in one single hydrogel was one of the primary limitations of the bioprinting technology utilized in earlier decades. Hydrogels often have poor mechanical strength, low viscosity, and lack of cell adhesion moieties, leading to structural instability of 3D printed structures, showing poor shape fidelity, and limiting their use for 3D bioprinting. A perfect bioink should have a few fundamental characteristics, like shear thinning behavior, a relatively high viscosity, quick crosslinking after printing, and the capacity to sustain shape integrity after multilayer 3D printing. (Gao, n.d) Therefore, researchers worldwide have begun employing composite bioink to overcome this restriction. Composite bioink is a blend of two or more biopolymers or filler materials that yield higher quality bioink that cannot be achieved with a single hydrogel. (Heid et al., n.d) Extrusion bioprinting technology is the primary method used to print cell-laden composite bioinks. Composite inks offer more versatility to get the required results. Adding bioactive molecules or biopolymer blends can produce a variety of printed structures, including fibrous tissue, soft tissue (vocal fold), and hard tissue (musculoskeletal system). These bioinks also provide more mechanical, electrical, and physiochemical tunability, allowing their use in 3D bioprinting technology for tissue engineering applications. Moreover, composite bioink can enable 4D bioprinting by incorporating shape-changing features. (Ravanbakhsh et al., n.d) Here, we have reviewed a few composite bioinks formulated using widely used biopolymers that significantly advance 3D bioprinting technology.

4.3.1   GelMA as base bioink

GelMA is a prominent bioink that has been extensively investigated in tissue engineering applications and has been used for various bioprinting applications. It is produced by adding methacrylic anhydride (MA) with gelatin. Gelatin facilitates cell attachment and remodeling, reduces immunogenicity, and improves solubility, while MA promotes on-demand photocrosslinking on exposure to photoinitiators and light sources . GelMA also has exceptional biocompatibility and a broad spectrum of physiochemical tunability. However, this bioink continues to be limited by low viscosity at room temperature, weak conductivity, poor mechanical strength, and other issues. As a result, it has been employed as a base ink, and numerous other active molecules have been incorporated to generate several composite bioinks that outperform GelMA. A recent study used blended bioink with gold nanorod, alginate, and GelMA to print cardiac tissue (Figure 4(A)). (Zhu, n.d) This study intended to increase this biomaterial's conductivity as high conductivity ensures better organization and spreading of cardiac cells. They optimized the gold nanorod and GelMA composite bioink concentration in a way that allowed them to simulate the local moduli of neonatal rat myocardium, which is around 4.0-11.4 KPa. This novel composite bioink has a relatively rough surface, promoting better cell membrane attachment and facilitating electrical signal propagation through cardiomyocytes encapsulated inside the matrices. Encapsulated cells with this composite bioink exhibit elevated expression of gap junction protein Connexin-43 and muscle calcium-binding and contraction protein troponin I. As a result, cardiomyocytes show synchronized beating after two days of culture with this gold nanorod/GelMA hydrogel.

Gianluca Cidonio et al. employed a nano clay called laponite (LPN) in conjunction with GelMA hydrogel to improve the viscous property of the composite bioink and overcome the issue of low viscous single-agent GelMA leading to low printability at room temperature. They discovered that increasing LPN concentration in the composite bioink enhanced the rheological properties of the bioink. Adding LPN also improved the printing shape fidelity of the bioprinted scaffold. SEM images of 3D-printed constructs indicated interconnected porous network. Human bone marrow mesenchymal stem cells exhibited high cellular viability and sustainable proliferation after a culture period of 21 days. This bioink could support osteogenic differentiation and extensive vascularization, as seen in Figure 4(B). (Cidonio, n.d). Guo-Liang Ying et al. employed polyethylene oxide (PEO) and GelMA to create a printed porous scaffold. Compared to dense biomaterials, interconnecting porous scaffolds can allow for more efficient oxygen, nutrient, and waste diffusion, increasing cell spreading, migration, and proliferation. They used 1.6% PEO droplets dispersed in a continuous 10% GelMA emulsion. PEO droplets were gradually removed to induce porosity by soaking them in PBS for 24 hours. It has been found that PEO content directly influences Young's modulus, and changes in volumetric ratio have a considerable effect on viscosity. The study showed that liver cancer cells, endothelial cells, and mouse fibroblasts had excellent cell viability, proliferation, and spreading following bioprinting. The composite bioink exhibited outstanding printability, structural integrity, and linked pores during multilayer printing, as seen in Figure 4(C). (Ying, n.d)

Haitei Cui et al. published a study with a GelMA-based composite bioink incorporating PEGDA and nHA (nano-hydroxyapatite). They employed this bioink to simulate the environment of human bones. Their primary goal was to examine the metastatic migration of breast cancer cells from a tumor microenvironment to colonization in bone via vessels. Further, they characterized the cell-cell interaction between breast cancer cells and osteoblasts. They printed the tumor matrix with GelMA, PEGDA, and breast cancer cell lines, whereas the vessels with just GelMA, and finally, the bone matrix with GelMA, PEGDA, nHA, and human fetal osteoblast cells as seen in Figure 4(D). Over a culture period of seven days, breast cancer cells invaded and migrated toward the bone matrix. Breast cancer cells invade and occupy the bone matrix after migration. (Cui, n.d)

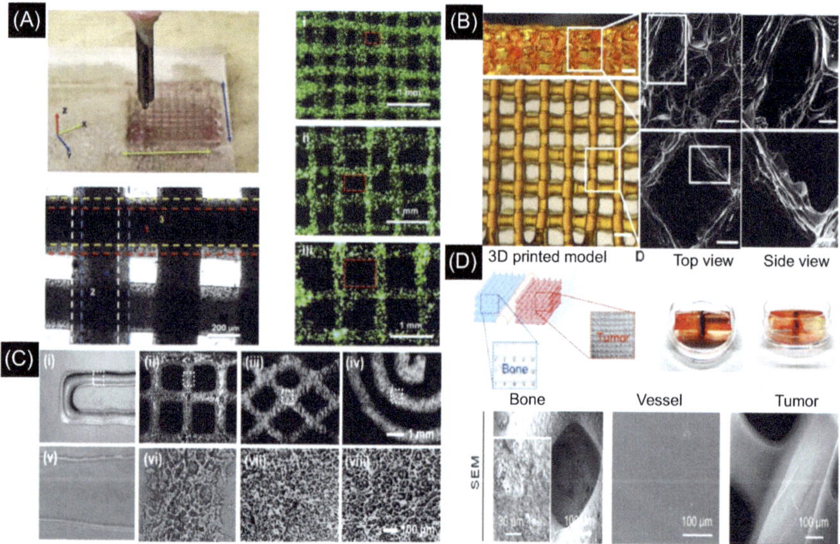

Fig. 4   GelMA based bioinks for 3D bioprinting application (A) Multilayer 3D bioprinting using Gold nanorod (GNR)/Alginate/GelMA composite bioink; 3D bioprinted construct has excellent cytocompatibility (green) (B) Interconnected porosity retention in 3D printed nanocomposite bioink composed of GelMA/Laponite (LPN) (C) Aqueous two-phase emulsion composite bioink composed of GelMA/Polyethylene oxide displaying 3D printed construct at low (i-iv) and high magnification (v-viii). (D) Breast cancer metastasis to bone: 3D printing of vascularized tissue model by using GelMA/PEGDA/nHA composite bioink. (Reproduced with permission from)

4.3.2   Alginate as base bioink

Alginate, a naturally found polysaccharide polymer, is unquestionably the most frequently used bioink in today's bioprinting technology. It is a cost-effective biomaterial derived from calcium, magnesium, and sodium alginate salts found in various brown algaes. Alginate is made up of (1-4)-linked β-d-mannuronic (M) and α-l-guluronic acids (G). The most notable feature of the alginate molecule is the sol-to-gel transition on exposure to ions, such as Ca^{2+}, making alginate-based hydrogels practically temperature-independent. It has shown strong printability and biocompatibility. It is commonly used to print vascular, cartilage, and bone tissue. However, the application of this polymer as a bioink is inadequate because of weak cellular adhesion, cellular proliferation, cellular differentiation, and slow breakdown rate. To address this, individuals have begun combining various biopolymers and growth factors with various filler materials to improve alginate's biocompatibility and mechanical strength. Alginate is not printable ink. Michael Muller *et al.*, used a sulfated version of alginate as base ink and mixed nano cellulose to make a composite printable bioink. Alginate sulfate can promote cell spreading through β1 integrin-dependent mechanisms. This mitogenic hydrogel can promote long-term chondrocyte proliferation and spreading and stimulate collagen II deposition by bovine chondrocytes. It was discovered that adding nanocellulose and alginate sulfate content can result in many-fold increases in viscosity. The cells were evenly distributed throughout the matrix, and a significant rise in proliferation and cell number was observed on days 14 and 28, respectively. Apart from collagen II, proteoglycans are produced and deposited throughout the matrix. (Axpe and Oyen, n.d)

Ellinor B. Heggset et al. developed another alginate-based composite 3D printable bioink containing cellulose nanofibril (CNF). They discovered that it is ideal for 3D bioprinting because it can keep structural integrity and shape fidelity even after printing. After printing, the entire printed scaffold was immersed in Ca^{+2} ion to increase mechanical strength. After mechanical testing, this printed structure had good viscoelastic properties and did not collapse. The rupture strength of the hydrogel was approximately 5-5.5 kg, and it also had good deformation ability when stretched or compressed, which was extremely useful for construction handling and replacement (Heggset et al., n.d). Duong Nguyen et al. conducted another study that demonstrated using nanofibrillated cellulose (NFC) and alginate composite bioink for cartilage tissue engineering applications. The group showcased that NFC simulated the mechanical, structural microenvironment, and bulk collagen matrix required for cartilage growth and development, at the same time, alginate mimicked the ECM proteoglycan component. Both components of this bioink are xenofree and FDA-approved. The group used irradiated human chondrocytes, and iPSC encapsulated in this bioink for 3D bioprinting. This material was suitable for cell proliferation, cartilage production, and even differentiation of iPSC (Ngyuen et al., n.d)

3D hydrogel composite bioink made up of sodium alginate mixed with laponite was designed by Yifei Jin et al. mainly for cartilage and bone tissue engineering applications. This composite could sustainably retain shape fidelity and good printability. This addition of nano clay enhanced mechanical strength due to hydrogen bonding, van der Waals , and ionic interactions between the polymer mixture and nanosilicate. In addition, due its plate-like shape, anisotropy, and high aspect ratio, the addition of laponite addition can boost Young's modulus by 7.4 fold, resulting in strong surface interaction between these two components. Furthermore, crosslinking can result in physical interaction between laponite particles and the hydrogel chain, increasing energy dissipation. A slow degradation rate of the printed construct could give enough stability throughout incubation, allowing a long-term window period for cell proliferation and tissue union (Jin et al., n.d)

4.3.3 Gelatin as base bioink

Gelatin is a popular biopolymer with several inherent cell-adhesive moieties present in their polymer chains and the property of enzyme mediated biodegradation which allows for cellular adhesion and proliferation. (Asim et al., n.d) This extremely biocompatible and biodegradable substance has extensive use in the tissue engineering field. Gelatin is formed by the denaturation process of the animal protein commonly known as collagen, which is the primary component of the extracellular matrix in the animal kingdom. Collagen and its derivative gelatin have triple helix structures that appear in gel form below 37°C due to the stabilization of the tertiary molecular structure. (Irmak et al., n.d) However, *in vitro* experiments are carried out at 37°C, which is higher than the gelation temperature of gelatin. So, gelatin is often chemically altered to produce covalent network formations after fabrication. (Bertlein et al., n.d) Several research groups have also combined gelatin with other biopolymers or filler materials to make composite bioinks.

Sahar Sultan et al., for instance, combined gelatin reinforced with cellular nanocrystal (CNC) and sodium alginate to generate one composite bioink. CNC can provide structural orientation, mechanical strength, and rheological qualities appropriate for bioprinting. The hydrogel's viscoelastic solid nature made it suitable for 3D bioprinting, and the hydrogel could retain dimensional stability

Table 2   Summary of Composite bioinks

Composite bioink			Cell	Crosslinking Technique	Stiffness (Young's/ Compressive) Modulus)	Applications	Ref
Polymer 1	Polymer 2	Additives					
GelMA		CaP	hiPSCs	UV -Irgacure	*Not mentioned*	Osteogenic differentiation in the absence of a growth agent	C.R. Alcala-Orozco et al.,
		Laponite	hMSCs	UV-Irgacure	12.9±1.3 KPa	Osteogenic differentiation is promoted and hydrogel stiffness is enhanced	J.R. Xavier
	κ-carrageenan	Laponite	hMSCs	UV-Irgacure	141±8KPa	Endochondral ossification	D. Chimene et al.,
	Me-HA	HA	hASCs	UV-LAP		Bone matrix deposition	A. Wenz et al.,
		CNT	Neonatal Rat cardiomyocyte	UV-irradiation	32KPa	Improved Mechanical Properties and Bioactution	S.R. Shin
Alginate	Gelatin	HA	hASCs	$CaCl_2$	Not mentioned	Osteogenic differentiation	X.-F. Wang et al.,
	Gelatin	Bioglass	SaOS-2	$CaCl_2$	Not mentioned	Post-printing Mineralization and Proliferation of cells	X. Wang
	Collagen		Chondrocytes	$CaCl_2$	Not mentioned	Mechanical stability and improved stiffness	X. Yang et al.,
	Pluronic		hMSCs	$CaCl_2$	Not mentioned	Porous hydrogel	J.P.K. Armstrong et al.,
	Gelatin microparticle		gMSCs	$Cacl_2$	Not mentioned	Controlled release of growth factor (BMP2) & influence osteogenecity	M.T. Poldervaart
Gelatin		Gas		Thermal	Not mentioned	Development of Porous hydrogel	M. Costantini
	Alginate	GO	MG-63		55MPa	Bone regeneration	S.D. Purohit et al.,
PCL		HA	hiBMSCs		4-11 MPa	Cellular differentiation and integration of construct with calvarial defect	A.E. Jakus
		HA, TC or DCB	hMSCs		30-80 MPa	Osteogenic gene expression	E. Nyberg et al.,
		β TCP			2-10 MPa	Induce bone growth	T. Kawai
		HAp	hMSCs		2.495 MPa	Improved Mechanical properties and degradation	A.H. Ambre et al.,
PEGDA		Laponite-XLG & RD	NIH-3T3	UV-irradiation	*Not mentioned*	Improvement of mechanical strength	Y. Jin et al.,
PEGDAMA		HA BG	hMSCs	UV-irradiation	358.91±48.05KPa	Osteogenesis	G. Gao et al.,

and structural integrity after ex-situ crosslinking. In addition, sequential crosslinking by ionic and covalent interaction has also contributed to the stability of the hydrogel. The printed constructs had uniform and gradient porosity ranging from 80 to 2125 μm. It has been shown that pore size substantially impacts cell interaction. For instance, chondrocytes and osteoblasts benefit from pore sizes between 380 and 405 μm, whereas fibroblasts and bone formation benefit from pore sizes between 290 and 310 μm, and chondrocyte proliferation and ECM secretion benefit from pore sizes between 250 and 500 μm. The group could imitate the graded mechanical properties of a native tissue environment by printing the multilayered construct with a regulated pore dimension and density gradation along the axis of printing (Sultan et al., n.d)

Another gelatin-based composite bioink was produced by Amir Sheikhi et al. as an injectable shear-thinning biomaterial using laponite. They studied the behavior of this ink in the presence of ions in phosphorus buffer saline (PBS) and cell culture media. They stated that the ink could maintain structural integrity up to 160 Pa of stress when prepared in Milli-Q water, but when created in salt solution, the ink became more susceptible to stress and broke down at lower-stress conditions. They also reported that the change in the ink's storage moduli depended on NaCl concentration. When the concentration of NaCl was 10 mM, the hydrogel could withstand high stress up to 160 Pa; however, if the ionic strength was increased past 100 mM, the storage modulus decreased even at a low stress. The storage moduli and loss modulus were comparatively smaller when the ink was made in Milli-Q instead of PBS and DMEM, which had ions that aided in the aggregation of ink (Sheiki et al., n.d). Recently, Yogendra Pratap Singh et al. developed a novel composite chemical crosslinker-free silk and gelatin blend based bioink for cartilage tissue printing. Their primary objective was to eliminate the need for chemical crosslinkers after printing because they are linked to cytotoxicity, complexity, and high cost. Because gelatin is a thermoresponsive substance, it can physically crosslink and produce hydrogels, but because this gel lacks sufficient mechanical strength, natural polymer silk is combined with gelatin to increase its mechanical strength. They have reported that the ink behaves as a liquid with the lowest viscosity at temperatures of 25-35°C, so they consider this temperature as the printing window for the ink. They reported that the ink behaves as a liquid with the lowest viscosity at temperatures in the range of 25 to 35°C, so they consider this temperature as the printing window for the ink. The temperature range and behavior of this bioink were highly beneficial for cell growth and sustainability. The printed construct exhibited dimensional solidity as well as shape fidelity. Cells within the bioprinted scaffold were highly viable and homogeneously distributed over two weeks. Chondrogenic marker Sox9 was upregulated, indicating the differentiation ability and cartilage-specific ECM production by encapsulated chondrocytes. To further evaluate *in vivo* biocompatibility, they performed subcutaneous implantation of the printed construct in a mouse model, and no prolonged immune response was found after a study over 14 days (Singh et al., n.d).

5. Commercially Available Bioinks

3D bioprinting is a junction of biology and engineering, reflecting the clinical need to create superior and viable biological constructs. The rising need for printable materials that can support cellular functions has prompted numerous companies to focus on developing and commercializing bioinks. Established in 2016, Cellink Life Sciences, a prominent Swedish company, is a key player in the commercial bioink sector. They offer a diverse range of bioinks tailored for various applications. These bioinks predominantly utilize common base polymers, including alginate, collagen, and gelMA, primarily focusing on crosslinking methods such as ionic gelation or photopolymerization. One of the bioinks, the alginate-cellulose-based CELLINK, is the first universal bioink designed explicitly for printing human tissue models. (Home, n.d) The American company Advanced Biomatrix (acquired by BICO) Offers DLP-based bioprinting and two-photon polymerization (2PP) techniques for printing bioinks. They provide lifeink® collagen bioinks, which come preformulated with a polymer and photoinitiator. Other similar examples include methacrylated gelatin or GelMA, methacrylated hyaluronic acid or HA-MA, methacrylated alginate, and PEGDA

Table 3 Summary of commercially available bioinks

Bioink	Components	Concentration	Gelation method	Bioprinting applications
Cellink Life Sciences				
A Series				
CELLINK A-RGD	RGD-functionalized alginate	NR	Ionic crosslinking	Cancer model (Vallulina, n.d)
CHITOINK	Chitosan, glucomannan thickener, and glycerol phosphate stabilizer	NR	Ionic crosslinking	
Cellink Series				
CELLINK	Alginate and hydrated cellulose nanofibrils	NR	Ionic crosslinking	3D *in vitro* cancer model, (Schmidt et al, n.d; Sbrana et al, 2021) Cellular reorganization, (Gao, n.d) Multi-branched hydrogel for vascular networks (Utagawa et al, n.d)
CELLINK RGD	RGD functionalized CELLINK alginate and cellulose nanofibrils	NR	Ionic crosslinking	
CELLINK Laminink+	CELLINK with laminins	NR	Ionic crosslinking	
Advanced Biomatrix				
Lifeink Series				
Lifeink® 200 Lifeink® 220	Bovine collagen type I	35 mg/mL 70 mg/mL	Thermal self-assembly	Nasal cartilage, (X. Lan) heart components, (Lee et al, 2019) (Maxson, n.d) meniscus (Stocco et al, n.d) (Filardo, n.d)
Lifeink® 240 Lifeink® 260	Acidified Bovine collagen	35 mg/mL 70 mg/mL	Thermal self-assembly	
PhotoGel®	GelMA, LAP	GelMA – 10 mg/mL, LAP – 0.25%	blue light crosslinking (405 nm)	
Humabiologics				
HumaDerm	Human skin collagen type I	3, 6, 10 mg/mL	Thermal self-assembly	Cell-matrix interaction (Schmitt, n.d)
HumaDerMA	Human skin collagen type I methacrylate	NR	Thermal self-assembly Photo-crosslinking	–
HumaMatrix	Native Human-Derived ECM	10, 20 mg/mL	Thermal self-assembly	*In vitro* tissue fibrosis model (Hewawasam et al, n.d)
Huma OsteoGelatin	Human bone-derived gelatin	NA (lyophilized)	NA	Photocrosslinkable hydrogel for cell-matrix interaction (Altunbek et al, n.d)

Contd.

Table 3   *Contd.*

Bioink	Components	Concentration	Gelation method	Bioprinting applications
Collplant				
Collink-3D				
Collink.3D^{TM} 50	Plant-based recombinant human type I collagen methacrylamide (50% functionalization)	13-17 mg/mL	Photo-crosslinking	Human ovarian grafting (Abir, n.d)
Collink.3D^{TM} 90	Plant-based recombinant Human type I collagen methacrylamide (90% functionalization)	13-17 mg/mL	Photo-crosslinking	
Jellagen				
JellaGel™	Type 0 collagen from marine jellyfish	3.7-4.3 mg/mL	Genipin	Cell-matrix interaction (Faruqui, n.d)
Axolotl Biosciences				
TissuePrint-HV	Fibrin-based bioink	NR	NR	Neural tissues (Chrenek et al, n.d)
TissuePrint-LV	Fibrin-based bioink	NR	NR	
Innoregen				
Gel4Cell®	GelMA-based bioink	NR	NR	*In vitro* bladder cancer model (Choi S.Y, n.d)
Gel4Tissue®	Pig's small intestinal submucosa extracellular matrix (SIS-ECM)-based bioink	NR	NR	–
Col4Cell	Collagen-based bioink	NR	NR	–
T&R Biofab				
deCelluid^{TM}	Bone/cartilage/skin dECM-based bioink	NR	Thermal self-assembly	rotator cuff regeneration, (Chae, n.d; Chae et al, n.d) *in vitro* vascularization (Kim et al, n.d)
3DBioFibR				
µCollaFibR^{TM}	Type I collagen bioink additive (50 µm fibers)	NA	NA	
Viscofan Bioengineering				
Fibercoll-Flex®	Type I collagen-based fibrillar bioink	5 mg/mL	Thermal self-assembly	Cell-matrix interaction (Garcia-Villen, n.d)

NA = Not applicable; NR = Not Reported

based biomaterial, which offers tunable hydrogels with exceptional features that can be prepared at numerous concentrations and crosslinked to form 3D scaffolds with varying stiffness. (https://www.cellink.com, n.d) Collplant is a company that focuses on developing rhCollagen-based bioinks for 3D bioprinting applications. They offer Collink.3D^{TM} 50L which is a recombinant human collagen (rhCollagen) derived bioink in lyophilized powder form for 3D bioprinting applications. CollPlant's rhCollagen is similar to the human type I collagen, making it an idyllic biomaterial for regenerative medicine. https://collplant.com/., n.d) Jellagen is a UK company specializing in collagen type 0-based bioinks/hydrogels sourced from marine jellyfish, which can be crosslinked using genipin for stable 3D gels supporting cell embodiment. They offer the formulation as a JellaGel solution, along with its buffer and crosslinker for ease of use. (https://jellagen.co.uk/., n.d) Axolotl Biosciences, a Canadian company, specializes in offering custom xeno-free fibrin-based bioinks. Their TissuePrint Low Viscosity (LV) bioink is optimized explicitly for microfluidic bioprinters, while TissuePrint High Viscosity (HV) is tailored for extrusion-based bioprinters. Alongside the bioink, Axolotl Biosciences provides a crosslinker that is essential in bioprinting. This crosslinker facilitates the creation of printable fibers, contributing to constructing intricate 3D constructs. (https://www.axolotlbiosciences.com., n.d)

Humabiologics stands as the pioneering company offering native human collagen, gelatin, and extracellular matrix (ECM) based bioinks tailored for extrusion-based 3D bioprinting. The company's product portfolio includes HumaDerm, featuring human skin collagen type I in both solution and lyophilized forms; HumaDerMA, presenting methacrylated HumaDerm in lyophilized form; HumaMatrix, providing native human-derived ECM in both solution and lyophilized formats; Huma OsteoGelatin, offering human bone gelatin, and its methacrylated counterpart OsteoGelMA in lyophilized forms, among others. Notably, Humabiologics collaborates with US FDA-registered and accredited tissue banks, ensuring rigorously screened donated human tissue is used. This strategic partnership helps navigate potential FDA regulatory challenges, expediting the progress of innovations in the field of life sciences. ((n.d.). https://www.axolotlbiosciences.com.)

6. Existing Challenges in Bioink Development

The aspiration in bioink development is to create bioink materials that entirely replicate the extracellular matrix's intricate biophysical and biochemical cues (ECM). However, this pursuit proves exceptionally challenging due to the present technical constraints of available biomaterials. With the purpose of catering to the varied requirements for mimicking specific tissue types, it is imperative that bioinks designed for different printing technologies exhibit fundamental properties that enable the fulfillment of complex prerequisites and the execution of intended functions. (Li et al, n.d; Xie et al, n.d; Fan et al, n.d; Bian, n.d; Veeravalli et al, n.d). Multiple challenges are faced concerning bioinks development and application in the bioprinting industry. First and foremost, ensuring that bioink materials are accurately deposited by printers with precise positioning and high resolution is a pivotal concern. Achieving this goal necessitates considering factors such as the crosslinking strategy (physical, chemical, and photo) and density of crosslinking, as well as the rheological properties of bioinks. The optimal parameters may vary contingent on the specific 3D bioprinting technology employed. For instance, inkjet printing demands rapid crosslinking for constructing and maintaining multilayer structures, while extrusion based printing requires bioinks with good rheological properties that showcase shear-thinning behavior. (Zhang et al., n.d; Lee et al., n.d) Secondly, ensuring that the printed constructs are non-toxic to the site of implantation and the surrounding native tissues and, to the greatest extent possible, they should not provoke immunogenic reactions after implantation is imperative. Controlling degradation rates to align with the nascent ECM deposition is also critical. (S.J. Bryant et al.,) Thirdly, incorporating biomimetic elements like proteins, peptides, and growth factors into the printed constructs is indispensable for regulating cellular behaviors. (K.J. Wolf et at., n.d.; R. Li et al., n.d.] This biofunctionalization can be achieved by integrating bioactive peptide residues within the hydrogels being used as bioinks. Next, printed structures must demonstrate appropriate biophysical characteristics, including the photoinitiator concentration, stiffness of the hydrogel, swelling index of the hydrogel, and permeability of the hydrogel. These properties substantially impact the structural strength of the bioprinted tissues, biotransport, and the biological activity of seeded or encapsulated cells. (Pradhan and Slater, 2019; Hsieh et al., n.d)

The biodegradation and remodeling property of the natural ECM proteins are crucial for numerous essential cellular events, including cellular spreading, cell viability and proliferation, cell invasion and migration, and cellular differentiation. (Gattazzo et al., n.d; Solomonov et al., n.d) In the context of cell-laden bioprinted structures, microscopic porous structures are essential for cellular adaptation within printed bioink structures. This facilitates effective cell-material interactions, intracellular signaling, and unobstructed three-dimensional cell proliferation and development. While current photocurable bioinks or ionically crosslinkable bioinks result in stiffer constructs after bioprinting, these structures lack dynamic crosslinking bonds.This is a drawback. The biodegradation of bioprinted constructs can be enhanced by microstructures over the long term. However, shortfalls in addressing the difficulties of fast cell growth during the initial phases are important for the development of bioprinted scaffolds. (Mondschein et al., n.d; Wang et al., n.d) Biodegradable bioinks are essential to guarantee long-term integration of bioprinted scaffolds with native host tissues during *in vivo* implantation.

Finally, bioinks must exhibit low batch-to-batch variations for scaled-up industrial level 3D bioprinting and lab-to-bench translational applications to maintain quality control. The challenge lies in the fact that current biomaterials used for bioink preparation for 3D bioprinting applications are derived from natural polymers, which can exhibit significant variations in molecular weights and compositions. Improving batch-to-batch consistency requires advances in the field of new biofabrication and synthesis technologies to enhance quality control. (Mondschein et al., n.d)

Conclusion and Outlook

In the field of tissue engineering and regenerative medicine, the invention of 3D bioprinting technology is a new frontier for exploration. Use of bioinks represents a cutting-edge technique that could significantly assist progress in bioprinting and change several sectors, such as tissue engineering, regenerative medicine, and pharmaceutical research. The advent of bioinks has made it easier to create intricate three-dimensional structures with fine control over cell viability, distribution, and functionality. This opens new possibilities for the fabrication of tissue constructions that closely mimic natural tissues and organs. Due to the compositional, rheological, and printability diversity of bioinks, scientists have been able to explore a variety of applications, ranging from the creation of basic tissue models to the construction of vascularized and organ-like structures. This adaptability has contributed to advancements in cell biology, biofabrication methods, and biomaterials design, propelling the field of bioprinting ahead. In terms of the future, bioinks and bioprinting have very bright prospects. By incorporating a variety of cell types and bioactive substances to encourage tissue maturation and functionality, scientists are actively attempting to improve bioink formulations to more closely resemble the complexity of native tissues. The capacities of bioinks are being increased, and the frontiers of tissue engineering and personalized medicine are being pushed by developments in bioprinting technologies like multi-material printing, organ-on-a-chip platforms, and in situ bioprinting. Furthermore, novel approaches to improving bioink characteristics, forecasting cell behavior, and creating patient-specific tissue constructs can be made possible by the integration of artificial intelligence (AI), machine learning (ML), and computational modeling with bioprinting procedures.

In conclusion, bioinks are the foundation of bioprinting technology. As novel bioinks continue to be developed and integrated with cutting-edge bioprinting platforms, they have the potential to fundamentally alter the course of medical research and practice by providing fresh approaches to pressing medical issues and enhancing patient outcomes everywhere.

References

A. Bandyopadhyay, B.B. Mandal, A three-dimensional printed silk-based biomimetic tri-layered meniscus for potential patient-specific implantation, Biofabrication. 12 (n.d.) 15003.

A. GhavamiNejad, N. Ashammakhi, X.Y. Wu, A. Khademhosseini, Crosslinking strategies for 3D bioprinting of polymeric hydrogels, Small. 16 (n.d.) 2002931.

A. Lee, A.R. Hudson, D.J. Shiwarski, J.W. Tashman, T.J. Hinton et al. 3D bioprinting of collagen to rebuild components of the human heart, Science (80-.). 365 (2019) 482–487. https://doi.org/10.1126/science.aav9051.

A. Moroni, L. Nakamura, M. Shu, W. Takeuchi, S. Vozzi et al. Biofabrication: reappraising the definition of an evolving field, Biofabrication. 8 (2016) 13001. https://doi.org/10.1088/1758-5090/8/1/013001.

A. Sheikhi, S. Afewerki, R. Oklu, A.K. Gaharwar, A. Khademhosseini et al. Effect of ionic strength on shear-thinning nanoclay–polymer composite hydrogels, Biomater Sci. 6 (n.d.) 2073–2083,. https://doi.org/10.1039/C8BM00469B.

A.C. Dell, G. Wagner, J. Own, J.P. Geibel, 3D Bioprinting Using Hydrogels: Cell Inks and Tissue Engineering Applications, Pharmaceutics. 14 (n.d.) 2596.

A.E. Jakus, Hyperelastic 'bone': A highly versatile, growth factor–free, osteoregenerative, scalable, and surgically friendly biomaterial, Sci Transl Med. 8 (n.d.). https://doi.org/10.1126/scitranslmed.aaf7704.

A.H. Ambre, D.R. Katti, K.S. Katti, Biomineralized hydroxyapatite nanoclay composite scaffolds with polycaprolactone for stem cell-based bone tissue engineering, J Biomed Mater Res A. 103 (n.d.) 2077–2101,. https://doi.org/10.1002/jbm.a.35342.

A.K. Valiullina, Cytotoxic effect of CAR-T cells against modified MCF-7 breast cancer cell line, Mol. Biol. Res. Commun. 12 (n.d.) 139–148,. https://doi.org/10.22099/mbrc.2023.47125.1820.

A.L. Rutz, E.S. Gargus, K.E. Hyland, P.L. Lewis, A. Setty et al. Employing PEG crosslinkers to optimize cell viability in gel phase bioinks and tailor post printing mechanical properties, Acta Biomater. (n.d.).

Advanced BioMatrix - Home, 13 (n.d.). https://advancedbiomatrix.com/.

B. Duan, L.A. Hockaday, K.H. Kang, J.T. Butcher, 3D bioprinting of heterogeneous aortic valve conduits with alginate/gelatin hydrogels, J. Biomed. Mater. Res. Part A. 101 (n.d.) 1255–1264.

B. Guillotin, Laser assisted bioprinting of engineered tissue with high cell density and microscale organization, Biomaterials. 31 (n.d.) 7250–7256,. https://doi.org/10.1016/j.biomaterials.2010.05.055.

B. Sarker, A.R. Boccaccini, Alginate utilization in tissue engineering and cell therapy, in: Alginates Their Biomed. Appl., n.d.: pp. 121–155.

B.A. Melo, Y.A. Jodat, E.M. Cruz, J.C. Benincasa, S.R. Shin et al. Strategies to use fibrinogen as bioink for 3D bioprinting fibrin-based soft and hard tissues, Acta Biomater. 117 (n.d.) 60–76.

B.K. Mann, A.S. Gobin, A.T. Tsai, R.H. Schmedlen, J.L. West et al, Smooth muscle cell growth in photopolymerized hydrogels with cell adhesive and proteolytically degradable domains: synthetic ECM analogs for tissue engineering, Biomaterials. 15; 22(22): (n.d.).

B.S. Kaith, A. Singh, A.K. Sharma, D. Sud, Hydrogels: synthesis, classification, properties, and potential applications—a brief review, J. Polym. Environ. 29 (n.d.) 3827–3841.

Bioink," Axolotl Biosciences, 14 (n.d.). https://www.axolotlbiosciences.com.

C. Piard, H. Baker, T. Kamalitdinov, J. Fisher, Bioprinted osteon-like scaffolds enhance in vivo neovascularization, Biofabrication. 11 (n.d.) 25013.

C. Stavarache, S.A. Gârea, A. Serafim, E. Olăreț, G.M. Vlăsceanu et al. Three-Dimensional-Printed Sodium Alginate and k-Carrageenan-Based Scaffolds with Potential Biomedical Applications, Polymers (Basel). 16 (n.d.) 305.

C. Tomasina, T. Bodet, C. Mota, L. Moroni, S. Camarero-Espinosa, Bioprinting vasculature: materials, cells and emergent techniques, Materials (Basel). 12 (n.d.) 2701.

C.C.L. Schuurmans, M. Mihajlovic, C. Hiemstra, K. Ito, W.E. Hennink et al. Hyaluronic acid and chondroitin sulfate (meth)acrylate-based hydrogels for tissue engineering: Synthesis, characteristics and pre-clinical evaluation, Biomaterials. 268 (n.d.) 120602. https://doi.org/10.1016/j.biomaterials.2020.120602.

C.R. Alcala-Orozco, X. Cui, G.J. Hooper, K.S. Lim, T.B.F. Woodfield et al. Converging functionality: Strategies for 3D hybrid-construct biofabrication and the role of composite biomaterials for skeletal regeneration, Acta Biomater. 132 (n.d.) 188–216,. https://doi.org/10.1016/j.actbio.2021.03.008.

Collplant, 13 (n.d.). https://collplant.com/.

D. Chimene, L. Miller, L.M. Cross, M.K. Jaiswal, I. Singh et al. Nanoengineered Osteoinductive Bioink for 3D Bioprinting Bone Tissue, ACS Appl Mater Interfaces. 12 (n.d.) 15976–15988,. https://doi.org/10.1021/acsami.9b19037.

D. Fan, U. Staufer, A. Accardo, Engineered 3d polymer and hydrogel microenvironments for cell culture applications, MDPI AG, Bioengineering, n.d.

D. Nguyen, Cartilage Tissue Engineering by the 3D Bioprinting of iPS Cells in a Nanocellulose/Alginate Bioink, Sci Rep. 7 (n.d.) 658. https://doi.org/10.1038/s41598-017-00690-y.

D.B. Kolesky, R.L. Truby, A.S. Gladman, T.A. Busbee, K.A. Homan et al. 3D bioprinting of vascularized, heterogeneous cell-laden tissue constructs, Adv. Mater. 26 (2014) 3124–3130. https://doi.org/10.1002/adma.201305506.

D.F.D. Campos, M. Rohde, M. Ross, P. Anvari, A. Blaeser et al. M. Fuest, Corneal bioprinting utilizing collagen-based bioinks and primary human keratocytes, (2019) 1945–1953. https://doi.org/10.1002/jbm.a.36702.

E. Axpe, M. Oyen, Applications of Alginate-Based Bioinks in 3D Bioprinting, Int J Mol Sci. 17 (n.d.). https://doi.org/10.3390/ijms17121976.

E. Hesse, T.E. Hefferan, J.E. Tarara, C. Haasper, R. Meller et al. Collagen type I hydrogel allows migration, proliferation, and osteogenic differentiation of rat bone marrow stromal cells, J. Biomed. Mater. Res. Part A. 94 (n.d.) 442–449.

E. Nyberg, A. Rindone, A. Dorafshar, W.L. Grayson, Comparison of 3D-Printed Poly-ε-Caprolactone Scaffolds Functionalized with Tricalcium Phosphate, Hydroxyapatite, Bio-Oss, or Decellularized Bone Matrix <sup/>, Tissue Eng Part A. 23 (n.d.) 503–514,. https://doi.org/10.1089/ten.tea.2016.0418.

E.B. Heggset, B.L. Strand, K.W. Sundby, S. Simon, G. Chinga-Carrasco et al. Viscoelastic properties of nanocellulose based inks for 3D printing and mechanical properties of CNF/alginate biocomposite gels, Cellulose. 26 (n.d.) 581–595,. https://doi.org/10.1007/s10570-018-2142-3.

E.E. Antoine, P.P. Vlachos, M.N. Rylander, Review of Collagen I hydrogels for bioengineered tissue microenvironments: characterization of mechanics, structure, and transport, Tissue Eng. Part B Rev. 20 (n.d.) 683–696.

E.E. Beketov, E. V Isaeva, N.D. Yakovleva, G.A. Demyashkin, N.V Arguchinskaya et al. Bioprinting of cartilage with bioink based on high-concentration Collagen and chondrocytes, Int. J. Mol. Sci. 22 (n.d.) 11351.

E.L. Maxson, In vivo remodeling of a 3D-Bioprinted tissue engineered heart valve scaffold, Bioprinting. 16 (n.d.) 59. https://doi.org/10.1016/j.bprint.2019.e00059.

E.O. Osidak, P.A. Karalkin, M.S. Osidak, V.A. Parfenov, D.E. Sivogrivov, F.D. Pereira, S.P. Domogatsky, Viscoll collagen solution as a novel bioink for direct 3D bioprinting, J. Mater. Sci. Mater. Med. 30 (n.d.) 1–12.

F. Garcia-Villen, Characterization and assessment of new fibrillar collagen inks and bioinks for 3D printing and bioprinting, Int. J. Bioprinting. 9 (n.d.). https://doi.org/10.18063/ijb.712.

F. Gattazzo, A. Urciuolo, P. Bonaldo, Extracellular matrix: A dynamic microenvironment for stem cell niche, Biochim. Biophys. Acta-Gen. Subj. Elsevier. 1840 (n.d.) 2506–19.

F. Mushtaq, Z.A. Raza, S.R. Batool, M. Zahid, O.C. Onder et al. Preparation, properties, and applications of gelatin-based hydrogels (GHs) in the environmental, technological, and biomedical sectors, Int. J. Biol. Macromol. (n.d.).

F. Pati, J. Jang, D.H. Ha, S. Won Kim, J.W. Rhie et al. Printing three-dimensional tissue analogues with decellularized extracellular matrix bioink, Nat. Commun. 5 (2014) 1–11. https://doi.org/10.1038/ncomms4935.

F.L.C. Morgan, L. Moroni, M.B. Baker, Dynamic Bioinks to Advance Bioprinting, Advanced Healthcare Materials. Wiley-VCH Verlag, n.d.

F.V. Sbrana, R. Pinos, F. Barbaglio, D. Ribezzi, F. Scagnoli et al. 3D Bioprinting Allows the Establishment of Long-Term 3D Culture Model for Chronic Lymphocytic Leukemia Cells, Front. Immunol. 12 (2021) 1–15. https://doi.org/10.3389/fimmu.2021.639572.

G. Cidonio, Osteogenic and angiogenic tissue formation in high fidelity nanocomposite Laponite-gelatin bioinks, Biofabrication. 11 (n.d.) 35027. https://doi.org/10.1088/1758-5090/ab19fd.

G. Egan, S. Phuagkhaopong, S.A. Matthew, P. Connolly, F.P. Seib et al., Impact of silk hydrogel secondary structure on hydrogel formation, silk leaching and in vitro response, Sci. Rep. 12 (n.d.) 3729.

G. Falcone, J.P. Real, S.D. Palma, R.P. Aquino, P. Del Gaudio et al. Floating ricobendazole delivery systems: a 3D printing method by co-extrusion of sodium alginate and calcium chloride, Int. J. Mol. Sci. 23 (n.d.) 1280.

G. Filardo, Patient-specific meniscus prototype based on 3D bioprinting of human cell-laden scaffold, Bone Jt. Res. 8 (n.d.) 101–106,. https://doi.org/10.1302/2046-3758.82.BJR-2018-0134.R1.

G. Gao, A.F. Schilling, T. Yonezawa, J. Wang, G. Dai et al. Bioactive nanoparticles stimulate bone tissue formation in bioprinted three-dimensional scaffold and human mesenchymal stem cells, Biotechnol J. 9 (n.d.) 1304–1311,. https://doi.org/10.1002/biot.201400305.

G. Gao, T. Yonezawa, K. Hubbell, G. Dai, X. Cui et al. Inkjet-bioprinted acrylated peptides and PEG hydrogel with human mesenchymal stem cells promote robust bone and cartilage formation with minimal printhead clogging, Biotechnol J. 10 (n.d.) 1568–77.

G. Irmak, T.T. Demirtaş, M. Gümüşderelioğlu, Highly Methacrylated Gelatin Bioink for Bone Tissue Engineering, ACS Biomater Sci Eng. 5 (n.d.) 831–845,. https://doi.org/10.1021/acsbiomaterials.8b00778.

G. Tang, B. Zhou, F. Li, W. Wang, Y. Liu et al. Advances of naturally derived and synthetic hydrogels for intervertebral disk regeneration, Front. Bioeng. Biotechnol. 8 (n.d.) 745.

G. Ying, Aqueous Two-Phase Emulsion Bioink-Enabled 3D Bioprinting of Porous Hydrogels, Adv. Mater. 30 (n.d.). https://doi.org/10.1002/adma.201805460.

H. Cui, Engineering a Novel 3D Printed Vascularized Tissue Model for Investigating Breast Cancer Metastasis to Bone, Adv Heal. Mater. 9 (n.d.). https://doi.org/10.1002/adhm.201900924.

H. Ding, N.P. Illsley, R.C. Chang, 3D bioprinted GelMA based models for the study of trophoblast cell invasion, Sci. Rep. 9 (n.d.) 18854.

H. Gao, Effects of Different Biomaterials and Cellular Status on Testicular Cell Self-Organization, Adv. Biosyst. 4 (n.d.) 1900292. https://doi.org/10.1002/adbi.201900292.

H. Gudapati, D. Parisi, R.H. Colby, I.T. Ozbolat, Rheological investigation of Collagen, fibrinogen, and thrombin solutions for drop-on-demand 3D bioprinting, Soft Matter. 16 (n.d.) 10506–10517.

H. Gudapati, J. Yan, Y. Huang, D.B. Chrisey, Alginate gelation-induced cell death during laser-assisted cell printing, Biofabrication. 6 (n.d.) 35022.

H. Gudapati, M. Dey, I. Ozbolat, A comprehensive review on droplet-based bioprinting: Past, present and future, Biomaterials. 102 (n.d.) 20–42,. https://doi.org/10.1016/j.biomaterials.2016.06.012.

H. Hong, Digital light processing 3D printed silk fibroin hydrogel for cartilage tissue engineering, Biomaterials. 232 (n.d.) 119679. https://doi.org/10.1016/j.biomaterials.2019.119679.

H. Ravanbakhsh, G. Bao, Z. Luo, L.G. Mongeau, Y.S. Zhang et al. Composite Inks for Extrusion Printing of Biological and Biomedical Constructs, ACS Biomater Sci Eng. 7 (n.d.) 4009–4026,. https://doi.org/10.1021/acsbiomaterials.0c01158.

H.H. Mishbak, G. Cooper, P.J. Bartolo, Development and characterization of a photocurable alginate bioink for three-dimensional bioprinting, Int. J. Bioprinting. 5 (n.d.).

Home, in: CELLINK, n.d. https://www.cellink.com/.

Humabiologics, Humabiologics, Humabiologics. 13 (n.d.). https://humabiologics.com/.

I. Lukin, I. Erezuma, L. Maeso, J. Zarate, M.F. Desimone et al. Progress in gelatin as biomaterial for tissue engineering, Pharmaceutics. 14 (n.d.).

I. Solomonov, E. Zehorai, D. Talmi-Frank, S.G. Wolf, A. Shainskaya et al. Distinct biological events generated by ECM proteolysis by two homologous collagenases, Proc Natl Acad Sci U S A. 27; 113(39) (n.d.).

J. Choi, Efficacy of recombinant Bacillus Calmette-Guérin containing dltA in in vivo three-dimensional bio-printed bladder cancer-on-a-chip and ex vivo orthotopic mouse model, Investig. Clin. Urol. 64 (n.d.) 296–305,. https://doi.org/10.4111/icu.20220293.

J. Chrenek, R. Kirsch, K. Scheck, S.M. Willerth, Protocol for printing 3D neural tissues using the BIO X equipped with a pneumatic printhead, STAR Protoc. 3 (n.d.) 101348. https://doi.org/10.1016/j.xpro.2022.101348.

J. Groll, Biofabrication: reappraising the definition of an evolving field, Biofabrication. 8 (n.d.) 13001. https://doi.org/10.1088/1758-5090/8/1/013001.

J. Lee, S. Park, S. Lee, H.Y. Kweon, Y.Y. Jo et al. Development of Silk Fibroin-Based Non-Crosslinking Thermosensitive Bioinks for 3D Bioprinting, Polymers (Basel). 15 (n.d.) 3567.

J. Lee, S.J. Oh, S.H. An, W.D. Kim, S.H. Kim et al. Machine learning-based design strategy for 3D printable bioink: Elastic modulus and yield stress determine printability, Biofabrication. (n.d.).

J. Li, C. Wu, P.K. Chu, M. Gelinsky, 3D printing of hydrogels: Rational design strategies and emerging biomedical applications, Materials Science and Engineering R: Reports. Elsevier Ltd, n.d.

J. Stepanovska, M. Supova, K. Hanzalek, A. Broz, R. Matejka et al. Collagen bioinks for bioprinting: a systematic review of hydrogel properties, bioprinting parameters, protocols, and bioprinted structure characteristics, Biomedicines. 9 (n.d.).

J. Yan, Y. Huang, D.B. Chrisey, Laser-assisted printing of alginate long tubes and annular constructs, Biofabrication. 5 (n.d.) 15002.

J.-H. Kim, M. Park, J.-H. Shim, W.-S. Yun, S. Jin, Multi-scale vascularization strategy for 3D-bioprinted tissue using coaxial core-shell pre-set extrusion bioprinting and biochemical factors, Int. J. Bioprinting. 9 (n.d.) 726. https://doi.org/10.18063/ijb.726.

J.R. Jangamreddy, M.K. Haagdorens, M.M. Islam, P. Lewis, A. Samanta et al. Short peptide analogs as alternatives to Collagen in pro-regenerative corneal implants, Acta Biomater. 69 (n.d.) 120–130.

J.Y. Hsieh, M.T. Keating, T.D. Smith, V.S. Meli, E.L. Botvinick et al. Matrix crosslinking enhances macrophage adhesion, migration, and inflammatory activation, APL Bioeng. (n.d.).

Jellagen, 13 (n.d.). https://jellagen.co.uk/.

K. Säljö, P. Apelgren, L. Stridh Orrhult, S. Li, M. Amoroso, P. et al. Long-term in vivo survival of 3D-bioprinted human lipoaspirate-derived adipose tissue: proteomic signature and cellular content, Adipocyte. 11 (n.d.) 34–46.

K. Zhang, Q. Fu, J. Yoo, X. Chen, P. Chandra et al. 3D bioprinting of urethra with PCL/PLCL blend and dual autologous cells in fibrin hydrogel: An in vitro evaluation of biomimetic mechanical property and cell growth environment, Acta Biomater. (n.d.).

K. Zhu, Gold Nanocomposite Bioink for Printing 3D Cardiac Constructs, Adv Funct Mater. 27 (n.d.). https://doi.org/10.1002/adfm.201605352.

K. Zhu, Gold Nanocomposite Bioink for Printing 3D Cardiac Constructs, Adv. Funct. Mater. 27 (n.d.) 1605352. https://doi.org/10.1002/adfm.201605352.

K.C. Kolan, J.A. Semon, B. Bromet, D.E. Day, M.C. Leu et al. Bioprinting with human stem cell-laden alginate-gelatin bioink and bioactive glass for tissue engineering, Int. J. Bioprinting. 5 (n.d.).

K.H. Schneider, B.J. Goldberg, O. Hasturk, X. Mu, M. Dötzlhofer et al. Silk fibroin, gelatin, and human placenta extracellular matrix-based composite hydrogels for 3D bioprinting and soft tissue engineering, Biomater. Res. 27 (n.d.) 117.

K.J. Wolf, S. Lee, S. Kumar, A 3D topographical model of parenchymal infiltration and perivascular invasion in glioblastoma, APL Bioeng. (n.d.).

L. Bian, Functional hydrogel bioink, a key challenge of 3D cellular bioprinting, APL Bioengineering. American Institute of Physics Inc, n.d.

L. Fan, Y. Ren, S. Emmert, I. Vučković, S. Stojanovic et al. The Use of Collagen-Based Materials in Bone Tissue Engineering, Int. J. Mol. Sci. 24 (n.d.) 3744.

L. Huang, X. Du, S. Fan, G. Yang, H. Shao et al. Bacterial cellulose nanofibers promote stress and fidelity of 3D-printed silk based hydrogel scaffold with hierarchical pores, Carbohydr. Polym. 221 (n.d.) 146–156.

L. Riacci, A. Sorriento, L. Ricotti, Genipin-Based Crosslinking of Jellyfish Collagen 3D Hydrogels, Gels. 7 (n.d.). https://doi.org/10.3390/gels7040238.

L. Sardelli, M. Tunesi, F. Briatico-Vangosa, P. Petrini, 3D-Reactive printing of engineered alginate inks, Soft Matter. 17 (n.d.) 8105–8117,. https://doi.org/10.1039/D1SM00604E.

L. Wei, Z. Li, J. Li, Y. Zhang, B. Yao et al. An approach for mechanical property optimization of cell-laden alginate–gelatin composite bioink with bioactive glass nanoparticles, J. Mater. Sci. Mater. Med. 31 (n.d.) 1–12.

L.E. Bertassoni, J.C. Cardoso, V. Manoharan, A.L. Cristino, N.S. Bhise et al. Ghaemmaghami, M.R. Dokmeci, A. Khademhosseini, Direct-write bioprinting of cell-laden methacrylated gelatin hydrogels, Biofabrication. 6 (2014). https://doi.org/10.1088/1758-5082/6/2/024105.

L.L. Wang, C.B. Highley, Y.C. Yeh, J.H. Galarraga, S. Uman et al. Three-dimensional extrusion bioprinting of single- and double-network hydrogels containing dynamic covalent crosslinks, J Biomed Mater Res A. 1;106(4):8 (n.d.).

M. Akhmanova, E. Osidak, S. Domogatsky, S. Rodin, A. Domogatskaya et al., Physical, spatial, and molecular aspects of extracellular matrix of in vivo niches and artificial scaffolds relevant to stem cells research, Stem Cells Int. (n.d.).

M. Altunbek, M. Gezek, P. Buck, G. Camci-Unal, Development of Human-Derived Photocrosslinkable Gelatin Hydrogels for Tissue Engineering, Biomacromolecules. 25 (n.d.) 165–176,. https://doi.org/10.1021/acs.biomac.3c00894.

M. Hibbert, J.M. Viljoen, L.H. Plessis, Print parameter optimisation for a Pluronic F-127 and alginate hybrid hydrogel, Bioprinting. (n.d.).

M. Hospodiuk, M. Dey, D. Sosnoski, I.T. Ozbolat, The bioink: A comprehensive review on bioprintable materials, Biotechnol Adv. 1;35(2):21 (n.d.).

M. Kotlarz, A.M. Ferreira, P. Gentile, S.J. Russell, K. Dalgarno et al. Droplet-based bioprinting enables the fabrication of cell–hydrogel–microfibre composite tissue precursors, Bio-Design Manuf. 5 (n.d.) 512–528.

M. Müller, E. Öztürk, Ø. Arlov, P. Gatenholm, M. Zenobi-Wong et al. Alginate Sulfate–Nanocellulose Bioinks for Cartilage Bioprinting Applications, Ann Biomed Eng. 45 (n.d.) 210–223,. https://doi.org/10.1007/s10439-016-1704-5.

M. Nowicki, W. Zhu, K. Sarkar, R. Rao, L.G. Zhang et al. 3D printing multiphasic osteochondral tissue constructs with nano to micro features via PCL based bioink, Bioprinting. (n.d.).

M. Zhou, B.H. Lee, L.P. Tan, A dual crosslinking strategy to tailor rheological properties of gelatin methacryloyl, Int. J. Bioprinting. 3 (n.d.). https://doi.org/10.18063/IJB.2017.02.003.

M.A. Ward, T.K. Georgiou, Thermoresponsive Polymers for Biomedical Applications, Polymers (Basel). 3 (n.d.). https://doi.org/10.3390/polym3031215.

M.C. Catoira, L. Fusaro, D. Francesco, M. Ramella, F. Boccafoschi et al, Overview of natural hydrogels for regenerative medicine applications, J. Mater. Sci. Mater. Med. 30 (n.d.) 1–10.

M.H. Kim, C.C. Lin, Poly(ethylene glycol)–Norbornene as a Photoclick Bioink for Digital Light Processing 3D Bioprinting, ACS Appl Mater Interfaces. 18;15(2):2 (n.d.).

M.L. Tomov, Bioprinted osteogenic and vasculogenic patterns for engineering 3D bone tissue, Adv. Heal. Mater. 8 (n.d.) 1900513. https://doi.org/10.1002/adhm.201900513.

N. Faruqui, Extracellular matrix type 0: From ancient collagen lineage to a versatile product pipeline–JellaGelTM, Mater. Today Bio. 22 (n.d.) 100786. https://doi.org/10.1016/j.mtbio.2023.100786.

N. Rajabi, A. Rezaei, M. Kharaziha, H.R. Bakhsheshi-Rad, H. Luo et al. Recent advances on bioprinted gelatin methacrylate-based hydrogels for tissue repair, Tissue Eng. Part A. 27 (n.d.) 679–702.

N.S. Bhise, A liver-on-a-chip platform with bioprinted hepatic spheroids, Biofabrication. 8 (n.d.) 14101. https://doi.org/10.1088/1758-5090/8/1/014101.

P. Jaipan, A. Nguyen, R.J. Narayan, Gelatin-based hydrogels for biomedical applications, Mrs Commun. 7 (n.d.) 416–426.

P.S. Gungor-Ozkerim, I. Inci, Y.S. Zhang, A. Khademhosseini, M.R. Dokmeci et al. Bioinks for 3D bioprinting: an overview, Biomater. Sci. 6 (n.d.) 915–946.

R. Abir, Novel extra cellular-like matrices to improve human ovarian grafting, J. Assist. Reprod. Genet. 37 (n.d.) 2105–2117,. https://doi.org/10.1007/s10815-020-01832-4.

R. Andreazza, A. Morales, S. Pieniz, J. Labidi, Gelatin-based hydrogels: potential biomaterials for remediation, Polymers (Basel). 15 (n.d.) 1026.

R. Khoeini, H. Nosrati, A. Akbarzadeh, A. Eftekhari, T. Kavetskyy et al. Natural and Synthetic Bioinks for 3D Bioprinting, Adv NanoBiomed Res. 1 (n.d.).

R. Levato, W.R. Webb, I.A. Otto, A. Mensinga, Y. Zhang et al. The bio in the ink: cartilage regeneration with bioprintable hydrogels and articular cartilage-derived progenitor cells, Acta Biomater. 61 (2017) 41–53. https://doi.org/10.1016/j.actbio.2017.08.005.

R. Li, S. Lin, M. Zhu, Y. Deng, X. Chen et al. Synthetic presentation of noncanonical Wnt5a motif promotes mechanosensing-dependent differentiation of stem cells and regeneration, Sci. Adv. 5 (2019).

R. Xie, W. Zheng, L. Guan, Y. Ai, Q. Liang et al. Engineering of Hydrogel Materials with Perfusable Microchannels for Building Vascularized Tissues, Small. Wiley-VCH Verlag, n.d.

R.J. Mondschein, A. Kanitkar, C.B. Williams, S.S. Verbridge, T.E. Long et al. Polymer structure-property requirements for stereolithographic 3D printing of soft tissue engineering scaffolds, Biomaterials. Elsevier Ltd, n.d.

R.N. Ghosh, J. Thomas, B.R. Vaidehi, N.G. Devi, A. Janardanan, P.K et al. An insight into synthesis, properties and applications of gelatin methacryloyl hydrogel for 3D bioprinting, Mater. Adv. 4 (n.d.) 5496–5529.

R.S. Hewawasam, R. Blomberg, P. Šerbedžija, C.M. Magin, Chemical Modification of Human Decellularized Extracellular Matrix for Incorporation into Phototunable Hybrid-Hydrogel Models of Tissue Fibrosis, ACS Appl. Mater. Interfaces. 15 (n.d.) 15071–15083,. https://doi.org/10.1021/acsami.2c18330.

R.S. Veeravalli, B. Vejandla, S. Savani, A. Nelluri, N.C. Peddi et al. Three-Dimensional Bioprinting in Medicine: A Comprehensive Overview of Current Progress and Challenges Faced, Cureus. (n.d.).

S. Anil Kumar, M. Alonzo, S.C. Allen, L. Abelseth, V. Thakur et al. A visible light-cross-linkable, fibrin–gelatin-based bioprinted construct with human cardiomyocytes and fibroblasts, ACS Biomater. Sci. Eng. 5 (n.d.) 4551–4563.

S. AnilKumar, S.C. Allen, N. Tasnim, T. Akter, S. Park et al. The applicability of furfuryl-gelatin as a novel bioink for tissue engineering applications, J. Biomed. Mater. Res. Part B Appl. Biomater. 107 (n.d.) 314–323.

S. Asim, T.A. Tabish, U. Liaqat, I.T. Ozbolat, M. Rizwan et al. Advances in Gelatin Bioinks to Optimize Bioprinted Cell Functions, Adv Heal. Mater. 12 (n.d.). https://doi.org/10.1002/adhm.202203148.

S. Bertlein, Thiol–Ene Clickable Gelatin: A Platform Bioink for Multiple 3D Biofabrication Technologies, Adv. Mater. 29 (n.d.). https://doi.org/10.1002/adma.201703404.

S. Chae, 3D cell-printing of gradient multi-tissue interfaces for rotator cuff regeneration, Bioact. Mater. 19 (n.d.) 611–625,. https://doi.org/10.1016/j.bioactmat.2022.05.004.

S. Chae, Y. Sun, Y.-J. Choi, D.-H. Ha, I. Jeon, D.-W. Cho, 3D cell-printing of tendon-bone interface using tissue-derived extracellular matrix bioinks for chronic rotator cuff repair, Biofabrication. 13 (n.d.) 35005. https://doi.org/10.1088/1758-5090/abd159.

S. Dinescu, M. Albu Kaya, L. Chitoiu, S. Ignat, D.A. Kaya et al. Collagen-based hydrogels and their applications for tissue engineering and regenerative medicine. Polymers and Polymeric Composites: A Reference Series, Springer, Cham, n.d.

S. Heid, A.R. Boccaccini, Advancing bioinks for 3D bioprinting using reactive fillers: A review, Acta Biomater. 113 (n.d.) 1–22,. https://doi.org/10.1016/j.actbio.2020.06.040.

S. Kumar, Synthetic polymer-derived single-network inks/bioinks for extrusion-based 3D printing towards bioapplications, Mater Adv. 2 (n.d.) 6928–41.

S. Pradhan, J.H. Slater, Tunable hydrogels for controlling phenotypic cancer cell states to model breast cancer dormancy and reactivation, Biomaterials. 215 (2019). https://doi.org/10.1016/j.biomaterials.2019.04.022.

S. Ramasamy, P. Davoodi, S. Vijayavenkataraman, J.H. Teoh, A.M. Thamizhchelvan et al. Optimized construction of a full thickness human skin equivalent using 3D bioprinting and a PCL/collagen dermal scaffold, Bioprinting. (n.d.).

S. Sakai, K. Ueda, E. Gantumur, M. Taya, M. Nakamura et al. Drop-On-Drop Multimaterial 3D Bioprinting Realized by Peroxidase-Mediated Cross-Linking, Macromol. Rapid Commun. 39 (n.d.) 1700534. https://doi.org/10.1002/marc.201700534.

S. Sultan, A.P. Mathew, 3D printed scaffolds with gradient porosity based on a cellulose nanocrystal hydrogel, Nanoscale. 10 (n.d.) 4421–4431,. https://doi.org/10.1039/C7NR08966J.

S. V. Murphy, A. Atala, 3D bioprinting of tissues and organs, Nat. Biotechnol. 32 (2014) 773–785. https://doi.org/10.1038/nbt.2958.

S. Vijayavenkataraman, N. Vialli, J.Y.H. Fuh, W.F. Lu, Conductive collagen/polypyrrole-b-polycaprolactone hydrogel for bioprinting of neural tissue constructs, Int J Bioprinting. Inval. date;5(1): (n.d.).

S. Xin, D. Chimene, E. Garza, K.G. J, L.A. A, D et al. Clickable PEG hydrogel microspheres as building blocks for 3D bioprinting, Biomater Sci. 7 (n.d.) 1179–87.

S.D. Purohit, R. Bhaskar, H. Singh, I. Yadav, M.K. Gupta et al. Development of a nanocomposite scaffold of gelatin–alginate–graphene oxide for bone tissue engineering, Int J Biol Macromol. 133 (n.d.) 592–602,. https://doi.org/10.1016/j.ijbiomac.2019.04.113.

S.H. Kim, H. Hong, O. Ajiteru, M.T. Sultan, Y.J. Lee et al. 3D bioprinted silk fibroin hydrogels for tissue engineering, Nat. Protoc. 16 (n.d.) 5484–5532.

S.J. Bryant, F.J. Vernerey, Programmable Hydrogels for Cell Encapsulation and Neo-Tissue Growth to Enable Personalized Tissue Engineering, Adv Heal. Mater. 10; 7(1 (n.d.).

S.K. Schmidt, R. Schmid, A. Arkudas, A. Kengelbach-Weigand, A.K. Bosserhoff et al, Tumor Cells Develop Defined Cellular Phenotypes After 3D-Bioprinting in Different Bioinks, Cells. 8 (n.d.). https://doi.org/10.3390/cells8101295.

S.N. Jayasinghe, A.N. Qureshi, P.A.M. Eagles, Electrohydrodynamic Jet Processing: An Advanced Electric-Field-Driven Jetting Phenomenon for Processing Living Cells, Small. 2 (n.d.) 216–219,. https://doi.org/10.1002/smll.200500291.

S.O. Sarrigiannidis, J.M. Rey, O. Dobre, C. González-García, M.J. Dalby et al. A tough act to follow: Collagen hydrogel modifications to improve mechanical and growth factor loading capabilities, Mater. Today Bio. 10 (n.d.) 100098.

S.Y. Choi, Enhanced Antitumor Effect of the Combination of Bacille Calmette-Guérin and an Immune Checkpoint Inhibitor in Bladder Cancer-On-a-Chip, BioChip J. 17 (n.d.) 496–506,. https://doi.org/10.1007/s13206-023-00125-z.

Scribd, Bioinks Review | PDF | Physical Sciences | Chemistry, (n.d.). https://www.scribd.com/document/671248694/Bioinks-review.

T. Gao, Optimization of gelatin–alginate composite bioink printability using rheological parameters: a systematic approach, Biofabrication. 10 (n.d.) 34106. https://doi.org/10.1088/1758-5090/aacdc7.

T. Hu, A.C. Lo, Collagen–alginate composite hydrogel: Application in tissue engineering and biomedical sciences, Polymers (Basel). 13 (n.d.).

T. Kawai, Customized, degradable, functionally graded scaffold for potential treatment of early stage osteonecrosis of the femoral head, J. Orthop. Res. 36 (n.d.) 1002–1011,. https://doi.org/10.1002/jor.23673.

T. Schmitt, N. Kajave, H.H. Cai, L. Gu, M. Albanna et al. In vitro characterization of xeno-free clinically relevant human collagen and its applicability in cell-laden 3D bioprinting, J. Biomater. Appl. 35 (n.d.) 912–923,. https://doi.org/10.1177/0885328220959162.

T.D. Stocco, M.C.M. Silva, M.A.F. Corat, G.G. Lima, A.O. Lobo et al. <p>Towards Bioinspired Meniscus-Regenerative Scaffolds: Engineering a Novel 3D Bioprinted Patient-Specific Construct Reinforced by Biomimetically Aligned Nanofibers</p>, Int. J. Nanomedicine. 17 (n.d.) 1111–1124,. https://doi.org/10.2147/IJN.S353937.

T.T. Demirtaş, G. Irmak, M. Gümüşderelioğlu, A bioprintable form of chitosan hydrogel for bone tissue engineering, Biofabrication. 9 (n.d.) 35003. https://doi.org/10.1088/1758-5090/aa7b1d.

W. He, J. Deng, B. Ma, K. Tao, Z. Zhang et al. Recent Advancements of Bioinks for 3D Bioprinting of Human Tissues and Organs, ACS Appl. Bio Mater. (2023). https://doi.org/10.1021/acsabm.3c00806.

X. Lan, In vitro maturation and in vivo stability of bioprinted human nasal cartilage, J. Tissue Eng. 13 (n.d.) 20417314221086368,. https://doi.org/10.1177/20417314221086368.

X. Wang, Effect of Bioglass on Growth and Biomineralization of SaOS-2 Cells in Hydrogel after 3D Cell Bioprinting, PLoS One. 9 (n.d.) 112497. https://doi.org/10.1371/journal.pone.0112497.

X.B. Chen, A.F. Anvari-Yazdi, X. Duan, A.Z.-B. Materials, undefined 2023, Biomaterials/bioinks and extrusion bioprinting, Elsevier. (n.d.). https://www.sciencedirect.com/science/article/pii/S2452199X23001809.

Y. Jin, C. Liu, W. Chai, A. Compaan, Y. Huang et al, Self-Supporting Nanoclay as Internal Scaffold Material for Direct Printing of Soft Hydrogel Composite Structures in Air, ACS Appl Mater Interfaces. 9 (n.d.) 17456–17465,. https://doi.org/10.1021/acsami.7b03613.

Y. Shi, T.L. Xing, H.B. Zhang, R.X. Yin, S.M. Yang et al. Tyrosinase-doped bioink for 3D bioprinting of living skin constructs, Biomed. Mater. 13 (2018) 1–14. https://doi.org/10.1088/1748-605X/aaa5b6.

Y. Utagawa, K. Ino, K. Hiramoto, H. Shiku, Simple, Rapid, and Large-Scale Fabrication of Multi-Branched Hydrogels Based on Viscous Fingering for Cell Culture Applications, Macromol. Biosci. 23 (n.d.) 2300069. https://doi.org/10.1002/mabi.202300069.

Y. Xu, Y. Hu, C. Liu, H. Yao, B. Liu et al. A Novel Strategy for Creating Tissue-Engineered Biomimetic Blood Vessels Using 3D Bioprinting Technology, Materials (Basel). (n.d.).

Y. Zhang, Y. Wang, Y. Li, Y. Yang, M. Jin et al., Application of Collagen-Based Hydrogel in Skin Wound Healing, Gels. 9 (n.d.) 185.

Y.P. Singh, A. Bandyopadhyay, B.B. Mandal, 3D Bioprinting Using Cross-Linker-Free Silk–Gelatin Bioink for Cartilage Tissue Engineering, ACS Appl Mater Interfaces. 11 (n.d.) 33684–33696. https://doi.org/10.1021/acsami.9b11644.

Z. Li, C. Ruan, X. Niu, Collagen-based bioinks for regenerative medicine: Fabrication, application and prospective, Med. Nov. Technol. Devices. 100211 (n.d.).

Z. Zhang, Y. Jin, J. Yin, C. Xu, R. Xiong et al. Evaluation of bioink printability for bioprinting applications, Appl Phys Rev. (n.d.).

Safety and Toxicity of 3D Printed Medical Products

Thamizharasan Sampath,[1]
Prakash Srinivasan Timiri Shanmugam,[2*]
Sandhiya Thamizharasan[3] *and Suresha KR*[4]

1. Introduction

Every day, 3D printers are becoming increasingly integrated into our lives. In 2018 alone, 1.42 million units were sold, and projections suggest that by 2027, this number will exceed eight million units. With their relatively affordable prices, starting at 140 euros, 3D printers have found their way into numerous industries, households, and even educational institutions. They offer the capability to produce prototypes of unique designs at minimal cost, and the availability of free downloadable models from the internet enables users to print various items, from games and figures to functional parts. The advent of 3D printing technology has heralded a new era in the field of medicine, offering unprecedented opportunities for innovation, customization, and patient-specific care. 3D printing, also known as additive manufacturing, enables the fabrication of intricate structures and complex geometries with precision and efficiency. In the realm of healthcare, this technology holds immense promise for the production of medical devices, implants, prosthetics, pharmaceuticals, and even tissue-engineered constructs. However, alongside these advantages, 3D printing also brings about a host of emerging risks, particularly concerning exposure to nanoparticles and volatile organic compounds (VOCs). Materials such as poly lactic acid (PLA) and acrylonitrile butadiene styrene (ABS) have been extensively studied due to their widespread usage. Nevertheless, as the market introduces new compounds and printing technologies, such as 3D resin printers, the scope of potential risks continues to evolve.

Furthermore, it is important to note that in many countries, there are no established occupational exposure limit values (OELVs) for nanoparticles. Nonetheless, there exist reference values to

[1]   Department of Pharmacology & Toxicology, VMCH, Dr.YSR University of health Sciences, Andhra Pradesh, India.
[2]   Global Product Safety & Toxicology, Avanos medical Inc, Alpharetta, USA.
[3]   The Tooth Doctor, Advanced Implant Centre, Vellapanchavadi, Chennai, India.
[4]   Department of Pharmacology, VMCH, Dr.YSR University of health Sciences, Andhra Pradesh, India
*   Corresponding author: thamizhpharma@gmail.com

aid in evaluating nanoparticle exposures originating from 3D printers. Regarding VOCs, not all compounds are regulated with an OELV, further complicating the assessment of associated risks.

By shedding light on these critical issues, this chapter seeks to inform healthcare professionals, researchers, policymakers, and industry stakeholders about the importance of prioritizing safety in the development and deployment of 3D printed medicinal products. Ultimately, our collective efforts in understanding and mitigating the risks associated with 3D printing will ensure the continued advancement and responsible integration of this transformative technology in healthcare.

2.   Materials used in 3D Printing

3D printing and bioprinting represent cutting-edge technologies in manufacturing and healthcare. In 3D printing, synthetic polymers like acrylonitrile, butadiene, styrene, polylactic acid, nylon, and metals serve as primary feedstocks. During the printing process, emissions of volatile organic compounds (VOCs) and nanoparticles can occur. Conversely, bioprinting predominantly employs natural polymers. However, exposure to these materials can pose direct and indirect toxic risks to individuals.

Plastics: The most common feedstock used in 3D printing.

- Polylactic acid (PLA)
- Acrylonitrile butadiene styrene (ABS)
- Polyvinyl Alcohol Plastic (PVA)
- Polycarbonate (PC)
- Polyamide (Nylon) – Powder

Metals: The second most common input used in 3D printing are metals or alloys; often used to print various parts of components and jewelry.

- Stainless-steel
- Bronze
- Gold
- Nickel
- Aluminum
- Titanium
- Alumide – powder

Resins: These have limited use that is often reserved for small figures and models.

- High-detail resins
- Paintable resin
- Transparent resin

Carbon Fiber: A composite used over plastic materials to increase strength.

Graphite and Graphene: Often used for devices, including touchscreens and solar panels, due to their strength, flexibility, and high electrical conductivity.

Nitinol: A highly flexible compound of titanium and nickel, often used in medical implants.

Paper: Used to print models and molds, often with recycled paper pulp mixed with a binding agent.

Off the materials used in 3D printing, plastics remain the most popular, particularly in PPE printing. These materials have been shown to release VOCs that include irritants as well as carcinogens. Yet even in cases where non-toxic materials, such as resins, are used, the AM process still releases potentially harmful particulates. According to a 2020 study by the Society for Risk Analysis, 3D printer particulate emissions were found to induce pronounced toxicological effects in small airway epithelial cells (SAEC) found in humans. These toxicological effects take place as particulates penetrating deep into the lungs.

Additives used in many of these materials, for color, shine, and other properties, have been shown to increase particulate and VOC generation during printing. Particulates and VOCs released during 3D printing can greatly impact indoor air quality and put occupants, especially children, at risk.

Most of the study findings indicate that fused deposition modeling often releases VOCs, while selective laser sintering emits ultra-fine particles. Occupational exposure to synthetic polymers has been linked to conditions such as asthma, chronic obstructive pulmonary disease, allergic rhinitis, and DNA damage. Moreover, metal nanoparticles present in certain printing processes can have adverse health effects on the respiratory and nervous systems.

2.1 Polylactic Acid (PLA)

PLA is one of the most popular FDM 3D printing materials . It is relatively inexpensive, easy to print and biodegradable. During the worldwide pandemic of COVID-19, a group of engineers created working ventilators using PLA plastic, a 3D printer and some off-the-shelf components for hospitals treating Coronavirus patients.

Table 1   Pros and Cons of PLA as 3D printing material

Pros	*Cons*
• Low cost • Easy to print • Rigid, stiff and good strength • Biodegradable • Odorless	• Low heat and chemical resistance • Less durable than ABS or PETG • Not suitable for outdoor (sunlight exposure)

Applications
- Personalized prostheses, such as limb sockets
- Biodegradable orthopedic devices, such as screws and fixation pins, plates, and suture anchors
- Bone scaffolds
- Drug delivery system

2.2 Acrylonitrile Butadiene Styrene (ABS)

ABS is another commonly used 3D printing material to date. It is strong, lightweight and allows for easy post-processing. ABS can be melted to form liquid and cooled to form solid, and this process can be repeated many times without any significant degradation in its properties.

However, ABS is slightly more difficult to print – it is prone to warping without an enclosed and heated build chamber. Also, ABS may have odors that could be uncomfortable or irritating for users. Printing shall thus be performed in a well-ventilated area and/or with an enclosure.

Table 2   Pros and Cons of ABS as 3D printing material

Pros	*Cons*
• Low cost • Tough, durable and light • Good heat resistance	• Heavy warping • Requires a heated bed or heated chamber. • Parts tend to shrink leading to dimensional inaccuracy. • Releases smelly and toxic chemicals during printing

Applications
- Surgical planning models
- Personalized prostheses
- Orthopedic corset

2.3 **Polyetheretherketone**

PEEK is considered as one of the world's highest performing engineering thermoplastics, offering exceptional chemical resistance and excellent mechanical properties. It is often used to replace certain metals. Since PEEK is sterilizable, it can be used for a number of medical applications including custom-made implants and medical devices. Medical grade PEEK is available in filament form for all FDM/FFF machines and is slowly becoming available in high quality powder form for medical device production with SLS processes. It is the ideal choice for low-volume production and specialist designs where it is difficult to create prototypes using metal and traditional techniques.

Table 3   Pros and Cons of PEEK as 3D printing material

Pros	*Cons*
• High impact strength and durability • Superior heat, water and chemical resistance • Greater design freedom • Biocompatible • Facilitate osteointegration, i.e.: bone ingrowth into an artificial implant • Shares properties similar to human bone	• Requires very high printing temperatures • Expensive • Requires measures against warping

Applications
- Customized medical devices
- Orthopedic implants

2.4 **Polyetherketoneketone (PEKK)**

Belonging to the same PAEK family as PEEK, PEKK has superior machinal, thermal, and chemical properties. It has a lower crystallization rate and PEKK is easier to print than PEEK.

PEKK is mainly found in filament form for high temperature FDM printers, but also in powder form for a very limited number of SLS 3D printers.

Table 4   Pros and Cons of PEKK as 3D printing material

Pros	*Cons*
• Excellent thermal, chemical and wear resistance • Easier to print than PEEK, less warping phenomenon • Better antibacterial properties than PEKK • Does not give out toxic fumes at high temperature	• Expensive • Requires very high printing temperature

Applications
- Customized medical devices
- Orthopedic implants

2.5 **Polycarbonate (PC)**

PC is extremely strong and resists deforming at higher temperatures unlike other common 3D printer filaments. PCs can be sterilized with various standard processes making it ideal for end-use parts and functional prototypes in the medical industries. However, the 3D printing of PC is more difficult since it requires a higher printing temperature than other standard FDM plastics (such as ABS and PLA) [**Society for Risk Analysis, 2020**]

Table 5   Pros and Cons of PC as 3D printing material

Pros	*Cons*
• Some of the best impact and thermal resistance of any common FDM plastics • High transparency • Bendable without breaking	• Require high printing temperature • Prone to warping • Absorb moisture from the air which can cause defects

Applications

- Medical equipment parts

2.6 Polymethyl Methacrylate

PMMA, also known as acrylic, is a strong, durable and transparent thermoplastic. PMMA has good impact strength, significantly higher than glass, but lower than some stronger and more expensive materials like polycarbonate (PC). It is applied as a PC substitute when an extremely high impact isn't necessary, but cost is an issue. Besides, PMMA is extremely biocompatible with human tissue and has a long history of use in dentures, bone implants and more. Biotech companies such as Ossfila have developed a Medical Grade PMMA Filament and Bonelcule, a PMMA-based Bioactive Filament with the addition of nano-hydroxyapatite coated copolymer, which offers bone-like properties and accelerates implant-to-bone integration as an alternative to non-bioactive PEEK.

Table 6   Pros and Cons of PMMA as 3D printing material

Pros	*Cons*
• Strong, lightweight, durable • High impact resistant and tensile strength; • Transparent • Inert, biocompatible • Affordable	• Require high printing temperature • May have odors that could be uncomfortable or irritating for users

Applications

- Surgical guides and tools
- Orthopedic implants

2.7 Bioceramics

Bioceramics are ceramic materials that are used to repair or replace damaged hard tissues like bone and teeth. The two bioceramics most explored within ceramic 3D printing are hydroxyapatite (HA) and tri-calcium phosphate (TCP). They are popular not only for their similarity to natural bone tissue but their prevalence within medicine. Extensive research on bioceramics 3D printing over the past 10 years highlighted its wide range of applications and potentials in bone tissue engineering. While a lot of applications can be accomplished in 3D printing of bioceramics, the development is still in its emerging stage.

Table 7   Pros and Cons of bioceramics as 3D printing material

Pros	*Cons*
• Good mechanical properties • Minimal risk of rejection • Osteoconductitve, induces bone growth on a surface	• Require high printing temperatures • Shrinkage may happen during heat treatment

Applications
- Medical devices
- Bone scaffolds
- Bone substitutes, such as intervertebral cages and tibial osteotomy wedges
- Cranial or jawbone implants

2.8 Titanium

Titanium has become one of the most commonly used metals in 3D printing, widely employed in aerospace, joint replacements and surgical tools, electronics, and other high-performance products. In the medical industry, 3D printed titanium implants, including those for spine, hip, knee, and extremity applications are widely applied due to the metal's inherent biocompatibility and good mechanical properties.

Table 8   Pros and Cons of titanium as 3D printing material

Pros	*Cons*
• High mechanical strength • Good corrosion resistance • Biocompatible	• Expensive • Printing time is longer than other 3D printing method

Applications
- Medical devices
- Implants

2.9 Polyethylene Glycol (PEG)

PEG is one of the most widely used hydrogels in cell research, tissue engineering scaffolds and drug delivery systems. It also plays a vital role in cell-filled 3D bioprinting. . PEG-based hydrogels mimic the physical and biochemical characteristics of natural extracellular matrix (ECM) and demonstrate good biocompatibility under both in vitro and in vivo conditions. PEG materials allow hydrogel to be photo-crosslinked, which provides better mechanical stability after bioprinting.

Table 9   Pros and Cons of PEG as 3D printing material

Pros	*Cons*
• Good mechanical stability • Biocompatible	• Synthetic material • Does not provide biological cues for cell proliferation • Relatively difficult to print

Applications
- Vascular tissue
- Bone tissue
- Cartilage tissue

3. Risks and Safety Considerations

3.1 Biological Hazards

3D printing has expanded into the medical field to include printing of biological materials, such as cells and frameworks for engineered tissue generation. Exposures to hazardous aerosols, infectious agents or bloodborne pathogens must be assessed and mitigated.

3.2   Compressed Gases

Inert gases (usually argon or nitrogen) are used to minimize contamination caused by reactive gases. Controls and exhaust ventilation are required to prevent low-oxygen environments.

4.   Flammable and Reactive Dusts

SLS employs a high-powered laser to meld powdered metals together. This technology utilizes reactive and pyrophoric metal powders like aluminum and titanium to craft alloy tools and metal parts. Additionally, stainless and nickel alloy steels can be utilized. Although particulate emissions from SLS printers are managed within a closed inert gas environment, such as argon, throughout the printing process, emissions may arise during filling, leveling, staging, filter changes, and cleanup. To ensure safety and prevent fires and explosions during SLS printing, stringent precautions are taken, including:

- Written standard operating procedures for proper handling and use of metal powders.
- Storing metal powders in cool, dry areas.
- Elimination of ignition sources and static grounding of equipment and personnel system safety interlocks.
- Class D fire extinguisher.
- Flame retardant clothing.
- Specialized wet HEPA vacuum.
- Meticulous housekeeping.
- Proper and timely waste disposal.

4.1   Physical Hazards

3D printers are intricate devices, comprising high-voltage power supplies, various moving components, hot surfaces, high-powered lasers, welding processes, and/or UV light, all of which entail risks if not properly managed in printer design and operation. Typically, printer manufacturers have implemented engineering controls to mitigate accidental exposures to physical hazards. It is crucial for users to refrain from tampering with interlocks or other safety mechanisms on 3D printers.

4.2   Printer Substrates

Thermoplastics and photopolymers can be flammable and toxic, and plastic monomers can cause irritation and skin sensitivity.

4.3   Ultrafine Particles

FDM and SLA printers produce UFPs having diameters less than 0.1 microns (um). The UFPs that are produced can penetrate and irritate the skin, lungs, nerves and brain tissues. Elevated UFP levels have been linked to adverse health effects, including cardiopulmonary mortality, strokes and asthma. Many users of 3D printers in poorly ventilated areas have reported eye, nose and throat irritation. MJM and SLS printers produce less ultrafine particulates during operation than other printers.

4.4   Volatile Organic Compounds

Research conducted by Steinle (2016) and Azimi et al. (2016) revealed a diverse array of volatile organic compounds (VOCs) emanating from FDM-style printers, also referred to as fused filament fabrication (FFF) printers. These studies documented over 50 organic vapor emissions from FFF printers, which vary depending on the filament material and operating temperatures. VOC emissions from ABS and PLA printers have been linked to symptoms such as headaches, respiratory irritation, and eye irritation. Similarly, MJM printers also release VOCs during operation. In inadequately ventilated spaces containing multiple printers, VOC levels could accumulate to potentially hazardous concentrations.

4.5   Chemical Risks

The process of both 3D printing and post-processing often requires the use of heat. This heat interaction with materials generates volatile organic compounds (VOCs), aerosols, and fine particles. The specific toxicity of these byproducts remains uncertain, underscoring the necessity for technicians to shield themselves from these airborne toxins to mitigate the risk of chronic toxicity or potential carcinogenic effects. Often categorized as ultra-fine particles (UFPs), these particles can penetrate biological barriers, posing challenges for the body's elimination mechanisms. Hence, appropriate safety equipment is indispensable. Moreover, exposure to toxic solvents and solvent vapors can pose significant risks. Direct contact with skin can result in irritation or burns, while prolonged or repeated exposure may lead to symptoms like skin rash, itching, dryness, and redness. Inhalation of solvent vapors can cause a range of effects, from nasal and throat irritation to dizziness, loss of coordination, and even unconsciousness.

4.6   Powder Risks

Certain types of 3D printing utilize polymer or metallic powders, which pose various risks during both printing and post-processing stages. Due to their fine texture, these powders can readily disperse into the air, presenting an inhalation hazard. Particularly, metal powders fused in specific 3D printing conditions can produce an elevated concentration of toxic emissions in the form of nanoparticles. Moreover, anoxia, caused by gases generated from various print technologies and solvents commonly employed in post-processing, is a significant concern. If the oxygen level in the room drops below 15%, the risk of asphyxia becomes pronounced.

4.7   Risk of Explosion/Fire

The risk of explosion comes from a multitude of components used in the additive process. For one, the powders used in many technologies (SLS, MJF, DMLS, SLM) can be volatile. Plastic dust and metal powders can increase the risk of fire or explosion in an additive setting. Traditional solvents used for resin removal, like IPA, can also cause a fire or explosion because of IPA's low flashpoint.

4.8   Musculoskeletal Disorders

Musculoskeletal disorders (MSDs) encompass a range of injuries affecting muscles, nerves, tendons, joints, cartilage, and spinal discs. These disorders include tendonitis, arthritis, bone fractures, and carpal tunnel syndrome, among others. Globally, an estimated 1.71 billion individuals suffer from musculoskeletal conditions. Specifically, tasks such as water blasting and sanding with sandpaper during post-processing for surface finishing can contribute to musculoskeletal injuries among technicians. Ergonomic workstation setups are crucial to prevent such adverse health effects. MSDs significantly impact the workforce, with approximately 100 million people affected in Europe alone, representing 60% of permanent work incapacity. Furthermore, MSDs have a substantial economic impact, affecting the gross domestic product (GDP) of both Europe and the US. In Europe, MSDs account for around 15% of total losses, with Germany experiencing losses of €17.2 billion in production costs and €30.4 billion in labor productivity. Similarly, in the US, MSDs impose significant financial burdens, estimated at $45-$54 billion annually in lost wages, compensation costs, and decreased productivity.

4.9 Psychosocial Considerations

Apart from physical risks, there are psychosocial hazards to address as well. Workers in the additive manufacturing field may encounter feelings of loneliness and isolation, particularly in confined, windowless environments aimed at regulating factors such as temperature. Prolonged use of respirators can also lead to significant discomfort for individuals. Additionally, the manual labor involved in traditional post-processing workflows can contribute to heightened stress levels among technicians. The need for consistent and precise post-processing quality across various materials, shapes, and batch sizes adds to this stress, requiring meticulous attention and effort. Burnout is another common psychosocial consequence of additive's traditionally labor-intensive post-processing step. Repetitive finishing is not only tough on technicians physically, but mentally as well.

5. 3D Printing Precautions and Good Practice

5.1 Adhere to Manufacturer's Safety Guidelines

It is imperative to follow all safety recommendations provided by the manufacturer when installing, operating, and maintaining 3D printers. Before acquiring a 3D printer, it is essential to request and thoroughly review information pertaining to pollutant generation, emission rates, exposure controls, and ventilation requirements. Any modified or unconventional use of 3D printers should be avoided unless explicitly approved in writing by both the manufacturer and Environmental Health and Safety (EHS) personnel.

5.2 Establish usage Protocols

Departments, principal investigators (PIs), supervisors, or course instructors utilizing 3D printers must establish clear guidelines and approval processes. Users are required to provide valid justifications for their intended creations, ensuring compliance with patent laws and avoiding the production of weapons or other hazardous materials. Additionally, users must demonstrate their capability to manage recognized hazards, and consideration may be given to controlling equipment operation duration.

5.3 Ensure Adequate Ventilation and Safety Measures

Most 3D printers lack built-in exhaust ventilation or filtration systems, making particulate, gas, and vapor emissions problematic in poorly ventilated environments. Therefore, areas where plastics, reactive metals, and toxic support materials are utilized must be adequately ventilated. A minimum of four air exchanges per hour is necessary to prevent occupant discomfort and mitigate the risk of fire or explosion, although a higher exchange rate may be warranted based on risk assessment considering the number of printers and their operating frequency and duration. Whenever feasible, utilize manufacturer-recommended exhaust ventilation and/or filtration kits, chemical fume hoods, or other local exhaust systems to manage hazardous emissions. Furthermore, areas where unreacted printing materials are handled or cured, and where caustic support materials are cleaned or removed, must also be properly ventilated to control hazardous emissions. Installation of an eyewash station is mandatory in areas where caustic chemicals are employed[8].

5.4 Machine Maintenance

It's important to keep your machines well-maintained and to conduct regular inspections. Inspections will help verify all parts of the machines are in good working order, including safety features.

5.5　*Prioritize Technology*

Prioritize technologies that remove dangerous materials and products from the additive process in favor of products with reduced impact on users and the environment. For example, machines can help eliminate harmful solvents in post-processing, automated systems that reduce the amount of technician time at the machine, and systems that use bio-sourced materials. Recent technological innovations that have come on the market for post-processing can also mitigate risks associated with traditional post processing methods.

5.6　*Collective Protective Equipment*

Collective Protective Equipment, or CPE, is a device that offers a safety precaution to several workers who are susceptible to certain hazards. CPE can help reduce the frequency of incidents or accidents in a work environment. For example, a ventilation system in the space where print operations and post-processing occur would alleviate hazards

5.7　*Personal Protective Equipment*

Personal Protective Equipment, also known as PPE, is another way to maintain a safe and healthy work environment. Common examples of PPE are gloves, safety glasses or goggles, fine dust filter masks, antistatic footwear, fireproof clothing, and lab coats or boiler suits. Each print technology and post-processing workflow will require a different level of PPE. An assessment should be made relative to the equipment, printer substrates, and procedures to determine the appropriate PPE. Follow any recommendations made by equipment manuals, SDS, or other hazard-specific documentation. PPE for 3D printing may include, but is not necessarily limited to the following:

5.8　*Eye Protection*

Safety glasses, goggles or face shields appropriate for the chemical hazards must be used, particularly when loading liquid monomer reservoirs or using caustic cleaners.

5.9　*Gloves*

3D processes may involve hot surfaces such as the print head block and UV lamp. Sharp or rough edges and pinch points may also be present. In addition to these physical hazards, resistance to irritant plastics and corrosive chemicals must also be considered when selecting glove(s) for 3D printing tasks.

5.10　*Chemical-resistant Lab Coat (or Apron)*

Lab coats, smocks or aprons should be worn when 3D printing or post-printing processes involve irritating or caustic chemicals. Selection is dependent on the materials and associated procedures.

5.11　*Flame-retardant lab Clothing*

Powdered metal printing with reactive metals or flammable polymers or monomers may present a fire or explosion risk. Flame-retardant gloves, lab coats, coveralls, head shrouds and face shields with appropriate static grounding may be needed.

5.12　*Respirators*

Powdered metal printer manufacturers recommend using powered air purifying respirators with a flame retardant hood, particularly when loading, leveling, changing filters, extracting or cleaning that involves pyrophoric and reactive materials. If negative pressure respirators are worn, they must be suitable for the emissions generated and users must be tested for fitness and trained to ensure protection.

5.13   Take Precautions when using Compressed Gases

Metal 3D printers commonly utilize inert gases such as argon or nitrogen to establish a noncombustible and non-explosive environment within the printing chamber during particle welding or sintering. While the controlled flow and ventilation of these gases during printer operation generally pose minimal risk of asphyxiation or toxic exposure, the potential for hazard arises in the event of a system leak, maintenance check, or equipment malfunction. In such instances, these gases may accumulate in confined areas such as printer chambers, floor pits, or other enclosed laboratory spaces, presenting a risk of asphyxiation. Even brief exposure to these low-oxygen environments could result in loss of consciousness and potential suffocation. Hence, it is crucial to identify and label all confined spaces within a 3D printing facility. Moreover, additional safety measures must be implemented whenever a gas leak or buildup is suspected in an enclosed area. These precautions may include opening doors, ports, or panels to allow for ventilation for several minutes before entering. Where appropriate, fans or blowers can be utilized to expedite the venting process[9].

5.14   Waste Disposal

Several different waste streams may be generated during the 3D printing process. Containment, labeling, and disposal of 3D printing wastes are outlined below.

5.15   Metal Powders

Metal powders collected in 3D printer collection containers should be covered/passivated with dry quartz sand or equivalent.

- Ensure the sand is completely dried in an oven before passivation, devoid of all water/moisture.
- Introduce dry quartz sand into the 3D printer system according to the manufacturer's recommendations (refer to the specific 3D printer operations manual for passivation instructions).
- Immediately place the lid on the metal powder collection container after passivation and securely fasten it.
- Monitor the lid and container for at least 48 hours to detect any gas generation (e.g., bulging lid or container sides).
- Affix a hazardous waste label to the container and fill it out completely, including details of the specific metal powder collected. Submit the labeled container to Environmental Health and Safety (EHS) as soon as possible.
- Utilize a specialized wet HEPA vacuum equipped with an inerting fluid to capture reactive metal powders during the cleaning of metal 3D printers.
- Adhere to the manufacturer's precautions for grounding, using, and emptying the vacuum.
- Avoid using standard shop vacuums for cleaning reactive metal powders to prevent fires and explosions.
- Label the vacuumed materials and dispose them off as hazardous waste following the described procedure.

5.16   Printer Cartridges

Empty printer cartridges should be disposed of according to the manufacturer's instructions (cartridge recycling, hazardous waste, or regular trash). Empty printer cartridges that can be returned to the manufacturer should not be disposed off as hazardous waste or disposed off in the regular trash. Recyclable cartridges must be empty prior to being returned g to the manufacturer. Original shipping boxes should be retained and used to return the cartridges whenever possible. Empty printer cartridges that cannot be returned to the manufacturer should be disposed off in accordance with EHS recommendations.

5.17 Vacuum Filters

The 3D printer cartridge filter and/or fine filter (if present) should be removed from the recirculating filter system. Consult the safety procedures outlined in the manufacturer's operation manual; be sure to follow all personal protective equipment recommendations when removing filters. The cartridge filters and fine filters should be placed in a container and immediately passivated with dry quartz sand (devoid of all water/moisture content by oven drying) or mineral oil as per the manufacturer's recommendations. Place a lid on the filter collection container immediately following passivation. Secure the lid. Observe the lid and container for at least 48 hours to determine if there is any gas generated (bulging lid or container sides). Affix a hazardous waste label to the container and fill it out completely, including the specific materials processed through the filters, and submit to EHS as soon as possible.

5.18 Base Bath Solution

Base bath solutions (e.g. sodium hydroxide, potassium hydroxide) used in the finishing steps of 3D printing process are to be collected as chemical waste when the solutions are spent or no longer utilized. Affix a hazardous waste label to the container(s) and fill out completely, including the full name of the chemical(s) used in the base bath solution, and submit to EHS as soon as possible[10].

5.19 Maintain Fire Extinguishers in (or Near) the 3D Printing Area

Contact EHS to ensure that proper fire extinguishers are available at the 3D printing location. Standard carbon dioxide (CO2) and dry chemical extinguishers are appropriate for most ink jet, thermoplastic or photopolymer printers. Class D extinguishers must be available where flammable or reactive metal powders are used[11].

5.20 Training

All persons working with 3D printers must receive training on the chemical, physical and biological hazards associated with the equipment as well the standard operating procedures (SOPs) implemented to mitigate those hazards.

- Manufacturer's representatives or procured hazard information should provide initial training upon equipment acquisition.
- Subsequent training for future users should be conducted by experienced individuals.
- Equipment manuals, online modules, and SOPs must be retained for continuous training.
- Departments and principal investigators (PIs) are responsible for ongoing safety and hazard communication training.
- Documentation of all training sessions, formal and informal, is essential.

5.21 Manage Chemical Risks

Properly storing chemicals and correctly labeling them in their original containers is also important. Safety DataSheets (SDS) should also be accessible to all employees. A system that captures pollutants at the source is essential to preserve your employee's health. Mitigating risks with additives will always be an ongoing process for any manufacturer. Familiarizing yourself with the rules and regulations in your region, along with implementing technology such as automation, especially with post-processing, will significantly improve working conditions for your employees[12].

6. Regulatory Compliance

The United States Food and Drug Administration (FDA) currently regulates 3D printed devices through existing medical device regulations. However, the FDA is increasingly interested in developing guidelines and regulations specifically for PoC 3D printing due to its rapid adoption across healthcare institutions. While the majority of 3D printed devices are regulated through the FDA's Center for Devices and Radiological Health (CDRH), the FDA's Center for Biologics Evaluation and Research (CBER) regulates all biological, cellular, or tissue-based applications of additive manufacturing, the FDA's Center for Drug Evaluation and Research (CDER) regulates all drug applications of additive manufacturing. The Office of Combination Products (OCP) regulates products that have components that would normally be regulated by different FDA centers[13]. The FDA has clarified in past workshops and documents that it does not regulate the use of raw 3D printing materials, final printing materials, or specific printing processes for unspecified uses. Instead, the FDA clears specific devices for particular clinical indications, regardless of whether they are designed through 3D printing and irrespective of the materials used (whether existing or novel). However, it may be beneficial in Premarket Notification submissions to include the names of previously cleared devices that utilize the same additive manufacturing process. This inclusion can help demonstrate substantial equivalence and strengthen the case for regulatory clearance.

6.1 FDA Device Classifications

The FDA classifies all medical devices based on the level of regulation necessary to ensure safety and efficacy. Among other things, this classification determines the type and degree of premarket submission necessary before the FDA clears the device to be marketed.

Class I devices, which present minimal risk of harm to the user, are typically exempt from Premarket Notification, though like all medical devices they still must follow a set of FDA provisions called General Controls which allow the FDA to ensure the safety of all medical devices.

Class II devices, which represent the majority of medical devices and pose a greater risk to users compared to Class I devices, typically require Premarket Notification (PMN), commonly known as a 510(k). A 510(k) submission is made to demonstrate that a device is substantially equivalent to a legally marketed device. The majority of 3D printed medical devices cleared by the FDA have followed this pathway.

Devices that lack a "substantial equivalent" but for which there is reasonable assurance of safety, as per specific FDA guidelines, can be classified as Class I or Class II devices through the "de novo" pathway. These devices can then be marketed and serve as predicate devices for future 510(k) submissions.

In contrast, Class III devices, which are a minority and either lack equivalents on the market, sustain or support life, or pose a relatively high risk of illness or injury, require the more rigorous Premarket Approval (PMA). They are not eligible for Premarket Notification through the 510(k) pathway. For most Class III devices, the FDA mandates clinical trial evidence demonstrating the device's safety and efficacy as part of the PMA requirements.

Most clinical applications for 3D printed devices which could be produced in the PoC setting fall into three categories: diagnostic use anatomic models, patient-specific surgical instruments, and patient-specific implants. Of these, diagnostic anatomic models are the most commonly produced in the PoC setting. Anatomic models are typically derived from patients' computed tomography (CT) imaging, allowing for visualization of patient-specific anatomy in three dimensions. Diagnostic use anatomic models sold by a manufacturer to a hospital typically fall under FDA Class II regulations[14]. All United States companies that currently manufacture and sell patient specific 3D printed anatomical models to physicians and to hospitals are required to follow the guidelines defined at a meeting jointly held by the RSNA and the FDA. Before the meeting jointly held by the RSNA and the FDA, there was a suggestion in the literature that could be interpreted so that PoC patient matched anatomic models could have been considered medical image hardcopies and not medical devices at all.

Patient-specific surgical instruments and patient-specific implants typically also fall under Class II regulations, but may require Class III regulations if they pose unique safety or efficacy considerations or lack a substantially equivalent predicate device. Though currently rarer in the PoC setting than diagnostic use anatomic models, these devices also face regulatory uncertainty[15].

6.2 Quality Systems Regulations

Legally marketed 3D printed devices are subject to the same regulatory requirements to which similar devices created without 3D printing are subject, including Quality Systems (QS) regulations. The purpose of these regulations is to ensure that medical devices consistently meet necessary requirements and specifications. Though it remains unclear exactly how they are to be regulated, it is still important that PoC centers manufacture safe devices. Outlined below are some QS regulations that medical device manufacturers must adhere to, and that PoC 3D printing centers should be particularly mindful of when creating their own "best practices."

6.3 Monitoring, Maintenance Protocols, and Control of Process Parameters

Parameters of the 3D printer system being used, such as calibration and maintenance protocols and environmental conditions, must be documented. If the device designer includes interactive steps in the patient matching workflow (e.g. outside transfer of patient data to create the 3D model), they must implement the FDA's Guidance on the "Content of Premarket Submissions for Management of Cybersecurity in Medical Devices".

6.4 Imaging

Imaging upon which patient-specific 3D-devices are modeled should be of sufficient resolution to properly capture the areas of interest. In general, the smallest anatomy of interest should be captured on at least 3 sequential DICOM images of a particular series. For small areas of interest, this may dictate the slice thickness of the computed tomography (CT) or magnetic resonance imaging (MRI) images[16].

6.5 Physical Device Manufacturing

- **Materials:** To ensure consistent starting material for each raw material used, the following documentation is essential: (i) Chemical name, common name, trade name, Chemical Abstracts Service (CAS) number, or recognized consensus material standard. (ii) Supplier information. (iii) Material certificates of analysis (COAs) and the test methods used for the COAs. Similarly, documentation should be maintained for all additives, processing aids, and cross-linkers used in the manufacturing process. If the device manufacturer intends to change a material, it is imperative to investigate and document the effect of this change on the build process, as well as the safety and efficacy of the final device. Furthermore, when reusing material (e.g., unsintered powder in powdered bed fusion or uncured resin in stereolithography), it is crucial to document the material reuse process and demonstrate that it does not negatively impact the performance of the final device.
- **Support material:** It's a common practice in the manufacturing of 3D printed devices to include support structures like struts to facilitate the printing of complex 3D builds. These support structures are necessary for features such as overhangs, high aspect ratio features protruding from the main body, internal channels, and thin features prone to distortion. After the printing process is complete, these supports are typically removed through either a physical or chemical process. Detailing when supportive materials will be utilized, how they will be

removed, and explaining that the final product isn't adversely affected by support removal is crucial. This ensures the integrity and functionality of the 3D printed device post-production.

- **Layering and Meshing:**   Layer thickness of the 3D printed device should be optimized for its intended use. Similar to the imaging selection stage, layer thickness should be determined such that the smallest area of interest is captured on at least three consecutive layers of the 3D printed device. 3D model files are frequently composed of a mesh of triangular faces and the number and size of these faces can affect model accuracy. The rationale behind the selected size and number of these triangles in the mesh should be documented.
- **Build paths:**   The build path utilized for printing a 3D printed device must undergo evaluation and documentation to ensure quality and consistency. For instance, variations in the delivery system's sweeping direction, such as alternating from left to right on one pass and right to left on the next, can result in uneven cooling or hardening, potentially leading to malorientation or distortion of the device. It's crucial to document such details about the build path and evaluate potential consequences.

Furthermore, the fill density of the device should be specified, especially for parts or components that are not fully dense (i.e., non-solid). If non-solid fill density is employed, documentation should indicate whether internal voids are externally accessible or externally sealed. In cases where internal voids are sealed but could potentially be breached during use, it's essential to report the material or gas filling the voids and the associated risks of patient exposure to these substances or gases. This thorough documentation ensures transparency and helps mitigate potential risks associated with the 3D printed device.

- **Post-processing:**   Post-processing steps should not affect the intended use or accuracy of the device, but should only enhance its utility. All post-processing steps should be documented, and a discussion of the effects of post-processing on the materials of the device should be included. For example, heat treatment with hot isostatic pressing (HIP) is used to reduce residual porosity and increase fatigue life in metal 3D printed implants, but has also been shown to reduce the strength of the material. Thus, the potential impact of HIP should be considered in the intended application for the implant[18].
- **Sterilization:**   Devices intended for use in the operative setting must also adhere to International Organization for Standardization (ISO) standards for sterility and biocompatibility. The sterilization process of additively manufactured devices may change the geometry of the printing material or cause crosslinking of this material, thereby affecting the shape and strength of the 3D printed device. QS regulations should, therefore, document sterility processes, and validation studies must be done to ensure that these sterility processes are compatible with the properties of the materials used in the 3D printed device.
- **Biocompatibility:**   If toxic chemical additives are used to create the 3D printed device, additional testing may be necessary. Common toxic additives include catalysts, binding and curing agents, uncured monomers, and plasticizers. In addition to assuring biocompatibility of these raw materials, manufactures must also assure biocompatibility of the final sterilized product. Furthermore, QS regulations documentation should include biocompatibility validation studies for patient-specific cutting guides (which may deposit debris onto the operative field when used with power tools) and patient-specific implants[19].

6.6 Labeling

Each 3D printed device should bear a patient identifier, detailing the intended use of the device, the device's design iteration number, and an expiration date. This information can either be directly marked on the device itself or documented on the accompanying packaging and labeling. For patient-specific devices, the expiration date may be determined based on the patient's date of imaging rather than the traditional shelf life determination, as patient anatomy can change over time, especially in cases involving pediatric or oncologic patients.

Additionally, events such as trauma may occur between the time of imaging used to model the 3D printed device and its actual use, potentially affecting the device's effectiveness or utility. Hence, the FDA recommends including a precaution in the labeling, advising healthcare providers to examine the patient for any anatomic changes prior to using the patient-specific device. This precautionary measure helps ensure patient safety and the efficacy of the 3D printed device[20].

7. Future Directions in Safety Enhancement

As we stand at the precipice of technological advancement, the future of 3D printed medical products brims with promise and possibility. The cutting-edge innovations and emerging trends are poised to revolutionize safety enhancement in 3D printing, shaping the landscape of healthcare for years to come.

One of the most transformative avenues of exploration lies in the realm of advanced materials. Researchers are pioneering the development of novel biomaterials with enhanced biocompatibility, mechanical properties, and degradation profiles tailored specifically for 3D printing applications. From biodegradable polymers to bioactive ceramics and smart materials, these innovations hold the potential to elevate the safety and efficacy of printed medical devices to unprecedented heights.

Moreover, the integration of additive manufacturing with advanced imaging technologies such as MRI, CT, and 3D scanning is opening new frontiers in patient-specific customization. By leveraging patient-specific anatomical data, clinicians can design and fabricate personalized medical devices with unparalleled precision, minimizing the risk of adverse reactions and optimizing therapeutic outcomes. Another promising area of exploration lies in the realm of computational modeling and simulation. Finite element analysis (FEA), computational fluid dynamics (CFD), and virtual prototyping techniques enable researchers to simulate and optimize the performance of 3D printed medical devices under a myriad of physiological conditions. By conducting virtual trials and predictive modeling, stakeholders can identify potential design flaws, optimize material properties, and refine printing parameters to enhance safety and efficacy[21].

Furthermore, advancements in artificial intelligence (AI) and machine learning are revolutionizing quality control and defect detection in 3D printing. AI algorithms can analyze real-time sensor data, monitor printing parameters, and identify deviations from optimal conditions, enabling proactive intervention to prevent defects and ensure consistency in product quality. In addition to technological innovations, interdisciplinary collaboration and knowledge sharing play a pivotal role in driving safety enhancement in 3D printing. By fostering partnerships between academia, industry, regulatory agencies, and healthcare providers, stakeholders can pool their expertise, share best practices, and accelerate the development of safe and effective 3D printed medical products.

Ultimately, the future of safety enhancement in 3D printing is imbued with boundless potential and transformative possibilities. By embracing innovation, collaboration, and a steadfast commitment to patient welfare, stakeholders can navigate the complex terrain of 3D printing with confidence, paving the way for a safer, more sustainable future in healthcare.

References

1. Garcia Gonzalez, H. and Teresa Lopez Pola, M. (2023). Health and Safety in 3D Printing. IntechOpen. doi: 10.5772/intechopen.109439.
2. Mohammadian Y, Nasirzadeh N. (2021) Toxicity risks of occupational exposure in 3D printing and bioprinting industries: A systematic review. Toxicology and Industrial Health. 37(9): 573-584. doi:10.1177/07482337211031691.
3. Davis, Aika Y., Zhang, Qian, Wonf, Jenny P.S., Weber, Rodney J., Black, Marilyn S et al., (2019) "Characterization of volatile organic compound emissions from consumer level material extrusion 3D printers," Building and Environment, no. 160.

4. Society for Risk Analysis, "3D Printers May Be Toxic for Humans," Lab manager, (December 2020). https://www.labmanager.com/news/3d-printers-may-be-toxic-for-humans-24664.

5. https://ehs.utk.edu/wp-content/uploads/2023/01/LS-023-3D-Printer-Safety.pdf

6. https://www.osha.gov/laws-regs/regulations/standardnumber/1910/1910.132

7. https://www.osha.gov/laws-regs/regulations/standardnumber/1910/1910.134

8. https://www.osha.gov/laws-regs/regulations/standardnumber/1910/1910.1200

9. Parham Azimi, Dan Zhao, Claire Pouzet, Neil E. Crain and Brent Stephens (2016) Emissions of Ultrafine Particles and Volatile Organic Compounds from Commercially Available Desktop Three Dimensional Printers with Multiple Filaments, Environmental Science & Technology, an ACS Publication.

10. Patrick Steinle (2016) Characterization of emissions from a desktop 3D printer and indoor air measurements in office settings, Journal of Occupational and Environmental Hygiene, 13:2, 121-132, DOI: 10.1080/15459624.2015.1091957.

11. https://osha.europa.eu/en/tools-and-publications/publications/3d-printing-new-industrial-revolution/view

12. https://blogs.cdc.gov/niosh-science-blog/2018/08/16/3d-printing/

13. Beitler, B.G., Abraham, P.F., Glennon, A.R. (2022) Interpretation of regulatory factors for 3D printing at hospitals and medical centers, or at the point of care. *3D Print Med* 8, 7.

14. Classify Your Medical Device. https://www.fda.gov/medical-devices/overview-device-regulation/classify-your-medical-device.

15. ISO. ISO 13485:2016 - Medical devices – Quality management systems – Requirements for regulatory purposes. Accessed March 15, 2024. https://www.iso.org/standard/59752.html

16. ASTM International. ASTM F2792-12(2018) - Standard Terminology for Additive Manufacturing Technologies. Accessed March 15, 2024. https://www.astm.org/Standards/F2792.htm

17. National Institutes of Health (NIH). 3D Print Exchange. Accessed March 15, 2024. https://3dprint.nih.gov/

18. European Medicines Agency (EMA). Regulatory framework for medicinal products for human use. Accessed March 15, 2024. https://www.ema.europa.eu/en/human-regulatory/overview/advanced-therapy-medicinal-products-overview

19. World Health Organization (WHO). Medical device regulations: Global overview and guiding principles. Accessed March 15, 2024. https://www.who.int/medical_devices/publications/global_overview_meddev-01-1_rev2_en.pdf

20. International Medical Device Regulators Forum (IMDRF). Accessed March 15, 2024. http://www.imdrf.org/.

21. National Institute of Standards and Technology (NIST). Additive Manufacturing (AM) - Research and Reports. Accessed March 15, 2024. https://www.nist.gov/topics/additive-manufacturing-am-research-and-reports.

3D Printing of Biomaterials

Jyotirmayee Sahoo,[1,2] *Drishya Prakashan*[1,2] *and
Sonu Gandhi*[1,2*]

1. Introduction

The field of three-dimensional (3D) bioprinting has shown promise in the development of functional tissues and organs. The imperative role of designing and fabricating intricate 3D biomedical devices is paramount in the field of tissue engineering (TE) and the timeline for their invention is depicted in Figure 1 (Murphy and Atala, 2014). This approach involves the meticulous arrangement of biological and biochemical constituents, and living cells in a layer-by-layer fashion (Fang et al., 2022). Unlike non-biological printing, 3D bioprinting introduces extra complexities and practical challenges stemming from the integration of living cells (Sun et al., 2020; Byakodi et al., 2022; Shah et al., 2024). This includes the need for suitable biomaterials which meet the criteria for both printability and functionality. The utilization of 3D biomedical devices extends to addressing the restoration of 3D anatomic defects, reconstructing intricate organs with 3D microarchitecture that are complex (such as the liver and lymphoid organs), and serving as scaffolds for guiding differentiation of stem cell (Gao et al., 2021; Zhang et al., 2016). An essential need for advanced medical interventions emerges when addressing anatomical defects in the craniomaxillofacial complex, which may be due to factors like cancer, trauma, or congenital anomalies. The successful restoration of these defects relies on the intricate reinstatement of functional nerves, vessels, muscles, bone, cartilage, ligaments, glands and lymph nodes (Lee et al., 2018). Current advancements in the domain have witnessed the exploration of diverse approaches grounded in tissue engineering principles to regenerate additional functional tissues pertinent to maxillofacial tissue rejuvenation (Agarwal et al., 2020; Roberts et al., 2022). In the field of tissue engineering, scaffolds play a crucial role by providing structural support for cell infiltration and proliferation. They create an environment conducive to the generation and remodeling of the extracellular matrix, offering biochemical cues to guide cellular behavior, and establish physical connections for injured tissue (Yildirimer L. et al., 2012; Zhu et al., 2013). During the development of scaffolds, meticulous attention to the architectural design at macro, micro, and nano levels prove essential for ensuring optimal structural integrity, facilitating nutrient transport,

[1] DBT-National Institute of Animal Biotechnology (NIAB), Hyderabad, India.
[2] DBT-Regional Centre for Biotechnology (RCB), Faridabad, India.
* Corresponding author: sonugandhi@gmail.com

and fostering meaningful interactions between cells and the extracellular matrix (Prakashan et al., 2024; Yasun et al., 2020; Kaushik et al., 2020). Through the utilization of image reconstruction based on computerized tomography (CT) scans and magnetic resonance imaging (MRI), it becomes feasible to model a specific tissue. This modeling process enables the creation of personalized devices, such as orthopedic instruments and implants tailored to individual patients, through 3D printing. These customized devices serve purposes related to surgical guidance and restoration (Ma et al., 2017).

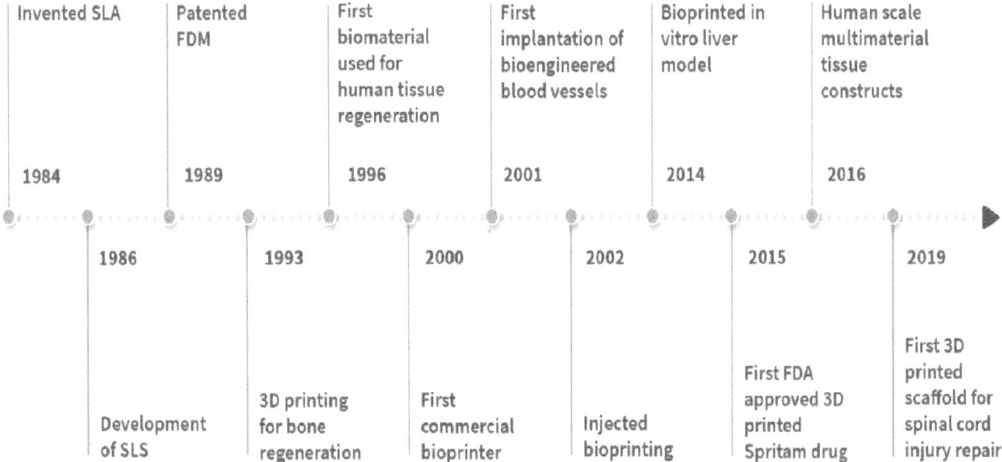

Fig. 1 Significant Achievements in 3D Printing: Ever since Charles Hull introduced 3D printing in 1984, this groundbreaking technology has found applications across a diverse spectrum, spanning from prosthetic components to the creation of tissue models, extending even to the regeneration of human tissue (Reprinted from with copyright permission of figure obtained from Elsevier).

In its early stages, 3D bioprinting primarily concentrated on producing acellular structures onto which cells were subsequently seeded for either *in-vitro* cultivation or *in-vivo* implantation. However, this method faces certain constraints, such as suboptimal seeding efficiency and challenges in achieving a heterogeneous distribution of cells (Eswaramoorthy et al., 2019). An alternative approach involves the direct encapsulation of living cells within a bioink, a substance employed in the 3D bioprinting process. Nonetheless, this method imposes constraints on the utilization of conventional 3D printing technologies due to stringent biocompatibility needed for both selection of ink materials and their processing. Hydrogels are frequently employed as carriers for cells for bioink formulations, offering an aqueous environment that emulates the extracellular matrix and facilitates the encapsulated cells (Fang et al., 2022). To address the pressing demand for the 3D printing of functional tissues, there has been a recent shift in the emphasis on bioink development. This shift involves transitioning from solely offering structural support to actively elicit the functionality of tissue (Tasnim et al, 2018).

Despite significant progress, the majority of 3D-printed tissues remain either in a preclinical stage or are distant from clinical application. Overcoming substantial challenges is crucial for bioprinting clinically relevant functional tissues (Fleischer et al., 2020). Addressing these challenges entails achieving tissue heterogeneity with a regulated distribution of various cell types and biomaterials at both micro and macro scales. It also involves the creation of essential functional components like vasculature, lymphatics and innervation, seamlessly combining them with the host tissues (Fang et al., 2022). This chapter focuses on 3D bioprinting technology, with a particular emphasis on integrating living cells during the process of manufacture. Furthermore, recent advancements in the technologies employed for 3D printing of cells and biomaterials, advanced bioinks, and different printing methods are discussed. Additionally, we explore the limitations of the field, indicating the future that involves applying 3D cell-printing in tissue engineering. To conclude, we offer insights into the designing of 3D printed tissues or organs and discuss their potential clinical applications.

2.　Methods Employed in the 3D Printing of Cells and Biomaterials

For the engineering of human tissue, 3D cell printing serves as a groundbreaking method for validating therapeutic efficacy and exploring disease mechanisms. Its recent surge in attention is attributed to its processing versatility, demonstrated by the precise control of variables and a range of process options. Furthermore, it takes a unique approach to establish tissue hierarchy, incorporating diverse bioinks, multi-scale active molecules, and cells (Kim et al., 2016; Park et al., 2016; Cho CS, Yoo JJ, 2016). The 3D printing procedure for a device often hinges on the choice of materials and the method in which the layers are interconnected to create the ultimate component (Mishra A, Srivastava V, 2021). 3D cell printing techniques are categorized into four different types based on the dispensing method such as- (a) inkjet bioprinting, (b) extrusion bioprinting and (c) light-assisted bioprinting (Zhu W et al. 2016) (Figure 2).

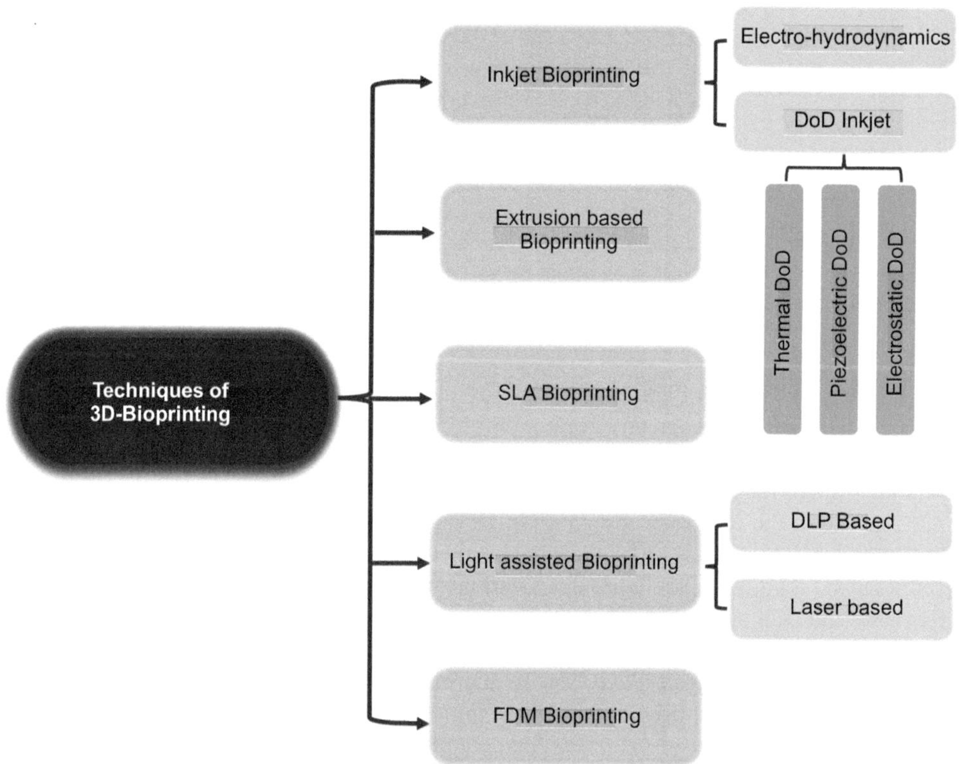

Fig. 2　Schematic presentation of diverse techniques of 3D bioprinting.

2.1　Inkjet Bioprinting

Inkjet printing emerges as a pioneering 3D printing technology uniquely tailored for printing cells with the goal of crafting desired tissues or organs. Furthermore, inkjet bioprinting entails the controlled manipulation, patterning, or assembly of biologically appropriate materials such as cells, different biomolecules and biomaterials using the inkjet technique. The objective is to achieve targeted biological functions through pre-designed arrangements. There are various types of inkjet bioprinters *(Figure-3A)* based on how they disperse the ink, such as- Drop-on-Demand (DoD), electrohydrodynamic inkjet bioprinting (Li et al., 2020).

2.1.1   Drop-on-Demand (DoD) inkjet bioprinting

The drop-on-demand inkjet device features several print heads, each housing a chamber with interconnected nozzles. Droplets are generated solely when the ejection signal is activated. The diameter of the nozzle may be as diminutive as 18 μm. Consequently, a regulated pressure pulse displaces the ink within the chamber (Figure-3A). Without a pressure pulse, the ink is retained by surface tension. When the pulse energy surpasses a specific threshold, a droplet is expelled out of the nozzle. (Wisshoff et al., 2010; Li et al., 2020).

2.1.1.1   Thermal inkjet bioprinting

In thermal inkjet printing, a heat actuator selectively warms the ink for a few microseconds, inducing rapid vaporization of the local ink and the formation of heat bubbles within the chamber. These bubbles rapidly expand until they reach a point of explosion that exerts pressure on the ink, creating a driving force to propel the ink out of the nozzle as a droplet. Usually, the diameter of the nozzle of the printer typically measures around 50 μm, with the resulting droplets having a diameter ranging from approximately 30 to 80 μm (Cu et al., 2012). To enhance the jet force during printing, a microchannel cavity usually integrates a cavity neck structure. This configuration ensures that the expanding bubble is guided away from the ink inlet and towards the outlet, thereby enhancing the overall jet force *(Figure-3A (a))*.

2.1.1.2   Piezoelectric Inkjet Bioprinting

Piezoelectric inkjet printing involves the deformation of the chamber wall by piezoelectric ceramics, ultimately causing the nozzle to expel the ink droplets (De Gans et al., 2013). The diameter of the piezo inkjet print head is within the range of 18 to 120 μm. In the printing process, the diameter of the generated droplets can vary and is generally observed within the range of 50 to 100 μm *(Figure-3A (b))*. After receiving a voltage pulse, the piezoelectric actuator undergoes chamber wall deformation, causing a rapid change in volume and subsequently ejecting a droplet (Li et al., 2020).

2.1.1.3   Electrostatic Inkjet Bioprinting

In electrostatic inkjet printing, the chamber wall has many deformations which cause the ink to get compressed inside the chamber. In a connected circuit, due to the influence of static electricity the pressure plate is drawn towards the electrode plate. This action causes the chamber to expand, (Li et al., 2020) allowing it to be refilled with ink. Subsequently, during disconnection of the circuit the plate promptly returns to its normal position *(Figure-3A (c))*. Here, the volume decreases, leading to the expulsion of ink in the form of droplets.

2.1.2   Electro-hydrodynamic inkjet bioprinting

In electrohydrodynamic jet printing, droplets are generated by harnessing an electric field instead of relying on thermal energy or chamber deformation to expel ink (Figure-3A (d)). Force is exerted on the ink within the chamber, leading to the creation of a conical ink meniscus at the nozzle orifice, commonly referred to as a "Taylor cone." The printing nozzles primarily consist of capillary tubes coated with metal. When a specified voltage is applied across the nozzle and the substrate, droplets are expelled (Li et al., 2020).

2.2   Extrusion Bioprinting

An extrusion-based bioprinting platform was established to layer-by-layer deposit pre-seeded alginate hydrogel, creating 3D pre-seeded living implants with arbitrary geometries (Zhu et al., 2016). In this method, a syringe loaded with bioink-containing cells is utilized, which is expelled via a nozzle using either a pneumatic or physical force generating device called piston (Jang et al., 2018). Recent technology *(Figure-3B)* shows nozzle-based bioprinting, particularly in a specific patterning of decellularized extracellular matrix (dECM), that emphasizes the possible capabilities of this bioprinting approach in exploiting biomimetic materials with intricate compositions. Notably, Mannoor et al. successfully crafted a bionic ear by 3D printing a hydrogel matrix seeded with cells, mirroring the anatomical geometry of a human ear. This innovative approach also integrated an interwoven conducting polymer infused with silver nanoparticles (Mannoor et al., 2013).

2.3　*Light assisted Bioprinting*

This system predominantly uses photo-polymerization of different biomaterials which can effectively print various types of cells while maintaining high cell viability. This can be categorized into two subgroups: DLP-based printers and laser-based printers.

2.3.1　*DLP-based printers*

DLP printers have experienced significant advancements with the implementation of a Dynamic Optical Projection Stereolithography (DOPsL) system, which utilizes a digital micromirror device (DMD) chip, comprising approximately a million micromirrors, for the precise control of UV light. This system extends an optical pattern onto a photopolymer solution based on a custom-designed Computer-Aided Design (CAD) model. The focal size of the emitted light beam from each micromirror determines the printer's resolution. The DLP based printer operates in parallel by expanding the total plane of the optical pattern towards the photopolymer solution *(Figure-3D)*, in contrast to the sequential printing processes of inkjet or extrusion printers (Zhang et al., 2012). This innovative approach significantly reduces the fabrication time. By constantly refreshing the expanded optical patterns and simultaneous moving of the printed object-containing stage, the DLP printer achieves the construction of smooth 3D objects without the occurrence of artificial interfaces commonly found between droplets or lines in inkjet or extrusion printers (Zhu et al., 2016).

2.3.2　*Laser-based printers*

Various types of laser-assisted printing methods exist, such as- laser-guided/directed writing (LDW) (Liao et al., 2012), laser-induced forward transfer (LIFT) (Koch et al., 2012), and matrix-assisted pulsed laser evaporation (MAPLE) (Doraiswamy et al., 2007). In these methodologies, to initiate polymerization/transfer of material on the sample slide, a beam of laser light is accurately concentrated via a higher-power objective lens. There is a specialized LDW system, identified as two-photon polymerization (TPP). It employs a concentrated 800 nm/ near-infrared femtosecond laser light, to produce a nonlinear optical phenomenon known as two-photon absorption. This phenomenon leads to the polymerization of the monomer solution, allowing TPP to achieve a remarkably high resolution that surpasses the diffraction limit, as illustrated in *(Figure-3C)* (Zhang et al., 2024). The LIFT system comprises a cell-containing bioink layer (ribbon) and a laser energy-absorbing layer. When coupled through the 3D motion of the stage with a sample, it becomes possible to produce intricate 3D structures with submicron resolution. As depicted in Figure 3a, LIFT was utilized to generate a multi-layered, fully cellularized skin substitute incorporating fibroblasts and keratinocytes.

Although light-assisted bioprinting presents several advantages, including biocompatibility, high resolution, and efficiency, certain challenges persist. Notably, material selection is restricted to photosensitive polymers, excluding a variety of biomaterials and necessitating additional modifications. Without nozzles, as in inkjet and extrusion printers, photo-polymers fill the entire reservoir, leading to material waste and increased costs. Addressing these challenges is crucial for further advancements in this technology (Zhu et al., 2016).

2.4   Stereolithography

Stereolithography (SLA) directly shapes a chosen 2D pattern by the solidification of a liquid photopolymer using visible light, ultraviolet (UV), or infrared (IR). The pre-designed 2D patterns undergo exposure in the reservoir of polymer solution containing the mixture of bioink (e.g., photocurable bioink, cells, and a photo-initiator). This 2D pattern that is solidified is incrementally stacked layer by layer to form a 3D structure. In the bottom-up method, following the curing of each layer, the platform carrying the solidified structure descends, and a fresh layer of liquid resin, yet to undergo curing, is evenly spread on top, preparing for the subsequent patterning cycle. On the contrary, the top-down approach involves projecting light onto a transparent plate situated close to the bottom of the resin container (Melchels et al., 2010). After patterning of the layer, the cured structure is detached, raised, and uncured resin fills the space for the next layer *(Figure-3F)*. To expedite curing, the masked lamp method can cure whole layers at once. After building the structure, draining removes unpolymerized resin, and postcuring in a UV oven enhances strength by converting any unreacted groups (Chia et al., 2024).

2.5   Fused Diffusion Modeling (FDM)

Fused deposition modeling (FDM) involves depositing molten thermoplastic materials using two heated extrusion heads, each equipped along with a small orifice, to adhere to a predetermined laydown pattern (Zein et al., 2002). In this traditional approach, there are two nozzles: one distributes the thermoplastic material, the other accumulates temporary material to provide support for cantilevers. The thermoplastic polymers melts to a semi-liquid state. Subsequently, the extrusion head loads the material onto the build platform *(Figure-3E)* (Van Noort et al., 2012). The part is constructed layer by layer, with the layers fused together. While FDM allows for the use of multiple extrusion nozzles, each with a different material, while theoretically allowing for compositional gradients in every dimension, this capability has not been achieved in practice (Chia et al., 2015).

3.   3D printable Biomaterials

Advancements in 3D printing methodologies over the last 15 years have extended the applicability of these technologies to diverse domains. Notably, the realm of medical devices and tissue engineering has witnessed substantial attention with the integration of 3D printing. The capability to manufacture patient-specific, adaptable devices within compressed time frames and at reduced expenses positions 3D printing as an ideal technological candidate for the imminent era of personalized medicine (Gopinathan J, Noh I, 2018). An exemplary bioink should exhibit specific physicochemical attributes encompassing mechanical, rheological, chemical, and biological characteristics. These attributes are crucial to achieving several key objectives: (i) fostering the development of tissue constructs that have sufficient mechanical strength and resilience, though concurrently preserving tissue-relevant mechanics, preferably in a modifiable manner; (ii) Enabling flexible gelation and stabilization to improve the bioprinting of structures while maintaining precise shape fidelity; (iii) ensuring biodegradability and biocompatibility to emulate the native tissue microenvironment; (iv) demonstrating responsiveness to meet tissue-specific requirements by chemical modification; and (v) demonstrating the capacity for extensive production with minimal variations from one batch to another (Hospodiuk et al., 2017; Fetah et al., 2016). Given that identifying the optimum formulation for cell-laden bioinks is pivotal for the success of bioprinting endeavors, a myriad of natural and synthetic biomaterials with distinct features have been employed as bioinks thus far. Furthermore, there is an urgent demand for standardized bioink formulations that permit their versatile application across diverse bioprinting scenarios (Ozbolat et al., 2016). The utilization of various biomaterials as inks has facilitated the formation of 3D structures characterized by a diverse range of dimensions and stiffness levels. Nevertheless, owing to their origins in industrial prototyping, the majority of 3D printing techniques face a limitation in the availability of highly evolved biocompatible materials

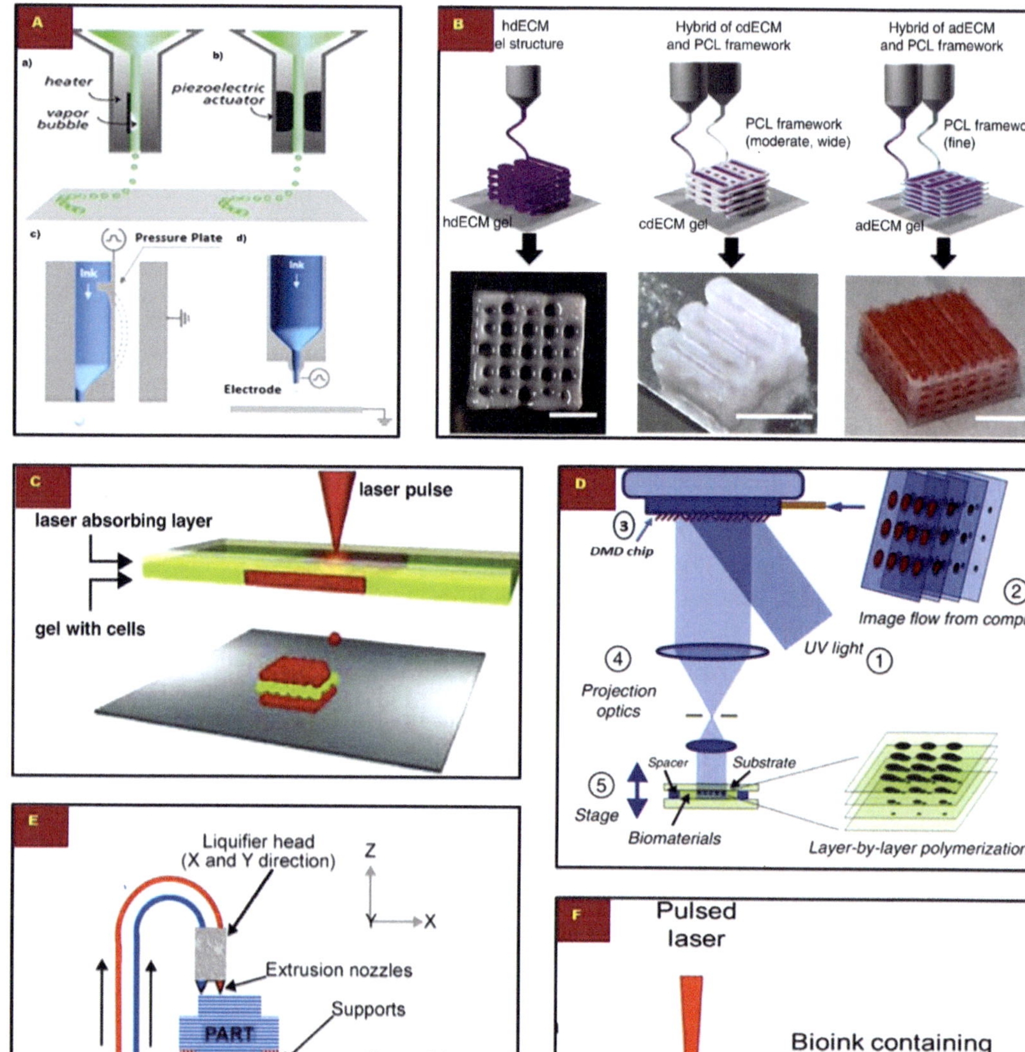

Fig. 3 Depicts techniques of 3D bioprinting, A-Inkjet Bioprinting, a-thermal drop-on-demand, b-piezoelectric (Reproduced from (Wang et al, 2020) which is an open access article under the Creative Commons Attribution License), c-Electrostatic, d-Electro-hydrodynamics (Reprinted with permission from (Li et al., 2020)); B-Extrusion based bioprinting of heart, cartilage and adipose tissue with their respective dECM; C-Laser based printer, D-DLP-based printer (Reprinted with permission from (Zhu et al., 2016)), E-Fused deposition modeling (FDM) (Reprinted from (Sidambe AT, Oh JK, 2014) which is an open access article under the Creative Commons Attribution License), F-Stereolithography (Reprinted with permission from (Jang et al., 2018).

that can rival conventional biomedical treatments (Shafiee A, Atala A, 2016). This section aims to delineate the essential material characteristics pivotal for the formulation of biomaterial inks tailored to each specific printing method. Additionally, an examination of presently employed biomaterial inks in 3D printing will be undertaken, encompassing a comprehensive analysis of their individual merits and shortcomings.

4.1 Polymer based Biomaterial Inks

4.1.1 Natural biopolymers

Polymers derived from natural sources and employed as biomaterials in the biomedical domain are termed natural biomaterials. These polymers offer distinct advantages compared to their synthetic counterparts, particularly in their ability to mimic the composition and structure of the extracellular matrix (ECM), self-assemble, and exhibit properties like biocompatibility and biodegradability (Shahdeo et al., 2022). The ensuing section provides a comprehensive discussion of various natural biomaterials utilized as bioinks in the context of 3D printing. Despite the merits of natural biomaterials, synthetic polymers contribute unique advantages that set them apart. These properties include the ability to control mechanical stability, photo-crosslinking capabilities, and responsiveness to pH and temperature changes. These attributes, absent in natural polymers, underscore the versatility of synthetic counterparts and their capacity to complement and enhance the overall toolkit of biomaterials, particularly in advanced applications like 3D printing within the biomedical landscape (Fatimi et al., 2022).

4.1.1.1 Agarose

Agarose, a natural polysaccharide obtained from red algae, consists of repeating disaccharide units of D-galactose and 3,6-anhydro-L-galactopyranose. Its widespread use in biomedical applications is credited to its abundance, biocompatibility, and distinctive natural gelling mechanism (López-Marcial et al., 2018). This mechanism involves the spontaneous transformation of a hot, aqueous solution into a hydrogel upon cooling, facilitated by robust hydrogen bonding. The resulting agarose hydrogel exhibits commendable mechanical toughness, adjustable stiffness, and permeability to water, rendering it highly desirable for a myriad of applications (Wenger et al., 2022; Gong et al., 2022). Their inherent properties make them a versatile and attractive option in the realm of biopolymers for biomedical purposes. In a study by Kreimendahl et al., an agarose-based bioink was employed, comprising distinct components of collagen and fibrinogen. The investigation showcased the capacity of these composite agarose-based biomaterials to effectively generate stable three-dimensional (3D) structures while concurrently fostering the growth of endothelial and fibroblast cells (Kreimendahl et al., 2017). A combination of different polymers such as alginate, carboxymethyl-chitosan, and agarose, was used to develop a method for 3D printing human neural stem cells that differentiate them to form functional neurons and supporting neuroglia. The substance solidifies, forming a porous 3D scaffold that encapsulates stem cells, allowing for their in-situ expansion and differentiation. The resulting tissues exhibit synaptic connections, network formation, spontaneous activity, and a predominant expression of gamma-aminobutyric acid. This approach facilitates the exploration of human neural development, function, and disease, with potential applications for engineering various 3D tissues using different stem cell types (Gu et al., 2024). Further, Ozler et al. in 2017 documented the utilization of multicellular aggregates for the direct 3D printing of cells, specifically involving smooth muscle, fibroblasts and endothelial cells. The study illustrated the capacity of these constructs to undergo fusion throughout the experimental duration with high cell viability. Despite exhibiting favorable gelation properties, it is emphasized that chemical modifications or blending interventions are imperative to sustain the structural integrity of the 3D printed constructs and to augment various cellular functionalities (Ozler et al., 2017).

4.1.1.2 Alginate

Alginate, a marine polysaccharide derived from brown seaweed, presents distinct characteristics that distinguish it from agarose. Its anionic nature is marked by the presence of a carboxylic acid in each uronic acid residue (Axpe et al., 2016). In its native form, alginate forms an insoluble alginic acid chain network which is interconnected through extensive hydrogen bonds. The aqueous-soluble sodium salt form of alginate is obtained through alkaline treatment, resulting in a dissolution of the aforementioned network (Pahlevanzadeh et al., 2020). Unlike materials like agarose, alginate does not exhibit a temperature-based sol-gel transition. Instead, it undergoes rapid ionic crosslinking reactions when exposed to multivalent cations, such as Ca^{2+}, Al^{3+}, and Ba^{2+}. The degree of ionic crosslinking varies between these blocks, leading to diverse mechanical properties in resulting alginate hydrogels. The gelation kinetics of alginate are facile and tunable, offering a versatile and attractive feature for biomedical applications. This, coupled with its biocompatibility and rich natural source, positions alginates as majorly embraced polymers in the field of biomedical research and applications (Jia et al., 2014). Alginate-based bioinks were employed in conjunction with cartilage cells to 3D print hollow constructs. These printable microfluidic channels, resembling vessels, exhibit the capability to facilitate the transport of oxygen, nutrients, and biomolecules within the construct, concurrently providing support for cellular growth (Zhang et al., 2013). Sodium alginate bioink containing fibroblast cells from mice was utilized for the fabrication of vascular-like structures employing a customized 3D printer, incorporating calcium chloride as a crosslinker (Christensen et al., 2015). Additionally, diverse polymers, including polycaprolactone (PCL), poloxamer, hydroxyapatite, and gelatin, were blended with alginate to generate a range of 3D printed constructs for tissue engineering applications (Prakashan et al., 2024a and Prakashan et al 2024b; Jang et al., 2016).

4.1.1.3 Hyaluronic acid (HA)

Hyaluronic acid (HA) stands out as a natural extracellular matrix (ECM) component abundantly present in cartilages and connective tissues. In the realm of 3D bioprinting for the development of intricate structures, HA has emerged as a prominent biomaterial (Noh et al., 2019; Petta et al., 2020). Numerous formulations of HA-based bioinks have been documented to date. Notably, a study focused on photo-crosslinked HA bioinks has garnered attention for its capacity to enhance rheological properties through chemical modifications (Highley et al., 2016). Despite the advantageous biomimetic properties of HA, akin to other natural polymers, it exhibits comparatively low mechanical strength and slow gelation behavior, especially when contrasted with synthetic polymer hydrogels (Hauptstein et al., 2020). Addressing these challenges, Ouyang et al. implemented a dual crosslinking strategy in a 3D printed construct utilizing HA. Their innovative approach showcased the efficacy of the HA-based dual crosslinked bioinks in 3D bioprinting, wherein post-printing, there was no discernible loss in mechanical properties. Furthermore, the bioink demonstrated commendable cellular adhesion properties, further augmented by the incorporation of cell-adhesive oligopeptides within the hydrogels. This multifaceted study not only highlighted the potential of HA in 3D bioprinting but also introduced a dual crosslinking methodology to overcome inherent limitations and enhance both structural and cellular aspects of the printed constructs (Ouyang et al., 2016).

4.1.1.4 Decellularized extracellular matrix (dECM)

An extensive exploration of biomaterials for biomedical applications has involved the thorough investigation of various synthetic and natural polymers, either individually or in both combinations (Zhang et al., 2022). Numerous engineering approaches have been devised to modulate their properties to cater to diverse requirements (Dzobo et al., 2019; Hoshiba et al., 2010). Despite these efforts, replicating the intricate cellular microenvironment solely through engineered biomaterials is inherently constrained and, in some cases, deemed practically impossible (Abaci et al., 2020; Zhang et al., 2021). To overcome this limitation, recent research efforts by Ott et al. propose an innovative methodology that involves utilizing the native Extracellular Matrix (ECM) in its unaltered state, with minimal disruption, achieved by selectively eliminating only the residing cells. Employing a cadaveric rat heart as a model, a mild liquid detergent was administered continuously till all cells were dissolved. Remarkably, this approach selectively removed cells while preserving the normal complex chemical compositions and structural intricacies, such as the vasculature of the ECM microenvironment (Ott et al., 2008). Subsequent reconstitution of this decellularized matrix (dECM) containing the cardiomyocytes demonstrated the restoration of mechanical and biochemical functionalities.

4.1.2   Synthetic polymers

Despite the ability of natural polymers or hydrogels to replicate the desired microenvironment conducive to cell attachment and proliferation, their inherent limitations lie in the relatively low tunability of their properties. Consequently, a strategic approach involves combining naturally derived polymers with synthetic counterparts or additional natural polymers (Guvendiren et al., 2013). This amalgamation aims to achieve more stable constructions endowed with tunable features, particularly crucial in the context of 3D bioprinting. Although these polymers may not inherently facilitate cellular adhesion or promotion to the extent of natural polymers, they emerge as promising candidates for tuning properties such as mechanical characteristics, printability, crosslinkng capabilities, and more (Gungor-Ozkerim et al., 2018). Among synthetic polymers, poly (ethylene glycol) (PEG) and Pluronic stand out as particularly prevalent choices in the realm of 3D bioprinting (Müller et al., 2015; Wu et al., 2011). Their utilization underscores the dynamic interplay between natural and synthetic components, strategically harnessed to enhance the overall performance and versatility of biomaterials for advanced bioprinting applications.

4.1.2.1   Poly (ethylene glycol) (PEG)

PEG stands out as a widely employed synthetic polymer widely used in the biomedical field and holds approval for medical use in numerous countries. Noteworthy for its cost-effectiveness, biocompatibility, hydrophilicity, and robust chemical and mechanical stability, PEG exhibits unique anti-fouling properties that set it apart from most other polymers (Knop et al., 2010). These attributes make PEG an ideal choice for implantable biomaterials, as it can effectively resist undesired physical adsorption of biological molecules. The process of conjugating PEG chains, commonly referred to as PEGylation, onto several materials such as drugs, has demonstrated efficacy in preventing protein and cellular adsorption, consequently delaying premature biodegradation (Skardal A et al., 2010). In contrast to natural polysaccharides capable of undergoing thermogelling and ionic crosslinking, hydrogels are not naturally formed through physical interactions in the case of PEG. Consequently, the development of PEG hydrogels requires the modification of PEG end groups with reactive functional groups capable of undergoing crosslinking reactions. This tailored approach enables the creation of PEG hydrogels with controlled properties, expanding the versatility of PEG as a biomaterial in biomedical research and applications (J. Zhu, 2010).

4.1.2.2   Pluronic polymers

Poloxamers, colloquially known as Pluronic, represent a distinctive category of synthetic tri-block copolymers characterized by central hydrophobic chains of polypropylene oxide flanked by two hydrophilic chains of polyethylene oxide. These polymers exhibit notable chemical attributes, including temperature-dependent self-assembly and thermo-reversible behavior. Coupled with their inherent biocompatible nature and physicochemical features, poloxamers emerge as highly promising biomaterials for biomedical applications, particularly in the domains of TE and drug delivery (Müller et al., 2015). Customization of tunable microstructure, bioactivity, and mechanical properties in poloxamers enables the emulation of the behavior found in different tissue types (Shamma et al., 2022). Poloxamers, recognized for their multifunctional properties, exhibit the capacity to form diverse structures including hydrogels and injectable hydrogels when 3D scaffolds, micro/nano-fibers, as well as constructs for cell carriers and drug micro/nano-carriers are integrated into blends and nanocomposites. This remarkable versatility positions poloxamer-based biomaterials as instrumental components across a broad spectrum of applications within tissue engineering. Notably, their utilization spans various realms including chondrogenesis, neurogenesis, angiogenesis, bone regeneration, and wound healing (Navara et al., 2022). Beyond their structural diversity, poloxamers also demonstrate notable attributes as inactive molecules, showcasing minimal cytotoxicity. This property renders them highly suitable for an array of pharmaceutical applications, particularly in the realm of gene and drug delivery systems (DDS) (Cui et al., 2022). The inherent biocompatibility and tunability of poloxamers make them integral contributors to advancing biomedical research and applications across diverse therapeutic domains (Müller et al., 2015).

5. Application: Tissue Engineering via 3D Cell-printing

One of the most robust aspects of bioprinting lies in its remarkable versatility. It can be applied across various domains, including fundamental research, investigations within the realms of TE and regenerative medicine, as well as drug testing (Cornelissen et al., 2017). In recent times, there has been a notable recognition of the utility of 3D models in the realms of both basic and translational research. This recognition is particularly evident in the development of cancer models, where 3D models prove invaluable for the effective screening of potential drug candidates. To enhance our understanding of the intricate mechanisms of action within the tumor microenvironment during pre-clinical drug testing, the implementation of a standardized 3D model is deemed essential (Kang et al., 2020).

The extracellular matrix (ECM) stands as a pivotal structural constituent, playing a crucial role in the organization of tissue and cell signaling. Given its significance, a more consistent focus was on conducting studies aimed at generating ECM scaffolds through 3D bioprinting, utilizing various biomaterials. Notably, hydrogels have emerged as a common choice for scaffolding due to their favorable printability and crosslinking properties. Biomaterials such as alginate, collagen, agarose, fibrin, and hyaluronic acid are frequently employed in this context. In a study conducted by Kreimendahl et al., type I collagen and fibrinogen are combined with agarose to fabricate onto the 3D bio-printed hydrogel blends. These blends exhibited remarkable mechanical stability, showcasing superior characteristics. Importantly, the engineered hydrogels demonstrated the capability to induce vascularization when exposed to human umbilical vein endothelial cells and human dermal fibroblasts, marking a significant advancement in the field (Kreimendahl et al., 2017). Monferrer and colleagues engineered bioprinted hydrogels using SK-N-BE(2) neuroblastoma cells, methacrylated gelatin, and methacrylated alginate. They conducted observations focused on assessing the rigidness of the hydrogels and the density of cell clusters (Monferrer et al., 2020). Nevertheless, bioprinted structures relying on scaffolds demand crucial attributes such as biocompatibility and biodegradability to facilitate their translation in clinical setup. In a study by Lee et al., a groundbreaking 3D printed glioblastoma model was showcased, employing a bioink consisting of fibrin, genipin, alginate, chitosan, and thrombin materials recognized for their biocompatible nature. Utilizing a specialized microfluidic printhead designed for drug screening applications, this groundbreaking system facilitated the 3D printing of neural tissue (Lee et al., 2019).

The blood vessel, being a pivotal player in tumor angiogenesis and metastatic progression within the tumor microenvironment, is identified as a crucial target for specific bioprinting efforts. Recent research has seen a surge in interest regarding novel bioprinting techniques that employ diverse cell types and biomaterials. For instance, Miller and colleagues delved into innovative approaches, where they used templates as carbohydrate glass for printing 3D filament networks. This template incorporated human umbilical vein endothelial cells (HUVECs) and facilitated blood flow, that resulted in the creation of perfused vascular channels embedded within several bulk ECM. In this methodology, cells encapsulated within the ECM were strategically arranged using sacrificial carbohydrate-glass lattices through extrusion bioprinting. This technique not only enabled the rapid but also reproducible fabrication of intricate microvascular architectures. Such advancements signify the potential of bioprinting in mimicking and studying the complex interactions within the tumor microenvironment, offering avenues for further exploration in cancer research and therapeutic development (Miller et al., 2012).

The applications of 3D bioprinting extend beyond the design of models for drug testing; they encompass groundbreaking potentials in diverse fields, including the 3D printing of SEVERAL scaffolds for bone TE. While bones possess a remarkable self-repair capability, they fall short in fully addressing extensive bone defects and articular cartilage damage caused by infection, trauma, and aging. Clinical bone repair and transplantation primarily target bone defects and osteoarthritis. Current transplantation methods encompass autologous, allogeneic, xenograft, and artificial bone transplantation. Allogeneic and artificial transplantation of bone are susceptible to immune rejection. Autologous bone, though ideal, is limited in supply and causes secondary damage to patients, posing challenges in meeting clinical demands (Zhang et al., 2023). 3D printing technology serves as an effective method for the fabrication of bone TE scaffolds. This technology is based on the discrete accumulation molding theory, which integrates numerical control technology, and biological materials by using CAD. This innovative digital molding approach enables the precise and swift creation of materials into a 1:1 model, employing the principles of layered manufacturing and layer-by-layer superposition. The scaffold preparation procedure involves acquiring 3-D data of the site of repair through CT scan or MRI. Subsequently, this 3-D model undergoes "slicing" using CAD software to extract data for each layer, which is then imported into the 3D printing system. Ultimately, the bone scaffold is constructed by layering constituents in accordance with the specified layered data using the device.

Research outcomes suggest that scaffolds made from polyester and inorganic particles offer notable benefits. In a study conducted by Schantz et al., a mixture of polycaprolactone and calcium phosphate served as the biomaterial for producing scaffolds using fusion lamination technology (Schantz JT et al., 2005). Comparative analysis with a standard polycaprolactone scaffold showed substantial enhancements in the mechanical strength and degradation rate of the hybrid scaffold. CT-guided FDM was used to construct a 3-D artificial bone composed of polycaprolactone/ hydroxyapatite, closely mimicking the natural structure of a goat femur. This method proves to be an easy, suitable, and cost-effective approach for artificial bone production (Xu N et al., 2014). Furthermore, the artificial bone produced with polycaprolactone/hydroxyapatite through this technology demonstrates mechanical properties more akin to natural bone, exhibiting favorable cell biocompatibility and in vitro biodegradability. Additionally, it displays an aptitude for inducing formation of new bone *in-vivo*. The polycaprolactone/hydroxyapatite 3-D artificial bone shows promise for treating clinical patients with bone defects. In recent days, the advancement of 4D printing technology has revolutionized the domain of 3D-printed constructs, introducing the capability for dynamic shape and functional modifications over time. The inherent self-remodeling and functional maturation capabilities of 4D-printed structures hold significant promise for the fabrication of complex hierarchical biological constructions that closely mimic native bone tissue. Moreover, employing various 4D-printed strategies enables the development of microvascular systems and nervous networks within bone constructs, which is imperative for the successful realization of large bone-graft substitutes (Wan et al., 2020).

6.   Future Challenges

The integration of 3D printing in clinical setups is progressing, as exemplified by the successful application of 3D-printed customized titanium prosthetics in personalized maxillofacial surgery in the UK (Mustafa et al., 2017). Expanding the achievement of this technique to 3D-printing tissues is a promising approach to transform transplantation and reconstructive surgery (Alderson et al., 2018). Recent reports express concerns about the integration of biological components in bioprinting, presenting significant challenges to 3D bioprinting. This process incorporates various cell types along with bioinks, and an advanced model of bioprinters. There are challenges in each of the sections such as-biological, technical, and ethical domains, with uncertainties regarding clinical and cost-effectiveness. The origin of cell sources and bioink materials, such as those for creating basic tissue structures like valves of heart, can be debated, with options including animals or humans. Clinically, valves of porcine are presently in use, illustrating the use of animal sources, allowing mass production but posing the risk of disease of Xeno-transmission due to allogenic material (Yoon J.K et al., 2015). On the other hand, human sources offer better biocompatibility and personalization opportunities, yet they face challenges of stricter regulation, longer production times, and higher costs. Prior to progressing to human trials, it is essential to conduct further research on the immunogenicity and toxicity of bioinks. Additional study is required to evaluate the potential risk of toxicity during the release of any by-products into the bloodstream and undergo renal or hepatic clearance. Designing clinical trials for tissue-engineered organ transplantation poses ethical challenges. Testing on healthy volunteers is unethical, and utilizing patient-specific cell populations requires patients to serve as their own controls, introducing significant heterogeneity when assessing treatment efficacy (Jovic T.H et al., 2020).

Conclusion

The applications of 3D bioprinting technology are wide-ranging, showcasing its capability to produce innovative constructs such as vessels, composite tissue, organoids, and intricate cellular and tissue models. The 3D bioprinting market has witnessed the emergence of companies specializing in various aspects, including desktop 3D bioprinters, bioinks, and scaffolds, with and without growth factors. This diversification has led to a multi-billion-dollar market. However, the challenge lies in the absence of "end-to-end" visibility by any single agency, highlighting the potential difficulty in fully harnessing the technology's true potential. Translating 3D printed constructs into clinical setups poses a considerable challenge. Achieving optimization of the translational pathway necessitates collaborative efforts from scientists, clinicians and engineers, operating within a robust infrastructure supported by an effective supply chain. Operating in isolated silos is no longer sufficient; a collaborative approach is essential to bring this technology into real-world clinical settings. To fully leverage the possibility of 3D printing in case of surgery, surgeons must remain informed about developments, identify applicable niches, and advocate for its incorporation into typical surgical practice. Anticipating gradual progress in 3D printing and bioprinting throughout the next century, there is a promising outlook for their transformative impact on future surgical procedures.

Author Contribution

Conceptualization, S.G, J.S, D.P; Writing—original draft preparation, J.S and D.P; Writing-review and editing, J.S and D.P; Supervision, S.G.

Conflict of Interest

The authors declare no conflict of interest.

Acknowledgement

The authors are grateful to the Science and Engineering Research Board (SERB), New Delhi (Grant Number-WEA/2020/000036 & CRG/2020/003014). The authors are grateful for the research endowment under the Intensification of Research in High Priority Area (IRHPA) program from Science and Engineering Research Board (SERB), New Delhi (Grant Number IPA/2020/000069). The authors are grateful for funding provided by the Department of Biotechnology (DBT), New Delhi (Grant number BT/PR34216/AAQ/1/765/2019). J.S. would like to acknowledge UGC Fellowship (221610016405) provided by the University Grants Commission (UGC), New Delhi, D.P. would like to acknowledge DBT Fellowships (DBT/2021-22/NIAB/1706) provided by the Department of Biotechnology (DBT), New Delhi.

References

Alderson D. The future of surgery. Br Surg. 2018;106(1): 9–10. https://dx.doi.org/10.1002/bjs.11086

Abaci A., Guvendiren M. Designing Decellularized Extracellular Matrix-Based Bioinks for 3D Bioprinting. Adv Healthc Mater. 2020; 9(24): 2000734. https://doi.org/10.1002/adhm.202000734

Agarwal S., Saha S., Balla V.K., Pal A., Barui A. et al. Current Developments in 3D Bioprinting for Tissue and Organ Regeneration–A Review. Front Mech Eng. 2020 (6): 589171. https://doi.org/10.3389/fmech.2020.589171

Antich C., de Vicente J., Jiménez G., Chocarro C., Carrillo E. et al. Bio-inspired hydrogel composed of hyaluronic acid and alginate as a potential bioink for 3D bioprinting of articular cartilage engineering constructs. Acta Biomater. 2020 (106): 114–23. https://doi.org/10.1016/j.actbio.2020.01.046

Axpe E., Oyen M.L. Applications of Alginate-Based Bioinks in 3D Bioprinting. Int J Mol Sci 2016; 17(12): 1976. https://doi.org/10.3390/ijms17121976

Byakodi M., Shrikrishna N. S., Sharma R., Bhansali S., Mishra Y. et al. Emerging 0D, 1D, 2D, and 3D Nanostructures for Efficient Point-of-Care Biosensing. Biosens Bioelectron X 2022; 12:100284. https://doi.org/10.1016/J.BIOSX.2022.100284.

Chia H.N., Wu B.M. Recent advances in 3D printing of biomaterials. J Biol Eng [Internet]. 2015 Mar 1 [cited 2024 Jan 8];9(1):1–14. Available from: https://jbioleng.biomedcentral.com/articles/10.1186/s13036-015-0001-4. https://doi.org/10.1186/s13036-015-0001-4

Cho C.S., Yoo J.J. Three-dimensional printing in tissue engineering and regenerative medicine. Tissue Eng Regen Med 2016; 13(6):611. https://doi.org/10.1007/s13770-016-9999-8

Christensen K., Xu C., Chai W., Zhang Z., Fu J. et al. Freeform inkjet printing of cellular structures with bifurcations. Biotechnol Bioeng. 2015; 112(5):1047–55. https://doi/full/10.1002/bit.25501

Cornelissen D.J., Faulkner-Jones A., Shu W. Current developments in 3D bioprinting for tissue engineering. Curr Opin Biomed Eng. 2017 (2): 76–82. https://doi.org/10.1016/j.cobme.2017.05.004

Cui N., Dai C.Y., Mao X., Lv X., Gu Y., Lee E.S., et al. Poloxamer-Based Scaffolds for Tissue Engineering Applications: A Review. Gels. 2022; 8(6): 360. https://doi.org/10.3390/gels8060360

Cui X., Breitenkamp K., Finn M.G., Lotz M., D'Lima D.D. et al. Direct Human Cartilage Repair Using Three-Dimensional Bioprinting Technology. Tissue Eng Part A. 2012; 18: 11–12: 1304–12. https://doi.org/10.1089/ten.tea.2011.0543

De Gans B.J., Duineveld P.C., Schubert U.S. Inkjet Printing of Polymers: State of the Art and Future Developments. Adv Mater. 2004; 16(3): 203–13. https://doi.org/10.1002/adma.200300385

Doraiswamy A., Narayan R.J., Harris M.L., Qadri S.B., Modi R. et al. Laser microfabrication of hydroxyapatite-osteoblast-like cell composites. J Biomed Mater Res A. 2007; 80A(3): 635–43. https://doi.org/10.1002/jbm.a.30969

Dzobo K., Motaung K.S.C.M., Adesida A. Recent Trends in Decellularized Extracellular Matrix Bioinks for 3D Printing: An Updated Review. 2019; 20(18):4628. https://doi.org/10.3390/ijms20184628

Eswaramoorthy S.D., Ramakrishna S., Rath S.N. Recent advances in three-dimensional bioprinting of stem cells. J Tissue Eng Regen Med. 2019; 13(6).908–24. https://onlinelibrary.wiley.com/doi/full/10.1002/term.2839

Fang Y., Guo Y., Ji M., Li B., Guo Y. et al. 3D Printing of Cell-Laden Microgel-Based Biphasic Bioink with Heterogeneous Microenvironment for Biomedical Applications. Adv Funct Mater. 2022; 32(13):2109810. https://doi.org/10.1002/adfm.202109810

Fang Y., Guo Y., Liu T., Xu R., Mao S. et al. Advances in 3D Bioprinting. Chinese Journal of Mechanical Engineering: Additive Manufacturing Frontiers. 2022; 1(1):100011. https://doi.org/10.1016/j.cjmeam.2022.100011

Fang Y., Sun W., Zhang T., Xiong Z. Recent advances on bioengineering approaches for fabrication of functional engineered cardiac pumps: A review. Biomaterials. 2022; 280:121298. https://doi.org/10.1016/j.biomaterials.2021.121298

Fatimi A., Okoro O.V., Podstawczyk D., Siminska-Stanny J., Shavandi A. et al. Natural Hydrogel-Based Bio-Inks for 3D Bioprinting in Tissue Engineering: A Review. Gels. 2022; 8(3):179. https://doi.org/10.3390/gels8030179

Fetah K., Tebon P., Goudie M.J., Potyondy T., Alfredo Uquillas J. et al. Bioink properties before, during and after 3D bioprinting. Biofabrication. 2016; 8(3):032002. https://doi.org/10.1088/1758-5090/8/3/032002

Fleischer S., Tavakol D.N., Vunjak-Novakovic G. From Arteries to Capillaries: Approaches to Engineering Human Vasculature. Adv Funct Mater. 2020; 30(37):1910811. https://doi.org/10.1002/adfm.201910811

Gao Q., Kim B.S., Gao G. Advanced Strategies for 3D Bioprinting of Tissue and Organ Analogs Using Alginate Hydrogel Bioinks. Marine Drugs. 2021; 19(12):708. https://doi.org/10.3390/md19120708

Gong C., Kong Z., Wang X. The Effect of Agarose on 3D Bioprinting. Polymers (Basel). 2021; 13(22): 4028. https://doi.org/10.3390/polym13224028

Gopinathan J., Noh I. Recent trends in bioinks for 3D printing. Biomaterials Research. 2018; 22(1):1–15. https://doi.org/10.1186/s40824-018-0122-1

Groll J., Burdick J.A., Cho D.W., Derby B., Gelinsky M. et al. A definition of bioinks and their distinction from biomaterial inks. Biofabrication. 2018; 11(1):013001. https://doi.org/10.1088/1758-5090/aaec52

Gu Q., Tomaskovic-Crook E., Lozano R., Chen Y., Kapsa R.M. et al. Functional 3D Neural Mini-Tissues from Printed Gel-Based Bioink and Human Neural Stem Cells. Adv Healthc Mater. 2016; 5(12):1429–38. https://doi.org/10.1002/adhm.201600095

Gungor-Ozkerim P.S., Inci I., Zhang Y.S., Khademhosseini A., Dokmeci M.R. et al. Bioinks for 3D bioprinting: an overview. Biomater Sci. 2018; 6(5): 915–46. https://doi.org/10.1039/C7BM00765E

Guvendiren M., Burdick J.A. Engineering synthetic hydrogel microenvironments to instruct stem cells. Curr Opin Biotechnol. 2013; 24(5): 841–6. doi: 10.1016/j.copbio.2013.03.009

Guvendiren M., Molde J., Soares R.M.D., Kohn J. Designing Biomaterials for 3D Printing. ACS Biomater Sci Eng [Internet]. 2016 Oct 10 [cited 2024 Jan 25]; 2(10):1679–93. Available from: https://pubs.acs.org/doi/abs/10.1021/acsbiomaterials.6b00121

Hauptstein J., Böck T., Bartolf-Kopp M., Forster L., Stahlhut P. et al. Hyaluronic Acid-Based Bioink Composition Enabling 3D Bioprinting and Improving Quality of Deposited Cartilaginous Extracellular Matrix. Adv Healthc Mater. 2020; 9(15):2000737. https://doi.org/10.1002/adhm.202000737

Highley C.B., Prestwich G.D., Burdick J.A. Recent advances in hyaluronic acid hydrogels for biomedical applications. Curr Opin Biotechnol. 2016; 40:35–40. https://doi.org/10.1016/j.copbio.2016.02.008

Hoshiba T., Lu H., Kawazoe N., Chen G. Decellularized matrices for tissue engineering. Expert Opin Biol Ther. 2010; 10(12): 1717–28. https://doi.org/10.1517/14712598.2010.534079

Hospodiuk M., Dey M., Sosnoski D., Ozbolat I.T. The bioink: A comprehensive review on bioprintable materials. Biotechnol Adv. 2017; 35(2): 217–39. https://doi.org/10.1016/j.biotechadv.2016.12.006

Jang C.H., Ahn S.H., Yang G.H., Kim G.H. A MSCs-laden polycaprolactone/collagen scaffold for bone tissue regeneration. RSC Adv. 2016; 6(8): 6259–65. https://doi.org/10.1039/C5RA20627H

Jang J., Park J.Y., Gao G., Cho D.W. Biomaterials-based 3D cell printing for next-generation therapeutics and diagnostics. Biomaterials. 2018; 156:88–106. https://doi.org/10.1016/j.biomaterials.2017.11.030

Jia J., Richards D.J., Pollard S., Tan Y., Rodriguez J. et al. Engineering alginate as bioink for bioprinting. Acta Biomater. 2014; 10(10):4323–31. https://doi.org/10.1016/j.actbio.2014.06.034

Jovic T.H., Combellack E.J., Jessop Z.M., Whitaker I.S. 3D Bioprinting and the Future of Surgery. Front Surg. 2020; 7:609836. https://doi.org/10.3389/fsurg.2020.609836

Kaushik S., Gandhi S., Chauhan M., Ma S., Das S., et al. Water-Templated, Polysaccharide-Rich Bioartificial 3D Microarchitectures as Extra-Cellular Matrix Bioautomatons. ACS Appl Mater Interfaces 2020; 12(18): 20912–20921. https://doi.org/10.1021/ACSAMI.0C01012.

Kim J.H., Yoo J.J., Lee S.J. Three-dimensional cell-based bioprinting for soft tissue regeneration. Tissue Eng Regen Med. 2016; 13(6):647. https://doi.org/10.3390/bioengineering10101232

Knop K., Hoogenboom R., Fischer D., Schubert U.S. Poly(ethylene glycol) in drug delivery: pros and cons as well as potential alternatives. Angew Chem Int Ed Engl. 2010; 49(36):6288–308. https://doi.org/10.1002/anie.200902672

Koch L., Deiwick A., Schlie S., Michael S., Gruene M. et al. Skin tissue generation by laser cell printing. Biotechnol Bioeng. 2012; 109(7):1855–63. https://doi.org/10.1002/bit.24455

Kreimendahl F., Köpf M., Thiebes A.L., Duarte Campos D.F., Blaeser A. et al. Three-Dimensional Printing and Angiogenesis: Tailored Agarose-Type I Collagen Blends Comprise Three-Dimensional Printability and Angiogenesis Potential for Tissue-Engineered Substitutes. Tissue Eng Part C Methods. 2017; 23(10):604–15. https://doi.org/10.1089/ten.tec.2017.0234

Lee C., Abelseth E., de la Vega L., Willerth S.M. Bioprinting a novel glioblastoma tumor model using a fibrin-based bioink for drug screening. Mater Today Chem. 2019; 12:78–84. https://doi.org/10.1016/j.mtchem.2018.12.005

Lee S.J., Esworthy T., Stake S., Miao S., Zuo Y.Y. et al. Advances in 3D Bioprinting for Neural Tissue Engineering. Adv Biosyst. 2018; 2(4):1700213. https://doi.org/10.1002%2Fadhm.202001600

Li X., Liu B., Pei B., Chen J., Zhou D. et al. Inkjet Bioprinting of Biomaterials. Chem Rev. 2020; 120(19):10793–833. https://doi.org/10.1021/acs.chemrev.0c00008

Liao Y., Song J., Li E., Luo Y., Shen Y. et al. Rapid prototyping of three-dimensional microfluidic mixers in glass by femtosecond laser direct writing. Lab Chip. 2012; 12(4):746–9. https://doi.org/10.1039/C2LC21015K

López-Marcial G.R., Zeng A.Y., Osuna C., Dennis J., García J.M. et al. Agarose-Based Hydrogels as Suitable Bioprinting Materials for Tissue Engineering. ACS Biomater Sci Eng. 2018; 4(10):3610–6. https://doi.org/10.1021/acsbiomaterials.8b00903

Ma L., Zhou Y., Zhu Y., Lin Z., Chen L. et al. 3D printed personalized titanium plates improve clinical outcome in microwave ablation of bone tumors around the knee. Sci Rep. 2017; 7(1):1–10. https://doi.org/10.1038/s41598-017-07243-3

Mannoor M.S., Jiang Z., James T., Kong Y.L., Malatesta K.A., et al. 3D printed bionic ears. Nano Lett. 2013; 13(6):2634–9. https://pubs.acs.org/doi/abs/10.1021/nl4007744

Melchels F.P.W., Feijen J., Grijpma D.W. A review on stereolithography and its applications in biomedical engineering. Biomaterials. 2010; 31(24):6121–30. https://doi.org/10.1016/j.biomaterials.2010.04.050

Miller J.S., Stevens K.R., Yang M.T., Baker B.M., Nguyen D.H.T. et al. Rapid casting of patterned vascular networks for perfusable engineered three-dimensional tissues. Nat Mater 2012; 11(9): 768–74. https://doi.org/10.1038/nmat3357

Mishra A., Srivastava V. Biomaterials and 3D printing techniques used in the medical field. J Med Eng Technol. 2021; 45(4):290–302. https://doi.org/10.1080/03091902.2021.1893845

Monferrer E., Martín-Vañó S., Carretero A., García-Lizarribar A., Burgos-Panadero R. et al. A three-dimensional bioprinted model to evaluate the effect of stiffness on neuroblastoma cell cluster dynamics and behavior. Sci Rep. 2020; 10(1):1–12. https://doi.org/10.1038/s41598-020-62986-w

Müller M., Becher J., Schnabelrauch M., Zenobi-Wong M. Nanostructured Pluronic hydrogels as bioinks for 3D bioprinting. Biofabrication. 2015; 7(3):035006. https://iopscience.iop.org/article/10.1088/1758-5090/7/3/035006

Murphy S.V., Atala A. 3D bioprinting of tissues and organs. Nat Biotechnol. 2014; 32(8): 773–85. https://doi.org/10.1038/nbt.2958

Mustafa S.F., Evans P.L., Sugar A.W., Key S.J. Streamlining the manufacture of custom titanium orbital plates with a stereolithographic three-dimensional printed model. Br J Oral Maxillofac Surg. 2017; 55(5): 546–7. https://doi.org/10.1016/j.bjoms.2016.03.003

Navara A.M., Kim Y.S., Xu Y., Crafton C.L. et al. A dual-gelling poly(N-isopropylacrylamide)-based ink and thermoreversible poloxamer support bath for high-resolution bioprinting. Bioact Mater. 2022; 14:302–12. https://doi.org/10.1016/j.bioactmat.2021.11.016

Noh I., Kim N., Tran H.N., Lee J., Lee C. et al. 3D printable hyaluronic acid-based hydrogel for its potential application as a bioink in tissue engineering. Biomater Res. 2019; 23(1):1–9. https://doi.org/10.1186/s40824-018-0152-8

Ott H.C., Matthiesen T.S., Goh S.K., Black L.D. et al. Perfusion-decellularized matrix: using nature's platform to engineer a bioartificial heart. Nat Med. 2008; 14(2):213–21. https://doi.org/10.1038/nm1684

Ouyang L., Highley C.B., Rodell C.B., Sun W., Burdick J.A. et al. 3D Printing of Shear-Thinning Hyaluronic Acid Hydrogels with Secondary Cross-Linking. ACS Biomater Sci Eng. 2016; 2(10):1743–51. https://doi.org/10.1021/acsbiomaterials.6b00158

Ozbolat I.T., Peng W., Ozbolat V. Application areas of 3D bioprinting. Drug Discov Today. 2016; 21(8):1257–71. https://doi.org/10.1016/j.drudis.2016.04.006

Ozler S.B., Bakirci E., Kucukgul C., Koc B. Three-dimensional direct cell bioprinting for tissue engineering. J Biomed Mater Res B Appl Biomater. 2017; 105(8):2530–44. https://doi.org/10.1002/jbm.b.33768

Pahlevanzadeh F., Mokhtari H., Bakhsheshi-Rad H.R., Emadi R., Kharaziha M. et al. Recent Trends in Three-Dimensional Bioinks Based on Alginate for Biomedical Applications. Materials. 2020; 13(18):3980. https://doi.org/10.3390/ma13183980

Park J.H., Jang J., Lee J.S., Cho D.W. Current advances in three-dimensional tissue/organ printing. Tissue Eng Regen Med. 2016; 13(6):612. https://doi.org/10.1007%2Fs13770-016-8111-8

Pati F., Jang J., Ha D.H., Won Kim S., Rhie J.W. et al. Printing three-dimensional tissue analogues with decellularized extracellular matrix bioink. Nat Commun. 2014; 5(1):1–11. https://doi.org/10.1038/ncomms4935

Petta D., D'Amora U., Ambrosio L., Grijpma D.W., Eglin D. et al. Hyaluronic acid as a bioink for extrusion-based 3D printing. Biofabrication. 2020; 12(3):032001. Available from: https://iopscience.iop.org/article/10.1088/1758-5090/ab8752

Prakashan D., Singh A., Deshpande A. D., Chandra V., Sharma G. T., et al. Bone Marrow Derived Mesenchymal Stem Cells Enriched PCL-Gelatin Nanofiber Scaffold for Improved Wound Healing. Int J Biol Macromol 2024; 274(2):133447. https://doi.org/10.1016/J.IJBIOMAC.2024.133447

Prakashan, D., Sahoo, J., Gandhi, S. Nanomaterial-Based Wound Therapy: Recent Advances and Future Perspectives. In: Javed, R., Chen, JT., Khalil, A.T. (eds) Nanomaterials for Biomedical and Bioengineering Applications. Springer, Singapore. 2024; pp.221–247. https://doi.org/10.1007/978-981-97-0221-3_9

Prakashan D., Sharma R., Halder S., Gandhi S. Nanomaterials for Tissue Engineering: Synthesis, Characterisation and Application, Nanoparticle Toxicity and compatibility, Material Research foundation LLC, USA, 2024; pp. 27-63. http://doi.org/10.21741/9781644902998-2.

Roberts A., Mahari S., Gandhi S. Cells and Organs on a Chip in Biomedical Sciences. Microfluidics and Multi Organs on Chip 2022; 219–245. https://doi.org/10.1007/978-981-19-1379-2_10

Schantz J.T., Brandwood A., Hutmacher D.W., Khor H.L., Bittner K. et al. Osteogenic differentiation of mesenchymal progenitor cells in computer designed fibrin-polymer-ceramic scaffolds manufactured by fused deposition modeling. J Mater Sci Mater Med. 2005; 16(9):807–19. https://doi.org/10.1007/s10856-005-3584-3

Shafiee A., Atala A. Printing Technologies for Medical Applications. Trends Mol Med. 2016 Mar 1; 22(3):254–65.

Shah M., Prakashan D., Gandhi S. Microfluidics, Organs-on-a-Chip, and 3D Printing. Human Organs-on-a-Chip Technology 2024; 91–112. https://doi.org/10.1016/B978-0-443-13782-2.00008-5

Shahdeo, D., Roberts, A., Kesarwani, V., Horvat, M., Chouhan, R. S. et al. Polymeric Biocompatible Iron Oxide Nanoparticles Labeled with Peptides for Imaging in Ovarian Cancer. Biosci Rep 2022; 42(2):BSR20212622. https://doi.org/10.1042/BSR20212622

Shamma R.N., Sayed R.H., Madry H., El Sayed N.S., Cucchiarini M. et al. Triblock Copolymer Bioinks in Hydrogel Three-Dimensional Printing for Regenerative Medicine: A Focus on Pluronic F127. 2022; 28(2):451–63. https://www.liebertpub.com/doi/10.1089/ten.teb.2021.0026

Sidambe A.T., Oh J.K. Biocompatibility of Advanced Manufactured Titanium Implants—A Review. Materials. 2014; 7(12):8168–88. https://doi.org/10.3390/ma7128168

Skardal A., Zhang J., Prestwich G.D. Bioprinting vessel-like constructs using hyaluronan hydrogels crosslinked with tetrahedral polyethylene glycol tetracrylates. Biomaterials. 2010; 31(24):6173–81. https://doi.org/10.1016/j.biomaterials.2010.04.045

Sun W., Starly B., Daly A.C., Burdick J.A., Groll J. et al., The bioprinting roadmap. Biofabrication. 2020; 12(2):022002. https://iopscience.iop.org/article/10.1088/1758-5090/ab5158

Tasnim N., De la Vega L., Anil Kumar S., Abelseth L., Alonzo M. et al. 3D Bioprinting Stem Cell Derived Tissues. Cell Mol Bioeng. 2018; 11(4): 219–40. https://doi.org/10.1007%2Fs12195-018-0530-2

Van Noort R. The future of dental devices is digital. Dental Materials. 2012 Jan 1; 28(1): 3–12. https://doi.org/10.1016/j.dental.2011.10.014

Wan Z., Zhang P., Liu Y., Lv L., Zhou Y. et al. Four-dimensional bioprinting: Current developments and applications in bone tissue engineering. Acta Biomater. 2020; 101:26–42. https://doi.org/10.1016/j.actbio.2019.10.038

Wang Y., Gao M., Wang D., Sun L., Webster T.J. et al. Nanoscale 3D Bioprinting for Osseous Tissue Manufacturing. Int J Nanomedicine. 2020; 15:215–26. https://doi.org/10.2147%2FIJN.S172916

Wenger L., Radtke C.P., Gerisch E., Kollmann M., Niemeyer C.M. et al. Systematic evaluation of agarose- and agar-based bioinks for extrusion-based bioprinting of enzymatically active hydrogels. Front Bioeng Biotechnol. 2022; 10:928878. https://doi.org/10.3389/fbioe.2022.928878

Wijshoff H. The dynamics of the piezo inkjet printhead operation. Phys Rep. 2010; 491(4–5):77–177. https://doi.org/10.1016/j.physrep.2010.03.003

Wu W., Deconinck A., Lewis J.A. Omnidirectional Printing of 3D Microvascular Networks. Advanced Materials. 2011; 23(24):H178–83. https://doi.org/10.1002/adma.201004625

Xu N., Ye X., Wei D., Zhong J., Chen Y. et al. 3D artificial bones for bone repair prepared by computed tomography-guided fused deposition modeling for bone repair. ACS Appl Mater Interfaces. 2014; 6(17):14952–63. https://pubs.acs.org/doi/abs/10.1021/am502716t

Yasun E., Gandhi S., Choudhury S., Mohammadinejad R., Benyettou F., Gozubenli N., Arami H. Hollow Micro and Nanostructures for Therapeutic and Imaging Applications. J Drug Deliv Sci Technol 2020; 60:102094. https://doi.org/10.1016/J.JDDST.2020.102094

Yildirimer L., Thanh N.T.K., Seifalian A.M. Skin regeneration scaffolds: a multimodal bottom-up approach. Trends Biotechnol. 2012; 30(12):638–48. https://doi.org/10.1016/j.tibtech.2012.08.004

Yoon J.K., Choi J., Lee H.J., Cho Y., Gwon Y.D. et al. Distribution of Porcine Endogenous Retrovirus in Different Organs of the Hybrid of a Landrace and a Jeju Domestic Pig in Korea. Transplant Proc. 2015 Jul 1; 47(6):2067–71. https://doi.org/10.1016/j.transproceed.2015.05.023

Zein I., Hutmacher D.W., Tan K.C., Teoh S.H. Fused deposition modeling of novel scaffold architectures for tissue engineering applications. Biomaterials. 2002; 23(4):1169–85. https://doi.org/10.1016/S0142-9612(01)00232-0

Zhang A.P., Qu X., Soman P., Hribar K.C., Lee J.W. et al. Rapid Fabrication of Complex 3D Extracellular Microenvironments by Dynamic Optical Projection Stereolithography. Adv Mater 2012; 24(31):4266–70. https://doi.org/10.1002/adma.201202024

Zhang C.Y., Fu C.P., Li X.Y., Lu X.C., Hu L.G. et al. Three-Dimensional Bioprinting of Decellularized Extracellular Matrix-Based Bioinks for Tissue Engineering. Molecules. 2022; 27(11): 3442. https://doi.org/10.3390/molecules27113442

Zhang Q., Zhou J., Zhi P., Liu L., Liu C et al. 3D printing method for bone tissue engineering scaffold. Med Nov Technol Devices. 2023; 17:100205. https://doi.org/10.1016%2Fj.medntd.2022.100205

Zhang W., Chen S. Femtosecond laser nanofabrication of hydrogel biomaterial. MRS Bull. 2011; 36(12):1028–33. https://doi.org/10.1557/mrs.2011.275

Zhang X., Liu Y., Luo C., Zhai C., Li Z. et al. Crosslinker-free silk/decellularized extracellular matrix porous bioink for 3D bioprinting-based cartilage tissue engineering. Mater Sci and Eng: C. 2021; 118:111388. https://doi.org/10.1016/j.msec.2020.111388

Zhang Y., Yu Y., Chen H., Ozbolat I.T. Characterization of printable cellular micro-fluidic channels for tissue engineering. Biofabrication. 2013; 5(2):025004. https://doi.org/10.1088/1758-5082/5/2/025004

Zhang Y.S., Arneri A., Bersini S., Shin S.R., Zhu K. et al. Bioprinting 3D microfibrous scaffolds for engineering endothelialized myocardium and heart-on-a-chip. Biomaterials. 2016; 110:45–59. https://doi.org/10.1016/j.biomaterials.2016.09.003

Zhao P., Gu H., Mi H., Rao C., Fu J. et al. Fabrication of scaffolds in tissue engineering: A review. Fron Mech Eng. 2018; 13(1):107–19. http://dx.doi.org/10.1007/s11465-018-0496-8

Zhu J. Bioactive modification of poly (ethylene glycol) hydrogels for tissue engineering. Biomaterials. 2010; 31(17):4639–56. https://doi.org/10.1016%2Fj.biomaterials.2010.02.044

Zhu N., Chen X. Biofabrication of Tissue Scaffolds. Advances in Biomaterials Science and Biomedical Applications. InTech. 2013; 570. https://www.intechopen.com/chapters/43739

Zhu W., Ma X., Gou M., Mei D., Zhang K. et al., Chen S. 3D printing of functional biomaterials for tissue engineering. Curr Opin Biotechnol. 2016; 40:103–12. https://doi.org/10.1016/j.copbio.2016.03.014

3D Printing in Prosthetic Devices

Prakash Srinivasan Timiri Shanmugam,[1*]
Thamizharasan Sampath,[2*]
Sandhiya Thamizharasan[3] *and Jayantha Saha*[4]

1. Introduction

1.1 Evolution of Prosthetic Devices

Prosthesis design can be dated back to the ancient Egyptian and Roman empires and has continued to develop across the world throughout the course of history. In the late 1800s, John Hanger's prosthesis, the Hanger Limb, was developed in response to the American Civil War, ushering prosthesis design into the modern era (Norton K, 2007). Medical advancements since the invention of the Hanger Limb have significantly reduced limb loss due to traumatic events. In 2005, an estimated 1.6 million people in the United States had a limb difference, and approximately 541,000 individuals had some level of upper-limb loss. Based on current projections, this value may double by 2050. Trauma remains the most significant cause of upper-limb amputation, predominantly for males, though the subsection of dysvascular-driven adult amputations is rapidly growing. Global monitoring for congenital limb loss is reported annually by the International Clearinghouse for Birth Defects Surveillance and Research Annual Report. It is reported that congenital and pediatric amputations account for a significant population of overall limb difference (Zuo K.J., Olson J.L. (2014)).

1.2 Overview of Prosthetic Devices

In the United States, more than 32,500 children have experienced a major pediatric amputation. The Centers for Disease Control and Prevention highlights an estimate that approximately 1500 children are born with upper-limb reductions each year, or approximately 4 of 10,000 live births.

[1] Global Product Safety & Toxicology, Avanos medical Inc, Alpharetta, Georgia, USA.
[2] Department of Pharmacology & Toxicology, VMCGH, Dr. YRS University of Health Sciences, Kurnool, India.
[3] The Tooth Doctor, Advanced Implant Centre, Vellapanchavadi, Chennai, India.
[4] Department of Physiology, SBIMS, University of Health Sciences, Raipur, India.
* Corresponding author: thamizhpharma@gmail.com

Internationally, limb reductions vary from 7.8/10,000 (France) to 13/10,000 (Finland), 21.1/10,000 (Netherlands), and 30.4/10,000 (Scotland). Due to the variety of complexities limiting both access and affinities to devices, usage rates by amputees with a prosthesis are still limited (Manero, A., Smith, P., Sparkman, et al., 2019). Substantial percentages of people with congenital limb loss or acquired limb loss choose not to use a device, despite having access to one. Usage rates have been reported for upper-limb devices between 37% and 56% among individuals with upper-limb loss. Lower-limb devices are often viewed as more of a necessity than upper-limb devices and have usage rates that vary in literature between 49% and 95%. This difference is particularly expressed among children with transverse upper-limb amputations, where usage rates fall between 44% and 66%. Low usage rates of upper-limb prostheses may result from a lack of aesthetic design, weight, availability of insurance and health care, and high costs. Additionally, device acceptance is complex at the user, provider, parental, and insurance levels. The combination of form and function in the design of prostheses has emerged to provide a higher degree of functionality patterned after the organic 21 degree of freedom of the human hand. Much of the design efforts have been prioritizing achieving a high degree of realism in comparison to the organic analog. Graham Pullin proposed in his book, Design Meets Disability that prostheses should not be limited to functional design and that duality should exist between aesthetics and functionality (Frontera W.R., Silver J.K. (2004)). Prosthetic devices have long been a cornerstone of rehabilitative medicine, providing essential support and functionality to individuals with limb loss or impairment. Over the years, significant strides have been made in prosthetic technology, leading to the development of increasingly sophisticated devices capable of mimicking natural movements and enhancing quality of life for users. However, traditional manufacturing methods often face limitations in producing customized, anatomically accurate prosthetics that seamlessly integrate with the human body.

1.3   3D Bioprinting

In recent years, the emergence of 3D bioprinting has revolutionized the field of prosthetics by offering a novel approach to design and fabrication. 3D bioprinting harnesses the power of advanced additive manufacturing techniques to create three-dimensional structures using living cells, biomaterials, and bioinks. This cutting-edge technology enables the precise deposition of biological materials layer by layer, allowing for the creation of complex tissue constructs with unparalleled precision and control. The convergence of 3D bioprinting and prosthetic device development holds immense promise for revolutionizing the field, offering the potential to overcome longstanding challenges and pave the way for the next generation of prosthetic solutions. By leveraging bioprinting techniques, researchers and clinicians can now create prosthetic devices that not only replicate the form and function of natural tissues but also exhibit enhanced biocompatibility, durability, and integration with the host organism (Elmansy R. (2015)).

This chapter explores the multifaceted intersection of 3D bioprinting and prosthetic devices, delving into the fundamental principles, materials, techniques, applications, challenges, and future directions of this rapidly evolving field. Through a comprehensive examination of recent advancements, case studies, and clinical applications, we aim to elucidate the transformative potential of 3D bioprinting in prosthetic device development, offering insights into how this groundbreaking technology is reshaping the landscape of rehabilitative medicine and patient care.

2.   Fundamentals of 3D Printing in Prothesis

3D bioprinting represents a groundbreaking approach to tissue engineering and regenerative medicine, seamlessly integrating principles of additive manufacturing with biological materials to construct intricate three-dimensional structures. Unlike conventional manufacturing techniques, 3D printing technology enables the fabrication of parts with complex geometries using minimal material. With 3D printing, there's no requirement for molding, and adjustments to the geometry of a part can be swiftly implemented. Objects conceived in a digital environment can be swiftly transitioned to the production process. This versatility makes three-dimensional printing particularly well-suited for creating objects with free-form surfaces. In the medical sector, 3D printing has found extensive application, notably in the fabrication of patient-specific biomedical devices, showcasing its potential to revolutionize personalized healthcare.

2.1   Stages of the 3D Printing Process

In the 3D printing process, the 3D model of the target object is first divided into layers using specialized software, often referred to as a 3D slicer. These layers are determined based on the desired surface precision, and the corresponding G-codes are generated. Subsequently, the data obtained in this stage is digitally transmitted to the 3D printer, where the first layer of the object is created according to these instructions. Successive layers are then added on top of the previous ones, gradually building up the object until its completion.

Generally, a 3D printing process involves several steps:

 (i) Obtaining the 3D model of the target object in a digital format, often through computer-aided design (CAD) software.
(ii) Converting the model file of the desired object into a digital file format compatible with the 3D printer, such as STL (stereolithography).
(iii) Slicing the model into layers using a 3D printer slicer software, which generates the necessary G-codes for printing.
(iv) Transmitting the G-codes to the 3D printer, typically via a computer or other digital interface.
 (v) Initiating the printing process, during which the object is constructed layer by layer according to the instructions provided by the G-codes.

This structured approach ensures precise and accurate fabrication of objects using additive manufacturing techniques, allowing for the creation of complex shapes and intricate designs with relative ease (Surmen et al., 2020).

2.2   3D Modeling

In the initial stage of the 3D printing process, acquiring a precise 3D model of the intended object is essential. This model can be obtained through various means, including computer-aided design (CAD) software or 3D scanning systems such as optical scanners, MRI scans, CT scans, or image-based techniques. Achieving optimal printing outcomes necessitates careful consideration of the design, considering the specific technology and capabilities of the 3D printer being utilized. Additionally, ensuring compatibility between the capabilities of the 3D printer and the intended assembly parts, as well as the desired clearance between moving components, is crucial for successful printing operations.

2.3   File Conversion

Once the 3D model has been obtained, it must be converted into a file format compatible with slicer software. The most prevalent format for 3D printing is STL, though other formats like OBJ and 3MF are also widely supported by various software. It's important to note that once the file format is converted, the geometry of the model cannot be altered, although adjustments to the size and orientation of the model remain possible.

2.4   3D Slicer Software

Models saved in an appropriate format are transferred to 3D slicer software before initiating the 3D printing process. The primary function of this software is to segment the model into individual layers and generate the G-codes necessary for the 3D printer's operation. Various parameters such as the object's placement on the printer bed, layer thickness, material selection, temperature settings, material density, and printing speed can be adjusted within the slicer software interface. Once the parameters are specified, the model is sliced accordingly, and the corresponding G-codes are generated. Additionally, slicer software allows for the simulation and monitoring of the printing process, akin to computer-aided manufacturing (CAM) programs. This capability enables the identification and rectification of potential errors or issues that may arise during the printing process. Numerous open-source and accessible 3D slicer software options are available to users, including Ultimaker Cura (Ultimaker B.V., The Netherlands), CraftWare (Craftunique, Hungary), and Z-Suite (Zortrax, Poland). Following the generation of G-codes, these instructions can be transferred to the 3D printer via a memory card or through a wired/wireless network connection, facilitating seamless communication between the slicer software and the printer for efficient and accurate fabrication of the desired object.

2.5 3D Printing

Once the file transfer is complete, the 3D printer, recognizing the G-codes, commences printing once it achieves the necessary temperature. Prior to printing, it's imperative to ensure that the printer is positioned on a level surface, calibration procedures are executed, and the printing material is adequately prepared. The duration of printing varies depending on factors such as the printer's technology, material density, model geometry and size, the quantity of support material required, and the desired resolution level. In 3D printing, the object's geometry directly influences the printing time. To ensure successful printing, the software generates support structures between the object and the printing tray in the sequence of the printing process. Therefore, it's crucial to position the object appropriately on the printing tray. By positioning the objects in a manner that minimizes the need for support structures, both printing time and post-processing time required for removing the model from the supports can be reduced. This optimization of positioning can significantly enhance efficiency in the printing process.

2.6 Post-processing

When printing is finished, the part is taken from the 3D printer tray and cleaned from the support structures. Support structures are of two types: standard and dissolvable. Standard support structures are removed from the workpiece using suitable hand tools. Dissolvable support structures are removed by immersing the workpiece in water or specific solutions developed for the material. After removal of the support structures, post-processing operations such as painting, polishing, sanding, gap filling, metal plating, epoxy coating, dipping, and vapor smoothing can be applied (Dombroski et al., (2014)).

3. Types of 3D Printing Technologies for Prosthetic Devices

3.1 Stereolithography (SLA)

The SLA technique operates on the principle of curing a photopolymer resin layer, which is in a liquid state at room temperature, through an ultraviolet laser beam based on geometric data of the target object. This process is rooted in the additive manufacturing approach, which underpins 3D printer technologies. Each layer is generated via G-code previously created using 3D slicer software. The laser beam scans the resin layer, initiating the curing process. Once the first layer solidifies, the building platform ascends to the specified layer height, a new resin layer is applied, and the curing process repeats. Through successive layering, the entire object is constructed. Consequently, highly detailed geometries can be achieved from the liquid resin contained in the pool, which lacks specific geometry. Renowned for its high precision and smooth surfaces, this 3D printing technology is well-suited for producing intricately shaped objects across various fields. SLA printing has demonstrated efficacy in manufacturing 3D ceramic components with desirable mechanical properties and 3D polymer parts in the biomedical device sector. Complex shapes can be attained by incorporating ceramic powder suspensions into the photopolymer and subsequently laser polymerizing the ceramic-resin mixture (Hull CW (1986)) (Fig. 1).

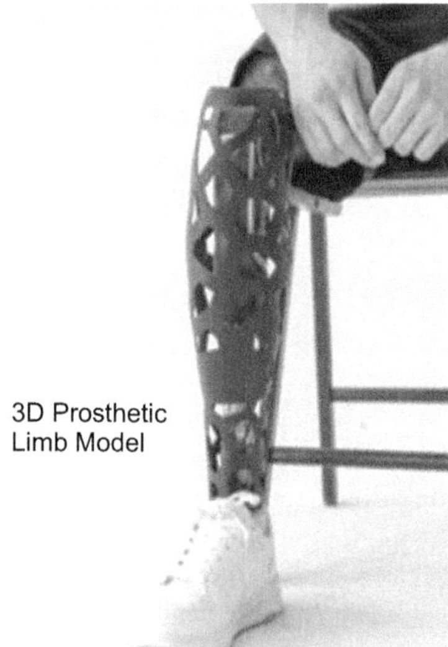

Fig. 1 3D Printing of Prosthetic limb

3.2 *Digital Light Processing (DLP)*

DLP and SLA technologies exhibit notable similarities, with their primary distinction lying in the light source utilized. DLP printing employs a projector positioned at the base of the resin pool instead of an ultraviolet laser, which is characteristic of SLA technology. In SLA, the laser beam scans each layer individually, whereas in DLP, the projector simultaneously illuminates the entire layer surface, leading to expedited print speeds. However, SLA remains preferable for parts demanding high resolution. In DLP, as the projected images of each layer are composed of pixels, small quadratic volumes emerge at the edges of the layers. The resolution of the projector directly impacts print quality and the printable volume in DLP technology (Chaput C, Chartier T (2007)).

3.3 *Binder Jetting*

In this technology, a liquid binding agent is employed to fuse materials together. The binder is applied onto the powdered material, forming a solid layer. Subsequently, the printer platform descends by one layer, and a new layer of powder material is deposited over the previously formed layer. This iterative process continues until the object's production is complete. Metallic, ceramic, and sand materials are compatible with this technology, making it suitable for manufacturing large parts. Unlike some other techniques, this method doesn't involve heating, thereby eliminating dimensional distortions caused by thermal effects. Similar to SLS technology, metal powders can serve as support, obviating the need for additional support structures. Additionally, binder jetting enables the creation of colored parts at a relatively low cost. However, parts produced via metal binder jetting may exhibit high porosity, which can compromise their mechanical properties. Furthermore, compared to alternative 3D printing methods, binder jetting offers a narrower range of compatible materials, constituting a limitation of this technology (Hornbeck LJ (1987)).

3.4   Polyjet

Another 3D printing technology utilized in fabricating objects with photopolymer resin material is PolyJet. Apart from its capacity to produce colored parts, PolyJet boasts of high-speed printing capabilities and can print multiple materials simultaneously. Consequently, it enables the manufacture of single-piece parts with diverse mechanical properties. This technology, renowned for its ability to produce parts with smooth surfaces and intricate geometries, can be seen as a fusion of 2D inkjet and SLA printing technologies. With PolyJet technology, which facilitates the simultaneous use of different materials, support materials can be easily removed, in a water-soluble form included. As a result, the removal of support structures is effortless, leaving no marks or residues on the fabricated part's surface upon completion of the removal process (Hanssen et al, 2014).

3.5   Selective Laser Melting (SLM)

SLM technology closely resembles SLS technology, albeit with a distinct feature: instead of sintering, SLM entails a complete melting process. Widely embraced in the aviation and medical sectors, SLM technology isn't viable for home users due to its high cost. Titanium, renowned for its high biocompatibility and corrosion resistance, finds extensive application in various biomedical fields within SLM technology (Masood S.H. (2014)). In addition to titanium, metals like stainless steel and aluminum can also be employed in SLM. However, materials such as plastic, glass, and ceramics, which are compatible with SLS, are incompatible with SLM. The precise control of the SLM process, which utilizes high-power lasers, presents challenges and necessitates meticulous temperature regulation throughout the operation (Meiners et al, 2001).

3.6   Electron Beam Melting (EBM)

EBM technology operates on the principle of fusing metal powders or filaments within a high-pressure atmosphere using a focused electron beam that generates intense energy and temperature. Geometric data guides the creation of a layer of fused powder, and once the current layer is exposed to the electron beam, the build platform descends. At each iteration, the top of the layer is replenished with metal powders, the fusion process repeats, and new layers are formed. Through the accumulation of these layers, 3D objects are fabricated. In EBM technology, the vacuum environment prevents electron collisions with gas molecules, thereby enhancing the efficiency of reactive metals processing while reducing energy consumption. EBM is highly favored for producing high-strength parts. Residual stresses can be mitigated by preheating the material and print bed, while adjusting beam parameters enables control over part porosity (Cui et al, 2012).

4.   3D Bioprinting

Three-dimensional bioprinting is the adaptation of 3D printing technology for printing living cell tissues, primarily aimed at tissue and organ transplantation in regenerative medicine applications. Thermal inkjet, microextrusion, and laser-assisted printing are the commonly employed technologies for this purpose. The choice of technology depends on factors such as material type, cell viability, and surface resolution, each with its own set of advantages and limitations.

Printers utilizing thermal inkjet technology offer low cost, high resolution, and rapid printing capabilities. However, they require materials to be in liquid form, and their printing density is relatively low. Microextrusion-based printers excel in depositing high cell densities and are commonly used for scaffold-free tissue spheroid bioprinting. Nevertheless, the cell viability ratio, inversely proportional to the applied extrusion pressure, tends to be lower compared to inkjet technology. Ongoing research aims to enhance printing speed and resolution in this technology (Panwar A, Tan LP (2016)).

Laser-assisted printing technology enables printing materials with varying viscosity ranges and eliminates nozzle clogging issues present in other technologies. However, achieving high resolution requires rapid gelation kinetics, posing a challenge for this method.

5.   Applications of 3D Bioprinting in Prosthetic Devices

Millions of people worldwide suffer from birth defects, trauma, or illness that affect their mental well-being, social interactions, professional life, finance, and life quality. Prosthesis revamps the standard of life for most affected people by restoring aesthetics and functions to anatomical parts where plastic surgery is unsuitable and costly. To overcome the issues of conventional fabrication such as lack of attachment, function, robustness, aesthetics, and cost, 3D printing could be a suitable technology to manufacture prosthesis products. However, 3D printing of prosthesis materials is currently in the very early phase of evolution and is facing various challenges, like limited 3D printing of compatible prosthesis materials, issues with printability, defects, and low mechanical strength in the printed parts (Anish Das et al., 2023).

5.1   Traditional Fabrication Process

In the traditional fabrication process, the journey begins with the prosthetist making an impression or "cast" of the residual limb to create an exact replica. This cast is then used by manufacturers to produce custom-molded sockets, tailored to fit each user's unique anatomy and range of motion. The thermoplastic material is heated and molded to conform to the shape of the patient's amputated area, forming the sockets. Once the sockets are ready, they are connected to off-the-shelf components that make up the artificial limbs. These components are designed for easy assembly and adjustment to ensure maximum comfort and functionality for each user. Finally, prosthetists fit the artificial limbs and make any necessary adjustments, including fine-tuning tension, releasing joints, and ensuring proper alignment of all components.

5.2   Digital Fabrication Process

In the realm of digital fabrication, the process begins with the acquisition of patient data, a crucial step. Advanced 3D medical imaging technologies, such as handheld 3D scanners, MRIs, or CT scans, are used to capture detailed anatomical information, laying the groundwork for subsequent phases. This data is then meticulously segmented and converted into digital surface meshes to facilitate downstream design operations. The subsequent phase involves design generation, where the blueprint of the device is created. Depending on the customization strategy, designers may opt for manual designs tailored to individual instances or embrace fully automated methodologies for patient-matched devices. The design process ensures not only functional efficacy but also regulatory compliance. Moving to manufacturing, the envisioned prostheses materialize into tangible form. 3D printing emerges as a versatile tool, enabling direct production of prostheses or, indirectly, through bespoke tooling creation. While direct 3D printing shines in realizing intricate design elements, the indirect route offers scalability advantages, especially in large-scale production scenarios. Regardless of the manufacturing approach, post-processing is crucial to ensure that each prosthesis meets stringent functional and aesthetic standards. Through meticulous attention to detail, the promise of digital fabrication is fully realized, ushering in a new era of personalized healthcare solutions.

5.2.1   Advantages of Digital Fabrication Process

Fully adopting digital fabrication offers numerous advantages in prosthetic component development. By beginning with a scan, providers can customize precise digital models ready for production, saving time and money. 3D printing enables the manufacturing of complex geometries impossible with other technologies, resulting in lower wait times, customized fit, and cost-savings.

Automation streamlines design operations, allowing quick exploration of design space and rapid iteration. Less technically adept users can run automated design processes using patient-specific data, freeing experienced designers for more complex tasks. Lattice structures for 3D-printed foams and data-driven design further enhance customization, comfort, and cost-effectiveness in prosthetics.

6.   3D Printing of Maxillofacial Prosthesis

The 3D printing of prosthesis materials is currently in its nascent stages of development and faces several challenges. These include limitations in the availability of compatible materials for 3D printing, issues related to printability, the occurrence of defects, and the low mechanical strength of printed parts. Conversely, the interface and software required for manufacturing maxillofacial prosthesis products are expensive. Furthermore, the successful implementation of additive manufacturing techniques in prosthesis will enhance its potential in large-scale biomedical applications and scalable customization. Maxillofacial prostheses, as defined by Ackerman in 1953, constitute a subspecialty of "Prosthodentistry" involving artificial substitutes to aid in reconstructing and repairing intraoral and extraoral structures. They serve to enhance appearance, protect defective tissue from the environment, and provide significant psychological benefits by improving patients' quality of life and self-esteem. Maxillofacial reconstruction broadly encompasses two branches: artificial replacements for intraoral structures like the temporomandibular joint (TMJ), maxilla, mandible, palate, tongue, and lips, as well as extraoral structures such as the ear, nose, eye, and other facial parts, tailored to the patient's needs. Prosthetic reconstruction techniques have evolved over centuries since ancient Egyptian civilization, with meticulous records by Ambrose Pare since 1541 detailing the use of handmade facial prostheses crafted from materials such as wood, ivory, and metals. The demand for maxillofacial prostheses surged during and after World War II (D.C. Miglani (1959)).

Materials for maxillofacial prostheses must meet standard criteria, including non-toxicity, biocompatibility, dimensional stability, lightness, low water absorption, color stability, tear strength, and resistance to skin secretions. Currently, polymers such as silicone block copolymers, polyphosphazenes, RTV silicone, polyvinyl chloride, siphenylenes, and polyurethane are commonly employed.

Traditionally, maxillofacial prostheses have been manufactured through subtractive methods like cast sculpture and mold-casting, which are time-consuming and labor-intensive. Computer-aided manufacturing (CAM), including 3-axis and 5-axis computer numerical control (CNC) machines, is used for more intricate designs, albeit at higher costs. However, advancements in biocompatible soft polymeric materials and additive manufacturing technologies, such as 3D printing, present opportunities to revolutionize maxillofacial prosthetics in terms of aesthetics, attachment, function, cost, and robustness. Additive manufacturing allows for the fabrication of precise prostheses, particularly beneficial for complex shapes and sizes of maxillofacial defects. Techniques like stereolithography (SLA), photopolymer jetting, selective laser sintering (SLS), fused deposition modeling (FDM), and liquid deposition modeling (LDM) offer promising avenues. Despite progress, there's a gap between performance needs and material availability, with silicone remaining the primary choice. Exploring new biocompatible materials with required properties is crucial for advancing direct 3D printed maxillofacial prostheses. Prospective solutions are thoroughly examined to inspire further research, potentially benefiting academia and businesses engaged in 3D printing of maxillofacial prosthetics (Goiato, 2014).

7.   Applications in Upper Limb Prosthetics

Upper limb prosthetics are artificial devices designed to restore the functions of missing limbs, enabling amputees to handle and manipulate objects for daily tasks. The mechanical structure, actuation method, sensing capability, and control features are key factors determining the functionality and performance of prosthetic devices. Emerging technologies like 3D printing and other additive manufacturing techniques are enhancing the design and manufacturing aspects of prosthetics. Hetherington and colleagues utilized additive manufacturing technology to design and produce a prosthetic limb. Their mechanically operated prosthetic hand, produced via 3D printing, was controlled by muscle activation recorded from electromyography (EMG) sensors, with actuation stimulated by forearm muscles. These assistive devices, crafted using modern production methods, are typically lightweight, affordable, customizable, and replaceable (Ten Kate et al., 2017).

The lightweight actuators, fabricated using 3D printing, facilitated compliant gripping with acceptable stress levels. Arjun et al. employed 3D printing to manufacture a low-cost, functional prosthetic hand capable of independently manipulating fingers and grasping various objects. This technique reduced the cost of customizable parts, enabling the prosthesis to grasp structures of different shapes such as cubes, spheres, and cylinders, with repeatable grip times and low standard deviations. Prosthetics for children necessitate frequent modifications due to ongoing anthropometric changes. Zuniga et al. developed a 3D-printed prosthetic hand for children with upper limb reductions, named "Cyborg Beast". They reported producing a low-cost prosthetic device that could significantly improve the quality of life for children from low-income, uninsured families (Kim H (2018)).

8.   Dental Indications and Applications of 3D Printing

Additive manufacturing using metal alloys has been successfully used in the dental sector since 2002. The use of laser sintering in the dental field represented a revolution in the processing of non-precious alloys at the time. Laser Sintering of Crowns and Bridges Made from Non-Precious Alloys Laser sintering has now become a standard process for the production of CoCr crowns and bridges. By optimizing post-processing after the actual building process, it is now possible to manufacture absolutely stress-free and accurately fitting non-precious alloy frameworks even for larger bridge spans. The large number of units that can be positioned on a single platform has reduced the production time per unit to a few minutes. The procedure is extremely cost-effective and is well established when it comes to fixed restorations made of non-precious alloys (Schweiger et al., 2021). To generate stress-free restorative frameworks, the build platforms are summarily subjected to a thermal post-treatment in a downstream processing step before the individual restorations are separated from the build platform. Most production centers automate this step. The support structures are then removed by manual finishing.

The physical and mechanical properties of laser-sintered non-precious alloy crown and bridge frameworks are comparable to cast restorations. The rougher surface compared to cast or milled restorations actually has a positive effect on the cementation of laser-sintered crowns and bridges. Inside the crown and at the crown margins, laser-sintered restorations exhibit small but macroscopically visible ledges parallel to the z-axis of the building process. Nevertheless, the fit of laser-sintered crowns is within the clinically acceptable range. Other studies have found that laser-sintered CoCr-alloy crowns have an even better marginal fit than casted CoCr-alloy crowns. Ceramic veneers are very easily applied to laser-sintered frameworks as their rougher surface makes them highly wettable by the opaquer. Direct 3D printing processes (material jetting, MJT) are also used in dental applications. A special process worth mentioning is multi-material 3D printing by Stratasys, which allows different colors and materials with different properties to be processed simultaneously in a single build. Material extrusion (MEX) processes such as fused-filament fabrication (FFF) or fused deposition modeling (FDM) are currently of lesser relevance on the dental market since they require long printing times and are restricted to lower resolutions. Off the technologies mentioned for the plastics sector, SLA, DLP, and MJT appear to be the most interesting from a technical and economic point of view.

Several intraoral 3D scanners now allow the digital capture of shade information in addition to surface data. Using Polyjet technology, it is possible to convert this data into physical models. The pertinent shade information is geometry-related, i.e., the two-dimensional shade information is uniquely assigned to 3D surfaces. Model builder software is used to generate a virtual shade model, which is then converted into a physical shade model using multi-material 3D printing (Polyjet technology; Stratasys, Rheinmünster, Germany). Since the transfer of shade information is not possible with analog impressions, graphic 3D models are a veritable "killer application." Data generation and model production mandate the use of a digital workflow. In the future, new possibilities will emerge here that will be associated with enormous improvements and simplified procedures, especially for highly aesthetic dental restorations (Tregermann et al., 2019). Another possible application of multi-material 3D printing in the dental field could be the fabrication of multi-layered dentures made from different materials. With regard to the identical reproduction of natural teeth by crowns or bridges, this technology is currently in the prototype phase. It is based on the tooth-structure database, according to Schweiger, which allows the multilayer structure of natural teeth to be copied and the data thus generated to be used in an additive manufacturing process. The ultimate aim is to produce biomimetic dental restorations that reflect the multi-layered three-dimensionality as well as the complex mechanical and optical properties of natural teeth. Considering the light-optical properties of the different tooth layers (pulp, dentin, enamel), an identical esthetic reproduction of natural teeth can be achieved (Jokusch J., Öczan M. (2020)).

9.   Patient-specific Facial Prosthesis

Microtia–anotia, a congenital birth deformity affecting approximately one in every 5,000 births worldwide, presents a challenge for affected individuals in terms of both functionality and aesthetics. While surgical reconstruction has been a traditional approach, prosthetic rehabilitation offers a less invasive alternative, particularly beneficial for those without access to surgical facilities or unable to undergo surgery. Anaplastology, the art of making cranio-facial prostheses, has evolved over time, utilizing various materials such as porcelain, polyethylene, wax, rubber, and papier-mâché. However, modern silicones have emerged as a breakthrough material due to their enhanced simulation of skin characteristics, including flexibility, pigmentation, and durability. The fabrication of prosthetics primarily relies on operator-dependent casting methods, which involve considerable labor and skill to achieve the desired outcome, often taking up to 14 hours for an ear prosthesis. Despite the advancements in prosthetic fabrication techniques, there has been relatively little exploration of 3D printing silicones directly for this purpose. While some studies have focused on printing moulds for prosthetic fabrication, the direct printing of silicones remains underexplored. This represents a potential area for innovation, as 3D printing technology continues to advance, offering opportunities for more efficient and customizable prosthetic solutions.

While prosthetic rehabilitation remains a valuable option for individuals with microtia–anotia, there is a need for further research and development in the area of 3D printing silicones for direct prosthetic fabrication. This could lead to improvements in efficiency, customization, and accessibility for individuals seeking prosthetic solutions for this congenital deformity. The prevailing method for producing prostheses involves the indirect mold-cast technique, largely due to the inherent challenges associated with working with highly viscous, non-Newtonian materials like various types of silicone (e.g., UV or thermal cross-linkable). These materials pose difficulties for many additive manufacturing techniques. For instance, SLA printers typically encounter maximum viscosities in the range of 300–5,000 mPa.s, while drop-on-demand inkjet printing operates within 10–100 mPa.s. However, extrusion-based dispensing has shown promise in handling materials with viscosities beyond these ranges.

Recent studies have explored 3D printing approaches for the aesthetic reconstruction of microtia, discussing direct printing of materials. For instance, researchers investigated the utilization of commercially available equipment (Connex 3500) and their proprietary material, Tango Plus (non-silicone), to produce a 3D printed ear from CT scans. Meanwhile, Picsima proposed a system capable of printing silicone, albeit requiring complex printing within a bath composed of silicone oil and a cross-linker, with Cartesian controlled extrusion of a catalyst and subsequent post-cleaning steps. Despite these advancements, there are no reported studies in the literature involving direct, free-standing 3D printing of silicone ear shapes using micro-extrusion techniques. The closest study involving PDMS and micro-extrusions for printing ears was conducted by Mannoor et al., but it was aimed at tissue engineering rather than prosthetics. Before employing 3D printing for prostheses, it's crucial to capture the necessary data to create the customized structure. Reviews of 3D scanning technologies have predominantly focused on sophisticated instruments available in centralized facilities, such as CT or MRI. However, access to this equipment, along with trained personnel and processing software, is prohibitively expensive. Recently, handheld scanners have emerged as a more affordable and portable alternative, ranging in price from $25,000 to $100,000, offering a solution for 3D imaging in regions where MRI or CT technologies may not be available.

While there have been reports of using conventional 3D printers for facial prostheses, primarily focusing on casting and molding approaches or utilizing different materials like wax, there hasn't been a reported study proposing an approach capable of 3D printing free-standing silicone-based complex structures, particularly ear shapes, via micro-extrusion in a cost-effective and portable manner.

10.   3D Printing an Ear Shape

The process began with the utilization of Matter Control software to fine-tune the printing parameters and meticulously slice the captured ear STL file. Recognizing the intricate curvatures and overhangs inherent in the ear model, support material, namely Vaseline or Petroleum Jelly, was strategically employed to fortify the structural integrity of the printed part. Simultaneously, the printer's three UV LEDs were engaged throughout the entirety of the printing process, ensuring continuous exposure to radiation. Following completion of the printing process, an additional 5-minute exposure to UV radiation was administered to ensure thorough cross-linking of the top layers. Subsequently, the support material was meticulously removed, and the part was delicately cleansed with soap and water to eliminate any residual Vaseline. To ascertain print accuracy, various sections of the 3D printed ear were meticulously examined under a microscope and meticulously compared with the original STL file. Leveraging the microscope's sophisticated software toolkit, measurements encompassing total dimensions, line spacing, strut size, and layer height were meticulously conducted. The resulting measurements of the printed ear part closely paralleled those of the original ear STL model. Any minor deviations observed could be attributed to variations in infill density within the printed ears. Altering infill density invariably affects line spacing, thereby potentially influencing geometric fidelity and spatial resolution due to increased diffusion between adjacent layers (Abdullah et al., 2019).

Microscopic analysis of the printed ear further unveiled the layer height of these intricate structures (measuring 0.58 ± 0.1 mm) in comparison to the preset printing value in the software (0.5 mm). This variance may be attributed to a multitude of factors including layer diffusion, die swelling of the PDMS during extrusion, and nozzle movement speed during printing. While concerted efforts were undertaken to optimize the 3D printing procedure to minimize defects and die swelling, a degree of swelling (characterized by an increase in the diameter of extruded struts due to material elasticity) remains inherent during the printing process. Overall, the printed ear exhibited striking similarity to the original STL model, with the printer adeptly capturing the intricate overhanging areas and curvatures. This success can be largely attributed to the meticulous adherence to optimized printing conditions and the meticulous inspection under a microscope for any potential defects. Notably, no discernible structural defects were identified throughout the examination process. One of the primary advantages of the developed solution is its portability and cost effectiveness. The developed printer is very compact and capable of being transported to a number of locations including within clinical environments and/or developing regions. This has the capacity to impact regions without access to centralized healthcare facilities to develop patient-specific prosthesis. The cost effectiveness of this printer is relatively high, and as a mobile platform it can immediately impact developing regions, allowing for mobile clinics to access it cheaply and quickly.

There are a number of other opportunities to examine. Considering that medical grade silicones are available for printing, other supracutaneous craniofacial prosthesis/structures that currently require ad hoc manufacturing are targeted for investigation, e.g. nose. Moreover, flexible subdermal structures required as a result of physical trauma or congenital disfigurement will be considered. In order for a prosthesis to successfully alleviate the emotional suffering of patients, it must be realistic in appearance. On that basis, another avenue for progression will be in the automatic coloring of the silicone during printing. Printing in the natural pigmentation color of a patient's skin is an important feature to possess for future consideration. Facial prostheses are required to possess good mechanical properties and high durability as they are subjected to tension by the users during daily care activities. Therefore, investigating the mechanical properties of fabricated prostheses is of great importance. Compression of the 3D printed ear in cycles can mimic the tensions applied to the ear by the users in real life conditions. In this work, we subjected the 3D printed ear to 100 cycles of a cyclic compression test with up to 70% strain. The ear showed a very negligible deformation after 100 cycles of compression, indicating that the 3D printed ear has a very low defect and a very high durability. Other mechanical properties tests such as impact and indentation tests can provide more information in this regard. Having appropriate viscosity and elasticity is a necessity for printing ink to ensure fabricating high-resolution structures. Materials with low viscosity cannot hold their shape after printing, while high viscous materials are hard to extrude. They have demonstrated the viscosity, elasticity, and shear thinning behavior of the ink can be tailored through utilizing a small amount of a silicone thickener to make the ink more suitable for printing high-resolution structures. Further optimization of the rheological properties of the ink should lead to higher fidelity printing.

There are several additional avenues for exploration within the realm of 3D printing for craniofacial prostheses and structures. One such area of interest involves leveraging medical-grade silicones for printing other supracutaneous craniofacial prostheses or structures that currently require ad hoc manufacturing, such as the nose. Furthermore, there is potential to explore the fabrication of flexible subdermal structures needed for addressing physical trauma or congenital disfigurement. It's crucial to recognize that for a prosthesis to effectively alleviate the emotional distress of patients, it must possess a realistic appearance. Therefore, one avenue for advancement lies in developing techniques for automatic coloring of silicone during the printing process, which could enable printing in the natural pigmentation color of a patient's skin.

Facial prostheses must also exhibit robust mechanical properties and high durability, as they are subjected to tension by users during daily use. Consequently, investigating the mechanical properties of fabricated prostheses is paramount. For instance, subjecting 3D printed ears to cyclic compression tests can mimic the tensions applied in real-life conditions. In the study, the 3D printed ear endured 100 cycles of cyclic compression with up to 70% strain, exhibiting minimal deformation. This suggests the 3D printed ear possesses low defects and high durability, indicating its suitability for facial prostheses fabrication. Further mechanical properties testing, such as impact and indentation tests, could provide additional insights. Ensuring the appropriate viscosity and elasticity of printing ink is imperative for fabricating high-resolution structures. Materials with low viscosity may struggle to maintain their shape post-printing, while highly viscous materials may pose challenges during extrusion (Abdullah et al., 2019).

11. Challenges and Future Directions

The future of 3D printing in prosthetics holds significant promise, but it also faces several challenges that need to be addressed for its widespread adoption and effectiveness. Let's delve into both aspects:

11.1   Customization and Personalization

3D printing enables the creation of prosthetic devices tailored to the unique anatomical features and functional requirements of each individual. This customization can lead to improved comfort, fit, and functionality, enhancing the overall quality of life for prosthetic users.

11.2   Complex Geometries and Design Flexibility

Additive manufacturing allows for the fabrication of prosthetic components with intricate geometries that are difficult or impossible to achieve using traditional manufacturing methods. This opens up possibilities for more ergonomic designs and innovative solutions to address specific challenges faced by prosthetic users.

11.3   Rapid Prototyping and Iteration

3D printing enables rapid prototyping and iteration of prosthetic designs, reducing the time and cost associated with traditional manufacturing processes. This facilitates quicker development cycles and allows for more efficient customization and optimization of prosthetic devices.

Integration of Advanced Materials: Advances in material science are expanding the range of materials available for 3D printing, including biocompatible polymers, metals, and composite materials. These materials offer improved durability, strength, and functionality, enhancing the performance and longevity of prosthetic devices.

11.4   Incorporation of Sensing and Feedback Systems

Integrating sensors and feedback systems into 3D printed prosthetic devices can provide real-time data on pressure, movement, and other parameters, allowing for more precise control and functionality. This can lead to prosthetic devices that respond more accurately to the user's intentions and provide a more natural and intuitive user experience.

11.5   Challenges

Material Properties and Biocompatibility: While there have been significant advancements in materials for 3D printing, ensuring that these materials are biocompatible, durable, and suitable for long-term use in prosthetic devices remains a challenge. Further research is needed to develop materials that meet the stringent requirements of prosthetic applications.

11.6   Quality and Consistency

Maintaining consistent quality and reliability in 3D printed prosthetic devices is essential for ensuring patient safety and satisfaction. Issues such as surface finish, dimensional accuracy, and structural integrity need to be addressed to achieve consistent results across different manufacturing processes and settings.

11.7   Regulatory and Standardization Issues

The regulatory landscape for 3D printed medical devices, including prosthetics, is still evolving, and there is a lack of standardized testing protocols and quality assurance guidelines specific to additive manufacturing. Clear regulatory pathways and industry standards are needed to ensure the safety and efficacy of 3D printed prosthetic devices.

11.8   Cost and Accessibility

While 3D printing has the potential to reduce costs and increase accessibility to prosthetic devices, initial investment in equipment and materials can be prohibitive for some healthcare providers and patients. Efforts to lower the cost of 3D printing technology and materials, as well as expand access to training and education, are needed to realize the full potential of additive manufacturing in prosthetics.

11.9 Education and Training

Healthcare professionals, including prosthetists and orthotists, require specialized training and expertise to effectively utilize 3D printing technology in prosthetics. There is a need for comprehensive education and training programs to ensure that healthcare providers have the knowledge and skills necessary to leverage 3D printing for the benefit of prosthetic users.

In conclusion, while the future of 3D printing in prosthetics holds immense potential to revolutionize the field and improve outcomes for prosthetic users, addressing the challenges outlined above will be essential to realize this potential fully. Continued research, innovation, collaboration, and investment are needed to overcome these challenges and drive forward the adoption and advancement of 3D printing in prosthetics.

References

Abdullah A., Mohamad D., Din T., Yahya S., Akil H., Rajion Z. (2019). Fabrication of nasal prosthesis utilizing an affordable 3d printer. Int J Adv Manuf Technol 100(5–8):1907–1912.

Anish Das, Pratiksha Awasthi, Veena Jain, Shib Shankar Banerjee, (2023). 3D printing of maxillofacial prosthesis materials: Challenges and opportunities, Bioprinting, Volume 32, e00282, ISSN 2405-8866.

Chaput C., Chartier T. (2007). Fabrication of ceramics by stereolithography. RTejournal-Forumfür Rapid Technologie 4(1).

Cui X., Boland T., DD'Lima D., Lotz M. (2012). Thermal inkjet printing in tissue engineering and regenerative medicine. Recent Pat Drug Deliv Formulation 6(2):149–155.

D.C. Miglani. (1959). Maxillofacial prosthesis and its role as a healing art, J. Prosthet. Dent.

Dombroski C.E., Balsdon M.E., Froats A. (2014). The use of a low-cost 3D scanning and printingtool in the manufacture of custom-made foot orthoses: a preliminary study. BMC Res Notes 7(1): 443.

Elmansy R. (2015). Designing the 3D Printed prosthetic hand. Des. Manag. Rev. 26:24–31.

Fay, C.D., Jeiranikhameneh, A., Sayyar, S. (2022). Development of a customised 3D printer as a potential tool for direct printing of patient-specific facial prosthesis. Int J Adv Manuf Technol 120, 7143–7155 https://doi.org/10.1007/s00170-022-09194-0.

Frontera W.R., Silver J.K. (2004). Fondamenti di Medicina Fisica e Riabilitativa. Verduci; Rome, Italy.

Hanssen J., Moe Z.H., Tan D., Chien O.Y. (2013). Rapid prototyping in manufacturing. In:Handbook of manufacturing engineering and technology, pp 1–16.

Hornbeck L.J. (1987). Spatial light modulator and method, 5 May. U.S. Patent No. 4,662,746.

Hull C.W. (1986). Apparatus for production of three-dimensional objects by stereolithography, 11 Mar. U.S. Patent No. 4,575,330.

Jokusch J., Öczan M. (2020). Additive manufacturing of dental polymers: An overview on processes, materials and applications. Dent. Mater. J;39:345–354.

Kim H. (2018). Market analysis and the future of sustainable design using 3D printing technology. Arch Des Res 31: 23–35.

M.C. Goiato, (2014). Implants in the zygomatic bone for maxillary prosthetic rehabilitation: a systematic review, Int. J. Oral Maxillofac. Surg.

Manero, A., Smith, P., Sparkman, J., Dombrowski, M., Courbin, D. et al. (2019). Implementation of 3D Printing Technology in the Field of Prosthetics: Past, Present, and Future. International journal of environmental research and public health, 16(9), 1641.

Masood S.H. (2014). Advances in fused deposition modeling. In: Comprehensive materials processing, pp 69–91.

Meiners W., Wissenbach K., Gasser A. (2001). Selective laser sintering at melting temperature,10 Apr. U.S. Patent No. 6,215,093.

Miglani, D.C. and Drane, J.B. (1959). Maxillofacial prosthesis and its role as a healing art. The Journal of Prosthetic Dentistry, 9(1), 159–168.

Norton K. (2007). A brief history of prosthetics. InMotion. 17: 11–13.

Panwar A., Tan L.P. (2016). Current status of bioinks for micro-extrusion-based 3D bioprinting. Molecules 21(6): 685.

Schweiger, J., Edelhoff, D. and Güth, J.F. (2021). 3D Printing in Digital Prosthetic Dentistry: An Overview of Recent Developments in Additive Manufacturing. Journal of clinical medicine, 10(9).

Surmen, Hasan and Ortes, Faruk and Arslan, Yunus Ziya, et al. (2020). Fundamentals of 3D Printing and Its Applications in Biomedical Engineering. 10.1007/978-981-15-5424-7_2.

Ten Kate J., Smit G., Breedveld P. (2017). 3D printed upper limb prostheses: a review. Disabil Rehabil Assistive Technol 12(3): 300–314.

Tregermann I., Renne W., Kelly A., Wilson D. (2019). Evaluation of removable partial denture frameworks fabricated using 3 differnet techniques. J. Prosthet. Dent; 122: 390–395.

Zuo K.J., Olson J.L. (2014). The evolution of functional hand replacement: From iron prostheses to hand transplantation. Plast. Surg. 22: 44–51.

3D Printing in Medicine

Thamizharasan Sampath,[1]
Prakash Srinivasan Timiri Shanmugam,[2*]
Sandhiya Thamizharasan[3] *and Krithaksha V*[4]

1. Introduction

In the ever-evolving landscape of healthcare, the integration of advanced technologies has become a catalyst for unprecedented innovation. Among these technological marvels, 3D printing stands out as a transformative force, offering novel solutions and redefining the way medical professionals approach patient care. 3D printing, also known as additive manufacturing, enables the creation of three-dimensional objects layer by layer from digital models. Its applications in medicine have become increasingly diverse and influential, touching various facets of patient diagnosis, treatment planning, and therapeutic interventions. One of the key strengths lies in the ability to produce highly detailed and patient-specific anatomical models, providing clinicians with invaluable tools for surgical preparation and training. This technology can be used to replace human organ transplants, speed up surgical procedures, produce cheaper versions of required surgical tools, and improve the lives of those reliant on prosthetic limbs (Paul et al., 2018).

3D printing in medicine encompasses a spectrum of groundbreaking applications. From the production of intricate models for surgical rehearsal to the customization of implants and prosthetics tailored to individual patients. In the field of bioprinting, where the possibility of constructing living tissues and organs holds promise for regenerative medicine and organ transplantation. Beyond its technical capabilities, 3D printing in medicine has the potential to democratize innovation, empowering healthcare professionals with tools to address unique patient needs. However, the integration of such cutting-edge technology into established medical practices is not without challenges. Ethical considerations, regulatory frameworks, and the need for standardization pose critical questions that demand careful reflection (Arslan-Yildiz A et al., 2016).

[1] Department of Pharmacology & Toxicology, VMCGH, Dr. YRS University of Health Sciences, Kurnool, India.
[2] Global Product Safety & Toxicology, Avanos medical Inc, Alpharetta, USA.
[3] The Tooth Doctor, Advanced Implant Centre, Vellapanchavadi, India.
[4] Georgian National University SEU, Tbilisi, U.S.A.
* Corresponding author: thamizhpharma@gmail.com

2. 3D Printing in Radiology

Magnetic resonance imaging (MRI) and ultrasound (US) are the first lines of investigation for the diagnosis and monitoring of pelvic pathologies. MRI and US are also used for pre-surgical planning of complex cases because they help a surgeon to visualize the patient's anatomy, and location and extent of the disease. Using medical imaging for pre-surgical planning of complex cases has been shown to reduce surgical complications and improve patient outcomes. However, for surgeons not experienced in reading 2D medical images, such as MRI and US, it can be difficult to appreciate complex anatomical structures and pathology in a way that can be applied to surgery (Silvina Zabala-Travers. (2021)). Recent technological advancements in imaging have made it possible to generate three-dimensional (3D) constructs from two-dimensional (2D) images. By using specialized software, 2D medical images such as MRI, can be converted to 3D digital models. Rendering of 2D images to 3D digital models has been shown to significantly improve anatomical comprehension by providing more accurate assessments of anatomical volumes, better perspective of structural orientations relative to adjacent structures, and improved visualization as transparency and colors can be modified to suit the user's needs.

Furthermore, these 3D digital models can be converted into tangible, physical models by way of 3D printing. Rather than 3D visualization where a volumetric model is viewed on a 2D computer screen, a 3D printed model can provide a real indication of depth and tactile feedback, thus allowing surgeons to develop a clearer understanding of surgical anatomy. With a better visualization of disease location relative to adjacent organs, surgeons utilizing 3D printed models for pre-operative planning have been shown to have greater surgical outcomes including, decreased operative time, blood loss, and incision length (Fletcher J, Miskovic D. (2021)).

3. Patient-Specific 3D Printing

The clinical benefits of using patient-specific 3D printed models for pre-surgical planning has been highlighted in the fields of orthopedics, cardiothoracic, and neurosurgery. In order to produce a patient specific and anatomically accurate 3D printed model, a high-resolution volumetric dataset is first required. Such datasets are typically stored as Digital Imaging and Communications in Medicine (DICOM) files. These files contain information about the medical image such as modality (type of imaging), contrast/gray values (in the form of 2D or 3D matrices), spacing between slices, spatial resolution, and anatomical orientation. Volumetric DICOM data can be acquired from MRI, US, or computed tomography (CT). From this, a labeling process called segmentation is used to identify and isolate anatomy of interest. Segmentation can be done automatically using algorithms such as thresholding, edge detection, and region growth, or manually by essentially tracing anatomy of interest on each image slice. Most often, segmentation requires a semi-automatic approach whereby a combination of algorithms is used and manually verified. Unfortunately, a reliance on manual or semi-automatic segmentation requires expertise and a significant time commitment on the part of the user (Kamio T et al., 2020).

4. 3D Printing in Gynecology

In the realm of gynecology, the integration of 3D printing technology with Magnetic Resonance Imaging (MRI) has paved the way for advanced visualization and understanding of intricate anatomical structures.

4.1 *Image Acquisition and Export*

De-identified cross-sectional MRI images post gadolinium, supplemented by additional 2 mm T2 weighted isometric sequenced images specifically acquired for 3D printing purposes, serve as the foundation for this transformative process. The images are exported in DICOM format, ensuring compatibility for further processing. Utilizing Materialize Mimics 20.0 software, a renowned tool in the field, the segmentation process unfolds under the meticulous supervision of trained radiologists. Employing a combination of signal thresholding, region growth, and mask splitting algorithms, basic masks of the relevant gynecologic structures and patient anatomy are created. Manual slice edits with interpolation, guaranteeing the accuracy of the masks. Once segmentation is complete, the 2D images metamorphose into 3D objects, resulting in a comprehensive 3D digital model. Given the nature of multi-organ segmentation, each anatomical structure of interest becomes a distinct 3D object. Subsequently, each object is exported to a separate STL file for further processing (Cooke, C.M. et al., 2023).

4.2   CAD Preparation for 3D Printing

The exported 3D objects undergo meticulous preparation in the computer-aided design (CAD) software 3-Matic from Materialize. Here, various operations such as wrapping, smoothing, and boolean operations (union, subtraction, and intersection) are performed. The boolean subtraction operation, in particular, plays a pivotal role in eliminating intersecting geometry among multiple 3D objects. This ensures the creation of cavities or negative spaces, such as removing the endometrial model from the uterus, preventing unwanted overlapped material deposition during the subsequent multi-material 3D printing process. The fusion of advanced imaging techniques with cutting-edge 3D printing technology in gynecology offers unprecedented insights into the intricacies of anatomical structures, thereby contributing to enhanced diagnostic and therapeutic approaches (Petric P. et al., 2019).

5.   3D Printing in Surgery

Uterine fibroids, prevalent gynecological tumors affecting up to 80% of women globally by age 50, present substantial challenges due to their symptomatic nature. While benign, nearly half of these women experience a significant impact on their quality of life, including heavy menstrual bleeding, dysmenorrhea, chronic pelvic pain, organ obstructions, bulk symptoms, and infertility, necessitating intervention. Best practice guidelines recommend conservative approaches for women wishing to preserve their uterus and fertility, encompassing medical, surgical, or interventional methods. Myomectomy, the surgical removal of fibroids, is a common approach, but complications can arise in 2–35% of cases due to the extent and complexity of the disease, leading to persistent symptoms and additional surgeries (Flaxman T.E. et al., 2021).

5.1   Leveraging 3D Printing for Surgical Planning

The integration of 3D printing as a complementary tool for myomectomy or hysterectomy planning in uterine fibroids has emerged as a novel approach beyond traditional 2D imaging. 3D printed models assist surgeons in assessing the relationship between uterine fibroids and surrounding anatomical structures, optimizing excisional courses. This additional knowledge minimizes surgical time, perceived blood loss, and helps preserve the integrity of the endometrial lining.

5.2   Improving Surgical Efficiency and Accuracy

3D rendered images significantly reduce the time required for pre-surgical planning and enhance the surgeon's accuracy in assessing disease complexity. Positive experiences have been reported in using 3D models for pre-surgical planning and patient education, particularly in cases of endometrial cancer requiring hysterectomy and complex cesarean deliveries with multiple fibroids.

5.3 Enhancing Visualization in Complex Cases

Patient-specific anatomical 3D printed models have the potential to improve a gynecologic surgeon's ability to prepare for highly complex surgical cases involving severe endometriosis. These models aid in visualizing patient-specific anatomy, the location and extent of endometriotic nodules, and suspicion for intraoperative complications, ultimately optimizing intra-operative performance and minimizing surgical complications.

5.4 Extending Utility to Various Gynecologic Surgeries

Beyond uterine fibroids, 3D printed models have demonstrated utility in multiple obstetrical and gynecologic surgeries, including cases of placenta accreta spectrum and urogynecology procedures. These models improve visualization of maternal, placental, and fetal anatomy, contributing to the development of appropriate multidisciplinary surgical teams and minimizing maternal and neonatal morbidity and mortality.

5.5 Applications in Patient Education and Surgical Training

3D printed models play a crucial role in patient education, providing a tangible understanding of pathology, surgical procedures, and potential complications. Additionally, these models benefit surgical trainees, offering opportunities for learning patient-specific anatomy, practicing surgical techniques, and simulating procedures outside the operating room.

5.6 The Future of Gynecologic Surgery

To minimize the risk of surgical complications and optimize patient outcomes, the integration of 3D printing in gynecologic surgery holds the potential to revolutionize surgical planning. By providing a three-dimensional understanding of patient-specific anatomy, 3D printing emerges as a valuable tool in achieving precision, minimizing complications, and ensuring the success of gynecologic interventions. The development of a 3D tool reflects the adage that "most surgery is done in your head," empowering surgeons to mentally rehearse their approach before making an incision (Semeniuk O et al., 2021).

6. 3D Printing Technology in Drug Delivery

3D printing technology has been explored to design different drug delivery systems by fabricating unique, novel, and specific geometries tuned with tailored drug release characteristics to achieve customized drug delivery profiles. 3D printing technology has been employed as an emerging tool to deliver API in different dosage forms as immediate-release tablets, sustained-release tablets, modified-release tablets, immediate-release films, pulsatile release capsular devices, controlled-release implants and controlled release transdermal patches. The 3D printing technology approach has been used for the delivery of both hydrophilic and lipophilic drugs. BCS class II and class IV drugs are also fabricated to improve the solubility and bioavailability profiles of these drugs via 3D printing technology (Abdul Aleem Mohammed, 2021).

6.1 Solid Oral Dosage Forms

3D printing technology has proven promising in the development of solid oral dosage forms. This technology allows the production of novel formulations that overcome many limitations associated with conventional drug manufacturing methods. 3D printing has the potential to develop different sizes and complicated shapes with tuned release characteristics to fulfill the demand for personalized medications. Among the 3D printing techniques, extrusion-based techniques are utilized the most in the development of oral dosage forms. The oral drug delivery approaches produced by 3D printing techniques have tuned the drug release characteristics of the API's according to patients' needs which led to the development of immediate-release systems, delayed-release systems, polypills containing a complete dosage regimen for a diabetic or hypertensive patient in a single pill, and gastro-retentive drug delivery systems. Oral dosage forms are the most convenient route to deliver API and have more patient compliance compared to the other route of administration. Great advances in the conventional manufacturing of oral dosage and a large library of excipients offer a versatile platform for drug delivery. However, the limited geometry and shapes that can be produced by conventional manufacturing have limited the flexibility of this technology. The principle underlying 3D printing, layer by layer formation, allows flexibility to produce geometric dimensions that cannot be produced by conventional methods.

With an approach to compare the conventional manufacturing method with 3D printing techniques, researchers developed an oral tablet by three different manufacturing techniques i.e. direct compression (DC), fused deposition modeling (FDM), and injection modeling (IM). The tablets were prepared with the same composition and are of the same dimensions. The physical and drug release characteristics of the tablets prepared by three different techniques showed a statistical variation. The drug release profile of the tablet prepared by direct compression (DC) method was immediate whereas the tablet prepared by injection modeling (IM) exhibited a sustained release profile for 48 h and similarly the tablet prepared by fused deposition modeling (FDM) exhibited both immediate and sustained release characteristics based on printing parameters. This concept provides evidence that 3D printing techniques have the capability to alter the drug release characteristics (Algathani et al., 2018).

6.2 Personalized Drug Delivery Devices

In another approach of delivering two different drugs in a single system to provide a time-delayed drug release profile, researchers developed a capsular device with two compartments, known as the modular Super-H capsule and can capsule. Dronedarone hydrochloride and ascorbic acid were used as the model drugs, and PVA was used to prepare the filament by using the FDM method (Fig. 1).

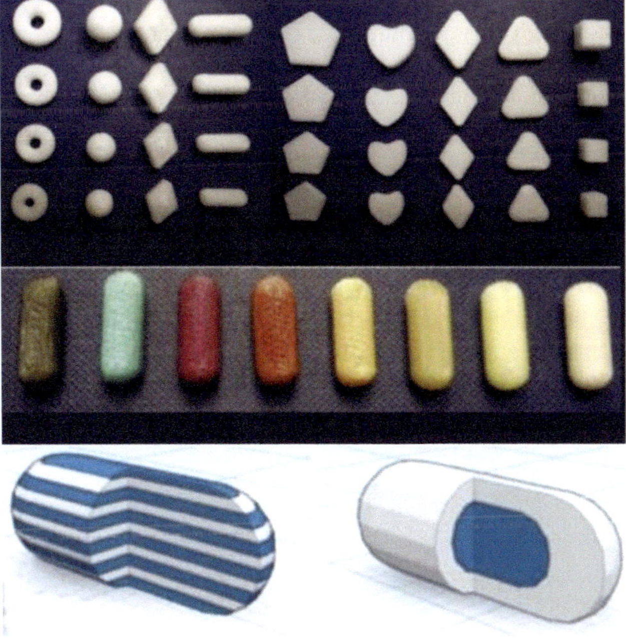

Fig. 1   Images of various tablets prepared by FDM technology.

The capsular device was developed with varying layer thicknesses. In vitro studies revealed that the Super-H capsule lag time in an acidic media depends on membrane thickness. The capsule demonstrated gastric resistance in acidic media for 2 hours and released the drug in alkaline media i.e. in the small intestine. This approach provides evidence that the 3D printing technique can be utilized to develop personalized drug delivery devices by encapsulating different drugs with delayed release profiles.

6.3   Transdermal Drug Delivery

The 3D printing technique has been focused on as a potential approach for transdermal drug delivery through the fabrication of complex and customized geometries for pharmaceutical drug products and medical devices. It has been successfully demonstrated in various transdermal formulation approaches, such as implants, micro-needles, masks, and patches, for the local and systemic delivery of API according to the patient's needs. An implant that can be administered to a specific application site can have its geometry tuned according to the application site using a 3D printing technique. This work demonstrated the formulation of an implant by using fluorescent dye quinine as a model drug. The method used to fabricate this implant was the extrusion-based FDM technique coupled with hot-melt extrusion of different polymers to form a drug-loaded filament. The polymers used in this method are polycaprolactone (PCL), Eudragit®RS, and ethyl cellulose (EC). The printed implant model was a hollow cylinder. The fluorescent dye quinine distribution was able to visualize the filament and implants. The results of this study showed the fastest drug release of 76% within 51 days from PCL implants, whereas only 5% drug release was achieved through Eudragit® RS and ethyl cellulose (EC) in 78 and 100 days, respectively[12]. In a similar approach, researchers developed a patient-tailored wound dressing nose and ear-shaped masks by employing FDM based 3D printing technique. In this approach zinc, silver, and copper metals were used as an antimicrobial agent. The Advantage of this approach was fixed adherence to custom-made wound dressings at the site of the application when compared with normal flat dressings. The PCL fabricated masks with silver and copper showed enhanced antimicrobial treatment.

7.   Respiratory Disease Treatment

3D printing (Haque, S. et al., 2018) as an emerging technology is used to treat respiratory diseases by fabricating 3D printed medical devices and models. 3D printed prototypes of lungs help the medical specialist to better understand the diseased condition and potentially provide a means to diagnose and treat respiratory organ diseases. These approaches will further aid in developing personalized inhaled medicines by using 3D printing techniques. The use of 3D printing in pulmonary treatment is demonstrated by Morrison et al., who fabricated 3D printed bioresorbable airway splints for the treatment of tracheobronchomalacia in pediatric patients. The 3D printed airway splints were found to be an effective alternative to reduce airway collapse in patients and provide a root map by fabricating customized devices for the treatment of life-threatening diseases. 3D printing technique also provides advancement in the development of medical devices for the treatment of asthma and breathing problems. A "sneezometer" was fabricated by using 3D printing technology by a group of researchers which measures the airflow and sneeze speed. This device is more precise and faster than a conventional spirometer. This device determines the airflow rate in patients suffering from asthma and other breathing problems and provides a means for better treatment by fabricating advanced design inhalers by using 3D printing technology. A 3D printed ergonomic and friendly asthma inhaler was designed which is an effective assistive solution to improve the usage of the inhaler devices by people suffering from asthma. This 3D printed object is an assistive technology designed to make asthma treatment more effective, convenient, and friendly by improving the ergonomy of any standard asthma inhaler available on the market (S. Kimura, et al., 2019).

8. Bioprinting and Organ Transplantation

Biomanufacturing of organs/tissues in vitro has been driven by two needs, i.e., organ transplantation and accurate tissue models. Bioprinting, also known as three-dimensional (3D) printing, is a technique used to develop many tissues/organs, such as the liver, skin, and heart. This technique is associated with printing structures using biomaterials, viable cells, and biomolecules. The creation of bioartificial organs has opened new avenues for future organ transplantation programs. The demand for organ transplants has increased rapidly worldwide. Organ transplants are required due to the increased incidence of vital organ failure and the higher success rate of post-transplant outcomes. Globally, a major organ shortage crisis has emerged due to higher demand and insufficient supply of organs for transplant. Owing to this crisis, the number of patients on transplant waiting lists is growing rapidly. Thousands of patients are deprived of a better quality of life due to the organ shortage crisis. It has also increased the cost of their medical care, such as dialysis. Several measures have been implemented to highlight the benefits of organ donation, including increased awareness through educational programs for the public and hospital staff. Although there is an increase in general willingness to donate organs, it is often not executed by family members due to varied reasons, such as the lack of prompt decision-making ability and emotional state (Ricci G et al., 2023).

8.1 Principles and Challenges

3D bioprinting is an extended application of additive manufacturing (AM) that involves the development of tissues or organs layer-by-layer. This is a versatile technique that uses a bottom-up approach. Bioprinting aims to mimic the natural cellular microstructure by depositing biomaterial and viable cells precisely. The newly developed organ/tissue by 3D printing looks and performs similarly to the complex natural organ/tissue. 3D bioprinting is based on three fundamental approaches: biomimicry, autonomous self-assembly, and mini-tissue building blocks. 3D bioprinting technology encounters multiple challenges that include gas and nutrient exchange, biocompatibility and biodegradability of the materials used as a substrate, tissue vascularization, shape-fidelity, and restoration of complex functionality of the printed tissue.

8.2 Steps and Concepts

3D bioprinting applies the concept of biomimicry or biomimetics, which is the process of studying nature to stimulate optimal solutions to human problems. In the 3D bioprinting process, the concept of biomimicry is used to choose cells based on an in depth understanding of the physiology and functions of different cells. These cells would be deposited on a substrate, layer-by-layer, to develop an organ with similar functions and properties. Autonomous self-assembly is a process that replicates a specific organ/tissue in vitro. This step is similar to embryonic organ development. In a developing tissue, early cellular components synthesize extracellular matrix components and cell signals that promote autonomous cellular organization and patterning of the desirable tissue/organ. The success of this step is strongly dependent on understanding the mechanism associated with embryonic organogenesis. Furthermore, it is crucial to identify and apply the parameters essential to regulate the embryonic mechanisms.

Materials play a crucial role in cell attachment. Cell type, size, and shape are essential features to regulate cell differentiation and proliferation in a scaffold. Nanoscale features that include ridges and grooves influence cellular attachment and cytoskeletal assembly. A scaffold, a highly porous 3D substrate, is the most essential component of tissue engineering. Cells grown in a culture medium are transferred to the scaffold. Subsequently, it adheres, proliferates, and produces an extracellular matrix of structural and functional saccharides and proteins that create living tissue. The biological properties of cells are modified and regulated based on the scaffolding material and its internal microstructure. 3D bioprinting techniques used in the creation of bioartificial organs. Different types of 3D bioprinting techniques and strategies are used to develop bioartificial organs. Some of the common techniques are discussed below:

8.3   *Bio-ink-based 3D Bioprinting*

As the name suggests, this 3D printing technique is based on bioink, a low-viscosity suspension biomaterial comprising viable cells. Bioink can be deposited on a "bio-paper" made of hydrogel substrate, a polymer construct, or a culture dish. This is a non-contact printing approach, which allows printing in a digitally controlled pattern. Ink-jet printing is conducted following any of the two methods, namely, a continuous manner and drop-on-demand (DOD) printing. The main advantage of bioink-based 3D printing is its non-contact nature and cost-effectiveness.

8.4   *Extrusion-based 3D Bioprinting*

This method involves direct ink writing (DIW) or pressure-assisted bioprinting methods. This is a material extrusion process where a nozzle continuously extrudes material to create a 3D architecture layer-by-layer. Optimal DIW material possesses rheological properties that promote bioprinting. Typically, polymer resins are blended with fillers, such as nano-clay or silica particles, to achieve suitable rheological properties.

8.5   *Laser-assisted 3D Bioprinting*

This method, also known as Laser Induced Forward Transfer, involves using a pulsed laser beam to deposit bioink onto the substrate. The use of a laser to deposit cells enables non-contact 3D printing of organs/tissues. The three key elements associated with this strategy are a ribbon coated with bioink, a pulsed laser source, and a substrate on which the bioink is to be deposited.

8.6   *Stereolithographic-based 3D Bioprinting*

This method of 3D printing is based on the height of the design instead of the structure complexity. The stereolithographic bioprinting method utilizes a photo-sensitive heat-curable bio-ink, which is deposited in a plane-by-plane fashion. The ink must have photocurable moieties since light is used as an agent for cross-linking. Common moieties used for photopolymerization of tissue engineering scaffolds are polyethylene glycol (PEG) and its derivatives (Rizzo M.L. et al., 2023).

9.   Biomanufacturing of Organs using Bioprinting Approach

Cardiovascular diseases are the most common cause of death across the world. 3D printing technology has made great progress in enabling heart transplantation, which could be the only option to survive for many patients. At present, 3D bioprinting technologies have been used to develop heart valves. Laser sintering 3D printers are typically used to create heart valve scaffolds and human umbilical cord blood vessel cells are deposited on the scaffold. Living heart tissues have also been developed using the extrusion printing method. Here, primary cardiomyocytes were obtained from young rats' hearts mixed with fibrin-based bioinks.

Recently, researchers have developed a cardiac model using 3D printing technology that mimics the realistic feel, mechanical properties, and elasticity of cardiac tissue (Fig. 2). This structure could be extremely useful for surgical training applications. 3D bioprinting technology has developed complex liver structures with higher cell density. Recently, scientists have bio-manufactured different hepatic tissues and organs based on hepatocytes and gelatin-based hydrogels. Skin is a complex, multi-layered organ, and the largest organ of the human body. It has been successfully regenerated via 3D bioprinting techniques. A large amount of autologous skin has been manufactured and transplanted in patients with extensive skin defects, including individuals with extensive burns or ulcers.

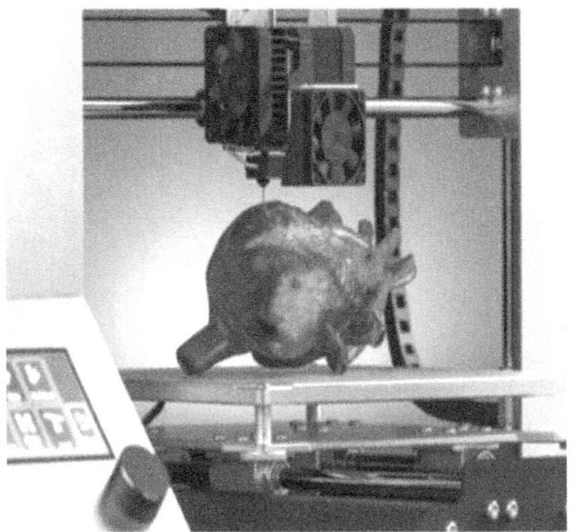

Fig. 2   3D Printing of Human heart model

10. 3D Printing in Dentistry

3D printing, or additive manufacturing (AM), has become a fixture in dental offices and practices around the world. Dental 3D printing creates dental parts for dentists as tools or fixtures to print parts and for patients to use. These parts can range from models of teeth and dental aligners to full sets of dentures. In the past, dental providers used scans, radiology, and teeth molds to obtain accurate images of patients' teeth. These images were then used to construct special, tailored implants for the patient. Now, with 3D printing, dental providers can both create more specialized implants and treat patients more rapidly. 3D printing in dentistry first arose in 1971 as "digital dentistry." In digital dentistry, dental providers use CT scans and other computer-based analyses to diagnose patients and assist in surgery. It wasn't until 1999 that 3D printing, as we know it today, really took hold in dentistry. At that point, it saw its first use in creating custom implants for patients. Today, continued advancements in 3D printing enable both faster turnaround and more accurate dental prints. Dental 3D printing is the use of additive manufacturing to create dental parts such as aligners, dentures, and crowns. To create custom parts that match a patient's anatomy, dental providers use a tool called an intraoral scanner. This creates images of a patient's teeth and records them in the form of a CAD file. Dentists then use this CAD file to create implants or dental molds through 3D printing. In the past, creating dental implants and molds was a cumbersome, invasive, and sometimes uncomfortable procedure. 3D printing has significantly simplified and improved the work of treating patients (3D Printing in Dentistry, (2022)).

Dental 3D printing makes use of all types of AM technology, including digital-light processing (DLP), selective laser melting (SLM), stereolithography (SLA), and selective laser sintering (SLS). 3D printing not only makes life easier for dental providers but also delivers significant benefits to patients: customized, affordable dental solutions (Fig. 3).

10.1 Implants

3D printers with high resolutions and printing accuracy (e.g., SLA and DLP printers) are exceptional at printing complex geometries like those associated with teeth. 3D-printed implants are biocompatible and have similar mechanical properties to human teeth. Additionally, maxillofacial dental implants can be 3D-printed as well. Maxillofacial dentistry is a specialized branch of oral surgery performed to correct injuries and defects of the jaws and mouth.

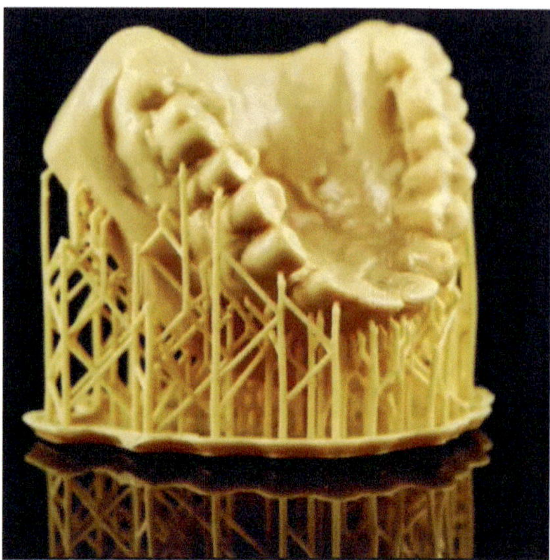

Fig. 3   3D printing of Dental anatomical model

10.2   Crowns and Bridges

Dental 3D printers can create precise crowns and bridges of both fixed and removable varieties. Burn-out resins can be printed to complete a lost-wax casting of a tooth. Patterns and geometries for casting are printed based on the results of an intraoral scanner. Dentists can then use these 3D printed patterns, burn them away, and be left with a cavity to be filled with resin. 3D printing has significantly improved the process to make crowns and bridges.

10.3   Surgical Guides

Dentists can use 3D printers to create surgical guides for drilling and cutting. These guides assist dentists to make surgery easier.

10.4   Anatomical Replicas and Models

Accurate anatomical replicas of a patient's mouth and jaw can be made with 3D printing. This gives the dentist a tangible model that can be seen and touched to better understand a patient's anatomy before beginning treatment. Materials used in dental 3D printing are not the same as those typically used in 3D printing of other industrial products. Dental 3D printing materials are designed specifically for biocompatibility, aesthetics, and safety in dental applications. Certain resins are explicitly used for anatomical models and replicas (referred to as model resins). Others are designed for implants (draft and castable resins). Additionally, there are resins that are used for creating temporary dental appliances, resins that print clearly for use in creating mouth guards, and resins that resemble gingiva for use with dental implants. Depending on the manufacturer, resins can have different chemical compositions. There is no prescribed standard for dental 3D printing materials, however. Dentists usually select the material they think is best for the patient's dental application. If several appropriate choices exist, the dentist may discuss them with the patient.

3D-printed dentures can be worn in the same way as normal dentures. They should be removed and cleaned with a denture cleaner daily. They should also be kept moist in a secured case when not in use. 3D-printed dentures can be expected to last about 5-7 years before possibly needing replacement. The traditional method of making crowns was remarkably slow and costly. 3D printing has enabled the creation of highly accurate crowns in a fraction of the time compared to traditional manufacturing methods. The ability to 3D print crowns saves time and money for dentists, allows for easy customization, and enables the creation of comfortable, long-wearing crowns.

Some 3D-printed crowns are made of ceramic, castable waxes, and 3D printable resins. Castable waxes and resins are composed of about 20% wax. The wax is what helps the crown stick to the patient's mouth and helps the crown have a similar density as actual teeth. For 3D printed crowns, however, many of the chemical compositions of materials are proprietary and vary from company to company. The technical data sheet of the resins should be reviewed to determine the specific material formulation for the resins. The appearance and disruptive development of 3D printing technologies bring favorable circumstances to the manufacturing of complex equipment in all walks of life. In the field of dentistry, 3D printing has a wide range of applications, making it possible to create new and more efficient methods for manufacturing dental products. The most common application is to create working models for diagnosis and surgery, followed by a variety of implantable devices, which can help dentists provide patients with more predictable, less invasive, and less costly procedures. For products with complex structures and fine details e that are difficult to produce using mechanical processing technology, 3D printing can utilize an increasing number of material types and rely on digital data to create complex geometric shapes. This allows for the accurate fulfillment of complex and personalized needs in the dental field. The application of 3D printing technology and CAD software based on 3D imaging and modeling can produce complex geometric shapes and has the advantage of high material utilization.

Three-dimensional printing transforms 3D manufacturing into simple 2D superposition, which greatly reduces the complexity of design and manufacturing; however, simultaneously, there will be many defects that affect the performance of products. First, the layer-by-layer superposition principle leads to anisotropy, which leads to different mechanical properties in different directions and restricts the long-term use of intraoral instruments such as occlusal splints. Second, the existence of layer thickness affects the consistency from the digital model to the entity, which makes the surface of the equipment with high surface smoothness requirements, such as ceramic restoration, non ideal. Future research should focus on reducing the negative impact of the 3D printing principle. It is also important to note that 3D printing requires a combination of digital file acquisition equipment and CAD software. The high cost of the equipment makes the popularization of 3D printing a challenge. In contrast, although current 3D printers can print out models in a relatively short period, acquiring digital files takes longer; therefore, 3D printing is not currently applicable to emergency cases. In addition, the accuracy of the printed models is somewhat reduced compared to that of digital files. Additionally, there are some challenges, such as high process, material cost, and time-consuming postprocessing. The lack of well-trained operators may also hinder the application of 3D printing in medical treatment. Moreover, 3D printing technology is suitable for many fields, and most of the machines currently used are not customized for dentistry, which causes some functions to be unsuitable to medical staff. Owing to these drawbacks, 3D printing is still at a competitive disadvantage compared to traditional methods for manufacturing products in bulk. Therefore, 3D printing technology in dentistry should aim to reduce the cost and production time, optimize the surface quality, and improve the process reliability and performance gradient in materials (Tian, Y. et al., 2021).

In the future, new materials and technologies that fulfill dental requirements should be further developed and applied. For example, the Co-Cr alloy material used in the restoration is one of the application materials for DMLS; however, its properties should be further studied to ensure the safety and applicability of the restoration. Additionally, in clinical applications, 3D scanners, CBCT, and CT will be better integrated with 3D printing technologies leveraging their advantages to further promote the development of digital processes. This integration will not only simplify traditional modeling and production process, but can also make products more accurate, streamline the production process and lower the labor cost. In recent years, 3D printing has progressed toward the cellular level, and 3D bioprinting provides unlimited possibilities for the creation of various tissues. The application of 3D printing in oral soft tissue biomaterials has transitioned from experimental to clinical stages. To improve the whole CAD/CAM process, machine learning (ML) has been applied to all aspects of technology. The application of ML algorithms covers all the main aspects that directly affect the quality of the final 3D printed parts, including 3D printing design and other aspects related to the efficiency of the design and manufacturing process. In the near future, ML will be more widely used in the field of 3D printing. Additionally, virtual reality design can interact with 3D printing technologies in the field of dentistry. For example, individuals can directly perform the 3D design of the restoration in the virtual world and observe the 3D restoration products to better estimate the feasibility of the products and reduce the wastage of time and resources.

11. 3D Printing in Prosthetics

Personalized medical devices, including prostheses, are becoming increasingly common, allowing healthcare providers to offer treatments tailored to each patient's unique physiology and needs. Customization is common in prosthetics, but traditional workflows are manual and rely on the technician having a high level of skill and expertise. Prostheses manufactured following a digital workflow are becoming more popular but still occupy a relatively small portion of the market. For patients needing a tailor-made prosthetic device, the design freedom associated with 3D printing technology provides endless opportunities for improved design and functionality. This means that 3D-printed prosthetic devices can offer superior comfort, customization, and cost-efficiency compared to traditionally manufactured devices.

11.1 Benefits of 3D Printing for Prostheses

3D printing enables you to create lighter designs, allowing patients to wear them more comfortably for extended periods. This is achievable because additive manufacturing enables you to create complex structures with minimal material consumption. Given that materials account for more than 40% of manufacturing costs, the opportunities for lightweighting can also result in cost savings. From a design viewpoint, another advantage of 3D printing prostheses is the ability to create "dynamic behaviors." For example, the socket can be stiff where needed and, at the same time, have flexible structures with foam-like behavior for cushioning or dampening. 3D-printed covers are another trending personalization use case for prostheses, as they offer unique aesthetics and high durability.

11.2 Traditional Fabrication Process

First, the prosthetist takes an impression or "cast" of the residual limb to make an exact copy of it. The manufacturer uses this cast to make custom-molded sockets with specific measurements tailored to fit each user according to their unique anatomy and range of motion. To create custom-molded sockets, the thermoplastic material is heated to conform to the shape of the patient's amputated area. Once the sockets are ready, they are connected to off-the-shelf components that make up the artificial limbs. These components are designed for easy assembly and can be adjusted to ensure maximum comfort and functionality for each user. Finally, prosthetists can fit the artificial limbs and make all necessary adjustments. This includes fine-tuning any tension or releasing joints and ensuring that all components are in alignment.

11.3 Digital Fabrication Process

In the realm of digital fabrication, the journey commences with the acquisition of patient data, a pivotal step in the process. Employing cutting-edge 3D medical imaging technologies such as handheld 3D scanners, MRIs, or CT scans, practitioners capture intricate anatomical details, thereby laying the foundation for subsequent phases. Following this, meticulous segmentation and conversion of this data into digital surface meshes pave the way for downstream design operations. The subsequent phase, design generation, marks a critical juncture wherein the device's blueprint is brought to life. Depending on the customization strategy at hand, designers may opt for manual designs tailored for singular instances or embrace fully automated methodologies to craft patient-matched devices. It's paramount to underscore that the intricacies of the design process bear profound implications, ensuring not only functional efficacy but also regulatory compliance. Transitioning to the realm of manufacturing, the third step in the sequence, the envisioned prostheses materialize into tangible form. Here, 3D printing emerges as a versatile tool, facilitating the direct production of prostheses or indirectly, through the creation of bespoke tooling for the primary manufacturing process. While the direct approach shines when realizing prostheses boasting intricate design elements achievable solely through additive manufacturing, the indirect route offers scalability advantages, particularly evident in large-scale production scenarios. Regardless of the manufacturing avenue pursued, a critical denouement awaits post-processing. This pivotal phase ensures that each prosthesis meets stringent functional requirements and aesthetic standards. It is through this meticulous attention to detail that the promise of digital fabrication is fully realized, ushering in a new era of personalized healthcare solutions (3D printing in prosthetics, 2023).

11.4   Advantages of the Digital Fabrication Process

Adopting a fully digital fabrication process offers many advantages in prosthetic component development. For medical device manufacturers, creating comfortable, well-fitted prostheses can be expensive and requires highly skilled experts. With the increasing demand for more complex products, healthcare providers are always trying to make production more efficient. Digital fabrication can help healthcare providers achieve this by reducing the number of processes and manual steps necessary to bridge the gap between the product and the patient. By beginning with a scan, providers can customize and create precise digital models ready for production, saving time and money. Once you have designed the prosthetic, 3D printing enables you to manufacture complex geometries that are impossible to create with other production technologies.

This digitalization process results in lower wait times for the patient, more comfortable and customized fit, and time and cost-savings for the provider. Moreover, by automating this process, the healthcare provider can spend more time with the patient, optimizing for fit and comfort. Digitalization also creates opportunities for developing new geometry, which can be easily adapted to meet a patient's personal wishes for aesthetics and function. Once approved, the design can be manufactured and iterated quickly. With traditional fabrication processes, on the other hand, the healthcare provider often needs to begin from scratch if alterations are necessary. Digital fabrication processes also help the industry evolve because they create opportunities and time for experts to innovate and develop new ideas.

11.5   Design Automation

In the research and development stage, design automation allows the exploration of available design space quickly, identifying important design variables, and lock in parameters. At the end of this stage, you should have an automated design workflow that only needs new inputs to generate new, pre-validated designs. Once the workflow is approved, you can deploy it in a production environment. A Graphic User Interface (GUI) allows less technically adept users to run the automated design process using patient-specific data as inputs. They can then inspect and troubleshoot the results without requiring the time or attention of more experienced designers. This frees them up for more complex tasks. Once the production volume has reached a critical threshold, automation via a programmatic environment facilitates economic viability. For instance, scripts running on a server or in the cloud can call upon design generation workflows to minimize design time and associated costs.

11.6   Lattice Structures for 3D-printed Foams

Lattice structures for 3D-printed foams can be precisely tuned to provide improved strength, flexibility, cushioning, and impact absorption compared to traditional foams. This can enable more comfortable, lightweight designs better suited to a wide range of users. The lattice structure also helps reduce the amount of material needed, making it possible to create prostheses at lower costs.

11.7   *Data-driven Design*

Using patient-specific data to drive design variables enables you to create prostheses tuned to each patient's unique physiology. Prosthetists can derive this data from either simulation data or direct measurements. Design automation allows the use of data to streamline and scale design operations quickly and efficiently. Customization is common in prosthetics, but traditional workflows are manual and rely on the technician having a high level of skill and expertise. Prosthetic devices manufactured following a digital workflow, which offers many benefits, are becoming more popular but still occupy a relatively small portion of the market. 3D printing has emerged as a transformative force in the field of medicine, offering unprecedented capabilities in patient-specific treatment modalities, prosthetics, and medical device manufacturing. Through the integration of advanced imaging technologies, streamlined design processes, and versatile manufacturing techniques, 3D printing has revolutionized the way medical practitioners approach diagnosis, treatment, and patient care.

Looking to the future, the potential of 3D printing in medicine is boundless. Continued advancements in material science, bioprinting, and precision manufacturing techniques hold promise for even greater levels of customization and sophistication in medical applications. As technologies mature and become more accessible, we can anticipate widespread adoption across diverse medical specialties, enabling tailored solutions for individual patient needs. Moreover, the synergy between 3D printing and other emerging technologies such as artificial intelligence, robotics, and nanotechnology will further expand the frontiers of medical innovation. From personalized implants and prosthetics to complex tissue engineering and drug delivery systems, the convergence of these disciplines will catalyze breakthroughs in patient care, disease management, and biomedical research.

It is imperative to address challenges related to regulatory frameworks, quality assurance, and ethical considerations to ensure the safe and responsible deployment of 3D printing technologies in healthcare. By fostering collaboration between industry stakeholders, healthcare providers, and regulatory agencies, we can harness the full potential of 3D printing to improve patient outcomes, enhance medical accessibility, and shape the future of medicine.

References

Abdul Aleem Mohammed, Mohammed S. Algahtani, Mohammad Zaki Ahmad, Javed Ahmad, Sabna Kotta et al. (2021). 3D Printing in medicine: Technology overview and drug delivery applications, Annals of 3D Printed Medicine, Volume 4, 100037.

Arslan-Yildiz A., El Assal R., Chen P., Guven S., Inci F. et al. (2016). Towards artificial tissue models: past, present, and future of 3D bioprinting. Biofabrication. 8(1): 014103.

Cooke, C.M., Flaxman, T.E., Sikora, L. (2023). Individualized medicine using 3D printing technology in gynecology: a scoping review. 3D Print Med 9, (6).

3D Printing in Dentistry, (2022). https://www.xometry.com/resources/3d-printing/3d-printing-in-dentistry/

3D printing in prosthetics: A design guide (2023). https://www.ntop.com/resources/blog/3d-printing-in-prosthetics-a-design-guide/

Flaxman T.E., Cooke C.M., Miguel O.X., (2021). A review and guide to creating patient specific 3D printed anatomical models from MRI for benign gynecologic surgery. 3D Print Med. 7:17.

Fletcher J., Miskovic D. (2021). Digital and 3D printed models for surgical planning. Cham: Springer; p. 95–110.

Haque, S., Md, S., Whittaker, M. and Kaminskas, L.M. (2018). The Applications of 3D Printing in Pulmonary Drug Delivery and Treatment of Respiratory Disorders. Current pharmaceutical design, 24(42),5072–5080.

Kamio T., Suzuki M., Asaumi R. (2020). DICOM segmentation and STL creation for 3D printing: a process and software package comparison for osseous anatomy. 3D Print Med 2020;17 6. doi: 10.1186/s41205-020-00069-2.

M.S. Algahtani, A.A. Mohammed, J. Ahmad. (2018). Extrusion-based 3D printing for pharmaceuticals: contemporary research and applications Curr Pharm Des, 24 (42), pp. 4991–5008.

Paul, G.M., Rezaienia, A., Wen, P., Condoor, S., Parkar, N. et al. (2018). Medical Applications for 3D Printing: Recent Developments. Missouri medicine, 115(1), 75–81.

Petric P., Fokdal L.U., Traberg Hansen A., (2019). 3D-printed tandem-needle-template for image guided adaptive brachytherapy in cervical cancer. Radiother Oncol. 2019; 133(1): S87.

Ricci, G., Gibelli, F. and Sirignano, A. (2023). Three-Dimensional Bioprinting of Human Organs and Tissues: Bioethical and Medico-Legal Implications Examined through a Scoping Review. Bioengineering (Basel, Switzerland), 10(9), 1052.

Rizzo M.L., Turco S., Spina F., Costantino A., Visi G. et al. (2023). 3D printing and 3D bioprinting technology in medicine: Ethical and legal issues. Clin. Ther. 1–11.

S. Kimura, T. Ishikawa, Y. Iwao, S. Itai, H. Kondo et al. (2019). Fabrication of zero-order sustained-release floating tablets via fused depositing modeling 3D printer, Chem Pharm Bull, 67 (9) pp. 992–999.

Semeniuk O, Cherpak A, Robar J. (2021). Design and evaluation of 3D printable patient-specific applicators for gynecologic HDR brachytherapy. Med Phys.20:20.

Silvina Zabala-Travers. (2021). Biomodeling and 3D printing: A novel radiology subspecialty, Annals of 3D Printed Medicine, Volume 4,100038, ISSN 2666–9641.

Tian, Y., Chen, C., Xu, X., Wang, J., Hou, X., et al. (2021). A Review of 3D Printing in Dentistry: Technologies, Affecting Factors, and Applications Scanning, 9950131

3D Printing in Food Technology

Mehmet Bozdag,[1] *Musa Ayran,*[1] *Esra Pilavci,*[1]
Sumeyye Cesur,[1] *Oguzhan Gunduz,*[1]
and *Canan Dogan*[1*]

1. Introduction

In the late 1990s and early 2000s, there was a broad trend toward industrialization and modernization that corresponded with the development of additive manufacturing, or 3D printing, particularly with the advent of Industry 4.0. During this time, conventional production methods were largely replaced by automated Technologies (Nodhi et al., 2022). Additive manufacturing played a crucial role in this transition by introducing innovative production techniques aligned with Industry 4.0 principles (Hassoun et al., 2022; Nodehi et al., 2022). The incorporation of additive manufacturing marked a departure from conventional practices, enabling more flexible, digitally-driven, and customizable production processes (Nodehi et al., 2022). The integration of 3D printing and the fourth industrial revolution has revolutionized the food manufacturing sector, specifically in digital gastronomy. This technology is recognized for providing innovative, sustainable, and futuristic solutions (K.H. Lee et al., 2021). 3D printing enables the customization of nutritional content, shapes, tastes, and colors of food, fostering the production of nutritious meals with natural ingredients (Derossi et al., 2020; K.H. Lee et al., 2021). Thanks to 3D printing, food products can be customized based on individual needs and there is a possibility of producing nutrient-dense foods with innovative shapes (Yang et al., 2017; J.Y. Zhang et al., 2022). This phenomenon permits the precise control of nutritional value (Yang et al., 2017). Functional components including probiotics, lipophilic bioactive substances, proteins and peptides, and algae can all be added to 3D-printed foods to increase the food items' nutritional content and health advantages. Additionally, the usage of hydrocolloids and hydrogels can improve the flow characteristics and viscosity of the paste used for 3D printing (Tomašević et al., 2021).

3D food printing (3DFP) has the potential to revolutionize business models with the ability to tailor nutrition, optimize supply chains, and reduce production costs. New niche markets can be created thanks to this technology, which makes it easy to create food products tailored to each

---

[1]   Center for Nanotechnology & Biomaterials Application and Research (NBUAM), Marmara University, Turkey. Department of Metallurgical and Materials Engineering, Faculty of Technology, Marmara University, Turkey.

*   Corresponding author: canan.dogan@marmara.edu.tr

customer's specific dietary requirements (Varvara et al., 2021a). Consumers can now produce personalized food products at home with inexpensive commercial 3D printers thanks to recent developments in automation and computing (Enfield et al., 2023a). 3DFP also increases productivity, reduces waste, and improves efficiency in the production process - all this helps companies become more profitable. In addition to reducing the reliance on large stocks and storage facilities, 3DFP also allows for on-demand production, radically changing the dynamics of the traditional supply chain (Varvara et al., 2021a). Food sustainability, which considers the effects of food production, distribution, and consumption on the environment, society, and economy, is a significant component of the food industry. With its ability to transform conventional methods and increase the utilization of already-existing resources 3DFP has the potential to improve the sustainability of food production (Panghal et al., 2023; Rogers and Srivastava, 2021). Food goods can now be made on demand and near the point of consumption thanks to 3D printing, eliminating the need for bulk production and storage. It may also lead to a decrease in the consumption of raw materials, energy, and water since it allows for precise control over the quantity and type of food products produced (Escalante-Aburto et al., 2021). By using innovative protein sources, reducing packing, and limiting waste, this technology makes production more environmentally friendly (Panghal et al., 2023). A notable benefit is the efficient utilization of food ingredients throughout storage, transit, preparation, and repurposing, leading to a significant reduction in food waste and enhanced environmental sustainability (Burke-Shyne et al., 2021; K. H. Lee et al., 2021).

A very creative and sensitive process is needed to create customized foods, and this is ideally suited to 3DFP technology. Food design programs are necessary for three-dimensional food printing technology before manufacturing can begin. The procedure algorithm can be designed and implemented with the help of this program. The printing device generates a layered procedure with continuous printing for layer accumulation, automatically recognizing the food design order (J. Lee, 2021). During the initial phase of the 3D printing process, using a three-dimensional computer-aided design (CAD) system to create a 3D model is the fundamental idea behind the 3DFP process. Before printing, the generated model file (.stl) is imported into slicing software (Mantihal et al., 2020). The quality of food materials should be taken into account while creating food ink formulations since the materials should have a high strength to meet printability requirements. While printing, several parameters, including line length, nozzle diameter, writing speed, laser power, number of layers, shape, and layer thickness—especially fast cooling and temperature management—should also be carefully taken into account (Yang et al., 2017). These properties affect the shape stability of printed food (Attarin and Attaran, 2020) It is difficult to post-process 3D-printed materials in a way that preserves the product's shape. Certain printed components, such as hydrogel, cheese, and chocolate, maintain their shape following material deposition since they do not need additional post-processing (Hussain et al., 2022). Additionally, if the printed food product was hot extruded or cooked before printing, it can be eaten immediately. If it is cold extruded, it can also be stored at freezing or refrigerator temperature for further processing, such as steaming, baking, or frying (Kewuyemi et al., 2022).

Understanding food rheology is crucial for the 3D printing of food, as it influences how food materials flow and deform under different conditions (Nodehi et al., 2022). It's critical to consider rheological qualities and printability variables, including viscosity, storage modulus, yield stress, phase angle, and shear recovery behavior (Maldonado-Rosas et al., 2022). The printing parameters and material properties governing 3D food printing applications are summarized in Figure 1. Viscosity plays a significant role in shaping texture, fidelity, and extrudability in printed food products. Increased viscosity can pose challenges in extrusion, requiring slower printing rates and more pressure, but it also enhances printing resolution and shape retention (Nodehi et al., 2022). Flow behavior (n) and consistency indexes (K) are essential measures of how easily materials can be extruded through a printer's nozzle. High-viscosity materials may lead to nozzle blockages and adhesion to extruder walls, impacting print results. Simplifying and optimizing these aspects is key to achieving successful 3D printing of food products (Maldonado-Rosas et al., 2022).

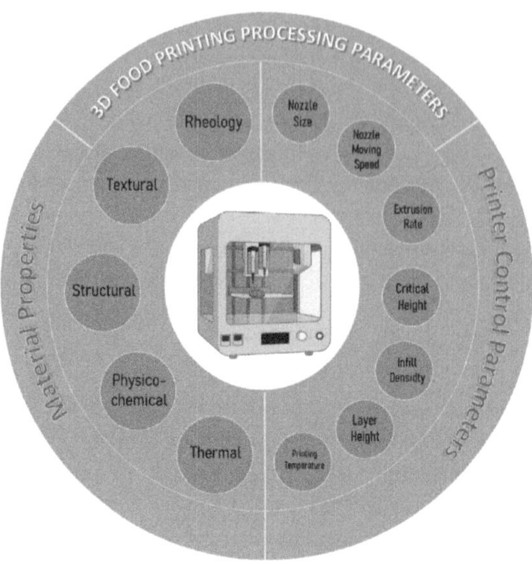

Fig. 1   Material properties and printing parameters that govern 3D food printing processes.

The present chapter is based on novel research and technologies in 3D printing for food technology. Food ink materials, process parameters, food printing techniques, and technologies were compiled. In the first section, food for 3D printing was mentioned. The second section contains 3DFP technologies that are extrusion-based printing, selective laser sintering, binder jetting, inkjet printing, fused deposition modeling, and miscellaneous technologies. The applications of 3DFP are featured in the next section. Furthermore, challenges and future aspects were evaluated in the last section of the chapter.

2.   Foods for 3D Printing Technology

As daily lives continue to change rapidly, the importance of convenient foods with health benefits increases. From the perspective of consumers, food products of any kind should be considered in terms of cost, convenience, nutrition, experience, and taste. Because of their low cost and fast effect on blood sugar (high glycemic index), convenient foods are frequently consumed worldwide (Singhal et al., 2020). With the increase in consumption, awareness about health concepts related to convenient foods has also increased among people. Food manufacturing techniques based on additive manufacturing principles have a great potential for fabricating customized food with economic and environmental benefits, tailored to the customer's preferences and needs (Singhal et al., 2020; J. Y. Zhang et al., 2022). Nowadays, various food manufacturing methods are being developed by using different principles of additive manufacturing. However, to achieve sustained production of 3D-printed foods, food inks must be understood first. To ensure the applicability of the printing process, the food-ink must be examined in terms of rheological and mechanical properties among other parameters. Today many different institutions and companies work on food-ink formulations, and characterization in order to find new printable recipes. Lille et al.(2018) mention a modified fruit-based puree food ink designed to create child snacks that can cover the needs of vitamin D, iron, and calcium intake of a 3-10-year-old child. Another novel work by Yang et al. (Yang et al., 2019) presents a simulation software, Polyflow to analyze the flow characteristics of the recipe inks before printing. By using the software, they were able to determine the effect of infill on swellings.

For sustainable optimized food printing, its essential to define the interactions between process, material, and functions involved . Parameters such as type of food-ink, concentration, and structural order influence printability, particularly rheological changes of the food-ink when exposed to stimuli such as temperature variations, shear, inclusion of gelation agents, and/or essential oils. However, to advance in such understanding, it's necessary to first comprehend the macronutrients,which are the main structures of the food constituents (Tejada-Ortigoza and Cuan-Urquizo, 2022; J.Y. Zhang et al., 2022). When selecting raw materials for 3D-printed food recipes, it's crucial to understand that the ingredients within will directly affect the printability of the recipe. After all, the material composition must firstly be capable of flowing through the nozzle of the extruder. Secondly,to ensure that the printed composition stays intact on the printing platform without collapsing or disturbances on the structure several factors need to be considered.Particularly, during raw material selection, glass transition, gelation, rheology, melting temperature, heat resistance, cooking, and mechanical properties of ingredients must be taken into account (Yang et al., 2017).

Materials for 3D-printed foods are considered in two groups overall: natively printable materials and non-printable traditional food materials. As the name indicates, natively printable materials can be easily modified for printing purposes. Examples include hydrogels, cake frostings, cheeses, chocolates, and hummus. These materials are easy to adjust in terms of flowability, taste, nutritional values, and 3D texture (Nachal et al., 2019a; Sun et al., 2015a). Sereno et al. (Serenó et al., 2012) demonstrate a recipe using two highly printable materials, chocolate, and peach jam, and perform syringe-type fabrication for the recipe via the fabrication system Fab@Home machine. This study showcases exemplary production through their open-source, versatile, and inexpensive Fab@Home system. Another demonstration by Le Tohic at al. (Le Tohic et al., 2018) presents the printing capabilities of cheese in 3D printing. Significant progress was also made by Blutinger et al. (Blutinger et al., 2023) who designed a seven-ingredient 3D-printed cake. The cake utilized Nutella, cherry drizzle, frosting, cracker pastes, banana puree, peanut butter, and strawberry jam all purchased from a local convenience store. This demonstrates that when the correct compositions and/or pretreatments are performed, natively printable materials are stable in terms of structure after printing, with no need for post-treatments and are already used in medical and space applications (Sun et al., 2015a). Meanwhile, natural non-printable standard food materials are not printable due to their properties. Rice, meat, fruits, vegetables, and many other dishes consumed daily are not printable. However, solid foods and demi-solid liquid dishes can be manipulated to make them more printable via gastronomic tricks and/or additives. By using organic-based additives like gelatin and xanthan gum, the structure can be maintained after printing. Kim et al. (Kim et al., 2017a) present the textural properties of different hydrocolloids in different concentrations such as gellan gum, methylcellulose, guar gum, locust bean gum, hydroxypropyl methylcellulose, and xanthan gum to estimate their suitability for 3D-printing. Nowadays, it is a rising idea to use natural food resources to make traditional foods more printable, such as the mentioned hydrocolloids, and alternative sources like algae, fungi, seaweeds, lupines, and even insects. These resources are considerably rich in proteins, bioactives, and fibers (Nachal et al., 2019a). Common food constituents such as carbohydrates, proteins, and fats have varied molecular and chemical properties which causes these macronutrients to affect the 3D printing process in various ways.

2.1 *Carbohydrates*

Carbohydrates are made from monosaccharides, and are commonly seen as sugars, starches, and non-starch polysaccharides in our diets. They commonly come across in plant-based foods such as, cereals, legumes, grains, edible seeds, vegetables, and fruits (Leong et al., 2019). Carbohydrates have significant importance in the human diet. Due to the importance of this macronutrient, many different trials have been performed to optimize different sources of carbohydrates to create sustainable food ink recipes. Sources include vegetables, fruits, isolated polysaccharides, chocolate, doughs, and mashed potatoes (Nachal et al., 2019a; J. Y. Zhang et al., 2022). However, most carbohydrate resources are not natively printable. The addition of water or designated gelation agents (hydrocolloids) to recipes can increase the printability of food ink. Dankar at al. (Dankar et al., 2018), presents their investigation of mashed potatoes with different additives. During their studies, four additives, alginate, agar, lecithin, and glycerol were used to improve the mechanical and internal straightness of potato puree and were able to succeed with alginate and agar samples. Another successful work presented by Yang et al. (Yang et al., 2018), shows the printability of a mashed potato and lemon juice mixture puree, showcasing a sustainable approach to 3D food printing. On the other hand, fruit and vegetable purees are on trial for food inks too. Severini et al. (Severini et al., 2018a), mention their banana and carrot-based food ink puree, but even with the addition of natural thickener pectin, the puree was not stable enough to print. In different cases carbohydrates, particularly starch, can increase the gelatinization and improve extruder-based 3D food printing and retention after printing (Nachal et al., 2019a). Lille et al. (Lille et al., 2018), present a study where the printability of faba bean, oat, milk powder, cellulose nanofiber, and starch was investigated via extrusion-based 3D food printing. Among various recipes, the finest outcomes were observed on semi-skimmed milk-based sample, which have 10% starch within. With such studies, our understanding of various carbohydrate-based 3D printed foods improves in many ways .

2.1.1   *Characteristics of carbohydrates as 3D food-Ink*

Most additive manufacturing systems designed for food printing commonly use a syringe, screw, or air pressure-driven extruder. The principle of this method requires raw materials to flow through the tip by maintaining a constant flow for the deposition and fabrication of the food structure. Extrusion-based 3D printing is considerably suitable for producing carbohydrate-based foods like cookies, pizza, and bread (Jiang et al., 2019). In terms of rheological and morphological properties, in most cases of carbohydrate-based printing the use of hydrocolloids and other organic additives is required in order to achieve a stable 3D food structure with desired properties (Jiang et al., 2019; Wu et al., 2023a). Dankar et al. (2018) present an exemplary study on mashed potato puree with four particular additives: lecithin, glycerol, alginate, and agar. The study examines the rheological properties and microstructural changes of starch molecules. Additives were examined in 0.5% and 1% concentrations with mashed potato. The findings Indicate that the addition of lecithin and glycerol cause a decrease in viscosity, while concentrated alginate increased the viscosity. Dankar et al. additionally mention the microscopic detection of large aggregations of starch granules in a mashed potato puree and the effect of additives on the granules. Glycerol and lecithin caused granules to expand while agar caused them to shrink. All additive samples were found to be non-Newtonian and exhibited shear-thinning behaviors. Among them, Dankar et al. indicate that agar and alginate were showed good implications on potato puree and can be used in further 3D food recipes. Another potato-based recipe presented by Liu et al. (Liu et al., 2018), shows the potential of potato starch as a gelation agent for 3D food printing. By adding 2% potato starch to mashed potato, Liu et al. were able to print sustainable, smoothed-shaped, and stable 3D food structures. The mixture of mashed potato and potato starch exhibited shear-thinning behavior, retained its shape after printing, and demonstrated outstanding extrudability and printability. Baking dough is also frequently used for 3D-printed foods, such as cookies and mini pizzas due to its printable nature. Yan et al. (Ahmed and Thomas, 2018), present an important study where they investigated the effects of processing parameters such as nozzle diameter, nozzle movement, filament diameter, nozzle height, and post-process fast-cooling to observe their effect on the rheological properties of baking dough and the accuracy of 3D printing. During the study, Yan et al. concluded that extrusion actions affect the viscous modulus of the dough and its flow behavior. Additionally, the dough's elastic modulus, gelation strength, rupture strength, and adhesiveness affect the shape retention of the final product (Ahmed and Thomas, 2018; Jiang et al., 2019).

The addition of polysaccharides, such as guar gum, xanthan gum, basil seed gum, and flaxseed gum is another method to manipulate the texture and rheology of food inks. Adding gum material to carbohydrate-based food inks can increase viscosity, exhibit gel-like behavior, and improve structural durability (Jiang et al., 2019). Ahmed and Thomas (Ahmed and Thomas, 2018), investigated the effects of xanthan and guar gums on brown wheat flour-based dough in terms of stickiness and pasting properties. They found a significant increase in dough viscosity with increasing concentrations of xanthan and guar gum. In another similar trial with different components, Cui et al. (Cui et al., 2022), conducted trials on potato starch for 3D food printing by adding xanthan gum, sodium alginate, and both together in various concentrations. The results indicated that the addition of polysaccharides resulted in more printable food ink with improved structural retention. Regarding thermal properties, carbohydrate-based food inks can be sensitive due to the cooking process, affecting the post-printing structure. Typically, starch-based food inks demand a heat treatment stage after the 3D printing, to have the final product cooked and in an edible form. After heating treatments, starch-based structures may expand and undergo changes in post-printing structure (Wu et al., 2023a). This necessitates control and knowledge about raw materials glass transition temperature Tg; for instance, high molecular weight carbohydrates usually have higher Tg values which can affect the post-printed structure (Nachal et al., 2019a).

In the case of most starch-based 3D printed foods, rapid heating such as high-heat ovens and/or microwaves can cause disturbances in the final form. To address these issues various recipes have been developed over the years. Teng et al.(Teng et al., 2022) address the problem of overpuffing of starch-based potato gel under rapid microwaves by including soybean insoluble dietary fibers (SIDF) in the recipe to modify the internal structure. They fabricated various microwave-puffed potato chips via 3D printing and found that, SIDF addition reduced over expansion, enhanced mechanical strength, and improved the formation ability of potato gel. Another innovative work by Maniglia et al.(Maniglia et al., 2020) presents cassava starch hydrogels for 3D printing via dry heating treatment (DHT). A 4-hour DHT-modified cassava starch showed changes in granular and molecular characteristics including a decrease in the peak apparent viscosity and an increase in the gel firmness. Using cassava starch instead of regular starch in food ink recipes can improve the after-heat treatment structure of the final product.

2.2 Proteins

Proteins are large polymer molecules made up of one or multiple long chains of amino acids. Proteins are vital macromolecules for body and cellular functions, such as enzymatic reactions, DNA replication, transportation, and cellular response duties (Jiang et al., 2019). Due to the human diet, we must obtain essential amino acids from other sources like plants or microorganisms. In natural form, only limited protein sources are suitable for 3D food printing applications, including protein denaturation due to stress making it harder to form new recipes (Z. Guo et al., 2022). Although, proteins possess an important place as raw material for extrusion-based 3D food printing applications Gelatin derived from collagen fibers is commonly used as a substrate in 3D protein-based food applications. Chen et al. (J. Chen et al., 2019), present their trials on soy protein isolate with sodium alginate and gelatin in order to find a new recipe for 3D food printing. They indicated that soy protein isolates with gelatin exhibit excellent printing properties with structural retention. 3D protein-based food fabrication requires additional cautions in pH and isoelectric point parameters. Using polysaccharide materials can help textural improvements, and prevent the external stress or compounds which may cause protein denaturation (Nachal et al., 2019a).

2.2.1 Characteristics of proteins as 3D food-Ink

To improve the rheology and textural properties of protein-based food inks, gelation, and hydrogel-forming mechanisms are commonly used for the printing process. This requires the addition of organic additives to the recipe. Wang et al.(L. Wang et al., 2018), demonstrate an important trial on another protein source used in 3D food printing applications, fish surimi gel. In their study, they used an extrusion-based 3D food printing system and investigated the rheological effects of NaCl on fish surimi gel. The addition of 1.5g/100g NaCl caused a decrease in fish surimi gel viscosity, which improved the printing process and structural retention. Another extensive research by Chen et al.(Y. Chen et al., 2021), presents a series of trials with drawing soy protein and textured soybean protein with various hydrocolloids such as hydroxyethyl cellulose, carboxymethyl cellulose, guar gum, sodium alginate, sodium, konjac gum and xanthan gum. The aim of their study was to fabricate a steak-like food through 3D food printing technologies. Among their trials, textured soybean protein with xanthan gum exhibits the best performance in terms of printability and structural integrity.

In terms of thermal properties proteins are more sensitive than other macronutrients due to fast denaturation and aggregation. However different sources of proteins may require pre and post-treatments to be used in 3D food printing applications. An exemplary study by Xu et al.(Xu et al., 2020), presents the impact of heat treatment on the rheological and microstructural properties of egg yolk for 3D food printing. The finest results were observed from the sample heated to 76°C for 8 minutes; the egg yolk paste was viscous enough to be 3D printed, and the formed 3D structure was rigid and stable. With this optimization, it may be possible to use egg yolk paste as a substrate for further studies in 3D protein-based food printing.

2.3   Lipids

Lipids are made up of different groups of molecules which makes them heterogeneous molecules. They are commonly hydrophobic and can dissolve in organic solvents. Like carbohydrates and proteins, lipids/fats are essential for a healthy human diet (Burdge and Calder, 2015). Lipids affect the physical properties of 3D food inks directly due to their lubricant effect. In this case, Lille et al. (Lille et al., 2018), mention during their 3D food printing trials with skim milk powder, that without the fat context, it was not possible to 3D print due to hardness and lack of lubrication. Such trials indicate that the fat and lipid context of 3D food inks can be used to manipulate rheology, and can be used as potential lubricant in food inks. However, the addition or removal of fat content will affect the melting range and crystalline structure of 3D printed food (Nachal et al., 2019a; Pérez et al., 2019a; J.Y. Zhang et al., 2022).

2.3.1   Characteristics of lipids as 3D food-Ink

Lipids, whether employed in bulk or emulsified forms, can serve as key components for the development of food inks. When utilized in bulk, lipids have the capacity to generate semi-solid structures. Particularly, when lipids exhibit partial crystallinity, their plastic rheological properties become conducive for applications in 3D food printing. To effectively comprehend and control the rheological properties of food ink, it is imperative to have a thorough understanding of the lipid source and its melting/crystallization profile. (J.Y. Zhang et al., 2022). Nowadays, it is possible to work with various lipid-based materials such as chocolate and cheese. Le Tohic et al. (Le Tohic et al., 2018), present their 3D food printing trial with processed cheese with 25% fat context. By melting the cheese at 75°C for 12 minutes they succeeded in 3D printing the cheese without any additives. Chocolate is another material with a high-fat content used in 3D food printing. In chocolate, cocoa butter acts as the main ingredient and due to the formation of fat crystals in various forms, it is possible to give chocolate different properties. The rheological properties of chocolate play a crucial role in the 3D food printing process and require control over the arrangement of fats and interactions to fabricate stable macrostructure (Afoakwa et al., 2007; Lanaro et al., 2018). Among other parameters such as temperature and shear rate, particle size is another parameter important to control the viscosity of chocolate during printing. Chocolate possesses semi-solid features due to the interactions of free liquid fat and solid particles. It is important to diminish the particle size to control the rheology and prevent the formation of gritty tastes in chocolate (Afoakwa et al., 2007; Lanaro et al., 2018).

2.4   Characteristics of Minerals & Vitamins as Fortifying Ingredients

In order to magnify certain properties of a food recipe it is possible to use specific fortifying constituents such as minerals, vitamins, probiotics, fibers, and other specific macromolecules/ingredients to ameliorate human health. For this purpose, nutrient-rich sources such as fruits, vegetables, nuts, seeds, and grains are commonly used to obtain vitamins A, C, B6, B12, E, and D including minerals such as magnesium, potassium, calcium, and others. With the progress in fortified foods and fabrication understandings, personalized 3D-printed food technology is advancing further for diverse food design and fabrication (Varvara et al., 2021a). These personalized 3D-printed foods can assist people with swallowing difficulties and could serve as a new sustainable nutrition source for teenagers and children, who may have specific needs such as increased iron and calcium intake (Zhao et al., 2021).

Fruits and vegetables have always been excellent sources of minerals and vitamins. Insufficient intake of these can lead to a deficiency of minerals and vitamins such as calcium, iron, and vitamin D. It is important to include such vitamins and minerals in personalized 3D-printed foods for patients who may have issues with regular food consumption (Zhao et al., 2021). Azam et al. (Azam et al., 2018), presented a blend of orange concentrate, wheat starch, and gum with additional liquid vitamin D to produce 3D printed food fortified with vitamin D. During their experiments, they found that among gum Arabic, guar gum, k-carrageenan gum, and xanthan gum; the best match for formulation was k-carrageenan gum. Azam et al. also observed that 3D constructs printed with k-carrageenan gum, orange concentrate, wheat starch, and liquid vitamin D exhibited the smoothest surface with a good microstructure and optimal chewing properties. Another innovative study by Scerra et al. (Scerra et al., 2018) demonstrated the addition of vitamin E acetate to peanut butter to improve its shelf life and investigate its impact on 3D printing. Throughout the fabrication and post-processing stages, the concentration of vitamin E decreased by 42%, indicating a significant loss due to thermal treatments.

In terms of mineral sources, calcium caseinate is a significant calcium provider. Zhang et al. (L. Zhang et al., 2018) developed a new recipe blending dough and calcium caseinate. They noted that the addition of calcium caseinate not only enhances the nutrition content but also improves the printability and post-printed stability of the dough. The water content, flour type, and number of additives affected the rheological and structural properties. During their trials, 3% Calcium caseinate provided the best printing results and structural retention after printing. Fruit-based inks for food printing have always been vital, due to their vitamins and minerals. Derossi et al. (Derossi et al., 2018), presented a 3D-printed snack for children made from canned white beans, dried non-fat milk, banana, dried mushrooms, and lemon juice, including ascorbic acid as an antioxidant. The goal was to formulate a healthy snack that provides an adequate amount of calcium, iron, and vitamin D.

2.5 *Additives for 3D Food-Ink*

Every ingredient in food-ink affects its materialistic properties, such as rheology and thermal behavior causing the printing parameters to change or vary depending on the printing process. Among these ingredients, the additives play crucial roles such as binding, coloring, and fortifying agents. To obtain tasty, colored, and designed 3D-printed food products, the effects of additives on food inks must be considered (Varvara et al., 2021a). Binding agents assist in maintaining the structural integrity and stability of the food ink during and after printing. Among many binding agents used in food-inks, xanthan gum, and pectin are among the most conventional (Varvara et al., 2021a). Xanthan gum is a polysaccharide produced via aerobic fermentation of the Xanthomonas bacterium and several other strains. Xanthan Gum is widely included in recipes as a thickener, emulsifier, and stabilizer due to its unique properties. Kim et al. (Kim et al., 2019), presented a trial of hydrocolloid effects on stability during 3D printable cookie fabrication, testing methylcellulose and xanthan gum . Samples with xanthan gum (0.5g/100g) solved deformation issues during post-treatments showing improved mechanical strength and better cooking performance than other blends. Another important study presented by Lee et al. (J.H. Lee et al., 2019), investigated the effects of particle size on the rheology and printing performance of a food-ink recipe made from spinach powder and xanthan gum (20 wt.% spinach powder in 10 wt.% xanthan gum gel). The results indicated that larger particle sizes of spinach powder caused more porous structures, and all formulations were printable.

Pectin is another natural polysaccharide obtained from plants and is often a by-product of various industrial food processes. It is used as a thickening, gelling, stabilizer, and texturizer agent [36]. Vancauwenberghe et al. (Vancauwenberghe et al., 2017), conducted a study investigating different amounts of pectin in a blend with sugar syrup, bovine serum albumin, and calcium chloride to formulate printable food ink. They successfully fabricated 43 edible 3D food structures with unchanged parameters and reported that increasing amounts of pectin enhanced the firmness and strength of printed objects. Coloring agents used in 3D food printing applications play a crucial role in the acceptability of the final food product by consumers . Natural coloring agents are more suitable and desired by consumers due to health concerns and their minor contributions to the functional properties of the final food product. Anthocyanins which are water-soluble organic pigments, are mainly found in flowers and fruits such as raspberries, eggplants, black-berries, and rose petals (Varvara et al., 2021a). Feng et al. (Feng et al., 2021), present a novel snack for 3D printed food blending rose petals with high anthocyanins concentrations and sodium alginate to create a unique food-ink. Various alginate concentrations were tested, resulting in the fabrication of 3D-printed stable food structures with stable purple and pink colors, depending on the rose petal concentration. Another organic coloring source for 3D food technologies is chlorophyll . Chlorophylls widespread among bacteria, algae, and plants, are considered good sources of antioxidants like vitamins A, C, and E (Varvara et al., 2021a). Uribe-Wandurraga et al. (Uribe-Wandurraga et al., 1947), present a cereal-based snack food ink formulated with various amounts of microalgae (Spirulina spp. and Chlorella spp.) for 3D food printing. The printed results exhibit various shades of green, which change according to the density of microalgae used . Spirulina algae, from Cyanobacterium species with their blue-green colors, can also be used for similar purposes in 3D food applications (Varvara et al., 2021a).

2.6 The Impact of Texture Influenced by Rheological and Mechanical Characteristics

In 3D food printing applications, the goal is not only to fabricate the food structure but also to ensure good texture, mouthfeel, and taste. Texture encompasses the mechanical, geometrical, and surface attributes of the entire structure (Tejada-Ortigoza and Cuan-Urquizo, 2022). When additive manufacturing methods are applied for production, rheology, and mechanical properties significantly affect the fabricated product . The impact of rheological properties on texture can be tested by using printable materials, which must be examined before and after printing. For mechanical properties, both printed and post-processed materials should be investigated to understand the effects. During formulation, model design, 3D printing, and post-processing, rheological and mechanical properties are crucial for ensuring the stable and accurate printing of design structure. The precision of texturing units in 3D printed food, and the complexity of the designed structure directly affect the mechanical properties. To maintain textural appeal, and visual attractiveness of inner structures can be refined during post-processing. This textural manipulation allows for the fabrication of 3D food products with reduced amounts of sugar, salt, and fat (Dankar, Pujolà, et al., 2018; Portanguen et al., 2019; Sungsinchai et al., 2019).

2.7 Nutrition and Moisture Content in 3D Printing Food Ink

Moisture content describes the water within the food-ink, which is a crucial parameter in order to fabricate high-quality and safe 3D food structures. The flowability, weight, shelf life, texture, and microbial safety of the food can be affected by the moisture content. The flowability of various food-ink formulations can alter with changes in moisture content. By controlling the moisture levels it is possible to manipulate the rheological properties of these materials, such as dough, during the fabrication of 3D food structures via controlled drying methods (Kim et al., 2018a; J. Y. Zhang et al., 2022). In the case of powder food materials, to enhance the printability of food the water content is crucial. Hydrocolloid-based food inks possess potential in terms of improving the flowability of the food ink (Kim et al., 2018a). Excessive amounts of moisture could also cause serious rheological changes in food ink and disturb printability. Severini et al. (Severini et al., 2018a) mention high moisture content in fruit and vegetable-based food inks and explain that during the formulation step, they had to separate the solid phase of fruits/vegetables from the liquid phase to reduce the moisture content. Otherwise, the viscosity of food material would be too high to print through extrusion-based 3D printing. Also, due to this separation, there was no need to use any hydrocolloids or proteins.

The nutritional content of additive manufactured-foods is of crucial importance to satisfy the needs of customers or even patients with specific dietary needs. In the additive manufacturing of food structures, various ingredients from different sources can be used. There are many applications of chocolate, cheese, sugar, and starch-based materials and a rising curiosity about the discovery of meat, fruit, and vegetable-based food inks. With such progress, practical applications of personalized 3D food printing are being tried to meet nutritional needs and protect human health (Burke-Shyne et al., 2021; Escalante-Aburto et al., 2021). Personalized 3D food printing systems are not only developed to satisfy the wishes of regular customers but also to cover the nutritional needs of serious patients who suffer from dietary illnesses like allergies, intolerances, swallowing disorders, and various digestive problems from the mouth to the anus (Escalante-Aburto et al., 2021). Hemsley et al. (Hemsley et al., n.d.), explain extensively the 3D food printing applications for people with swallowing disorders, and dysphagia, and mention that covering a patient's nutritional needs must consider the customer's age, health risks, allergies, and intolerances. In this context, Pant et al. (Pant et al., 2021a) presented a 3D food ink recipe for dysphagia patients made from garden peas, carrots, and bok choy. The raw materials turned to puree and tried with various gums to fabricate an aesthetic and palatable 3D printed food structure. Many samples were fabricated successfully and it was concluded that such fabrication methods can be utilized in daycare centers, nursing homes, and hospitals for people with specific nutrition needs.

3. 3D food Printing Emerging Technologies

The application of three-dimensional printing technology in the realm of food industries introduces novel prospects for augmenting the nutritional content, accessibility, and aesthetic appeal of food products. This nascent technology streamlines the process of crafting personalized meals that align with individual caloric intake and distinct nutritional prerequisites. Figure 2 illustrates several 3D printing techniques, encompassing extrusion printing, powder binding deposition, inkjet printing, and bioprinting.

3.1 Extrusion Printing

In 3D food printing, Fused Deposition Modelling (FDM) relies on a moving syringe nozzle to build objects layer by layer. Hot material extruded from the syringe forms each layer, which cools and fuses with the one below. Employing a syringe nozzle in motion, this technique carefully deposits layers. Material, supplied by the syringe, is extruded to form each layer. As the layers undergo the cooling process, a seamless fusion takes place, ensuring the integration of each successive layer with the one that precedes it (Godoi et al., 2016). This versatile and user-friendly approach is suitable for printing both liquid and semi-solid materials. An essential stage in the extrusion printing procedure, beyond the capacity to extrude ink from the nozzle, is the aptitude to produce a robust 3D structure and attain precise shape fidelity. This is crucial for imparting the printed object with aesthetic appeal and the intended characteristics. (Pant et al., 2021b). One crucial factor to be considered in food printing is rheological properties, which strongly influence the printing accuracy of food. Therefore, edible food materials need to be easily extruded through the nozzle without requiring excessive pressure or exhibiting flow instabilities. Once deposited, they should retain their shape, resisting gravitational collapse and preserving the intended geometry of the printed structure (Kim et al., 2017b). Despite the conditions being met by only a handful of foods, processing food materials to make them suitable for FDM remains challenging. This difficulty stems from the fact that FDM technology is tailored for thermoplastic materials, characterized by consistent properties, in contrast to food materials that display highly variable rheological properties both pre and post the 3D printing. (Severini et al., 2018b). However, the past few years have witnessed a growing trend towards the adaptation of FDM technology for 3D food printing applications.

A study employing an extrusion-based printing compared various food materials with 3D-printed chocolates, expanding the potential applications beyond dehydrated powders (Hao et al., 2010a). Utilizing the Fab@home™ platform, researchers successfully printed cake frostings and processed cheeses, demonstrating the versatility of extrusion-based printing beyond dry food powders (Periard et al., 2007). Despite the predominance of dehydrated and freeze-dried food powders in current 3D food printing approaches, recent explorations have yielded novel food-ink systems. These systems, combining vegetable powder materials with a continuous hydrocolloid framework, show promise for integration with FDM techniques (Kim et al., 2018b).

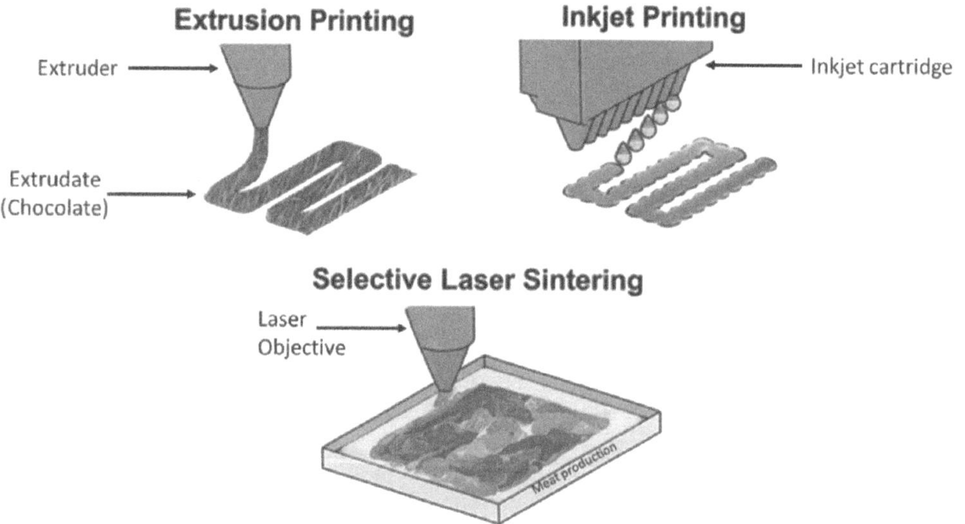

Fig. 2   Illustrations of three types of 3D printing technology for food printing.

3.2 *Powder Binding Deposition*

Following extrusion processes, powder binding deposition stands as the second most widely adopted system in the field of 3D food printing. This classification can be segmented into three subtypes: Selective Laser Sintering (SLS), Selective Hot Air Sintering and Melting (SHASAM), and Liquid Binding (LB). SLS and SHASAM achieve layer bonding through heat-induced fusion: SLS with an infrared laser and SHASAM with hot air. Liquid binding, conversely, uses a non-melting adhesive deposited onto powder layers sequentially (Wegrzyn et al., 2012). SLS employs a laser as the energy source for sintering powder particles. A coherent structure is built by directing the laser to predetermined points outlined by a 3D model. The laser methodically merges specific regions within the particulate powder bed by scanning cross-sections. Following this, the powder bed is gradually lowered by one layer thickness, a new layer of particles is introduced, and the iterative process persists until the object is fully formed. This methodology is adaptable for generating multiple layers of a food matrix, with each layer accommodating distinct components of food material (Godoi et al., 2016). Acting as a controlled heat source, the laser strategically melds powdered material through a cross-sectional scanning process, guided by the 3D digital description encoded in the accompanying software. The successful fabrication of a product is contingent upon various raw material properties such as particle size, shape, density, coarseness, porosity, and powder texture (Leontiou et al., 2023). Moreover, the arrangement and temperature-sensitive behavior of particles play a pivotal role in influencing powder flowability. Significantly, SLS holds advantages over alternative techniques, particularly in processing intricate macroscopic designs. This is attributed to the inherent support provided by the unsintered powder, which accommodates designs featuring voids and protrusion (Jonkers et al., 2022).

The Netherlands Organization for Applied Scientific Research (TNO) leveraged SLS for innovative food fabrication, incorporating both nutrition and flavor into the printed products. SLS relies on melting sugars or fats to fuse the powder layers, acting as a built-in binding agent (Nachal et al., 2019b; Noort et al., 2016). In the SHASAM procedure, a meticulously controlled and gentle airflow of heated air is precisely applied to a powdered medium, such as sugar, for the intricate construction of a two-dimensional image. Subsequent to the formation of this image, the powder bed undergoes a gradual descent, and a thin layer of powder is applied to envelop the initial layer. Following this, the same hot air process selectively fuses the new layer. This cyclic procedure continues based on the design specifications outlined in the 3D model until the comprehensive formation of the 3D object is achieved. Within the SHASAM process, the heated air beam is directed onto the powder bed, with the X-axis and Y-axis of the beam alternating in movement. This coordinated motion facilitates the formation of the product by shaping the sintered powder, while the unsintered powder retains its viability for subsequent reuse. It is noteworthy that SLS has demonstrated efficacy in fabricating intricate 3D structures using sugar-rich powders (*Looking to the Future: Creating Novel Foods Using 3D Printing*, n.d.). This method is also distinguished by its capability to sinterize any material to a powdered state (Kruth et al., 2003). However, it is imperative to recognize the limitation of this process to materials in a powder-based form (Lai, 2007).

In the liquid binding approach, a drop-on-demand printing head accurately dispenses a binder onto a thin layer of powder, adhering to a sliced 2D profile derived from a computer-generated 3D model.The binder assumes a vital function, serving to unite neighboring particles and thereby constructing a three-dimensional framework. This bonding process can manifest through either the dissolution-fusion or interlinking of particle exteriors (Peltola et al., 2008). The advantages of binder binding 3D printing, compared to alternative 3D printing technologies, primarily encompass the capability to craft products with an elevated material density, the flexibility to utilize various material compositions, and the ease of achieving color variations across different components (Zhu et al., 2022). One drawback associated with this technique is the less-than-ideal surface texture of the printed food, necessitating subsequent post-treatment procedures such as high-temperature curing. The food, typically composed of sugar and starch powders, undergoes these additional steps to enhance its overall texture and quality (He et al., 2020).

3.3   Inkjet Printing

This technique is primarily employed for the adornment and surface embellishment of food items. Small droplets of food ink are generated and meticulously applied to the surfaces of edible substrates, such as cakes, cookies, or candies, in order to replicate an image sourced from a digital file. Described as a non-contact methodology, inkjet printing serves to safeguard the food from potential contamination during the printing process, as the print-head maintains physical separation from the food substrate(Varvara et al., 2021b). In 2015, TNO incorporated Inkjet technology into microencapsulation processes. Their printhead, comprising of 500 nozzles with a capacity of 100 L/h, facilitates the generation of highly monodisperse droplets that subsequently undergo powder formation during the drying process. This versatile printing technology is compatible with a broad spectrum of materials, including waxes, polymers, aqueous solutions, emulsions, and dispersions. It enables the creation of core-shell microcapsules and particles suitable for encapsulating aqueous flavor and colorant solutions. Furthermore, the method permits the production of calcium alginate gel particles through the precise printing of alginate drops within a calcium chloride solution

(Gholamipour-Shirazi et al., 2020; Godoi et al., 2019). De Grood Innovations™ employed pneumatic membrane nozzle jets in a Drop-on-Demand (DoD) mode to perform surface filling of pizza bases and biscuits utilizing the Foodjet™ printer (Nachal et al., 2019b).

3.4 Bioprinting

Bioprinting involves the systematic layer-by-layer deposition of biological materials and the cultivation of living cells. It is widely considered as the prospective frontier for the development of complex and heterogeneous plant-based food products. Among 3D-bioprinting methodologies for soft hydrogels, FRESH printing stands out as a pioneering and technologically sophisticated platform, offering remarkable advantages in precision and material compatibility (Ianovici et al., 2022). Researchers have employed this methodology to produce tissues without the reliance on a bio-material substrate. The process begins by selecting a suitable bio-compatible platform for depositing the bio-material, which is subsequently transferred to a bioreactor. During the maturation period within the bioreactor, the necessary bio-mechanical properties develop. Through this innovative approach, a team at the University of Missouri successfully engineered an edible porcine tissue strip (Marga et al., 2012; Norotte et al., 2009). This approach, acknowledged as a sustainable substitute for conventional meat production, holds the capacity to influence ethical, religious, and societal viewpoints pertaining to the consumption of animal-derived meat. Another inquiry delved into a process of producing cultured meat, emphasizing the emerging paradigm of 3D bioprinting. This innovative technique exhibits distinctive advantages, displaying potential for elevating quality and yield, diminishing production expenses, and augmenting the ecological sustainability of cultured meat. The examination of 3D bioprinting within the study posits its prospective contribution to addressing the escalating demand for meat in a more sustainable manner(X. Guo et al., 2023).

4. Applications of 3D Food Printing

4.1 Tailor-made Food Designs

Food printing emerges as a transformative digital fabrication process, merging 3D printing with cutting-edge culinary techniques to manufacture customized food items. This technology empowers individuals to conceive and manufacture foods with personalized attributes encompassing color, shape, flavor, texture, and nutritional profiles, thereby transcending conventional gastronomic boundaries (van Bommel and Spicer, 2011). Presently, extrusion-based printing stands as the predominant method in food printing, serving as an engineering solution to translate digitized food designs into tangible entities while ensuring precise control over nutritional content. This technology holds significant potential for addressing the specific needs of populations with dietary restrictions or difficulties, such as elderly individuals with swallowing or chewing challenges (*3ders.Org - EU Develops PERFORMANCE 3D Printed Food for Elderly and Patients with Dysphagia | 3D Printer News & 3D Printing News*, n.d.). This promising technology also unlocks the potential for fabricating personalized and complex food structures, offering unprecedented control over texture, appearance, and even nutritional composition, paving the way for a new era of culinary customization and dietary optimization.

The procedural sequence initiates with the generation of a virtual 3D model, which undergoes segmentation into discrete layer patterns through specialized software. These patterns are subsequently transformed into machine codes that dictate the parameters of the printing process. Upon uploading the codes and specifying the desired food recipe, the printer initiates its operation. Adhering to the predetermined layer patterns, the printer facilitates the extrusion of the food material, either by mobilizing the nozzle above a motorized stage or reciprocally, systematically depositing each layer atop the preceding one. This incremental layer-by-layer deposition culminates in the realization of the intended 3D structure. (Sun et al., 2015b). To facilitate food printing design and development, researchers have adapted open-source commercial printers like the Fab@Home system (Cohen et al., n.d.). However, user interfaces should prioritize user knowledge and context. For example, 3D Systems' ChefJet series uses Digital Cookbook software, catering to users unfamiliar with complex modeling tools. Platform design must also consider the intended environment, whether household, factory, or laboratory. In essence, interfaces for customized shapes, personalized nutrition, and product prototyping need distinct approaches(Sun et al., 2015b).

4.2 Printing Parameters

Factors such as powder density and compressibility necessitate meticulous attention due to their substantial impact on the flow characteristics of powder within the container. This, in turn, assumes a pivotal role in the patterning process when the heat source is applied to the powder bed. (Berretta et al., 2014; Schmid et al., n.d.). The significance of flowability in achieving uniform powder distribution for the construction of thin layers is crucial. Insufficient flowability impedes effective recoating, while excessive flowability introduces instability to the powder bed. Additionally, the wettability of particles plays a vital role, influencing both the volume of binder dispersed in the powder bed and the degree of binder absorption by the particles. Insufficient wetting of fine particles contributes to the reorganization of the powder bed, while heightened wettability, coupled with a slow powder reaction, may constrain the attainable minimum feature size.

The quality of the produced food items is intricately linked to several process parameters. An investigation aimed at comprehending this relationship identified nozzle diameter, deposition height, and the speed of stage movement as pivotal factors influencing the geometrical precision of chocolate deposition. (Hao et al., 2010a). However, the existing body of literature predominantly focuses on the fabrication of food items, with comparatively limited emphasis on the optimization of process parameters. While chocolate has been well-studied, crafting unique 3D structures using dark chocolate offers a fascinating frontier. Several researchers are exploring its printability, focusing on parameters like nozzle diameter, printing speed, and nozzle height accuracy for optimal printing. Although valuable insights have been gained, existing chocolate printing parameters are constrained by the limitations of individual 3D printers. To unlock the full potential of chocolate 3D printing for a wider range of machines, further research is crucial to optimize parameters for specific printer configurations (Hao et al., 2010b; Lanaro et al., n.d.).

4.3 3D Food Printing in Space

3D food printing has witnessed significant strides, transforming from a novelty to a promising technology capable of producing innovative food products in space missions. Material extrusion, the prevailing approach in 3D printing food, involves the expulsion of a fluid or semi-solid food substance through a nozzle, subsequently undergoing solidification. The application of this method demonstrates promise for space missions, as it allows for the production of diverse food items within confined spaces using a limited set of inks. This attribute becomes particularly significant in the context of prolonged missions characterized by constrained resources. 3D food printing technology in space differs from traditional processing methods, as it reduces reliance on engineering equipment for raw material pre-treatment, packaging, and sterilization. Additionally, this technology allows the independent design of product specifications, shapes, and flavors tailored to astronauts' preferences, enhancing the acceptability of food.

In the space industry, 3D printing technology offers rapid production of specialized parts, cost-effective prototyping, and potential self-sustainability through on-demand printing during space voyages. Researchers are exploring polymer and metal materials for in-space 3D printing, allowing adaptive responses to unforeseen circumstances. Several additive manufacturing techniques demonstrate exceptional adaptability to zero-gravity environments, achieving comparable print quality to terrestrial operations (Sacco and Moon, 2019). The successful deployment of 3D printers on the International Space Station, resulting in the fabrication of a minimum of 115 components in orbit (*Solving the Challenges of Long Duration Space Flight with 3D Printing - NASA*, n.d.), underscores the technology's efficacy for applications beyond the realm of food in space.

In the pursuit of exploring the potential applications of 3D food printing, research sponsored by the National Aeronautics and Space Administration (NASA) concentrated on mitigating micronutrient degradation in dehydrated and prepackaged foods. Initiated in 2013, the project aimed to formulate protein and starch pastes with diverse textures, presenting experimental recipes featuring a well-balanced amalgamation of protein, starch, fat, flavors, and micronutrients. Beyond the realm of food design, the project encompassed the development of a system for nutrient preservation and transportation, a mixing station tailored for environments with low or microgravity, and an adapted 3D printing system (Enfield et al., 2023b). Subsequently, a mechanical engineer and the founder of Beehex LLC, assumed a leading role in the conceptual phase of Space Mission Resource Control (SMRC) proposals in September 2019. During this stage, a zero-G 3D printer was employed to fabricate a 12-inch pizza in a mere 12 minutes. The implications of this endeavor extended beyond space missions, serving as a global introduction to heighten awareness regarding the vast potential of 3D printing technology (*Deep-Space Food Science Research Improves 3D-Printing Capabilities | NASA Spinoff*, n.d.).

In 2016, as part of the Green Space Interstellar Project, China utilized a food 3D printer to create moon cakes, showcasing the ability to prepare a diverse range of novel foods through 3D printing technology. In September 2019, Israeli startup "Aleph Farms" achieved a milestone by presenting the first 3D-printed meat in space. The process involved extracting cow meat cells, growing them in vials, and printing the beef on the space station. Despite potential water constraints, this breakthrough showcased the viability of 3D bioprinting technology for meat production in challenging environments, providing a competitive alternative to lab-grown meat (*In a First, Astronauts 3D-Print Meat in Space - Times of India*, n.d.). Adopting a bioprinting-inspired methodology, Beehex has devised a technique wherein designated bacteria facilitate the conversion of plastic waste into biomass within a spacecraft. Subsequently, this biomass is employed in the production of 3D-printed meals through a specialized printer (*3D Printed Meals From Plastic Waste Ready for Space - 3Dnatives*, n.d.). Nonetheless, a comprehensive examination is imperative to comprehend the potential physiological implications on human health subsequent to the consumption of such printed biomass.

In contrast to terrestrial 3D printing, the application of this technology in space encounters distinctive challenges primarily arising from the zero-gravity (zero-G) environment. The specific conditions prevailing in space introduce complexities during the printing process, manifesting in the tendency of molten materials to assume spherical droplet forms, thereby compromising the performance of 3D printing. Particularly within the domain of extrusion 3D printing, challenges manifest in layer deposition, leading to potential inconsistencies and unsuccessful print outcomes. Mitigating these challenges necessitates the development of specialized 3D printers tailored for microgravity environments. Furthermore, the printing process itself must undergo modifications to accommodate the absence of gravity in a space setting (Santhoshkumar et al., 2024).

4.4 *Food Packaging*

Food packaging functions as a safeguarding barrier, shielding against tampering and contamination originating from physical, chemical, and biological sources. This role contributes to the extension of shelf life and guarantees the provision of high-quality food to consumers. Additionally, packaging assumes a crucial role in conveying brand elements, disseminating nutritional information, and facilitating marketing initiatives. Polymers find extensive application in food packaging owing to their facile manufacturing process, robust molecular structures or crosslinking, and exceptional performance characteristics, encompassing strength, oxygen and moisture barrier capabilities, as well as resistance to the degradation caused by food components (Kovačević et al., 2022). Commonly utilized in active food packaging, non-biodegradable polymers encompass polypropylene (PP), polyethylene (PE), polyethylene-co-vinyl acetate (EVA), polyvinyl chloride (PVC), and polyethylene terephthalate (PET). Biodegradable natural-based polymers, such as cellulose, chitosan, starch, agar, gelatin, soy protein, and whey protein (Díez-Pascual, 2020; Nilsen-Nygaard et al., 2021), offer distinct advantages over petroleum-based counterparts, aligning with both consumer preferences and environmental considerations.

Caro et al. pioneered an innovation in the creation of active packaging films employing chitosan and chitosan/quinoa protein. They integrated chitosan-tripolyphosphate-thymol nanoparticles into the films through the application of thermal inkjet printing (Caro et al., 2016). The results indicated that these films demonstrated enhanced water vapor barrier properties, served as proficient mediums for the controlled release of active compounds, and exhibited heightened antimicrobial efficacy against notable microorganisms, including Staphylococcus aureus, Escherichia coli, and Pseudomonas aeruginosa. This technological progression holds potential for the development of inventive packaging materials, with the prospect of prolonging the shelf life of fresh fruits. The increasing demand for packaged food and beverages has spurred advancements in packaging systems, propelled by the growing complexity of products, the globalization of food markets, and consumer preferences favoring environmentally sustainable packaging. This trend has given rise to specific classifications in the global market, namely smart packaging, active packaging, and intelligent packaging. Smart packaging systems find extensive applications across diverse sectors, encompassing food and beverages, healthcare products, and personal care, among others. These systems demonstrate the capacity to survey physicochemical factors, such as environmental conditions, and preemptively manage microbiological alterations (Biji et al., 2015; Schaefer and Cheung, 2018). The subsequent sections provide indepth discussions on active packaging and intelligent packaging, both of which represent specialized forms within the realm of smart packaging.

5. Challenges and Future Perspectives for 3D Food Printing Technologies

In the context of 3DFP, much is still to be learned and many obstacles have to be overcome, particularly about materials and procedures. Some of these aspects—such as factors to be considered while selecting food inks and preparatory process steps required for food safety—are outlined below.

5.1 *Food Quality and Safety in 3D Food Printing*

Food and nutrition security should be achieved through food safety. Increasing the use of current resources and research to support evidence-based decision-making is a major obstacle to scaling up nutrition, public health, and food security/safety internationally. The process of averting harmful chemicals and microbes from getting into, developing, or existing within the country's food supply chain is known as food safety. (Uyttendaele et al., 2016). As with any new technology, it's crucial to confirm that food that has been 3D printed is safe to eat. To guarantee that the materials used in 3D printing are safe and that no hazardous pollutants are introduced during the printing process, researchers and food manufacturers must take the necessary precautions. Figure 3 schematically illustrates food safety and quality requirements in 3D-printed food production.

Food deterioration or spoilage due to various chemical, biological, and/or physical changes is a major issue that arises during production, distribution, and storage operations. When the aforementioned characteristics change, food loses its nutritional content, chemical and biological activity, tissue integrity, and other qualities that make it unfit for human ingestion. In addition to making food unsafe and hazardous for human and public health, spoilage also results in financial losses (Baykara et al., 2021). In order to protect public health and consumer confidence, food safety and quality evaluation are essential for identifying hazards such as spoilage, contamination, and allergies (dos Santos et al., 2022). Ensuring the safety and longevity of 3D-printed foods is

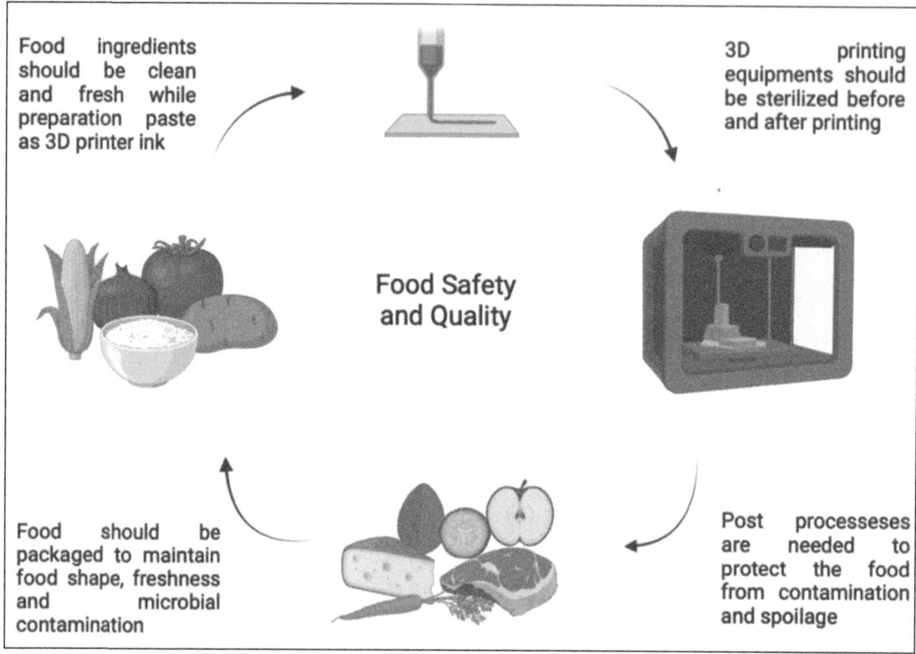

Fig. 3   Food safety and quality requirements in the process of production of 3D printed food.

a major challenge in the food industry (M. Wang et al., 2022). Protecting food quality involves addressing various factors throughout the production, handling, and storage processes. In order to preserve ingredients' quality and safety during the printing process, proper procurement, storage, and handling are significant stages (Hamilton et al., 2024).

Packaging plays a crucial role in maintaining the quality and preventing contamination of 3D-printed food. The growth of mold, bacteria, and other microorganisms that can cause spoilage can be stopped by using the right packaging materials and practices (J. Wang and Zhang, 2023). However, conventional packing methods can only separate food from the outside environment; they cannot assure producers, distributors, or customers about the food's freshness. Smart packaging, which blends intelligent elements with conventional packaging methods, is one of the newest advancements in package technology. Information sensing, storing, transmission, and feedback tasks are handled by intelligent packaging, starting with the supply of raw materials, and continuing through product manufacturing, packaging, and the removal of packaging waste when processing food (Shao et al., 2021). Post-3D printing processes, such as cooking (e.g., frying, baking, drying), are important for further enhancing the quality of printed food products and enabling their storage by preventing contamination and spoiling (Hamilton et al., 2024; J. Wang and Zhang, 2023). Storage is an important aspect of protecting 3D-printed food. Proper storage conditions, such as temperature and humidity control, can help to extend the shelf-life of the food and prevent spoilage (J. Wang and Zhang, 2023).

When using 3D printing to process food, some considerations need to be made. The components of a 3D printer that come into contact with food must meet the same standards as conventional food equipment. They should be strong, resistant to rust, non-absorbent, accessible for inspection, safe under typical operating conditions, and easily cleaned. Additionally, they should lack breaks and sharp internal angles. As a result, the type of 3D printer used, and the use of efficient cleaning techniques determine the safety of printed food (Baiano, 2022a). Maintaining the food quality of 3D-printed food requires adherence to food safety laws and guidelines. To ensure food safety, customer confidence, and industry compliance, laws that cover the entire 3D food printing process including materials, equipment, and processes need to be developed (Hamilton et al., 2024).

5.2   *Alteration of Food Matrix Properties*

The size, shape, microstructure, and texture of 3D-printed food can be altered by a variety of chemical processes that occur during post-processing, including the Maillard reaction, protein denaturation, and moisture content decrease (M. Wang et al., 2022) The growth of food 3D printing depends largely on the quantification of food ingredients' printability since many meals lack the necessary qualities to be printed without first being processed. The rheological behavior of the food system and food additives are two elements that affect printability (Lipton et al., 2010). Understanding the rheological characteristics of food formulas and optimizing printing conditions are essential for producing sophisticated 3D structures (Pérez et al., 2019b). Primarily, optimizing 3D printing entails modifying printing parameters such as writing speed, line length, laser power, number of layers, thickness, form, and shape in addition to temperature and cooling rates. Important aspects to consider are the design and process characteristics, such as the deposition rate, nozzle diameter, depth of nozzle, suck-back and push-back timings, radiation intensity, hot air temperature, and layer spacing (Nachal et al., 2019c).

The qualities of food materials restrict the speed at which existing food printers can print, making the use of 3D printing as a tool for on-demand food production in consumer settings challenging. Robust food printers with integrated software controls are required to make the creation of customized foods easier. These control systems are essential for adjusting printing parameters according to the characteristics of the food material (Jayaprakash et al., 2020). Materials can be layered and extruded into desired shapes using hot extrusion 3D printing technology, which emphasizes the accuracy, shape-recovery ability, and structural support performance of the molded sample. This process is based on 3D models. As a result, 3D printing is a cutting-edge technique for preparing food that has very high standards for raw materials that can be easily extruded and retain their shape while exhibiting favorable rheological behavior (Rong et al., 2023). Viscosity and consistency are crucial factors that determine a material's ability to flow through a nozzle in the extrusion printing process. This has to do with the printed food structures' textural qualities and their capacity to hold their shape following the deposition process (Nachal et al., 2019c). Researchers have looked into ways to preserve texture and shape during post-processing, such as adding components to increase dimensional stability and using other cooking techniques such as direct infrared radiation. By addressing the challenges associated with post-processing, researchers aim to enhance the properties of printed food matrices, paving the way for more sophisticated and appealing culinary creations (M. Wang et al., 2022). Consequently, the use of 3D printing technology to modify the properties of the food matrix presents intriguing prospects for the creation of new food products with personalized features and improved nutritional content (Waghmare et al., 2023) The extensive development of functional food inks has made it possible for 3D printing to alter the sensory qualities and look of food, potentially catering to consumer preferences and influencing eating habits (Ma and Zhang, 2022).

5.3   *Economic & Financial Concerns of 3D Printed Food*

The production cost, consumer demand, and regulatory issues are only a few of the many economic and financial issues surrounding 3D-printed food. Research and development expenditures, together with the purchase of specialist equipment, are critical to the development of 3D printing technology for food production. Important economic factors to consider are the price of edible ink ingredients and the effectiveness of mass production through clever transformation (Yu et al., 2023). It has been observed that 3D food printing could change the food sector in a number of ways and close the gap between small and large-scale firms, which could have a substantial impact on the global economy. It should be mentioned, too, that 3D printing technology—meant for professional use—is now highly costly. This might prevent smaller companies or individuals from adopting it (Baiano, 2022b). Researchers developed an economic model using the system thinking technique to assess how the advent of additive manufacturing technology might affect small-batch production firms including restaurants, bakeries, and confectionery in the food business. The model predicts that the demand for food capsules will rise as 3D printing technology becomes more widely used. As a result, manufacturing volumes rise and the production costs and food capsule selling prices drop because of economies of scale enabled by the implementation of novel machinery or processes (Dabbene et al., 2018).

Unlike other technologies where the cost of highly intrinsic molds must be added to the production cost in order to get the necessary geometry and design, the cost of complicated designs using 3D printing technology solely depends on the amount of material utilized. However, because most printed meals have a short shelf life and processing might change the texture in ways that the consumer would find undesirable, the shelf-stability of 3D-printed food products is an issue. Therefore, the upfront expenses of the technology, continuing production costs, and the possible effects on consumer perception and marketability are the economic and financial considerations around 3D printed food (Agunbiade et al., 2022). Scalability is another economic challenge with 3D-printed food. Due to technological restrictions and the time required to print each food item individually, 3D printing may not be appropriate for large-scale production, even though it does allow for customization and individualized food products. In addition, the continuous expenses associated with maintaining and running 3D printing machinery may pose a financial risk. The expense of hiring qualified staff to run and oversee the 3D printing process is another issue. The cost to firms of employing and training staff members with the requisite knowledge of 3D printing technology can increase (Praveena et al., 2022). All things considered, even if 3D-printed food has the potential to have a huge impact on the food industry and economy, smaller firms or individuals may not be able to adopt it due to its expensive cost (Baiano, 2022b).

5.4 *Future Perspectives*

The composition of 3D printing inks used for printing may become more consistent in the future thanks to advancements in control parameters, which should cut down on the amount of time needed to print intricate patterns (Wu et al., 2023b). Molecular gastronomy and 3D food printing can be combined to give functional nutrients to regular food, improving both its nutritional profile and look. Furthermore, the food industry stands to gain a great deal from the application of 3D printing to produce aesthetically pleasing and nutritionally optimal meals (Xie et al., 2023). Among the main benefits provided by this technology is the ability to print structures in desired sizes quickly and precisely, as well as the ability to do so. Even with these technological advances, creating printer ink compositions that work well for a given purpose is still difficult (Agarwal et al., 2021). Modern 3D printers are becoming more and more sophisticated and affordable, which means that personalized and customized foods may be produced using them on a large scale in the future. However, the use of 3D printing in the food industry also helps the sector grow more intelligently and mechanistically. For example, it's feasible that, similar to many homes presently owning microwave ovens, many homes in the future will own 3D printers (Y. Chen et al., 2022). Researchers' recent technological advancements in the creation of pharmaceutical foods and plant and insect-based meat substitutes made possible by 3D printing, were notable highlights. It is widely held that in the pandemic era, personalization and customization of 3D-printed foods may play a significant role in addressing unmet nutritional needs and eliminating a number of chronic diseases (Eswaran et al., 2023). With the use of 3D printing technology, new business model development opportunities may arise. Printed foods, however, are still in the early stages of development and require further optimization tests before commercialization. It is necessary to investigate factors of printed food safety as well as the feasibility of printing heterogeneous food components with varying textures (Nachal et al., 2019c).

Conclusions

In terms of design, nutrition, and formulation, 3D food printing applications have great potential for new and innovative food customization. With the development of 3D food technologies and recipes, and the necessity of new personalized nutritious foods, 3D food-printing has become more widespread and studied. Even the general concept of 3D food printing has become more available for some food-markets and mid-sized businesses. However, the economic reality of 3D food printing becomes clearer and requires investigation considering its effectiveness on large-scale productions and implementation for larger firms. However, finding a sustainable source of balanced-nutritious food adapted to new lifestyles will be a major challenge due to the continued population growth, pandemics, climate change, diminishing resources, environmental challenges, and public health. With innovations in additive manufacturing methods and 3D food printing technologies, it could be possible to find safer, more nutritious, delicious, and sustainable food in the future.

References

3D Printed Meals From Plastic Waste Ready for Space-3 Dnatives. (n.d.). Retrieved January 30, 2024, from https://www.3dnatives.com/en/3d-printed-food-nasa-plastic-waste-19012023/

3ders.org - EU develops PERFORMANCE 3D printed food for elderly and patients with dysphagia | 3D Printer News & 3D Printing News. (n.d.). Retrieved January 30, 2024, from https://www.3ders.org/articles/20151026-eu-develops-performance-3d-printed-food-for-elderly-and-patients-with-dysphagia.html

Afoakwa, E.O., Paterson, A. and Fowler, M. (2007). Factors influencing rheological and textural qualities in chocolate - a review. *Trends in Food Science and Technology*, 18(6), 290–298. https://doi.org/10.1016/j.tifs.2007.02.002

Agarwal, T., Costantini, M. and Maiti, T.K. (2021). Extrusion 3D printing with Pectin-based ink formulations: Recent trends in tissue engineering and food manufacturing. *Biomedical Engineering Advances*, 2. https://doi.org/10.1016/j.bea.2021.100018

Agunbiade, A.O., Song, L., Agunbiade, O.J., Ofoedu, C.E., Chacha et al. (2022). Potentials of 3D extrusion-based printing in resolving food processing challenges: A perspective review. In *Journal of Food Process Engineering* (Vol. 45, Issue 4). https://doi.org/10.1111/jfpe.13996

Ahmed, J. and Thomas, L. (2018). Effect of xanthan and guar gum on the pasting, stickiness and extensional properties of brown wheat flour/β-glucan composite doughs. *LWT*, 87, 443–449. https://doi.org/10.1016/j.lwt.2017.09.017

Attarin, S. and Attaran, M. (2020). Food Printing: Evolving Technologies, Challenges, Opportunities and Best adoption Strategies. *Journal of International Technology and Information Management*, 29(1), 25–55. https://doi.org/10.58729/1941-6679.1442

Azam, R.S.M., Zhang, M., Bhandari, B. and Yang, C. (2018). Effect of Different Gums on Features of 3D Printed Object Based on Vitamin-D Enriched Orange Concentrate. *Food Biophysics*, 13(3), 250–262. https://doi.org/10.1007/s11483-018-9531-x

Baiano, A. (2022a). 3D Printed Foods: A Comprehensive Review on Technologies, Nutritional Value, Safety, Consumer Attitude, Regulatory Framework, and Economic and Sustainability Issues. In *Food Reviews International* (Vol. 38, Issue 5). https://doi.org/10.1080/87559129.2020.1762091

Baiano, A. (2022b). 3D Printed Foods: A Comprehensive Review on Technologies, Nutritional Value, Safety, Consumer Attitude, Regulatory Framework, and Economic and Sustainability Issues. In *Food Reviews International* (Vol. 38, Issue 5). https://doi.org/10.1080/87559129.2020.1762091

Baykara, D., Pilavci, E., Meran, M. and Onur Caliskaner, Z. (2021). Antimicrobial properties and application of fig seed oil as an additive for chitosan-based films. *Ukrainian Food Journal*, 10(2). https://doi.org/10.24263/2304-974X-2021-10-2-7

Berretta, S., Ghita, O., ... K.E.-... R. in V. and 2013, undefined. (2014). Size, shape and flow of powders for use in Selective Laser Sintering (SLS). *Books.Google.ComS Berretta, O Ghita, KE Evans, A Anderson, C NewmanHigh Value Manufacturing: Advanced Research in Virtual and Rapid, 2013•books.Google.Com.*

Biji, K.B., Ravishankar, C.N., Mohan, C.O. and Srinivasa Gopal, T.K. (2015). Smart packaging systems for food applications: a review. *Journal of Food Science and Technology*, 52(10), 6125–6135. https://doi.org/10.1007/S13197-015-1766-7/TABLES/2

Blutinger, J.D., Cooper, C.C., Karthik, S., Tsai, A., Samarelli, N. et al. (2023). The future of software-controlled cooking. *Npj Science of Food*, 7(1). https://doi.org/10.1038/s41538-023-00182-6

Burdge, G.C. and Calder, P.C. (2015). Introduction to fatty acids and lipids. In *World Review of Nutrition and Dietetics* (Vol. 112, pp. 1–16). S. Karger AG. https://doi.org/10.1159/000365423

Burke-Shyne, S., Gallegos, D. and Williams, T. (2021). 3D food printing: nutrition opportunities and challenges. *British Food Journal*, 123(2), 649–663. https://doi.org/10.1108/BFJ-05-2020-0441

Caro, N., Medina, E., Díaz-Dosque, M., López, L., Abugoch, L. et al. (2016). Novel active packaging based on films of chitosan and chitosan/quinoa protein printed with chitosan-tripolyphosphate-thymol nanoparticles via thermal ink-jet printing. *Food Hydrocolloids, 52*, 520–532. https://doi.org/10.1016/J.FOODHYD.2015.07.028

Chen, J., Mu, T., Goffin, D., Blecker, C., Richard, G. et al. (2019). Application of soy protein isolate and hydrocolloids based mixtures as promising food material in 3D food printing. *Journal of Food Engineering, 261*, 76–86. https://doi.org/10.1016/j.jfoodeng.2019.03.016

Chen, Y., McClements, D.J., Peng, X., Chen, L., Xu, Z et al. (2022). Starch as edible ink in 3D printing for food applications: a review. In *Critical Reviews in Food Science and Nutrition*. https://doi.org/10.1080/10408398.2022.2106546

Chen, Y., Zhang, M. and Bhandari, B. (2021). 3d printing of steak-like foods based on textured soybean protein. *Foods, 10*(9). https://doi.org/10.3390/foods10092011

Cohen, D.L., Lipton, J.I., Cutler, M., Coulter, D., Vesco, A et al. . *Hydrocolloid Printing: A Novel Platform for Customized Food Production.*

Cui, Y., Li, C., Guo, Y., Liu, X., Zhu, F et al. (2022). Rheological & 3D printing properties of potato starch composite gels. *Journal of Food Engineering, 313*. https://doi.org/10.1016/j.jfoodeng.2021.110756

Dabbene, L., Ramundo, L. and Terzi, S. (2018). Economic Model for the Evaluation of 3D Food Printing. *2018 IEEE International Conference on Engineering, Technology and Innovation, ICE/ITMC 2018 - Proceedings.* https://doi.org/10.1109/ICE.2018.8436285

Dankar, I., Haddarah, A., El Omar, F., Sepulcre, F. and Pujolà, M. et al. (2018). Assessing the microstructural and rheological changes induced by food additives on potato puree. *Food Chemistry, 240*, 304–313. https://doi.org/10.1016/j.foodchem.2017.07.121

Dankar, I., Pujolà, M., El Omar, F., Sepulcre, F. and Haddarah, A. et al. (2018). Impact of Mechanical and Microstructural Properties of Potato Puree-Food Additive Complexes on Extrusion-Based 3D Printing. *Food and Bioprocess Technology, 11*(11), 2021–2031. https://doi.org/10.1007/s11947-018-2159-5

Deep-Space Food Science Research Improves 3D-Printing Capabilities | NASA Spinoff. (n.d.). Retrieved January 30, 2024, from https://spinoff.nasa.gov/Spinoff2019/ip_2.html

Derossi, A., Caporizzi, R., Azzollini, D. and Severini, C. (2018). Application of 3D printing for customized food. A case on the development of a fruit-based snack for children. *Journal of Food Engineering, 220*, 65–75. https://doi.org/10.1016/j.jfoodeng.2017.05.015

Derossi, A., Husain, A., Caporizzi, R. and Severini, C. (2020). Manufacturing personalized food for people uniqueness. An overview from traditional to emerging technologies. In *Critical Reviews in Food Science and Nutrition* (Vol. 60, Issue 7, pp. 1141–1159). Taylor and Francis Inc. https://doi.org/10.1080/10408398.2018.1559796

Díez-Pascual, A.M. (2020). Antimicrobial Polymer-Based Materials for Food Packaging Applications. *Polymers 2020, Vol. 12, Page 731, 12*(4), 731. https://doi.org/10.3390/POLYM12040731

dos Santos, D.M., Cardoso, R.M., Migliorini, F.L., Facure, M.H.M., Mercante, L.A. et al. (2022). Advances in 3D printed sensors for food analysis. In *TrAC - Trends in Analytical Chemistry* (Vol. 154). https://doi.org/10.1016/j.trac.2022.116672

Enfield, R.E., Pandya, J.K., Lu, J., McClements, D.J. and Kinchla, A.J. et al. (2023a). The future of 3D food printing: Opportunities for space applications. In *Critical Reviews in Food Science and Nutrition* (Vol. 63, Issue 29, pp. 10079–10092). Taylor and Francis Ltd. https://doi.org/10.1080/10408398.2022.2077299

Enfield, R.E., Pandya, J.K., Lu, J., McClements, D.J. and Kinchla, A.J. et al. (2023b). The future of 3D food printing: Opportunities for space applications. *Critical Reviews in Food Science and Nutrition, 63*(29), 10079–10092. https://doi.org/10.1080/10408398.2022.2077299

Escalante-Aburto, A., Trujillo-de Santiago, G., Álvarez, M.M. and Chuck-Hernández, C. (2021). Advances and prospective applications of 3D food printing for health improvement and personalized nutrition. *Comprehensive Reviews in Food Science and Food Safety, 20*(6), 5722–5741. https://doi.org/10.1111/1541-4337.12849

Eswaran, H., Ponnuswamy, R.D. and Kannapan, R.P. (2023). Perspective approaches of 3D printed stuffs for personalized nutrition: A comprehensive review. In *Annals of 3D Printed Medicine* (Vol. 12). https://doi.org/10.1016/j.stlm.2023.100125

Feng, C., Zhang, M., Bhandari, B., Wang, Y. and Wang, B. et al. (2021). Improvement of 3D printing properties of rose-sodium alginate heterogeneous gel by adjusting rose material. *Journal of Food Process Engineering, 44*(1). https://doi.org/10.1111/jfpe.13583

Gholamipour-Shirazi, A., Kamlow, M.A., Norton, I.T. and Mills, T. (2020). How to Formulate for Structure and Texture via Medium of Additive Manufacturing-A Review. *Foods 2020, Vol. 9, Page 497, 9*(4), 497. https://doi.org/10.3390/FOODS9040497

Godoi, F.C., Bhandari, B.R., Prakash, S. and Zhang, M. (2019). An Introduction to the Principles of 3D Food Printing. *Fundamentals of 3D Food Printing and Applications*, 1–18. https://doi.org/10.1016/B978-0-12-814564-7.00001-8

Godoi, F.C., Prakash, S. and Bhandari, B.R. (2016). 3d printing technologies applied for food design: Status and prospects. *Journal of Food Engineering, 179*, 44–54. https://doi.org/10.1016/J.JFOODENG.2016.01.025

Guo, X., Wang, D., He, B., Hu, L. and Jiang, G. et al. (2023). 3D Bioprinting of Cultured Meat: A Promising Avenue of Meat Production. *Food and Bioprocess Technology 2023*, 1–22. https://doi.org/10.1007/S11947-023-03195-X

Guo, Z., Arslan, M., Li, Z., Cen, S., Shi, J. et al. (2022). Application of Protein in Extrusion-Based 3D Food Printing: Current Status and Prospectus. In *Foods* (Vol. 11, Issue 13). MDPI. https://doi.org/10.3390/foods11131902

Hamilton, A.N., Mirmahdi, R.S., Ubeyitogullari, A., Romana, C.K., Baum, J.I. et al. (2024). From bytes to bites: Advancing the food industry with three-dimensional food printing. *Comprehensive Reviews in Food Science and Food Safety, 23*(1), 1–22. https://doi.org/10.1111/1541-4337.13293

Hao, L., Mellor, S., Seaman, O., Henderson, J., Sewell, N. et al. (2010a). Material characterisation and process development for chocolate additive layer manufacturing. *Virtual and Physical Prototyping, 5*(2), 57–64. https://doi.org/10.1080/17452751003753212

Hao, L., Mellor, S., Seaman, O., Henderson, J., Sewell, N. et al. (2010b). Material characterisation and process development for chocolate additive layer manufacturing. *Virtual and Physical Prototyping, 5*(2), 57–64. https://doi.org/10.1080/17452751003753212

Hassoun, A., Bekhit, A.E.D., Jambrak, A.R., Regenstein, J.M., Chemat, F. et al. (2022). The fourth industrial revolution in the food industry—part II: Emerging food trends. In *Critical Reviews in Food Science and Nutrition*. Taylor and Francis Ltd. https://doi.org/10.1080/10408398.2022.2106472

He, C., Zhang, M. and Fang, Z. (2020). 3D printing of food: pretreatment and post-treatment of materials. *Critical Reviews in Food Science and Nutrition, 60*(14), 2379–2392. https://doi.org/10.1080/10408398.2019.1641065

Hemsley, B., Palmer, S., Kouzani, A., Adams, S. and Balandin, S. (n.d.) et al. *Review Informing the Design of 3D Food Printing for People with Swallowing Disorders: Constructive, Conceptual, and Empirical Problems.* https://hdl.handle.net/10125/60009

Hussain, S., Malakar, S. and Arora, V.K. (2022). Extrusion-Based 3D Food Printing: Technological Approaches, Material Characteristics, Printing Stability, and Post-processing. In *Food Engineering Reviews* (Vol. 14, Issue 1, pp. 100–119). Springer. https://doi.org/10.1007/s12393-021-09293-w

Ianovici, I., Zagury, Y., Redenski, I., Lavon, N. and Levenberg, S. et al. (2022). 3D-printable plant protein-enriched scaffolds for cultivated meat development. *Biomaterials, 284*, 121487. https://doi.org/10.1016/J.BIOMATERIALS.2022.121487

In a first, astronauts 3D-print meat in space - Times of India. (n.d.). Retrieved January 30, 2024, from https://timesofindia.indiatimes.com/home/science/in-a-first-astronauts-3d-print-meat-in-space/articleshow/71535842.cms

Jayaprakash, S., Paasi, J., Pennanen, K., Ituarte, I.F., Lille, M. et al. (2020). Techno-economic prospects and desirability of 3d food printing: Perspectives of industrial experts, researchers and consumers. *Foods, 9*(12). https://doi.org/10.3390/foods9121725

Jiang, H., Zheng, L., Zou, Y., Tong, Z., Han, S. et al. (2019). 3D food printing: main components selection by considering rheological properties. In *Critical Reviews in Food Science and Nutrition* (Vol. 59, Issue 14, pp. 2335–2347). Taylor and Francis Inc. https://doi.org/10.1080/10408398.2018.1514363

Jonkers, N., van Dommelen, J.A.W. and Geers, M.G.D. (2022). Selective Laser Sintered food: A unit cell approach to design mechanical properties. *Journal of Food Engineering, 335*, 111183. https://doi.org/10.1016/J.JFOODENG.2022.111183

Kewuyemi, Y.O., Kesa, H. and Adebo, O.A. (2022). Trends in functional food development with three-dimensional (3D) food printing technology: prospects for value-added traditionally processed food products. In *Critical Reviews in Food Science and Nutrition* (Vol. 62, Issue 28, pp. 7866–7904). Taylor and Francis Ltd. https://doi.org/10.1080/10408398.2021.1920569

Kim, H.W., Bae, H. and Park, H.J. (2017a). Classification of the printability of selected food for 3D printing: Development of an assessment method using hydrocolloids as reference material. *Journal of Food Engineering, 215*, 23–32. https://doi.org/10.1016/j.jfoodeng.2017.07.017

Kim, H.W., Bae, H. and Park, H.J. (2017b). Classification of the printability of selected food for 3D printing: Development of an assessment method using hydrocolloids as reference material. *Journal of Food Engineering, 215*, 23–32. https://doi.org/10.1016/J.JFOODENG.2017.07.017

Kim, H.W., Lee, I.J., Park, S.M., Lee, J.H., Nguyen, M.H et al. (2019). Effect of hydrocolloid addition on dimensional stability in post-processing of 3D printable cookie dough. *LWT, 101*, 69–75. https://doi.org/10.1016/j.lwt.2018.11.019

Kim, H.W., Lee, J.H., Park, S.M., Lee, M.H., Lee, I.W. et al. (2018a). Effect of Hydrocolloids on Rheological Properties and Printability of Vegetable Inks for 3D Food Printing. *Journal of Food Science, 83*(12), 2923–2932. https://doi.org/10.1111/1750-3841.14391

Kim, H.W., Lee, J.H., Park, S.M., Lee, M.H., Lee, I.W. et al. (2018b). Effect of Hydrocolloids on Rheological Properties and Printability of Vegetable Inks for 3D Food Printing. *Journal of Food Science, 83*(12), 2923–2932. https://doi.org/10.1111/1750-3841.14391

Kovačević, K., Karadžić, M., Banjac, K., Yan, M.R., Hsieh et al, S. (2022). Innovative Food Packaging, Food Quality and Safety, and Consumer Perspectives. *Processes 2022, Vol. 10, Page 747, 10*(4), 747. https://doi.org/10.3390/PR10040747

Kruth, J.P., Wang, X., Laoui, T. and Froyen, L. (2003). Lasers and materials in selective laser sintering. *Assembly Automation, 23*(4), 357–371. https://doi.org/10.1108/01445150310698652/FULL/XML

Lai. (2007). *Manufacturing method of three-dimensional food by rapid prototyping.*

Lanaro, M., Desselle, M.R. and Woodruff, M.A. (2018). 3D printing chocolate: Properties of formulations for extrusion, sintering, binding and ink jetting. In *Fundamentals of 3D Food Printing and Applications* (pp. 151–173). Elsevier. https://doi.org/10.1016/B978-0-12-814564-7.00006-7

Lanaro, M., Forrestal, D., Scheurer, S., ... D. S.-J. of F., and 2017, undefined. (n.d.) et al. 3D printing complex chocolate objects: Platform design, optimization and evaluation. *Elsevier.*

Le Tohic, C., O'Sullivan, J.J., Drapala, K.P., Chartrin, V., Chan et al. (2018). Effect of 3D printing on the structure and textural properties of processed cheese. *Journal of Food Engineering, 220*, 56–64. https://doi.org/10.1016/j.jfoodeng.2017.02.003

Lee, J. (2021). A 3d food printing process for the new normal era: A review. In *Processes* (Vol. 9, Issue 9). MDPI. https://doi.org/10.3390/pr9091495

Lee, J.H., Won, D.J., Kim, H.W. and Park, H J. (2019). Effect of particle size on 3D printing performance of the food-ink system with cellular food materials. *Journal of Food Engineering, 256*, 1–8. https://doi.org/10.1016/j.jfoodeng.2019.03.014

Lee, K.H., Hwang, K.H., Kim, M. and Cho, M. (2021). 3D printed food attributes and their roles within the value-attitude-behavior model: Moderating effects of food neophobia and food technology neophobia. *Journal of Hospitality and Tourism Management, 48*, 46–54. https://doi.org/10.1016/j.jhtm.2021.05.013

Leong, S.Y., Duque, S.M., Muhammad Abduh, S.B. and Oey, I. (2019). Carbohydrates. In *Innovative Thermal and Non-Thermal Processing, Bioaccessibility and Bioavailability of Nutrients and Bioactive Compounds* (pp. 171–206). Elsevier. https://doi.org/10.1016/B978-0-12-814174-8.00006-8

Leontiou, A., Georgopoulos, S., Karabagias, V.K., Kehayias, G., Karakassides, A. et al. (2023). Three-Dimensional Printing Applications in Food Industry. *Nanomanufacturing 2023, Vol. 3, Pages 91-112, 3*(1), 91–112. https://doi.org/10.3390/NANOMANUFACTURING3010006

Lille, M., Nurmela, A., Nordlund, E., Metsä-Kortelainen, S. and Sozer, N. et al. (2018). Applicability of protein and fiber-rich food materials in extrusion-based 3D printing. *Journal of Food Engineering, 220*, 20–27. https://doi.org/10.1016/j.jfoodeng.2017.04.034

Lipton, J., Arnold, D., Nigl, F., Lopez, N., Cohen, D. et al. (2010). Multi-Material Food Printing With Complex Internal Structure Suitable for file:///Users/Exodus/Downloads/1-s2.0-S092422441500045X-main.pdf Conventional Post-Processing. *Solid Freeform Fabrication Symposium.*

Liu, Z., Zhang, M., Bhandari, B. and Yang, C. (2018). Impact of rheological properties of mashed potatoes on 3D printing. *Journal of Food Engineering, 220*, 76–82. https://doi.org/10.1016/j.jfoodeng.2017.04.017

Looking to the future: Creating novel foods using 3D printing. (n.d.). Retrieved January 30, 2024, from https://www.foodnavigator.com/Article/2010/12/23/Looking-to-the-future-Creating-novel-foods-using-3D-printing

Ma, Y. and Zhang, L. (2022). Formulated food inks for extrusion-based 3D printing of personalized foods: a mini review. In *Current Opinion in Food Science* (Vol. 44). https://doi.org/10.1016/j.cofs.2021.12.012

Maldonado-Rosas, R., Tejada-Ortigoza, V., Cuan-Urquizo, E., Mendoza-Cachú, D., Morales-de la Peña, M. et al. (2022). Evaluation of rheology and printability of 3D printing nutritious food with complex formulations. *Additive Manufacturing, 58*. https://doi.org/10.1016/j.addma.2022.103030

Maniglia, B.C., Lima, D.C., Matta Junior, M.D., Le-Bail, P., Le-Bail, A. et al. (2020). Preparation of cassava starch hydrogels for application in 3D printing using dry heating treatment (DHT): A prospective study on the effects of DHT and gelatinization conditions. *Food Research International, 128*. https://doi.org/10.1016/j.foodres.2019.108803

Mantihal, S., Kobun, R. and Lee, B.B. (2020). 3D food printing of as the new way of preparing food: A review. In *International Journal of Gastronomy and Food Science* (Vol. 22). AZTI-Tecnalia. https://doi.org/10.1016/j.ijgfs.2020.100260

Marga, F., Jakab, K., Khatiwala, C., Shepherd, B., Dorfman, S. et al. (2012). Toward engineering functional organ modules by additive manufacturing. *Biofabrication, 4*(2). https://doi.org/10.1088/1758-5082/4/2/022001

Nachal, N., Moses, J.A., Karthik, P. and Anandharamakrishnan, C. (2019a). Applications of 3D Printing in Food Processing. In *Food Engineering Reviews* (Vol. 11, Issue 3, pp. 123–141). Springer New York LLC. https://doi.org/10.1007/s12393-019-09199-8

Nachal, N., Moses, J.A., Karthik, P. and Anandharamakrishnan, C. (2019b). Applications of 3D Printing in Food Processing. *Food Engineering Reviews, 11*(3), 123–141. https://doi.org/10.1007/S12393-019-09199-8/FIGURES/4

Nachal, N., Moses, J.A., Karthik, P. and Anandharamakrishnan, C. (2019c). Applications of 3D Printing in Food Processing. In *Food Engineering Reviews* (Vol. 11, Issue 3). https://doi.org/10.1007/s12393-019-09199-8

Nilsen-Nygaard, J., Fernández, E.N., Radusin, T., Rotabakk, B.T., Sarfraz, J. et al. (2021). Current status of biobased and biodegradable food packaging materials: Impact on food quality and effect of innovative processing technologies. *Comprehensive Reviews in Food Science and Food Safety, 20*(2), 1333–1380. https://doi.org/10.1111/1541-4337.12715

Nodehi, M., Aguayo, F., Nodehi, S.E., Gholampour, A., Ozbakkaloglu, T. et al. (2022). Durability properties of 3D printed concrete (3DPC). In *Automation in Construction* (Vol. 142). Elsevier B.V. https://doi.org/10.1016/j.autcon.2022.104479

Noort, M.W.J., Diaz, J., Bommel, K.J.C. van, Renzetti, S., Henket, J. et al. (2016). *Method for the production of an edible object using SLS.*

Norotte, C., Marga, F.S., Niklason, L.E. and Forgacs, G. (2009). Scaffold-free vascular tissue engineering using bioprinting. *Biomaterials, 30*(30), 5910–5917. https://doi.org/10.1016/J.BIOMATERIALS.2009.06.034

Panghal, A., Vern, P., Mor, R.S., Panghal, D., Sindhu, S. et al. (2023). A study on adoption enablers of 3D printing technology for sustainable food supply chain. *Management of Environmental Quality: An International Journal, 34*(4), 943–961. https://doi.org/10.1108/MEQ-03-2022-0056

Pant, A., Lee, A.Y., Karyappa, R., Lee, C.P., An, J. et al. (2021a). 3D food printing of fresh vegetables using food hydrocolloids for dysphagic patients. *Food Hydrocolloids, 114.* https://doi.org/10.1016/j.foodhyd.2020.106546

Pant, A., Lee, A.Y., Karyappa, R., Lee, C.P., An, J., Hashimoto, M., Tan, U.X., Wong, G., Chua, C.K. and Zhang, Y. (2021b). 3D food printing of fresh vegetables using food hydrocolloids for dysphagic patients. *Food Hydrocolloids, 114*, 106546. https://doi.org/10.1016/J.FOODHYD.2020.106546

Peltola, S.M., Melchels, F.P.W., Grijpma, D.W. and Kellomäki, M. (2008). A review of rapid prototyping techniques for tissue engineering purposes. *Annals of Medicine, 40*(4), 268–280. https://doi.org/10.1080/07853890701881788

Pérez, B., Nykvist, H., Brøgger, A.F., Larsen, M.B. and Falkeborg, M.F. et al. (2019a). Impact of macronutrients printability and 3D-printer parameters on 3D-food printing: A review. *Food Chemistry, 287*, 249–257. https://doi.org/10.1016/j.foodchem.2019.02.090

Pérez, B., Nykvist, H., Brøgger, A.F., Larsen, M.B. and Falkeborg, M.F et al. (2019b). Impact of macronutrients printability and 3D-printer parameters on 3D-food printing: A review. *Food Chemistry, 287*. https://doi.org/10.1016/j.foodchem.2019.02.090

Periard, D., Schaal, N., Schaal, M., Malone, E. and Lipson, H. et al. (2007). *Printing Food.* https://doi.org/10.26153/TSW/7242

Portanguen, S., Tournayre, P., Sicard, J., Astruc, T. and Mirade, P.S. et al. (2019). Toward the design of functional foods and biobased products by 3D printing: A review. In *Trends in Food Science and Technology* (Vol. 86, pp. 188–198). Elsevier Ltd. https://doi.org/10.1016/j.tifs.2019.02.023

Praveena, B.A., Lokesh, N., Buradi, A., Santhosh, N., Praveena, B.L. et al. (2022). A comprehensive review of emerging additive manufacturing (3D printing technology): Methods, materials, applications, challenges, trends and future potential. *Materials Today: Proceedings, 52.* https://doi.org/10.1016/j.matpr.2021.11.059

Rogers, H. and Srivastava, M. (2021). Emerging sustainable supply chain models for 3d food printing. *Sustainability (Switzerland), 13*(21). https://doi.org/10.3390/su132112085

Rong, L., Chen, X., Shen, M., Yang, J., Qi, X. et al. (2023). The application of 3D printing technology on starch-based product: A review. In *Trends in Food Science and Technology* (Vol. 134). https://doi.org/10.1016/j.tifs.2023.02.015

Sacco, E. and Moon, S.K. (2019). Additive manufacturing for space: status and promises. *International Journal of Advanced Manufacturing Technology, 105*(10), 4123–4146. https://doi.org/10.1007/S00170-019-03786-Z

Santhoshkumar, P., Negi, A. and Moses, J.A. (2024). 3D printing for space food applications: Advancements, challenges, and prospects. *Life Sciences in Space Research, 40*, 158–165. https://doi.org/10.1016/J.LSSR.2023.08.002

Scerra, M., Barrett, A., Eswaranandam, S. and Okamoto, M. (2018). Effects of 3D Printing and Thermal Post Processing on the Stability of Vitamin E Acetate. *Journal of the Academy of Nutrition and Dietetics, 118*(10), A148. https://doi.org/10.1016/j.jand.2018.08.101

Schaefer, D. and Cheung, W.M. (2018). Smart Packaging: Opportunities and Challenges. *Procedia CIRP, 72*, 1022–1027. https://doi.org/10.1016/J.PROCIR.2018.03.240

Schmid, M., Amado, F., … G.L.-… : A.R. in, and 2013, undefined. (n.d.) et al. Flowability of powders for selective laser sintering (SLS) investigated by round robin test. *Books.Google.ComM Schmid, F Amado, G Levy, K*

WegenerHigh Value Manufacturing: Advanced Research in Virtual and Rapid, 2013•books.Google.Com. https://doi.org/10.3929/ethz-a-010057806

Serenó, L., Vallicrosa, G., Delgado, J. and Ciurana, J. (2012). A new application for food customization with additive manufacturing technologies. *AIP Conference Proceedings, 1431*, 825–833. https://doi.org/10.1063/1.4707640

Severini, C., Derossi, A., Ricci, I., Caporizzi, R. and Fiore, A. et al. (2018a). Printing a blend of fruit and vegetables. New advances on critical variables and shelf life of 3D edible objects. *Journal of Food Engineering, 220*, 89–100. https://doi.org/10.1016/j.jfoodeng.2017.08.025

Severini, C., Derossi, A., Ricci, I., Caporizzi, R. and Fiore, A. et al. (2018b). Printing a blend of fruit and vegetables. New advances on critical variables and shelf life of 3D edible objects. *Journal of Food Engineering, 220*, 89–100. https://doi.org/10.1016/J.JFOODENG.2017.08.025

Shao, P., Liu, L., Yu, J., Lin, Y., Gao, H. et al. (2021). An overview of intelligent freshness indicator packaging for food quality and safety monitoring. In *Trends in Food Science and Technology* (Vol. 118). https://doi.org/10.1016/j.tifs.2021.10.012

Singhal, S., Rasane, P., Kaur, S., Garba, U., Bankar, A. et al. (2020). 3D food printing: Paving way towards novel foods. *Anais Da Academia Brasileira de Ciencias, 92*(3), 1–26. https://doi.org/10.1590/0001-3765202020180737

Solving the Challenges of Long Duration Space Flight with 3D Printing - NASA. (n.d.). Retrieved January 30, 2024, from https://www.nasa.gov/missions/station/solving-the-challenges-of-long-duration-space-flight-with-3d-printing/

Sun, J., Peng, Z., Zhou, W., Fuh, J.Y.H., Hong, G.S. et al. (2015a). A Review on 3D Printing for Customized Food Fabrication. *Procedia Manufacturing, 1*, 308–319. https://doi.org/10.1016/j.promfg.2015.09.057

Sun, J., Peng, Z., Zhou, W., Fuh, J.Y.H., Hong, G.S. et al. (2015b). A Review on 3D Printing for Customized Food Fabrication. *Procedia Manufacturing, 1*, 308–319. https://doi.org/10.1016/J.PROMFG.2015.09.057

Sungsinchai, S., Niamnuy, C., Wattanapan, P., Charoenchaitrakool, M. and Devahastin, S. et al. (2019). Texture Modification Technologies and Their Opportunities for the Production of Dysphagia Foods: A Review. In *Comprehensive Reviews in Food Science and Food Safety* (Vol. 18, Issue 6, pp. 1898–1912). Blackwell Publishing Inc. https://doi.org/10.1111/1541-4337.12495

Tejada-Ortigoza, V. and Cuan-Urquizo, E. (2022). Towards the Development of 3D-Printed Food: A Rheological and Mechanical Approach. In *Foods* (Vol. 11, Issue 9). MDPI. https://doi.org/10.3390/foods11091191

Teng, X., Zhang, M. and Mujumdar, A.S. (2022). Strategies for controlling over-puffing of 3D-printed potato gel during microwave processing. *LWT, 153*. https://doi.org/10.1016/j.lwt.2021.112508

Tomašević, I., Putnik, P., Valjak, F., Pavlić, B., Šojić, B. et al. (2021). 3D printing as novel tool for fruit-based functional food production. In *Current Opinion in Food Science* (Vol. 41, pp. 138–145). Elsevier Ltd. https://doi.org/10.1016/j.cofs.2021.03.015

Uribe-Wandurraga, Z.N., Zhang, L., Noort, M.W.J., Schutyser, M.A.I., García-Segovia, P. et al. (1947). *Printability and Physicochemical Properties of Microalgae-Enriched 3D-Printed Snacks.* https://doi.org/10.1007/s11947-020-02544-4/Published

Uyttendaele, M., De Boeck, E. and Jacxsens, L. (2016). Challenges in Food Safety as Part of Food Security: Lessons Learnt on Food Safety in a Globalized World. *Procedia Food Science, 6.* https://doi.org/10.1016/j.profoo.2016.02.003

van Bommel, K. and Spicer, A. (2011). Hail the Snail: Hegemonic Struggles in the Slow Food Movement. *Http://Dx.Doi.Org/10.1177/0170840611425722, 32*(12), 1717–1744. https://doi.org/10.1177/0170840611425722

Vancauwenberghe, V., Katalagarianakis, L., Wang, Z., Meerts, M., Hertog, M. et al. (2017). Pectin based food-ink formulations for 3-D printing of customizable porous food simulants. *Innovative Food Science and Emerging Technologies, 42*, 138–150. https://doi.org/10.1016/j.ifset.2017.06.011

Varvara, R.A., Szabo, K. and Vodnar, D.C. (2021a). 3D food printing: Principles of obtaining digitally-designed nourishment. In *Nutrients* (Vol. 13, Issue 10). MDPI. https://doi.org/10.3390/nu13103617

Varvara, R.A., Szabo, K. and Vodnar, D.C. (2021b). 3D Food Printing: Principles of Obtaining Digitally-Designed Nourishment. *Nutrients, 13*(10). https://doi.org/10.3390/NU13103617

Waghmare, R., Suryawanshi, D. and Karadbhajne, S. (2023). Designing 3D printable food based on fruit and vegetable products—opportunities and challenges. In *Journal of Food Science and Technology* (Vol. 60, Issue 5). https://doi.org/10.1007/s13197-022-05386-4

Wang, J. and Zhang, X. (2023). The big food view and human health from the prospect of bio-manufacturing and future food. In *Frontiers in Nutrition* (Vol. 10). https://doi.org/10.3389/fnut.2023.1160743

Wang, L., Zhang, M., Bhandari, B. and Yang, C. (2018). Investigation on fish surimi gel as promising food material for 3D printing. *Journal of Food Engineering, 220*, 101–108. https://doi.org/10.1016/j.jfoodeng.2017.02.029

Wang, M., Li, D., Zang, Z., Sun, X., Tan, H. et al. (2022). 3D food printing: Applications of plant-based materials in extrusion-based food printing. In *Critical Reviews in Food Science and Nutrition* (Vol. 62, Issue 26). https://doi.org/10.1080/10408398.2021.1911929

Wegrzyn, T.F., Golding, M. and Archer, R.H. (2012). Food Layered Manufacture: A new process for constructing solid foods. *Trends in Food Science & Technology, 27*(2), 66–72. https://doi.org/10.1016/J.TIFS.2012.04.006

Wu, H., Sang, S., Weng, P., Pan, D., Wu, Z. et al. (2023a). Structural, rheological, and gelling characteristics of starch-based materials in context to 3D food printing applications in precision nutrition. In *Comprehensive Reviews in Food Science and Food Safety* (Vol. 22, Issue 6, pp. 4217–4241). John Wiley and Sons Inc. https://doi.org/10.1111/1541-4337.13217

Wu, H., Sang, S., Weng, P., Pan, D., Wu, Z. et al. (2023b). Structural, rheological, and gelling characteristics of starch-based materials in context to 3D food printing applications in precision nutrition. In *Comprehensive Reviews in Food Science and Food Safety* (Vol. 22, Issue 6). https://doi.org/10.1111/1541-4337.13217

Xie, Y., Liu, Q., Zhang, W., Yang, F., Zhao, K. et al. (2023). Advances in the Potential Application of 3D Food Printing to Enhance Elderly Nutritional Dietary Intake. In *Foods* (Vol. 12, Issue 9). https://doi.org/10.3390/foods12091842

Xu, L., Gu, L., Su, Y., Chang, C., Wang, J. et al. (2020). Impact of thermal treatment on the rheological, microstructural, protein structures and extrusion 3D printing characteristics of egg yolk. *Food Hydrocolloids, 100*. https://doi.org/10.1016/j.foodhyd.2019.105399

Yang, F., Guo, C., Zhang, M., Bhandari, B. and Liu, Y. et al. (2019). Improving 3D printing process of lemon juice gel based on fluid flow numerical simulation. *LWT, 102*, 89–99. https://doi.org/10.1016/j.lwt.2018.12.031

Yang, F., Zhang, M. and Bhandari, B. (2017). Recent development in 3D food printing. *Critical Reviews in Food Science and Nutrition, 57*(14), 3145–3153. https://doi.org/10.1080/10408398.2015.1094732

Yang, F., Zhang, M., Bhandari, B. and Liu, Y. (2018). Investigation on lemon juice gel as food material for 3D printing and optimization of printing parameters. *LWT, 87*, 67–76. https://doi.org/10.1016/j.lwt.2017.08.054

Yu, Q., Zhang, M., Bhandari, B. and Li, J. (2023). Future perspective of additive manufacturing of food for children. In *Trends in Food Science and Technology* (Vol. 136). https://doi.org/10.1016/j.tifs.2023.04.009

Zhang, J.Y., Pandya, J.K., McClements, D.J., Lu, J. and Kinchla, A.J et al. (2022). Advancements in 3D food printing: a comprehensive overview of properties and opportunities. In *Critical Reviews in Food Science and Nutrition* (Vol. 62, Issue 17, pp. 4752–4768). Taylor and Francis Ltd. https://doi.org/10.1080/10408398.2021.1878103

Zhang, L., Lou, Y. and Schutyser, M.A.I. (2018). 3D printing of cereal-based food structures containing probiotics. *Food Structure, 18*, 14–22. https://doi.org/10.1016/j.foostr.2018.10.002

Zhao, L., Zhang, M., Chitrakar, B. and Adhikari, B. (2021). Recent advances in functional 3D printing of foods: a review of functions of ingredients and internal structures. In *Critical Reviews in Food Science and Nutrition* (Vol. 61, Issue 21, pp. 3489–3503). Taylor and Francis Ltd. https://doi.org/10.1080/10408398.2020.1799327

Zhu, S., Vazquez Ramos, P., Heckert, O. R., Stieger, M., van der Goot, A.J. et al. (2022). Creating protein-rich snack foods using binder jet 3D printing. *Journal of Food Engineering, 332*, 111124. https://doi.org/10.1016/J.JFOODENG.2022.111124

CHAPTER

16

3D Bioprinted Scaffolds

Ashtami J,[1] Manjoosha RY,[2] Greeshma N,[2]
*Renu John[2] and Mohanan PV[1]**

1. Introduction

Tissue or organ grafts are in high demand in curative medicine. The allograft, autograft or xenograft substitutes hold a few complications like low availability, immune rejections, disease transmission, and more (Giannoudis et al., 2005). Initially developed alternative solutions like freeze-drying or solvent-casting yielded scaffolds with low control over important structural features such as geometry, pore size, shape and distribution (Yazdanpanah et al., 2022). A more advanced option is 3D bioprinting, a subset of additive manufacturing (Singh, D., 2018). 3D bioprinting enables the achievement of scaffold fabrication in specific morphology and geometry as per personalized demands (Włodarczyk-Biegun et al., 2017). One important reason for the relevance of 3D bioprinting is the gap between organ demand v/s actual availability (He, Y et al., 2019). 3D bioprinting opened an opportunity to construct organs via layer-by-layer construction of required 3D structures of transplantable quality, biocompatibility, adaptability to microenvironments and proper functioning. 3D bioprinting also enables a better platform to learn about drug screening, tissue engineering and disease mechanisms compared to 2D methods.

The foremost case of 3D printing involved the stereolithographic technique, way back in 1986 (Singh, D., 2018). Initially, 3D structures were constructed from ultra-violet (UV) light-cured single layers by the stereolithographic technique. Over the years 3D printing has evolved and 3D scaffolds of biological materials were fabricated using stereolithographic technique (Murphy, S.V. and Atala, A., 2014). Later on, with further advancement in biology, chemistry and 3D printing techniques, the 3D bioprinting technique was developed (He, Y et al., 2019). The first bioprinter was reported to be invented at Clemson University by Thomas Boland and was instrumental in printing cells (Thayer, P. et al., 2020). 3D bioprinting makes possible the construction of 3D structures with biomaterials, cells and other biofactors with better control over the composition and distribution (Mao et al., 2020). A 3D bioprinted scaffold enables it to mimic the structure and functionalities required at the target site. 3D bioprinting helps to fabricate biocompatible structures as per personalized demands

[1] Toxicology Division, Biomedical Technology Wing, Sree Chitra Tirunal Institute of Medical Science and Technology, Trivandrum, Kerala.

[2] Department of Biomedical Engineering, Indian Institute of Technology Hyderabad, Sangareddy, India.

* Corresponding author: mohananpv10@gmail.com

with the help of computer-aided design and modeling (Antezana et al., 2022). 3D bioprinting is done either directly or indirectly. In the direct approach, layer-by-layer deposition of layers to form a 3D structure is followed. The direct approach facilitates multi-cell type deposition and the use of biomaterial combinations as per target site demands. Indirect 3D bioprinting is done using molds to construct the required 3D structures followed by the removal of molds (Zhang et al., 2017).

3D bioprinting uses natural biomaterials or synthetic ones. Natural biomaterials are better at mimicking the target microenvironment and functionality but show poorer mechanical strength. Natural biomaterials are also preferred for 3D bioprinting because of their biocompatibility (Mao H et al., 2020). Synthetic materials on the other-hand offer better mechanical strength and materialistic properties, though they have some disadvantages related to their degradation products and cytocompatibility (Mao et al., 2020). An important requisite for 3D bioprinting is bioink. Basically, bio inks are printable formulations developed for 3D printing depending on the 3D structures constructed. Bioinks can either be cell-alone or hydrogel-based ones that contain natural, synthetic or decellularized hydrogels (Ashammakhi et al., 2019). Hydrogels are formed by reversible or irreversible crosslinking of natural or synthetic polymer units via chemical, physical or biochemical methods (Liu et al., 2018). The selection of bioinks is based on their chemical characteristics, mechanical strength, rheological properties and biological features (Figure 1) (Loo, Y. et al., 2015). The bioink should exhibit a feasible formulation with good printability with appreciable mechanical strength (Gungor-Ozkerim et al., 2018). The choice of the proper bioink is therefore critical for successful 3D bioprinting.

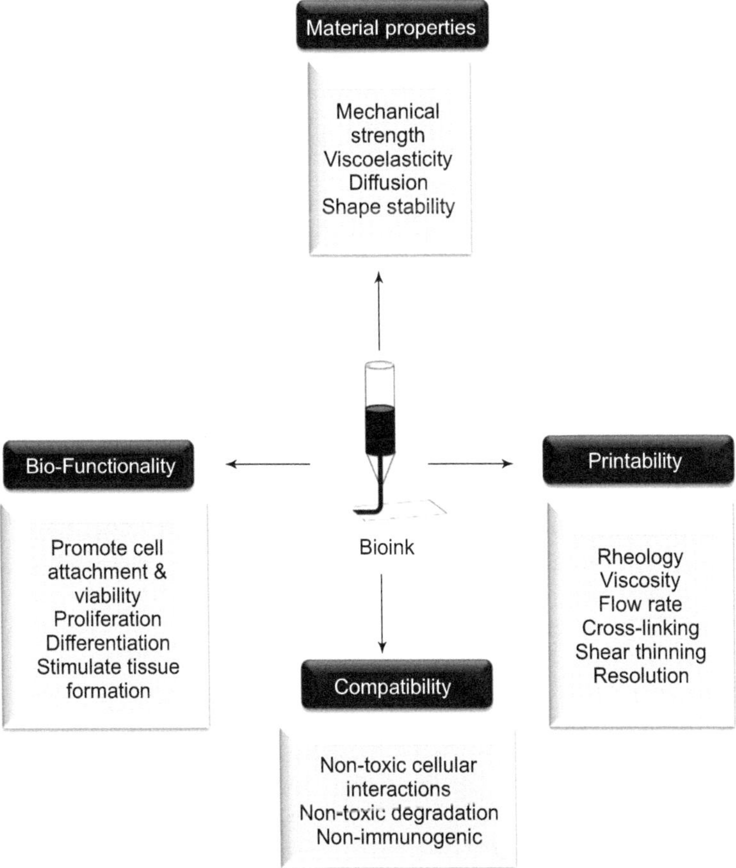

Fig. 1   Characteristics of bioink in 3D bioprinting

2. 3D Bioprinting

3D bioprinting utilizes computer-aided design (CAD) in the pre-processing step to design the construct of interest (Gu et al., 2020). Previous literature outlines the 3D printing in 4 steps: Initial data acquisition, material selection, bio-printing and finally functionalization (Figure 2). In the data acquisition step, the target spot data is collected by various imaging techniques such as X-rays, magnetic resonance imaging (MRI), computed tomography or designed using the CAD technique. Then, the proper choice of biomaterials, bioink and cells is made depending on the target organ or tissue. The target organ being bone demands a high mechanical strength biomaterial while soft tissues may need one with lower mechanical strength. But other properties like viscoelasticity and shear modulus are more important parameters for soft tissues (Iram et al., 2019). Some organs like extracellular matrices require heterogeneity thereby requiring multiple biomaterial types for the 3D construct. Also, depending on the target, cell choice may vary from single-cell to multiple-cell types. The combination of biomaterials/polymers and cells forms the bioink. Bioink selection is also an important decisive factor in 3D bioprinting and the characteristics of the selected bioink influence the the 3D bio-construct's quality.

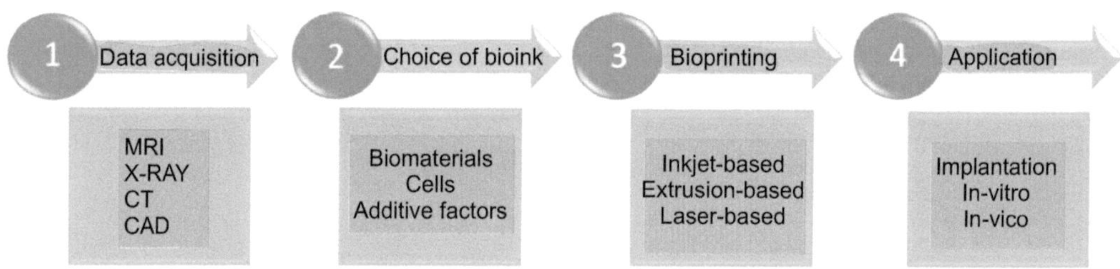

Fig. 2   Steps involved in working of 3D bioprinting

The three check points of bioink are (1) printability (2) mechanical properties, (3) biocompatibility and degradation profile (Gu et al., 2020). Some of the listed characteristics of bioink are: biocompatibility, printability, degradation profile, permeability, biostability, sterilizability, suturabilty and storage (Abassov 2022). The proper selection of material is followed by the most important step-printing. Bioprinting requires the optimization of different factors like resolution and speed (Thayer et al., 2020). After bioprinting, the post-processing step includes the functionalization of scaffolds to attain the desired function of the target tissue/organ. Successful performance of the 3D scaffold at the target site demands matching up with the microenvironment, attaining the structural framework and meeting the desired functionality. In this context, 3D bioprinting provides many advantages like better control over the microarchitecture of the fabricated scaffold, maintaining cellular composition and tunable size. (Peng et al., 2016). Most of the tissue structures require multiple cell types and the use of 3D bioprinting for fabrication reduces the chances of cross-contamination (Donderwinkel et al., 2017).

3D bioprinting is being used for both soft and hard tissues. A few major applications of 3D bioprinting are bone scaffold printing, cartilage printing and skin printing (Zhang et al., 2018), Most interestingly, 3D bioprinting makes possible 3D construction of tumour models enabling drug testing, disease mechanism and progression. This facilitates personalized cancer therapy. The three major approaches in 3D printing are (1) Inkjet-based bioprinting, (2) Extrusion-based bioprinting, and (3) Laser-assisted bioprinting (Figure 3) (Y. et al., 2020).

2.1 *Inkjet-based Bioprinting*

Inkjet-based bioprinting is a non-contact printing approach. With this approach, droplets in the size range of picoliters are released on the substrate (Hölzl 2016). It is then subdivided into the continuous

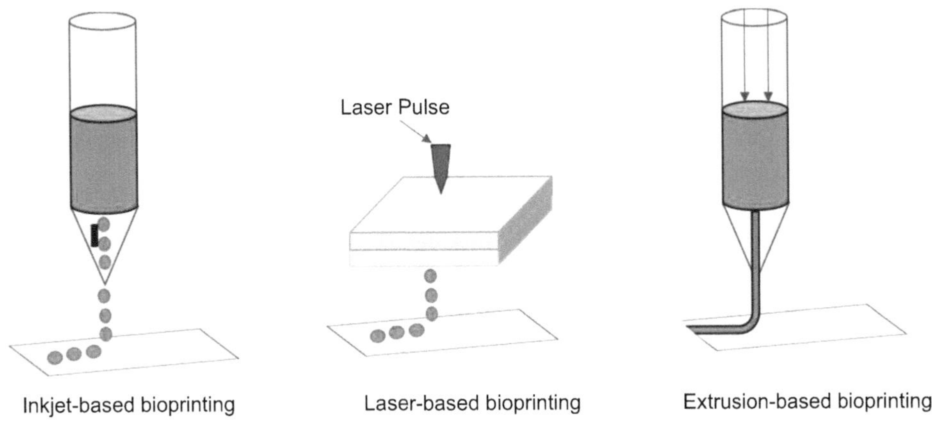

Fig. 3 Different 3D bioprinting approaches

droplet method and the drop-on-demand method (Li, 2020). The continuous inkjet printing method was developed before the drop-on-demand method. In continuous inkjet bioprinting, droplet flow of controllable size is achieved at high speed (Schneider, Hendricks, 1964). On the other hand, the droplet is released only upon receiving a digital signal in case of the drop-on-demand method (Li, 2020). Drop-on demand-based inkjet bioprinting is preferred more for biomaterials. The drop-on demand-based inkjet bioprinter can produce lower volumes of droplets thereby giving better resolution. Continuous inkjet printers produce droplets of about double the size of the orifice (Saunders and Derby 2014). Also, continuous inkjet printers cause disadvantages like low sterility since the method recirculates bioink and also involves higher wastage of bioink . Henceforth, as mentioned earlier, for healthcare applications drop-on-demand printers are preferred.

The usually chosen methods for inkjet printing are (1) piezoelectric bioprinting and (2) thermal inkjet bioprinting. In piezoelectric inkjet printers, the droplets are forced from the nozzle with the help of waves created using piezoelectric crystals (Pereira and Bártolo 2015). In thermal inkjet systems, droplets are produced by vaporizing the bioink using a heating element (Hölzl et al., 2016). Inkjet bioprinters are cost-effective for scaffold printing and advantageous for printing multiple cell types from different nozzles all at once (Saunders and Derby 2014). This approach is not very suitable for highly viscous liquids because of the chances of sedimentation and clogging of nozzles.

2.2 *Extrusion-based Bioprinting*

In extrusion-based bioprinting, the bioink is delivered on the substrate through the nozzle by applying pneumatic or mechanical pressure (Kačarević et al., 2018). The extrusion-based approach is also considered as a direct bioprinting method (Gu et al., (2020). Extrusion-based bioprinters produce continuous strands of bioink, unlike droplets in case of inkjet bioprinters (Bishop et al., (2017). As previously mentioned, inkjet-based bioprinters have a limitation in using highly viscous fluids and therefore confine bioink to lower cell densities to avoid clogging. This limitation is solved in extrusion-based bioprinting where high cell density extrusion is possible (Bishop et al., 2017). However, the resolution in the case of extrusion-based bioprinters is lower in comparison to other approaches. Lower resolution limits its application for soft tissues but still holds potential usage for hard tissues (Falguni, P. et al., 2015). Two major points noted while choosing materials for extrusion-based bioprinting is its thermal crosslinking capacity and shear thinning character (Murphy and Atala 2014). The bioink flow/extrusion depends on the rheological properties of bioink. Hydrogels are highly recommended for extrusion-based bioprinters since they are non-Newtonian fluids. Non-Newtonian fluids exhibit properties of varying viscosity with shear stress. The bioink flow in extrusion-based bioprinters also depends on the diameter of the nozzle, the height of dispersion, speed, volume and adhesion to the substrate (Kačarević et al., 2018).

Three sub-categorizations of extrusion-based bioprinting based on the force exerted are: screw-driven, piston-driven and pneumatic type (Khoeini et al., 2021). In the screw-driven type of extrusion bioprinters, the extrusion is obtained by rotational mechanical force. For the piston type, the force acting is vertical mechanical force, while extrusion is made possible with the help of air pressure in pneumatic-type extrusion bioprinters (He et al., 2016). One of the disadvantages of extrusion-based bioprinters, other than resolution issues, is the mechanical stress faced by cells because of the shear stress (Boularaoui et al, 2020).

2.3 Laser-assisted Bioprinting

The laser-assisted printing method is also a non-contact-based bioprinting approach. Laser-assisted bioprinters have a donor slide, laser pulse and a receiver slide. The donor slide consists of a transparent glass, bioink and a metal layer underneath. The metal layer underneath is evaporated using a laser pulse and the bioink is then transferred from the donor slide to the receiver slide/substrate (Kačarević et al., 2018). This approach is appreciated for its ability to print even a single cell (Keriquel et al., 2017). Major applications of laser-assisted bioprinters are for cell printing and tissue regeneration scaffold printing (Liu et al., 2022). Laser-assisted printing is reported to yield scaffolds with control over the positioning of cells, facilitating repair and regeneration. This approach also yields high cell viability and resolution (Xiong et al., 2017). Laser-assisted bioprinting is also nozzle-free, which reduces the chances of clogging of cells leading to cellular damage (Hopp et al., 2005). The cell viability, cellular integrity and functionality are not compromised in laser-assisted bioprinting (Zorlutuna et al., 2012 and Guillemot et al., 2010). This approach enables high-resolution bioprinting at appreciably high speeds. The types of crosslinking mostly associated with laser-assisted bioprinting are chemical crosslinking and photo-crosslinking (Murphy and Atala 2014).

Skin cells types like fibroblasts, keratinocytes and even human mesenchymal cells printed using laser-assisted bioprinters showed a high survival rate post-printing and similar performance as control cells. Laser-assisted bioprinting holds potential applicational scope in the area of regenerative skin (Koch et al., 2010). Micheal *et al.* printed a 3D structure of a completely cellularized skin substituent (Michael et al., 2013). Fibroblast and keratinocytes were loaded onto the top of the matrix. In the study, different types of cells were successfully positioned to form the target 3D scaffold. The printed 3D structure was planted onto the wound of the mice model to evaluate the performance. The laser-printed skin substituent stimulated tissue formation *in vivo*. The printed keratinocytes formed multi-layered epidermis. Evidence for blood vessel formation and collagen production by printed fibroblast was also observed.

This approach successfully fabricates scaffolds that are architecturally similar to the target organ and have homogeneous cell distribution. Laser-assisted bioprinted scaffolds show enhanced vascularization, lesser body rejection risk and higher regeneration (Ventura 2021). One of the demerits associated with laser-assisted bioprinters is their high cost (Jones, N, 2012). Another drawback associated with laser-assisted bioprinters is their low productivity (Dou, et al., 2021).

3. 3D Bioprinted Scaffolds

3D bioprinting of tissue scaffolds is done in two ways. (Giannoudis et al, 2005) Using a scaffold with cells produces the matrix at the implanted site and the implanted scaffold is replaced by the neo-tissue (Jin and Dijkstra 2010). In this method, the scaffold acts as a cell support system (Fontes and Marcomini 2020). On the other hand, the scaffold is utilized as a delivery vector that could actively release growth factors and drug molecules. The released growth factors or drugs indeed recruit needed cells to the target spot and trigger new matrix formation (Howard et al., 2008). Ideally, a porous structure is preferred since the scaffold should aid in cell attachment, proliferation and differentiation. Also, an interconnected pore system is needed to aid in the flow of essential nutrients in and out. Importantly, the scaffold should be such that the selected material shows compatibility with the microenvironment and has non-toxic degradation products (Howard et al., 2008). Another important characteristic of the scaffold material is the mechanical strength and that should be comparably matching to the target tissue/organ. The biomaterials opted for scaffold fabrication are either natural or synthetic polymers. Examples of natural polymers are collagen, cellulose, gelatin, chitosan, hyaluronic acids and more. The commonly used synthetic biomaterials are polyethylene glycol (PEG), poly(ε-caprolactone) (PCL) and poly(lactic-co-glycolic acid) (Aljohani et al., 2018); Zorlutuna et al., 2012). Hydrogels are a preferred bioink formulation for bioprinting.

Natural polymers have several advantages including bioactivity, similarity to human extracellular matrices and compatibility. Yet, the low mechanical strength of natural polymers limits its applicability. On the other hand, synthetic polymers are reported to exhibit better tunable mechanical properties than natural polymers. Poor compatibility and toxic degradation products are drawbacks of synthetic polymers (Murphy and Atala 2014). Among various materials chosen for 3D bioprinting, hydrogels are highly preferred bioink material (He et al., 2016). The hydrophilic and adsorbent nature of hydrogels is chosen since they provide a more compatible environment for cells. Crosslinking is an important step in scaffold fabrication to maintain the structural integrity of the scaffold. Physical and chemical options are available for scaffold crosslinking. Physical crosslinking involves ionic interactions, hydrogen bonding, hydrophobic interactions π–π stacking and dipole-dipole interactions (Ghavami Nejad et al., 2020). Physical crosslinking is therefore reversible and displays lower mechanical strength. Chemical crosslinking is irreversible and exhibits withstanding capacity. Scaffolds can be irreversibly crosslinked using click chemistry, photoinduced polymerization, enzymatic reactions, hydrazide-aldehyde coupling, Diels–Alder linkage and Michael-type addition reactions (Hölzl et al., 2016 and Ghavami et al., 2020). Crosslinking through chemical reactions raises concerns about toxicity in cells. Therefore, attention needs to be taken while choosing reagents and chemical crosslinking agents. Enzymatic crosslinking is comparatively mild and scaffolds crosslinked using enzymes are found to exhibit cytocompatibility. Scaffolds crosslinked using different enzymes like tyrosinases, transferases and lysyl oxidases also exhibited sustained release kinetics (Teixeira et al., 2012).

4. Major Applications of 3D Bio-printed Scaffolds

The regenerative medicinal application demands scaffolds capable of mimicking the complex architecture of target tissues, compactable in an *in-vivo* environment and exhibiting desired biological functionality. In this context, 3D bio-printed scaffolds are considered meritorious for tissue regeneration applications. 3D bioprinting enables us to achieve the complex architecture of organs compared to conventional scaffold preparation. 3D bioprinted scaffolds exhibit comparable porosity, cell distribution, and interconnections to that of target organs (Sundaramurthi 2016). Over the years, 3D bioprinted scaffolds have been reported to be widely suitable for a range of organs like bone, skin, heart, cartilage, and liver (Assad et al., 2023).

4.1 Osteo Applications

Bone grafts are in high demand for the treatment of fractures, osteodegenerative conditions and tumors. The ability to induce osteoconductivity, the capacity to host osteogenic cells from the donor site and the presence of osteoinductive factors are important characteristics favourable for the ideal performance of bone grafts (Calori et al., 2011). Autografts possess these characteristics and remain the most opted for choice. Morbidity and donor site availability are concerning issues associated with its applications. As mentioned before, allografts and xenograft bone remedies often encounter body rejection and unwanted immune responses. Synthetic bone grafts are fabricated with osteointegration properties but have issues like poor compatibility, and toxic degradation products (Moore et al., 2001 and Alaribe et al., 2016). 3D printing stands as a reliable option to overcome the limitations associated with alternative choices. In case of bone substituents which are hard tissues, apart from the biological function it is equally important to have mechanical strength. 3D bioprinting technique is chosen to design and fabricate bone grafts with osteointegration, osteoinduction, and desired mechanical properties as per the type of bone. It is also desirable for the bioprinted scaffold to be biocompatible and have safe degradation products (Ashammakhi et al., 2018). Micro-extrusion-based bioprinting is the most chosen approach to construct bone scaffolds, followed by inkjet and laser-based bioprinting (Ashammakhi et al., 2019).

Kondiah *et al.* reported making bone scaffolds using CAD software, fabricated using MATLAB software and artificial neural network (Kondiah et al., 2020). The bone scaffold was bioprinted using a polymer composite of pluronics, polypropylene fumarate and polyethylene glycol-polycaprolactone. The bioprinted scaffold successfully endorsed cellular adhesion. The fabricated scaffold loaded with simvastatin showed sustained release and promoted healing. Bone scaffold bioprinted with a polymer combination of graphene oxide (GO)/alginate/gelatin and human mesenchymal stem cells promoted osteoblastic/osteocytic cell differentiation and ECM mineralization (Zhang et al., 2021).

Successful bone regeneration and repair demands proper vascularization. Therefore, attaining vascularization is one of the target objectives of 3D bioprinted scaffolds for bone defects. Byambaa et al. fabricated 3D bioprinted Gelma hydrogels loaded with human mesenchymal stem cells, vascular endothelial growth factor and silicate nanoparticles to achieve the target functions-osteogenesis and vascularization (Byambaa et al., 2017). The loaded cells in 3D bioprinted hydrogel scaffold differentiated, promoted vascularization and new bone formation. However, the scaffold was found to lose its mechanical strength after 21 days. Similarly, alginate-polyvinyl alcohol-hydroxyapatite hydrogel constructed using extrusion-based bioprinting showed well-laid MC3T3 cells, high cell viability and appreciable osteoconductive and biodegradation profile but showed disintegration after 14 days (Bendtsen et al., 2017). Improving the materialistic properties of scaffolds to maintain their structural integrity until complete regeneration is a current area of focus.

4.2 *Wound-healing Applications*

Skin is the largest organ of our body and an important component of protection against external factors (Ghosh et al., 2021). Therefore, any threat to the integrity of skin raises concerns. Wound healing is the body's mechanism of addressing injury and restoring a healthy skin barrier (Smandri et al., 2020). Scaffolds are explored for skin regeneration and wound healing applications (Ghosh et al., 2021). The scaffolds for this purpose are made to exhibit similar skin structure and function. Anticipated features for an efficient skin scaffold are (1) well-distributed interconnected pores for cellular migration, proliferation and vascularization, (2) having wound healing promoting factors, (3) the possibility for personalization, (4) on-demand manufacturing (Tan et al., 2022). Even though autografts and allografts remain the standard option, large wounds are difficult to amend with conventional methods. Shortage of available healthy removable skin, chances of rejection and disease transmission are some concerns with autograft and allograft choices (Manita et al., 2021). 3D bioprinting makes possible the construction of skin scaffolds of desirable size, shape, and functionality as per customer need (Deptuła et al., 2023).

The performance and functionality of 3D bioprinted scaffolds greatly depend on the type of material chosen as the bioink (Masri et al., 2022). Collagen is used as bioink in 3D printing and is reported to promote cell adhesion and migration. However, collagen shows poor mechanical properties, gelation difficulties and shape fidelity. Opting for composite collagen-based bioinks helps improve the performance of collagen-based bioinks. For example, collagen–fibrinogen bioink enable improved wound-re-epithelialization (Mathew-Steiner et al., 2021). Biomaterials other than collagen have also been tried as bioink and showed appreciable results. For example, 3D extrusion-based bioprinting using silk-gelatin bioink yielded physiological, biochemical performance and mechanical characteristics similar to human skin (Admane et al., 2019).

Wu *et al.* fabricated gelatine-sodium alginate hydrogel-based 3D scaffold using an extrusion-based bioprinting approach and studied its wound healing performance in a severe burn model (Figure 4). The bio-printed hydrogel scaffold loaded with adipose-derived mesenchymal stem cells and nitric oxide showed enhanced expression of collagen and angiogenesis in the tested model (Wu, Yu et al., 2021). Similarly, 3D bio-printed sodium alginate/gelatin/collagen-based full-thickness skin scaffold efficaciously accomplished wound healing in the *in vivo* test model (pig) (Velnar et al., 2009). The gradient pore structure in the fabricated skin scaffold leads to three layers-dense layer, epidermis layer, and dermis layer with different ratios of bioinks. The scaffold also exhibited high cell viability and most importantly was effective for re-epithelialization. Wound healing is dynamic and involves multiple cell types and ECM (Velnar et al., 2009). 3D bioprinting helps to construct skin scaffolds using different biomaterials to mimic the natural ECM. Though 3D bioprinting puts forward the opportunity to fabricate skin constructs with similar anatomical features, the approach still has limitations in achieving effective vascularization and minimizing cost (He et al., 2018).

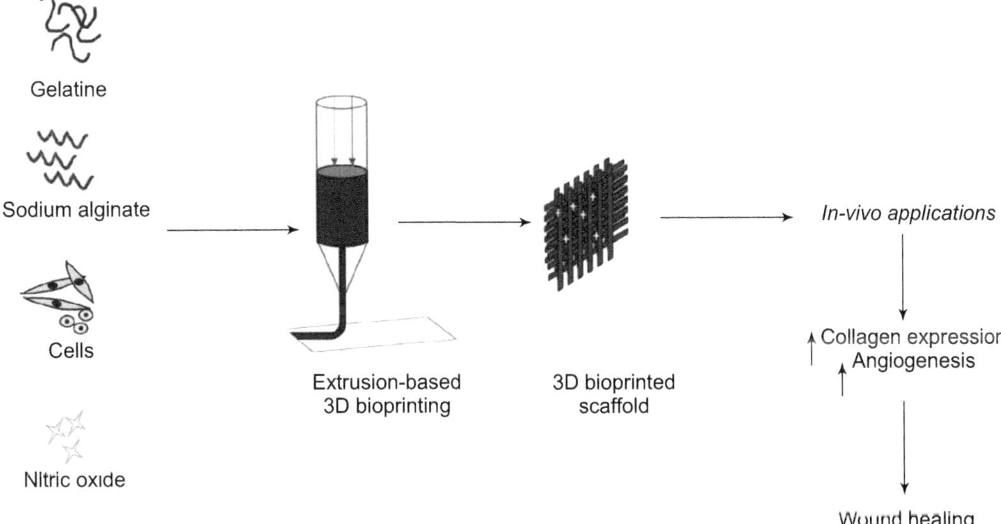

Fig. 4 Gelatine-sodium alginate hydrogel-based 3D scaffold in wound healing

4.3 Neuro-applications

The central nervous system has a complex architecture and therefore mimicking the microstructural features of CNS is a bit of a challenge. Hence, the possibility of precise and controlled scaffold fabrication with 3D bioprinting is beneficial in constructing neural structures (Lee et al., 2018). As per previous reports, characteristics searched for a perfect neural regeneration scaffold are (1) facilitating cell attachments, proliferation and differentiation, (2) non-toxic degradation products, (3) capacity for neural transmission, (4) structurally mimicking ECM, (5) mechanical characteristics, and (6) vascularization (Bedir et al., 2020). Spinal cords show very low regeneration from injuries. Therefore, spinal cord injuries are a major health concern. Jiang *et al.* successfully bioprinted collagen/silk fibroin-based scaffold incorporated with neural stem cells. The fabricated scaffold showed inhibition of scars and regeneration of the spinal cord (Liu et al., 2022). A 3D bioprinted scaffold made using sodium alginate/gelatin bioink was reported by Liu et al. The bio-printed scaffold loaded with neural stem cells and oligodendrocytes when tested on rat models showed that the scaffold mediated hindlimb motor function and promoted nerve regeneration (Jiang et al., 2020).

4.4 Cardiac Tissue Applications

Cardiovascular diseases are a major concern in healthcare worldwide (Benjamin et al., 2017). Regenerative scaffolds are a relatively newer solution explored to address the lack of heart donors compared to the demand for transplantation (Furman 2013). 3D bioprinting scaffolds have also been tried for cardiac tissue regeneration engineering (Liu et al., 2021). 3D bioprinting holds the potential to attain complex architecture, microstructure and functions of the cardiovascular system. Bioink containing biomaterials along with heart cells are chosen, designed and optimized to attain the cardiac microstructures. The most common cells used for 3D bioprinting of scaffolds for cardiac tissue applications are bone marrow-derived stem cells, cardiac stem cells, induced pluripotent stem cells, progenitor cells, myocytes and adipose-derived stem cells (Jafari et al., 2022). Zhang *et al.* reported bioprinting of a multilayer microfibrous scaffold made of alginate and gelatin methacryloyl (GelMA). The alginate-GelMA scaffold with a well-distributed population of human umbilical vein endothelial cells caused the development of endothelialized human myocardium (López et al., 2018). Alginate-agarose scaffold printed using extrusion-based 3D bioprinting showed good mechanical properties and printability (López-Marcial et al., 2018). The 3D bio-printed alginate-agarose scaffold showed high cell viability and enhanced glycosaminoglycan production.

Conclusion

Over the last few years, 3D bioprinting has been a field of discussion in regenerative medicine. 3D bioprinting is being explored for the fabrication of scaffolds mimicking the microstructure of tissues. 3D bio-printed scaffolds are favourable for tissue regeneration applications since 3D bioprinting enables us to achieve the complex architecture of organs compared to conventional scaffold preparation. 3D bioprinted scaffolds exhibit comparable porosity, cell distribution, and interconnected pores mimicking target tissues/organs. 3D bioprinted scaffolds are being constructed and examined for their performance as different organs like bone, skin, heart, cartilage and liver. Though 3D bioprinting scaffolds exhibit promising advantages, they also have certain limitations currently. Many reports noted the degradation of scaffolds within a few days. Further upgradation of bioink formulations capable of retaining the mechanical strength of scaffolds post-implantation needs to be achieved. Another concern with the performance of bioprinted scaffolds is their failure so far to attain sufficient *in vivo* vascularization. Research has been focussed on fine-tuning scaffold fabrication to achieve vascular networks *in vivo*. 3D bioprinting of scaffolds also raises concerns about sterilization issues which need to be taken care of. Scaffold making by 3D bioprinting has a long way to reach a successful translation from the bench to the patient. Extensive research and development in the area of bioink and bioprinting techniques will enable 3D bioprinted scaffolds to outperform conventional options and make a remarkable impact in medicine.

Acknowledgments

The authors wish to express their thanks to the Director Sree Chitra Tirunal Institute for Medical Sciences and Technology (Govt. of India), Trivandrum, Kerala, India, and the Director, Indian Institute of Technology Hyderabad for their support and for providing the infrastructure facility for carrying out this work.

References

Abbasov, I.B. (2022). Three-Dimensional Bioprinting of Organs: Modern Trends. *Critical Reviews™ in Biomedical Engineering*, *50*(3).

Admane, P., Gupta, A.C., Jois, P., Roy, S., Chandrasekharan Lakshmanan, C., Kalsi, G., ... and Ghosh, S. (2019). Direct 3D Bioprinted Full-thickness Skin Constructs Recapitulate Regulatory Signaling Pathways and Physiology of Human Skin. Bioprinting, 15: e00051.

Alaribe, F.N., Manoto, S.L. and Motaung, S.C. (2016). Scaffolds from biomaterials: advantages and limitations in bone and tissue engineering. *Biologia, 71*(4), 353–366.

Aljohani, W., Ullah, M. W., Zhang, X. and Yang, G. (2018). Bioprinting and its applications in tissue engineering and regenerative medicine. *International journal of biological macromolecules, 107*, 261–275.

Antezana, P. E., Municoy, S., Álvarez-Echazú, M. I., Santo-Orihuela, P. L., Catalano et al. (2022). The 3D bioprinted scaffolds for wound healing. *Pharmaceutics, 14*(2), 464.

Ashammakhi, N. and Kaarela, O. (2018). Three-dimensional bioprinting can help bone. *Journal of Craniofacial Surgery, 29*(1), 9–11.

Ashammakhi, N., Ahadian, S., Xu, C., Montazerian, H., Ko, H. et al. (2019). Bioinks and bioprinting technologies to make heterogeneous and biomimetic tissue constructs. *Materials Today Bio, 1*, 100008.

Ashammakhi, N., Hasan, A., Kaarela, O., Byambaa, B., Sheikhi, A., Gaharwar, A.K. and Khademhosseini, A. (2019). Advancing frontiers in bone bioprinting. *Advanced healthcare materials, 8*(7), 1801048.

Assad, H., Assad, A. and Kumar, A. (2023). Recent developments in 3D bio-printing and its biomedical applications. *Pharmaceutics, 15*(1), 255.

Bedir, T., Ulag, S., Ustundag, C.B. and Gunduz, O. (2020). 3D bioprinting applications in neural tissue engineering for spinal cord injury repair. *Materials Science and Engineering: C, 110*, 110741.

Bendtsen, S. T., Quinnell, S.P. and Wei, M. (2017). Development of a novel alginate-polyvinyl alcohol-hydroxyapatite hydrogel for 3D bioprinting bone tissue engineered scaffolds. *Journal of Biomedical Materials Research Part A, 105*(5), 1457–1468.

Benjamin, E.J., Blaha, M.J., Chiuve, S.E., Cushman, M., Das, S.R., Deo, R., ... and Muntner, P. (2017). Heart disease and stroke statistics—2017 update: a report from the American Heart Association. *circulation, 135*(10), e146-e603.

Bishop, E.S., Mostafa, S., Pakvasa, M., Luu, H.H., Lee, M.J., Wolf, J.M., ... and Reid, R.R. (2017). 3-D bioprinting technologies in tissue engineering and regenerative medicine: Current and future trends. *Genes & diseases, 4*(4), 185–195.

Boularaoui, S., Al Hussein, G., Khan, K.A., Christoforou, N. and Stefanini, C. (2020). An overview of extrusion-based bioprinting with a focus on induced shear stress and its effect on cell viability. *Bioprinting, 20*, e00093.

Byambaa, B., Annabi, N., Yue, K., Trujillo-de Santiago, G., Alvarez, M.M., Jia, W., ... and Khademhosseini, A. (2017). Bioprinted osteogenic and vasculogenic patterns for engineering 3D bone tissue. *Advanced healthcare materials, 6*(16), 1700015.

Calori, G.M., Mazza, E., Colombo, M. and Ripamonti, C. (2011). The use of bone-graft substitutes in large bone defects: any specific needs?. *Injury, 42*, S56–S63.

Deptuła, M., Zawrzykraj, M., Sawicka, J., Banach-Kopeć, A., Tylingo, R. and Pikuła, M. (2023). Application of 3D-printed hydrogels in wound healing and regenerative medicine. *Biomedicine & Pharmacotherapy, 167*, 115416.

Donderwinkel, I., Van Hest, J.C. and Cameron, N.R. (2017). Bio-inks for 3D bioprinting: recent advances and future prospects. *Polymer Chemistry, 8*(31), 4451–4471.

Dou, C., Perez, V., Qu, J., Tsin, A., Xu, B. and Li, J. (2021). A state- of- the- art review of laser-assisted bioprinting and its future research trends. *ChemBioEng Reviews, 8*(5), 517–534.

Falguni, P., Jinah, J., Lee, J.W. and Dong-Woo, C. (2015). Extrusion bioprinting. *Essentials of 3D Biofabrication and Translation; Elsevier: Amsterdam, The Netherlands*, 123–152.

Fontes, A.B. and Marcomini, R.F. (2020). 3D bioprinting: a review of materials, processes and bioink properties. *The Journal of Engineering and Exact Sciences, 6*(5), 0617–0639.

Furman, E. (2013). The dynamic state of patents in regenerative medicine. *Tissue Engineering and Regenerative Medicine, 10*(5), 230–233.

GhavamiNejad, A., Ashammakhi, N., Wu, X.Y. and Khademhosseini, A. (2020). Crosslinking strategies for 3D bioprinting of polymeric hydrogels. *Small, 16*(35), 2002931.

Ghosh, S., Kaushik, G., Roy, P. and Lahiri, D. (2021). Application of 3D Bioprinting in Wound Healing: A Review. *Trends in Biomaterials & Artificial Organs, 35*(5).

Giannoudis, P.V., Dinopoulos, H. and Tsiridis, E. (2005). Bone substitutes: an update. *Injury, 36*(3), S20–S27.

Gu, Z., Fu, J., Lin, H. and He, Y. (2020). Development of 3D bioprinting: From printing methods to biomedical applications. *Asian Journal of Pharmaceutical Sciences, 15*(5), 529-557.

Guillemot, F., Souquet, A., Catros, S. and Guillotin, B. (2010). Laser-assisted cell printing: principle, physical parameters versus cell fate and perspectives in tissue engineering. *Nanomedicine, 5*(3), 507–515.

Gungor-Ozkerim, P.S., Inci, I., Zhang, Y.S., Khademhosseini, A. and Dokmeci, M.R. et al. (2018). Bioinks for 3D bioprinting: an overview. *Biomaterials science, 6*(5), 915–946.

He, P., Zhao, J., Zhang, J., Li, B., Gou, Z., Gou, M. and Li, X. (2018). Bioprinting of skin constructs for wound healing. *Burns & trauma, 6*.

He, Y., Gu, Z., Xie, M., Fu, J. and Lin, H. (2020). Why choose 3D bioprinting? Part II: methods and bioprinters. *Bio-Design and Manufacturing, 3*, 1–4.

He, Y., Xie, M., Gao, Q. and Fu, J. (2019). Why choose 3D bioprinting? Part I: a brief introduction of 3D bioprinting for the beginners. *Bio-Design and Manufacturing, 2*, 221–224.

He, Y., Yang, F., Zhao, H., Gao, Q., Xia, B. and Fu, J. (2016). Research on the printability of hydrogels in 3D bioprinting. Sci. Rep. 6, 29977.

Hölzl, K., Lin, S., Tytgat, L., Van Vlierberghe, S., Gu, L. and Ovsianikov, A. (2016). Bioink properties before, during and after 3D bioprinting. *Biofabrication, 8*(3), 032002.

Hopp, B., Smausz, T., Kresz, N., Barna, N., Bor, Z., Kolozsvári, L., ... and Nógrádi, A. (2005). Survival and proliferative ability of various living cell types after laser-induced forward transfer. *Tissue engineering, 11*(11-12), 1817–1823.

Howard, D., Buttery, L.D., Shakesheff, K.M. and Roberts, S.J. (2008). Tissue engineering: strategies, stem cells and scaffolds. *Journal of anatomy, 213*(1), 66–72.

Iram, D., Riaz, R. and Iqbal, R.K. (2019). 3D Bioprinting: An attractive alternative to traditional organ transplantation. *Biomed. Sci. Eng, 5*(1), 7–18.

Jafari, A., Ajji, Z., Mousavi, A., Naghieh, S., Bencherif, S.A. and Savoji, H. (2022). Latest advances in 3D bioprinting of cardiac tissues. *Advanced materials technologies, 7*(11), 2101636.

Jiang, J.P., Liu, X.Y., Zhao, F., Zhu, X., Li, X.Y., Niu, X. G., ... and Zhang, S. (2020). Three-dimensional bioprinting collagen/silk fibroin scaffold combined with neural stem cells promotes nerve regeneration after spinal cord injury. *Neural regeneration research, 15*(5), 959–968.

Jin, R. and Dijkstra, P.J. (2010). Hydrogels for tissue engineering applications. *Biomedical applications of hydrogels handbook*, 203–225.

Jones, N. Science in three dimensions: the print revolution. Nature 487, 22–23 (2012).

Kačarević, Ž.P., Rider, P.M., Alkildani, S., Retnasingh, S., Smeets, R., Jung, O., ... and Barbeck, M. (2018). An introduction to 3D bioprinting: possibilities, challenges and future aspects. *Materials, 11*(11), 2199.

Keriquel, V., Oliveira, H., Rémy, M., Ziane, S., Delmond, S., Rousseau, B., ... and Fricain, J.C. (2017). In situ printing of mesenchymal stromal cells, by laser-assisted bioprinting, for in vivo bone regeneration applications. *Scientific reports, 7*(1), 1778.

Khoeini, R., Nosrati, H., Akbarzadeh, A., Eftekhari, A., Kavetskyy, T., Khalilov, R., ... and Ozbolat, I.T. (2021). Natural and synthetic bioinks for 3D bioprinting. *Advanced NanoBiomed Research, 1*(8), 2000097.

Koch, L., Kuhn, S., Sorg, H., Gruene, M., Schlie, S., Gaebel, R., ... and Chichkov, B. (2010). Laser printing of skin cells and human stem cells. *Tissue Engineering Part C: Methods, 16*(5), 847–854.

Kondiah, P. J., Kondiah, P.P., Choonara, Y.E., Marimuthu, T. and Pillay, V. (2020). A 3D bioprinted pseudo-bone drug delivery scaffold for bone tissue engineering. *Pharmaceutics, 12*(2), 166.

Lee, S.J., Esworthy, T., Stake, S., Miao, S., Zuo, Y.Y., Harris, B.T. and Zhang, L.G. (2018). Advances in 3D bioprinting for neural tissue engineering. *Advanced Biosystems, 2*(4), 1700213.

Li, X., Liu, B., Pei, B., Chen, J., Zhou, D., Peng, J., ... and Xu, T. (2020). Inkjet bioprinting of biomaterials. *Chemical Reviews, 120*(19), 10793–10833.

Liu, F., Chen, Q., Liu, C., Ao, Q., Tian, X. et al. (2018). Natural polymers for organ 3D bioprinting. *Polymers, 10*(11), 1278.

Liu, N., Ye, X., Yao, B., Zhao, M., Wu, P., Liu, G., ... and Zhu, P. (2021). Advances in 3D bioprinting technology for cardiac tissue engineering and regeneration. *Bioactive Materials, 6*(5), 1388–1401.

Liu, N., Zhang, X., Guo, Q., Wu, T. and Wang, Y. (2022). 3D bioprinted scaffolds for tissue repair and regeneration. *Frontiers in Materials, 9*, 925321.

Liu, S., Yang, H., Chen, D., Xie, Y., Tai, C., Wang, L., ... and Wang, B. (2022). Three-dimensional bioprinting sodium alginate/gelatin scaffold combined with neural stem cells and oligodendrocytes markedly promoting nerve regeneration after spinal cord injury. *Regenerative Biomaterials, 9*, rbac038.

Loo, Y., Lakshmanan, A., Ni, M., Toh, L.L., Wang, S. et al. (2015). Peptide bioink: self-assembling nanofibrous scaffolds for three-dimensional organotypic cultures. *Nano letters, 15*(10), 6919–6925.

López-Marcial, G.R., Zeng, A.Y., Osuna, C., Dennis, J., García, J.M. and O'Connell, G.D. (2018). Agarose-based hydrogels as suitable bioprinting materials for tissue engineering. *ACS biomaterials science & engineering, 4*(10), 3610–3616.

Manita, P.G., Garcia-Orue, I., Santos-Vizcaino, E., Hernandez, R.M. and Igartua, M. (2021). 3D bioprinting of functional skin substitutes: From current achievements to future goals. *Pharmaceuticals, 14*(4), 362.

Mao, H., Yang, L., Zhu, H., Wu, L., Ji, P. et al. (2020). Recent advances and challenges in materials for 3D bioprinting. *Progress in Natural Science: Materials International, 30*(5), 618–634.

Masri, S., Zawani, M., Zulkiflee, I., Salleh, A., Fadilah, N.I.M., Maarof, M., ... and Fauzi, M.B. (2022). Cellular interaction of human skin cells towards natural bioink via 3D-bioprinting technologies for chronic wound: A comprehensive review. *International Journal of Molecular Sciences, 23*(1), 476.

Mathew-Steiner, S.S., Roy, S. and Sen, C.K. (2021). Collagen in wound healing. *Bioengineering, 8*(5), 63.

Michael, S., Sorg, H., Peck, C.T., Koch, L., Deiwick, A., Chichkov, B., ... and Reimers, K. (2013). Tissue engineered skin substitutes created by laser-assisted bioprinting form skin-like structures in the dorsal skin fold chamber in mice. *PloS one, 8*(3), e57741.

Moore, W.R., Graves, S.E. and Bain, G.I. (2001). Synthetic bone graft substitutes. *ANZ journal of surgery, 71*(6), 354–361.

Murphy, S.V. and Atala, A. (2014). 3D bioprinting of tissues and organs. *Nature biotechnology, 32*(8), 773–785.

Niu, C., Wang, L., Ji, D., Ren, M., Ke, D., Fu, Q., ... and Yang, X. (2022). Fabrication of SA/Gel/C scaffold with 3D bioprinting to generate micro-nano porosity structure for skin wound healing: A detailed animal in vivo study. *Cell Regeneration, 11*(1), 10.

Peng, W., Unutmaz, D. and Ozbolat, I.T. (2016). Bioprinting towards physiologically relevant tissue models for pharmaceutics. *Trends in biotechnology, 34*(9), 722–732.

Pereira, R.F. and Bártolo, P.J. (2015). 3D bioprinting of photocrosslinkable hydrogel constructs. *Journal of Applied Polymer Science, 132*(48).

Saunders, R.E. and Derby, B. (2014). Inkjet printing biomaterials for tissue engineering: bioprinting. *International Materials Reviews, 59*(8), 430–448.

Schneider, J.M. and Hendricks, C.D. (1964). Source of uniform-sized liquid droplets. *Review of scientific Instruments, 35*(10), 1349–1350.

Singh, D. (2018). 3D bioprinting for scaffold fabrication. In *3D Bioprinting for Reconstructive Surgery* (pp. 89–123). Woodhead Publishing.

Smandri, A., Nordin, A., Hwei, N.M., Chin, K.Y., Abd Aziz, I. and Fauzi, M.B. (2020). Natural 3D-printed bioinks for skin regeneration and wound healing: A systematic review. *Polymers, 12*(8), 1782.

Sundaramurthi, D., Rauf, S. and Hauser, C. (2016). 3D bioprinting technology for regenerative medicine applications. *International Journal of Bioprinting, 2*(2).

Tan, S.H., Ngo, Z.H., Leavesley, D. and Liang, K. (2022). Recent advances in the design of three-dimensional and bioprinted scaffolds for full-thickness wound healing. *Tissue Engineering Part B: Reviews, 28*(1), 160–181.

Teixeira, L.S.M., Feijen, J., van Blitterswijk, C.A., Dijkstra, P.J. and Karperien, M. (2012). Enzyme-catalyzed crosslinkable hydrogels: emerging strategies for tissue engineering. *Biomaterials, 33*(5), 1281–1290.

Thayer, P., Martinez, H. and Gatenholm, E. (2020). History and trends of 3D bioprinting. *3D Bioprinting: Principles and Protocols*, 3–18.

Velnar, T., Bailey, T. and Smrkolj, V. (2009). The wound healing process: an overview of the cellular and molecular mechanisms. *Journal of international medical research, 37*(5), 1528–1542.

Ventura, R.D. (2021). An overview of laser-assisted bioprinting (LAB) in tissue engineering applications. *Medical Lasers; Engineering, Basic Research, and Clinical Application, 10*(2), 76–81.

Włodarczyk-Biegun, M.K. and Del Campo, A. (2017). 3D bioprinting of structural proteins. *Biomaterials, 134*, 180–201.

Wu, Yu, Tangzhao Liang, Ying Hu, Shihai Jiang, Yuansen Luo, Chang Liu, Guo Wang, Jing Zhang, Tao Xu and Lei Zhu. "3D bioprinting of integral ADSCs-NO hydrogel scaffolds to promote severe burn wound healing." *Regenerative biomaterials* 8, no. 3 (2021): rbab014.

Xiong, R., Zhang, Z., Chai, W., Chrisey, D.B. and Huang, Y. (2017). Study of gelatin as an effective energy absorbing layer for laser bioprinting. *Biofabrication, 9*(2), 024103.

Yazdanpanah, Z., Johnston, J.D., Cooper, D.M. and Chen, X. (2022). 3D bioprinted scaffolds for bone tissue engineering: State-of-the-art and emerging technologies. *Frontiers in bioengineering and biotechnology, 10*, 824156.

Zhang, B., Luo, Y., Ma, L., Gao, L., Li, Y. et al. (2018). 3D bioprinting: an emerging technology full of opportunities and challenges. *Bio-Design and Manufacturing, 1*, 2–13

Zhang, J., Eyisoylu, H., Qin, X.H., Rubert, M. and Müller, R. (2021). 3D bioprinting of graphene oxide-incorporated cell-laden bone mimicking scaffolds for promoting scaffold fidelity, osteogenic differentiation and mineralization. *Acta Biomaterialia, 121*, 637–652.

Zhang, Y.S., Arneri, A., Bersini, S., Shin, S.R., Zhu, K., Goli-Malekabadi, Z., ... and Khademhosseini, A. (2016). Bioprinting 3D microfibrous scaffolds for engineering endothelialized myocardium and heart-on-a-chip. *Biomaterials, 110*, 45–59.

Zhang, Y.S., Yue, K., Aleman, J., Mollazadeh-Moghaddam, K., Bakht, S.M. et al. (2017). 3D bioprinting for tissue and organ fabrication. *Annals of biomedical engineering, 45*, 148–163.

Zorlutuna, P., Vrana, N.E. and Khademhosseini, A. (2012). The expanding world of tissue engineering: the building blocks and new applications of tissue engineered constructs. *IEEE reviews in biomedical engineering, 6*, 47–62.

17

3D Bioprinting and Tissue Engineering

Vidhi Mathur,[1] *Mrunmayi Gadre,*[1]
Amit Panwar[2] *and Kirthanashri S Vasanthan*[1]*

1. Introduction

A world-wide emerging technique known as three-dimensional bioprinting has been playing an important role in the field of health care along with various *in vitro* applications. Different health care branches such as reconstruction of organs and tissue regeneration and repair have been widely explored and applied in various therapies (Nyberg E.L. et al., 2017; Fahmy M.D. et al., 2016; Ricci J.L. et al., 2012; Hull C.W. [n.d]). The term tissue engineering was introduced in the late 1980s, and the concept was widespread due to its application in repair and regeneration. The first ever skin grafting was described in a Sanskrit text around 3000 BCE India. Following this the next autologous skin grafting was carried out in 1794 by Bunger, Raverdin and Baronio in Europe and in 1881 by Girdner for allografting cadaveric skin (Herman A. R., 2002). In 1944, the preservation of the skin allografts was performed by Webster by refrigeration (Webster J.P. 1944). Further the ideology for preserving cells and skins at subzero and lower temperatures was developed by (Polge C. et al., 1949) and (Billingham R.E., Medawar, P.B., 1952) respectively. In 1975, the concept of cultivating keratinocytes *in vitro* was invented by (Rheinwatd J.G., Green, H., 1975) and in 1979, the culturing of the autologous epithelium layer was developed by Genzyme (Green H. et al., 1979). By the 1980s, commercial skin grafts were available in the market for various applications such as Apligraf (composite living skin) by Organogenesis (Bell E. et al., 1981) and dermal regeneration template (collagen-glycosaminoglycans based dermal matrix) by Integra life sciences (Yannas I.V. et al., 1982). The concept of cellular transplantation on biodegradable polymers was well known by 1988 which gave rise to new methods of using cell-based transplantation for different applications (Vacanti, J.P. et al., 1988).

The first bioartificial bladder was cultured *in vitro* and then successfully transplanted *in vivo* (Atala A. et al., 2006) and in 2008 the use of tissue engineered trachea composed of decellularized

---

[1] Manipal Centre for Biotherapeutics Research, Manipal Academy of Higher Education, Manipal, India.
[2] School of Biological Sciences, Amity University Punjab, Mohali, India.
* Corresponding author: kirthanashri.sv@manipal.edu

extracellular matrix along with human derived stem cells was fabricated. Over time, new and better bioactive substances have been implemented for the development of scaffolds for different applications, including s cases where there is no treatment available (Berthiaume F. et al., 2011). At present, in the 2020s the application of tissue engineered scaffolds have a wide range of use. Recently, Bhere et al., fabricated a patient-specific scaffold composed of purified collagen type I and decellularized extracellular matrix from skeletal muscles; this scaffold helped the patient in the regeneration of tissues and recover volumetric muscle loss (Behre A. et al., 2022). With the improvement in technology and manufacturing methods, more diverse techniques under tissue engineering have been emerging. One of the main goals of tissue engineering is the fabrication of 3D models that are able to closely mimic the microenvironment of the host site (Kruth JP. et al., 1991). These engineered models have been studied and research has revealed that they are able to provide the internal as well as the external architecture which provides an essential framework for cellular attachment, proliferation and migration (Klimek K. et al., 2020; He Y. et al., 2021). The different techniques in tissue engineering have also provided an added advantage of the ability to produce custom-made models that can be applied in the required impaired site (Ma X. et al., 2021; Yang J. et al., 2021; Tang Y.C., 2022). Added ingredients like stem cells and signalling molecules during the fabrication of these models have provided successful results post transplantation in the intended defects (Gaharwar A.K. et al., 2020; Nakamura M. et al., 2010).

An important prerequisite of these scaffold-based models is that they must biodegrade post their implied function i.e., after the tissue is repaired or regenerated (Gaharwar A.K. et al., 2016; Zhang J. et al., 2021). Main conventional methods for fabrication of the models are 3D bioprinting (Sun Y. et al., 2020; Ravanbakhsh H. et al., 2022; Hollister SJ. et al., 2005), casting/particulate leaching (van Bochove B. et al., 2021; Zhu N., Chen X., 2013), gas foaming (Nam Y.S. et al., 2000; Januariyasa I.K., Yusuf Y., 2020), melt moulding (Oh S.H. et al., 2003; Brooks-Richards T.L. et al., 2022), phase separation (Nam Y.S., 1999; Park T.G., 1999; Yao Q., 2020), freeze-drying (Sultana N., Wang M., 2008; Skardal A. et al., 2016), and electrospinning (Li C. et al., 2006; Taymour R. et al., 2022). Most of these techniques are able to successfully fabricate structures which are porous in nature that brings them closer to the native porosity present naturally (Park J.Y. et al., 2017). 3D bioprinting is considered to be the most attractive biofabrication methodology as it provides the precise deposition of the cells added in the bioink on predefined coordinates (Jang J., Yi H.G., Cho D.W., 2016; Wüst S. et al., 2011; Melchels F.P. et al., 2012). Different terminologies have been used for describing 3D bioprinting such as additive manufacturing, solid freeform fabrication and rapid prototyping. Over all the other tissue engineering techniques, 3D bioprinting when compared to other techniques offers four different printing techniques based on varying working principles, mainly (a) Inkjet-droplet based, (b) Micro-extrusion based, (c) laser-assisted, and (d) stereolithography techniques. The key element of this technique involves the selection and standardization of bioink. Bioink consists mainly of biomaterial, crosslinking agents and cellular components. An ideal bioink is known to meet few requirements which includes biocompatibility, biodegradability, bioprintability, and mechanical stability post 3D bioprinting (Guillemot F. et al., 2012; Guvendiren M. et al., 2016; Ji S., Guvendiren M., 2017).

The biomaterials that have been used are majorly natural or synthetic polymers and hybrid polymers as a base material along with the other required components. Based on the requirement of the application, the bioink can be formulated which involves a cocktail of biopolymers and sometimes signalling molecules and various cells (Costantini M. et al., 2021). During 3D bioprinting, bioink turns into hydrogel and finally into stable 3D structures (Benwood C. et al., 2021). Crosslinking can be achieved either through chemical or physical agents, which again is chosen based on the application and mechanism of action. In most of the cases the crosslinking agents that are implied are chemical agents as they favor a wide range of tunability and stability (Li X. et al., 2018; Akhtar M.F. et al., 2016). Selection of the right crosslinking agent is crucial as it depends on various factors like the backbone of the polymer, functional side groups present in the polymer, mechanism of crosslinking, and requirement of additional supplementary chemicals (Kim S.Y. et al., 2021; Ghavami Nejad A. et al., 2020; Lim K.S. et al., 2020). Once the bioink components are finalized, another initial step involved in 3D bioprinting remains i.e., the making of a good blueprint of the 3D model from a method known as computer aided design (CAD). The CAD models provide the arrays in a layer-by-layer manner and the exact coordinates for the bioink deposition (Horn T.J., Harrysson O.L., 2012). The information that is required to make CAD can be fed in either by Computer-aided manufacturing (CAM) tools or computed tomography (CT) or magnetic resonance imaging (MRI). The raw data acquired from these sources is then analyzed and reconstructed to make a volumetric 3D model (Moreau J.L. et al., 2007; Kasturi M. et al., 2024). In this chapter, we will discuss the basics of tissue engineering, the evolution of 3D bioprinting and the various strategies and bioinks used for 3D bioprinting. We also talk about the commercially available tissue engineered constructs and various applications in the biomedical field.

2.   Tissue Engineering

Over the past decade, there has been an immense advancement in personalized medicine which effectively addresses the complexities in disease which is specific to patients. The rise in therapeutic strategies has developed a wide range of patients that require characterization using the pathology results and clinical observations (Gorshkov K. et al., 2019). Different therapeutic approaches including personalized medications have been designed in order to recognize the variability of efficacy and adverse effects in the patients. It has been observed that there is a gap in the regeneration medicine and organ transplantation due to the rejection caused by the HLA and minor antigen causing histocompatibility which can be overcome with the developing technology of tissue engineering (Li Y. et al., 2022). This has given birth to personalized medicines in health care that utilize an individual's genetic profile that is unique to the individual, helping directly in prevention, diagnosis and finally the treatment (Ho D. et al., 2020). The personalized medication has helped in tailoring personalized plans based on the response, which provides overall efficacy, safety and enhanced outcomes which not only helps the patient and the health care facilitators but also the industries to benefit in reducing the healthcare cost and patient favourable outcomes (Mathur S., Sutton J., 2017). The major discoveries over the decade are depicted in the figure. The discovery of stem cells and culturing of the human embryonic stem cells dates back to the 1990s, which was later revolutionized by modifying these cells by the Yamanaka factors that had turned the focus towards personalized medicine in the 2000s. During the same period the invention of the first tissue engineering technique known as stereolithography took place (Takahashi K. et al., 2008). Post this the focus turned towards the use of induced pluripotent stem cells without the use of embryos to eliminate the ethical concerns (Robertson J.A., 2001).

Over time, the U.S. FDA approved the world's first 3D-printed drug, Spritam, for treating partial-onset seizures in epilepsy (Reddy C.V. et al., 2021). This marks a significant milestone in personalized medicine. Particularly the emergence of tissue engineering led to the fabrication of *in vitro* models via 3D bioprinting. These provide the best available technology for making personalised medications. The primary objective of 3D bioprinting is to create three dimensional structures with multiple functions incorporating both structural and mechanical properties. The production of these 3D bioprinted models is carefully performed using layer by layer positioning of the bioink that consists of the polymers and cells along with other biological cues (Murphy S.V., Atala A., 2014). 3D models apart from personalized medicines have been applied for studying drug mechanisms, toxicology and development (Mazzocchi A. et al., 2019). Further advancements in the awareness and utilization of tissue engineering techniques like the above-mentioned methods reduce the cost of personalized medicines as they provide accurate results and outcomes (Lam EH. et al., 2023).

There are numerous fabrication techniques available for developing 3D models and each method has benefits and drawbacks resulting in different features of scaffolds like the pore size and the mechanical and structural characteristics.

2.1   *Solvent Casting and Particulate Leaching*

This method employs the dissociation of polymers in the desired solvent along with insoluble salts. The solvent is then evaporated from the mixture to form a salt-polymer composite, after which the composite is immersed in water to leach the salt out from the composite resulting in a structure with high porosity (Hutmacher D.W. et al., 2000; Bajaj P. et al., 2014). Thermal energy is used for fabricating models. The advantage of using thermal energy is that the pore size is adjustable within the range of 50-90% and it is cost efficient (Prasad A. et al., 2017; Li Z. et al., 2016). Sim and others combined polyurethane coated scaffolds with collagen resulted to achieve uniform cellular distribution which is beneficial for cardiac tissue engineering (Sin D. et al., 2010). However, it's important to note that this technique results in structurally simple scaffolds. Additionally, any residual solvent in the model can lead to cytotoxicity post fabrication (Subia B. et al., 2010).

2.2   *Freeze Drying*

The other term used for freeze drying is lyophilization, this process includes the dissolution of the polymer present in solvent. The mixture is then poured on to a mould which is cooled below its freezing point which results in a solidified polymer-solvent compound that undergoes sublimation leading to formation of countless porous scaffolds. The pore formation takes place when the solution starts cooling and the solute gets separated in the ice-phase and the size of the pore can be changed by controlling the temperature that usually ranges from $-20°C$ and $-80°C$ (Roseti L. et al., 2017; Aranaz I. et al., 2014). The advantage of this technique is that high temperatures are not used which helps in preserving the biological factors present in the scaffolds (Thavornyutikarn B. et al., 2014; Valencia C. et al., 2018). Kordjamshidi and colleuges fabricated scaffolds composing of sodium alginate and magnetite nanoparticles further designed with calcium silicate along with celecoxib (pain relieving medication). This scaffold is a potential model for applying as a graft in bone cancer for easy drug delivery (Kordjamshidi A. et al., 2019).

2.3   *Thermal Induced Phase Separation*

This method engages the use of temperature to separate the homogenous polymer mixture in different phases by reducing the solubility of components resulting in the formation of two phases called polymer-poor and polymer rich phases (Aram E. et al., 2019; Conoscenti G. et al., 2017). The polymer-poor phase is discarded whereas the polymer-rich phase is further solidified forming a nanofiber-like structure with high porosity (Graham P.D. et al., 1997; Ma W. et al., 2023). This technique can be applied to fabricate a crystalline polymer scaffold, giving which has the advantage of incorporating bioactive molecules (Eltom A. et al., 2019). Another significant advantage of this method is the tunable porosity.By employing freeze drying after fabricating the scaffold using phase separation, its possible to achieve porosity levels exceeding 95% (Kim K.O. et al., 2014; Zhang H. et al., 2015). Jing et al., developed scaffolds by combining thermoplastic polyurethane and graphene oxide. These scaffolds exhibited good porosity creating a highly supportive environment for cell proliferation (Jing X. et al., 2014).

2.4   *Gas Foaming*

This technique involves the use of inert gases as a foaming agent that generates pressure and is applied on the polymers suspended in a solvent at a high temperature. The pressure is exerted until it reaches the saturation point to produce gas bubbles in the polymer, this results in the formation of a spongy structure with about 80-85% porosity (Rao F. et al., 2019). Few of the commonly used gases include nitrogen, hydrogen, carbon dioxide and methane (Rao F. et al., 2019). The main drawback of this method is the involvement of high temperature throughout the procedure; this was later overcome by use of particulate leaching which resulted in a scaffold with about 97% porosity

(Harris et al., 1998). Some researchers, fabricated scaffolds composed of agarose and chitosan matrix using gas foaming further reinforced with nanohydoxyapatite during freeze drying. This scaffold had unique porosity with open and interconnected macropores with potential use in bone related applications. The scaffold when studied *in vitro* showed no cytotoxicity and good adhesion and growth properties with additional formation of apatite layer that confirmed excellent bioactivity as an implant (Nee AY. et al., 2014).

2.5   *Electrospinning*

This method employs the use of an electric field generated with high voltage resulting in the fabrication of fine fibres from a polymeric solution. The structural morphology and the diameter of fibres depends on the viscosity, molecular weight and the charge density of the polymer apart from the strength of the electrical field (Pham Q.P. et al., 2006; Babu P.J. et al., 2017). This technique is highly versatile as it provides a platform to process a large variety of materials and fibres ranging in microns and nanometres (Yang X. et al., 2009; Xu L. et al., 2017). The main drawback of electrospinning is the use of organic solvents and uniform distribution of the fibres to produce complex architecture (Afsharian YP. et al., 2021; Lu et al., 2013). Pezeshki et al., fabricated scaffolds composed of gelatin and chitosan and the biocompatibility of the scaffolds was assessed for application as a skin implant. The scaffold provided good biocompatibility and the nanofibers maintained the structure after exposure in the medium containing chemical and physical properties required for cell growth (Pezeshki-Modaress M. et al., 2018). 3D bioprinting is the advanced technology for scaffold fabrication.

3.   3D Bioprinting

3D bioprinting has emerged as the latest addition to additive manufacturing. It is a convergence between tissue engineering, biofabrication, regenerative medicine and additive manufacturing. This technique has advanced in the previous years and is becoming one of the most promising therapeutic applications for transplantations and regenerative medicine. In 3D bioprinting, a 3D structure is modelled using computer aided designing followed by the utilization of bioinks. Bioinks consist of biomaterials, cells and other growth factors; the scaffold is fabricated as shown in Figure 1. The advantages of the technique are that it offers control over the organization of cells within the construct and repeatability of the fabrication units (Dey M., 2020).

3.1   *CAD Designing*

When it comes to 3D bioprinting for any application, specialized software plays a crucial role. It focuses on aspects such as complexity, arrangement, organization and accuracy. There are specific tools for CAD, control, and converting the medical data to CAD formats. Different companies are manufacturing their own specific software based on the graphical user interfaces. One of the softwares developed by GeSim company, Bioscaffolder, is a stereolithography based which has two parts-generator and interface (Chua C.K., Leong K.F., 2014). Another software is NovoGen MMX developed by the Organovo company that provides all the essential functions like selection of materials, cell type to be used, printing speed, and printer head movements. Organovo is also collaborating with Autodesk for controller software development (Pakhomova C. et al., 2020). CELLINK has developed a user friendly software package (HeartOS, DNA studio and DNA cloud) for control over the bioprinting. It also provides layer-by-layer printing and slicing preview to see how the print will occur in reality (https://www.regenhu.com/3d-bioprinters/software). BioPrint Pro, developed by Allevi, can be accessed from any computer and it also has an integrated slicing function (https://www.cellink.com/software). Another company, RegenHU Ltd, developed a software package representing a bioprinting software suite consisting of BIOCAD, BIOCAM and BIOCUT. BIOCAD focusses on drawing designs of scaffolds. BIOCAM has a specific slicer

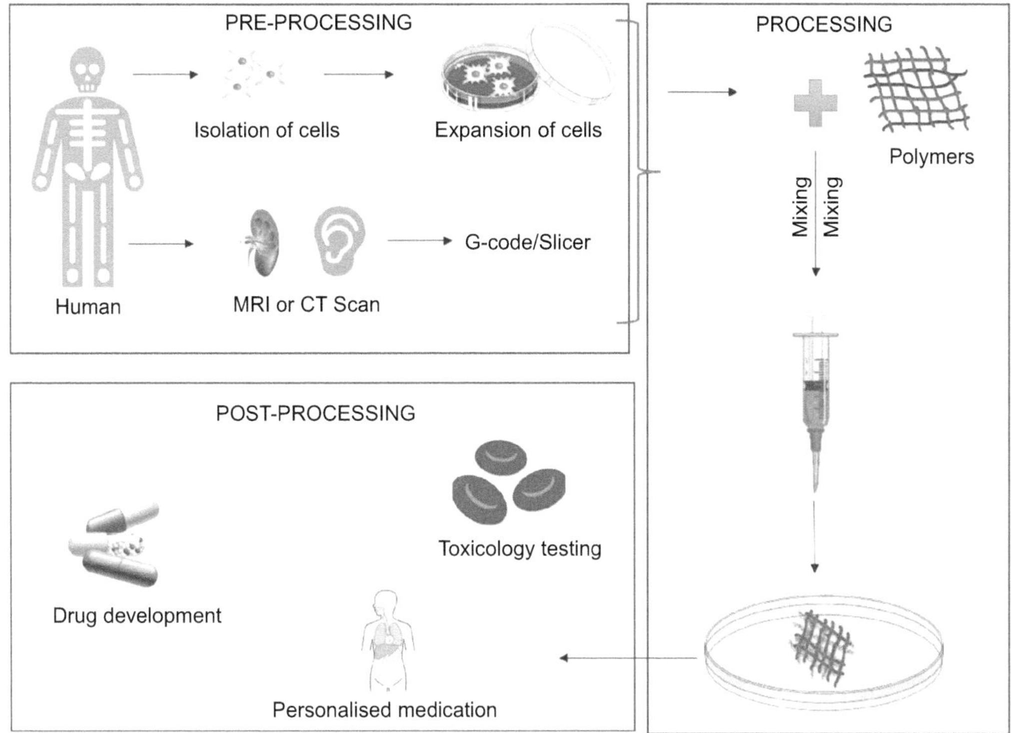

Fig. 1 Overall process of 3D bioprinting

function for RegenHU bioprinters. BIOCUT helps in creating models from medical images (https://www.3dnatives.com/en/allevi-software-bioprinting-050920195).

G-code operation-focused software helps users specify movements of the machine more accurately and precisely. These software applications are based on C# and python (Gulyas M. et al., 2018). The graphical user interfaces used include gCode editor, PetriPrinters, and gCodeAPLNET. These interfaces allow for printer movements in culture dishes with collision-safe movement. The printing temperature and start height can be set. Using CAD-based software for bioprinting is the most general approach. TinkerCAD is one of the user friendly CAD systems that does not require very specific knowledge of modelling systems. Many structures such as cuboids, cylinders, letters and lattices were developed using TinkerCAD. The STL file produced by the software is made of a triangular mesh and requires mesh processing. Software like Meshmixer has been developed for processing meshes, allowing for the filling inside the 3D model. Many open-source software tools are available for slicing the model into layers. Simplify 3D is one such software that provides preprocessing simulations, mesh analysis, and support for multiple machines (https://www.simplify3d.com). Cura, a large open-source project, offers many software options for slicing and preprocessing, such as CuraEngine and Slic3r (https://www.ultimaker.com/software/ ultimaker-cura; https://www.github.com/ultimaker/ curaengine.).

3.2 Strategies for 3D Bioprinting

3D bioprinting utilizes three approaches for fabricating products that help achieve maturation and functionality similar to native tissue. The first approach, biomimicry involves replicating the cellular and extracellular components of the tissue or organ. The second approach, autonomous self-assembly, uses stem cells or embryonic cells that develop the desired architecture as required by the native tissue. The last approach is mini tissue, which refers to the building blocks of organs that can be used by the above-mentioned approaches (Howard D. et al., 2008). There are three main strategies used for bioprinting: inkjet, extrusion based and, laser assisted.

Inkjet bioprinting is inspired by the conventional technique used in desktop printers, where individual droplets are used to create a pattern. In the early 1950s, Epson, Hewlett-Packard and Canon developed inkjet printing technology, and in 2003, a patent was granted for inkjet based bioprinting with viable cells (Doyle K., 2014). The structure is formed when the bioink is continuously deposited in the form of droplets at predetermined points (Xia Z. et al., 2018). Inkjet based bioprinting practices either the thermal or acoustic approach to deposit the bioink on the printing surface. Thermal inkjet bioprinting uses electrical heating systems to eject the bioink from the nozzle, whereas acoustic inkjet bioprinting creates pulses in the printer heads that break the bioink into droplets and then force it to come out of the nozzle (Roth EA. et al., 2004; Agarwal P. et al., 2023). Xu et al., used fibrin collagen to make hydrogel and an electrospun PCL matrix to form a scaffold on which rabbit articular chondrocytes were added. The presence of PCL helped increase the mechanical properties of the hydrogel. Post *in vitro* analysis, the scaffold was implanted in rats, and it was observed that there was dense organized, collagen present in the treated mice, which was absent in the control group (Xu T. et al., 2012). Lorber et al., printed with adult neural cells, which are more challenging to work with as they are prone to damage and have less regenerative potential. They used a high-speed image capture system to print glial cells and observed that the cells did not undergo major distortion and that the cell survival rate was similar between printed and non-printed cells (Lorber B. et al., 2013). Lee et al., used collagen type I and rat tail gel and printed dermal fibroblasts and keratinocytes between the gel using a microvalve bioprinting process. The inner layer comprised fibroblasts and the outer layer had keratinocytes. They observed that there was no significant difference between printed cells and seeded cells in terms of viability and morphology (Lee W. et al., 2009; Lee V. et al., 2014).

Extrusion based bioprinting, developed in the 1980s by Scott Crump of Stratasys Ltd is the most commonly used bioprinting technique (Pranzo D. et al., 2018). The construct is fabricated in a layer-by-layer manner by extruding ink from the printhead, either by piston, screw or using pneumatic pressure (Ozbolat I.T., Hospodiuk M., 2016). The advantages of extrusion based bioprinting include control over the deposition and distribution of cells, and the ability to print a high number of cells with a high fabrication speed (Bishop E.S. et al., 2017; Marga F. et al., 2012). However, a significant issue with this technique is the potential for cell apoptosis due to the pressure drop when printing using a micro-nozzle (Pati F. et al., 2015). Adjusting printing parameters, such as material concentration, nozzle diameter and pressure, can help mitigate the issue of cell apoptosis. Fedorovich et al., used endothelial progenitor cells and multipotent stromal cells combined with Matrigel and Matrigel-alginate to study cellular responses. Post implantation in mice, it was observed that cells showed better migration in Matrigel-only scaffold compared to the Matrigel-alginate scaffold, and bone-like tissue developed at the implantation site. To study load bearing applications, another material would need to be added to the Matrigel to explore its potential in bone tissue engineering (124). Schuurman et al., used GelMA mixed with chondrocytes, hyaluronic acid, and PCL to study the potential of the scaffold for cartilage. It was observed that the cell viability was higher in the composite scaffold in comparison to the GelMA-scaffolds and post implantation, cartilaginous tissue forming after 4 weeks (Schuurman W. et al., 2013). Jang et al., developed patches to study cardiac functions using decellularized porcine heart and human c-kit cardiac progenitor cells. To provide support to patch, PCL was printed over it, and the patches were implanted in rat myocardial infarction model. It was seen that the patches improved epicardial activation and also enhanced angiogenesis. There was the formation of tissue matrix along with proper vascularization, which enhanced cardiac functions. These bioprinted patches show potential as a therapeutic method for heart diseases (Jang et al., 2017).

Laser assisted bioprinting uses high pressure to generate bubbles to propel the bioink onto the surface (Bohandy et al., 1986). The bubble formation begins with the creation of a ribbon consisting of an energy-absorbing layer that takes in the high energy laser pulses, resulting in the vaporization of the layer at the focus point. This bioprinting technique provides excellent cellular viability since there is no contact between the dispensing nozzle and the surface. However, due to its cost, this method has not been widely utilized (Li J. et al., 2016; Dababneh A.B., 2015). Koch et al., used LAB to print fibroblasts and keratinocytes along with hMSCs. Cell viability was assessed for printed and non-printed cells and it was found to be similar in terms of apoptotic activity and proliferation rate. hMSCs maintained the same morphology throughout the experimentation, suggesting that there was no up regulation of surface markers. Biopapers which are natural receivers help enhance cell viability in LAB (Koch L. et al., 2009). Kawecki et al., used laser assisted bioprinting to position human umbilical vein endothelial cells on the biopaper to provide pre-vascularization. On the osseous biopaper, the orientation of HUVECs was aligned, and tubule-like endothelial cells were observed (Kawecki F. et al., 2010).

3.3 Bioinks

3D bioprinting techniques require bioinks to print the 3D construct to facilitate cell proliferation. These bioinks are formulations that consist of cells, biomaterials and biological molecules as shown in Figure 2. They provide an environment that aids maintenance of cell viability and functionality. Developing bioinks requires the performance of several series of assays to for performance assessment that includes optimization of pre-printing and post printing. The most important and first step in the development of bioink is that consideration of the tissue of interest. The bioink developed should have mechanical properties similar to the target tissue and possess cell motifs that help in adherence (O'Connell C. et al., 2020). Cytocompatibility and degradation of the material and byproducts of bioink production must be considered. Next comes the evaluation of the printing parameters, specifically determining if the developed bioink can address resolution and clogging issues. We will discuss the bioinks requirement further. The structures printed using the bioink should be able to maintain their integrity post printing and be effective in terms of biological performance. The bioprinted constructs must be cytocompatible, biocompatible and bioactive. Once transplanted the constructs must be non-toxic to the host body and should provide an environment conducive to cell proliferation. Printability and viscosity are two main criteria that must be optimal for bioprinting. The controlled deposition of bioink is known as printability and is influenced by rheological properties, printing parameters, and the viscosity of the bioink. The materials used in

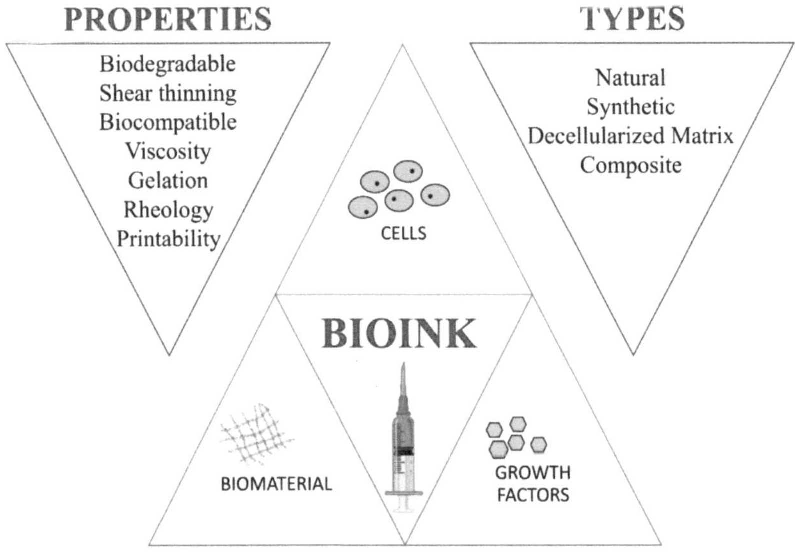

Fig. 2   Bioink-properties and types

bioinks should have properties similar to the native tissue and its ECM; otherwise they may result in low cell viability and activity (Groll J. et al., 2018).

The mechanical properties are different for the materials that are used for 3D bioprinting. Natural polymers typically exhibit poor mechanical strength compared to synthetic polymers. However, crosslinking can be employed to tune these properties, chemically modifying the polymer to make it more stable and stronger. Choosing the right crosslinking agent is crucial as it depends on various factors such as the backbone of the polymer, the functional side groups present in the polymer, mechanism of crosslinking, and the requirement for additional supplementary chemicals. Another important consideration is the impact of the crosslinking agents on the cytocompatibility, physio-chemical, physico-mechanical, and cellular behaviour in the 3D construct. Gelation also affects stability, as it involves the phase change of bioink from liquid to gel. Rapid gelation of the bioink is required to avoid structure collapse and spreading (Malda J. et al., 2013). The biodegradation rate of the construct should align with the production of the ECM *in vivo* and the by-products of degradation should be non-toxic and harmless to the host body. An ideal degradation rate is important because too rapid degradation may lead to loss of scaffold function before repair is complete, while too slow degradation may reduce cell proliferation and differentiation. Optimal degradation at the site of defect will help in release of drugs and other therapeutic molecules loaded in the construct (Gasperini L. et al., 2014).

There are various types of bioinks developed and formulated for use in tissue engineering and regenerative medicine. It is divided into four main types-decellularized extracellular matrix based, natural polymers based, synthetic polymers based and hybrid bioinks.

Decellularized matrix based bioinks

For production of such bioink the process of decellularization has to take place which removes the cellular content either using the physical, chemical and biological method and retains the ECM. ECM comprises of many proteins such as collagen, fibronectin, laminin, and proteoglycans and the microenvironment of ECM helps in the functionality of the tissue (Subbiah R., Guldberg R.E., 2019). Sometimes to increase the stability different polymers are also added to the dECM inks (Mewhort H.E. et al., 2017). To formulate dECM based inks, first, the tissue is processed, followed by cleaning, the tissue is further sliced into tiny pieces and given a thorough washing with either phosphate buffer saline or water. Depending on the tissue type, ECM composition, cell density, etc., the tissue decellularization process uses the suitable decellularizing agent. This primary goal is to eliminate all cellular contents while maintaining the integrity of the original extracellular matrix. Ultimately, post-decellularization entails sterilizing the tissue using ethanol or peracetic acid and eliminating any remaining substances from the tissue to prevent cytotoxicity. The decellularized tissue is lyophilized and ground to a powder after sterilization. To obtain the liquid dECM for 3D bioprinting, the resulting tissue can be solubilized using pepsin or papain. Different forms of crosslinking are applied to the dECM bioinks in order to promote cell adhesion and proliferation. A 3D cell printing technique with a heating modulus was created by Ahn et al., who also demonstrating its aid accurate stacking of the dECM-based construct (Ahn G. et al., 2017). The heating module enabled simultaneous crosslinking of the bioink. Kim et al. developed a cornea-derived dECM bioink using human turbinate mesenchymal stem cells (hTMSCs) and dECM with biochemical characteristics similar to the original cornea (Kim H. et al., n.d). The hTMSCs in the bioink demonstrated good cell survival, lineage development into keratinocytes, and stable 3D architectures upon heat crosslinking. Jang et al. created heart constructs with improved mechanical properties and stable structures made up of ten layers using two-step crosslinking. Vitamin B2 was utilized as a photoinitiator, and the dECM solution digested by pepsin produced three-dimensional structures. Each layer was then photocrosslinked with ultraviolet (UV) light and stabilized by thermal cross-linking. Similar mechanical characteristics to the original heart tissue were demonstrated by the design, along with improved cardiomyogenic differentiation (Cho DW, 2009). Gao et al. used both thermal and ionic crosslinking to create blood vessels (Jang J. et al., 2016). Coaxial printing of the

CPF-127 solution was done after mixing and printing alginate and vascular tissue-derived dECM. Alginate was crosslinked ionically when both substances were deposited at the same time. Ionic crosslinking was created with the original shape fidelity and tubular architectures using calcium chloride ($CaCl_2$) solution (CPF127) as the inner circle and dECM and alginate as the outside shell. The constructs were incubated at 37°C for thermal crosslinking following the printing of the final structure. After the CPF127 solution was eliminated, an *in vivo* observation of the artificial bio-blood artery was made. It was shown that the rate of ischemia injury recovery had improved.

Polymer based bioinks

Naturally occurring polymers that are found in large amounts include collagen, gelatin, keratin, silk, and elastin. Their biocompatible, biodegradable, and controllable physiochemical, biological, and mechanical characteristics make them suitable candidates for use as biomaterials in 3D bioprinting (Gao G. et al., 2017). These have better biocompatibility, higher degradability, and lower immunogenicity when compared to synthetic polymers; these characteristics all point to the potential advantages of natural polymer-based inks in the creation of hierarchical constructions. The viscosity and its modification, printability, and form integrity are all improved by the proteins in the inks. These renewable, eco-friendly materials contribute to a decrease in the usage of synthetic polymers generated from fossil fuels (Khoeini R. et al., 2021).

Collagen makes up almost 30% of the total mass of proteins in mammals, making it one of the most common proteins. It is primarily obtained from porcine, bovine, murine, or marine sources (Mirzaei M. et al., 2021). They belong to the hydrophilic fibrous glycoprotein family and are an essential part of the extracellular matrix (ECM). They are made up of three polypeptide chains: triple helical domains, alpha chains, and beta chains. There are about 28 distinct forms of collagens based on the combinations of these domains. The most prevalent form of collagen, called type I collagen, is found in skin, tendons, and bones. It is a member of the fibril-forming collagen family and has a triple helical structure made up of three alpha helices. Type II collagen is found in cartilage. The source and kind of tissue determine the collagen extraction procedure (Khan R., Khan M.H., 2013). Because collagen is stabilized by crosslinking and intermolecular interactions, it dissolves relatively slowly. Since there are numerous non-collagenous elements present that could cause impurities in the isolated collagen, pre-treating the collagen before the hydrolysis process is crucial.

Collagen can be isolated using either chemical hydrolysis or enzymatic hydrolysis. Acids are used in chemical hydrolysis to dissolve collagen fibers at low pH levels. In order to disrupt the open inter-chain cross links in collagen, acetic acid is the chosen solubilizer for uncrosslinked collagens (Rajan N. et al., 2006; Fratzl P., 2008). Trypsin, chymotrypsin, pepsin, alcalase, papain, and other enzymes are frequently utilized in enzymatic hydrolysis. Enzymatic separation and enzymes can be used in low-lying environments, and the degree of hydrolysis and specificity can be adjusted. In order to replicate skin tissue, Koch et al. printed a three-dimensional construct with fibroblasts and keratinocytes embedded in collagen. After applying 20 layers of fibroblasts to the surface and 20 layers of keratinocytes to the collagen hydrogel, the cells were arranged in 3D using the laser-aided bioprinting approach. After the hydrogel that produced the dermis and epidermis was examined, it was cultured for ten days to check the viability and activity of the cells. Both cell adhesion and proliferation were increased (Koch L. et al., 2010).

Human hair, wool, nails, hooves, horns, and other tissues are rich in keratin, a protein that is made up of several amino acids, such as cystine, glycine, proline, and serine. There is relatively little histidine, methionine, or lysine present. Because keratin has processing issues, there is relatively little work being done in tissue engineering with this material. It is an inexpensive material that forms hydrogels by self-assembly and has good stability and low solubility (Gómez-Guillén M.C. et al., 2011). Leucine-aspartic acid-valine (LDV) and arginine-glycine (RGD) are two cell binding motifs that are known to enhance cell attachment. These motifs are binding motifs for proteins, and their presence contributes to a reduction in manufacturing process complexity by eliminating the need for an extra post-processing step to incorporate them (Qiu J. et al., 2020; Horvath A.L.,

1983). Keratin and PCL were used to create an electrospun skin substitute, and keratinocytes and fibroblasts were cultivated to resemble natural skin tissue. To prevent unintentional folding and tearing, support material for PCL was printed in between the layers of fibroblast and keratinocyte nanofibers. Animals were given a scaffold containing cells and merely PCL scaffold as a skin substitute for wound healing; the former demonstrated superior wound healing compared to the latter (Nelson W.G., Sun T.T. et al., 1983).

Silk is one of the many naturally occurring polymers and is a popular textile material because of its lustrous appearance, dyeability, and breathability. Its superior mechanical strength, biocompatibility, flexibility, and hierarchical structure also led researchers to consider using silk in tissue engineering and biomedical applications. It is possible to separate silk from the arthropod species that construct their webs, cocoons, and nests. Spiders, crickets, bees, silkworms, fleas, glowworms, and other insects are among the species that produce silk (Choi W.S. et al., 2021). Fibrin and sericin are the two structural proteins found in silk thread. Fibroin, the primary constituent of silk, serves as the inner core and contributes to its mechanical strength, whilst sericin functions as a covering akin to glue. Because SF has characteristics like biocompatibility, lack of immunogenicity, mechanical strength, and native extracellular matrices, it is regarded as a potential scaffold material for use in biomedical applications. For the purpose of bone tissue creation, SF and hydroxyapatite were combined to create a scaffold. Because silk provided the elasticity and flexibility and HA provided the brittle osteogenic bioceramic, the resulting scaffold had a structure substantially similar to that of genuine bone. These hybrid systems have the ability to promote both osteogenesis and angiogenesis. The system can be developed into films, hydrogels, or 3D-printed scaffolds, according to the final result of the study (Porter D. et al., 2009; Cacciotti I., 2019). Sun et al. created 3D scaffolds with graduated pore diameters. BMP-2 was added to SF scaffolds in order to study the osteogenic response to bone repair. One powerful osteoinductive cytokine model is BMP-2. According to the study, the BMP-s/SF scaffold can repair acute damage without the use of hMSCs since it has a higher bone volume and mechanical strength (Sun L. et al., 2012).

The most common synthetic biomaterial used to create 3D printed constructs is Polyethylene glycol (PEG), yet because of its hydrophilicity, the characteristics are not ideal for construct creation. The mechanical qualities are improved by combining it with synthetic materials. Joas et al. created a hydrogel with diacrylate of PEG, anionic and cationic monomers 3-sulfopropyl acrylate, and (2-(acryloyloxy)-ethyl)-trimethylammonium chloride by employing an extrusion-based printing approach. The hydrogel was then crosslinked with visible light (Chung J.H. et al., 2013). By creating a triblock copolymer of poly (ethylene glycol)-polycaprolactone and diacrylated polycaprolactone, Xu et al. looked into this further (PCL-PEG-PCL). Cellular proliferation was seen, accompanied by higher survival rates (Xia Z. et al., 2018). A polyethylene glycol (PEG) hydrogel and methacrylated poly(N-(2-hydroxypropyl) methacrylamide mono/dilactate) (pHPMA-lac) were made for cartilage constructions. They also included methacrylated hyaluronic acid to improve printability (Joas S. et al., 2018). A pH-sensitive, thermoresponsive hydrogel was made using methylated poly(ethylene oxide)-poly(propylene oxide)-poly(ethylene oxide) (PEO-PPO-PEO). The hydrogels were printed using stereolithography, which allowed for the demonstration of reversible swelling and deswelling responses (Mouser V.H. et al., 2017). Using acrylic acid monomer, polyethylene glycol diacrylate, and 2,4,6-trimethylbenzoyl-diphenylphosphine oxide (TPO) nanoparticles, Larush et al. developed a drug-loaded system with unique drug release characteristics and pH responsive features (Dutta S., Cohn D., 2017).

Hybrid bioinks

As hydrogels lack the necessary mechanical qualities to aid in the engineering of tissues such as bone and cartilage, several biomaterials are mixed with other materials to enable hydrogels to perform as best they can. In one study, alginate and gelatin were mixed to create Alg-Gel. The results showed that while temperature-controlled Alg-Gel had a higher viscosity and consistency that improved printability, pre-crosslinked Alginate bioink was too liquid to print. Even when printing at high pressures, bioink did not appear to have any influence on the viability of the cells in *in vitro* experiments using myoblasts (Larush L. et al., 2017). Law et al. examined the vitality, stability, and rheological behaviour of mesenchymal stem cells in hydrogels containing methylcellulose and hyaluronic acid (HAMC). Higher HAMC concentrations have been found to work best for cell encapsulation (Das S. et al., 2015). GelMA, the most popular hybrid bioink, aids in creating the ideal environment for cell migration, differentiation, and proliferation. Gelatin and methacryloyl react to generate it; the former contributes biocompatibility while the latter gives mechanical strength. Duan et al. created trileaflet heart valves using gelatin methacrylate to preserve human aortic valve interstitial cells and improve their cell adhesion characteristics. For digital light processing, chitosan and acrylamide were mixed to create a bioink. The 3D hydrogels that were created might be used to create tissues and organs since they had improved mechanical and biological qualities (Law N. et al., 2018). A medication delivery device was created using 3D printing methods using alginate and PLGA.

Hydrogels can have their mechanical, chemical, and electrical characteristics improved by certain nanomaterials. To boost the viscosity and improve the mechanical characteristics of cell-laden carboxymethyl cellulose (CMC), PEG-made microparticles were added. However, it was found that the extra stress had a significant negative impact on the survivability of the cells. Silicates are being introduced to biomaterials to address shear thinning, self-healing, and mechanical property tuning. Poly(N-isopropyl acrylamide) was crosslinked using clay nanosheets, and the resulting hydrogel stretched 1424 percent further than it had originally been, although it remained brittle and robust (Do AV et al., 2017). In bone tissue engineering, hydroxyapatite—a naturally occurring substance in native osseous tissue is employed.

Various cells that are used for development of bioinks targeting different organs/tissues are shown in Figure 3.

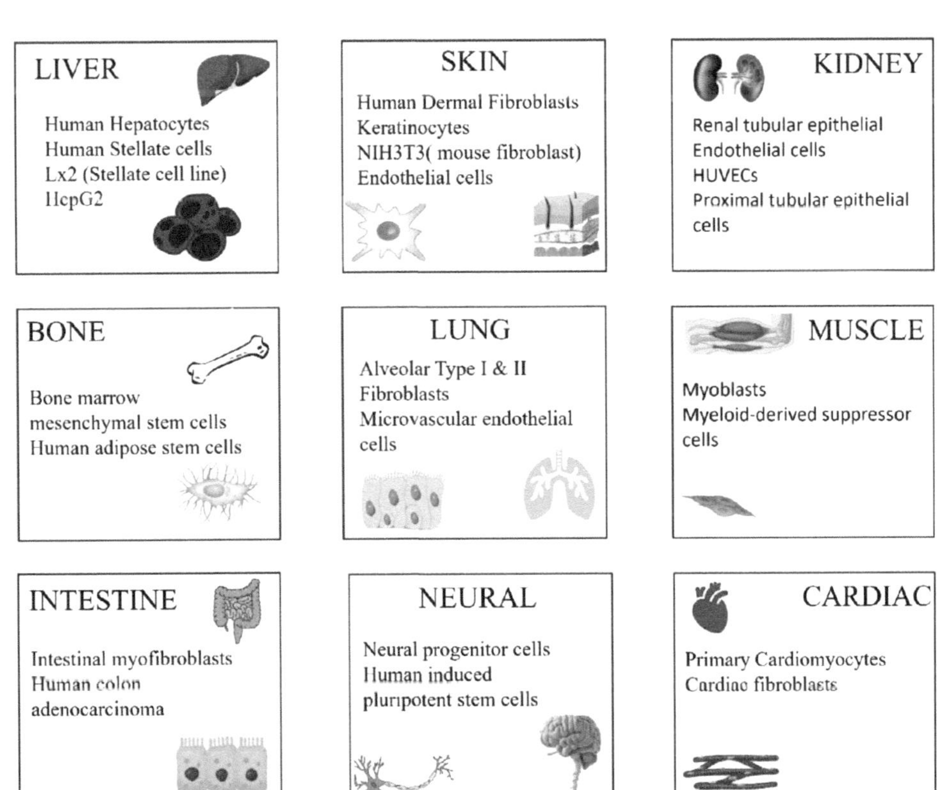

Fig. 3   Different types of cells used for development of bioink

3.4 Applications of 3D Bioprinting

The advancement in formulation of bioinks and in 3D bioprinting techniques have aided the generation of constructs with high potential for carrying bioactive components. These constructs have been proven to have successful applications as drug-development and tissue regenerating models (Haraguchi K., Takehisa T., 2002). Such technology has not only helped in providing potential outcomes in clinical trials but also added an alternative platform for animal models. 3D bioprinting has offered numerous applications in tissue engineering, pharmaceuticals and regenerative medicine as shown in Figure 4.

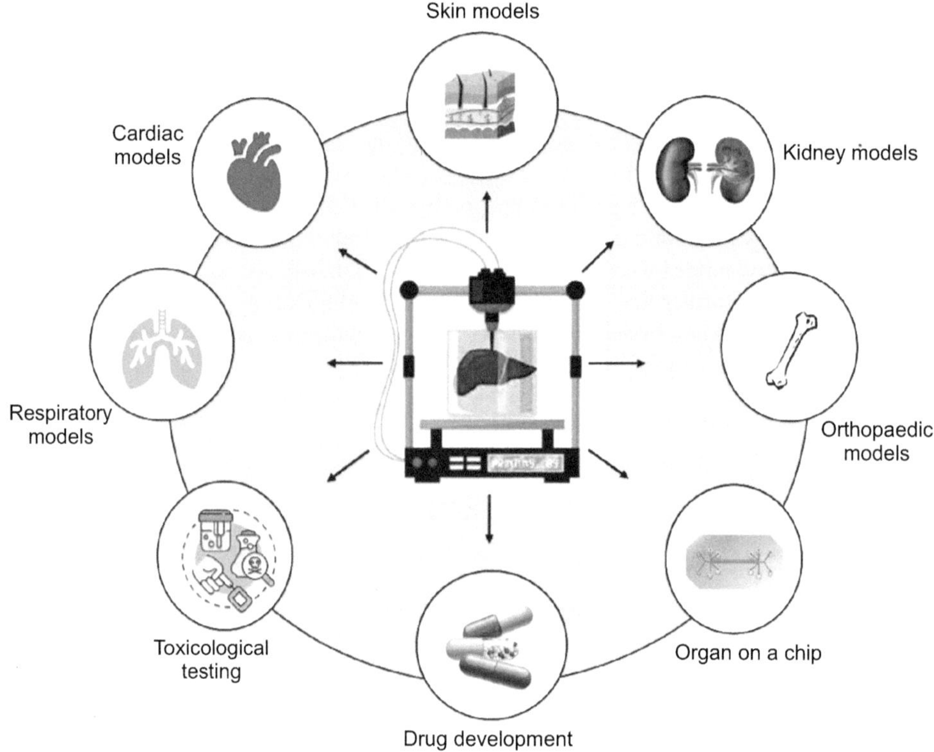

Fig. 4   Various applications of 3D bioprinting

3.4.1 Cancer research

Cancer is one most studied multifactorial disease that is caused by unregulated cell divisions. The cases of cancer have increased progressively in the past decade with the most common being breast cancer, lung cancer, colorectal cancer and prostate cancer. Tumor progression and metastasis are promoted by collaboration between tumor cells and other multiple cells. Tumor comprises a microenvironment that helps in tumorigenesis with the help of stromal components like fibroblasts, immune cells, vasculature and cancer cells. The tumor microenvironment (TME) is constantly evolving to different stages of tumor progression and the crosstalk between the cells in TME helps in cancer progression. The cancer cells also secrete various ECM proteins like collagen, glycoproteins, proteoglycans and secretory factors (Youhanna S. et al., 2022). The conventional techniques used for studying cancer involved 2D cell culture of monolayer cells and xenograft animal models (Liotta L.A., Kohn E.C., 2001). 2D culture easily provided availability of cells and cost-effectiveness but was unable to deliver the spatial arrangement of cancer cells and the extracellular environment. The drug development process was severely affected by this issue, as drugs often surpass the preclinical trials but fail in the clinical phase. In recent times, the conventional practices have been accompanied with 3D culture that helps in studying cancer in three dimensional planes and serves as a step before clinical studies for detection of action of anti-cancer drugs more accurately (Padrón J.M. et al., 2000; Kim J.B., 2005).

It is important to fabricate the native human tissue as tumor models to study tumors. 3D bioprinted scaffolds are developed by emphasising on the TME that helps in defining the functionality. 3D constructs mimic the heterogeneity and the complexity of the tumor and serve as a bridge between the *in vitro* and *in vivo* (Mak I.W. et al., 2014). Using different 3D bioprinting strategies and biomaterials, the desired mechanical property and cell support can be achieved post printing. There are two strategies that can be approached for the fabrication of the cancer model. The first one includes creating the 3D printed scaffold and then seeding the cells onto it. The other approach involves 3D bioprinting with cell laden bioink either directly on a platform or within a cancer-on-chip model. 3DP cancer models are used in studying the crosstalk between the cancer cells, efficacy of anti-cancer drugs, gene expressions and invasion characteristics. Using 3D bioprinting, researchers have come a long way in developing a cost effective and precise disease model that is helping disease management (Wang C. et al., 2014).

Zhao et al., printed HeLa cells along with hydrogel made up of gelatin, alginate and fibrinogen to fabricate cervical tumor models. They compared the 2D culture model and 3D printed tumor model by measuring cell proliferation, matrix metalloproteinase and chemoresistance. It was observed that the rate of proliferation was higher in 3D printed models; MMP expression and chemoresistance were also increased (Shukla P. et al., 2022). In one study, a decellularized extracellular matrix from brain tissue was used to fabricate a glioblastoma tumor model by adding patient derived tumor cells and vascular endothelial cells. They fabricated an anatomically similar model by depositing cancer and vascular cells along with BdECM onto a glass slide providing proper spatial tissue organization. The fabrication of glioblastoma on the chip model helped in analyzing the precision medicine concept for the patient by screening the drugs and its efficacy on the patient's cells (Zhao Y. et al., 2014). Zhou et al., fabricated a biomimetic bone matrix to study the interaction between breast cancer cells and bone stromal cells. Using stereolithography, bone matrices were fabricated with hydroxyapatite nanocrystalline and GelMA hydrogel in which osteoblasts were encapsulated. In these cell laden matrices, BrCa cells were introduced and it was observed that their growth was enhanced and that of osteoblasts was inhibited. They also observed that there was an increase in vascular endothelial growth factor in the 3D model in comparison to the 2D BrCa culture. This model has potential to study the interactions between multiple cells involved in metastatic cancer progression in bone (Yi H.G. et al., 2019).

3.4.2   *Drug discovery and development*

Drug launching is a time intensive process divided into two major stages, drug discovery and drug development. The former focuses on identifying suitable compounds from multiple molecular compounds which are compatible with the biochemical target and the latter addresses the safety and efficacy validation through different phases of trails (Amir-Aslani A. et al., 2010). In drug discovery, the main emphasis is on the *in vitro* assays to screen the lead molecules and exclude the toxic compounds. Traditionally, the *in vitro* tests are performed on a 2D monolayer cells culture which may not replicate the conditions present *in vivo* and thus, it is difficult to assess the drug effects accurately (Amir-Aslani A., Mangematin V., 2010). Hence, there is a requirement of developing models that can mimic the *in vivo* environment helping in identifying drugs correctly and avoiding misleading results. 3D culture systems developed to overcome the limitations of 2D assays are 3D scaffold based in which cell sheets, aggregated cells or individual cells are seeded in a matrix. The matrix assembles the ECM-like structure and helps in providing space for cell attachment, growth and migration. To fabricate 3D models many techniques are being used such as the hanging drop method (Wrzesinski K., J Fey S, 2015), microfluidics (Wissing M.D. et al., 2014), 3D bioprinting (Shin Y. et al., 2012), and hydrogel culture (Gurkan U.A. et al., 2012; Blehm B.H. et al., 2015).

Different techniques of bioprinting have been adopted to deliver plasmids, genes and growth factors to the cells. The thermal inkjet technique was utilized to create pores in the cell membrane so that the DNA plasmids entered the cells due to the shear stress and heat available at the printhead. Once the plasmids entered the cells, they got printed as droplets containing genetically modified cells (Lam V.Y., Wakatsuki T., 2011; Xu T. et al., 2009; Cui X. et al., 2010). In one study, the vascular endothelial growth factor was encapsulated in gelatin microparticles and then implanted in scaffolds fabricated by 3D bioprinting human endothelial progenitor cells and Matrigel/alginate biomaterial. For three weeks, continuous release of VEGF was observed and when the scaffolds were implanted in nude mice it was observed that slow release from the microparticles helped in more vessel formation in comparison to VEGF added to the media (Owczarczak A.B. et al., 2012).

3.4.3 Organ on a chip

The intricacy of the human tissues in terms of complexity and uniqueness is regulated by microenvironment and the organization mimicking the physiology. This intricacy helps in maintaining the homeostasis and tissue remodelling. Organ on a chip system (OoC) comes into play to replicate this physiology *in vitro*. OoC has enormous potential in showcasing the microarchitecture of human physiology helping understand the mechanisms, functionalities, and other biological processes of the body (Poldervaart MT et al., 2014). The principle behind the system is the culturing of the cells on the chip to mimic the mechanical and physiological responses and characteristics of the organs (Park J.Y. et al., 2018). A combination of tissue engineering and microfluidics helps in creating OoC by adding the complexity of media flow and electrical stimuli on the *in vitro* models. This technique uses different biomaterials along with multiple cell types to develop complex architecture.

The new advancement in OoC research is the addition of 3D bioprinting, as it helps in fabricating *in vitro* models having similar functionality as that of native tissue and also providing spatial arrangement of cells. Earlier, while fabricating OoC chips, biomaterials were used as coating materials and cells were added for adhesion but the limitation with this prototype was the difficulty to stimulate the complex structures. 3D bioprinting overcomes this limitation by providing a means for patterning the chip for single or multiple cell types. 3D printing can fabricate multiple cells array in one step and along with microfluidics, the structure can be used to study new drugs and biological processes. A liver OoC was developed to study drug toxicity, in which three chambers were created and connected by fluidic channels. PDMS was used to create chambers and channels and using 3D bioprinting, spheroids of HepG2/C3A were created within GelMA hydrogel and added to the channels.

Hepatic functional proteins were studied by observing the spheroids sustaining the continuous perfusion (Li X et al., 2000). Skardal et al., developed a multi-tissue OoC focussing on liver, heart and lung spheroids. They were 3D printed into the microfluidic bioreactors and normal expression of biomarkers was reported in single tissue organoids with long term viability. They also studied the interconnection of the three systems by introducing bleomycin to target lung inhibition. It was seen that in the interconnected model, heart organoids changed morphologically and also, they ceased beating but when bleomycin was added to only the heart system, the cells were beating normally. This suggests that when introduced in multi tissue OoC, bleomycin may release some factors affecting other organ systems. This demonstrates the value of integrated devices to study the efficacy and side effects of drugs (Bhise NS et al., 2016). Lind et al., utilised 3D bioprinting to fabricate microphysiological devices for functional cardiac tissue models. They used six different biocompatible inks which were piezo resistive, having high conductance. The device also contained strain gauge sensors to measure the contractile forces while performing *in vitro* drug screening. They validated that the sensors embedded in the devices helped in providing electronic readouts of stresses observed by the tissue contractility inside the cells (Skardal A et al., 2017).

Overall, 3D bioprinting helps advance OoC technology, but several limitations still need to be addressed. These include the development of biomaterials that provide good printability and biocompatibility, effective co-culturing of cells and processes that can accurately biomimic natural tissues. 3D bioprinting provides fabrication of cell-laden microfluidics and biosensor systems and can also be used for patient specific tissue model construction.

3.4.4   Organ systems

This particular section highlights various 3D bioprinted models that have been applied for various tissues and organs like neural, skin, liver, cardiac and bone (Lind JU et al., 2017; Rouwkema Jeroen et al., 2011). instance, the only available tool as a translational brain model was the differentiation of induced pluripotent stem cells into neural-like cells. However, the 3D bioprinted model fabricated by Tang et al.,which utilized hyaluronic acid combined with various cells (macrophages, neural cells, glioblastoma and astrocytes) it was possible to successfully mimic a brain tumour. This model has the potential to study drug sensitivity, cell invasion and immune cell interactions (https:// rokithealthcare.com/tag/bio printing/[Accessed 5 October 2021]). Salaris et al. developed a bioink composed of matrigel along with alginate and cells (glial cells and cortical neurons). Once bioprinted, the construct exhibited molecular, structural and functional properties characteristic of a neuron-like network. This model can be further applied for neuronal disease modelling and drug screening (M. Tang et al., 2020). Skin plays an important role in protection and is generally vulnerable to wounds. For various reasons, wound healing may be slow or even irreversible. A 3D bioprinted construct aids in providing a customized, and precise platform forthe biofabrication of tissue-engineered dressings. Wan et al. fabricated a scaffold consisting of 2 layers: one loaded with silver-gelatin cryogel and the other with platelet-derived growth factor. This model was instrumental in delivering growth factors from the silver nanoparticles in the top layer and providing protection from infection in the lower layer. The results of implantation in mice demonstrated neovascularization, an accelerated rate of collagen deposition and, tissue formation (Salaris, F. et al., 2019).

Li et al., developed a skin dressing scaffold made up of polydopamine-modified bioceramic. The skin scaffolds showed promising results in preventing inflammatory infiltration and promoting sufficient collagen deposition and vascular regeneration making it an ideal model for healing diabetic wounds (Wan W. et al., 2019). The liver, being the largest organ and with the capability to regenerate, can have its capacity hindered after reaching a highly damaged stage. The only way to cure this end-stage liver condition is through transplantation. However, the lack of donor availability and the high chances of rejection make 3D bioprinted constructs as the only potentially successful alternative. Gravina et al., formulated bioink consisting of sodium alginate and gelatin blend along with decellularized extracellular matrix from porcine liver and cells (human mesenchymal stem cells) and bioprinted to form an *in vitro* liver model for regeneration efficiency testing. This construct was demonstrated to produce a hepatic microenvironment ,which could potentially be applicable for *in vivo* liver regeneration (Li T. et al., 2019). Another well-known application of 3D liver models is in drug development and testing, Ma et al., developed a triculture 3D bioprinted model composed of gelatin methacrylate and glycidyl methacrylate-hyaluronic acid, along with cells (human induced pluripotent stem cells-derived hepatic progenitor cells) that demonstrated an increase in catabolic and anabolic activity of key cytochrome enzyme expressions indicating potential for drug interaction studies. This construct has shown promise as a model for drug screening and model evaluation (Di Gravina G.M. et al., 2023).

The heart, a vital organ, is susceptible to tissue damage due to adverse drug reactions. While there have been many attempts to generate heart tissues using stem-cell therapy, they have, not been consistently successful. Yeung et al fabricated a 3D bioprinted model that was biomaterial-free and was composed of spheroids enriched with human-induced pluripotent stem cell-derived cardiomyocytes, fibroblasts, and endothelial cells. This bioprinted model showed improved cardiac tissue regeneration and promoted angiogenesis in damaged tissues. As this construct reduced scar formation when implanted *in vivo*, it shows potential for application in cardiac tissue regeneration (Ma X. et al., 2016). In another study, Shevach et al., developed a 3D model consisting of patient-derived omentum decellularized extracellular matrix along with silver nanoparticles loaded with cardiac cells isolated from the same patient. The matrix, when implanted, proved to have superior functioning when compared to pristine patches by showing stronger contractile forces, low excitation threshold and quicker calcium transients, which are all important for heart tissue transplantation (Yeung E. et al., 2019). Bone damage, primarily resulting from trauma and accidents, often leads to a prolonged recovery stage. However, the availability of 3D bioprinted scaffolds has significantly reduced this recovery period by aiding in the delivery of the required bioactive components for regeneration and repair. Diomede et al., fabricated a 3D construct composing of polylactic acid with polyethyleneimine-engineered extracellular vesicles and human gingival mesenchymal stem cells. This study provided promising results for treating the cranial bone in patients experiencing surgery trauma as it promoted osteogenic inductivity when implanted *in vivo* (Shevach M. et al., 2014). Another study conducted by Teixeira et al., used polylactic acid to 3D bioprint scaffolds coated with polydopamine along with Bone marrow-derived mesenchymal stem cells. This model when implanted *in vitro* promoted osteoinductivity and hence can be considered for bone tissue engineering for regeneration (Diomede, F. et al., 2018). Many such studies conducted by groups all over the globe has led to alternative and improved methods for regeneration, repair and regeneration of tissues and organs (Teixeira B.N. et al., 2019; Fransen M.F. et al., 2021; Chuah J.K., Zink D., 2017; Tang M., 2020).

3.5   *Challenges of 3D Bioprinting*

Challenges associated with 3D bioprinting are multiple and multifold especially regarding commercialization and clinical translation. Bioprinting is a slow process and when scalability is in focus, it is very difficult to maintain cells without damaging their integrity. The possibility of cell survival in the long bioprinting process is a challenge. although, the upcoming volumetric bioprinting technology has been known to reduce the time taken for printing (You S et al., 2023). *In situ* monitoring of the cells happens post printing and that can be a challenge when it comes to fabrication of tissue/organs at a human scale (Bliley J.M. et al., 2022). Time, cost and effort can be saved if process parameters assessed early and necessary amendments are made.

Addressing the accessibility of bioprinters for clinicians is a significant challenge. Current bioprinters lack user-friendliness requiring. basic knowledge and skill sets to manage and setup the bioprinting process. Clinicians typically cannot handle the whole process independently and need technical staff to operate the equipment. Isolating and culturing cells from the biopsies, developing 3D models and designs, and optimizing printing parameters are complex tasks for clinicians. Consequently, there is a growing demand for clinician-friendly 3D bioprinters that are easy to maintain, use, and meet medical requirements.

Bioinks used generally for 3D bioprinting are either from a natural source or synthetic. Both have their own set of advantages and challenges. For synthetic polymers based bioinks, the pros are the tunable mechanical properties and limited batch to batch variation but they do not have bioactive molecules sites or sites where cells can adhere (Tashman J.W., 2022). In the case of natural polymers, the source is the problem. Polymers like gelatin, collagen, and chitosa are isolated from different animals and can cause immunological reactions that can be potentially fatal. In terms of cellular architecture or cultivated meat, using animal sourced polymers is a mockery as the whole point is to reduce the usage of animals. Another challenge with natural polymers is the batch-to-batch variations. Each animal consists of ECM that differs from that of other animals. It also depends on the age of the animal as it can affect the structural, mechanical and biological properties leading to variations in the batch. Other factors that contribute to batch-to-batch variations are molecular weight, rheological properties, degree of substitution and chemical structure. The bioinks developed and made available are very tissue specific and it takes a lot of time to optimize recipes. The concept of universal bioink is still very farfetched. The commercially available bioinks undergo only basic assays like cell viability and biocompatibility and do not consider the cellular functions that can be affected by the bioink (Li J. et al., 2020).

In extrusion based printing, parameters like extrusion pressure and speed are crucial, while in inkjet printing, heat and voltage play significant roles (Vijayavenkataraman S., 2023). These parameters not only affect the printing process and the cell viability but also affect the mechanical strength, and stability of the printed structure. There are few other parameters that determine the properties of the bioprinted tissue like the temperature, humidity, and nozzle size. Therefore, optimizing the printing parameters is essential for advancing the field of 3D bioprinting (Kesti M. et al., 2016). When it comes to clinical translation, bioprinting faces many hurdles. Firstly, sourcing cells is a significant challenge. The processes of cell harvesting of cells, expansion in the laboratory and subsequent bioprinting to the required scale, are full of uncertainties. Additionally, clinical translation faces hurdles in long-term storage and transportation. Given the critical nature of timing for transplantation, developing technologies that ensure prolonged storage and viability is imperative. There are various legal, ethical and social aspects associated with bioprinting. As such there are no regulatory guidelines created especially for the use and approval of bioprinted products and there is no specific document regarding the regulatory guidelines in bioprinting. In conclusion, there are various aspects of 3D bioprinting that have to be optimized and looked into for better progress in the field of biomedical and regenerative medicine (Li J. et al., 2020).

4.   Commercial/Clinical Trial of Tissue Engineered Scaffolds

Research has increasingly focused on 3D bioprinting, which serves as a pivotal tool for fabricating 3D models used in a range of preclinical and clinical studies by leading pharmaceutical companies (Soman S.S., Vijayavenkataraman S., 2020). Numerous companies have begun to invest heavily in this sector fostering a surge of ideas for the efficient and effective fabrication of 3D models (https://www.drugdiscoverytrends.com/pharma-50-the-50-largest-pharmaceutical-companies-in-the-world, 2022; Nguyen, D.G, 2016). A majority of the 3D models in preclinical/clinical trials are aiming for either tissue repair and reconstruction or development of drugs and drug testing models. Most of the models that have been used in the above applications focus on organs like liver, kidney, lung, heart, intestine, eye, skin, neural tissues and bone tissues (Janani G. et al., 2022). A few of the recent 3D bioprinted scaffolds that have been proven as potential models for preclinical trials with different applications are mentioned in this section as well as detailed information regarding various studies conducted are listed in Table 1. Janani et al., fabricated a 3D bioprinted scaffold using an extrusion based bioprinter, incorporating an extra cellular matrix-based hydrogel with various cell types (human umbilical vein endothelial cells, hematopoietic progenitor and mature cells and human hepatocyte-like cells). This scaffold emulates the liver's native structure, featuring alternate cords of hepatocytes and a functional network with sinusoidal lumen. This model holds promise as a high-throughput ee *in vitro* model for drug screening and toxicological studies (Lau C S. et al., 2023).

Lau et al., fabricated a 3D bioprinted bone graft using a fused deposition modelling bioprinter. The graft composed of polycaprolactone–tricalcium phosphate with adipose-derived mesenchymal stem cells was designed for alveolar ridge augmentation in a porcine lateral alveolar defect model. Conducted over a 3 month period in pigs, the study suggests that the model holds potential for bone regeneration and could be a viable alternative for alveolar ridge augmentation treatments (Lau, C.S. et al., 2023). Li/Xu et al., fabricated a 3D bioprinted model using a micro-extrusion printer, employing poly(d,l-lactide-co-glycolide)/nano-hydroxyapatite with bioactive lentiviral vectors (LV-pdgfb) for bone tissue regeneration. The study conducted over an 8 week period in mice demonstrated that the scaffold successfully enhanced bone regeneration bone with angiogenic properties making it a promising model for various bone tissue engineering applications (Li, J. et al., 2016). Smeets et al., fabricated a 3D bioprinted model using selective laser sintering, incorporating poly (d,l-lactide) and β-tricalcium phosphate with mesenchymal stem cells for bone regeneration. The study conducted over a 4 week period in rats, demonstrated. enhanced bone replacement. This suggests that the scaffold could be a viable alternative for treating bone defects in humans (Smeets, R. et al., 2017). Kundu et al., fabricated a 3D bioprinted model using a multi-head deposition

Table 1 Comparison of different 3D cell culture models

	2D cell culture	Spheroids	Organoids	Organ on chip	3D bioprinted models
BIOLOGICAL COMPLEXITIY					
Compositions of cells in the model	●○○○○	●●●○○	●●○○○	●●○○○	●●●●○
Capacity to develop ECM composition	●○○○○	●○○○○	●●○○○	●○○○○	●●●○○
Capability to remodel the microenvironment	●○○○○	●○○○○	●○○○○	●●○○○	●●●○○
Architecture	●○○○○	●○○○○	●●○○○	●●○○○	●●●●○
Physiological function	●○○○○	●○○○○	●●○○○	●●●○○	●●●●○
High-throughput screening	●○○○○	●○○○○	●●○○○	●●●○○	●●●●●
PHYSICAL CUES					
Physical stiffness	●○○○○	●●○○○	●●●○○	●●●●●	●●●●○
Tunability	●○○○○	●●○○○	●●○○○	●●○○○	●●●●○
Durability	●○○○○	●○○○○	●●○○○	●●●○○	●●●○○
Genetic variation	●○○○○	●○○○○	●○○○○	●○○○○	●●●○○
TECHNICAL CHALLENGES					
Ease in the development	●●●●●	●●○○○	●●○○○	●●●○○	●●●○○
Relative complexity	●○○○○	●○○○○	●○○○○	●●○○○	●●●●○
Expense in the development	●○○○○	●○○○○	●●○○○	●●●○○	●●●○○
Level of maintenance	●○○○○	●○○○○	●○○○○	●●●○○	●●○○○

system, employing polycaprolactone (PCL) and chondrocyte cell-encapsulated alginate hydrogel for cartilage regeneration. The study conducted over a 4 week period on mice, found that the scaffolds post-implantation promoted enhanced cartilage tissue growth and type II collagen fibril formation, thereby establishing it as a suitable model for cartilage regeneration studies (Kundu J. et al., 2015). X. Liu et al., fabricated a 3D bioprinted model using a micro-extrusion based bioprinter, combining methacrylated gelatin and acrylate β-cyclodextrin with neural stem cells. Aimed at promoting neuronal regeneration, the study spanned 8 weeks on mice. The inclusion of a small molecule drug laden construct positions this model as a potential therapeutic strategy for treating spinal cord injuries (Liu X., 2022).

Clinical trials of 3D bioprinted models are being conducted due to the significant interest from candidates requiring treatment for various conditions. For example, traumatic spinal cord injury is a devastating neurological disorder, has seen an increase in incidence, with rates ranging from 11 to 16 cases per 1,00,000 people worldwide (Howard D. et al., 2008). With few available treatments for irreversible spinal cord injuries, there is a significant demand for various tissue engineered products. Clinical trials typically progress through five stages, beginning with the pre-clinical stage, where *in vitro* and *in vivo* experiments are conducted. Phase I follows, involving upto 10 participants to assess the initial treatment's effects in humans. If successful, phase II commences with a larger group of upto 50 participants to evaluate the treatment's efficacy and the safety. Upon satisfactory results, phase III starts, involving upto 200 participants to confirm the initial phases' findings. If the initial phases yield satisfactory results, phase IV commences involving over 200 participants to monitor and record the treatment's long-term effects. Upon a successful clinical trial, the product is then launched into the market for public use. A few of the products that currently have a market presence are CartiMax (CorMatrixCardiovascularSciences), AlloDerm (LifeCell), Osteocel (NuVasive), VascuCel (LeMaitreVascular), DuraMatrix (Stryker), CryoPatch (Cryolife), Matrion (LifeNetHealth), Axi (Coloplast), Permacol Surgical Implant (Medtronic), Strattic (Strattice Reconstructive Tissue Matrix), Tutopatch (RTISurgical), Veritas (Baxter) (Alizadeh A. et al., 2019).

Recent advances in various branches of tissue engineering have emerged as the most effective treatments for irreversible tissue and organ damage. The number of emergency cases have been rising ever since due to trauma injuries and road accidents. This has led to the alarming demand for products fabricated from tissue engineered procedures as they have the added advantage of covering patient-specific requirements. Moreover inactive lifestyles have led to an increase in widespread chronic diseases like cardiovascular disorders, obesity, diabetes and most frequently, cancer. A recent report suggests that annually there are 250,000-500,000 individuals worldwide suffering from spinal cord injury and tissue engineering is the only promising treatment for this condition. One of the primary drivers of growth in the tissue engineered scaffold market is the advancement in creating efficient implants for various body parts. Additionally, the expansion of applied 3D bioprinted scaffolds in health care has been significantly supported by both government and private sector funding for research and development.

There has been an exponential increase in consumer healthcare awareness, normalizing surgeries for replacement and reconstruction (Global Tissue Engineering Market by Product, 2028) When examining the global tissue engineering market, it is been estimated to reach upto 8.9 billion US dollars by 2028, up from 4.4 billion US dollars in 2023. The synthetic materials sector has captured the largest market share in tissue engineering due to its widespread use. The market for synthetic materials is expected to grow alongside advancements in the tissue engineering and the rising demand for regenerative medicines. Major countries contributing to this growth include the U.S., Canada, UK, Germany, France, Italy, Spain, Denmark, Sweden, Norway, China, Japan, India, Australia, South Korea, Thailand, Brazil, Mexico, Argentina, Saudi Arabia, South Africa, UAE and Kuwait. Few of the key players in the glpbal tissue engineering market include Organogenesis (US), AbbVie Corporation (US), Baxter (US), BD (US), B. Braun (Germany), TEIJIN Limited (Japan), Institut Straumann AG (Switzerland), Integra Lifesciences (US), Johnson & Johnson Services,

Table 2   Commercial/ clinical trials for tissue engineered 3D bioprinted scaffolds

Sl. No.	Study design	Tissue/ organ focused	Major outcome	References
1	The study had thirteen patients and were divided randomly in a test group ($n=6$) where PCL scaffolds were inserted inside the tooth socket and control ($n=7$) where no implant was inserted. Two things were measured (alveolar ridge width and height) at the initial time point and later at the end of 6 months post the extraction. Using the micro-tomographic and histological tests, the results were analyzed. Another surgery was performed using fresh implants in the test group after 4 to 6 months.	BONE	The test group showed lesser resorption in the vertical ridge when compared with the control group. The statistical significance of $P = 0.008$ in the mesio buccal aspect. The micro-tomographic and histological tests showcased bone formation in the test group except for one patient. Hence these PCL scaffolds could help in normal bone healing and better ridge height maintenance.	Tissue Engineering Market Size, Share Analysis Report 2030
2	The study had twenty-six patients and were divided randomly in two groups, one group (n=13) where scaffolds were custom-made bone using computer-aided design technique, another group (n=13) where commercial titanium meshes implant was used. Few of the clinical aspects analyzed during the trial was time of the operation, mucosal rupture, infection, retaining screw.	BONE	The operation time recorded to implant the custom-made group was 75.4 ± 11.6 min which when compared to the conventional group was significantly shorter 111.9 ± 17.8 min with $p < 0.01$. There was no mucosal rupture in the test group with significant difference ($p = 0.27$), Infection was found higher in the test group with 23.1% and lesser in the other group with 7.7%. The use of retaining screw was significantly less in the custom-made group than another group with $p < 0.01$. This study provides a novel protocol with simple and safe fabrication of implants for bone regeneration.	Goh B.T. et al., 2015
3	The study had twenty-one patients and underwent an operation for replacement of the implant. The head implants were fabricated using the computed tomography technique and skull shape with symmetry were constructed. There was additional use of autologous bone grafts for the treatment.		The patients were satisfied and had no recurrent wound problems. good fixation of titanium implants.	Sumida T. et al., 2015

Contd.

Table 2 *Contd.*

Sl. No.	Study design	Tissue/organ focused	Major outcome	References
4	The study had twenty-three patients and underwent an operation for replacement of the mandibular for maxillofacial defects repair. The implants were fabricated using the computed tomography technique to obtain individual custom-made mandibular angles. Few of the clinical aspects analyzed during the trial were infection, mandibular symmetry, difficulty in opening the mouth.	BONE	After three months, the primary result from the operation i.e., the healing of incisions was seen in all the patients along with no infection, hematoma and no individual had difficulty in opening the mouth. Each patient had symmetrical mandibular reconstruction and a perfect integration of 3D fabricated bone.	Park E.K. et al., 2016
5	The study had eight patients and underwent an operation for replacement of the skull implant. It made use of the stereolithography technique to fabricate implants made of ceramic and hydroxyapatite. The implants were fabricated using the computed tomography technique to obtain individual custom-made implants to cure defects in craniofacial bone. Few of the clinical aspects analyzed during the trial was infection, fracture in implants.	SKULL	After twelve months, the primary result from the operation i.e., the defect in craniofacial bone was rectified and there were no major complications or infections or fractures due to the implant. This study developed a novel concept of custom-made ceramic implants in hydroxyapatite in order to reconstruct large and complex craniofacial bone defects	Shen C. et al., 2014
6	The study had twenty-six patients who suffered with infertility and included for non-controlled, phase I clinical trials. The implant scaffolds were fabricated using collagen along with the mesenchymal stem cells and transplanted into the uterine cavity. Few of the clinical aspects analyzed during the trial was endometrial thickness, intrauterine adhesion score and other biological molecules related to proliferation and differentiation in endometrial line before and three months after the procedure.	UTERUS	On average the observations found in the trial was the thickness of endometrium increased and intra-uterine adhesion score decreased. There was an upregulation in the expression of genes like ERα, Ki67 and vWF that indicated improvement in neovascularization, proliferation and differentiation in the endometrium. Ten of the patients had pregnancy and delivered healthy babies.	Bric J. et al., 2013

Contd.

Table 2 *Contd.*

Sl. No.	Study design	Tissue/ organ focused	Major outcome	References
7	The study had eighteen patients who suffered from infertility with unresponsive endometrium were included for self-control prospective study. The implant scaffolds were fabricated using collagen along with the mesenchymal stem cells were transplanted into the uterine cavity in two consecutives menstrual cycles. Few of the clinical aspects analyzed during the trial were thickness in endometrium, receptivity of uterus, hormone responses, proliferation and the angiogenesis in endometrial lining before and three months after the procedure.	UTERUS	There was an increase in the thickness in the endometrium line by an average of 4.08 ± 0.26 mm to 5.87 ± 0.77 mm with $P < 0.001$. There was an upregulation in the expression of genes like ERα, Ki67 and vWF that indicated improvement in neovascularization, proliferation and differentiation in endometrium. Immunohistochemistry test revealed an increased density of micro-vessel. Out of eighteen patients three were pregnant; two of them delivered healthy babies and one had a miscarriage.	Cao Y. et al., 2018
8	The study had twenty patients who had caudal septal who had undergone septoplasty, they were subjected to printed mesh composed of polycaprolactone. The only inclusion criteria were that the nasal obstruction symptom score was supposed to be greater than 20. Few of the clinical aspects analyzed during the trial were the change in the score, the change in the nasal cross-sectional area and the angle.	NOSE	There were changes in the score; the change in the nasal obstruction symptom score, cross-sectional area and the angle after the 4th week and the 12th week proving the scaffolds were able to improve the defect.	Zhang Y. et al., 2021
9	The study had twenty-eight patients who had malignant oral tumours, undergone unilateral segment resection of mandible. These patients were treated with a pre-bent reconstructed plate. The models were designed with the MRI scan and then designed by CAD individually for all the patients. Few of the clinical aspects analyzed during the trial were to check the reconstruction of the mandible when compared with traditional surgery methods.	MANDIBLE	The symmetry observed in the mandibular where the patients received a scaffold had had better results having improved reconstruction when compared to the patients who underwent conventional surgery.	Yun W.S. et al., 2018

Contd.

Table 3   Tissue engineered 3D bioprinted scaffolds

S. No.	Tissue/organ focused	Method of 3D bioprinting	Biomaterials used	Cells used	Animal model used	Study duration	Application	Reference
1	Lungs	Extrusion bioprinting	alginate, collagen, gelatin	adenocarcinoma human alveolar basal epithelial cells, human lung fibroblasts, THP-1	–	–	transplantation	Azuma M. et al., 2014
2	Heart	3D bioprinting spheroids	hyaluronic acid macomers	cardiomyocytes and human mesenchymal stem cells and induced pluripotent stem cells derived cardiomyocytes	–	–	pro-regenerative microRNA treatment	Berg J. et al., 2021
3	Heart	Droplet based bioprinter	sodium alginate, PRONOVA®	human induced pluripotent stem cells derived cardiomyocytes	–	–	drug testing	Daly A.C. et al., 2021
4	Small intestine	Extrusion bioprinting	collagen-I, decellularized porcine small intestine submucosa	colorectal adenocarcinoma cell	–	–	transplantation	Faulkner-Jones A. et al., 2022
5	Cornea	Extrusion bioprinting	collagen, gelatin, sodium alginate	human corneal keratocytes	–	–	repair and regeneration	Kim W., Kim GH, 2020
6	Skin	Droplet based bioprinter		normal human keratinocytes	–	–	reconstruction	Kutlehria S et al., 2020
7	Jawbone	vat photopolymerization bioprinting	GelMA, PEGDA3400, hyaluronic acid	serous adenocarcinoma	–	–	transplantation	Madiedo-Podvrsan, et al., 2021
8	Alveolar ridge	Ready to use	polycaprolactone-tricalcium phosphate	mesenchymal stem cells	Dog	8 weeks	regeneration	Amler A.K., 2021

Contd.

Table 3   *Contd.*

S. No.	Tissue/organ focused	Method of 3D bioprinting	Biomaterials used	Cells used	Animal model used	Study duration	Application	Reference
9	Lateral ridge	Modeler RP system bioprinter	polycaprolactone-tricalcium phosphate	–	Micropig	6 months	Repair	Khojasteh A. et al., 2013
10	Bone	Deposition modelling bioprinter	polycaprolactone-tricalcium phosphate	–	Monkey	6 months	regeneration	Yeo A. et al., 2012
11	Calvarial bone	Ready to use	Polycaprolactone and plasma rich platelets	dental pulp stem cells	Rat	10 weeks	Repair	Goh B.T. et al., 2014
12	Bone	Laser printer	polyetherketoneketone	bone marrow-derived human and sheep mesenchymal stem cells	Sheep	12 weeks	repair	Li J. et al., 2017
13	alveolar bone	micro-extrusion bioprinting	β-tricalcium phosphate, wollastonite, and bredigite	–	Rabbit	16 weeks		Adamzyk C. et al., 2016
14	Bone	Ready to use	polycaprolactone-nanometric hydroxyapatite	–	Sheep	12 weeks	translational model for bone reconstruction	Ciocca L. et al., 2017
15	cartilage tissues	extrusion based 3D printing	atelocollagen, hyaluronic acid and polycaprolactone	human mesenchymal stromal	Rabbit	8 weeks	regeneration	Shim JH. et al., 2016
16	articular cartilage bone	preconstructed bench-based bioprinter	gelatin-metacryloyl and methacrylated hyaluronic acid	sheep derived mesenchymal stem cell	Sheep	8 weeks	regeneration	Shim J.H. et al., 2016
17	Spinal cord	Ready to use	collagen and silk fibroin	(human umbilical mesenchymal stem cells	rat	8 weeks	repair	Di Bella C. et al., 2018
18	Neurons	Ready to use	hydroxypropyl chitosan, thiolated hyaluronic acid, vinyl sulfonated hyaluronic acid and Matrigel	neural stem cell	rat	12 weeks	neural tissue engineering model	Chen C. et al., 2022
19	spinal cord	extrusion based bioprinter	collagen and silk fibroin	neural stem cell	rat	8 weeks	Repair and reconstruction	Liu X. et al., 2021
20	spinal cord	Ready to use	collagen/silk fibroin	neural stem cell	rat	8 weeks	repair and reconstruction	Li X.H. et al., 2021

Contd.

Table 3 *Contd.*

S. No.	Tissue/organ focused	Method of 3D bioprinting	Biomaterials used	Cells used	Animal model used	Study duration	Application	Reference
21	spinal cord	extrusion based bioprinter	methacrylated gelatin and poly(ethylene glycol) diacrylate	neural stem cell	rat	24 weeks	reconstruction	Jiang J.P. et al., 2020
22	spinal cord	extrusion based bioprinter	collagen and chitosan	–	rat	8 weeks	Repair and reconstruction	Koffler J. et al., 2019
23	kidney	extrusion based bioprinter	Matrigel- or GelTrex-	induced pluripotent stem cells	–	–	renal replacement therapy	Sun Y. et al., 2019
24	kidney	extrusion based bioprinter	sodium alginate and decellularized kidney ECM	human umbilical vein endothelial cells and human renal proximal tubule epithelial cells	mice	4 weeks	renal subcapsular transplantation	Lawlor K.T. et al., 2021
25	bone	Ready to use	polycaprolactone–tricalcium phosphate along with platelet-rich plasm	–	rat	12 weeks	repairing orthotopic defects	Singh N.K. et al., 2019
26	bone	fused deposition modelling bioprinter	polycaprolactone-20% tricalcium phosphate	–	rabbit	12 weeks	replacement	Rai B. et al., 2007
27	bone	Ready to use	polycaprolactone–hyaluronic acid-tricalcium phosphate	one marrow-derived mesenchymal stromal cells and dental pulp-derived stromal cells custom-made from each pig	pig	5 weeks	regeneration	Yeo A. et al., 2010
28	bone	micro-extrusion bioprinting	pure calcium silicate and dilute Mg-dcped CSi	–	rabbit	12 weeks	osteoconduction and bone repair	Jensen J. et al., 2016
29	bone	micro-extrusion bioprinting	polycaprolactone and polycaprolactone/β-tricalcium phosphate	–	dog	8 weeks	regeneration	J.H. Shim. et al., 2017

Contd.

Table 3 *Contd.*

S. No.	Tissue/organ focused	Method of 3D bioprinting	Biomaterials used	Cells used	Animal model used	Study duration	Application	Reference
30	mandible	inkjet bioprinting	β-tricalcium phosphate and polycaprolactone	porcine bone marrow progenitor cells	pig	8 weeks	treatment of mandibular defects	J.H. Shim et al., 2017
31	articular cartilage	extrusion based bioprinter	polycaprolactone and alginate	ATDC 5 chondrogenic cell	mouse	3 weeks	regeneration	Konopnicki S. et al., 2015
32	articular cartilage	Ready to use	poly (ethylene glycol) methyl ether methacrylate	Bone marrow derived mesenchymal stem cells	mouse	3 weeks	repair	Olubamiji A.D. et al., 2016
33	Spinal cord	digital light processing	Gelatin–methacryloyl	human amniotic epithelial	rat	8 weeks	regenerative medicine	Gao G. et al., 2017
34	Spinal cord	micro-extrusion based bioprinter	gelatin	neural stem cell and oligodendrocytes	rat	8 weeks	repair	Qiu C. et al., 2022

Corporation (US), Medtronic (Ireland), NuVasive, Corporation (US), Stryker (US), Terumo Corporation (Japan), W.L. Gore & Associates Corporation(US), Zimmer Biomet (US), Smith & Nephew plc (UK), MIMEDX Group, Corporation(US), BioTissue (US), CollPlant Biotechnologies Limited (Israel), Sumitomo Pharma Company, Limited (Japan), Matricel GmbH (Germany), Mallinckrodt (US), Regrow Biosciences private limited (India), Vericel Corporation (US), Tecnoss S.R.L. (Italy), Tegoscience (South Korea), and Tissue Regenix (UK), Becton Dickinson and Company (US), ACell Corporation (US), Athersys Corporation (US), RTI Surgical Corporation (US) and ReproCell Corporation (Japan) (https://www.who.int/news-room/fact-sheets/detail/spinal-cord-injury). There has been increasing collaborations seen in the recent times between the leading biopharmaceutical companies and industries working in the field of tissue engineering. For example, Sartorius (Biopharma, Laboratory, Applied & Life Sciences), Germany has collaborated with BICO formerly known as Cellink-a Swedish bioconvergence-startup- and has made an acquisition worth approximately 49.91 million in 2023. Looking ahead, the successful application of major tissue engineered products have been observed in orthopaedics, particularly in muscle and spine segments. In 2022, this segment accounted for 59.75% of the tissueengineering market's revenue, which is more than half of the total share. According to the WHO, millions of individuals are affected by rheumatoid arthritis with a global incidence rate of 460 per 1000,000 people suffering due to the lack of adequate medication. Tissue engineering, with its multifaceted use of elements including stem cells and other bioactive compounds, has the potential to create solutions to effectively treat rheumatoid arthritis (Tissue Engineering Market Size, Share and Forecast 2024-2032 [imarcgroup. com]).

Conclusion

The field of tissue engineering and 3D bioprinting offers transformative solutions to the multiple challenges in healthcare and research. It can help in fabrication of complex tissue constructs and also patient specific disease models to understand the human body and simultaneously improve the possible outcomes. Throughout this chapter we have discussed the principles, categories and applications of advanced technologies along with the various commercially available tissue engineered constructs. Looking ahead, the future of tissue engineering and bioprinting holds immense potential to address the unmet healthcare needs like organ transplantation and also escort the era of personalized medicine. Innovation, collaboration and making patient specific needs as the center of attention, we can fully unleash the great realm of possibilities this field holds.

Acknowledgements

The authors wish to acknowledge Manipal Centre for Biotherapeutics Research, MAHE for infrastructural support

References

Adamzyk C., Kachel P., Hoss M., Gremse F., Modabber A. et al. Bone tissue engineering using polyetherketoneketone scaffolds combined with autologous mesenchymal stem cells in a sheep calvarial defect model. Journal of Cranio-Maxillofacial Surgery. 2016 Aug 1; 44(8): 985–94. https://doi.org/10.1016/j.jcms.2016.04.012.

Afsharian Y.P., Rahimnejad M. Bioactive electrospun scaffolds for wound healing applications: A comprehensive review. Polymer Testing. 2021 Jan 1; 93: 106952. https://doi.org/10.1016/j.polymertesting.2020.106952.

Agarwal P., Arora G., Panwar A., Mathur V., Srinivasan V. et al. Diverse Applications of Three-Dimensional Printing in Biomedical Engineering: A Review. 3D Printing and Additive Manufacturing. 2023 Oct 1; 10(5): 1140–63. https://doi.org/10.1089/3dp.2022.0281.

Ahn G., Min K.H., Kim C., Lee J.S., Kang D. et al. Precise stacking of decellularized extracellular matrix based 3D cell-laden constructs by a 3D cell printing system equipped with heating modules. Scientific reports. 2017 Aug 17; 7(1): 1–1. http://doi.org/10.1038/s41598-017-09201-5.

Akhtar M.F., Hanif M., Ranjha N.M. Methods of synthesis of hydrogels… A review. Saudi Pharmaceutical Journal. 2016 Sep 1; 24(5): 554–9. https://doi.org/10.1016/j.jsps.2015.03.022.

Alizadeh A., Dyck S.M., Karimi-Abdolrezaee S.. Traumatic spinal cord injury: an overview of pathophysiology, models and acute injury mechanisms. Frontiers in neurology. 2019 Mar 22; 10: 441408. https://doi.org/10.3389/fneur.2019.00282.

Amir-Aslani A., Mangematin V. The future of drug discovery and development: shifting emphasis towards personalized medicine. Technological Forecasting and Social Change. 2010 Feb 1; 77(2): 203–17.

Amler A.K., Thomas A., Tüzüner S., Lam T., Geiger M.A. et al. 3D bioprinting of tissue-specific osteoblasts and endothelial cells to model the human jawbone. Scientific Reports. 2021 Mar 1; 11(1): 4876. https://doi.org/10.1038/ s41598-021-84483-4.

Aram E., Mehdipour-Ataei S. A review on the micro-and nanoporous polymeric foams: Preparation and properties. International journal of polymeric materials and polymeric biomaterials. 2016 May 2; 65(7): 358–75. https://doi.org/10.1080/00914037.2015.1129948.

Aranaz I., Gutiérrez M.C., Ferrer M.L., Del Monte F. Preparation of chitosan nanocompositeswith a macroporous structure by unidirectional freezing and subsequent freeze-drying. Marine Drugs. 2014 Nov 24; 12(11): 5619–42. https://doi.org/10.3390/md12115619.

Atala A., Bauer S.B., Soker S., Yoo J.J., Retik A.B. et al. Tissue-engineered autologous bladders for patients needing cystoplasty. The lancet. 2006 Apr 15; 367(9518): 1241–6. https://doi.org/10.1016/S0140-6736(06)68438-9.

Azuma M., Yanagawa T., Ishibashi–Kanno N., Uchida F., Ito T. et al. Mandibular reconstruction using plates prebent to fit rapid prototyping 3-dimensional printing models ameliorates contour deformity. Head & face medicine. 2014 Dec; 10(1): 1–8.

Babu P.J., Doble M., Raichur A.M. Silver oxide nanoparticles embedded silk fibroin spuns: Microwave mediated preparation, characterization and their synergistic wound healing and anti-bacterial activity. Journal of colloid and interface science. 2018 Mar 1; 513: 62–71. https://doi.org/10.1016/j.jcis.2017.11.001.

Bajaj P., Schweller R.M., Khademhosseini A., West J.L., Bashir R. 3D biofabrication strategies for tissue engineering and regenerative medicine. Annual review of biomedical engineering. 2014 Jul 11; 16: 247–76.A. https://doi.org/10.1146/annurev-bioeng-071813-105155.

Behre A., Tashman J.W., Dikyol C., Shiwarski D.J., Crum R.J. et al. 3D Bioprinted Patient-Specific Extracellular Matrix Scaffolds for Soft Tissue Defects. Advanced Healthcare Materials. 2022 Dec; 11(24): 2200866. https://doi.org/10.1002/adhm.202200866

Bell E., Ehrlich H.P., Buttle D.J., Nakatsuji T. Living tissue formed in vitro and accepted as skin-equivalent tissue of full thickness. Science. 1981 Mar 6; 211(4486): 1052–4. https://doi.org/10.1126/science.7008197.

Benwood C., Chrenek J., Kirsch R.L., Masri N.Z., Richards H. et al. Natural biomaterials and their use as bioinks for printing tissues. Bioengineering. 2021 Feb 20; 8(2): 27. https://doi.org/10.3390/bioengineering8020027.

Berg J., Weber Z., Fechler-Bitteti M., Hocke A.C., Hippenstiel S. et al. Bioprinted multi-cell type lung model for the study of viral inhibitors. Viruses. 2021 Aug 11; 13(8): 1590. https://doi.org/10.3390/v13081590.

Berthiaume F., Maguire T.J., Yarmush M.L. Tissue engineering and regenerative medicine: history, progress, and challenges. Annual review of chemical and biomolecular engineering. 2011 Jul 15; 2: 403–30. https://doi.org/10.1146/annurev-chembioeng-061010-114257.

Bhise N.S., Manoharan V., Massa S., Tamayol A., Ghaderi M. et al. A liver-on-a-chip platform with bioprinted hepatic spheroids. Biofabrication. 2016 Jan 12; 8(1): 014101. 10.1088/1758-5090/8/1/014101.

Billingham R.E., Medawar P.B. The freezing, drying and storage of mammalian skin. Journal of Experimental Biology. 1952 Sep 1; 29(3): 454–68. https://doi.org/10.1242/jeb.29.3.454.

Bioprinting | ROKIT Healthcare, INC., (n.d.). https://rokithealthcare.com/tag/bio printing/(Accessed 5 October 2021).

Bishop E.S., Mostafa S., Pakvasa M., Luu H.H., Lee M.J. et al. 3-D bioprinting technologies in tissue engineering and regenerative medicine: Current and future trends. Genes & diseases. 2017 Dec 1; 4(4): 185–95. http://doi.org/10.1016/j.gendis.2017.10.002.

Blehm B.H., Jiang N., Kotobuki Y., Tanner K. Deconstructing the role of the ECM microenvironment on drug efficacy targeting MAPK signaling in a pre-clinical platform for cutaneous melanoma. Biomaterials. 2015 Jul 1; 56: 129–39. https://doi.org/10.1016/j.biomaterials.2015.03.041.

Bliley J.M., Shiwarski D.J., Feinberg A.W. 3D-bioprinted human tissue and the path toward clinical translation. Science Translational Medicine. 2022 Oct 12; 14(666): eabo7047. https://doi.org/10.1126/scitranslmed.abo7047.

Bohandy J., Kim B.F., Adrian F.J. Metal deposition from a supported metal film using an excimer laser. Journal of Applied Physics. 1986 Aug 15; 60(4): 1538–9. http://doi.org/10.1063/1.337789.

Brie J., Chartier T., Chaput C., Delage C., Pradeau B. et al. A new custom made bioceramic implant for the repair of large and complex craniofacial bone defects. Journal of Cranio-Maxillofacial Surgery. 2013 Jul 1; 41(5): 403–7.

Brooks-Richards T.L., Paxton N.C., Allenby M.C., Woodruff M.A. Dissolvable 3D printed PVA moulds for melt electrowriting tubular scaffolds with patient-specific geometry. Materials & Design. 2022 Mar 1; 215: 110466. https://doi.org/10.1016/j.matdes.2022.110466.

Cacciotti I. Multisubstituted hydroxyapatite powders and coatings: The influence of the codoping on the hydroxyapatite performances. International Journal of Applied Ceramic Technology. 2019 Sep; 16(5): 1864–84. https://doi.org/10.1111/ijac.13229.

Cao Y., Sun H., Zhu H., Zhu X., Tang X. et al. Allogeneic cell therapy using umbilical cord MSCs on collagen scaffolds for patients with recurrent uterine adhesion: a phase I clinical trial. Stem cell research & therapy. 2018 Dec; 9(1): 1–0.

Characterization of cornea-specific bioink: high transparency, improved in vivo safety. Journal of tissue engineering. 2019 Jan; 10: 2041731418823382. http://doi.org/10.1177/2041731418823382.

Chen C., Xu H.H., Liu X.Y., Zhang Y.S., Zhong L. et al. 3D printed collagen/silk fibroin scaffolds carrying the secretome of human umbilical mesenchymal stem cells ameliorated neurological dysfunction after spinal cord injury in rats. Regenerative Biomaterials. 2022; 9: rbac014. https://doi.org/10.1093/rb/rbac014.

Choi W.S., Kim J.H., Ahn C.B., Lee J.H., Kim Y.J. et al. Development of a Multi-Layer Skin Substitute Using Human Hair Keratinic Extract-Based Hybrid 3D Printing. Polymers. 2021 Aug 4; 13(16): 2584. https://doi.org/10.3390/polym13162584.

Chua C.K., Leong K.F. 3D Printing and additive manufacturing: Principles and applications (with companion media pack)-of rapid prototyping. World Scientific Publishing Company; 2014 Aug 6.

Chuah J.K., Zink D. Stem cell-derived kidney cells and organoids: Recent breakthroughs and emerging applications. Biotechnology advances. 2017 Mar 1; 35(2): 150-67. https://doi.org/10.1016/j.biotechadv.2016.12.001.

Chung J.H., Naficy S., Yue Z., Kapsa R., Quigley A. et al. Bio-ink properties and printability for extrusion printing living cells. Biomaterials Science. 2013; 1(7): 763–73. DOI: https://doi.org/10.1039/C3BM00012E.

Ciocca L., Lesci I.G., Mezini O., Parrilli A., Ragazzini S. et al. Customized hybrid biomimetic hydroxyapatite scaffold for bone tissue regeneration. Journal of Biomedical Materials Research Part B: Applied Biomaterials. 2017 May; 105(4): 723–34. https://doi.org/10.1002/jbm.b.33597.

Conoscenti G., Schneider T., Stoelzel K., Pavia F.C., Brucato V. et al. PLLA scaffolds produced by thermally induced phase separation (TIPS) allow human chondrocyte growth and extracellular matrix formation dependent on pore size. Materials science and engineering: C. 2017 Nov 1; 80: 449–59. https://doi.org/10.1016/j.msec.2017.06.011.

Costantini M., Barbetta A., Swieszkowski W., Seliktar D., Gargioli C. et al. Photocurable biopolymers for coaxial bioprinting. Computer-Aided Tissue Engineering: Methods and Protocols. 2021: 45–54. https://doi.org/10.1007/978-1-0716-0611-7_4.

Cui X., Dean D., Ruggeri Z.M., Boland T. Cell damage evaluation of thermal inkjet printed Chinese hamster ovary cells. Biotechnology and bioengineering. 2010 Aug 15; 106(6):963-9. https://doi.org/10.1002/bit.22762.

Dababneh A.B., Ozbolat I.T. Bioprinting technology: a current state-of-the-art review. Journal of Manufacturing Science and Engineering. 2014 Dec 1; 136(6): 061016. http://doi.org/10.1115/1.4028515.

Daly A.C., Davidson M.D., Burdick J.A. 3D bioprinting of high cell-density heterogeneous tissue models through spheroid fusion within self-healing hydrogels. Nature communications. 2021 Feb 2; 12(1): 753. https://doi.org/10.1038/s41467-021-21029-2.

Das S., Pati F., Choi Y.J., Rijal G., Shim J.H. et al. Bioprintable, cell-laden silk fibroin gelatin hydrogel supporting multilineage differentiation of stem cells for fabrication of three-dimensional tissue constructs. Acta biomaterialia. 2015 Jan 1; 11: 233–46. https://doi.org/10.1016/j.actbio.2014.09.023.

Dey M., Ozbolat I.T. 3D bioprinting of cells, tissues and organs. Scientific reports. 2020 Aug 18; 10(1): 14023. https://doi.org/10.1038/s41598-020-70086-y.

Di Bella C., Duchi S., O'Connell C.D., Blanchard R., Augustine C. et al. In situ handheld three-dimensional bioprinting for cartilage regeneration. Journal of tissue engineering and regenerative medicine. 2018 Mar; 12(3): 611–21. https://doi.org/10.1002/term.2476.

Di Gravina G.M., Bari E., Croce S., Scocozza F., Pisani S. et al. Design and development of a hepatic lyo-dECM powder as a biomimetic component for 3D-printable hybrid hydrogels. Biomedical Materials. 2023 Dec 4; 19(1): 015005. https://doi.org/10.1088/1748-605X/ad0ee2.

Diomede, F., Gugliandolo, A., Cardelli, P. Three-dimensional printed PLA scaffold and human gingival stem cell-derived extracellular vesicles: a new tool for bone defect repair. *Stem Cell Res Ther* 9, 104 (2018). https://doi.org/10.1186/s13287-018-0850-0.

Do A.V., Akkouch A., Green B., Ozbolat I., Debabneh A. et al. Controlled and sequential delivery of fluorophores from 3D printed alginate-PLGA tubes. Annals of biomedical engineering. 2017 Jan; 45(1): 297–305. doi: 10.1007/s10439-016-1648-9.

Doyle K. Bioprinting: from patches to parts. Genetic Engineering & Biotechnology News. 2014 May 15; 34(10): 1–34. http://doi.org/10.1089/gen.34.10.01.

Dutta S., Cohn D. Temperature and pH responsive 3D printed scaffolds. Journal of Materials Chemistry B. 2017; 5(48): 9514–21. https://doi.org/10.1039/C7TB02368E.

Eltom A., Zhong G., Muhammad A. Scaffold techniques and designs in tissue engineering functions and purposes: a review. Advances in materials science and engineering. 2019 Mar 7; 2019. https://doi.org/10.1155/2019/3429527.

Fahmy M.D., Jazayeri H.E., Razavi M., Masri R., Tayebi L. et al. Three-dimensional bioprinting materials with potential application in preprosthetic surgery. Journal of Prosthodontics. 2016 Jun; 25(4): 310–8. https://doi.org/10.1111/jopr.12431.

Faulkner-Jones A., Zamora V., Hortigon-Vinagre M.P., Wang W., Ardron M. et al., Smith G.L., Shu W. A bioprinted heart-on-a-chip with human pluripotent stem cell-derived cardiomyocytes for drug evaluation. Bioengineering. 2022 Jan 13; 9(1): 32. https://doi.org/10.3390/bioengineering9010032.

Fedorovich N.E., Wijnberg H.M., Dhert W.J., Alblas J. Distinct tissue formation by heterogeneous printing of osteo- and endothelial progenitor cells. Tissue Engineering Part A. 2011 Aug 1; 17(15-16): 2113–21. http://doi.org/10.1089/ten.TEA.2010.0623.

Fransen M.F., Addario G., Bouten C.V., Halary F., Moroni L. et al. Bioprinting of kidney in vitro models: cells, biomaterials, and manufacturing techniques. Essays in biochemistry. 2021 Aug; 65(3): 587–602. https://doi.org/10.1042/EBC20200158.

Fratzl P. Collagen: structure and mechanics, an introduction. InCollagen 2008 (pp. 1-13). Springer, Boston, MA.

Gaharwar A.K., Arpanaei A., Andresen T.L., Dolatshahi-Pirouz A. 3D biomaterial microarrays for regenerative medicine: current state- of- the- art, emerging directions and future trends. Advanced Materials. 2016 Jan; 28(4): 771–81. https://doi.org/10.1002/adma.201503918.

Gaharwar A.K., Singh I., Khademhosseini A. Engineered biomaterials for in situ tissue regeneration. Nature Reviews Materials. 2020 Sep; 5(9): 686–705. https://doi.org/10.1038/s41578-020-0209-x.

Gao G., Lee J.H., Jang J., Lee D.H., Kong J.S. et al. Tissue engineered bio-blood-vessels constructed using a tissue-specific bioink and 3D coaxial cell printing technique: a novel therapy for ischemic disease. Advanced functional materials. 2017 Sep; 27(33): 1700798. https://doi.org/10.1002/adfm.201700798.

Gao G., Zhang X.F., Hubbell K., Cui X. NR2F2 regulates chondrogenesis of human mesenchymal stem cells in bioprinted cartilage. Biotechnology and Bioengineering. 2017 Jan; 114(1): 208–16. https://doi.org/10.1002/bit.26042.

Gasperini L., Mano J.F., Reis R.L. Natural polymers for the microencapsulation of cells. Journal of the royal society Interface. 2014 Nov 6; 11(100): 20140817. http://doi.org/10.1098/rsif.2014.0817.

GhavamiNejad A., Ashammakhi N., Wu X.Y., Khademhosseini A. Crosslinking strategies for 3D bioprinting of polymeric hydrogels. Small. 2020 Sep; 16(35): 2002931. https://doi.org/10.1002/smll.202002931.

Global Tissue Engineering Market by Product (Scaffolds (Collagen, Stem Cell), Tissue Grafts [Allograft, Autograft, Xenograft]), Material (Biological, Synthetic), Application (Orthopedics, Dermatology, Wound Care, Cardiovascular) - Forecast to 2028 (researchandmarkets.com) ID: 5917837.

Goh B.T., Chanchareonsook N., Tideman H., Teoh S.H., Chow J.K. et al. The use of a polycaprolactone–tricalcium phosphate scaffold for bone regeneration of tooth socket facial wall defects and simultaneous immediate dental implant placement in Macaca fascicularis. Journal of Biomedical Materials Research Part A. 2014 May; 102(5): 1379–88. https://doi.org/10.1002/jbm.a.34817.

Goh B.T., Teh L.Y., Tan D.B., Zhang Z., Teoh S.H. et al. Novel 3 D polycaprolactone scaffold for ridge preservation–a pilot randomised controlled clinical trial. Clinical oral implants research. 2015 Mar; 26(3): 271–7.

Gómez-Guillén M.C., Giménez B., López-Caballero M.A., Montero M.P. Functional and bioactive properties of collagen and gelatin from alternative sources: A review. Food hydrocolloids. 2011 Dec 1; 25(8): 1813–27. https://doi.org/10.1016/j.foodhyd.2011.02.007.

Gorshkov K., Chen C.Z., Marshall R.E., Mihatov N., Choi Y. et al. Advancing precision medicine with personalized drug screening. Drug discovery today. 2019 Jan 1; 24(1): 272–8. https://doi.org/10.1016/j.drudis.2018.08.010.

Graham P.D., Pervan A.J., McHugh A.J. The dynamics of thermal-induced phase separation in PMMA solutions. Macromolecules. 1997 Mar 24; 30(6): 1651–5. https://doi.org/10.1021/ma961720m.

Green H., Kehinde O., Thomas J. Growth of cultured human epidermal cells into multiple epithelia suitable for grafting. Proceedings of the National Academy of Sciences. 1979 Nov; 76(11): 5665–8. https://doi.org/10.1073/pnas.76.11.5665.

Groll J., Burdick J.A., Cho D.W., Derby B., Gelinsky M. et al. A definition of bioinks and their distinction from biomaterial inks. Biofabrication. 2018 Nov 23;11(1): 013001. http://doi.org/10.1088/1758-5090/aaf8a4.

Guillemot F., Mironov V., Nakamura M. Bioprinting is coming of age: report from the International Conference on Bioprinting and Biofabrication in Bordeaux (3B'09). Biofabrication. 2010 Mar 25; 2(1): 010201. https://doi.org/10.1088/1758-5082/2/1/010201.

Gulyas M., Csiszer M., Mehes E., Czirok A. Software tools for cell culture-related 3D printed structures. PLoS One. 2018 Sep 4; 13(9): e0203203. http://doi.org/10.1371/journal.pone.0203203.

Gurkan U.A., Sung Y., El Assal R., Xu F., Trachtenberg A. et al. Bioprinting anisotropic stem cell microenvironment. InJournal of Tissue Engineering and Regenerative Medicine 2012 Sep 1 (Vol. 6, pp. 366-366). 111 RIVER ST, HOBOKEN 07030-5774, NJ USA: WILEY-BLACKWELL. https://doi.org/10.1021/mp400573g.

Guvendiren M., Molde J., Soares R.M., Kohn J. Designing biomaterials for 3D printing. ACS biomaterials science & engineering. 2016 Oct 10; 2(10): 1679-93. https://doi.org/10.1021/acsbiomaterials.6b00121.

Haraguchi K., Takehisa T. Nanocomposite hydrogels: A unique organic-inorganic network structure with extraordinary mechanical, optical, and swelling/de-swelling properties. Advanced materials. 2002 Aug 16; 14(16): 1120-4. DOI:10.1002/1521-4095(20020816)14:163.0.CO;2-9.

Harris L.D., Kim B.S., Mooney D.J. Open pore biodegradable matrices formed with gas foaming. Journal of Biomedical Materials Research: An Official Journal of The Society for Biomaterials, The Japanese Society for Biomaterials, and the Australian Society for Biomaterials. 1998 Dec 5; 42(3): 396-402. https://doi.org/10.1002/(SICI)1097-4636(19981205)42:3%3C396::AID-JBM7%3E3.0.CO;2-E.

He Y., Wang F., Wang X., Zhang J., Wang D. et al. A photocurable hybrid chitosan/acrylamide bioink for DLP based 3D bioprinting. Materials & Design. 2021 Apr 1; 202: 109588. https://doi.org/10.1016/j.matdes.2021.109588

Herman A.R. The history of skin grafts. Journal of drugs in dermatology: JDD. 2002 Dec 1; 1(3): 298-301. PMID: 12851989.

Ho D., Quake S.R., McCabe E.R., Chng W.J., Chow E.K. et al. Enabling technologies for personalized and precision medicine. Trends in biotechnology. 2020 May 1; 38(5): 497-518. https://doi.org/10.1016/j.tibtech.2019.12.021.

Hollister S.J. Porous scaffold design for tissue engineering. Nature materials. 2005 Jul 1; 4(7): 518-24. https://doi.org/10.1038/nmat1421.

Horn T.J., Harrysson O.L. Overview of current additive manufacturing technologies and selected applications. Science progress. 2012 Sep; 95(3): 255-82. https://doi.org/10.3184/003685012X13420984463047.

Horvath A.L. Solubility of structurally complicated materials: 3. Hair. TheScientificWorldJOURNAL. 2009 Jan 1; 9: 255-71. https://doi.org/10.1100/tsw.2009.27.

Howard D., Buttery L.D., Shakesheff K.M., Roberts S.J. Tissue engineering: strategies, stem cells and scaffolds. Journal of anatomy. 2008 Jul; 213(1): 66-72. https://doi.org/10.1111/j.1469-7580.2008.00878.x

https://www.3dnatives.com/en/allevi-software-bioprinting-050920195.

https://www.cellink.com/software.

https://www.github.com/ultimaker/ curaengine.

https://www.regenhu.com/3d-bioprinters/ software.

https://www.simplify3d.com

https://www.ultimaker.com/software/ ultimaker-cura.

https://www.who.int/news-room/fact-sheets/detail/spinal-cord-injury.

Hull C.W., inventor; UVP Inc, assignee. Apparatus for production of three-dimensional objects by stereolithography. United States patent US 4,575,330.

Hutmacher D.W. Scaffolds in tissue engineering bone and cartilage. Biomaterials. 2000 Dec 15; 21(24): 2529-43. https://doi.org/10.1016/S0142-9612(00)00121-6.

Janani G., Priya S., Dey S., Mandal B.B. Mimicking native liver lobule microarchitecture in vitro with parenchymal and non-parenchymal cells using 3D bioprinting for drug toxicity and drug screening applications. ACS Applied Materials & Interfaces. 2022 Feb 16; 14(8): 10167-86. https://doi.org/10.1021/acsami.2c00312.

Jang J., Kim T.G., Kim B.S., Kim S.W., Kwon S.M. et al. Tailoring mechanical properties of decellularized extracellular matrix bioink by vitamin B2-induced photo-crosslinking. Acta biomaterialia. 2016 Mar 15; 33: 88-95. doi: 10.1016/j.actbio.2016.01.013.

Jang J., Park H.J., Kim S.W., Kim H., Park J.Y. et al. 3D printed complex tissue construct using stem cell-laden decellularized extracellular matrix bioinks for cardiac repair. Biomaterials. 2017 Jan 1; 112: 264-74. http://doi.org/10.1016/j.biomaterials.2016.10.026.

Jang J., Yi H.G, Cho D.W. 3D printed tissue models: present and future. ACS biomaterials science & engineering. 2016 Oct 10; 2(10): 1722-31. https://doi.org/10.1021/acsbiomaterials.6b00129.

Januariyasa I.K., Yusuf Y. Porous carbonated hydroxyapatite-based scaffold using simple gas foaming method. Journal of Asian Ceramic Societies. 2020 Jul 2; 8(3): 634-41. https://doi.org/10.1080/21870764.2020.1770 938.

Jensen J., Tvedesøe C., Rölfing J.H., Foldager C.B., Lysdahl H. et al. Dental pulp-derived stromal cells exhibit a higher osteogenic potency than bone marrow-derived stromal cells in vitro and in a porcine critical-size bone defect model. Sicot-j. 2016; 2. https://doi.org/10.1051%2Fsicotj%2F2016004.

Ji S., Guvendiren M. Recent advances in bioink design for 3D bioprinting of tissues and organs. Frontiers in bioengineering and biotechnology. 2017 Apr 5; 5: 23. https://doi.org/10.3389/fbioe.2017.00023.

Jiang J.P., Liu X.Y., Zhao F., Zhu X., Li X.Y. et al. 3-D bioprinting collagen/fibroin scaffold combined with neural stem cells promotes nerve regeneration after spinal cord injury. Chinese Neural Regeneration Research. 2020 May 15; 15(5): 959. https://doi.org/10.4103/1673-5374.268974.

Jing X., Mi H.Y., Salick M.R., Peng X.F., Turng L.S. et al. Preparation of thermoplastic polyurethane/graphene oxide composite scaffolds by thermally induced phase separation. Polymer composites. 2014 Jul; 35(7): 1408–17. https://doi.org/10.1002/pc.22793.

Joas S., Tovar G.E., Celik O., Bonten C., Southan A. et al. Extrusion-based 3D printing of poly (ethylene glycol) diacrylate hydrogels containing positively and negatively charged groups. Gels. 2018 Aug 14; 4(3): 69. https://doi.org/10.3390/gels4030069.

Kasturi M., Mathur V., Gadre M., Srinivasan V., Vasanthan K.S. et al. Three Dimensional Bioprinting for Hepatic Tissue Engineering: From In Vitro Models to Clinical Applications. Tissue Engineering and Regenerative Medicine. 2024 Jan; 21(1): 21–52. https://doi.org/10.1007/s13770-023-00576-3.

Kawecki F., Clafshenkel W.P., Auger F.A., Bourget J.M., Fradette J. et al. Self-assembled human osseous cell sheets as living biopapers for the laser-assisted bioprinting of human endothelial cells. Biofabrication. 2018 Apr 30; 10(3): 035006. http://doi.org/10.1088/1758-5090/aab78b.

Kesti M., Fisch P., Pensalfini M., Mazza E., Zenobi-Wong M. et al. Guidelines for standardization of bioprinting: a systematic study of process parameters and their effect on bioprinted structures. BioNanoMaterials. 2016 Sep 1; 17(3-4): 193–204. https://doi.org/10.1515/bnm-2016-0004.

Khan R., Khan M.H. Use of collagen as a biomaterial: An update. Journal of Indian Society of Periodontology. 2013 Jul 1; 17(4): 539–42. https://doi.org/10.4103/0972-124X.118333.

Khoeini R., Nosrati H., Akbarzadeh A., Eftekhari A., Kavetskyy T. et al. Natural and synthetic bioinks for 3D bioprinting. Advanced NanoBiomed Research. 2021 Aug; 1(8): 2000097. https://doi.org/10.1002/anbr.202000097.

Khojasteh A., Behnia H., Hosseini F.S., Dehghan M.M., Abbasnia P. et al. The effect of PCL-TCP scaffold loaded with mesenchymal stem cells on vertical bone augmentation in dog mandible: a preliminary report. Journal of Biomedical Materials Research Part B: Applied Biomaterials. 2013 Jul; 101(5): 848–54. https://doi.org/10.1002/jbm.b.32889.

Kim H, Park MN, Kim J, Jang J, Kim HK, Cho DW. Characterization of cornea-specific bioink: high transparency, improved in vivo safety. Journal of tissue engineering. 2019 Jan;10:2041731418823382. http://doi.org/10.1177/2041731418823382

Kim J.B. Three-dimensional tissue culture models in cancer biology. In Seminars in cancer biology 2005 Oct 1 (Vol. 15, No. 5, pp. 365–377). Academic Press.

Kim K.O., Lee Y., Hwang J.W., Kim H., Kim S.M. et al. Wound healing properties of a 3-D scaffold comprising soluble silkworm gland hydrolysate and human collagen. Colloids and Surfaces B: Biointerfaces. 2014 Apr 1; 116: 318–26. https://doi.org/10.1016/j.colsurfb.2013.12.004.

Kim S.Y., Han G., Hwang D.B., Won D.H., Shin Y.S. et al. Design and Usability Evaluations of a 3D-Printed Implantable Drug Delivery Device for Acute Liver Failure in Preclinical Settings. Advanced Healthcare Materials. 2021 Jul; 10(14): 2100497. https://doi.org/10.1002/adhm.202100497.

Kim W., Kim G.H. An intestinal model with a finger-like villus structure fabricated using a bioprinting process and collagen/SIS-based cell-laden bioink. Theranostics. 2020; 10(6): 2495. https://doi.org/10.7150/thno.41225.

Klimek K., Ginalska G. Proteins and peptides as important modifiers of the polymer scaffolds for tissue engineering applications—a review. Polymers. 2020 Apr 6; 12(4): 844. https://doi.org/10.3390/polym12040844.

Koch L., Kuhn S., Sorg H., Gruene M., Schlie S. et al. Laser printing of skin cells and human stem cells. Tissue Engineering Part C: Methods. 2010 Oct 1; 16(5): 847–54. http://doi.org/10.1089/ten.tec.2009.0624.

Koffler J., Zhu W., Qu X., Platoshyn O., Dulin J.N. et al. Biomimetic 3D-printed scaffolds for spinal cord injury repair. Nature medicine. 2019 Feb; 25(2): 263–9. https://doi.org/10.1038/s41591-018-0296-z.

Konopnicki S., Sharaf B., Resnick C., Patenaude A., Pogal-Sussman T. et al. Tissue-engineered bone with 3-dimensionally printed β-tricalcium phosphate and polycaprolactone scaffolds and early implantation: an in vivo pilot study in a porcine mandible model. Journal of Oral and Maxillofacial Surgery. 2015 May 1; 73(5): 1016-e1. https://doi.org/10.1016/j.joms.2015.01.021.

Kordjamshidi A., Saber-Samandari S., Nejad M.G., Khandan A. Preparation of novel porous calcium silicate scaffold loaded by celecoxib drug using freeze drying technique: Fabrication, characterization and simulation. Ceramics International. 2019 Aug 1; 45(11): 14126–35. https://doi.org/10.1016/j.ceramint.2019.04.113.

Kruth J.P. Material incress manufacturing by rapid prototyping techniques. CIRP annals. 1991 Jan 1; 40(2): 603–14. https://doi.org/10.1016/S0007-8506(07)61136-6.

Kundu J., Shim J.H., Jang J., Kim S.W., Cho D.W. et al. An additive manufacturing-based PCL–alginate–chondrocyte bioprinted scaffold for cartilage tissue engineering. Journal of tissue engineering and regenerative medicine. 2015 Nov; 9(11): 1286–97. https://doi.org/10.1002/term.1682.

Kutlehria S., Dinh T.C., Bagde A., Patel N., Gebeyehu A. et al. High-throughput 3D bioprinting of corneal stromal equivalents. Journal of Biomedical Materials Research Part B: Applied Biomaterials. 2020 Oct; 108(7): 2981–94. https://doi.org/10.1002/jbm.b.34628.

Lam E.H., Yu F., Zhu S., Wang Z. 3D Bioprinting for Next-Generation Personalized Medicine. International Journal of Molecular Sciences. 2023 Mar 28; 24(7): 6357. https://doi.org/10.3390/ijms24076357.

Lam V.Y., Wakatsuki T. Hydrogel tissue construct-based high-content compound screening. Journal of biomolecular screening. 2011 Jan; 16(1): 120–8. https://doi.org/10.1177/1087057110388269.

Larush L., Kaner I., Fluksman A., Tamsut A., Pawar A.A. et al. 3D printing of responsive hydrogels for drug-delivery systems. Journal of 3D printing in medicine. 2017 Oct; 1(4): 219–29. https://doi.org/10.3390/gels9120960.

Lau C.S., Chua J., Prasadh S., Lim J., Saigo L. et al. Alveolar Ridge Augmentation with a Novel Combination of 3D-Printed Scaffolds and Adipose-Derived Mesenchymal Stem Cells—A Pilot Study in Pigs. Biomedicines 2023, 11, 2274. https://doi.org/10.3390/ biomedicines11082274.

Law N., Doney B., Glover H., Qin Y., Aman Z.M. et al. Characterisation of hyaluronic acid methylcellulose hydrogels for 3D bioprinting. Journal of the mechanical behavior of biomedical materials. 2018 Jan 1; 77: 389–99. https://doi.org/10.1016/j.jmbbm.2017.09.031.

Lawlor K.T., Vanslambrouck J.M., Higgins J.W., Chambon A., Bishard K. et al. Cellular extrusion bioprinting improves kidney organoid reproducibility and conformation. Nature materials. 2021 Feb; 20(2): 260–71. https://doi.org/ 10.1038/s41563-020-00853-9.

Lee V., Singh G., Trasatti J.P., Bjornsson C., Xu X., Tran TN et al. Design and fabrication of human skin by three-dimensional bioprinting. Tissue Engineering Part C: Methods. 2014 Jun 1; 20(6): 473–84. http://doi.org/10.1089/ten.TEC.2013.0335.

Lee W., Debasitis J.C., Lee V.K., Lee J.H., Fischer K. et al. Multi-layered culture of human skin fibroblasts and keratinocytes through three-dimensional freeform fabrication. Biomaterials. 2009 Mar 1; 30(8): 1587–95. http://doi.org/10.1016/j.biomaterials.2008.12.009.

Li C., Vepari C., Jin H.J., Kim H.J., Kaplan D.L. Electrospun silk-BMP-2 scaffolds for bone tissue engineering. Biomaterials. 2006 Jun 1; 27(16): 3115–24. https://doi.org/10.1016/j.biomaterials.2006.01.022.

Li J., Chen M., Fan X., Zhou H. Recent advances in bioprinting techniques: approaches, applications and future prospects. Journal of translational medicine. 2016 Dec; 14: 1–5. http://doi.org/10.1186/s12967-016-1046-6.

Li J., Chen M., Wei X., Hao Y., Wang J. et al. Evaluation of 3D-printed polycaprolactone scaffolds coated with freeze-dried platelet-rich plasma for bone regeneration. Materials. 2017 Jul 19; 10(7): 831. https://doi.org/10.3390/ ma10070831.

Li J., Wu C., Chu P.K., Gelinsky M. 3D printing of hydrogels: Rational design strategies and emerging biomedical applications. Materials Science and Engineering: R: Reports. 2020 Apr 1; 140:100543. https://doi.org/10.1016/j.mser.2020.100543.

Li J., Xu Q., Teng B., Yu C., Song L. et al. Investigation of angiogenesis in bioactive 3-dimensional poly (d, l-lactide-co-glycolide)/nano-hydroxyapatite scaffolds by in vivo multiphoton microscopy in murine calvarial critical bone defect. Acta biomaterialia. 2016 Sep 15; 42: 389–99. https://doi.org/10.1016/j.actbio.2016.06.024.

Li T., Ma H., Ma H. Mussel-inspired nanostructures potentiate the immunomodulatory properties and angiogenesis of mesenchymal stem cells. *ACS Appl Mater Interfaces*. 2019; 11(19): 17134–17146. https://doi.org/10.1021/ acsami.8b22017.

Li X., Kolltveit K.M., Tronstad L., Olsen I. Systemic diseases caused by oral infection. Clinical microbiology reviews. 2000 Oct 1, 13(4): 547–58. https://doi.org/10.1128/cmr.13.4.547.

Li X., Sun Q., Li Q., Kawazoe N., Chen G. Functional hydrogels with tunable structures and properties for tissue engineering applications. Frontiers in chemistry. 2018 Oct 22; 6: 499. https://doi.org/10.3389/ fchem.2018.00499.

Li X.H., Zhu X., Liu X.Y., Xu H.H., Jiang W. et al. The corticospinal tract structure of collagen/silk fibroin scaffold implants using 3D printing promotes functional recovery after complete spinal cord transection in rats. Journal of Materials Science: Materials in Medicine. 2021 Apr; 32: 1–3. https://doi.org/10.1007/s10856-021-06500-2.

Li Y., Nieuwenhuis L.M., Keating B.J., Festen E.A., de Meijer V.E. et al. The impact of donor and recipient genetic variation on outcomes after solid organ transplantation: a scoping review and future perspectives. Transplantation. 2022 Aug 1; 106(8): 1548–57. https://doi.org/10.1097/TP.0000000000004042.

Li Z., Xie M.B., Li Y., Ma Y., Li J.S. et al. Recent progress in tissue engineering and regenerative medicine. Journal of Biomaterials and Tissue Engineering. 2016 Oct 1; 6(10): 755–66. https://doi.org/10.1166/jbt.2016.1510.

Lim K.S., Galarraga J.H., Cui X., Lindberg G.C., Burdick J.A. et al. Fundamentals and applications of photo-crosslinking in bioprinting. Chemical reviews. 2020 Apr 17; 120(19): 10662–94. https://doi.org/10.1021/acs.chemrev.9b00812.

Lind J.U., Busbee T.A., Valentine A.D., Pasqualini F.S., Yuan H. et al., Instrumented cardiac microphysiological devices via multimaterial three-dimensional printing. Nature materials. 2017 Mar; 16(3): 303–8. https://doi.org/10.1038/nmat4782.

Liotta L.A., Kohn E.C. The microenvironment of the tumour–host interface. Nature. 2001 May 17; 411(6835): 375–9. https://doi.org/10.1038/35077241.

Liu S., Yang H., Chen D., Xie Y., Tai C. et al. Three-dimensional bioprinting sodium alginate/gelatin scaffold combined with neural stem cells and oligodendrocytes markedly promoting nerve regeneration after spinal cord injury. Regenerative Biomaterials. 2022; 9:rbac038. https://doi.org/10.1093/rb/rbac038.

Liu X., Hao M., Chen Z., Zhang T., Huang J. et al. 3D bioprinted neural tissue constructs for spinal cord injury repair. Biomaterials. 2021 May 1; 272: 120771. https://doi.org/10.1016/j.biomaterials.2021.120771.

Liu X., Song S., Chen Z., Gao C., Li Y. et al. Release of O-GlcNAc transferase inhibitor promotes neuronal differentiation of neural stem cells in 3D bioprinted supramolecular hydrogel scaffold for spinal cord injury repair. Acta biomaterialia. 2022 Oct 1; 151: 148–62. https://doi.org/10.1016/j.actbio.2022.08.031.

Lorber B., Hsiao W.K., Hutchings I.M., Martin K.R. Adult rat retinal ganglion cells and glia can be printed by piezoelectric inkjet printing. Biofabrication. 2013 Dec 17; 6(1): 015001. http://doi.org/10.1088/1758-5082/6/1/015001.

Ma W., Zhou Z., Ismail N., Tocci E., Figoli A. et al. Membrane formation by thermally induced phase separation: Materials, involved parameters, modeling, current efforts and future directions. Journal of Membrane Science. 2023 Mar 5; 669: 121303. https://doi.org/10.1016/j.memsci.2022.121303.

Ma X., Liu J., Zhu W., Tang M., Lawrence N. et al. 3D bioprinting of functional tissue models for personalized drug screening and in vitro disease modeling. Advanced drug delivery reviews. 2018 Jul 1; 132: 235–51. https://doi.org/10.1016/j.addr.2018.06.011.

Ma X., Qu X., Zhu W., Li Y.S., Yuan S. et al. Deterministically patterned biomimetic human iPSC-derived hepatic model via rapid 3D bioprinting. Proceedings of the National Academy of Sciences. 2016 Feb 23; 113(8): 2206–11. https://doi.org/10.1073/pnas.1524510113.

Madiedo-Podvrsan S., Belaïdi J.P., Desbouis S., Simonetti L., Ben-Khalifa Y. et al., Collin-Djangone C, Soeur J, Rielland M. Utilization of patterned bioprinting for heterogeneous and physiologically representative reconstructed epidermal skin models. Scientific Reports. 2021 Mar 18; 11(1): 6217.. https://doi.org/10.1038/s41598-021-85553-3.

Mak I.W., Evaniew N., Ghert M. Lost in translation: animal models and clinical trials in cancer treatment. American journal of translational research. 2014; 6(2): 114.

Malda J., Visser J., Melchels F.P., Jüngst T., Hennink W.E. et al. 25th anniversary article: engineering hydrogels for biofabrication. Advanced materials. 2013 Sep; 25(36): 5011–28. http://doi.org/10.1002/adma.201302042.

Manavitehrani I., Le T.Y., Daly S., Wang Y., Maitz P.K. et al., Formation of porous biodegradable scaffolds based on poly (propylene carbonate) using gas foaming technology. Materials Science and Engineering: C. 2019 Mar 1; 96: 824–30. https://doi.org/10.1016/j.msec.2018.11.088.

Marga F., Jakab K., Khatiwala C., Shepherd B., Dorfman S. et al. Toward engineering functional organ modules by additive manufacturing. Biofabrication. 2012 Mar 12; 4(2): 022001. http://doi.org/10.1088/1758-5082/4/2/022001.

Mathur S., Sutton J. Personalized medicine could transform healthcare. Biomedical reports. 2017 Jul 1; 7(1): 3–5. https://doi.org/10.3892/br.2017.922.

Mazzocchi A., Soker S., Skardal A. 3D bioprinting for high-throughput screening: Drug screening, disease modeling, and precision medicine applications. Applied Physics Reviews. 2019 Mar 1; 6(1). https://doi.org/10.1063/1.5056188.

Melchels F.P., Domingos M.A., Klein T.J., Malda J., Bartolo P.J. et al. Additive manufacturing of tissues and organs. Progress in polymer science. 2012 Aug 1; 37(8): 1079–104. https://doi.org/10.1016/j.progpolymsci.2011.11.007.

Mewhort H.E., Svystonyuk D.A., Turnbull J.D., Teng G., Belke D.D. et al. Bioactive extracellular matrix scaffold promotes adaptive cardiac remodeling and repair. Basic to Translational Science. 2017 Aug 1; 2(4): 450–64. http://doi.org/10.1016/j.jacbts.2017.05.005.

Mirzaei M., Okoro O.V., Nie L., Petri D.F., Shavandi A. et al. Protein-based 3D biofabrication of biomaterials. Bioengineering. 2021 Apr 16; 8(4): 48. https://doi.org/10.3390/bioengineering8040048.

Moreau J.L., Caccamese J.F., Coletti D.P., Sauk J.J., Fisher J.P. et al. Tissue engineering solutions for cleft palates. Journal of Oral and Maxillofacial Surgery. 2007 Dec 1; 65(12): 2503–11. https://doi.org/10.1016/j.joms.2007.06.648.

Mouser V.H., Abbadessa A., Levato R., Hennink W.E., Vermonden T. et al. Development of a thermosensitive HAMA-containing bio-ink for the fabrication of composite cartilage repair constructs. Biofabrication. 2017 Mar 23; 9(1): 015026. https://doi.org/10.1088/1758-5090/aa6265.

Murphy S.V., Atala A. 3D bioprinting of tissues and organs. Nature biotechnology. 2014 Aug; 32(8): 773-85. https://doi.org/10.1038/nbt.2958.

Nakamura M., Iwanaga S., Henmi C., Arai K., Nishiyama Y. et al. Biomatrices and biomaterials for future developments of bioprinting and biofabrication. Biofabrication. 2010 Mar 10; 2(1): 014110. https://doi.org/10.1088/1758-5082/2/1/014110.

Nam Y.S., Park T.G. Porous biodegradable polymeric scaffolds prepared by thermally induced phase separation. Journal of Biomedical Materials Research: An Official Journal of The Society for Biomaterials, The Japanese Society for Biomaterials, and The Australian Society for Biomaterials and the Korean Society for Biomaterials. 1999 Oct; 47(1): 8–17. https://doi.org/10.1002/(SICI)1097-4636(199910)47:1%3C8::AID-JBM2%3E3.0.CO;2-L.

Nam Y.S., Yoon J.J., Park T.G. A novel fabrication method of macroporous biodegradable polymer scaffolds using gas foaming salt as a porogen additive. Journal of Biomedical Materials Research: An Official Journal of The Society for Biomaterials, The Japanese Society for Biomaterials, and The Australian Society for Biomaterials and the Korean Society for Biomaterials. 2000; 53(1): 1–7. https://doi.org/10.1002/(SICI)1097-4636(2000)53:1%3C1::AID-JBM1%3E3.0.CO;2-R.

Nee A.Y. Handbook of manufacturing engineering and technology. Springer Publishing Company, Incorporated; 2014 Oct 15. https://doi.org/10.1007/978-1-4471-4976-7_23-5.

Nelson W.G., Sun T.T. The 50-and 58-kdalton keratin classes as molecular markers for stratified squamous epithelia: cell culture studies. The Journal of cell biology. 1983 Jul; 97(1): 244–51. https://doi.org/10.1083/jcb.97.1.244

Nguyen, D.G., 2016. Bioprinted 3D primary liver tissues allow assessment of organ-level response to clinical drug induced toxicity in vitro. PLoS One 11 (7), e0158674. https://doi.org/10.1371/journal.pone.0158674.

Nyberg E.L., Farris A.L., Hung B.P., Dias M., Garcia J.R. et al. 3D-printing technologies for craniofacial rehabilitation, reconstruction, and regeneration. Annals of biomedical engineering. 2017 Jan; 45: 45–57. https://doi.org/10.1007/s10439-016-1668-5.

O'Connell C., Ren J., Pope L., Li Y., Mohandas A. et al. Characterizing bioinks for extrusion bioprinting: printability and rheology. 3D Bioprinting: Principles and Protocols. 2020: 111–33. http://doi.org/10.1007/978-1-0716-0837-5_7.

Oh S.H., Kang S.G., Kim E.S., Cho S.H., Lee J.H. et al. Fabrication and characterization of hydrophilic poly (lactic-co-glycolic acid)/poly (vinyl alcohol) blend cell scaffolds by melt-molding particulate-leaching method. Biomaterials. 2003 Oct 1; 24(22): 4011–21. https://doi.org/10.1016/S0142-9612(03)00284-9.

Olubamiji A.D., Zhu N., Chang T., Nwankwo C.K., Izadifar Z. et al. Traditional invasive and synchrotron-based noninvasive assessments of three-dimensional-printed hybrid cartilage constructs in situ. Tissue Engineering Part C: Methods. 2017 Mar 1; 23(3): 156–68. https://doi.org/10.1089/ten.tec.2016.0368.

Owczarczak A.B., Shuford S.O., Wood S.T., Deitch S., Dean D. et al. Creating transient cell membrane pores using a standard inkjet printer. JoVE (Journal of Visualized Experiments). 2012 Mar 16(61): e3681. https://dx.doi.org/10.3791/3681-v.

Ozbolat I.T., Hospodiuk M. Current advances and future perspectives in extrusion-based bioprinting. Biomaterials. 2016 Jan 1; 76: 321–43. http://doi.org/10.1016/j.biomaterials.2015.10.076.

Padrón J.M., van der Wilt C.L., Smid K., Smitskamp-Wilms E., Backus H.H. et al. The multilayered postconfluent cell culture as a model for drug screening. Critical reviews in oncology/hematology. 2000 Nov 1; 36(2-3): 141–57. https://doi.org/10.1016/S1040-8428(00)00083-4.

Pakhomova C., Popov D., Maltsev E., Akhatov I., Pasko A. et al. Software for bioprinting. International Journal of Bioprinting. 2020; 6(3). https://doi.org/10.18063/ijb.v6i3.279.

Park E.K., Lim J.Y., Yun I.S., Kim J.S., Woo S.H. et al. Cranioplasty enhanced by three-dimensional printing: custom-made three-dimensional-printed titanium implants for skull defects. Journal of Craniofacial Surgery. 2016 Jun 1; 27(4): 943–9.

Park J.Y., Choi Y.J., Shim J.H., Park J.H., Cho D.W. et al. Development of a 3D cell printed structure as an alternative to autologs cartilage for auricular reconstruction. Journal of Biomedical Materials Research Part B: Applied Biomaterials. 2017 Jul; 105(5): 1016–28. https://doi.org/10.1002/jbm.b.33639.

Park J.Y., Jang J., Kang H.W. 3D Bioprinting and its application to organ-on-a-chip. Microelectronic Engineering. 2018 Nov 15; 200: 1–1. https://doi.org/10.1016/j.mee.2018.08.004.

Pati F., Jang J., Lee J.W., Cho D.W. Extrusion bioprinting. InEssentials of 3D biofabrication and translation 2015 Jan 1 (pp. 123–152). Academic Press. http://doi.org/10.1016/B978-0-12-800972-8.00007-1.

Pezeshki-Modaress M., Zandi M., Rajabi S. Tailoring the gelatin/chitosan electrospun scaffold for application in skin tissue engineering: an in vitro study. Progress in biomaterials. 2018 Sep; 7: 207–18. https://doi.org/10.1007/s40204-018-0094-1.

Pham Q.P., Sharma U., Mikos A.G. Electrospinning of polymeric nanofibers for tissue engineering applications: a review. Tissue engineering. 2006 May 1; 12(5): 1197–211. https://doi.org/10.1089/ten.2006.12.1197.

Pharma 50: The 50 largest pharmaceutical companies in the world. Drug Discovery and Development. https://www.drugdiscoverytrends.com/pharma-50-the-50-largest-pharmaceutical-companies-in-the-world/(accessed Aug. 23, 2022).

Poldervaart M.T., Gremmels H., van Deventer K., Fledderus J.O., Öner F.C. et al. Prolonged presence of VEGF promotes vascularization in 3D bioprinted scaffolds with defined architecture. Journal of controlled release. 2014 Jun 28; 184: 58–66. https://doi.org/10.1016/j.jconrel.2014.04.007.

Polge, C., Smith, A. U., & Parkes, A. S. (1949). Revival of spermatozoa after vitrification and dehydration at low temperatures. Nature, 164(4172), 666. https://doi.org/10.1038/164666a0.

Porter D., Vollrath F. Silk as a biomimetic ideal for structural polymers. Advanced Materials. 2009; 21(4): 487–92. https://doi.org/10.1002/adma.200801332.

Pranzo D., Larizza P., Filippini D., Percoco G. Extrusion-based 3D printing of microfluidic devices for chemical and biomedical applications: A topical review. Micromachines. 2018 Jul 27; 9(8): 374. http://doi.org/10.3390/mi9080374.

Prasad A., Sankar M.R., Katiyar V. State of art on solvent casting particulate leaching method for orthopedic scaffoldsfabrication. Materials Today: Proceedings. 2017 Jan 1; 4(2): 898–907. https://doi.org/10.1016/j.matpr.2017.01.101.

Qiu C., Sun Y., Li J., Xu Y., Zhou J. et al. Therapeutic effect of biomimetic scaffold loaded with human amniotic epithelial cell-derived neural-like cells for spinal cord injury. Bioengineering. 2022 Oct 9; 9(10): 535. https://doi.org/10.3390/bioengineering9100535.

Qiu J., Wilkens C., Barrett K., Meyer A.S. Microbial enzymes catalyzing keratin degradation: Classification, structure, function. Biotechnology Advances. 2020 Nov 15; 44: 107607. https://doi.org/10.1016/j.biotechadv.2020.107607.

Rai B., Oest M.E., Dupont K.M., Ho K.H., Teoh S.H. et al. Combination of platelet-rich plasma with polycaprolactone-tricalcium phosphate scaffolds for segmental bone defect repair. Journal of biomedical materials research Part A. 2007 Jun 15; 81(4): 888–99. https://doi.org/10.1002/jbm.a.31142.

Rajan N., Habermehl J., Coté M.F., Doillon C.J., Mantovani D. et al. Preparation of ready-to-use, storable and reconstituted type I collagen from rat tail tendon for tissue engineering applications. Nature protocols. 2006 Dec; 1(6): 2753–8. https://doi.org/10.1038/nprot.2006.430.

Rao F., Yuan Z., Li M., Yu F., Fang X. et al., Expanded 3D nanofibre sponge scaffolds by gas-foaming technique enhance peripheral nerve regeneration. Artificial cells, nanomedicine, and biotechnology. 2019 Dec 4; 47(1): 491–500. https://doi.org/10.1080/21691401.2018.1557669.

Ravanbakhsh H., Luo Z., Zhang X., Maharjan S., Mirkarimi H.S. et al. Freeform cell-laden cryobioprinting for shelf-ready tissue fabrication and storage. Matter. 2022 Feb 2; 5(2): 573–93. https://doi.org/10.1016/j.matt.2021.11.020.

Reddy C.V., Venkatesh M.P., Kumar P., First FDA approved 3D printed drug paved new path for increased precision in patient care. Applied Clinical Research, Clinical Trials and Regulatory Affairs. 2020 Aug 1; 7(2): 93–103. https://doi.org/10.2174/2213476X07666191226145027.

Rheinwatd J.G., Green H. Seria cultivation of strains of human epidemal keratinocytes: the formation keratinizin colonies from single cell is. Cell. 1975 Nov 1; 6(3): 331–43. https://doi.org/10.1016/S0092-8674(75)80001-8.

Ricci J.L., Clark E.A., Murriky A., Smay J.E. Three-dimensional printing of bone repair and replacement materials: impact on craniofacial surgery. Journal of Craniofacial Surgery. 2012 Jan 1; 23(1): 304–8. https://doi.org/10.1097/SCS.0b013e318241dc6e.

Robertson J.A. Human embryonic stem cell research: ethical and legal issues. Nature Reviews Genetics. 2001 Jan 1; 2(1): 74–8. https://doi.org/10.1038/35047594.

Roseti L., Parisi V., Petretta M., Cavallo C., Desando G. et al. Scaffolds for bone tissue engineering: state of the art and new perspectives. Materials Science and Engineering: C. 2017 Sep 1; 78: 1246–62. https://doi.org/10.1016/j.msec.2017.05.017.

Roth E.A., Xu T., Das M., Gregory C., Hickman J.J. et al. Inkjet printing for high-throughput cell patterning. Biomaterials. 2004 Aug 1; 25(17): 3707–15. http://doi.org/10.1016/j.biomaterials.2003.10.058.

Rouwkema Jeroen, Susan Gibbs, Matthias P. Lutolf In vitro platforms for tissue engineering: implications for basic research and clinical translation, J. Tissue Eng. Regen. Med 5(8) (2011) e164–e167, https://doi.org/10.1002/term.414.

Salaris F., Colosi C., Brighi C., Soloperto A., de Turris, V. et al. 3DBioprinted Human Cortical Neural Constructs Derived from Induced Pluripotent Stem Cells. J. Clin. Med. 2019, 8, 1595.

Schuurman W., Levett P.A., Pot M.W., van Weeren P.R., Dhert W.J. et al. Gelatin-methacrylamide hydrogels as potential biomaterials for fabrication of tissue-engineered cartilage constructs. Macromolecular bioscience. 2013 May; 13(5): 551–61.http://doi.org/10.1002/mabi.201200444.

Shao H., Ke X., Liu A., Sun M., He Y. et al. Bone regeneration in 3D printing bioactive ceramic scaffolds with improved tissue/material interface pore architecture in thin-wall bone defect. Biofabrication. 2017 Apr 12; 9(2): 025003. https://doi.org/10.1088/1758-5090/aa663c.

Shao H., Sun M., Zhang F., Liu A., He Y. et al. Custom repair of mandibular bone defects with 3D printed bioceramic scaffolds. Journal of dental research. 2018 Jan; 97(1): 68–76. https://doi.org/10.1177/0022034517734846.

Shen C., Zhang Y., Li Q., Zhu M., Hou Y. et al. Application of three-dimensional printing technique in artificial bone fabrication for bone defect after mandibular angle ostectomy. Zhongguo xiu fu chong jian wai ke za zhi=

Zhongguo xiufu chongjian waike zazhi= Chinese journal of reparative and reconstructive surgery. 2014 Mar 1; 28(3): 300–3.

Shevach M., Fleischer S., Shapira A., Dvir T. Gold nanoparticle-decellularized matrix hybrids for cardiac tissue engineering. Nano letters. 2014 Oct 8; 14(10): 5792–6. https://doi.org/10.1021/nl502673m.

Shim J.H., Jang K.M., Hahn S.K., Park J.Y., Jung H. et al. Three-dimensional bioprinting of multilayered constructs containing human mesenchymal stromal cells for osteochondral tissue regeneration in the rabbit knee joint. Biofabrication. 2016 Feb 4; 8(1): 014102. http://dx.doi.org/10.1088/1758-5090/8/1/014102.

Shin Y., Han S., Jeon J.S., Yamamoto K., Zervantonakis I.K., Sudo R. et al. Microfluidic assay for simultaneous culture of multiple cell types on surfaces or within hydrogels. Nature protocols. 2012 Jul; 7(7): 1247–59. https://doi.org/10.1038%2Fnprot.2012.051.

Shim J.H., Won J.Y., Park J.H., Bae J.H., Ahn G. et al. Effects of 3D-Printed Polycaprolactone/ beta-Tricalcium phosphate membranes on guided bone regeneration, Int. J. Mol. Sci. 18 (5) (2017). https://doi.org/10.3390/ijms18050899.

Shukla P., Yeleswarapu S., Heinrich M.A., Prakash J., Pati F. et al. Mimicking tumor microenvironment by 3D bioprinting: 3D cancer modeling. Biofabrication. 2022 May 31; 14(3): 032002. 10.1088/1758-5090/ac6d11.

Sin D., Miao X., Liu G., Wei F., Chadwick G. et al. Polyurethane (PU) scaffolds prepared by solvent casting/ particulate leaching (SCPL) combined with centrifugation. Materials Science and Engineering: C. 2010 Jan 1; 30(1): 78–85. https://doi.org/10.1016/j.msec.2009.09.002.

Singh N.K., Han W., Nam S.A., Kim J.W., Kim J.Y. et al. Three-dimensional cell-printing of advanced renal tubular tissue analogue. Biomaterials. 2020 Feb 1; 232: 119734. https://doi.org/10.1016/j.biomaterials.2019.119734.

Skardal A., Devarasetty M., Kang H.W., Seol Y.J., Forsythe S.D. et al. Bioprinting cellularized constructs using a tissue-specific hydrogel bioink. JoVE (Journal of Visualized Experiments). 2016 Apr 21(110):e53606. https://dx.doi.org/10.3791/53606.

Skardal A., Murphy S.V., Devarasetty M., Mead I., Kang H.W. et al. Multi-tissue interactions in an integrated three-tissue organ-on-a-chip platform. Scientific reports. 2017 Aug 18; 7(1): 8837. https://doi.org/10.1038/s41598-017-08879-x.

Smeets R., Barbeck M., Hanken H., Fischer H., Lindner M. et al. 2017. Selective laser-melted fully biodegradable scaffold composed of poly (d, l-lactide) and β-tricalcium phosphate with potential as a biodegradable implant for complex maxillofacial reconstruction: In vitro and in vivo results. Journal of Biomedical Materials Research Part B: Applied Biomaterials, 105(5), pp.1216–1231. https://doi.org/10.1002/jbm.b.33660.

Soman S.S., Vijayavenkataraman S.. Applications of 3D bioprinted-induced pluripotent stem cells in healthcare. International journal of bioprinting. 2020; 6(4).1 https://doi.org/10.18063/ijb.v6i4.280.

Subbiah R., Guldberg R.E. Materials science and design principles of growth factor delivery systems in tissue engineering and regenerative medicine. Advanced healthcare materials. 2019 Jan; 8(1): 1801000. http://doi.org/10.1002/adhm.201801000.

Subia B., Kundu J., Kundu S.C. Biomaterial scaffold fabrication techniques for potential tissue engineering applications. Tissue engineering. 2010 Mar 1; 141: 13–8. DOI: 10.5772/8581.

Sultana N., Wang M.. Fabrication of HA/PHBV composite scaffolds through the emulsion freezing/freeze-drying process and characterisation of the scaffolds. Journal of Materials Science: Materials in Medicine. 2008 Jul; 19: 2555–61. https://doi.org/10.1007/s10856-007-3214-3.

Sumida T., Otawa N., Kamata Y.U., Kamakura S., Mtsushita T. et al. Custom-made titanium devices as membranes for bone augmentation in implant treatment: clinical application and the comparison with conventional titanium mesh. Journal of Cranio-Maxillofacial Surgery. 2015 Dec 1; 43(10): 2183–8.

Sun L., Parker S.T., Syoji D., Wang X., Lewis J.A. et al. Direct-write assembly of 3D silk/hydroxyapatite scaffolds for bone co-cultures. Advanced healthcare materials. 2012 Nov; 1(6): 729–35. https://doi.org/10.1002/adhm.201200057.

Sun Y., Yang C., Zhu X., Wang J.J., Liu X.Y. et al. 3D printing collagen/chitosan scaffold ameliorated axon regeneration and neurological recovery after spinal cord injury. Journal of Biomedical Materials Research Part A. 2019 Sep; 107(9): 1898–908. https://doi.org/10.1002/jbm.a.36675.

Sun Y., You Y., Jiang W., Wang B., Wu Q. et al. 3D bioprinting dual-factor releasing and gradient-structured constructs ready to implant for anisotropic cartilage regeneration. Science advances. 2020 Sep 9; 6(37): eaay1422. https://doi.org/10.1126/sciadv.aay1422.

T. Lu, Y. Li, T. Chen, Techniques for fabrication and construction of three dimensional scaffolds for tissue engineering, Int. J. Nanomed. 8 (2013) 337. https://doi.org/10.2147/IJN.S38635.

Takahashi K., Tanabe K., Ohnuki M., Narita M., Ichisaka T. et al. Induction of pluripotent stem cells from adult human fibroblasts by defined factors. Obstetrical & Gynecological Survey. 2008 Mar 1; 63(3): 153. https://doi.org/10.1097/01.ogx.0000305204.97355.0d.

Tang M., Xie Q., Gimple R.C., Zhong Z., Tam T., et al. Three-dimensional bioprinted glioblastoma microenvironments model cellular dependencies and immune interactions, Cell Res. 30 (2020) 833–853, https://doi.org/10.1038/s41422-020-0338-1.

Tang Y.C., Powell R.T., Gottlieb A. Molecular pathways enhance drug response prediction using transfer learning from cell lines to tumors and patient-derived xenografts. Scientific Reports. 2022 Sep 27; 12(1): 16109. https://doi.org/10.1038/s41598-022-20646-1.

Tashman J.W., Shiwarski D.J., Coffin B., Ruesch A., Lanni F. et al. In situ volumetric imaging and analysis of FRESH 3D bioprinted constructs using optical coherence tomography. Biofabrication. 2022 Oct 31; 15(1): 014102. 10.1088/1758-5090/ac975e.

Taymour R., Chicaiza-Cabezas N.A., Gelinsky M., Lode A. Core–shell bioprinting of vascularized in vitro liver sinusoid models. Biofabrication. 2022 Sep 27; 14(4): 045019. https://doi.org/10.1088/1758-5090/ac9019.

Teixeira B.N., Aprile P., Mendonca R.H., Kelly D.J., Thiré R.M. et al. Evaluation of bone marrow stem cell response to PLA scaffolds manufactured by 3D printing and coated with polydopamine and type I collagen. Journal of Biomedical Materials Research Part B: Applied Biomaterials. 2019 Jan; 107(1): 37–49. https://doi.org/10.1002/jbm.b.34093.

Thavornyutikarn B., Chantarapanich N., Sitthiseripratip K., Thouas G.A., Chen Q. Bone tissue engineering scaffolding: computer-aided scaffolding techniques. Progress in biomaterials. 2014 Dec; 3: 61–102. https://doi.org/10.1007/s40204-014-0026-7.

Tissue Engineering Market Size, Share Analysis Report 2030 (grandviewresearch.com) Report ID: 978-1-68038-768-1.

Tissue Engineering Market Size, Share and Forecast 2024-2032 (imarcgroup.com) Report ID: SR112024A4880.

Vacanti J.P., Morse M.A., Saltzman W.M., Domb A.J., Perez-Atayde A. et al. Selective cell transplantation using bioabsorbable artificial polymers as matrices. Journal of pediatric surgery. 1988 Jan 1; 23(1): 3–9. https://doi.org/10.1016/S0022-3468(88)80529-3.

Valencia C., Valencia C.H, Zuluaga F, Valencia M.E., Mina J.H. et al. Synthesis and application of scaffolds of chitosan-graphene oxide by the freeze-drying method for tissue regeneration. Molecules. 2018 Oct 16; 23(10): 2651. https://doi.org/10.3390/molecules23102651.

van Bochove B., Grijpma D.W. Mechanical properties of porous photo-crosslinked poly (trimethylene carbonate) network films. European polymer journal. 2021 Jan 15; 143: 110223. https://doi.org/10.1016/j.eurpolymj.2020.110223.

Vijayavenkataraman S. 3D bioprinting: challenges in commercialization and clinical translation. Journal of 3D printing in medicine. 2023 Jun; 7(2): 3DP8. https://doi.org/10.2217/3dp-2022-0026.

Wallmanderco, 2020. CELLINK announces collaboration with AstraZeneca to utilize CELLINKs' 3D-bioprinting technology for liver organoid culture. CELLINK. https://www.cellink.com/cellink-announces-collaboration-with-astrazeneca-to-utilize-cellinks-3d-bioprinting-technology-for-liver-organoid-culture/(accessed Aug. 23, 2022).

Wan W., Cai F., Huang J. A skin-inspired 3D bilayer scaffold enhances granulation tissue formation and anti-infection for diabetic wound healing. *J Mater Chem B*. 2019; 7(18): 2954–2961. https://doi.org/10.1039/c8tb03341b.

Wang C., Tang Z., Zhao Y., Yao R., Li L. et al. Three-dimensional in vitro cancer models: a short review. Biofabrication. 2014 Apr 14; 6(2): 022001. 10.1088/1758-5082/6/2/022001.

Wang X., Yang C., Yu Y., Zhao Y.. In situ 3D bioprinting living photosynthetic scaffolds for autotrophic wound healing. Research. 2022 Mar 20. https://doi.org/10.34133/2022/9794745.

Webster J.P. Refrigerated skin grafts. Annals of surgery. 1944 Oct;120(4):431. https://doi.org/10.1097%2F00000658-194410000-00002.

Wissing M.D., Dadon T., Kim E., Piontek K.B., Shim J.S. et al. Small-molecule screening of PC3 prostate cancer cells identifies tilorone dihydrochloride to selectively inhibit cell growth based on cyclin-dependent kinase 5 expression. Oncology reports. 2014 Jul 1; 32(1): 419-24.

Wrzesinski K., J. Fey S. From 2D to 3D-a new dimension for modelling the effect of natural products on human tissue. Current Pharmaceutical Design. 2015 Nov 1; 21(38): 5605–16. 10.2174/1381612821666151002114227.

Wüst S., Müller R., Hofmann S. Controlled positioning of cells in biomaterials—approaches towards 3D tissue printing. Journal of functional biomaterials. 2011 Aug 4; 2(3): 119–54. https://doi.org/10.3390/jfb2030119.

Xia Z., Jin S., Ye K. Tissue and organ 3D bioprinting. SLAS TECHNOLOGY: Translating Life Sciences Innovation. 2018 Aug; 23(4): 301–14. http://doi.org/10.1177/2472630318761797.

Xu L., Wang S., Sui X., Wang Y., Su Y. et al. Mesenchymal stem cell-seeded regenerated silk fibroin complex matrices for liver regeneration in an animal model of acute liver failure. ACS Applied Materials & Interfaces. 2017 May 3; 9(17): 14716–23. https://doi.org/10.1021/acsami.7b02805.

Xu T., Binder K.W., Albanna M.Z., Dice D., Zhao W. et al. Hybrid printing of mechanically and biologically improved constructs for cartilage tissue engineering applications. Biofabrication. 2012 Nov 21; 5(1): 015001. http://doi.org/10.1088/1758-5082/5/1/015001.

Xu T., Rohozinski J., Zhao W., Moorefield E.C., Atala A. et al. Inkjet-mediated gene transfection into living cells combined with targeted delivery. Tissue Engineering Part A. 2009 Jan 1; 15(1): 95–101. https://doi.org/10.1089/ten.tea.2008.0095.

Yang J., Huang S., Cheng S., Jin Y., Zhang N. et al. Application of ovarian cancer organoids in precision medicine: key challenges and current opportunities. Frontiers in cell and developmental biology. 2021 Aug 2; 9: 701429. https://doi.org/10.3389/fcell.2021.701429.

Yang X., Chen X., Wang H. Acceleration of osteogenic differentiation of preosteoblastic cells by chitosan containing nanofibrous scaffolds. Biomacromolecules. 2009 Oct 12; 10(10): 2772–8. https://doi.org/10.1021/bm900623j.

Yannas I.V., Burke J.F., Orgill D.P., Skrabut E.M. Wound tissue can utilize a polymeric template to synthesize a functional extension of skin. Science. 1982 Jan 8; 215(4529): 174–6. https://doi.org/10.1126/science.7031899.

Yao Q., Liu Y., Pan Y., Miszuk J.M., Sun H. et al. One-pot porogen free method fabricated porous microsphere-aggregated 3D PCL scaffolds for bone tissue engineering. Journal of Biomedical Materials Research Part B: Applied Biomaterials. 2020 Aug;108(6): 2699–710. https://doi.org/10.1002/jbm.b.34601.

Yeo A., Cheok C., Teoh S.H., Zhang Z.Y., Buser D. et al. Lateral ridge augmentation using a PCL-TCP scaffold in a clinically relevant but challenging micropig model. Clinical oral implants research. 2012 Dec; 23(12): 1322–32. https://doi.org/10.1111/j.1600-0501.2011.02366.x.

Yeo A., Wong W.J., Teoh S.H. Surface modification of PCL-TCP scaffolds in rabbit calvaria defects: Evaluation of scaffold degradation profile, biomechanical properties and bone healing patterns. Journal of Biomedical Materials Research Part A: An Official Journal of The Society for Biomaterials, The Japanese Society for Biomaterials, and The Australian Society for Biomaterials and the Korean Society for Biomaterials. 2010 Jun 15; 93(4): 1358–67. https://doi.org/10.1002/jbm.a.32633.

Yeung E., Fukunishi T., Bai Y., Bedja D., Pitaktong I. et al. Cardiac regeneration using human-induced pluripotent stem cell-derived biomaterial-free 3D-bioprinted cardiac patch in vivo. Journal of tissue engineering and regenerative medicine. 2019 Nov; 13(11): 2031–9. https://doi.org/10.1002/term.2954.

Yi H.G., Jeong Y.H., Kim Y., Choi Y.J., Moon H.E. et al. A bioprinted human-glioblastoma-on-a-chip for the identification of patient-specific responses to chemoradiotherapy. Nature biomedical engineering. 2019 Jul; 3(7): 509–19. https://doi.org/10.1038/s41551-019-0363-x.

Youhanna S., Kemas A.M., Preiss L., Zhou Y., Shen J.X. et al. Organotypic and microphysiological human tissue models for drug discovery and development—current state-of-the-art and future perspectives, Pharmacol. Rev. 74 (2022) 141–206, https://doi.org/10.1124/pharmrev.120.000238.

You S., Xiang Y., Hwang H.H., Berry D.B., Kiratitanaporn W. et al. High cell density and high-resolution 3D bioprinting for fabricating vascularized tissues. Science advances. 2023 Feb 22; 9(8): eade7923. https://doi.org/10.1126/sciadv.ade7923.

Yun W.S., Shim J.H., Park K.H., Choi D., Park M. et al. Clinical application of 3-dimensional printing technology for patients with nasal septal deformities: a multicenter study. JAMA Otolaryngology–Head & Neck Surgery. 2018 Dec 1; 144(12): 1145–52.

Zhang H., Liu X., Yang M., Zhu L. Silk fibroin/sodium alginate composite nano-fibrous scaffold prepared through thermally induced phase-separation (TIPS) method for biomedical applications. Materials Science and Engineering: C. 2015 Oct 1; 55: 8–13. https://doi.org/10.1016/j.msec.2015.05.052.

Zhang J., Wehrle E., Rubert M., Müller R. 3D Bioprinting of human tissues: Biofabrication, bioinks, and bioreactors. International Journal of Molecular Sciences. 2021 Apr 12; 22(8): 3971. https://doi.org/10.3390/ijms22083971

Zhang Y., Shi L., Lin X., Zhou F., Xin L. et al. Unresponsive thin endometrium caused by Asherman syndrome treated with umbilical cord mesenchymal stem cells on collagen scaffolds: a pilot study. Stem Cell Research & Therapy. 2021 Dec; 12(1): 1–4.

Zhao Y., Yao R., Ouyang L., Ding H., Zhang T. et al. Three-dimensional printing of Hela cells for cervical tumor model in vitro. Biofabrication. 2014 Apr 11;6(3):035001. 10.1088/1758-5082/6/3/035001.

Zhou X., Zhu W., Nowicki M., Miao S., Cui H. et al., 3D bioprinting a cell-laden bone matrix for breast cancer metastasis study. ACS applied materials & interfaces. 2016 Nov 9; 8(44): 30017–26. https://doi.org/10.1021/acsami.6b10673.

Zhu N., Chen X. Biofabrication of tissue scaffolds. In Advances in biomaterials science and biomedical applications 2013 Mar 27 (Vol. 319). London, UK: InTech. https://doi.org/10.5772/54125.

3D Printing of Composite Materials for Bone Tissue Engineering

Renold Elsen Selvam,[1][*] *Umanath Puthillam*[1] and *Deepan Karuppan*[1]

1. Introduction

Bone is a living tissue made of calcium, phosphate, protein, collagen, and minerals capable of remodelling. The collagen and calcium phosphate provide a framework for the bone which consists of 2 layers, the inner layer which has low density and reduced strength called cancellous bone and the outermost layer which is highly dense and has high strength called cortical bone (Yazdanpanah Z. et al., 2022). The bone has the ability to self-heal small defects but cannot regenerate if the defect is very large which is termed as "Critical sized defect". A critical size defect is not yet properly defined and depends on the location of the injury. An injury to bone is categorized as a critical size defect if the size of the defect is greater than 1 cm (Schemitsch, E.H. 2017) or if the injury size is 50% of the diameter of cortical bone (Court-Brown, C.M. 1998). The critical size defects may arise due to accidents, diseases such as osteoporosis, osteogenesis imperfecta, tumor resection, osteoarthritis, and insufficient nutrients. Some other factors like the patient's age and health also influence the self-healing capability of bone (Schmitz and Hollinger, 1986). External interventions are necessary in such situations and the traditional treatment methods include casting, splinting, traction, open reduction, and internal fixation. These traditional methods are not an ideal treatment practice due to slow integration and poor remodelling (Migliorini, F. et al, 2021; Adel, I.M. et al, 2022). The modern treatment involves grafting and scaffolding as shown in Figure 1.

The grafting method consists of autografts (bone from different locations of the same patient), Allografts (bone tissue from another individual) or xenografts (bone tissue from another species). The autograft provides the osteoinductive growth factor, osteogenic progenitor cells and osteoconductive

[1] School of Mechanical Engineering. Vellore Institute of Technology, Vellore.
[*] Corresponding author: renoldelsen.s@vit.ac.in

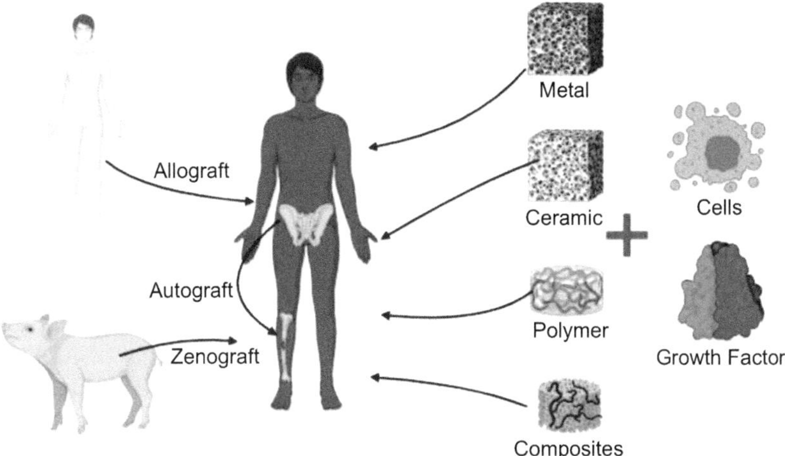

Fig. 1   Current trends in the treatment of Critical size bone defects

matrices (Fomby, P. 2010; Wang, W. 2023; Albrektsson, T. et al., 2023). Even though they are considered the gold standard, autografts have limitations due to the availability of donor sites, the complexity at the donated site and demand for additional surgery on the same person. Allograft is the next best option where the mechanical and biological properties are similar to autograft but with the possibility of transmitting diseases and the limited number of suitable donors (Schieker, M. et al., 2006). Moreover, it is difficult to match the shape of defects in grafting technology which varies from person to person. This can be easily achieved in scaffolds made of metals, polymers or ceramics and their composites developed using additive manufacturing technology. This chapter explores the scaffolds made of composite materials developed using various additive manufacturing technologies specifically designed for bone tissue engineering.

1.1   What is Additive Manufacturing?

Additive manufacturing is also known as rapid prototyping or 3D printing technology. The definition of additive manufacturing by American Society for Testing and Materials (ASTM) is "a process of joining materials to make objects from 3D model data, usually layer upon layer, as opposed to subtractive manufacturing methodologies" (Committee F42 on Additive Manufacturing Technologies). Additive manufacturing is commonly used in various fields like aerospace, automobile, construction, and biomedical industries. The additive manufacturing technique is capable of handling a wide range of materials such as metals, ceramics, polymers, and their composites which makes them suitable for bone tissue engineering applications. Incorporation of cells and growth factors like Bone Morphogenic Proteins (BMP) can also be done using this technology.

1.2   Historical Overview of 3D Printing in Bone Tissue Engineering

During the year 1933, concepts of tissue engineering were introduced and tumour cells were successfully incorporated with a polymeric membrane into the abdominal cavity of a pig and successfully introduced tumour cells into the artificial organ in 1964 (Kim, H.S. et al., 2019). The tissue engineering modern concepts were introduced by Langer and Vacanti in 1993 as "an interdisciplinary field that applies the principle of engineering and life sciences towards the development of biological substitutes that restore, maintain or improve tissue function" (Fisher, J.P. et al., 1993). Bone tissue engineering has been one of the major benefactors of the emerging 3D printing technique. This technique is useful for creating complex structures with high precision and minimum material wastage. Compared to subtractive manufacturing techniques, the additive manufacturing technique is capable of designing complex shapes and structures since a component is fabricated layer by layer through a predefined slicing code (Kalsoom, U. et al., 2016). In 1986, 3D printing technology was first introduced to the world by Chuck Hull who is the co-founder of 3D systems. He invented the photopolymer-based 3D printer machine and named it as stereolithography. A year later, he invented another manufacturing technology at Carl Deckard University and developed the selective laser sintering (SLS) technique, which is capable of printing metal, ceramics, and plastics (Mateti, T. et al., 2023). In 1989 the founder of Stratasys, Scott Crump invented the extrusion-based 3D printing technique. The sheet lamination technique was introduced by Helisys Company in 1990. In 1996, the Sandia National Laboratory released a new method of additive manufacturing machine named Direct Ink writing (DIW) (Qu, H. 2020). At the end of 1999, the Wake Forest Institute of Regenerative Medicine (WFIRM) successfully developed a 3D-printed tissue, which drove the entire biomedical industry towards the next era of tissue engineering with the help of additive manufacturing. Additive manufacturing was used in biomedical engineering and revolutionized the treatment techniques and materials in ophthalmology, orthopaedics, and cardiovascular treatments (Schubert, C. et al., 2014).

The 21st century produced tremendous progress in additive manufacturing. In the year 2005, Adrian Bowyer introduced a low-cost 3D printer called RepRap (Romero, L. et al., 2014). One of the most famous 3D printer manufacturers, "Objet", released a multi-material 3D printer machine in 2007. The Makerbot released the first consumer-grade 3D printer by Bre Pettis, Adam Mayer, and Zach Smith in 2009. The Prusa research company was founded in 2011 to develop a 3D printer based on earlier work on RepRap. Finally, the Prusa i3 company successfully manufactured low-cost 3D printers. In 2012, Stratasys and Objet combined to form Stratasys Ltd. which has emerged as the world's largest 3D printing manufacturer. Additive manufacturing has been focusing on the bone tissue engineering field and providing extensive benefits over traditional manufacturing methods since 1980 (Haleem, A. et al., 2020). In the case of bone defects, obtaining grafts which can match the shape and size of the defect was a tedious task. This issue was easily addressed with the introduction of additive manufacturing where the scaffolds were developed using the CT scan data to exactly replicate the defects.

Figure 2 illustrates the freedom of design in additive manufacturing where a scaffold was printed in the shape of a femur bone section with tailored porosity. The porosity and material can be selected accordingly to match the mechanical and biological properties of the defective bone area.

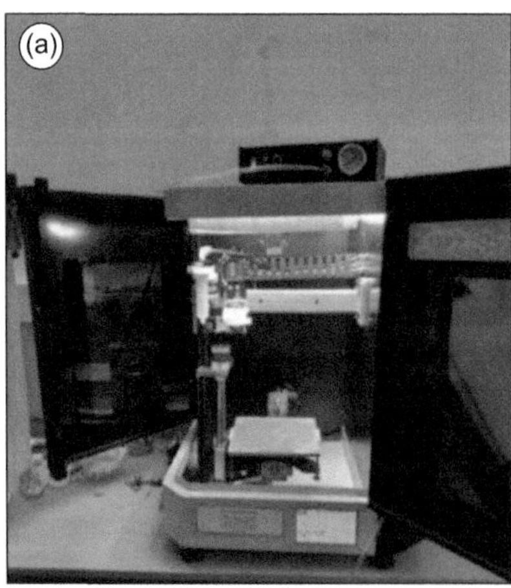
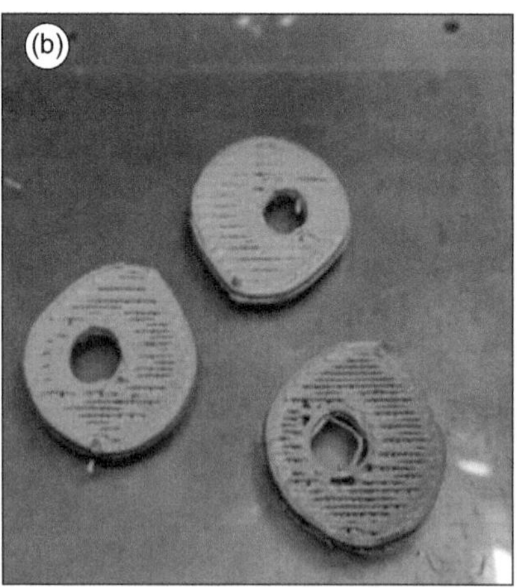

Fig. 2   (a) robocasting 3D printing machine and (b) scaffolds printed in the shape of the femur bone

1.3 What are Composite Materials?

A biomaterial is any object that can interact with biological systems and does not cause any harmful effect while restoring functions and facilitating the healing of damaged tissue. Biomaterials are classified into metals, polymers and ceramics. Metals are used as biomaterials where excellent electrical and thermal conductivity and mechanical properties are required. Examples are bone implants, surgical equipment and dental implants. Polymeric biomaterials are light weight and easy to manufacture and they are used as disposable or degradable implants. Ceramics are refractory and polycrystalline which include silicates, metal oxides and carbides. Ceramics which can be used for biomedical applications are termed bioceramics and are used as implants due to their inertness in body fluids and high compressive strength (Park, J.B. et al., 2002). Composites are a class of materials developed by the combination of two or more different materials, generally a matrix and reinforcement. It offers a combination of properties that can address the limitations of traditional bone grafting material. In bone tissue engineering, different types of composite materials are used such as polymer matrix composites, Metal matrix composites, Ceramic matrix composites and hybrid matrix composites. Table 1 shows the various bio-composite materials used for bone tissue engineering and the additive manufacturing technology used to develop the scaffold.

Table 1 Various bio-composite materials used for bone tissue engineering with the application of additive manufacturing

AM techniques	*Author and Year*	*Matrix*	*Reinforcement*	*Observation from the study*	*Ref*
Binder Jetting (BJ)	Polley et al., 2023	Barium Titanate	45S5 Bioactive glass	• Enhance Piezoelectric constant	Polley, C. 2023
Material Extrusion (ME)	Zerankeshi et al., 2023	Polylactic acid	Graphite and Magnesium	• Enhance Mechanical strength • Control degradation rate	Mohammadi-zerankeshi, M. and Alizadeh, R. 2022
	Wang et al., 2023	Polylactic acid	β-Tri Calcium Phosphate	• Improve Biological performance	Wang, W. 2023
		Poly(L-lactide)	Hydroxyapatite	• Biocompatible and bioactivity	Zhang, H. 2016
	Tan et al., 2023	Poly Lactic-co-glycolic acid	Magnesium Oxide	• Enhance hydrophilicity	Tan, L. 2023
	Jirofti et al., 2023	Chitosan	Collagen Hydroxyapatite Crocin	• Crocin increased Strength • Decrease degradation rate	Jirofti, N. et al., 2023
	Du et al., 2019	Mesoporous Bioactive glass	Silk Fibroin	• Good mechanical strength	Du, X. et al., 2019
Powder Bed fusion (PBF)	Yang et al., 2020	Poly L lactic acid	Barium Titanate and graphene	• Promote piezoelectric response	Yang, Y. 2020
	Xu et al., 2018	Ti6Al4V	Copper	• Copper addition enhances the rate of metal ion release	Xu, X. 2018
	Shuai et al., 2020	Barium Titanate	Polyvinylidene Fluoride and Silver	• Enhanced output voltage promotes cell proliferation and differentiation	Shuai, C. 2020

1.4 Why are 3D-printed Composite Materials Ideal for Bone Tissue Engineering?

The bone requires a 3-dimensional solid structure that can provide mechanical support and aid in osseointegration to heal critical bone defects (Schmitz and Hollinger, 1986). A bone scaffold is a 3-dimensional and interconnected porous structure which fills the voids developed due to fractured bone and offers mechanical support and the pores on the scaffolds allow nutrient transfer and fibrogenesis (Kemppi, H., et al., 2001). The scaffolds can be developed using conventional and modern techniques. In conventional scaffolds, the scaffolds are fabricated using methods like particulate leaching, electro-spinning, freeze casting and more. (T.L.D.A. Montanheiro, 2022; Deb, P. et al., 2018). It is impossible to fabricate complicated and conforming shapes using these techniques while additive manufacturing possesses a high degree of freedom in design and manufacturing. There is no single material that can be used to develop a scaffold which can fulfil all the demanding properties. Hence a combination of different materials can be developed to match the bone properties and facilitate bone regeneration. The properties of an ideal scaffold material are discussed in section 3. Additive manufacturing is capable of printing a wide range of materials including composite materials, which can be tailored to meet desired mechanical and biological properties (Suamte, L. et al., 2022).

1.5 Current State of the Field and Future Outlook

Additive manufacturing gives excellent control in the manufacturing of complex structures and is a cost-effective production method. The scope of additive manufacturing in bone tissue engineering to introduce a biocompatible material to stimulate the desired responses and nano printing of multi-materials is currently being studied widely (Mirzaali, M.J., et al., 2022). The future of scaffolds in tissue engineering is bright as nanotechnology is being explored for scaffold integration. In tissue engineering, the development of organoids and biofluids and the inclusion of organ on-chips are expected to provide better treatment with the help of additive manufacturing technology. The 4D printing technology could successfully implant the printed object into the donor site which changes the shape with respect to time (Adel, I.M. et al., 2022). Additive manufacturing technology offers high resolution, flexibility, reproducibility, and reliability. However, traditional tissue engineering approaches, which involve scaffold development and the use of growth factors, have shown limited success in producing 3D shapes for *in vivo* organ regeneration. This has made them non-feasible for clinical application. Recently, the introduction of 3D bioprinting offers an extended application opportunity of additive manufacturing for tissue engineering.

2. 3D Printing Technologies for Bone Tissue Engineering

As per ASTM standard 52900-21 additive manufacturing is classified into the following categories; Vat Polymerization, Material Jetting, Binder Jetting, Material Jetting, Material Extrusion, Powder Bed Fusion, Sheet Lamination and Direct Energy Deposition ('Defining Additive Manufacturing| Symmetry Electronics, 2022'). Based on the type of technology and material used for printing, the additive manufacturing techniques can be classified into three categories as shown in Table 2.

2.1 Bioprinting

3D bioprinting is one of the most advanced technologies developed in the field of tissue engineering. It enables the building of complex 3D structures producing precise geometrical structures through controlled printing parameters with the help of generated computer graphics (Agarwal, S. et al., 2020). Customized skin shapes with cells can be printed using 3D bioprinting for wound repair and regeneration (Weng, T. 2021). This technology was initially developed as an organ printing technology to utilize the fusing and morphing property of cells to a supporting structure where cells or

Table 2   The categories of additive manufacturing (Mirzaali, M.J. et al., 2022), (de Camargo, I.L. et al.).

	Techniques	*Advantages*	*Disadvantages*

Material Deposition	• Material Extrusion
	  • *Hydrogel*
	  • *Thermoplastics*
	  • *Ceramics*
	  • *Bio-Inks*
		• Widely known process
		• Low cost
		• Accessible
		• Fast
			• Low resolution
			• Require post-process

	• Direct Energy Deposition • *Metal*	• Fast • Density • Composite material	• Expensive • Low resolution

	• Material Jetting
	  • *Photopolymers*
	  • *Bio-Inks*
		• Good resolution
		• Good Surface Finish
			• Material wastage
			• Limited Fabrication Size

Powder based	• Powder Bed Fusion
	  • *Thermoplastics*
	  • *Ceramics*
	  • *Metals*
		• Overhanging structure without secondary support material
		• High resolution
		• Strength
			• Most Expensive
			• Require more material

	• Binder Jetting
	  • *Metal*
	  • *Polymers*
	  • *Ceramics*
		• Low cost
		• Fast
		• Multi-colour printing
		• No support material required
			• Low strength
			• Low resolution
			• Require post-process

Liquid Based	• Vat Polymerization
	  • *Photopolymer*
	  • *Ceramic resin*
		• High resolution
		• Fast
		• Complex
		• Overhanging
			• Limited material
			• Limited size

cell aggregates in gel form were printed layer by layer until the desired shape was obtained (Mironov, V. 2003). Although additive manufacturing has been used to create living tissue in regenerative medicine, these structures lack the dynamic functionality required to mimic the behaviours of living systems. The 3D printing technology combines with smart materials such as shape memory polymers, hydrogels, and bio-inks that can change the shape and properties by external stimuli, which creates dynamic structures (Ramezani, M. 2023). Bioprinting follows the same steps as in a 3D printing process. While the former can seed cells in the printing ink called the "bioink" and are usually printed in gel form, the latter cannot seed cells and are usually printed in a solid state or molten state which quickly turns solid. Bioprinting is sometimes carried out in a contactless manner with the droplet printing method. Usually, microtissues are used to prepare the bioink and have the advantage of automation in cell seeding to a scaffold and high concentration of cells. Even though bioprinting puts forward the idea of manufacturing tissues in bulk, the current technology is limited to *in vitro* tests and real-life application needs further studies and proof. Presently, bioprinting is used to develop heart valves for treating some defects (Bhandari, S. 2023). 4D bioprinting is also attracting attention in the research community as it can develop organs that can change shape with time according to the healing pattern (An, J. et al., 2015).

3. Composite Materials for 3D Printing in Bone Tissue Engineering

An ideal scaffold should be able to replicate the bone properties in terms of healing and regeneration. The ideal properties that a scaffold should possess are biocompatibility, mechanical strength, biodegradability and resorbability, ability to match the shape and porosity of bone, ability to sterile the material to remove germs before implanting and ability to carry and deliver drugs if required. The first quality to be fulfilled by a scaffold material is biocompatibility. That is, it should perform the repair operation without causing adverse reactions in the host environment. This is common to all biomaterials used for implants, dental applications, and stents. Many types of materials such as metals, polymers and ceramics are used as biomaterials. For the scaffold application, it should be biodegradable as the bone would regenerate and replace the shape occupied by the scaffold. In an ideal condition, the degradation rate of the scaffold should match the regeneration rate of bone. Even though the scaffolds are temporary structures, they are expected to experience various types of loads during their life span and hence should be capable of bearing them. The scaffold should be designed considering the implant location and the porosity, pore size and shape and should facilitate bone regeneration and nutrient transportation. The biomaterials is sterilized before insertion into the host environment to get rid of harmful life forms and biological agents using UV rays, alcohol or hot water. During this process, the material should not lose any of its inherent properties and bioactivity. Bioactive materials are those which actively take part or aid in bone regeneration. Finally, the scaffold should be able to release the drugs, growth factors or bone regeneration-facilitating ions like Mg^{2+} Si^{2+} etc. at a controlled rate to help the healing process (Ghassemi, T. et al., 2018).

Metals like Titanium (Ti), and Stainless Steel (SS316L) are biocompatible and have high load bearing capacity, and sterilizability among others, but do not degrade quickly to facilitate bone regeneration. On the other hand, polymers could be manufactured to degrade at a specific rate to match the bone regeneration, however, the load-carrying capacity is limited and could fail quickly in hostile environments. Ceramics are well suited for bone scaffolds compared to polymers and metals and are commonly used in bone tissue engineering. However, the brittle nature of ceramics could lead to abrupt failure of bone scaffolds. Hence composite materials are used to 3D print the scaffolds where each material fulfils a particular function. The following chapters emphasize different types of scaffolds used in bone tissue engineering at the moment.

3.1 *Metal-based Composites*

Metals are commonly used for bone repairs. What makes metals stand out compared to polymers and ceramics is their stiffness and fracture toughness which is essential for load-bearing scenarios. The metals are biocompatible, but not as bioactive as ceramic and polymer counterparts. Titanium and its alloys, Stainless Steel and Cobalt Chromium alloys are the most common metals used in Bone Tissue Engineering (BTE). Among the metals, Titanium and its alloys are most suited for bone regeneration applications since they have low density, Their Young's modulus (100-110 GPa) is closer to natural bone (4-30 GPa) than other metals and alloys and the osseointegration is better (Geetha, M. et al., 2009). The possibility of metal scaffolds for segmental defects which require longer healing periods is investigated. The metal scaffolds are usually coated with bioactive materials like HAP and CS rather than developing a composite scaffold since the metal alone can provide the mechanical properties (Tsai, C.H. et al., 2019; Graziani, G. 2021; Nuswantoro, N.F. 2021).

Porous metal scaffolds are developed using additive manufacturing techniques to overcome the 'stress shielding effect' by reducing the Young's Modulus (E) and improving osseointegration. The relationship between porosity and reduction in E was investigated by many scientists. Some suggested that the relationship is linear and depends on porosity and Poisson ratio while some other reports state that it can be exponential or quadratic depending on the pore size, shape and structure (Choren J.A. et al., 2013). While designing, the size, shape and morphology of the porous structure are very important for achieving the required properties (Sun, C. 2022). The porosity can be controlled to develop metal scaffolds having properties similar to trabecular bone or cortical bone in the SLM technique for different metals (Čapek, J. 2016; Weißmann, V. et al., 2016). Mg is a metal which has similar mechanical properties to a cortical bone and is biocompatible. However, faster degradation hinders their application in BTE since it could fail prematurely. The latest reports indicate that the Mg produced using the SLM technique has better corrosion resistance than conventional methods due to grain refinement and minimal composition segregation due to rapid cooling and solidification (Shuai, C. 2017). This is still not sufficient to use them as dependable scaffolds and the reactive nature of Mg makes it difficult to process the scaffold at bulk level (Yang, Y. 2019). Titanium and its alloys are the next best option available as Young's Moduli of SS316 and Co-Cr alloys are close to 200GPa. The cp-Ti and Ti6Al4V demonstrate similar mechanical and biological compatibility from short-term studies. Some studies demonstrate that cp Ti has better biomechanical capabilities, further long-term trials are required to arrive at a conclusion (Shah, F.A. 2016). It is evident that Ti and its alloys are the most suitable materials for bone repair owing to their physical, mechanical, electrochemical and biological characteristics (Geetha, M. et al., 2009; Nouri, A. et al., 2010).

The mismatch of mechanical properties leads to stress shielding effect, additional bone loss, bone relaxation and osteoporosis. Moreover, the release of toxic ions to the surroundings, corrosion, and high rigidity limits their standalone application in BTE. They are either mixed with polymers, ceramics or both (Zerankeshi, M. Mohammadi et al., 2021; Lopez - Heredia, M.A. et al., 2008; Zhu, C. 2021) to overcome the limitations or the scaffold is designed in such a way that the properties are matched with the natural bone while reducing the release of toxic substances. The slow degradation rate makes the metals more suitable for implants rather than scaffolds which should remain inside the patient for a longer period (Zheng, Y.F. et al. 2014).

3.2 *Polymer-based Composites*

The biocompatibility and ability to control the biomechanical properties make natural and synthetic polymers an excellent choice in bone scaffolding (N'Gatta, K.M. 2022). Polymers are suitable for developing scaffolds for cancellous bone defects for their similarities in properties. The properties like strength, degradation rate, porosity, pore structure and pore shape can be controlled during the production stage and the degradation can be controlled to match the bone regeneration rate. Polymers can be classified into natural and synthetic polymers. Synthetic polymers like polyglycolic acid (PGA), polycaprolactone (PCL) and polylactic acid (PLA) are biocompatible and their properties can be controlled easily (Ma, P.X. 2004). Yet the hydrophobicity and faster degradation limit their applications. These synthetic polymers can be mixed with natural polymers such as gelatine, keratin, cellulose, chitosan and alginate to overcome the limitations. The incorporation of cellulose nanofiber (CNF) into the PLA and scaffold developed through screw extrusion improved the mechanical strength and the combination displayed biological activities required for biomedical applications (Jonoobi, M. et al., 2010; Patel, D.K. et al., 2020). Similarly, the addition of chitosan to PLA improved the cell viability and alkaline phosphatase (ALP) activity. The Young's Modulus of the scaffold was around 0.5 GPa with a compressive strength of 20 MPa which is sufficient for cancellous bones (Geetha, M. et al., 2009; Pon-On, W. et al., 2018). Another synthetic polymer Poly Vinyl Alcohol (PVA) also displayed favourable properties for bone tissue engineering when incorporated with sodium alginate and cellulose (Kumar, A. 2017). Silk fibroin is a naturally occurring material produced by silkworms and spiders. It has excellent mechanical properties and tuneable degradation properties and the ability to aid in osteogenic differentiation makes it an excellent option for a filler in BTE. It can be mixed with bioceramics like TCP, and HAP to improve the bone regeneration rate and control the degradation rate (Peifen, M. 2023; Logeshwaran et al., 2023; Zhang, Y et al., 2009). Collagen is another polymer which is a primary component in natural bone and is helpful in maintaining the structural integrity of the Extracellular Matrix of the bone. The poor mechanical properties of collagen make them unsuitable for BTE applications directly. They are used with other polymers like PCL or ceramics like TCP and HAP to improve the cytocompatibility of matrix material (Zhang, D. et al., 2018; Kiany, F. 2024; Xu, J. 2024).

Collagen PLGA hybrid scaffold was tested on the dorsa of athymic nude mice and displayed excellent capability to treat the defects. The cytoplasm of osteoprogenitor cells contains a type of polymer called Hyaluronic Acid. This can reduce the immunogenicity at the implant site (M. van Beek et al., 2008). Chitosan (CHI) is a polymer derived from chitin which is found on the exoskeleton of animals like shrimp and lobster. CHI is bioactive, biodegradable and hydrophilic which makes it an excellent choice for bone repair applications. The cell-seeded 3D scaffold could repair bone

Table 3   Classification of bioceramics (J. Huang, 2017)

Bioceramics		
Bioinert	*Bioactive*	*Bioresorbable*
Neither take part in bone regeneration nor degrade inside the host environment	Will actively take part in bone healing process	Will get degraded and resorbed to the body fluid
Will remain inside the body for a long period	May or may not remain inside the body for a long period	Will not remain inside the body for a long period
Form a non-adherent fibrous membrane around the tissue	Form an interfacial bond between tissue and scaffold	The scaffold will be replaced by newly formed tissues
Example: Alumina (Al_2O_3), Zirconia (ZrO_2)	Example: Bioactive glass, Hydroxyapatite (HAP)	Example: Tricalcium Phosphate (TCP)

defects as the studies were successful in treating cranial bone defects in mice. CHI can be mixed with other polymers like collagen, Hyaluronic Acid, SF and ceramics like TCP, HAP to treat bone defects (Tang, S. et al., 2021; Bi, L. et al., 2010). However, most of the polymer-based scaffolds do not have the mechanical properties to be used as scaffolds, especially in load-bearing scenarios and poor cellular response of polymers limits their extensive usage in bone tissue engineering. Research is still going on to develop better methods for polymer-based materials as they are robust, cost-effective and can be easily engineered to the required degradability.

3.3 Ceramic-based Composites

Ceramics, on the other hand, have an excellent cellular response and match the mechanical composition of the natural bone. This makes bioceramics ideal candidates for treating bone defects (Baino, F. et al., 2015). The ceramics used as biomaterials are known as bioceramics. They are classified into 3 groups as shown in Table 3 based on their performance inside the host environment.

Bioinert ceramics are those materials which remain stable inside the human body and they neither show any harmful responses nor take part in bone regeneration activities. Alumina (Al_2O_3) and Zirconia (ZrO_2) are examples of bioinert materials. Bioactive ceramics connect directly with the bone without the formation of fibrillar tissue which is formed in the case of bioinert materials. Bioactive glass or Bioglass is an example of a bioactive material. These materials remain inside the body unless they are removed through clinical procedures. On the other hand, Bioresorbable materials are gradually resorbed in the body. These resorbed materials are already present inside the body as trace elements and do not trigger any cellular response or defence mechanism from the immune system. HAP, TCP are bioresorbable materials used in bone treatment (Ishikawa, K. et al., 2003). The natural bone consists of water (25% in volume), organic components such as collagen (35% in volume) and inorganic components like hydroxyapatite (HAP, $(Ca_3(PO_4)_2)_3Ca(OH)_2$) (40% in volume) (Fraile-martínez, O. 2021). Element-wise analysis of bone reveals that 62% per cent of cortical bone is Ca and 37% is P while cancellous bone consists of 53% of Ca and 38% of P. The remaining % consists of trace elements like Fe, Mn, Cu and Zn (Lin, S. 2022). The bioceramics can be classified as Calcium-based ceramics and other ceramics since they constitute more than half of the bone.

Hydroxyapatite (HAP) is a ceramic material and it is the source of Calcium (Ca) and Phosphate (P) in the bone. It is an osteoinductive material since it can release calcium and phosphate ions to help cell differentiation (Tripathy, N. et al., 2018; Barradas, A.M.C. et al., 2011). Even though dense HAP have excellent mechanical strength, mimicking the bone geometry will bring them down considerably (Woodard, J.R. 2007). There have been attempts to improve the strength of HAP-based scaffolds using reinforcements and other processing techniques. The addition of Multi-Walled Carbon Nanotubes (MWCNT) improved the compressive strength as well as the biological response of the scaffold (Lawton, K. et al., 2019). However, the slow degradation rate of HAP makes them unsuitable for scaffold applications (Huang. Y.Z. et al., 2020). To overcome this issue, another calcium and phosphate-based ceramic is used which is β-Tricalcium Phosphate (β-TCP). It has a similar elemental composition compared to HAP which makes it a rich source of Ca and P ions required for bone regeneration. At the same time, β-TCP also possesses high porosity compared to HAP and they degrade up to twelve times faster than HAP (Cohn, M.R. 2017). This can be controlled and brought down up to three times faster (Lu, J. 2002). Reinforcements like Multi-Walled Carbon Nanotube (MWCNT), Graphene and Graphene Oxide (GO) can be used to improve the mechanical strength of the ceramic scaffolds (Shuai, C. et al., 2014; Li, Z. et al., 2017; Ravoor, J. et al., 2022). MWCNT is the most common reinforcement since it is Graphene rolled into cylindrical structures and has better mechanical properties. The addition of MWCNT to TCP improved the mechanical as well as biological properties of the scaffold developed using an extrusion-based robocasting technique. In this method, CAD models of the scaffolds are developed and then sliced using Simplify 3D software which is custom-designed for an in-house developed Fabforge printer.

The MWCNT and ceramic powder are mixed together using a tumbler machine for homogeneous mixing. A slurry is prepared by mixing the composite powder in the carboxy methyl cellulose (CMC) binder (2.5 wt% of CMC dissolved in distilled water using a magnetic stirrer to prepare the binder) and the powder : the slurry ratio was finalized based on the extrudability of the slurry. The samples were then printed and sintered using a microwave furnace in an inert atmosphere to prevent oxidation of MWCNT. Studies revealed that the argon atmosphere successfully retained the MWCNT and incorporation of 0.5 wt% of MWCNT improved the mechanical strength by 38%, displayed better cell viability and proliferation. Further addition of reinforcement produced detrimental effects due to agglomeration of low density MWCNT particles (Puthillam U. et al., 2022). Figure 3 shows the 3D printed scaffolds, the FESEM image of the scaffold and Raman Spectroscopy data. The arrow mark highlights the MWCNT traces in the FESEM image and the Raman spectroscopy data confirms the presence of TCP with characteristic peaks around 843 cm^{-1}, 1360 cm^{-1}, 1580 cm^{-1}, 1610 cm^{-1}, 2700 cm^{-1} and 2930 cm^{-1}.

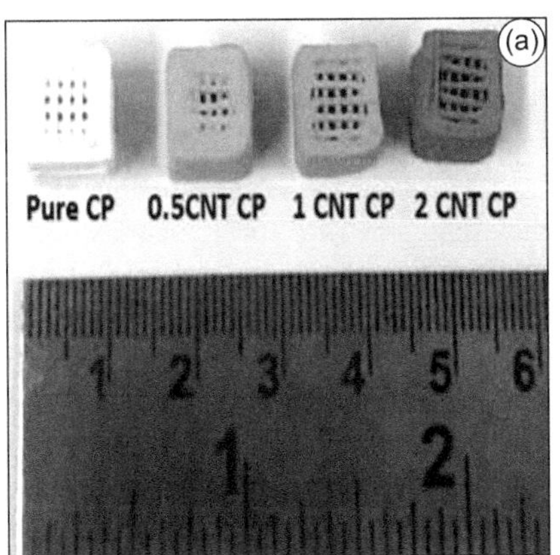

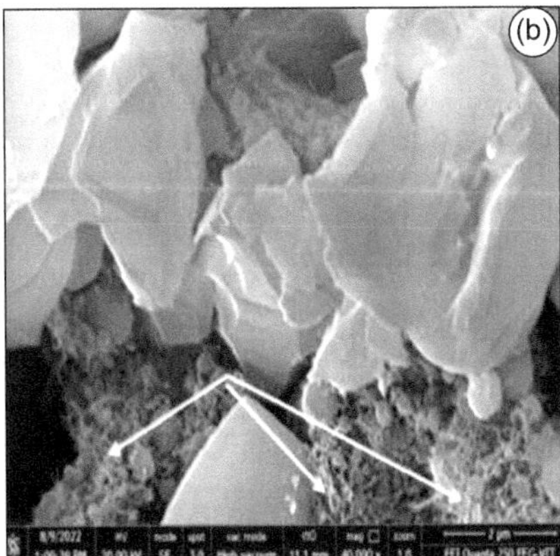

Fig. 3   (a) scaffold printed using robocasting and sintered at 1200°C using microwave furnace in argon atmosphere, (b) FESEM image showing the presence of MWCNT

A combination of HAP and β-TCP is also used which is known as Bi-phasic Calcium Phosphate (BCP) to engineer the degradation rate and bioactivity (Hu, X. 2020). A BCP scaffold developed using DLP printing technology and tested on rabbits indicated bone refrigeration and the rate of regeneration was influenced by the pore size (Lim, H.K. 2020). The ratio of Ca to P is critical in bone regeneration and a ratio of 1:1.67 (Ca:P) is considered as an ideal ratio which is present in HAP. Calcium-deficient and Calcium-rich variants of Calcium Phosphate ceramics are also used based on the application. For example, the Ca:P ratio of β-TCP is 1.5 and used when faster degradation rates are required. The variation in the Ca/P ratio could produce inconsistencies in the biological performance. A study conducted to analyze the importance of the Ca/P ratio found that if the ratio is above 2, the bioactivities will be reduced after 72 hours and a value between 1.5 and 1.7 promotes osteogenic differentiation (Liu H. et al., 2008). α-TCP is another Calcium and phosphate-based bioceramic with a very high degradation rate and can be used to control the degradation of the scaffolds (Cao, Q. 2019).

Similar ceramic materials such as Calcium Silicate [CS, ($CaSiO_3$)] can be used to develop bone scaffolds which will facilitate bone regeneration with its inherent properties and are bioresorbable while Bioglass, Bentonite, Magnesium Phosphate (MgP, $Mg_3(PO4)_2$) etc. are some other ceramics which are gaining interest in bone scaffold research. are used in bone tissue engineering since they can induce favourable properties like angiogenesis (Baino, F. et al., 2015; Vargas, G.E. 2013). CS is a Ca-based ceramic and is better than CaP-based ceramics in angiogenesis osteogenic differentiation of pre-osteoblasts by secreting odontogenic Dentin Sialo Phosphor Protein (DSPP) and Dentin Matrix Protein 1 (DMP-1) and angiogenic von Willebrand factor (vWF) and Angiopoietin (ang-1) (Chen, Y.W. et al., 2016). The Silicate ion (SiO_2^+) released from the scaffold accelerates the proliferation differentiation and mineralization of osteoblasts (Deng, F. et al., 2021; T.-T. H. et al., 2020; Shie, M. et al., 2017; Ding, Z. et al., 2021). These bioceramics are doped with some functional materials to improve bone regeneration and differentiation. $CaSiO_3$ doped with Magnesium and Strontium indicates a better response in *in vivo* conditions than the base material scaffold (Lin, Y. et al., 2021). Graphene-reinforced $CaSiO_3$ developed using the SLS technique improved the fracture toughness by 46% and compression strength by 142%. (Shuai, C. et al., 2014) whereas incorporation of MWCNT improved the strength while maintaining the biocompatibility. Bentonite is an aluminosilicate nanoplatelet used in pharmaceutical products. Studies found that it can be an ideal candidate for BTE owing to its low cost, availability and non-toxicity, and presence of minerals like Mg, Silica, Ca, P and more (Naeini, S.A. et al., 2012; Chakraborty, S. et al., 2020). The scaffold developed using Bentonite along with HAP displayed excellent mechanical and biological compatibility (Logeshwaran, A. et al., 2023). Apart from BTE, they are used in treating skin burns and drug release studies. Bioactive Glasses or Bioglasses (Na_2O-CaO-SiO_2-P_2O_5) are highly biocompatible and have excellent bonding with the bone. The availability of ions that promote bone regeneration, controllable degradability etc. make them excellent choices for bone scaffolds. The borate-based BG degrades much faster than silicate-based ones and forms HAP-like products on their surface when exposed in *vivo* quickly (Ning, J. 2007). However, the low stiffness and fracture toughness limit their use in load-bearing applications. The MgP-based scaffolds are gaining more attention due to the presence of Mg^{2+} ions which can facilitate the production of collagen which in turn improves cell differentiation and mineralization (Pahlevanzadeh, F. et al., 2023). The MgP incorporated with Strontium and PCL and extrusion 3D printed composite scaffold displayed excellent osteogenic activities on the *in vivo* model indicating that they are ideal candidates for BTE (Golafshan, N. 2020).

However, none of these were helpful in improving the overall toughness of the scaffolds. For this purpose, ceramics like Zirconia and Alumina are used. The addition of 6% ZrO_2 to the HAP scaffold developed using DLP techniques improved the tensile strength by 29.4% and the bending moment by 23.9% (Zhang, J. 2019). The biocompatibility of Al_2O_3 and ZrO_2 is often utilized to develop bone scaffolds for load-bearing applications. The Al_2O_3 scaffold developed using the foaming technique had enough mechanical strength with porosity above 90% (Soh, E. 2015). However, the biocompatibility of the sample was not tested. The yttria-stabilized zirconia doped with Zn/HAP was developed using the bioprinting method and found that the scaffold had strength comparable to cortical bone and the bioactivity was boosted with the coating (Sakthiabirami, K. 2020). The Zirconia-toughened alumina (ZTA) scaffolds were developed using the robocasting method and found suitable for bone regeneration applications (Stanciuc, A.M. 2018). The fracture toughness of bioceramic scaffolds can be improved using whiskers of the matrix material. Multiple 3D printing techniques like Stereolithography (SLA), Laser Engineered Net Shaping (LENS), Selective Laser Sintering (SLS) and Direct Ink Writing (DIW) were successful in developing whisker-reinforced bioceramic scaffolds (Sun, J. 2023). 20% HAP whiskers in $CaSiO_3$ are found to improve the compressive strength by 50% and fracture toughness by 20% while the flexural strength rose to 15.64 MPa from 2.83 MPa in the SLS process (Feng, P. et al., 2014). Similarly, Carbon fibres and Silicon Carbide fibres can be incorporated into bone scaffolds with the help of additive manufacturing technologies. These reinforced scaffolds can resist catastrophic failures and have good damage tolerance (Guo, S. 2017; Baker, B. 2019). The biocompatibility of these reinforced scaffolds is, however, yet to be verified.

3.4 Hybrid Composites

Hybrid composites are those composites that consist of more than 1 reinforcement material in the matrix. Multiple materials are added to improve the functionality and bone regeneration of the composite. The HAP and ZrO_2 reinforced Ti scaffold displayed better hardness, fracture toughness and corrosion resistance than the Ti and Ti/HAP scaffold. However, the composite was supposed to increase the sintering capability and the load-bearing capacity, though it produced a low compressive strength of 3.80 MPa compared to those of 18.83 and 11.25 MPa possessed by Ti and Ti/HAP composites (Topuz, M. et al., 2021). This is due to the improper sintering of the matrix material which was covered by the reinforcements. Hence proper mixing of the composite is mandatory for achieving the expected results and the mixing method is crucial and should be optimized. A combination of the metal-ceramic—polymer was used to develop a hybrid scaffold where MgP was the matrix and strontium and PCL were added as reinforcements to the matrix. The printed scaffold had mechanical properties similar to trabecular bone. The release of Mg^{2+} and Sr^{2+} facilitated bone regeneration in the *in vivo* analysis carried out on the bone defect in female ponies (Golafshan, N. 2020). Silk fibroin-TCP-Gelatin-hyaluronic acid hybrid composite scaffolds developed using bioprinting were found suitable for bone regeneration applications. Incorporating platelet-rich plasma could further improve the utility and regeneration rate, but further studies are required to find an effective method to incorporate the PRP into the scaffolds (Wei, L. 2019).

Proper selection of material and design parameters can develop scaffolds with properties similar to cortical bones using cost-effective 3D printing methods like Robocasting and Direct ink writing. A scaffold developed by direct ink writing method using a combination of strontium (Sr) doped hardystonite ($Ca_2ZnSi_2O_7$), gahnite ($ZnAl_2O_4$) bioglass developed a compressive strength greater than 100MPa which is equivalent to that of cortical bones. This experiment further established the importance of design features like pore size and shape that had a critical impact on the mechanical properties of the final product.

4. Design and Fabrication of 3D-printed Composite Scaffolds for Bone Tissue Engineering

Additive manufacturing has enormous potential in the field of biomedical engineering due to its versatility in developing scaffolds which demands unique characteristics which cannot be fulfilled by normal production techniques. It can easily develop structures based on lattice designs, auxetic designs and interconnected porosity easily and quickly without much material wastage. The pore size can be controlled at the micro level.

4.1 Scaffold Design Principles

Theoretically, additive manufacturing can develop scaffold designs of any shape, structure and dimensions. This is not completely true at the application level, especially for those methods which require support structures and post-processing to obtain the final product. The most common limitations are in wall thickness, printing orientation and in the case of designs with overhanging parts (Wang, X. 2016). Hence an ideal design should avoid or reduce the requirement of support materials and overhanging parts.

4.2   Scaffold Fabrication Parameters

The fabrication parameters vary from method to method. For instance, in the PBF method, the overhanging parts can cause undesirable effects on the lattice (Calignano, F. 2014). Hence the orientation of the printing becomes very important and should be printed in a manner where overhanging structures are minimal. This could change the total material consumption and printing time. The size of support material that can be removed depends on the pore size and orientation. The best option is to remove the necessity of support material by changing the direction or orientation of the printing (Xu-bin, S.U. et al., 2012). This may not be always a viable option since the printing direction can influence the mechanical properties of the final product. The removal of support material is easy in methods like FDM and SLA, compared to SLM and SLS, but the design freedom is limited in the former techniques. In the case of closed lattice designs, it is impossible to remove the support materials inside the lattice which is why open lattices are more common (Mirzaali, M.J. et al., 2022). After the design limitations, the quality of the final product is determined by part bed temperature, energy of the power source, scan speed and the material used for printing (An, J. et al., 2015). In the case of extrusion-based printing methods, the nozzle diameter, consistency of printing ink or filament quality will influence the final product. Table 4 shows the common printing techniques used in bone tissue engineering and major printing parameters that influence the final quality of the product like surface roughness, dimensional accuracy, and energy consumption.

Table 4   Printing parameters of common 3D printing techniques

FDM (Raja, S., 2022)	Robocasting/DIW (Lamnini, S. et al. 2022)	SLS (Rahman, M. 2023)	SLA/DLP (Romli, D.P.P. et al. 2021)	SLM (Nandhakumar, R. et al. 2023)	EBM (Barbagallo, R. et al. 2022)
Bed temperature	Printing speed.	Laser power	Light-off (Delay)	Laser power	Speed function
Extruder temperature	Distance between nozzle tip and bed	Part bed temperature	Bottom Layers Count	Layer thickness	Focus offset
Layer height	Printing pressure	Layer thickness	Lift Distance	Scanning speed	Line offset
Printing speed	Layer height	Scan speed	Lift Speed	Hatch spacing	Number of contours
Travel speed	Nozzle diameter	Scan mode and count	Retract Speed		
Infill (density/ pattern)	Ink viscosity	Spot size.			
Shell count	Strut spacing	Hatch spacing and length			

5.   Bioactive Factors and Cellularization of 3D-printed Composite Scaffolds for Bone Tissue Engineering

5.3   Incorporation of Bioactive Factors into 3D-printed Scaffolds

It is already proven that incorporating trace elements of bone into the scaffold improves the biological performance of the scaffold. The addition of elements like Magnesium and Silicon to the scaffold accelerates the recovery process by improving bone regeneration and differentiation. Another method to improve the integration of scaffold is to include proteins like bone morphogenetic protein (BMP), silk fibrin, platelet-derived growth factors, transforming growth factor beta (TGF-β), and fibroblast growth factors (FGF) (Janssens, K. et al., 2005; Luu, H.H. 2007). Reinforcement materials like CNT, graphene and graphene oxides have also been found to promote quick bone healing techniques in *in vitro* test conditions and clinical proofs are required to confirm the same (C. Gao, et al., 2017).

5.4 Cell Seeding and Culture Techniques

Cell seeding and culture is an important step in biological characterization studies. The most commonly followed seeding technique is called static seeding where the cell is deposited in a suspension droplet onto the construct's surface and the seeding solution penetrates the scaffold over time. This is followed by cell culture techniques which include cell observation, medium exchange and passaging. Then the scaffold is observed using a microscope to confirm the cell detachment and proliferation.

5.5 Coculture of Different Cell Types

Many types of cells are used for cell culture techniques like mesenchymal stem cells (MSCs), embryonic stem cells (ESCs), adult stem cells, and induced pluripotent stem cells (iPSCs). The efficacy of the scaffold depends on the ability of the material to differentiate the seeded cells from bone cells which is essential for adequate scaffold-bone integration. MSCs are multipotent cells which have the ability to differentiate into different cell types like osteoblasts, adipocytes, or chondrocytes and have become the favourite source of cell-based therapy (Hu, L. et al., 2018).

6. In vitro and in vivo Evaluation of 3D-printed Composite Scaffolds for Bone Tissue Engineering

6.1 In vitro Cell Culture Studies

In vitro is the study of the biological behaviours of implants and their interaction with host tissue under a controlled atmosphere rather than living bodies. The main goal of in vitro studies is to understand/predict future responses in vivo. The in-vitro studies confirm the cytotoxicity of samples. Standard protocols should be followed to confirm the acceptance of testing material. The International Organization for Standardization (ISO) standard is usually followed to test biomedical devices and scaffolds. ISO 10993 explains the procedures to be followed while testing a biomedical device or material. In this standard, section 1 explains the procedures for biocompatibility testing of devices, section 3 explains the procedure to test genotoxicity, carcinogenicity and reproductive toxicity, and section 5 explains the cytotoxicity testing methods. The cytotoxicity can be carried out by two different methods, direct and indirect. Direct cytotoxicity is observed as harmful to cell growth by the direct contact of implantation. Indirect cytotoxicity is also known as the agar diffusion test. The cells are seeded into the samples containing plates and sterilized for growing confluent. This result, indicates the leeching of substances from the tested objects due to the cytotoxic effects (Li, W. et al., 2015). Wang et al., 2022 compared the direct and indirect cytotoxicity assays for a SLM 3D printed lattice structure made of SS316L material. The indirect assay demonstrated greater cell viability 20-30% more efficient than the direct cytotoxicity assay, caused due to potentially harmful effects caused by the direct exposure to high dosages (Wang, N. et al., 2022). Furthermore, cell proliferation, cell adhesion, and differentiation assays can be conducted in in-vitro studies. Hassanajili et al., 2019 conducted cytotoxicity to confirm the cell viability and proliferation on the prepared samples (Hassanajili, S. et al., 2019).

6.2 *In vivo Animal Studies*

Unlike In vitro, in vivo analyses are carried out on living animals. In vivo analyses are mandatory before experimenting with the samples on humans and the results should be positive. The In vivo tests usually assess the interaction with blood, the effect of the implant on the implant site, identify and quantify degradation products, skin irritation sensitization and material toxicity. These are explained in ISO 10993 sections 4, 6, 9, 10 and 11 respectively. Usually, the tests are carried out on rats, rabbits, mice, pigs, and sheep. Animal selection is based on the condition that it should be appropriate as an analogue to humans, transferability of information, genetic uniformity, information on biological properties, cost and availability, ease of generalization and adaptation, ecological effects and ethical implications (Davidson, M.K. et al., 1987). A study conducted on sheep using a HAP scaffold revealed that the defects were completely cured in 4 months. The micro CT scan indicates that void spaces were completely filled with new bone ingrowths as shown in Figure 4 (Lovati, A.V. 2016). The addition of collagen and CNT to the HAP could improve the healing capacity as the defects were cured within 12 weeks in an experiment conducted on rat bones (Jing, A. 2017).

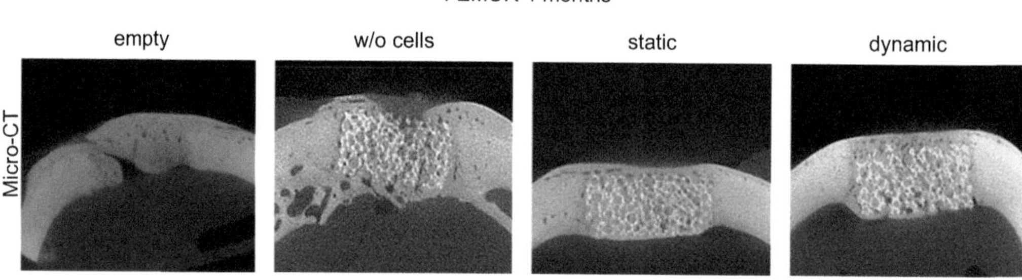

Fig. 4 New bone ingrowth on HAP scaffold inserted on sheep after 4 months (Lovati, A.B. 2016)

Treatment of spinal defects using spongy and porous titanium alloy (Ti6Al4V) + apatite composite scaffold developed using the SLS technique on sheep proved effective as it cured the defect but took 6 months to do so (Vlad, M.D. 2020). The longer period indicates that metals are not as effective as ceramic counterparts but are essential in the case of load-bearing applications. After in vivo analysis, clinical trials are carried out to confirm the efficacy of the technique on humans.

6.3 *Clinical Trials*

Clinical trials are those studies which focus on the safety and efficacy of a product on human beings. This could be either in vitro or in vivo. The In vivo clinical trials of 3D printed bone scaffolds are not common yet. The main reason is that the 3D printing technology is still in its infancy period and great leaps are required in optimizing the printing parameters. The accuracy and precision are very important for bone scaffolds which is not yet achieved in additive manufacturing technologies. Collagen, HAP and TCP scaffolds are more familiar in clinical trials than other materials mentioned above (Zeng, J.H. 2018). The reason for this is that these materials are basic constituents of natural bone and are FDA-approved while some others are not like $CaSiO_3$ even though their bioactivities are proven at the laboratory level (Gillman, C.E. et al., 2021).

Conclusion

Additive manufacturing has emerged as a pathbreaking technique in tissue engineering which is capable of handling patient-specific designs with great precision and scalability. It has evolved from scaffold fabrication to the bioprinting of complex tissue structures and organs. It has revolutionized the research in the tissue engineering field quickly. Innovations in biomaterials research along with improvements in the precision and accuracy of 3D printing techniques will bring great achievements to mankind and engineered tissues will be a reality in the near future. However, the emphasis should not be only on the replication of bone to treat but on finding better materials that can cure the defects easily. The clinical trials on 3D-printed bone scaffolds could shed light on and navigate us in the right direction in material selection and manufacturing methods.

References

Adel, I.M., Elmeligy, M.F. and Elkasabgy, N.A. "Conventional and Recent Trends of Scaffolds Fabrication : A Superior Mode for Tissue Engineering," 2022.

Agarwal, S., Saha, S., Balla, V.K., Pal, A., Barui, A. et al, "Current Developments in 3D Bioprinting for Tissue and Organ Regeneration–A Review," *Front. Mech. Eng.*, vol. 6, no. October, 2020, doi: 10.3389/FMECH.2020.589171.

Albrektsson, T. and Johansson, C. "Osteoinduction, osteoconduction and osseointegration," *Eur. Spine J.*, vol. 10, pp. S96–S101, 2001, doi: 10.1007/s005860100282.

An, J., Teoh, J.E.M., Suntornnond, R. and Chua, C.K. "Design and 3D Printing of Scaffolds and Tissues," *Engineering*, vol. 1, no. 2, pp. 261–268, 2015, doi: 10.15302/J-ENG-2015061.

Baino, F., Novajra, G. and Vitale-Brovarone, C. "Bioceramics and scaffolds: A winning combination for tissue engineering," *Front. Bioeng. Biotechnol.*, vol. 3, no. December, pp. 1–17, 2015, doi: 10.3389/fbioe.2015.00202.

Baker, B. "Development of a slurry injection technique for continuous fibre ultra-high temperature ceramic matrix composites," *J. Eur. Ceram. Soc.*, vol. 39, no. 14, pp. 3927–3937, 2019, doi: 10.1016/j.jeurceramsoc.2019.05.070.

Barbagallo, R., Di Bella, S., Mirone, G. and La Rosa, G. "Study of the Electron Beam Melting Process Parameters' Influence on the Tensile Behavior of 3D Printed Ti6Al4V ELI Alloy in Static and Dynamic Conditions," 2022.

Barradas, A.M.C., Yuan, H., Blitterswijk, C.A. van and Habibovic, P. "Osteoinductive biomaterials: current knowledge of properties, experimental models and biological mechanisms.," *Eur. Cell. Mater.*, vol. 21, pp. 407–429, 2011, doi: 10.22203/eCM.v021a31.

Beek, M. van, Weeks, A., Jones, L. and Sheardown, H. "Immobilized hyaluronic acid containing model silicone hydrogels reduce protein adsorption," *J. Biomater. Sci. Polym. Ed.*, vol. 19, no. 11, pp. 1425–1436, Jan. 2008, doi: 10.1163/156856208786140364.

Bhandari, S. "Trends and Challenges in the Development of 3D-Printed Heart Valves and Other Cardiac Implants: A Review of Current Advances.," *Cureus*, vol. 15, no. 8, p. e43204, Aug. 2023, doi: 10.7759/cureus.43204.

Bi, L., Cheng, W., Fan, H. and Pei, G. "Reconstruction of goat tibial defects using an injectable tricalcium phosphate/chitosan in combination with autologous platelet-rich plasma," *Biomaterials*, vol. 31, no. 12, pp. 3201–3211, 2010, doi: https://doi.org/10.1016/j.biomaterials.2010.01.038.

Calignano, F. "Design optimization of supports for overhanging structures in aluminum and titanium alloys by selective laser melting," *Mater. Des.*, vol. 64, pp. 203–213, 2014, doi: https://doi.org/10.1016/j.matdes.2014.07.043.

Cao, Q. "Improvement of calcium phosphate scaffold osteogenesis in vitro via combination of glutamate-modified BMP-2 peptides," *Mater. Sci. Eng. C*, vol. 96, no. October 2018, pp. 412–418, 2019, doi: 10.1016/j.msec.2018.11.048.

Čapek, J. "Highly porous, low elastic modulus 316L stainless steel scaffold prepared by selective laser melting," *Mater. Sci. Eng. C*, vol. 69, pp. 631–639, 2016, doi: 10.1016/j.msec.2016.07.027.

Chakraborty, S. and Pimentel, C.J.M., "Bentonite reinforced chitosan scaffold: Effect of bentonite exfoliation on scaffold properties," *Philipp. J. Sci.*, vol. 149, no. 4, pp. 1127–1133, 2020, doi: 10.56899/149.04.11.

Chen, Y.W., Hsu, T.T., Wang, K. and Shie, M.Y. "Preparation of the fast setting and degrading Ca-Si-Mg cement with both odontogenesis and angiogenesis differentiation of human periodontal ligament cells," *Mater. Sci. Eng. C*, vol. 60, pp. 374–383, 2016, doi: 10.1016/j.msec.2015.11.064.

Choren, J.A., Heinrich, S.M. and Silver-thorn, B. "Young's modulus and volume porosity relationships for additive manufacturing applications Young's modulus and volume porosity relationships for additive manufacturing applications," no. December, 2013, doi: 10.1007/s10853-013-7237-5.

Cohn, M.R., Unnanuntana, A., Pannu, T.J., Warner, S.J. and Lane J.M. et al, "7.16 Materials in Fracture Fixation," *Compr. Biomater. II*, pp. 278–297, Jan. 2017, doi: 10.1016/B978-0-12-803581-8.10109-2.

"Committee F42 on Additive Manufacturing Technologies." https://www.astm.org/committee-f42 (accessed Mar. 18, 2024).

Court-Brown, C.M. "External casting of diaphyseal fractures of the tibia and fibula," *Curr. Orthop.*, vol. 12, no. 4, pp. 262–272, 1998, doi: https://doi.org/10.1016/S0268-0890(98)90046-9.

Davidson, M.K., Lindsey, J.R. and Davis, J.K. "Requirements and selection of an animal model.," *Isr. J. Med. Sci.*, vol. 23, no. 6, pp. 551–555, Jun. 1987.

de Camargo, I.L., Fortulan, C.A. and Colorado, H.A. "A review on the ceramic additive manufacturing technologies and availability of equipment and materials," *Ceramica*, vol. 68, no. 387, pp. 329–347, 2022, doi: 10.1590/0366-69132022683873331.

Deb, P., Deoghare, A.B., Borah, A., Barua, E. and Das Lala S. et al, "Scaffold Development Using Biomaterials: A Review," *Mater. Today Proc.*, vol. 5, no. 5, pp. 12909–12919, 2018, doi: 10.1016/j.matpr.2018.02.276.

"Defining Additive Manufacturing | Symmetry Electronics," 2022.

Deng, F., Zhai, W., Yin, Y., Peng, C. and Ning, C. et al, "Advanced protein adsorption properties of a novel silicate-based bioceramic: A proteomic analysis," *Bioact. Mater.*, vol. 6, no. 1, pp. 208–218, 2021, doi: 10.1016/j.bioactmat.2020.08.011.

Ding, Z., Xi, W., Ji, M., Chen, H., Zhang, Q. et al, "Developing a biodegradable tricalcium silicate/glucono-delta-lactone/calcium sulfate calcium sulfate dihydrate composite cement with high preliminary mechanical property for bone filling," *Mater. Sci. Eng. C*, vol. 119, no. March 2020, p. 111621, 2021, doi: 10.1016/j.msec.2020.111621.

Du, X. Wei, D. Huang, L. Zhu, M. Zhang Y. et al, "3D printing of mesoporous bioactive glass/silk fibroin composite scaffolds for bone tissue engineering," *Mater. Sci. Eng. C*, vol. 103, no. May, p. 109731, 2019, doi: 10.1016/j.msec.2019.05.016.

Feng, P., Wei, P., Li, P., Gao, C., Shuai, C., et al, , "Calcium silicate ceramic scaffolds toughened with hydroxyapatite whiskers for bone tissue engineering," *Mater. Charact.*, vol. 97, pp. 47–56, 2014, doi: 10.1016/j.matchar.2014.08.017.

Fisher, J.P., Mikos, A.G. and Bronzino, J.D. "Tissue Engineering," *Science (80-.).*, pp. 1–583, Jan. 1993, doi: 10.1126/SCIENCE.8493529.

Fomby P. "Stem cells and cell therapies in lung biology and diseases: Conference report," *Ann. Am. Thorac. Soc.*, vol. 12, no. 3, pp. 181–204, 2010, doi: 10.1002/term.

Fraile-martínez, O. "Applications of polymeric composites in bone tissue engineering and jawbone regeneration," *Polymers (Basel).*, vol. 13, no. 19, pp. 1–17, 2021, doi: 10.3390/polym13193429.

Gao, C., Feng, P., Peng, S. and Shuai, C. "Carbon nanotube, graphene and boron nitride nanotube reinforced bioactive ceramics for bone repair," *Acta Biomater.*, vol. 61, pp. 1–20, 2017, doi: https://doi.org/10.1016/j.actbio.2017.05.020.

Geetha., M., S. A.K, A. R, and Gogia, A.K. "Ti based biomaterials , the ultimate choice for orthopaedic implants – A review," *Prog. Mater. Sci.*, vol. 54, no. 3, pp. 397–425, 2009, doi: 10.1016/j.pmatsci.2008.06.004.

Ghassemi, T., Shahroodi, A., Ebrahimzadeh, M.H., Mousavian, A. Movaffagh, J. et al, "Current concepts in scaffolding for bone tissue engineering," *Archives of Bone and Joint Surgery*, vol. 6, no. 2. pp. 90–99, 2018. doi: 10.22038/abjs.2018.26340.1713.

Gillman, C.E. and Jayasuriya, A.C. "FDA-approved bone grafts and bone graft substitute devices in bone regeneration," *Mater. Sci. Eng. C*, vol. 130, no. July, p. 112466, 2021, doi: 10.1016/j.msec.2021.112466.

Golafshan, N. "Tough magnesium phosphate-based 3D-printed implants induce bone regeneration in an equine defect model," *Biomaterials*, vol. 261, no. February, 2020, doi: 10.1016/j.biomaterials.2020.120302.

Graziani, G. "Ionized jet deposition of antimicrobial and stem cell friendly silver-substituted tricalcium phosphate nanocoatings on titanium alloy," *Bioact. Mater.*, vol. 6, no. 8, pp. 2629–2642, 2021, doi: 10.1016/j.bioactmat.2020.12.019.

Guo, S. "Fiber size effects on mechanical behaviours of SiC fibres-reinforced Ti3AlC2 matrix composites," *J. Eur. Ceram. Soc.*, vol. 37, no. 15, pp. 5099–5104, 2017, doi: 10.1016/j.jeurceramsoc.2017.07.023.

H., T.-T. and H., C.-C., Kao, Chia-Tze, Chen, Yen-Jen, Huang, Tsui-Hsien et al, "Assessment of the Release Profile of Fibroblast Growth Factor-2-Load Mesoporous Calcium Silicate/Poly-ε-caprolactone 3D Scaffold for Regulate Bone Regeneration," 2020.

Haleem, A., Javaid, M., Khan, R.H. and Suman, R. "3D printing applications in bone tissue engineering," *J. Clin. Orthop. Trauma*, vol. 11, no. December, pp. S118–S124, 2020, doi: 10.1016/j.jcot.2019.12.002.

Hassanajili, S., Karami-Pour, A., Oryan, A. and Talaei-Khozani, T. "Preparation and characterization of PLA/PCL/HA composite scaffolds using indirect 3D printing for bone tissue engineering," *Mater. Sci. Eng. C*, vol. 104, no. July, p. 109960, 2019, doi: 10.1016/j.msec.2019.109960.

Hu, L., Yin, C., Zhao, F., Ali, A., Ma, J. et al, "Mesenchymal Stem Cells: Cell Fate Decision to Osteoblast or Adipocyte and Application in Osteoporosis Treatment.," *Int. J. Mol. Sci.*, vol. 19, no. 2, Jan. 2018, doi: 10.3390/ijms19020360.

Hu, X., Zhang, W. and Hou, D. "Synthesis, microstructure and mechanical properties of tricalcium phosphate – hydroxyapatite (TCP/HA) composite ceramic," *Ceram. Int.*, vol. 46, no. 7, pp. 9810–9816, 2020, doi: 10.1016/j.ceramint.2019.12.254.

Huang, J. "Design and Development of Ceramics and Glasses," A. Vishwakarma and J.M.B. T.-B. and E. of S.C.N. Karp, Eds. Boston: Academic Press, 2017, pp. 315–329. doi: https://doi.org/10.1016/B978-0-12-802734-9.00020-2.

Huang, Y.-Z., Xie, H.-Q. and Li, X. *Scaffolds in Bone Tissue Engineering: Research Progress and Current Applications*. Elsevier Inc., 2020. doi: 10.1016/b978-0-12-801238-3.11205-x.

Ishikawa, K., Matsuya, S., Miyamoto, Y. and Kawate, K. "9.05 - Bioceramics," *Compr. Struct. Integr. Nine Vol. Set*, vol. 1–9, pp. 169–214, 2003, doi: 10.1016/B0-08-043749-4/09146-1.

Janssens, K., Ten Dijke, P., Janssens, S. and Van Hul, W. "Transforming growth factor-β1 to the bone," *Endocr. Rev.*, vol. 26, no. 6, pp. 743–774, 2005, doi: 10.1210/er.2004-0001.

Jing, Z. "Carbon Nanotube Reinforced Collagen/Hydroxyapatite Scaffolds Improve Bone Tissue Formation In Vitro and In Vivo," *Ann. Biomed. Eng.*, vol. 45, no. 9, pp. 2075–2087, 2017, doi: 10.1007/s10439-017-1866-9.

Jirofti, N., Hashemi, M., Moradi, A. and Kalalinia, F. "Fabrication and characterization of 3D printing biocompatible crocin-loaded chitosan/collagen/hydroxyapatite-based scaffolds for bone tissue engineering applications," *Int. J. Biol. Macromol.*, vol. 252, no. April, p. 126279, 2023, doi: 10.1016/j.ijbiomac.2023.126279.

Jonoobi, M., Harun, J., Mathew, A.P. and Oksman, K. "Mechanical properties of cellulose nanofiber (CNF) reinforced polylactic acid (PLA) prepared by twin screw extrusion," *Compos. Sci. Technol.*, vol. 70, no. 12, pp. 1742–1747, Oct. 2010, doi: 10.1016/J.COMPSCITECH.2010.07.005.

Kalsoom, U., Nesterenko, P.N. and Paull, B. "3," *RSC Adv.*, vol. 6, no. 65, pp. 60355–60371, 2016, doi: 10.1039/c6ra11334f.

Kemppi, H. "Design and development of poly-L/D-lactide copolymer and barium titanate nanoparticle 3D composite scaffolds using breath figure method for tissue engineering applications," *Colloids Surfaces B Biointerfaces*, vol. 199, 2021, doi: 10.1016/j.colsurfb.2020.111530.

Kiany, F. "Bone repair potential of collagen-poly(3-hydroxybutyrate)-carbon nanotubes scaffold loaded with mesenchymal stem cells for the reconstruction of critical-sized mandibular defects," *J. Stomatol. Oral Maxillofac. Surg.*, vol. 125, no. 2, p. 101670, 2024, doi: https://doi-org.egateway.vit.ac.in/10.1016/j.jormas.2023.101670.

Kim, H.S., Sun, X., Lee, J.H., Kim, H.W., Fu, X. et al. "Advanced drug delivery systems and artificial skin grafts for skin wound healing," *Adv. Drug Deliv. Rev.*, vol. 146, pp. 209–239, 2019, doi: 10.1016/j.addr.2018.12.014.

Kumar, A. "Effect of crosslinking functionality on microstructure, mechanical properties, and in vitro cytocompatibility of cellulose nanocrystals reinforced poly (vinyl alcohol)/sodium alginate hybrid scaffolds," *Int. J. Biol. Macromol.*, vol. 95, pp. 962–973, Feb. 2017, doi: 10.1016/J.IJBIOMAC.2016.10.085.

Lamnini, S., Elsayed, H., Lakhdar, Y., Baino, F., Smeacetto, F. et al, "Robocasting of advanced ceramics : ink optimization and protocol to predict the printing parameters-A review Heliyon Robocasting of advanced ceramics : ink optimization and protocol to predict the printing parameters-A review," *Heliyon*, no. September, p. e10651, 2022, doi: 10.1016/j.heliyon.2022.e10651.

Lawton, K., Le, H., Tredwin, C. and Handy, R.D. "Carbon nanotube reinforced hydroxyapatite nanocomposites as bone implants: Nanostructure, mechanical strength and biocompatibility," *International Journal of Nanomedicine*, vol. 14. pp. 7947–7962, 2019. doi: 10.2147/IJN.S218248.

Li, W., Zhou, J. and Xu, Y. "Study of the in vitro cytotoxicity testing of medical devices," *Biomed. reports*, vol. 3, no. 5, pp. 617–620, Sep. 2015, doi: 10.3892/br.2015.481.

Li, Z., Khun, N.W., Tang, X.Z., Liu, E. and Khor, K.A. et al, "Mechanical, tribological and biological properties of novel 45S5 Bioglass® composites reinforced with in situ reduced graphene oxide," *J. Mech. Behav. Biomed. Mater.*, vol. 65, pp. 77–89, 2017, doi: 10.1016/j.jmbbm.2016.08.007.

Lim, H.K. "3D-printed ceramic bone scaffolds with variable pore architectures," *Int. J. Mol. Sci.*, vol. 21, no. 18, pp. 1–12, 2020, doi: 10.3390/ijms21186942.

Lin, S., Chen, C., Cai, X. and Yang, F. "The concentrations of bone calcium , phosphorus and trace metal elements in elderly patients with intertrochanteric hip fractures," no. December, pp. 1–12, 2022, doi: 10.3389/fendo.2022.1005637.

Lin, Y., Lee, A.K., Ho, C., Fang, M. and Kuo, T. et al, "The effects of a 3D-printed magnesium-/strontium-doped calcium silicate scaffold on regulation of bone regeneration via dual-stimulation of the AKT and WNT signaling pathways," *Mater. Sci. Eng. C*, no. August 2021, p. 112660, 2022, doi: 10.1016/j.msec.2022.112660.

Liu, H., Yazici, H., Ergun, C., Webster, T.J. and Bermek, H. et al, "An in vitro evaluation of the Ca/P ratio for the cytocompatibility of nano-to-micron particulate calcium phosphates for bone regeneration," *Acta Biomater.*, vol. 4, no. 5, pp. 1472–1479, 2008, doi: https://doi-org.egateway.vit.ac.in/10.1016/j.actbio.2008.02.025.

Logeshwaran, A., Elsen, R. and Nayak, S. "Mechanical and biological characteristics of 3D fabricated clay mineral and bioceramic composite scaffold for bone tissue applications," *J. Mech. Behav. Biomed. Mater.*, vol. 138, no. October 2022, p. 105633, 2023, doi: 10.1016/j.jmbbm.2022.105633.

Logeshwaran, A., Srinivas, C. K., Venkatesh, V. and Nayak, S. (2023). Silk fibroin infilled 3D printed polymer-ceramic scaffold to enhance cell adhesion and cell viability. Materials Letters, 347, 134607.

Lopez-Heredia, M.A., Sohier, J., Gaillard, C., Quillard, S., Dorget, M. et al, "Rapid prototyped porous titanium coated with calcium phosphate as a scaffold for bone tissue engineering," *Biomaterials*, vol. 29, no. 17, pp. 2608–2615, 2008, doi: 10.1016/j.biomaterials.2008.02.021.

Lovati, A.B. "In Vivo Bone Formation With in Engineered Hydroxyapatite Scaffolds in a Sheep Model," *Calcif. Tissue Int.*, vol. 99, no. 2, pp. 209–223, 2016, doi: 10.1007/s00223-016-0140-8.

Lu, J. "The biodegradation mechanism of calcium phosphate biomaterials in bone," *J. Biomed. Mater. Res.*, vol. 63, no. 4, pp. 408–412, Jan. 2002, doi: 10.1002/JBM.10259.

Luu, H.H. "Distinct roles of bone morphogenetic proteins in osteogenic differentiation of mesenchymal stem cells," *J. Orthop. Res.*, vol. 25, no. 5, pp. 665–677, 2007, doi: 10.1002/jor.20359.

Ma, P.X. "Scaffolds for tissue fabrication," *Mater. Today*, vol. 7, no. 5, pp. 30–40, May 2004, doi: 10.1016/S1369-7021(04)00233-0.

Mateti, T., Jain, S., Ananda Shruthi, L., Laha, A. and Thakur, G. et al. "An overview of the advances in the 3D printing technology," *3D Print. Technol. Water Treat. Appl.*, pp. 1–37, Jan. 2023, doi: 10.1016/B978-0-323-99861-1.00002-3.

Migliorini, F., La Padula, G., Torsiello, E., Spiezia, F., Oliva, F. et al., "Strategies for large bone defect reconstruction after trauma, infections or tumour excision: a comprehensive review of the literature," *Eur. J. Med. Res.*, vol. 26, no. 1, pp. 1–11, 2021, doi: 10.1186/s40001-021-00593-9.

Mironov, V., Boland, T., Trusk, T., Forgacs, G. and Markwald, R.R. et al, "Organ printing: Computer-aided jet-based 3D tissue engineering," *Trends Biotechnol.*, vol. 21, no. 4, pp. 157–161, 2003, doi: 10.1016/S0167-7799(03)00033-7.

Mirzaali, M.J., Moosabeiki, V., Rajaai, S.M. and Zhou, J. "Additive Manufacturing of Biomaterials — Design Principles and Their Implementation," 2022.

Mirzaali, M.J., Moosabeiki, V., Rajaai, S.M., Zhou, J. and Zadpoor, A.A. et al, "Additive Manufacturing of Biomaterials—Design Principles and Their Implementation," *Materials (Basel).*, vol. 15, no. 15, 2022, doi: 10.3390/ma15155457.

Mohammadi Zerankeshi, M., Bakhshi, R. and Alizadeh, R. "Polymer/metal composite 3D porous bone tissue engineering scaffolds fabricated by additive manufacturing techniques: A review," *Bioprinting*, vol. 25, no. November 2021, p. e00191, 2022, doi: 10.1016/j.bprint.2022.e00191.

Mohammadi-zerankeshi M. and Alizadeh, R. "3D-printed PLA-Gr-Mg composite scaffolds for bone tissue engineering applications," *J. Mater. Res. Technol.*, vol. 22, pp. 2440–2446, 2022, doi: 10.1016/j.jmrt.2022.12.108.

Montanheiro, T.L.D.A. "Recent progress on polymer scaffolds production: Methods, main results, advantages and disadvantages," *Express Polym. Lett.*, vol. 16, no. 2, pp. 197–219, 2022, doi: 10.3144/EXPRESSPOLYMLETT.2022.16.

N'Gatta, K.M. "3D printing of cellulose nanocrystals based composites to build robust biomimetic scaffolds for bone tissue engineering," *Sci. Rep.*, vol. 12, no. 1, pp. 1–14, 2022, doi: 10.1038/s41598-022-25652-x.

Naeini, S.A., Naderinia, B. and Izadi, E. "Unconfined compressive strength of clayey soils stabilized with waterborne polymer," *KSCE J. Civ. Eng.*, vol. 16, no. 6, pp. 943–949, 2012, doi: 10.1007/s12205-012-1388-9.

Nandhakumar, R. and Venkatesan, K. *A process parameters review on selective laser melting-based additive manufacturing of single and multi-material : Microstructure, physical properties, tribological, and surface roughness*, vol. 35, no. February. Elsevier Ltd, 2023. doi: 10.1016/j.mtcomm.2023.105538.

Ning, J. "Synthesis and in vitro bioactivity of a borate-based bioglass," *Mater. Lett.*, vol. 61, no. 30, pp. 5223–5226, 2007, doi: 10.1016/j.matlet.2007.04.089.

Nouri, A., P. D. and We, C. "Biomimetic Porous Titanium Scaffolds for Orthopedic and Dental Applications," *Biomimetics Learn. from Nat.*, pp. 415–451, 2010, doi: 10.5772/8787.

Nuswantoro, N.F. "Hydroxyapatite coating on titanium alloy TNTZ for increasing osseointegration and reducing inflammatory response in vivo on Rattus norvegicus Wistar rats," *Ceram. Int.*, vol. 47, no. 11, pp. 16094–16100, 2021, doi: 10.1016/j.ceramint.2021.02.184.

Pahlevanzadeh, F., Emadi, R., Kharaziha, M., Poursamar, S.A., Nejatidanesh, F. et al, "Amorphous magnesium phosphate-graphene oxide nano particles laden 3D-printed chitosan scaffolds with enhanced osteogenic potential and antibacterial properties," *Biomater. Adv.*, vol. 158, no. December 2023, p. 213760, 2024, doi: 10.1016/j.bioadv.2024.213760.

Park, J.B. and Bronzino, J.D. *BIOMATERIALS: PRINCIPLES and APPLICATIONS*, 1st ed. CRC PRESS, 2002.

Patel, D.K., Dutta, S.D., Hexiu, J., Ganguly, K. and Lim, K.T. et al, "Bioactive electrospun nanocomposite scaffolds of poly(lactic acid)/cellulose nanocrystals for bone tissue engineering," *Int. J. Biol. Macromol.*, vol. 162, pp. 1429–1441, Nov. 2020, doi: 10.1016/J.IJBIOMAC.2020.07.246.

Peifen, M. "New skin tissue engineering scaffold with sulfated silk fibroin/chitosan/hydroxyapatite and its application," *Biochem. Biophys. Res. Commun.*, vol. 640, pp. 117–124, 2023, doi: https://doi-org.egateway.vit.ac.in/10.1016/j.bbrc.2022.11.086.

Polley, C. "3D printing of piezoelectric and bioactive barium titanate-bioactive glass scaffolds for bone tissue engineering." *Mater. Today Bio*, vol. 21, no. July, p. 100719, 2023, doi 10.1016/j.mtbio.2023.100719.

Pon-On, W., Suntornsaratoon, P., Charoenphandhu, N., Thongbunchoo, J., Krishnamra, N. et al, "Synthesis and investigations of mineral ions-loaded apatite from fish scale and PLA/chitosan composite for bone scaffolds," *Mater. Lett.*, vol. 221, pp. 143–146, Jun. 2018, doi: 10.1016/J.MATLET.2018.03.063.

Puthillam, U., Ravoor, J., Elsen Selvam, R., Karuppan, D., Bakthavachalam, B. et al, "Physical, mechanical, and biological characterization of robocasted carbon nanotube reinforced microwave sintered calcium phosphate scaffolds for bone tissue engineering," *J. Mech. Behav. Biomed. Mater.*, vol. 136, no. October, p. 105523, 2022, doi: 10.1016/j.jmbbm.2022.105523.

Qu, H. "Additive manufacturing for bone tissue engineering scaffolds," *Mater. Today Commun.*, vol. 24, no. February 2020, p. 101024, 2020, doi: 10.1016/j.mtcomm.2020.101024.

Rahman, M. "Optimization of Selective Laser Sintering Three-Dimensional Printing of Thermoplastic Polyurethane Elastomer : A Statistical Approach," 2023.

Raja, S. "Optimization of 3D Printing Process Parameters of Polylactic Acid Filament Based on the Mechanical Test," vol. 2022, 2022.

Ramezani, M. and Mohd Ripin, Z. "4D Printing in Biomedical Engineering: Advancements, Challenges, and Future Directions," *J. Funct. Biomater.*, vol. 14, no. 7, 2023, doi: 10.3390/jfb14070347.

Ravoor, J. and R.E. S, "A study on retention of MWCNT in robocasted MWCNT-HAP scaffold structures using vacuum sintering technique and their characteristics," *Ceram. Int.*, no. May, 2022, doi: 10.1016/j.ceramint.2022.06.204.

Ravoor, J. and Selvam, R.E. "Microwave sintering and characterization of robocasted HA, CNT-HA scaffold structures for bone regeneration applications," *Ceram. Int.*, vol. 49, no. 8, pp. 12585–12595, 2023, doi: 10.1016/j.ceramint.2022.12.121.

Ravoor, J., Selvam, R.E., Karuppan, D. and Puthillam, U. "Development of robocasted MWCNTS-calcium silicate 3D structures for bone regeneration applications with retention of MWCNTS using vacuum sintering technique," *J. Mater. Res.*, vol. 38, no. 9, pp. 2389–2400, 2023, doi: 10.1557/s43578-023-00968-0.

Romero, L., Guerrero, A., Espinosa, M.M., Jiménez, M., Domínguez I.A. et al. "Additive manufacturing with RepRap methodology: Current situation and future prospects," *25th Annu. Int. Solid Free. Fabr. Symp. � An Addit. Manuf. Conf. SFF 2014*, no. August, pp. 120–131, 2014.

Romli, D.P.P., Seprianto, M.Y.D. and Hasan, A.N. "Optimization of Production Process Parameters of DLP Type 3D Printer Design for Product Roughness Value," vol. 7, pp. 179–183, 2021.

Roohani-Esfahani, S.I., Newman, P. and Zreiqat, H. "Design and Fabrication of 3D printed Scaffolds with a Mechanical Strength Comparable to Cortical Bone to Repair Large Bone Defects," *Sci. Rep.*, vol. 6, no. February, 2016, doi: 10.1038/srep19468.

Sakthiabirami, K. "Hybrid porous zirconia scaffolds fabricated using additive manufacturing for bone tissue engineering applications," *Mater. Sci. Eng. C*, vol. 123, no. October 2020, p. 111950, 2021, doi: 10.1016/j.msec.2021.111950.

Schemitsch, E.H. "Size Matters: Defining Critical in Bone Defect Size!," *J. Orthop. Trauma*, vol. 31, 2017, (Online). Available: https://journals.lww.com/jorthotrauma/fulltext/2017/10005/size_matters__defining_critical_in_bone_defect.5.aspx

Schieker, M., Seitz, H., Drosse, I., Seitz, S. and Mutschler, W. et al, "Biomaterials as Scaffold for Bone Tissue Engineering," *Eur. J. Trauma*, vol. 32, no. 2, pp. 114–124, 2006, doi: 10.1007/s00068-006-6047-8.

Schmitz, J.P. and Hollinger, J.O. (1986). The critical size defect as an experimental model for craniomandibulofacial nonunions. Clinical Orthopaedics and Related Research (1976-2007), 205, 299–308.

Schubert, C., van Langeveld, M.C. and Donoso, L.A. "Innovations in 3D printing: a 3D overview from optics to organs.," *Br. J. Ophthalmol.*, vol. 98, no. 2, pp. 159–161, Feb. 2014, doi: 10.1136/bjophthalmol-2013-304446.

Shah, F.A., Trobos, M., Thomsen, P. and Palmquist, A. "Commercially pure titanium (cp-Ti) versus titanium alloy (Ti6Al4V) materials as bone anchored implants - Is one truly better than the other?," *Mater. Sci. Eng. C*, vol. 62, pp. 960–966, 2016, doi: 10.1016/j.msec.2016.01.032.

Shie, M., Chiang, W., Chen, I.P., Liu, W. and Chen, Y. et al, "Synergistic acceleration in the osteogenic and angiogenic differentiation of human mesenchymal stem cells by calcium silicate – graphene composites," *Mater. Sci. Eng. C*, vol. 73, pp. 726–735, 2017, doi: 10.1016/j.msec.2016.12.071.

Shuai, C. "A strawberry-like Ag-decorated barium titanate enhances piezoelectric and antibacterial activities of polymer scaffold," *Nano Energy*, vol. 74, no. April, p. 104825, 2020, doi: 10.1016/j.nanoen.2020.104825.

Shuai, C. "Laser rapid solidification improves corrosion behavior of Mg-Zn-Zr alloy," *J. Alloys Compd.*, vol. 691, pp. 961–969, 2017, doi: 10.1016/j.jallcom.2016.09.019.

Shuai, C., Gao, C., Feng, P. and Peng, S. "Graphene-reinforced mechanical properties of calcium silicate scaffolds by laser sintering," *RSC Adv.*, vol. 4, no. 25, pp. 12782–12788, 2014, doi: 10.1039/C3RA47862A.

Soh, E., Kolos, E. and Ruys, A.J. "Foamed high porosity alumina for use as a bone tissue scaffold," *Ceram. Int.*, vol. 41, no. 1, pp. 1031–1047, 2015, doi: 10.1016/j.ceramint.2014.09.026.

Stanciuc, A.M. "Robocast zirconia-toughened alumina scaffolds: Processing, structural characterisation and interaction with human primary osteoblasts," *J. Eur. Ceram. Soc.*, vol. 38, no. 3, pp. 845–853, 2018, doi: 10.1016/j.jeurceramsoc.2017.08.031.

Suamte, L., Tirkey, A., Barman, J. and Jayasekhar Babu, P. "Various manufacturing methods and ideal properties of scaffolds for tissue engineering applications," *Smart Mater. Manuf.*, vol. 1, no. November 2022, p. 100011, 2023, doi: 10.1016/j.smmf.2022.100011.

Sun, C. "The Promotion of Mechanical Properties by Bone Ingrowth in Additive-Manufactured Titanium Scaffolds," *J. Funct. Biomater.*, vol. 13, no. 3, 2022, doi: 10.3390/jfb13030127.

Sun, J. "A review on additive manufacturing of ceramic matrix composites," *J. Mater. Sci. Technol.*, vol. 138, pp. 1–16, 2023, doi: 10.1016/j.jmst.2022.06.039.

Tan, L., "3D printed PLGA/MgO/PDA composite scaffold by low-temperature deposition manufacturing for bone tissue engineering applications," *Regen. Ther.*, vol. 24, pp. 617–629, 2023, doi: 10.1016/j.reth.2023.09.015.

Tang, S. and Wang, W. "Preparation and characterization of a novel composite membrane of natural silk fiber/nano-hydroxyapatite/chitosan for guided bone tissue regeneration," *e-Polymers*, vol. 21, no. 1, pp. 671–680, 2021, doi: doi:10.1515/epoly-2021-0068.

Topuz, M., Dikici, B. and Gavgali, M. "Titanium-based composite scaffolds reinforced with hydroxyapatite-zirconia: Production, mechanical and in-vitro characterization," *J. Mech. Behav. Biomed. Mater.*, vol. 118, no. January, p. 104480, 2021, doi: 10.1016/j.jmbbm.2021.104480.

Tripathy, N., Perumal, E., Ahmad, R., Song, J.E. and Khang G. et al, *Hybrid Composite Biomaterials.* Elsevier Inc., 2018. doi: 10.1016/B978-0-12-809880-6.00040-0.

Tsai, C.H., Hung, C.H., Kuo, C.N., Chen, C.Y., Peng, Y.N. et al, "Improved bioactivity of 3D printed porous titanium alloy scaffold with chitosan/magnesium-calcium silicate composite for orthopaedic applications," *Materials (Basel).*, vol. 12, no. 2, 2019, doi: 10.3390/ma12020203.

Vargas, G.E. "Effect of nano-sized bioactive glass particles on the angiogenic properties of collagen based composites," *J. Mater. Sci. Mater. Med.*, vol. 24, no. 5, pp. 1261–1269, May 2013, doi: 10.1007/S10856-013-4892-7/METRICS.

Vlad, M.D. "Novel titanium-apatite hybrid scaffolds with spongy bone-like micro architecture intended for spinal application: In vitro and in vivo study," *Mater. Sci. Eng. C*, vol. 110, no. January, 2020, doi: 10.1016/j.msec.2020.110658.

Wang, N., Meenashisundaram, G.K., Chang, S., Fuh, J.Y.H., Dheen, S.T. et al, "A comparative investigation on the mechanical properties and cytotoxicity of Cubic, Octet, and TPMS gyroid structures fabricated by selective laser melting of stainless steel 316L," *J. Mech. Behav. Biomed. Mater.*, vol. 129, no. November 2021, p. 105151, 2022, doi: 10.1016/j.jmbbm.2022.105151.

Wang, W. "3D printing of lithium osteogenic bioactive composite scaffold for enhanced bone regeneration," *Compos. Part B Eng.*, vol. 256, no. February, p. 110641, 2023, doi 10.1016/j.compositesb.2023.110641.

Wang, W. "Fused Deposition Modeling Printed PLA/Nano β-TCP Composite Bone Tissue Engineering Scaffolds for Promoting Osteogenic Induction Function," *Int. J. Nanomedicine*, vol. 18, pp. 5815–5830, 2023, doi: 10.2147/IJN.S416098.

Wang, X. "Topological design and additive manufacturing of porous metals for bone scaffolds and orthopaedic implants: A review," *Biomaterials*, vol. 83, pp. 127–141, 2016, doi: 10.1016/j.biomaterials.2016.01.012.

Wei, L. "3D printing of silk fibroin-based hybrid scaffold treated with platelet rich plasma for bone tissue engineering," *Bioact. Mater.*, vol. 4, no. July 2019, pp. 256–260, 2019, doi: 10.1016/j.bioactmat.2019.09.001.

Weißmann, V., Bader, R., Hansmann, H. and Laufer, N. "Influence of the structural orientation on the mechanical properties of selective laser melted Ti6Al4V open-porous scaffolds," *Mater. Des.*, vol. 95, pp. 188–197, 2016, doi: 10.1016/j.matdes.2016.01.095.

Weng, T. "3D bioprinting for skin tissue engineering: Current status and perspectives," *J. Tissue Eng.*, vol. 12, no. 88, 2021, doi: 10.1177/20417314211028574.

Woodard, J.R. "The mechanical properties and osteoconductivity of hydroxyapatite bone scaffolds with multi-scale porosity," vol. 28, pp. 45–54, 2007, doi: 10.1016/j.biomaterials.2006.08.021.

Xu, J. "Incorporating strontium enriched amorphous calcium phosphate granules in collagen/collagen-magnesium-hydroxyapatite osteochondral scaffolds improves subchondral bone repair," *Mater. Today Bio*, vol. 25, p. 100959, 2024, doi: https://doi-org.egateway.vit.ac.in/10.1016/j.mtbio.2024.100959.

Xu, X. "Copper-modified Ti6Al4V alloy fabricated by selective laser melting with pro-angiogenic and anti-inflammatory properties for potential guided bone regeneration applications," *Mater. Sci. Eng. C*, vol. 90, no. April, pp. 198–210, 2018, doi: 10.1016/j.msec.2018.04.046.

Xu-bin, S.U., Yong-qiang, Y., Peng, Y.U. and Jian-feng, S.U.N. "Development of porous medical implant scaffolds via laser additive manufacturing," *Trans. Nonferrous Met. Soc. China*, vol. 22, pp. s181–s187, 2012, doi: 10.1016/S1003-6326(12)61706-3.

Yang, Y. "Additive manufacturing of bone scaffolds," *Int. J. Bioprinting*, vol. 5, no. 1, pp. 1–25, 2019, doi: 10.18063/IJB.v5i1.148.

Yang, Y. "Graphene-assisted barium titanate improves piezoelectric performance of biopolymer scaffold," *Mater. Sci. Eng. C*, vol. 116, no. May, p. 111195, 2020, doi: 10.1016/j.msec.2020.111195.

Yazdanpanah, Z., Johnston, J.D., Cooper, D.M.L. and Chen, X. "3D Bioprinted Scaffolds for Bone Tissue Engineering: State-Of-The-Art and Emerging Technologies," *Front. Bioeng. Biotechnol.*, vol. 10, no. April 2022, doi: 10.3389/fbioe.2022.824156.

Zeng, J.H. "Scaffolds for the repair of bone defects in clinical studies: a systematic review," *J. Orthop. Surg. Res.*, vol. 13, no. 1, Feb. 2018, doi: 10.1186/S13018-018-0724-2.

Zhang, D., Wu, X., Chen, J. and Lin, K. "The development of collagen based composite scaffolds for bone regeneration," *Bioact. Mater.*, vol. 3, no. 1, pp. 129–138, 2018, doi: https://doi.org/10.1016/j.bioactmat.2017.08.004.

Zhang, H., "Three dimensional printed macroporous polylactic acid/hydroxyapatite composite scaffolds for promoting bone formation in a critical-size rat calvarial defect model," *Sci. Technol. Adv. Mater.*, vol. 17, no. 1, pp. 136–148, 2016, doi: 10.1080/14686996.2016.1145532.

Zhang, J. "Zirconia toughened hydroxyapatite biocomposite formed by a DLP 3D printing process for potential bone tissue engineering," *Mater. Sci. Eng. C*, vol. 105, no. August, p. 110054, 2019, doi: 10.1016/j.msec.2019.110054.

Zhang, Y., Wu, C., Friis, T. and Xiao, Y. "The osteogenic properties of CaP/silk composite scaffolds," *Biomaterials*, vol. 31, no. 10, pp. 2848–2856, 2010, doi: https://doi.org/10.1016/j.biomaterials.2009.12.049.

Zheng, Y.F., Gu, X.N. and Witte, F. "Biodegradable metals," *Mater. Sci. Eng. R Reports*, vol. 77, pp. 1–34, 2014, doi: 10.1016/j.mser.2014.01.001.

Zhu, C. "Titanium-interlayer mediated hydroxyapatite coating on polyetheretherketone: a prospective study in patients with single-level cervical degenerative disc disease," *J. Transl. Med.*, vol. 19, no. 1, pp. 1–8, 2021, doi: 10.1186/s12967-020-02688-z.

19

3D Bioprinted Organs for Toxicity Evaluation

*Manjoosha RY,[1] Greeshma N,[1] Megha KB,[2] Mohanan PV[2] and Renu John[1]**

1. Introduction

Drug toxicity evaluation is a crucial step in the drug development process, wherein different processes such as dose selection, primary and secondary toxicity, genotoxicity, reproductive and developmental toxicity are investigated. Toxicity to tissues and safety concerns, in addition to basic interspecies differences between animals and humans, are the primary causes of high failure rates in clinical trials of potential drugs. 96% of the developed drugs fail during initial clinical trials, and the probability of failure is even higher if the diseases are not well studied, target new mechanisms of action, or the cure has not been developed yet (Hingorani et al., 2019; Szűcs et al., 2023). Assessment of drug potency and safety requires a thorough, long term and accurate analysis. Though there have been several advances in the pharmaceutical industry, the high attrition rate remains the primary reason for the high cost and time involved in pharmaceutical research (Waring et al., 2015).

The major organs involved in toxicological evaluation of drugs are the liver, kidney, heart, blood vessels, brain, skin, and other tissues. The existing practices rely on *in vitro* cell culture analysis and animal studies. Traditional 2D cell culture models have several shortcomings – the major factor being that the nutrient medium is static (is at rest) and uniform, and that multiple biochemical and physical culture conditions cannot be studied simultaneously. Also, other parameters such as the vascularization and extent of diffusion of signaling molecules/nutrients cannot be replicated. The resultant cell morphology is unnatural, with altered signalling behaviour, often accompanied by loss of tissue specific functions and tissue complexity, thus making the model physiologically less relevant. To date, animal models are the gold standard for preclinical drug evaluation, wherein experimental animals like mice, rabbits, and monkeys are used. These models offer physiological similarity to humans, allowing us to observe them as a complete complex entity. It is thus possible

[1] Department of Biomedical Engineering, Indian Institute of Technology Hyderabad, Sangareddy, India.
[2] Division of Toxicology, Sree Chitra Tirunal Institute of Medical Science and Technology, Thiruvananthapuram, India.
* Corresponding author: renujohn@bme.iith.ac.in

to study biological processes and disease conditions while mimicking human conditions. Animal studies are often expensive, time-consuming, require specialized facilities and expertise, and are subject to ethical concerns.

3D bioprinting is a method that involves automated and spatially controlled deposition of cells, biomaterials or cell-contained biomaterials (known as bioink) in defined three-dimensional patterns (Roskos et al., 2015). Based on the working principles, there are several 3D bioprinting techniques, namely, inkjet printing, extrusion bioprinting, laser polymerization-based bioprinting, and digital light processing-based printing. Several natural-derived and synthetic biomaterials have been employed in bioprinting, including alginate, gelatin, collagen, chitosan, agarose, fibrin, hyaluronic acid, polyethylene glycol, and polyurethane (Fu et al., 2022). The important considerations for the bioprinting method and biomaterials used include sterility, compatibility with the cellular support, feature size and shape, cell transfer efficiency and post-print cell viability (Nguyen and Pentoney, 2017).

With the advances in 3D bioprinting and microfabrication strategies, it is now possible to develop 3D tissue and organ models with greater structural complexity. These models are designed to replicate the *in vivo* conditions, mimicking the native tissue architecture, allowing for cell-cell and cell-microenvironment interactions, thus providing physiologically relevant models to study drug interactions. An extension of these 3D models are the organ-on-a-chip and multi-organ-on-chip devices, which use microfluidic technology to integrate different organs, while mimicking physiological fluid flow, barrier functions and the biochemical microenvironment thus providing high throughput 3D models to evaluate toxicological response to dose-dependent drug treatment. (Fitzgerald et al., 2015). In the following sections, an overview of some exclusive 3D printed tissue/organ models for toxicological evaluation is provided, followed by a discussion on the challenges associated with them.

2.   Organs in Toxicity Evaluation

As mentioned previously, one of the primary reasons for the high failure rates of new drugs during pre-clinical trials is due to the insufficient understanding of fundamental human pathophysiological mechanisms. 3D models that can closely mimic the tissue microarchitecture and physiological functions can provide a better understanding of the underlying phenomena in a controllable and traceable manner, relative to 2D and animal models (C. Ma et al., 2021). Toxic effects of drug products can potentially affect various organs, but the most commonly investigated organs include liver, heart, kidney and skin. The liver and kidney also play a significant role in the processing and excretion of the drug metabolites after administration. Figure 1 represents the various toxicity evaluation methods for polymers employed in 3D printing techniques (Anju et al., 2020). This section presents several studies on toxicological evaluation of drug effects on these organs, with a special focus on 3D bioprinted organ models.

2.1   Liver

The liver, the largest solid organ in the human body, is the primary site for metabolism and detoxification of initial doses of drugs, contaminants and xenobiotics. The hepatic lobule is its basic structural unit, which is made of hexagonally organized hepatocytes perforated with the liver sinusoid network. Nutrient and oxygen-rich blood enter the liver through the portal vein and hepatic artery, respectively, and based on the spatial location along the portal vein axis, the hepatic functions are highly specialized. Parameters such as liver zonation, shear stress due to hepatic blood flow through the sinusoids, and cross-talk between hepatocytes, sinusoidal endothelial cells, Kupffer cells and hepatic stellate cells affect the various hepatic functions (Malarkey et al., 2005). The heterogeneity and specificity of various cells lead to more than 500 vital functions being associated with the liver (Messelmani et al., 2022).

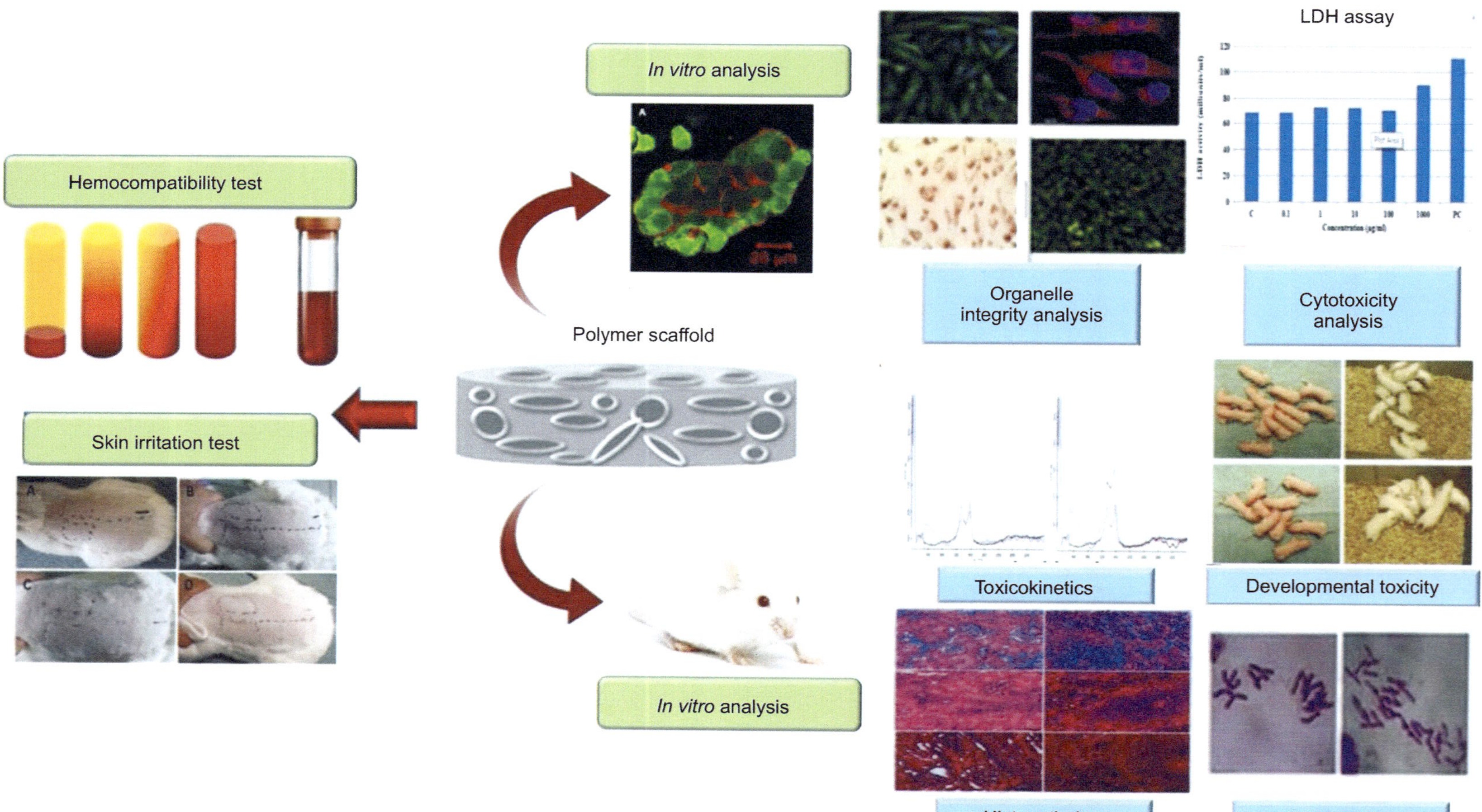

Fig. 1   Toxicity evaluation techniques for polymers used in 3D bioprinting. Reproduced with permission (Anju et al., 2020).

Hepatotoxicity is one of the major safety concerns for the pharmaceutical industry. Drug-induced liver injury and adverse drug reactions are the causes of high attrition rates of new drugs, and post-marketing withdrawals (Hay et al., 2014; Stevens and Baker, 2009). 3D *in vitro* liver models can replicate the complex architecture and cellular diversity of the liver, and thus offer a superior option compared to monolayer cultures for hepatotoxicity testing. Different biomaterials such as alginate, gelatin, hyaluronan, collagen, and gelatin methacryloyl (GelMA) in various combinations, and various cell sources such as primary and stem-cell derived hepatocytes, non-parenchymal cells (like Kupffer and stellate cells) and liver cancer cell lines have been reported to be used for creating biomimetic 3D liver structures (L. Ma et al., 2020; Xiang et al., 2022).

There have been several reports of the fabrication of 3D bioprinted liver tissue models with the purpose of replicating the hepatic lobular and vascular architecture (Kang et al., 2020; C. Yu et al., 2019), for liver regeneration (Yang et al., 2021). In addition to understanding the physiological processes, 3D-printed liver tissues have also been developed for modeling liver diseases and drug-induced hepatotoxicity. Ma et al. (2015) developed a 3D bioprinted model with human induced pluripotent stem cells (hiPSCs)-derived hepatic cells and supporting cells into a liver lobule model. The expression of key enzymes involved in drug metabolism, with and without the presence of hepatotoxic agents were compared and analyzed (X. Ma et al., 2016). Ngyuyen et al. (2016) developed a bioprinted human liver tissue with a defined architecture, composed of patient-derived hepatocytes and non-parenchymal cells (endothelial and hepatic stellate cells) for studying drug-induced liver injury. Herein, the dose-response of a potential hepatotoxic drug Trovafloxacin and structurally-related non-toxic drug Levofloxacin were compared. Based on histological, biochemical and metabolic characterization, it was observed that Trovafloxacin induced significant toxicity at clinically relevant doses (Nguyen et al., 2016). Schmidt et al. (2020) developed an alginate/gelatin/Matrigel-based 3D printed liver tissue model to analyze the cytotoxicity of aflatoxin B1 (Schmidt et al., 2020). Similarly, Massa et al. (2017) developed a vascularized GelMA-based 3D liver model with perfusions and an endothelial layer that acts as a barrier for the diffusion of nutrients and drugs. This model has been evaluated for acetaminophen toxicity, which is known to affect the sinusoidal endothelial cells (Massa et al., 2017). Hong and Song (2021) developed a 3D-bioprinting based HepG2 liver spheroid culture model, and compared it with 2D culture models for assessing nefazodone-induced hepatotoxicity. It was observed that the 3D spheroids were more resistant to the nefazodone-induced mitochondrial permeability transition, indicating that the 3D culture system provides enhanced resistance to hepatotoxic drugs (Hong and Song, 2021).

Drug and chemical exposure, metabolic disease or alcoholism can result in liver fibrosis, leading to stiffening of the liver causing cirrhosis and failure. Norona et al. (2016) developed a 3D bioprinted liver tissue model with hepatic and non-parenchymal cells to analyze drug-induced fibrosis. The tissues were treated with methotrexate and thioacetamide, which are known fibrogenic compounds, and the fibrogenic responses at histological, cellular, and molecular levels were observed (Norona et al., 2016). Further, the tissue model was exposed to methotrexate for 28 days, to analyze the role of Kupffer cells in fibrogenesis (Norona et al., 2019).

3D bioprinting combined with microfluidics is also a developing field, as microfluidics can improve the complexity of the models, while the cells can be cultured with minimum shear stress. For example, Bhise et al. (2016) fabricated a perfusable microfluidic bioreactor with 3D printed HepG2/C3A hepatic spheroid-laden GelMA constructs for assessing acetaminophen toxicity (Bhise et al., 2016). In another study, a 3D-cell printed liver-on-chip model with liver vascular and biliary microchannels was fabricated. It was observed that acetaminophen toxicity was detected more effectively in this model than 2D or 3D cell cultures (Lee et al., 2019). These 3D bioprinted liver tissues and liver-on-chips are thus promising models for accurate prediction of clinically relevant hepatotoxicity, or decreasing the risk of drug-induced liver injury and subsequent drug development failure.

2.2 Cardiovascular System

The heart and the circulatory system working together provide a continuous, unidirectional nutrient-rich blood flow to all organs. The heart is composed of four chambers, enclosed by a thick, robust wall that can withstand continuous beating and the associated shear forces. Parameters such as the multiple cell types making up the wall, shear forces caused by the movements, and electrical stimulation system affect the development of a suitable system for cardiotoxicity assessments. Cardiovascular toxicity is a major concern during pre-clinical and clinical drug development, and is the most serious adverse drug reaction causing post-marketing withdrawals of drugs (Ferri et al., 2013).

3D bioprinting can mimic the complex structural, functional and physiological features of the native cardiovascular structures. Various polymers such as collagen, hyaluronic acid, gelatin, fibrin, chitosan, agarose, Matrigel, and polycaprolactone, have been used as biomaterials in bioprinting the 3D heart tissue models (Liu et al., 2021). The cell sources include human coronary artery smooth muscle cells, endothelial cells, hiPSC-derived smooth muscle and vascular cells, and human umbilical vein endothelial cells (HUVECs) (Marei et al., 2022).

3D bioprinting of cardiac tissues to develop systems replicating the anisotropic cardiomyocyte orientation (Chikae et al., 2019; Noor et al., 2019; Zou et al., 2020), or the synchronous contractile function (Polonchuk et al., 2021; Tsukamoto et al., 2020) are commonly found in the literature. Lind et al. (2017) reported a novel device, wherein, six bioinks that were conductive, piezo-resistive and biocompatible were prepared for 3D bioprinting. Soft-strain gauge sensors were integrated in the matrix that guided the self-assembly of cardiac tissues. Also, these embedded sensors provided a real-time non-invasive, electronic readout of the contractile stresses. The spontaneously beating constructs were treated with two different drugs; Verapamil induced a negative chronotropic effect while isoproterenol showed a positive chronotropic effect. (Lind et al., 2017). Arai et al. (2020) developed a cardiac model by bioprinting cardiac spheroids onto a needle array in the desired 3D design which further showed contractility and responded to electrical stimulation. The cytotoxic effect of doxorubicin on the cells was evaluated in the concentration range of 0.1–10 μM, and a decrease in cell viability was observed after 48 hours, with no contractions observed beyond 72 hours (Arai et al., 2020).

Microfluidic organ-on-chip devices in combination with 3D-printed cardiac tissues can provide better control of the flow and shear stress, by incorporating blood vessels and functional endothelial barriers. Zhang et al. (2016) developed a 3D printed, endothelialized myocardium with controlled anisotropy and synchronized contractions, in a microfluidic bioreactor for cardiotoxicity studies. The dose-dependent response towards doxorubicin, an anticancer drug, was assessed, and it was observed that the beating of cardiomyocytes reduced from 94.5% in the control, to 66% and 2.78% for 10 μM and 100 μM doxorubicin, respectively (Zhang et al., 2016). Skardal et al. (2017) developed a multi-organ-on-chip model, with both cardiac and liver organoids bioprinted in separate bioreactors interconnected through a microfluidic circulatory perfusion system. The drug epinephrine generally increases the cardiac beating rate, while the drug propranolol has the opposite effect. However, when both drugs were simultaneously administered into the dual organoid system, the liver tissues could metabolically deactivate the propranolol, while the cardiac beating rate was increased due to epinephrine (Skardal et al., 2017).

2.3 Kidney

The kidney functions to maintain the homeostasis of the body, fluid and electrolyte balance, acid-base balance, and retains essential serum proteins and amino acids. In addition, their major role is in the excretion of water-soluble waste products, toxins, and xenobiotics. Various cell types such as podocytes, mesangial, parietal epithelial, glomerular endothelial, juxtaglomerular, special cells of the proximal and distal tubules, collecting ducts and loops of Henle, and the cells of the basic structural unit nephron, are all involved in performing various activities. Kidney toxicity is the second-leading cause of attrition of new drugs, and drug-induced kidney toxicity accounts for around 25% of the reported adverse drug reactions (Perazella, 2009). Multiple conditions can cause drug-induced nephrotoxicity, which include inflammation, renal tubular cytotoxicity, crystal nephropathy, altered glomerular hemodynamics and crystal nephropathy (P. Yu et al., 2021). 3D printed tissue and organ models can reproduce the anatomical complexity of the kidney in a better way, allowing improved modelling of the physiological pathways. It has also been reported in a study that when treated with nephrotoxins, 3D tissues are more sensitive to lower drug concentrations in comparison to the same cells grown in 2D (DesRochers et al., 2013). Different biomaterials such as gelatin, agarose, fibrin, alginate, pectin, and decellularized extracellular matrix have been used for bioprinting the scaffolds of 3D models (Fransen et al., 2021). The common cell sources include renal fibroblasts, human primary kidney cells, HUVECs, renal proximal tubular epithelial cells, and adult renal progenitor cells (Sochol et al., 2016).

3D printed kidney models have been designed to model various segments of the nephron, including the proximal and distal tubule, the glomerulus and the collecting duct. Particularly, the proximal tubule (PT) is the site of active renal secretion and reabsorption, in addition to the accumulation of drugs and xenobiotics (Dekant, 1996; Perazella, 2009). In combination with microfluidics and organ-on-chip technology, several inherent features such as the polarization of the epithelial cells, and the physiological fluidic shear stress can be reproduced. Homan et al. (2016) developed 3D bioprinted models of convoluted PT made of PT epithelial cells and consisting of a perfusable lumen, exhibiting significantly enhanced epithelial morphology and physiological properties relative to 2D controls. Upon treatment with the nephrotoxic Cyclosporine A, and subsequent analysis of the histological and diffusional permeability, a dose-dependent disruption of the epithelial barrier was observed (Homan et al., 2016). Similarly, King et al. (2017) developed a 3D printed PT model comprising renal fibroblasts, endothelial cells, and primary human PT epithelial cells, which subsequently demonstrated tight junction formation and polarized localization, and the expression of uptake and efflux transporters. Treatment with nephrotoxic cisplatin induced dose-dependent loss of epithelial cells and tissue viability, while the treatment with cimetidine rescued these effects (King et al., 2017). Table 1 presents an overview of the various reports of 3D-printed organ models used in toxicity evaluation.

2.4 *Skin*

Skin is one of the largest organs in the human body, making up around 15% of the total body mass. The skin has a crucial role in thermoregulation, water homeostasis, synthesis of pigments for protection against sunlight, removal of waste products through sweat and in energy storage. It is also a sensory organ for the perception of touch, heat, cold, pain and pressure, as it is equipped with specialized nerve endings. Its architecture is multi-layered, consisting of epidermis, dermis and hypodermis, with the skin barrier composed of various cells such as the corneocytes, keratinocytes, melanocytes, fibroblasts, adipocytes, endothelial cells, sensory cells and immunological cells such as T-cells and Langerhans cells (Albers and Davis, 2007; Rauma et al., 2013). Skin is the primary target organ for exposure to toxicants, via environmental and cosmetic agents (Alépée et al., 2014). The development of *in vitro* skin models for toxicology assessment is probably more advanced compared to other organ models, possibly due to the ban on *in vivo* and animal testing of cosmetic ingredients by the European Union (Fritsche et al., 2021). Regulatory authorities have classified model test guidelines into four different types, which are skin absorption, skin corrosion, skin irritation and skin sensitization (Ng and Yeong, 2019). For the fabrication of 3D printed skin models, different scaffolding biomaterials that have been reported including gelatin, chitosan, fibrin, alginate and collagen, while the cell sources include fibroblasts, keratinocytes, epidermal and dermal cell lines (Yun et al., 2018).

Table 1   3D-printed organ models for toxicity evaluation

Organ model	3D printing strategy	Cells used	Toxicity tested with	Ref.
Liver	Continuous deposition microextrusion	Patient-derived hepatocytes Hepatic stellate cells HUVEC	Trovafloxacin Levofloxacin	(Nguyen et al., 2016)
Liver	Extrusion-based	HepaRG	Aflatoxin B1	(Schmidt et al., 2020)
Liver	Extrusion-based sacrificial bioprinting	HepG2/C3A HUVEC	Acetaminophen	(Massa et al., 2017)
Liver	Extrusion-based	HepG2	Nefazodone	(Hong and Song, 2021)
Liver	Extrusion-based	Human hepatocytes Hepatic stellate cells HUVEC	Methotrexate Thoacetamide	(Norona et al., 2016)
Liver	Extrusion-based	HepG2/C3A	Acetaminophen	(Bhise et al., 2016)
Liver		HepaRG HUVEC	Acetaminophen	(Lee et al., 2019)
Heart	Extrusion-based	hiPSC cardiomyocytes	Verapamil Isoproterenol	(Lind et al., 2017)
Heart		Normal human dermal fibroblasts HUVEC	Doxorubicin	(Arai et al., 2020)
Heart	Extrusion-based	HUVEC Neonatal rat cardiomyocytes hiPSC cardiomyocytes	Doxorubicin	(Zhang et al., 2016)
Heart, Liver and Lung	Extrusion-based	Hepatic stellate cells Primary human hepatocytes Kupffer cells hiPSC cardiomyocytes Human primary cardiomyocytes Lung microvascular endothelial cells Airway stromal mesenchymal cells Bronchial epithelial cells	Epinephrine Propranolol	(Skardal et al., 2017)
Kidney	Extrusion-based	Human proximal tubule epithelial cells	Cyclosporine A	(Homan et al., 2016)
Kidney	Extrusion-based	Renal fibroblasts HUVEC Human proximal tubule epithelial cells	Cisplatin	(King et al., 2017)
Skin	Extrusion-based		Triton X-100 SDS	(Nguyen and Pentoney, 2017)

HUVECs: Human umbilical vein endothelial cells
hiPSC: human induced pluripotent stem cells

Several studies on 3D bioprinted skin models have been investigated for wound dressing and healing, 3D skin constructs and toxicology applications. Nguyen et al. (2017) reported a 3D-printed full-thickness skin tissue that exhibited epidermal stratification. Upon exposure to the skin irritant 1% Triton X-100 and the corrosive agent 5% SDS, the tissues showed a decline and complete loss of viability, respectively (Nguyen and Pentoney, 2017).

3.   Challenges with 3D Printed Models for Toxicity Evaluation

3D in vitro tissue models are becoming increasingly popular as an advanced approach for toxicology printing, as they can provide the advantage of closely mimicking the physiology of the native organ, while achieving controllable manipulation of the microenvironment. As discussed in the various reports mentioned previously, 3D models show a marked difference in toxicity responses compared to 2D studies. 3D printing of tissue and organ models can offer better control over the replication of the complex architecture while providing an improved, functionally biomimetic tissue for the specific application. Though 3D bioprinting offers several advantages, there is still room for improvement, with several challenges and limitations to be overcome. For example, in the case of kidney models, modelling the different functional nephron sections with their complex architectures, including cellular interactions, presence of capillaries, shear stress, and differences in oxygen tensions *in vitro* remains challenging. The basic challenge with 3D printed models is replicating the complex tissue architecture. Several factors such as the complex cellular composition within an organ, control over the biochemical cues, dynamic nature of the extracellular matrix and surrounding fluids have to be taken into consideration. For example, 3D printing an *in vitro* cardiac tissue model is challenging due to the non-proliferative nature of cardiomyocytes, and the requirement for high cardiomyocyte density, that complicate the replication of a large model with integrated anatomical structures (Xiang et al., 2022). With the limited resolution of bioprinting, recreating the microarchitecture of the organs is challenging. For example, the alveoli of the lungs are air sacs that are held and entangled by a network of capillaries (Huh et al., 2012). This sophisticated structure, which functions as a center for the exchange of oxygen and carbon dioxide between the circulatory and pulmonary systems, is difficult to fabricate. Modelling vasculatures and perfusions is another challenging aspect in the development of larger 3D models. The current commonly used approach is to design a sacrificial template, which is removed later by perfusions (Xiang et al., 2022).

From a toxicological perspective, the source of the cells and polymeric scaffold materials used in fabricating the 3D models are of particular concern. Since the drugs being assessed are intended for human use, it is essential that the cell source is also of human origin. The polymers used in bioprinting are expected to have suitable mechanical properties and biocompatibility to support the cells to maintain their morphological and phenotypic functions. In addition, the breakdown of the polymeric materials should not leach out toxic by-products that can interfere with toxicology studies. Long-term toxicological studies require that the stability and functionality of the 3D-printed organ is maintained for long periods, which is also a challenging task. The pharmaceutical and cosmetic industries are constantly on the lookout for *in vitro* models for pre-clinical trials, and early detection of toxicological effects, as an alternative to animal testing. The toxicological effects of any drug or cosmetic product are generally due to several parallel mechanisms operating in multistep and multicellular processes. To realize this, Serras et al. (2021) proposed a systematic tiered strategy, wherein, a set of well-characterized 3D models, with well-defined purposes can be used in a multistep manner to evaluate the toxicity. Ultimately, the data obtained from these multiple systems can be integrated, to deliver robust information to pharmaceutical regulators to improve the decision-making process (Serras et al., 2021). Finally, the pharmaceutical industry requires high-throughput *in vitro* models, while also considering the cost and efficiency of the system. Microfluidic technology has made it possible to control the flow and drug dosage precisely, to achieve continuous, real-time and high throughput assessment systems. With the integration of 3D bioprinting and microfluidic organ-on-chip technology, multi-drug screening, and multi-organ interaction can also be realized, which can bring about significant developments in toxicity evaluation.

Conclusions

The significant advances in 3D bioprinting have made it possible to generate 3D tissues and organ models that can closely mimic the native architecture and function. For performing toxicological evaluations, 3D organ models are a better alternative to 2D models and *in vivo* animal models which are fraught with ethical issues. As presented in this chapter, appropriate fabrication strategies have resulted in a close replication of the cellular composition, tissue microarchitecture and functionality of several organs such as the liver, heart, kidney and skin. Despite the encouraging outcomes, 3D-bioprinted models are still marginalized in the pharmaceutical industry due to several challenges that exist with the practical implementation of these models for preclinical toxicity evaluations. Future work should focus on improving the accuracy of tissue microarchitecture, with the inclusion of the complete cellular repertoire in each organ. In addition, efforts must be made to achieve high-throughput, cost-effective, efficient, and reproducible models that can be reliably used by the pharmaceutical and cosmetic industries. In combination with microfluidic technology, multi-organ-on-chip devices for evaluating systemic toxicity can also be made feasible.

References

Albers, K.M. and Davis, B.M. (2007). The Skin as a Neurotrophic Organ. *The Neuroscientist, 13*(4), 371–382. https://doi.org/10.1177/10738584070130040901

Alépée, N., Bahinski, A., Daneshian, M., De Wever, B., Fritsche, E. et al. (2014). State-of-the-art of 3D cultures (organs-on-a-chip) in safety testing and pathophysiology. *Altex, 31*(4), 441–477. https://doi.org/10.14573/altex1406111

Anju, S., Prajitha, N., Sukanya, V.S. and Mohanan, P.V. (2020). Complicity of degradable polymers in health-care applications. *Materials Today Chemistry, 16*, 100236. https://doi.org/10.1016/j.mtchem.2019.100236

Arai, K., Murata, D., Takao, S., Nakamura, A., Itoh, M. et al. (2020). Drug response analysis for scaffold-free cardiac constructs fabricated using bio-3D printer. *Scientific Reports, 10*(1), 8972. https://doi.org/10.1038/s41598-020-65681-y

Bhise, N.S., Manoharan, V., Massa, S., Tamayol, A., Ghaderi, M. et al. (2016). A liver-on-a-chip platform with bioprinted hepatic spheroids. *Biofabrication, 8*(1), 014101. https://doi.org/10.1088/1758-5090/8/1/014101

Chikae, S., Kubota, A., Nakamura, H., Oda, A., Yamanaka, A. et al. (2019). Three-dimensional bioprinting human cardiac tissue chips of using a painting needle method. *Biotechnology and Bioengineering, 116*(11), 3136–3142. https://doi.org/10.1002/bit.27126

Dekant, W. (1996). *Biotransformation and Renal Processing of Nephrotoxic Agents* (pp. 163–172). https://doi.org/10.1007/978-3-642-61105-6_17

DesRochers, T.M., Suter, L., Roth, A. and Kaplan, D.L. (2013). Bioengineered 3D Human Kidney Tissue, a Platform for the Determination of Nephrotoxicity. *PLoS ONE, 8*(3), e59219. https://doi.org/10.1371/journal.pone.0059219

Ferri, N., Siegl, P., Corsini, A., Herrmann, J., Lerman, A. et al (2013). Drug attrition during pre-clinical and clinical development: Understanding and managing drug-induced cardiotoxicity. *Pharmacology & Therapeutics, 138*(3), 470–484. https://doi.org/10.1016/j.pharmthera.2013.03.005

Fitzgerald, K.A., Malhotra, M., Curtin, C.M., O' Brien, F.J. and O' Driscoll, C.M. et al. (2015). Life in 3D is never flat: 3D models to optimise drug delivery. *Journal of Controlled Release, 215*, 39–54. https://doi.org/10.1016/j.jconrel.2015.07.020

Fransen, M.F.J., Addario, G., Bouten, C.V.C., Halary, F., Moroni, L. et al. (2021). Bioprinting of kidney in vitro models: cells, biomaterials, and manufacturing techniques. *Essays in Biochemistry, 65*(3), 587–602. https://doi.org/10.1042/EBC20200158

Fritsche, E., Haarmann-Stemmann, T., Kapr, J., Galanjuk, S., Hartmann, J. et al. (2021). Stem Cells for Next Level Toxicity Testing in the 21st Century. *Small, 17*(15). https://doi.org/10.1002/smll.202006252

Fu, Z., Ouyang, L., Xu, R., Yang, Y. and Sun, W. et al. (2022). Responsive biomaterials for 3D bioprinting: A review. *Materials Today, 52*, 112–132. https://doi.org/10.1016/j.mattod.2022.01.001

Hay, M., Thomas, D.W., Craighead, J.L., Economides, C. and Rosenthal, J. et al. (2014). Clinical development success rates for investigational drugs. *Nature Biotechnology, 32*(1), 40–51. https://doi.org/10.1038/nbt.2786

Hingorani, A.D., Kuan, V., Finan, C., Kruger, F.A., Gaulton, A. et al. (2019). Improving the odds of drug development success through human genomics: modelling study. *Scientific Reports, 9*(1), 18911. https://doi.org/10.1038/s41598-019-54849-w

Homan, K.A., Kolesky, D.B., Skylar-Scott, M.A., Herrmann, J., Obuobi, H. et al. (2016). Bioprinting of 3D Convoluted Renal Proximal Tubules on Perfusable Chips. *Scientific Reports, 6*(1), 34845. https://doi.org/10.1038/srep34845

Hong, S. and Song, J.M. (2021). A 3D cell printing-fabricated HepG2 liver spheroid model for high-content in situ quantification of drug-induced liver toxicity. *Biomaterials Science*, 9(17), 5939–5950. https://doi.org/10.1039/D1BM00749A

Huh, D., Leslie, D.C., Matthews, B.D., Fraser, J.P., Jurek, S. et al. (2012). A Human Disease Model of Drug Toxicity–Induced Pulmonary Edema in a Lung-on-a-Chip Microdevice. *Science Translational Medicine*, 4(159). https://doi.org/10.1126/scitranslmed.3004249

Kang, D., Hong, G., An, S., Jang, I., Yun, W. et al. (2020). Bioprinting of Multiscaled Hepatic Lobules within a Highly Vascularized Construct. *Small*, 16(13). https://doi.org/10.1002/smll.201905505

King, S.M., Higgins, J.W., Nino, C.R., Smith, T.R., Paffenroth, E.H. et al. (2017). 3D Proximal Tubule Tissues Recapitulate Key Aspects of Renal Physiology to Enable Nephrotoxicity Testing. *Frontiers in Physiology*, 8. https://doi.org/10.3389/fphys.2017.00123

Lee, H., Chae, S., Kim, J.Y., Han, W., Kim, J. et al. (2019). Cell-printed 3D liver-on-a-chip possessing a liver microenvironment and biliary system. *Biofabrication*, 11(2), 025001. https://doi.org/10.1088/1758-5090/aaf9fa

Lind, J.U., Busbee, T.A., Valentine, A.D., Pasqualini, F.S., Yuan, H. et al. (2017). Instrumented cardiac microphysiological devices via multimaterial three-dimensional printing. *Nature Materials*, 16(3), 303–308. https://doi.org/10.1038/nmat4782

Liu, N., Ye, X., Yao, B., Zhao, M., Wu, P. et al. (2021). Advances in 3D bioprinting technology for cardiac tissue engineering and regeneration. *Bioactive Materials*, 6(5), 1388–1401. https://doi.org/10.1016/j.bioactmat.2020.10.021

Ma, C., Peng, Y., Li, H. and Chen, W. (2021). Organ-on-a-Chip: A New Paradigm for Drug Development. *Trends in Pharmacological Sciences*, 42(2), 119–133. https://doi.org/10.1016/j.tips.2020.11.009

Ma, L., Wu, Y., Li, Y., Aazmi, A., Zhou, H. et al. (2020). Current Advances on 3D-Bioprinted Liver Tissue Models. *Advanced Healthcare Materials*, 9(24). https://doi.org/10.1002/adhm.202001517

Ma, X., Qu, X., Zhu, W., Li, Y.S., Yuan, S. et al. (2016). Deterministically patterned biomimetic human iPSC-derived hepatic model via rapid 3D bioprinting. *Proceedings of the National Academy of Sciences of the United States of America*, 113(8), 2206–2211. https://doi.org/10.1073/pnas.1524510113

Malarkey, D.E., Johnson, K., Ryan, L., Boorman, G. and Maronpot, R.R. et al. (2005). New Insights into Functional Aspects of Liver Morphology. *Toxicologic Pathology*, 33(1), 27–34. https://doi.org/10.1080/01926230590881826

Marei, I., Abu Samaan, T., Al-Quradaghi, M.A., Farah, A.A., Mahmud, S.H. et al. (2022). 3D Tissue-Engineered Vascular Drug Screening Platforms: Promise and Considerations. *Frontiers in Cardiovascular Medicine*, 9. https://doi.org/10.3389/fcvm.2022.847554

Massa, S., Sakr, M.A., Seo, J., Bandaru, P., Arneri, A. et al. (2017). Bioprinted 3D vascularized tissue model for drug toxicity analysis. *Biomicrofluidics*, 11(4). https://doi.org/10.1063/1.4994708

Messelmani, T., Morisseau, L., Sakai, Y., Legallais, C., Le Goff, A. et al. (2022). Liver organ-on-chip models for toxicity studies and risk assessment. *Lab on a Chip*, 22(13), 2423–2450. https://doi.org/10.1039/D2LC00307D

Ng, W.L. and Yeong, W.Y. (2019). The future of skin toxicology testing – Three-dimensional bioprinting meets microfluidics. *International Journal of Bioprinting*, 5(1). https://doi.org/10.18063/ijb.v5i2.1.237

Nguyen, D.G., Funk, J., Robbins, J.B., Crogan-Grundy, C., Presnell, S.C. et al. (2016). Bioprinted 3D Primary Liver Tissues Allow Assessment of Organ-Level Response to Clinical Drug Induced Toxicity In Vitro. *PLOS ONE*, 11(7), e0158674. https://doi.org/10.1371/journal.pone.0158674

Nguyen, D.G. and Pentoney, S.L. (2017). Bioprinted three dimensional human tissues for toxicology and disease modeling. *Drug Discovery Today: Technologies*, 23, 37–44. https://doi.org/10.1016/j.ddtec.2017.03.001

Noor, N., Shapira, A., Edri, R., Gal, I., Wertheim, L. et al. (2019). 3D Printing of Personalized Thick and Perfusable Cardiac Patches and Hearts. *Advanced Science*, 6(11). https://doi.org/10.1002/advs.201900344

Norona, L.M., Nguyen, D.G., Gerber, D.A., Presnell, S.C. and LeCluyse, E.L et al. (2016). Modeling Compound-Induced Fibrogenesis In Vitro Using Three-Dimensional Bioprinted Human Liver Tissues. *Toxicological Sciences*, 154(2), 354–367. https://doi.org/10.1093/toxsci/kfw169

Norona, L.M., Nguyen, D.G., Gerber, D.A., Presnell, S.C., Mosedale, M. et al., (2019). Bioprinted liver provides early insight into the role of Kupffer cells in TGF-β1 and methotrexate-induced fibrogenesis. *PLOS ONE*, 14(1), e0208958. https://doi.org/10.1371/journal.pone.0208958

Perazella, M.A. (2009). Renal Vulnerability to Drug Toxicity. *Clinical Journal of the American Society of Nephrology*, 4(7), 1275–1283. https://doi.org/10.2215/CJN.02050309

Polonchuk, L., Surija, L., Lee, M.H., Sharma, P., Liu Chung Ming, C. et al. (2021). Towards engineering heart tissues from bioprinted cardiac spheroids. *Biofabrication*, 13(4), 045009. https://doi.org/10.1088/1758-5090/ac14ca

Rauma, M., Boman, A. and Johanson, G. (2013). Predicting the absorption of chemical vapours. *Advanced Drug Delivery Reviews*, 65(2), 306–314. https://doi.org/10.1016/j.addr.2012.03.012

Roskos, K., Stuiver, I., Pentoney, S. and Presnell, S. (2015). Bioprinting: An Industrial Perspective. In *Essentials of 3D Biofabrication and Translation* (pp. 395–411). Elsevier. https://doi.org/10.1016/B978-0-12-800972-7.00024-4

Schmidt, K., Berg, J., Roehrs, V., Kurreck, J. and Al-Zeer, M.A. et al. (2020). 3D-bioprinted HepaRG cultures as a model for testing long term aflatoxin B1 toxicity in vitro. *Toxicology Reports, 7*, 1578–1587. https://doi.org/10.1016/j.toxrep.2020.11.003

Serras, A.S., Rodrigues, J.S., Cipriano, M., Rodrigues, A.V., Oliveira, N.G. et al. (2021). A Critical Perspective on 3D Liver Models for Drug Metabolism and Toxicology Studies. *Frontiers in Cell and Developmental Biology, 9.* https://doi.org/10.3389/fcell.2021.626805

Skardal, A., Murphy, S.V., Devarasetty, M., Mead, I., Kang, H.-W et al. (2017). Multi-tissue interactions in an integrated three-tissue organ-on-a-chip platform. *Scientific Reports, 7*(1), 8837. https://doi.org/10.1038/s41598-017-08879-x

Sochol, R.D., Gupta, N.R. and Bonventre, J.V. (2016). A Role for 3D Printing in Kidney-on-a-Chip Platforms. *Current Transplantation Reports, 3*(1), 82–92. https://doi.org/10.1007/s40472-016-0085-x

Stevens, J.L. and Baker, T.K. (2009). The future of drug safety testing: expanding the view and narrowing the focus. *Drug Discovery Today, 14*(3–4), 162–167. https://doi.org/10.1016/j.drudis.2008.11.009

Szűcs, D., Fekete, Z., Guba, M., Kemény, L., Jemnitz, K. et al. (2023). Toward better drug development: Three-dimensional bioprinting in toxicological research. *International Journal of Bioprinting, 9*(2), 663. https://doi.org/10.18063/ijb.v9i2.663

Tsukamoto, Y., Akagi, T. and Akashi, M. (2020). Vascularized cardiac tissue construction with orientation by layer-by-layer method and 3D printer. *Scientific Reports, 10*(1), 5484. https://doi.org/10.1038/s41598-020-59371-y

Waring, M.J., Arrowsmith, J., Leach, A.R., Leeson, P.D., Mandrell, S. et al. (2015). An analysis of the attrition of drug candidates from four major pharmaceutical companies. *Nature Reviews Drug Discovery, 14*(7), 475–486. https://doi.org/10.1038/nrd4609

Xiang, Y., Miller, K., Guan, J., Kiratitanaporn, W., Tang, M. et al. (2022). 3D bioprinting of complex tissues in vitro: state-of-the-art and future perspectives. *Archives of Toxicology, 96*(3), 691–710. https://doi.org/10.1007/s00204-021-03212-y

Yang, H., Sun, L., Pang, Y., Hu, D., Xu, H. et al. (2021). Three-dimensional bioprinted hepatorganoids prolong survival of mice with liver failure. *Alépée, N. (2014). State-of-the-Art of 3D Cultures (Organs-on-a-Chip) in Safety Testing and Pathophysiology. ALTEX, 441–477. Https://Doi.Org/10.14573/Altex1406111Gut, 70*(3), 567–574. https://doi.org/10.1136/gutjnl-2019-319960

Yu, C., Ma, X., Zhu, W., Wang, P., Miller, K.L. et al. (2019). Scanningless and continuous 3D bioprinting of human tissues with decellularized extracellular matrix. *Biomaterials, 194*, 1–13. https://doi.org/10.1016/j.biomaterials.2018.12.009

Yu, P., Duan, Z., Liu, S., Pachon, I., Ma, J. et al. (2021). Drug-Induced Nephrotoxicity Assessment in 3D Cellular Models. *Micromachines, 13*(1), 3. https://doi.org/10.3390/mi13010003

Yun, Y.E., Jung, Y.J., Choi, Y.J., Choi, J.S. and Cho, Y.W. et al. (2018). Artificial skin models for animal-free testing. *Journal of Pharmaceutical Investigation, 48*(2), 215–223. https://doi.org/10.1007/s40005-018-0389-1

Zhang, Y.S., Arneri, A., Bersini, S., Shin, S.-R., Zhu, K. et al. (2016). Bioprinting 3D microfibrous scaffolds for engineering endothelialized myocardium and heart-on-a-chip. *Biomaterials, 110*, 45–59. https://doi.org/10.1016/j.biomaterials.2016.09.003

Zou, Q., Grottkau, B.E., He, Z., Shu, L., Yang, L. et al. (2020). Biofabrication of valentine-shaped heart with a composite hydrogel and sacrificial material. *Materials Science and Engineering: C, 108*, 110205. https://doi.org/10.1016/j.msec.2019.110205

3D Bioprinting in Vascular Tissue Engineering

Purnimajayasree Ramesh,[1,2] *Rohin Shyam,*[1,2]
and *Arunkumar Palaniappan*[2*]

1. Introduction

The human vascular system comprises vessels that carry blood and lymph fluid throughout the body and play a very important role in the sustenance of the physiological homeostasis. Importantly, blood vessels deliver oxygen and nutrients to various organs and in turn remove metabolic wastes from the organs. Due to the current inappropriate lifestyle modifications as well as increase in geriatric population, there is an increased incidence of diseases due to dysfunction of vascular systems. Some of these diseases include atherosclerosis, aneurysms, congenital vascular malformations, deep vein thrombosis (DVT), peripheral arterial diseases, and stroke (Conte, 2013; Garg et al., 2023; Tuohy et al., 2023). In most of the arterial diseases, autograft is the gold standard. However, infection in the donor site and morbidity are limitations (Veith et al., 1979). In other eligible cases, allografts, xenografts, and synthetic grafts are also used, which are not free from limitations. Allografts and xenografts suffer from problems due to disease transmission and untoward immune reactions. On the other hand, synthetic grafts too fail due to clotting and other immune rejection-based issues and most importantly they are synthetic and do not really mimic the native vascular tissue. Moreover, these synthetic grafts are not suitable for paediatric patients as they do not grow with the patients (Harskamp et al., 2013; Klinkert et al., 2004). One strategy to counter these limitations is to build tissue-mimics combining biomaterials, appropriate cells, and factors, which are constituently, structurally, and functionally very similar to vascular tissues-resulting in the birth of a new field-vascular tissue engineering (VTE). VTE could result in two applications:

1. Fabrication of bioengineered vascular grafts for implantation.
2. Developing vascularization inside tissue engineered constructs, which is crucial for the survival of cells in thicker tissue constructs (Maina et al., 2018).

[1] School of Biosciences and Technology.
[2] Human Organ Manufacturing Engineering (HOME) Lab, Centre for Biomaterials, Cellular and Molecular Theranostics, Vellore Institute of Technology, Vellore, India.
* Corresponding author: arunkumar.p@vit.ac.in

Conventionally, VTE is classified as scaffold-based VTE techniques, decellularization-based VTE strategies, molding techniques, and cell-sheet engineering. Scaffold based VTE methods are limited by non-homogenous cell distribution during the seeding process, longer processing times and poor control of porosity and microstructures (Ong et al., 2017; K. Wang et al., 2016). High costs and increased risk of immune rejection are limitations of decellularization-based VTE techniques (Xiong et al., 2013). Molding techniques lack the ability to develop patient-specific vascular tissue. Finally, cell-sheet engineering methods possess limitations like high cost, long maturation time and more importantly poor scalability. Thus, to overcome the above-mentioned challenges, 3D bioprinting, an advanced additive manufacturing technology, is currently being explored for the fabrication of vascular tissues (Ahn et al., 2015; Koens et al., 2015).

In 3D bioprinting, vascular tissues can be built layer-by-layer using the right combination of biomaterials, cells, and factors. The bioprinting technique has various process parameters which help to control geometry, spatial distributions, and cellular orientation of the tissue to mimic the structure and function of the native vascular tissues (Song et al., 2018). Numerous printing technologies have been employed to fabricate complex vascular tissues which include extrusion bioprinting, inkjet bioprinting, laser assisted bioprinting, co-axial printing, and light-mediated stereolithography (Fazal et al., 2021). Hyaluronic acid, alginate, and gelatin methacryloyl (GelMA), collagen are some of the common biomaterials used in the fabrication of vascular tissues. Furthermore, the incorporation of time into the bioprinting process known as four dimensional (4D) bioprinting results in variations in biophysical parameters of tissue models in response to environmental stimuli (Miri et al., 2019). This chapter is mainly focussed on the utilization of 3D bioprinting technique for the fabrication of vascular constructs. The chapter begins with a concise introduction of the anatomy and physiology of vascular tissues followed by an elaborative discussion on types of 3D bioprinting techniques employed, as well as the biomaterials and cells used for the fabrication of bioprinted vascular constructs.

2. Anatomy and Physiology of Vascular Tissues

The human vascular system maintains physiological homeostasis by supplying oxygen and nutrients to the tissues/cells while removing metabolic wastes away from the tissues/organs. The vascular system consists of five classes of blood vessels: arteries, arterioles, veins, venules, and capillaries. Figure 1 depicts the different types of blood vessels and their role in gas transportation. Arteries are branching or bifurcating vessels that branch off into smaller arteries and arterioles and are responsible for transporting oxygenated blood, nutrients, and hormones from the heart to all parts of the body. Veins are tubular vessels that help in transportation of blood from the heart to other parts of the body. Capillaries are the smallest blood vessels in the human body which helps in the transportation of blood, nutrients, and oxygen through their thin walls at cellular level. Table 1

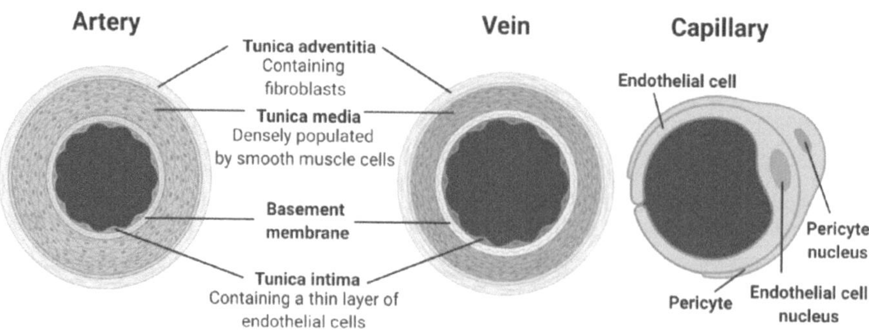

Fig. 1   The composition of blood vessels. Reprinted with permission from (Jouda et al., 2022) under the creative commons licence. Copyright authors, MDPI, Basal Switzerland 2021, Schöneberg et al., 2018).

provides a brief function of the 5 major blood vessels. Table 2 provides the main components of the Extracellular matrix (ECM) of the blood vessels and their functions. Figure 1 shows the differences between the different blood vessels (Elaine N and Katja, 2019).

The blood vessels, except the smallest one, are made up of three layers: the inner tunica interna/intima, middle tunica media, and outer tunica externa/adventia. The tunica interna/intima is composed of endothelial cells and is in direct contact with blood and offers very little resistance to blood flow (Elaine N and Katja, 2019). The endothelial cells adhere on the surface of a thin connective tissue composed of elastin and collagen and anchors the tunica interna to the tunica media. The endothelial cells are aligned longitudinally in the direction of blood flow and help in preventing blood coagulation. The tunica media is composed of densely populated smooth muscle cells (SMCs) that are arranged in a concentric manner. SMCs with the help of innervating sympathetic nerves play a vital role in vasodilation/constriction with respect to the modifications in blood flow properties. The outermost tunica externa/adventitia is composed primarily of connective tissue fibres that protect the blood vessels and attach them to the surrounding tissue. They have fibroblasts that are arranged randomly which secrete extracellular matrices that help in protecting the integrity of the blood vessel structure.

The blood vessels within the vasculature network work in tandem with the heart in a closed circuit to deliver oxygenated blood to cells and tissues while transporting metabolic waste. The varying physiological features and anatomical features of the veins, arteries and capillaries allow them to function and perform their role correctly as shown in Table 1.

Table 1   Different type of blood vessels found in the vascular network and their functions.

Vessel Type	*Function*
Arteries	Transportation of high-pressure and oxygenated blood to smaller arteries and arterioles
Arterioles	Connecting arteries and capillaries
Veins	Transportation of low-pressure and de-oxygenated blood from venules to heart
Venules	Connecting veins and capillaries
Capillaries	Allows the exchange of gases, nutrients and metabolic wastes between the blood and tissue fluid

Table 2   Components and function of ECM in a healthy vascular tissue

S.No.	*Component*	*Function*	*Reference*
1	Collagen (Type I: 80%, Type III: 10% & Type VI ~ 5%)	Fibrous networks that are the bulk of the ECM.	(Horn and Trafford, 2016)
2	Hyaluronic acid	Regulating cellular function	(Bonafè et al., 2014)
3	Glycosaminoglycans (Glycoprotein, Proteoglycans)	Organize the matrix structure and activate fibroblasts and space fillers	(Christensen et al., 2019)
4	Endothelial Cells (45%)	Responsible for regulating angiogenesis	(Talman and Kivelä, 2018)
5	Fibroblasts (11%)	Produce structural proteins of the ECM	(Talman and Kivelä, 2018)
6	Fibronectin	Mediates cellular behaviour	(Lockhart et al., 2011)
7	Other cells (6-8%) Pericytes, smooth muscle cells.	Pericytes and smooth muscle cells help in blood flow regulation.	(Talman and Kivelä, 2018).

3. 3D Bioprinting of Vascular Tissues

3D bioprinting is an emerging and advanced additive manufacturing technique that is used to build vascular tissues layer-by-layer with excellent spatial control of the deposition process. Bioprinting uses a combination of hydrogel biomaterials and cells, together called bioinks. The bioprinting technique has various process parameters which help to control geometry, spatial distributions, and cellular orientation of the tissue to mimic the structure and function of the native vascular tissues. The bioprinting process involves the following steps:

- *Pre-bioprinting* In this step, 3D models that are recognizable and executable by the printer need to be developed. This might involve either building the 3D model from scratch or conversion of processed 3D medical images (MRI / CT images) into STL format.
- *Bioprinting* This is the actual printing step where bioinks are used to build vascular tissues layer-by-layer. Printability and rheometric analyses are performed to optimize the process parameters involved in the 3D bioprinting.
- *Post-bioprinting* After printing the desired 3D structure, crosslinking is performed to improve the stability of the bioprinted structures. The crosslinking could be through chemical reactions (eg. Schiff's reaction) or through physical stimuli such as UVrays or temperature.

3.1 Bioinks

The successful bioprinting of vascular tissue is highly dependent on the choice of bioink with the right physicochemical, rheological, and biological properties. In case of physicochemical properties, suitable crosslinking chemistries could lead to stable structures after printing with reasonable crosslinking times. For rheological properties, the hydrogel should exhibit atleast good shear thinning and thixotropic properties, along with appropriate flow characteristics, for extrusion-based bioprinting. The biological properties mainly include biocompatibility. The bioprinted structures should incorporate the appropriate factors that can positively affect the proliferation and migration of vascular cells, as well as differentiation, followed by proliferation or migration of vascular cells when stem cells are utilized. Some of the most common biomaterials that are explored in the bioprinting of vascular tissues are listed in Table 3.

3.2 Cells used for the 3D Bioprinting of Vascular Tissues

The choices of cells play a crucial role in the performance of the bioprinted vascular tissue/grafts. Some of the principal cells that are used in vascular tissue engineering are vascular associated cells and stem/progenitor cells. The vascular associated cells include endothelial cells (ECs), SMCs and pericytes. These cells are present in three different layers in the blood vessels. Some of the most used ECs include human umbilical cord vein endothelial cells (HUVECs), human dermal microvascular endothelial cells (HDMECs). Similarly, most used SMCs are human umbilical vein smooth muscle cells (HUVSMC).

In case of stem/progenitor cells, human pluripotent stem cells (hPSCs) such as human induced PSCs (hiPSCs) and human embryonic stem cells (hESCs) are commonly used. These cells are differentiated towards either arterial or venous endothelial cells based on the blood vessels that are bioprinted. Also, another type of progenitor cells that are used include endothelial colony-forming cells (ECFC), which are typically obtained from tissue-resident vascular endothelium, human umbilical cords or peripheral blood, or could be derived from human induced pluripotent stem cells (Jiang et al., 2023).

3.3 Bioactive Factors

In addition to the primary constituents such as biomaterials and cells that are discussed in the above section, there are few important bioactive factors that are found to impart better tissue-mimicking

Table 3   Biomaterials used in the fabrication of 3D bioprinted vascular models. The table is reproduced as such from (Fazal et al., 2021).

S. No	Biomaterial Used	Printing Method	Printing Resolution	Outcome	Source of cells
1.	Agarose	Extrusion	Moderate	Limited cell attachment and slow degradation rate, effective porosity, low gelling temperature	—
2.	Alginate	Extrusion	Moderate	Cell viability is more than 90% immediately after bioprinting	Cartilage progenitor cells
3.	Fibrin	Inkjet	High	Cell viability is 90%	HMVEC, primary neonatal human dermal fibroblasts (HDF-n)
4.	Fibrin	Extrusion drop-based	Moderate	Shape retention and integrity	HMVECs
5.	Collagen	Extrusion drop-based	Moderate	Stable tubular structure, Mimic blood vessel composition	SMCs
6.	Collagen	Extrusion drop-based	Moderate	Angiogenic intravasation Long-term stability	HUVECs
7.	Gelatin	Extrusion	Moderate	Cell survival rate more than 90%	NIH 3T3
8.	Gelatin	Extrusion	Moderate	Cell viability is 97%	Normal human dermal fibroblast cells (NHDF) and human umbilical vein endothelial cells (HUVEC)
9.	GelMA, alginate, PEGDA, alginate lyase	Extrusion	Moderate	Steady cell proliferation. Perfusable properties under various conditions of flow velocity, flow viscosity, and temperature	VSMC and HUVEC
10.	Gelatin and pluronic F127	Stereolithography	High	Good *in vitro* cytocompatibility and was suitable for cell attachment and for proliferation	HUVEC
11.	Gelatin–poly(ethylene glycol)–tyramine (GPT)	Extrusion	Moderate	Cell viability above 90%	Human dermal neonatal fibroblasts, NIH-3T3, RFP-HUVEC, GFP-HDF
12.	NovoGel (Organovo)	Inkjet	High	Cell viability above 82%	NIH 3T3 mouse fibroblast

properties for the 3D bioprinted vascular tissue, as shown in **Table 4.** Some of the key bioactive factors reported include growth factors, factors that help in the differentiation of stem cells, cell adhesion molecules, and other key constituents of extracellular matrix (ECM).

Table 4   Role of Growth Factors during vascularization (Jiang et al., 2023)

S.No	Growth Factors	Functions
1.	Vascular endothelial growth factor (VEGF)	• Angiogenic bud formation • VEGF-A: transform EC into tip/stalk cells
2.	Platelet-derived growth factor (PDGF)	• Recruiting pericytes and SMCs • Stimulating vessel growth and maturation while also attenuating the response to anti-VEGF therapy
3.	Fibroblast growth factors (FGF)	• FGF-2: stimulating ECs barrier integrity • bFGF: promoting migration, proliferation, and survival of ECs and SMCs
4.	Transforming growth factor-β (TGF-β)	• Inhibiting ECs invasion and capillary lumen formation • Limiting ECs apoptosis and block EC migration • Stabilizing blood vessels
5.	Angiotensin (Ang)	• Ang1: promoting ECs survival and vascular stabilization and tightness • Ang2: regulating angiogenesis and regression, promote pericyte separation and vascular permeability

4.   Various 3D Bioprinting Methods for Vascular Tissue Engineering

4.1   *Sacrificial Bioprinting*

Sacrificial bioprinting involves the use of sacrificial bioink that can be washed away at a later stage. This feature is used for the generation of hollow structures typically associated with blood vessels and enables the formation of a lumen. There are a variety of ways the lumen can be formed. In this approach, sacrificial materials such as agarose or pluronic F127 or gelatin are used to fabricate channels and then covered with hydrogel matrices. The next stage involves removal of the fabricated channels either by washing with cold PBS or dissolved with sterile water. This bioprinting strategy can achieve rapid fabrication of perfusable blood vessels with complex vascular patterns. However, a drawback of such a method is that it is limited in its ability to print spatially distributed complex vascular patterns due to lack of support in the 3D volume and therefore cannot be used in sophisticated 3D vasculature designs.

Extrusion-based systems are the most commonly used method in 3D bioprinters. Bioinks are deposited in a way that allows precise deposition of cylindrical filaments. There are three typical types of extrusion-based bioprinters: pneumatic, piston, and screw. Extrusion based bioprinting allows the use of a wide range of biomaterials, however, a key aspect is that the material have viscoelastic properties, specifically shear thinning and thixotropy(Sánchez-Sánchez et al., 2023). Viscoelastic behaviour allows the fluid to maintain properties of a fluid while having structural properties of an elastic solid. When a deformation force such as pneumatic pressure is applied, the material undergoes a change in viscosity and flows out of nozzles with small diameters and once the extrusion process is complete, recovers the energy absorbed as a result of its elastic nature and maintains a consistent 3D structure. This property also allows the incorporation of cells into bioactive materials and the generation of tissue analogues for therapeutic purposes or mimicking the microenvironment of tissue for development of human reconstructed tissue models (Zhang et al., 2021). A few major benefits of using extrusion based bioprinting systems is the low costs, wide range of biomaterials available, high throughput and repeatability, and ability to print with cells. However, a few limitations include the lower resolution of printing when compared to other bioprinting methods, nozzles that are prone to clogging, and crosslinkers that are limited for bioprinting.

The methods that are reported under extrusion-based bioprinting for vascular tissues can be categorized into the following types: support bath method, coaxial printing method, mandrel-based method, and direct-bioprinting method.

4.1.1   FRESH (Freeform Reversible Embedding of Suspended Hydrogel) Printing

FRESH printing was used to print the cell laden hydrogel in a supportive bath containing gelatin microparticles which have mechanical resistance as the nozzle passes through the bath. After printing the gelatin dissolves by incubating at 37°C thereby resulting in the scaffold. Using a coacervation method, the resolution of the FRESH printing can be enhanced in the supporting bath, leading to a vasculature with smaller diameters and denser networks, including perfusable arteries with a diameter of about 100 mM (Kong and Wang, 2023). Kreimendahl et al, has fabricated a tubular structure using fibrinogen and hyaluronic acid ink containing HUVEC and human dermal fibroblasts. The bioink was crosslinked using calcium chloride and thrombin. The printing parameters of the tubular structure includes: printer velocity of 8 mm/s, a fill density of 1.5 mL, a layer height of 0.2 mm, and a grid fill pattern. The fibrinogen-HA constructs were printed in a tubular form with a height of 2 mm and a diameter of 8 mm. At room temperature, all printed structures were polymerized for 20 mins post printing. Finally the developed structure was analyzed for the CD 31 angiogenic marker expression (Kreimendahl et al., 2021).

4.1.2   Coaxial bioprinting

Co-axial printing (CP) is used for the fabrication of continuous tubular structures with the help of two layered nozzles. The bioink can be extruded from the two different nozzles to make a core-shell layer of the tubular structure. The three main components of CP are co-axial nozzles, propulsion, and print bed . The nozzles are stacked together to attain printing of inks in different layers. When the nozzle diameter is less its rate of extrusion and shear rate will be high thus there will be a change in the shape of the extrusion. Also if the shear rate is high, it has its influence on the cell viability. The propulsion is the key component as the thickness of the sample is dependent on the printing pressure. The final component printing bed needs to be adjusted according to the inbuilt program. The optimum nozzle, printing rate, speed, and viscosity of the bioink needs to be optimized before bioprinting (Xu et al., 2022).

Ozbolat et al have used coaxial bioprinting to create vessel-shaped tubular microchannels using co-axial bioprinting. Alginate encapsulated human umbilical vein smooth muscle cells (HUVSMCs) were injected through the coaxial nozzle's outer channel, and the crosslinker solution was injected through the inner channel. The constructed vascular conduit not only ensured structural integrity but also allowed fluid to pass through the lumen (Zhang et al., 2015). In one study, the perfusable biomimetic blood vessels were developed by a flexible coaxial 3D bioprinting technique. In brief, gelatin methacryloyl (GelMA), sodium alginate, and 4-arm poly (ethylene glycol)-tetra-acrylate (PEGTA) encapsulated HUVECs bioink were co-axially printed to form a tubular structure. To create a stable construct, this blend bioink was covalently photocrosslinked (GelMA and PEGTA) after being ionically crosslinked by calcium ions (Jia et al., 2016). Using vascular tissue derived extracellular matrix and HUVECs as a bioink, Gao et al. has developed a co-axial printed vascular construct with a diameter of 247 ± 31 μm and a thickness of 49 ± 21 μm. The fabricated vessel exhibits preliminary endothelialization including permeability, leukocyte adhesion, self-remodelling to shear stress and improved pro-angiogenic signals. Therefore this CP method helps in the development of an intricate vascular network (G. Gao et al., 2018).

Zhou et al, developed the biomimetic vascular construct using vascular smooth muscle cells (VSMC) in the shell and vascular endothelial cells (VEC) in the core using co-axial 3D bioprinting with lumen dimensions of 0.3mm thickness and 1mm diameter. The author has used the GelMA/PEGDA/alginate/lyase along with VSMC as a bioink for the shell region. The core region was printed with the pluronic F-127. The wire-like blood vessels were dual crosslinked using calcium chloride (alginate) and photocrosslinking (GelMA/PEGDA). The fabricated vessel was then placed in a medium with gentle shaking at 15°C for 5mins to remove the F-127 and to create the hollow tube-like structure. Finally, the lumen of the vessel was filled with gelatin solution containing VEC. On day 6 upon proliferation and differentiation of the VSMC and VEC, the vessel like structure was analyzed for its proliferation using cell tracker and expression of maturation of VSMC and angiogenesis using immunostaining with α-SMA (VSMC maturation) and CD31(angiogenesis) (Zhou et al., 2020). So, coaxial bioprinting can be used to construct a small blood vessel, however this method is limited for developing a continuous bifurcated blood vascular structure.

4.1.3 Mandrel based bioprinting

Mandrel based bioprinting has been employed in the fabricating vascular grafts. This technique utilizes a rod to create a hollow tubular structure and the bioink is printed on a rotating rod to form a tubular structure. In a study conducted by Gao et al, the blood vessel was printed using a coaxial nozzle containing SMC and fibroblast cells on a rotating rod. Post printing the HUVEC cells were added to the hollow channel upon rod removal **Figure 2**. The fabricated structure also contains perfusable micro and macro channels for the delivery of nutrients and oxygen to the cells. Freeman et al employed gelatin and fibrinogen for printing a vascular graft on a polystyrene rod pre-treated with pluronic F-127. Within 60 days, collagen deposition and a burst pressure of about 1000 mmHg. This is significantly lower than the pressure in the native blood vessels (Q. Gao et al., 2017).

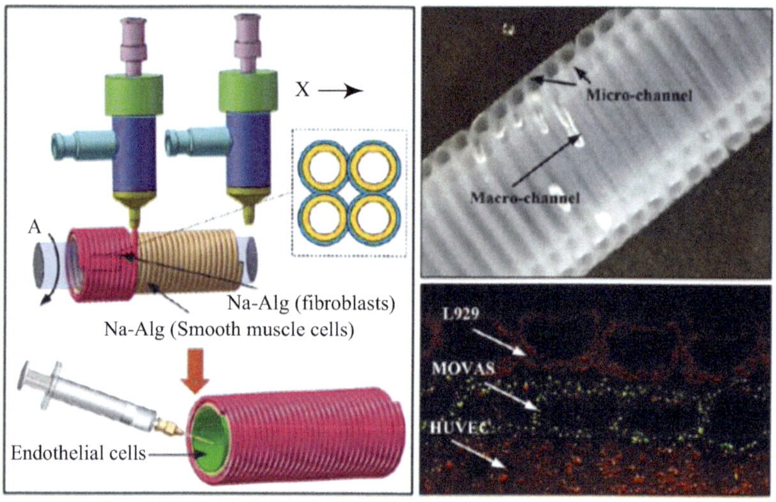

Fig. 2   Schematic illustration of mandrel and co-axially 3D bioprinted biomimetic blood vessel (Q. Gao et al., 2017).

4.2 Light Based Bioprinting

Light based bioprinting has been categorized into two types : (1) laser based bioprinting and (2) digital light processing based bioprinting. In this chapter LAB based vascular bioprinting has been discussed as there are no studies on DLP based vascular bioprinting

4.2.1 Laser Assisted bioprinting (LAB) and Stereolithography based bioprinting

Laser assisted bioprinting (LAB) has been developed from laser direct writing and laser induced forward transfer technique. LAB is based on the energy absorption of the donor layer consisting of titanium and gold on the top and bioink on the bottom. During the printing process, the laser pulse vaporizes the donor layer and penetrates deep into the bioink solution using high pressure thereby creating droplets. The droplets are then collected by the receiving substrate and crosslinked (Kong and Wang, 2023). LAB avoids direct contact with the bioink, and it also prevents the cells from shear stress. Only limited studies are carried out using the LAB for vascular bioprinting (Dikyol et al., 2021).

Wu et al. used a laser-based bioprinter to fabricate blood vessels that mimick native structures using HUVECs and HUVSMC (human vascular smooth muscle cells) within an encapsulated hydrogel. The process began with the deposition of endothelial cells using laser power followed by a period of incubation to allow for cell communication and differentiation into luminal structures. Subsequently, th HUVSMCs were printed atop the endothelial layer to further replicate the native blood vessel architecture. The study demonstrated that LAB printing has the special ability to regulate cell-cell interactions in three-dimensional hydrogel scaffolds through the simultaneous deposition of both HUVECs and HUVSMCs. This co-deposition promotes a proliferative state in SMCs adjacent to the printed EC network and supports the HUVECs in maintaining the differentiated lumen structure (Wu and Ringeisen, 2010). Guillotin et al, mixed human umbilical vein endothelial cell line Eahy 926 and rabbit cancer cell line B16 with different concentrations of glycerol, sodium alginate, or thrombin (MatrigelTM). The bioink was printed onto a fibrinogen sheet using LIFT to create a network with microvasculature dimensions. The authors were able to control the droplet size and, consequently, the diameter of the printed vasculature by varying the concentration of alginate. Alginate additionally served as an extracellular matrix replacement (Hauser et al., 2021).

The stereolithography (SLA) technique prints the polymers in a layer-by-layer manner and utilizes UV or visible light to crosslink the polymers with photocurable moieties. It is an additive manufacturing (AM) technique with several advantages like high resolution, scalability, quick printing, and precise geometry to fabricate the extremely intricate 3D constructs (Kačarević et al., 2018; Kumar and Kim, 2020). The SLA working mechanism is similar for both 3D printing and 3D bioprinting as it is based on the computer aided laser beam for photocrosslinking. The bioink can be cured onto a vertically driven (z-direction) print bed upon exposure to a raster-scanning laser. The platform is shifted away from the printing location to restock liquid bioink for the preparation of the second layer's photocuring after the first layer's photocrosslinking. In case of the bioprinted samples, it may require additional photocuring in order to make the sample stable (Li et al., 2023). Based on the photopolymerization process, the SLA is categorized into two types namely single photon and multiphoton SLA. The single photon method was employed by mask-based SLA and direct laser writing based SLA. The photoinitiator in the polymer undergoes single photon linear absorption for the polymerization to take place. The drawback of this method is that light penetration of inadequate depth for the photocuring to occur. Whereas, the multiphoton SLA utilizes few low intensity photons and ultra-short high intensity lasers to generate radicals for photocuring. Usually, two photo based SLA (TP-SLA) were used in the tissue engineering applications. The TP-SLA works on the principle of using highly intense lasers with non-optical absorption (Zennifer et al., 2022).

In this chapter, SLA based 3D bioprinting of complex vascular networks has been explained. Thomas et al, has fabricated an enzymatic degradable sacrificial bioink using a multimaterial SLA bioprinter (Figure 2). Methacrylated gelatin and hyaluronic acid were used as a base polymer for bioprinting. The author has 3D bioprinted HUVEC on a perfusable channel with dimensions of 720 to 360 µm diameter and 360 µm height. The fabricated sample remained stable for 28 days and the angiogenesis was confirmed using endothelial marker CD 31 (A. Thomas et al., 2020).

4.3　Inkjet Based Bioprinting

Inkjet based bioprinting is a 2D non-contact printing technique, where the printing is carried out in a digitally controlled pattern. This printing method utilizes low viscosity bioink which is squeezed out of the cartridge either using thermal or piezoelectric process. Inkjet printing is categorized into two types based on the extrusion of the ink: continuous and drop-on demand. In the continuous method, constant pressure is applied to extrude the droplets continuously. Whereas, the drop on demand (DOD) method is performed only when there is a need to extrude droplets. DOD is the most preferred type in tissue engineering applications and is categorized into thermal and piezoelectric DOD methods (Agarwal et al., 2020; Kong and Wang, 2023). In the piezoelectric DOD method, the microfluidic chamber located above the nozzle employs the piezoelectric transducer to produce the transient pressure for droplet generation. in the thermal DOD method, a pulsed electric current is applied onto a heating element in the microfluidic chamber, which then vaporizes the ink to generate droplets. The pressure produced by the vapor bubble forces the ink droplet onto the substrate's surface through the nozzle. In this method, the cells are subjected to very short-term exposure to high-temperature which does not damage the cells. In both types of printing systems, the rheological characteristics of the bioink plays a vital role in printing. Although the precise specifications for the ink varies based on the system, 30 mPa/s is often the required viscosity (Agarwal et al., 2020).

A trilayered blood artery was bioprinted in the drop on demand printing technique. In this study, ECs were encapsulated in the sacrificial gelatin core, SMCs in fibrinogen were cross-linked by thrombin, and fibroblast cells in collagen solution were printed using a specially constructed printing apparatus. After a few hours, the sacrificial layer was taken off to guarantee that the ECs adhered to the lumen surface properly (Fazal et al., 2021). Cui et al. printed cells in a quasi-3D structure using a modified thermal inkjet printer. The bioink consists of human microvascular ECs (HMVECs) and fibrin. The bioprinted HMVECs align on the fibrin channel as depicted in Figure 3, and the cells proliferate on day 21. With the advancement of their inkjet printer, it was believed that the HMVECs on the thin grid build may generate actual 3D blood arteries (Cui and Boland, 2009).

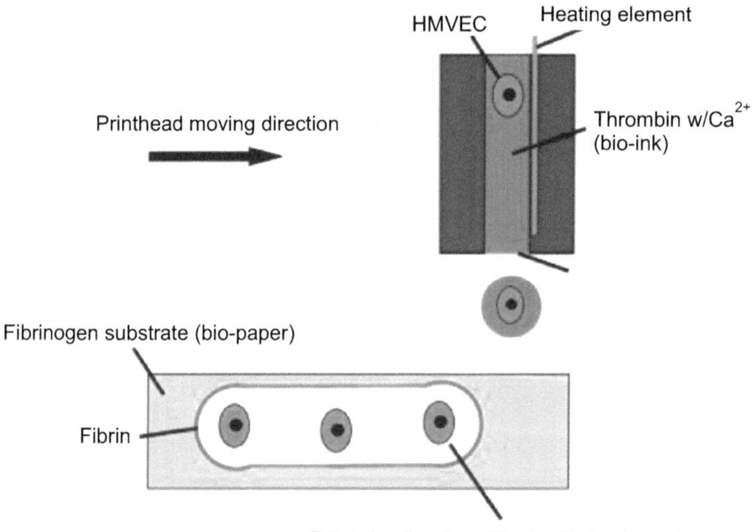

Fig. 3   Schematic illustration of thermal inkjet based bioprinting of HMVEC on fibrin scaffold (Cui and Boland, 2009).

5.   Advanced Methods of Fabricating Vascular Tissue Models

5.1   4D Bioprinting

4D bioprinting is an advanced version of the 3D bioprinting technique which utilizes stimuli responsive materials for the fabrication of tissue mimicing models. The 4th dimension is the time which allows the smart biomaterials to mimic the tissue dynamics and structural changes of the engineered tissues. 4D printing is carried out using stimuli responsive polymers along with or without cells. For instance, the hydrogel is water responsive and undergoes deformation in the presence of moisture. Similarly other stimuli include pH (collagen), electric fields (polyelectrolytes), magnetic fields (platelets) (Zeenat et al., 2023) (Figure 4). There are no available reports on 4D bioprinted vascular conduits.

Kirillova et al. used a 4D printing strategy to create tubes with a diameter of only 20 µm, smaller than the 3D printed vascular graft. The tubular structure was fabricated by taking a layer of mouse bone marrow stromal cells and mixing it with a methacrylated alginate and hyaluronic acid hydrogel and printed on a glass slide. In the second phase green light was used to crosslink the polymer. The polymer sheets, which were sensitive to Ca2+ ions, altered shape and rolled up to form a tubular structure once placed in solution. The ability to construct tubes with small diameters makes this approach perfect for creating miniature vascular systems (Kirillova et al., 2017).

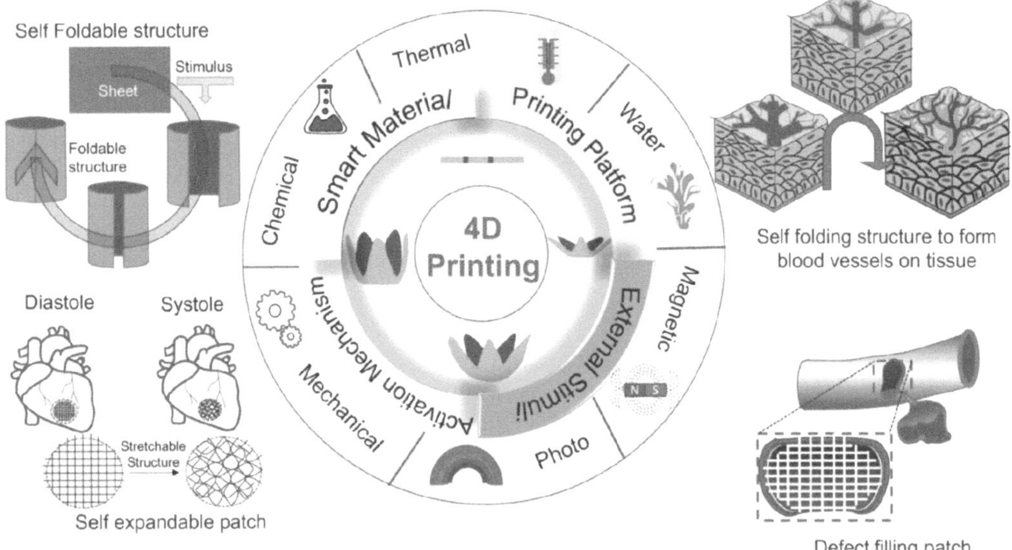

Fig. 4   Schematic illustration of 4D bioprinting in vascular tissue engineering (Zeenat et al., 2023).

5.2 *Microfluidics Based Bioprinting*

The ability of organ-on-a-chip technologies to mimic essential components of human physiology is vital for comprehending disease causes and medication effects, enhancing preclinical safety, and carrying out efficacy testing. Microfluidic chips, in contrast to other 3D cell culture models, can replicate the biomechanical parameters found in the human body. These biomechanical signals are essential for the development of certain tissues and organs, including kidney infiltration, skeletal muscle, cardiac tissue, and vasculature (Abudupataer et al., 2020). Abudupataer et al, has fabricated a bioprinted vessel on a chip to establish an *in vitro* vascular model. In this work, the 3D printed vessels were fabricated using GelMA containing endothelial cells (ECs) and smooth muscle cells (SMCs) on a microfluidic chip. The developed vessel on a chip was perfused with a continuous medium to mimic the native blood flow. The coculture exhibited decreased CD31 expression and increased SM22, αSMA expression which might be due to the SMC and EC interaction (Abudupataer et al., 2020).

Wang et al fabricated a venous and arteries like structure using microfluidic bioprinting. The hydrogel is made up of elastic enzyme crosslinked gelatin and ionically cross-linked alginate. The double crosslinked hydrogel has robust mechanical properties which help in the formation and stability of tubular structures. Two different methods were used in conjunction with microfluidic bioprinting to create venous and arterial synthetic vasculature that closely resembled their native blood vessels. In particular, monolayered hydrogel tubes were bioprinted to create venous conduits, which were then seeded with human umbilical vein smooth muscle cells (HUVSMCs) on the exterior and human umbilical vein ECs (HUVECs) in the lumens. On the other hand, arterial conduits were created by directly bioprinting the shell of the tubular structure using human umbilical artery SMC (HUASMC) and core hydrogel layer, and human umbilical artery ECs (HUAECs) were seeded into the lumens. Key characteristics of blood vessels, such as stretchability, perfusability, and barrier performance, were present in both venous and arterial conduits. In response to a vasoconstrictor and vasodilator, respectively, the arterial conduits showed constriction and dilatation (D. Wang et al., 2022).

6.   Future Perspective and Conclusion

Establishing a vascular network is crucial for the survival of engineered constructs by providing nutrients and oxygen to cells. Creating a vascular network remains a significant challenge in tissue engineering despite its importance. 3D bioprinting has become a promising tool for creating biomimetic tissue constructs and organs for clinical use. Furthermore, advanced techniques for generating *in vitro* models for drug testing, metabolism, and toxicity screening can be achieved through 3D bioprinting. This method offers unmatched benefits for replicating anatomical characteristics and functions of the original tissue (Datta et al., 2017).

In this chapter, we have elaborated advanced methods of fabrication of ideal vascular grafts. The conventional methods have several limitations in developing small diameter blood vessels. 3D bioprinting is an advanced method of developing a patient specific implant. Among the above explained methods of fabrication, extrusion is one of the commonly used methods in the fabrication of tubular structures. Despite its advantages, the extrusion-based bioprinted tubular structures have not succeeded in translation towards clinical application, mainly due to their poor mechanical properties. To address this issue, recent reports have highlighted the significant role of the mechanical stiffness of matrices in influencing the differentiation of progenitor or stem cells. Also, the recent research indicates promising outcomes in creating a graft with bifurcation and comparable properties to native arteries. Several investigations lack the biomechanical characterization data recommended by ISO and FDA. Hence, further research is required to determine if materials with adjustable mechanical properties can be created and if these mechanical properties can be incorporated into bioprinting on a large scale. Another crucial aspect to consider is establishing a vascular network and ensuring its stability while maintaining the desired shape (Zeenat et al., 2023). After following the ISO and FDA guidelines, the vascular transplant can be advanced to clinical trials and long-term *in vivo* testing. Given recent improvements, vascular surgeons may employ hand-held bioprinters or bio-pens to quickly restore injured vascular tissues, as has been done in cartilage and bone restoration treatments.

In 4D bioprinting, the fourth dimension integrates the "time" factor, enabling cells and materials to adapt their functionalities and shape in response to external stimuli. Therefore, printed structures can be rearranged to enhance their performance. It is essential to consider that the native vasculature is multi-scalar, and future bioprinting technologies need to create vascularization at various scale dimensions, from arteries and veins to capillaries. Yet, using current bioprinting methods, it remains challenging to bioprint capillaries at a sub-micron scale. Thus, upcoming projects should aim to print micro-vascular networks alongside macro-sized tissue (An et al., 2015).

In addition to the challenges in the field, 3D bioprinting technology will also need to address regulatory and intellectual property issues. Currently, bioprinting technology is not officially categorized as such; however, it must be classified under the device/biological category, necessitating the standardization of bioprinted constructs. For the benefit of investors seeking commercial gains, it is essential to have appropriate intellectual property protection. Bioprinting processes and products differ from natural tissues or tissue formation processes. They require human intellectual input and could be eligible for intellectual property protection. These details are essential for successful clinical translation (Datta et al., 2017).

References

Abudupataer, M., Chen, N., Yan, S., Alam, F., Shi, Y. et al. (2020). Bioprinting a 3D vascular construct for engineering a vessel-on-a-chip. *Biomedical Microdevices*, *22*(1), 10. https://doi.org/10.1007/s10544-019-0460-3

Agarwal, S., Saha, S., Balla, V.K., Pal, A., Barui, A. et al. (2020). Current Developments in 3D Bioprinting for Tissue and Organ Regeneration–A Review. *Frontiers in Mechanical Engineering*, *6*. https://www.frontiersin.org/articles/10.3389/fmech.2020.589171

Ahn, H., Ju, Y.M., Takahashi, H., Williams, D.F., Yoo, J.J. et al. (2015). Engineered small diameter vascular grafts by combining cell sheet engineering and electrospinning technology. *Acta Biomaterialia*, *16*, 14–22. https://doi.org/10.1016/j.actbio.2015.01.030

An, J., Chua, C. and Mironov, V. (2015). A Perspective on 4D Bioprinting. *International Journal of Bioprinting*, *2*. https://doi.org/10.18063/IJB.2016.01.003

Bertassoni, L.E., Cecconi, M., Manoharan, V., Nikkhah, M., Hjortnaes, J. et al. (2014). Hydrogel bioprinted microchannel networks for vascularization of tissue engineering constructs. *Lab on a Chip*, *14*(13), 2202–2211. https://doi.org/10.1039/C4LC00030G

Bonafè, F., Govoni, M., Giordano, E., Caldarera, C.M., Guarnieri, C. et al. (2014). Hyaluronan and cardiac regeneration. In *Journal of Biomedical Science* (Vol. 21, Issue 1, pp. 31–48). BioMed Central Ltd. https://doi.org/10.1186/s12929-014-0100-4

Christensen, G., Herum, K.M. and Lunde, I.G. (2019). Sweet, yet underappreciated: Proteoglycans and extracellular matrix remodeling in heart disease. In *Matrix Biology* (Vols. 75–76, pp. 286–299). Elsevier B.V. https://doi.org/10.1016/j.matbio.2018.01.001

Conte, M.S. (2013). Critical appraisal of surgical revascularization for critical limb ischemia. *Journal of Vascular Surgery*, *57*(2), 8S-13S. https://doi.org/10.1016/j.jvs.2012.05.114

Cui, X. and Boland, T. (2009). Human microvasculature fabrication using thermal inkjet printing technology. *Biomaterials*, *30*(31), 6221–6227. https://doi.org/10.1016/j.biomaterials.2009.07.056

Datta, P., Ayan, B. and Ozbolat, I.T. (2017). Bioprinting for vascular and vascularized tissue biofabrication. *Acta Biomaterialia*, *51*, 1–20. https://doi.org/10.1016/j.actbio.2017.01.035

Dikyol, C., Altunbek, M., Bartolo, P. and Koc, B. (2021). Multimaterial bioprinting approaches and their implementations for vascular and vascularized tissues. *Bioprinting*, *24*, e00159. https://doi.org/10.1016/j.bprint.2021.e00159

Elaine N., M. and Katja, H. (2019). *Human Anatomy Physiology*.

Fazal, F., Raghav, S., Callanan, A., Koutsos, V. and Radacsi, N. et al. (2021). Recent advancements in the bioprinting of vascular grafts. *Biofabrication*, *13*(3), 032003. https://doi.org/10.1088/1758-5090/ac0963

Gao, G., Park, J.Y., Kim, B.S., Jang, J. and Cho, D.-W. et al. (2018). Coaxial Cell Printing of Freestanding, Perfusable, and Functional In Vitro Vascular Models for Recapitulation of Native Vascular Endothelium Pathophysiology. *Advanced Healthcare Materials*, *7*(23), 1801102. https://doi.org/10.1002/adhm.201801102

Gao, Q., Liu, Z., Lin, Z., Qiu, J., Liu, Y. et al. (2017). 3D Bioprinting of Vessel-like Structures with Multi-level Fluidic Channels. *ACS Biomaterials Science & Engineering*, *3*. https://doi.org/10.1021/acsbiomaterials.6b00643

Garg, I., Grist, T.M. and Nagpal, P. (2023). MR Angiography for Aortic Diseases. *Magnetic Resonance Imaging Clinics of North America*, *31*(3), 373–394. https://doi.org/10.1016/j.mric.2023.05.002

Harskamp, R.E., Lopes, R.D., Baisden, C.E., de Winter, R.J. and Alexander, J.H. et al. (2013). Saphenous Vein Graft Failure After Coronary Artery Bypass Surgery: Pathophysiology, Management, and Future Directions. *Annals of Surgery*, *257*(5), 824. https://doi.org/10.1097/SLA.0b013e318288c38d

Hauser, P.V., Chang, H.-M., Nishikawa, M., Kimura, H., Yanagawa, N. et al. (2021). Bioprinting Scaffolds for Vascular Tissues and Tissue Vascularization. *Bioengineering*, *8*(11), Article 11. https://doi.org/10.3390/bioengineering8110178

Horn, M.A. and Trafford, A.W. (2016). Aging and the cardiac collagen matrix: Novel mediators of fibrotic remodelling. In *Journal of Molecular and Cellular Cardiology* (Vol. 93, pp. 175–185). Academic Press. https://doi.org/10.1016/j.yjmcc.2015.11.005

Hu, N. and Zhang, Y.S. (2018). 18—3D bioprinting blood vessels. In D. J. Thomas, Z.M. Jessop and I.S. Whitaker (Eds.), *3D Bioprinting for Reconstructive Surgery* (pp. 377–391). Woodhead Publishing. https://doi.org/10.1016/B978-0-08-101103-4.00018-1

Jia, W., Gungor-Ozkerim, P.S., Zhang, Y.S., Yue, K., Zhu, K. et al. (2016). Direct 3D bioprinting of perfusable vascular constructs using a blend bioink. *Biomaterials*, *106*, 58–68. https://doi.org/10.1016/j.biomaterials.2016.07.038

Jiang, H., Li, X., Chen, T., Liu, Y., Wang, Q. et al. (2023). Bioprinted vascular tissue: Assessing functions from cellular, tissue to organ levels. *Materials Today Bio*, *23*, 100846. https://doi.org/10.1016/j.mtbio.2023.100846

Kačarević, Ž., Rider, P., Alkildani, S., Retnasingh, S., Smeets, R. et al. (2018). An Introduction to 3D Bioprinting: Possibilities, Challenges and Future Aspects. *Materials*, *11*(11), 2199. https://doi.org/10.3390/ma11112199

Kirillova, A., Maxson, R., Stoychev, G., Gomillion, C.T. and Ionov, L. et al. (2017). 4D Biofabrication Using Shape–Morphing Hydrogels. *Advanced Materials*, *29*(46), 1703443. https://doi.org/10.1002/adma.201703443

Klinkert, P., Post, P.N., Breslau, P.J. and Bockel, J.H. van. (2004). Saphenous Vein Versus PTFE for Above-Knee Femoropopliteal Bypass. A Review of the Literature. *European Journal of Vascular and Endovascular Surgery*, *27*(4), 357–362. https://doi.org/10.1016/j.ejvs.2003.12.027

Koens, M.J.W., Krasznai, A.G., Hanssen, A.E.J., Hendriks, T., Praster, R. et al. (2015). Vascular replacement using a layered elastin-collagen vascular graft in a porcine model: One week patency versus one month occlusion. *Organogenesis*, *11*(3), 105–121. https://doi.org/10.1080/15476278.2015.1038448

Kong, Z. and Wang, X. (2023). Bioprinting Technologies and Bioinks for Vascular Model Establishment. *International Journal of Molecular Sciences*, *24*(1), 891. https://doi.org/10.3390/ijms24010891

Kreimendahl, F., Kniebs, C., Tavares Sobreiro, A.M., Schmitz-Rode, T., Jockenhoevel, S. et al. (2021). FRESH bioprinting technology for tissue engineering – the influence of printing process and bioink composition on cell behavior and vascularization. *Journal of Applied Biomaterials & Functional Materials*, *19*, 228080002110288. https://doi.org/10.1177/22808000211028808

Kumar, H. and Kim, K. (2020). Stereolithography 3D Bioprinting. In J.M. Crook (Ed.), *3D Bioprinting* (Vol. 2140, pp. 93–108). Springer US. https://doi.org/10.1007/978-1-0716-0520-2_6

Li, W., Wang, M., Ma, H., Chapa-Villarreal, F.A., Lobo, A.O. et al. (2023). Stereolithography apparatus and digital light processing-based 3D bioprinting for tissue fabrication. *iScience*, *26*(2), 106039. https://doi.org/10.1016/j.isci.2023.106039

Lockhart, M., Wirrig, E., Phelps, A. and Wessels, A. (2011). Extracellular matrix and heart development. In *Birth Defects Research Part A - Clinical and Molecular Teratology* (Vol. 91, Issue 6, pp. 535–550). https://doi.org/10.1002/bdra.20810

Maina, R.M., Barahona, M.J., Finotti, M., Lysyy, T., Geibel, P. et al. (2018). Generating vascular conduits: From tissue engineering to three-dimensional bioprinting. *Innovative Surgical Sciences*, *3*(3), 203–213. https://doi.org/10.1515/iss-2018-0016

Mir, A., Lee, E., Shih, W., Koljaka, S., Wang, A. et al. (2023). 3D Bioprinting for Vascularization. *Bioengineering*, *10*(5), 606. https://doi.org/10.3390/bioengineering10050606

Miri, A.K., Khalilpour, A., Cecen, B., Maharjan, S., Shin, S.R. et al. (2019). Multiscale bioprinting of vascularized models. *Biomaterials*, *198*, 204–216. https://doi.org/10.1016/j.biomaterials.2018.08.006

Ong, C.S., Fukunishi, T., Liu, R.H., Nelson, K., Zhang, H. et al. (2017). Bilateral Arteriovenous Shunts as a Method for Evaluating Tissue-Engineered Vascular Grafts in Large Animal Models. *Tissue Engineering Part C: Methods*, *23*(11), 728–735. https://doi.org/10.1089/ten.tec.2017.0217

Sánchez-Sánchez, R., Rodríguez-Rego, J.M., Macías-García, A., Mendoza-Cerezo, L. and Díaz-Parralejo, A. et al. (2023). Relationship between shear-thinning rheological properties of bioinks and bioprinting parameters. *International Journal of Bioprinting*, *9*(2), 687. https://doi.org/10.18063/ijb.687

Schöneberg, J., De Lorenzi, F., Theek, B., Blaeser, A., Rommel, D. et al. (2018). Engineering biofunctional in vitro vessel models using a multilayer bioprinting technique. *Scientific Reports*, *8*(1), 10430. https://doi.org/10.1038/s41598-018-28715-0

Song, H.-H.G., Rumma, R.T., Ozaki, C.K., Edelman, E.R. and Chen, C.S. et al. (2018). Vascular Tissue Engineering: Progress, Challenges and Clinical Promise. *Cell Stem Cell*, *22*(3), 340–354. https://doi.org/10.1016/j.stem.2018.02.009

Talman, V. and Kivelä, R. (2018). Cardiomyocyte—Endothelial Cell Interactions in Cardiac Remodeling and Regeneration. *Frontiers in Cardiovascular Medicine*, *5*. https://doi.org/10.3389/fcvm.2018.00101

Thomas, A., Orellano, I., Lam, T., Noichl, B., Geiger, M.-A. et al. (2020). Vascular bioprinting with enzymatically degradable bioinks via multi-material projection-based stereolithography. *Acta Biomaterialia*, *117*, 121–132. https://doi.org/10.1016/j.actbio.2020.09.033

Tuohy, M.C., Hillman, E.M.C., Marshall, R. and Agalliu, D. (2023). The age-dependent immune response to ischemic stroke. *Current Opinion in Neurobiology*, *78*, 102670. https://doi.org/10.1016/j.conb.2022.102670

Veith, F.J., Moss, C.M., Sprayregen, S. and Montefusco, C. (1979). Preoperative saphenous venography in arterial reconstructive surgery of the lower extremity. *Surgery*, *85*(3), 253–256.

Wang, D., Maharjan, S., Kuang, X., Wang, Z., Mille, L.S. et al. (2022). Microfluidic bioprinting of tough hydrogel-based vascular conduits for functional blood vessels. *Science Advances*, *8*(43), eabq6900. https://doi.org/10.1126/sciadv.abq6900

Wang, K., Zheng, W., Pan, Y., Ma, S., Guan, Y. et al. (2016). Three-Layered PCL Grafts Promoted Vascular Regeneration in a Rabbit Carotid Artery Model. *Macromolecular Bioscience*, *16*(4), 608–618. https://doi.org/10.1002/mabi.201500355

Wu, P.K. and Ringeisen, B.R. (2010). Development of human umbilical vein endothelial cell (HUVEC) and human umbilical vein smooth muscle cell (HUVSMC) branch/stem structures on hydrogel layers via biological laser printing (BioLP). *Biofabrication*, *2*(1), 014111. https://doi.org/10.1088/1758-5082/2/1/014111

Xiong, Y., Chan, W.Y., Chua, A.W.C., Feng, J., Gopal, P. et al. (2013). Decellularized Porcine Saphenous Artery for Small-Diameter Tissue-Engineered Conduit Graft. *Artificial Organs*, *37*(6), E74–E87. https://doi.org/10.1111/aor.12014

Xu, H., Su, Y., Liao, Z., Liu, Z., Huang, X. et al. (2022). Coaxial bioprinting vascular constructs: A review. *European Polymer Journal*, *179*, 111549. https://doi.org/10.1016/j.eurpolymj.2022.111549

Zeenat, L., Zolfagharian, A., Sriya, Y., Sasikumar, S., Bodaghi, M. et al. (2023). 4D Printing for Vascular Tissue Engineering: Progress and Challenges. *Advanced Materials Technologies*, *8*(23), 2300200. https://doi.org/10.1002/admt.202300200

Zennifer, A., Manivannan, S., Sethuraman, S., Kumbar, S.G. and Sundaramurthi, D. et al. (2022). 3D bioprinting and photocrosslinking: Emerging strategies & future perspectives. *Biomaterials Advances*, *134*, 112576. https://doi.org/10.1016/j.msec.2021.112576

Zhang, Y., Kumar, P., Lv, S., Xiong, D., Zhao, H. et al. (2021). Recent advances in 3D bioprinting of vascularized tissues. *Materials & Design*, *199*, 109398. https://doi.org/10.1016/j.matdes.2020.109398

Zhang, Y., Yu, Y., Akkouch, A., Dababneh, A., Dolati, F. et al. (2015). In vitro study of directly bioprinted perfusable vasculature conduits. *Biomaterials Science*, *3*(1), 134–143. https://doi.org/10.1039/C4BM00234B

Zhou, X., Nowicki, M., Sun, H., Hann, S.Y., Cui, H. et al. (2020). 3D Bioprinting-Tunable Small-Diameter Blood Vessels with Biomimetic Biphasic Cell Layers. *ACS Applied Materials & Interfaces*, *12*(41), 45904–45915. https://doi.org/10.1021/acsami.0c14871

3D Bioprinting of Liver Tissue

Haleema Sabia,[1] *Sandhya Sharma*[2]
and *Radha Chaube**

1. Introduction

Drugs that have been consumed enter the bloodstream and first reach the liver. There is a pressing need to develop in vitro liver models for preclinical and clinical testing since drug-induced liver injuries are common. Liver-on-chip techniques are useful for tracking medication effectiveness and toxicity, identifying foodborne infections and diseases, examining the impact of dietary supplements and cosmetics on human organs, and comprehending liver function and disease impairment (Deng et al., 2019; Fetah et al., 2019). Recent advancements in CAD and fabrication technology have accelerated the development of 3D printing. Charles Hull invented 3D printing, also known as additive manufacturing (AM), rapid prototyping (RP), and free form fabrication (FFF), in 1986. His proposal was based on the idea of applying consecutive layers of a base material on top of another to 'print' items. Since its debut, 3D printing has had an impact on many disciplines, including engineering, industry, and medicine. In recent years, biocompatible 3D printing techniques have shown great promise for tissue engineering applications. Tissue engineering often involves growing cells, seeding them into biocompatible scaffolds, and enabling them to grow and mature in vitro or in a bioreactor to generate desired tissues.3D bioprinting involves precisely layering cells, scaffolds, and factors to replicate a biological tissue. Compared to classic tissue engineering approaches, 3D bioprinting devices provide more precise spatial relationships between tissue elements. 3D bioprinting shows enormous potential for regenerative medicine applications (E.S.Bishop et al. (2017).

The liver is in charge of several bodily metabolic functions as well as the creation of various vital substances as it is engaged in more than 500 metabolic reactions. The liver performs a variety of vital processes, including the metabolism of harmful xenobiotics, the synthesis of sterols and albumin, and the central metabolism of energy. Though the liver can regenerate itself remarkably, liver illnesses are a leading cause of morbidity and mortality globally in recent decades (Li, C., Jiang, Z. and Yang, H. (2022). This chapter will cover the most recent developments in the creation

[1] Department of Zoology, Institute of Science, Banaras Hindu University, Varanasi, India.
[2] Department of Zoology, Institute of Science, Banaras Hindu University, India.
* Corresponding author: chauberadha@rediffmail.com

of vascularized liver tissues, including cutting-edge techniques, materials, and applications. We'll start out by talking about printing blood vessels and work our way through the state of bioprinting tissue and organoids. Along with some of the exciting new places this 3D Bioprinting technique may lead us to, we will also examine and talk about the present drawbacks of vascularized tissue engineering.

1.1 *General Approach*

3D printing refers to any of various technologies for creating three-dimensional things by building two-dimensional cross sections on top of each other. The phrase 3D printing initially referred to a specific technology called 3DP, which was developed by scientists at the Massachusetts Institute of Technology (MIT) in 1993 and licenced it to various firms.

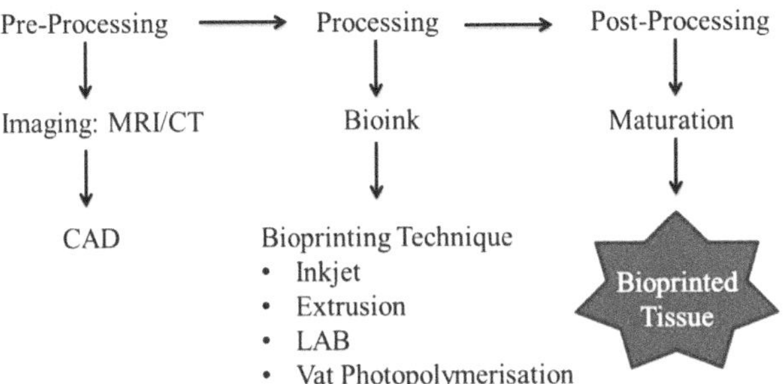

Fig. 1   Bioprinting overview schematic (E.S.Bishop et al. (2017))

Bioprinting is a technology that builds intricate biological tissue and organ structures precisely by layering cells with bioink using a computer-controlled process i.e; CAD based on Pre-processing. An overview of Bioprinting has been presented in Figure 1. This innovative method has been effective in developing several organs. To overcome issues like lack of organs and other associated problems, this technology which has arisen from engineering, biomaterial science, cell biology, physics, and medicine is an important milestone and 3D bioprinting has made significant progress towards functional tissue printing as a consequence. The method of 3D bioprinting is based on additive manufacturing, in which a digital file serves as a blueprint for printing an object layer by layer. Although bioprinting is a new technique, it has already demonstrated significant benefits in the fields of regenerative and personalised medicine, tissue engineering, drug discovery, and cosmetics. In other words, 3D bioprinting refers to the use of 3D printing concepts to create biological entities like tissues and organs. Bioprinting is essentially based on existing printing technologies, such as ink-jet or laser printing, but employs "bioink" (suspensions of living cells and cell growth media), which can be created in micropipettes or other equipment that function as printer cartridges. Cells are subsequently deposited in specified patterns onto culture plates or other sterile surfaces using a computer-controlled printing process. Valve-based printing, which allows for fine control over cell deposition and increased cell survivability, has been utilized to print human embryonic stem cells in preprogrammed patterns that encourage their aggregation into spheroids. Such human tissue models like ear and liver were created by using these types of techniques. Whole or partial liver substitutes can be created using 3D printing, hydrogel-based tissue fabrication, or by using native decellularized liver extracellular matrix as a scaffold.

The fundamental goal of bioprinting has been to address the organ donor crisis by developing the ability to print living organs and other body parts. For future patients, this means a shorter wait time for their organ transplant, as well as an organ that is suited to their specific genetic and physiological profile, lowering the likelihood of rejection. However, the human body, particularly 3D printing organs, is a difficult topic that will require more investigation in the coming years and decades. Isolating and cultivating primary hepatocytes in vitro, along with optimising 3D bioprinting, has the ability to preserve hepatocyte transcriptional characteristics and biological activity. The concept has significant implications for regenerative medicine, personalized drug testing, and liver disease research. This process has been fully explained in Figure 2.

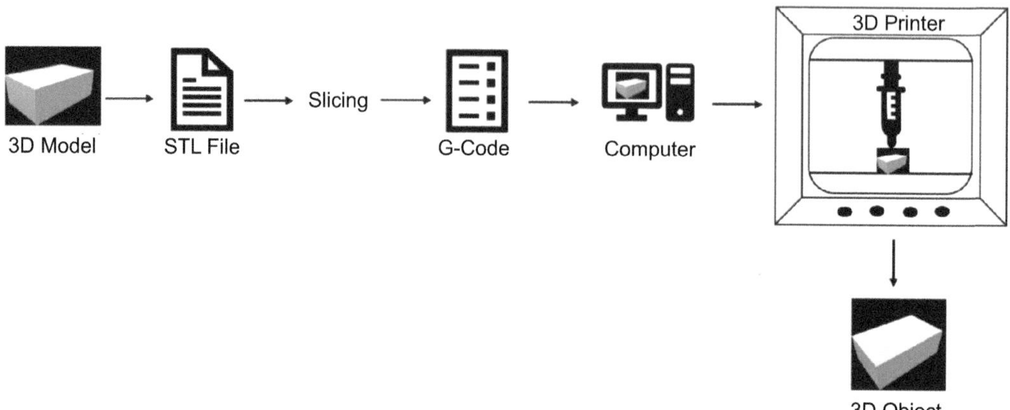

Fig. 2   Flow chart for 3D Bioprinting

Presently the goal is to create a completely developed bile duct and a non-leaky endothelium in order to establish a functional liver graft. Compared to transplantation, the use of cell therapy is less intrusive and expensive; yet, challenges remain, such as the dearth of readily available cell sources with low or no immunogenicity and inconsistent clinical trial results (Acun, A., et al. (2019). With a limited supply of organ donors and available organs for transplantation, the aim of tissue engineering with three-dimensional (3D) bioprinting technology is to construct fully functional and viable tissue and organ replacements for various clinical applications. 3D bioprinting allows for the customization of complex tissue architecture with numerous combinations of materials and printing methods to build different tissue types, and eventually fully functional replacement organs. The main challenge of maintaining 3D printed tissue viability is the inclusion of complex vascular networks for oxygen supply, nutrient transport and waste disposal. Rapid development and discoveries in recent years have taken huge strides toward perfecting the incorporation of vascular networks in 3D printed tissue and organs. In this review, we will discuss the latest advancements in fabricating vascularized tissue and organs including novel strategies and materials, and their applications. Our discussion will begin with the exploration of printing vasculature, progress through the current status of bioprinting tissue/organoids from bone to muscles to organs, and conclude with relevant applications for in vitro models and drug testing. We will also explore and discuss the current limitations of vascularized tissue engineering and some of the promising future directions this technology may bring.

With the advancement of technology and emergence of sophisticated tools, 3D Printing acts as an important tool in the form of 3D Bioprinting in the biological world which is actually the cousin of 3D Printing. Due to the limited number of organ donors, there is a massive need for transplants. There is an urgent need for artificial organs with biocompatible properties, a challenge that can be addressed through tissue engineering. The objective of employing three-dimensional (3D) bioprinting technology in tissue engineering is to create fully functional and viable substitutes for tissues and organs. This approach is particularly crucial given the scarcity of organ donors and the limited availability of organs suitable for transplantation. The goal of tissue engineering using three-dimensional (3D) bioprinting technology is to create completely functional and viable tissue and organ substitutes for diverse clinical purposes, given the limited number of organ donors and available organs for transplantation. Many metabolic, endocrine, and exocrine functions are performed by the liver. Liver failure is responsible for around 2 million fatalities per year. The scope of three-dimensional printing is quickly expanding, with novel approaches leading to the development of cutting-edge 3D bioprinting (3DbioP) techniques for solving problems in bioengineering and biopharmaceutical research.

2. Evolution of 3D Printing Technologies

Currently, 3D bioprinting of completely functional organs for transplantation is not feasible. It is undeniable, nonetheless, that bioprinting methods have advanced dramatically.

Many pioneers, including Vladimir Mironov, Gabor Forgacs, and Thomas Boland, saw decades ago that it was natural to combine technologies like commercial inkjet printing with cell patterning to create living structures that might one day be used in organ transplantation (Gu, Z., Fu, J., Lin, H. and He, Y. (2020). An idea of the evolution of 3D Bioprinting provides us information about the first liver tissue 3D print made in 2014. The 3D structure was a glimpse but that was a landmark discovery in the field of 3D hepatic modeling.

3. 3D Bioprinting Methods

One of the most exciting and innovative sectors of the 21st century is 3D bioprinting, a highly innovative manufacturing process that tackles the constraints of traditional manufacturing methods. This is especially true in the realm of biomedical research. 3D bioprinting has been used in organs-on-chips and organ engineering because it can create extremely intricate 3D patterns with living cells that resemble organ level functionality. A number of layer-by-layer manufacturing technologies are referred to as 3D printing. Each has a different method for forming metal and plastic components. They might also differ in terms of durability, surface quality, choice of materials, speed, and cost of manufacture. Over the last decade, multiple bioprinting technologies have been created and adapted to produce various tissues or organs. Mechanical-based technologies, such as inkjet and extrusion bioprinting, are the most established and well-developed. Laser-assisted bioprinting, including LIFT, SLA, DLP, SLS, and 2-PP, is a rapidly evolving technology.

4. Bioinks for 3D Bioprinting

Bioinks play a crucial role in the 3DbioP method by promoting cell growth and function. Furthermore, bioinks assist minimizing the impact of printing on the viability of cells while maintaining the resolution form and stiffness of the construct. The primary material used as a foundation for 3D bioprinting is called Bioink, and it is made of Biomaterial (Natural i.e. Collagen, Alginate, Gelatin, etc and Synthetic i.e. PLA, PVG, etc), Cells (Kuffer cells, Hepatocytes, Hepatic Stellate Cells, Endothelial cells) and other additives like temperature, concentration, pH, growth factor etc. Research on biomaterials and variation in the cell type has advanced, providing a strong basis for the creation of accurate, repeatable, and biologically supportive liver tissue engineering (LTE). For 3D bioprinting, dECM, agar (or agarose), alginate, silk, gelatin, collagen, hyaluronan, fibrinogen, and chitosan are the most often utilized natural polymeric hydrogel-based bioinks. (Liu, F. et al. (2018).

Here for the sake of 3D bioprinting of liver tissue we will focus on the cells dedicated for liver i.e. Hepatic nonparenchymal cells (hepatic stellate cells, hepatic sinusoidal endothelial cells, and Kupffer cells) and hepatic parenchymal cells (hepatocytes). Cell selection is categorized as single or multicellular printing based on the number of cell types. The most commonly utilised cells for single cell printing are HepG2, HepaRG, and PMH. Some research employs single cells to assess the bioink's biocompatibility. Multicellular printing typically uses two types of cells: primary cells and co-culture cells. Main cells are hepatocytes or can develop into them. There are four main categories: cell line, primary cell, stem cell, and induced hepatocyte. Co-culture cells are combined with or printed near primary cells to better simulate the cellular environment in vivo. They primarily consist of HUVEC, fibroblast cells, and Kupffer cells and so on (Jin, B., et al. (2022).

Table 1   Summary of the current 3D bioprinting technologies (Sun, L., et al. (2023)).

Technology Type	Working Principle	Advantage	Limitation
Mechanical based- Inkjet-based 3D bioprinting	• Similar to a typical 2D desktop inkjet printer, the bioink is discharged from the nozzle in droplet form by varying the pressure.	• Affordable, • Feasible	• Only applied to low-viscosity and low-populated bioink.
Extrusion-based 3D bioprinting	• The printer moves using mechanical or pneumatic drive in response to preprogrammed orders. • The nozzle disperses bioink in the desired pattern.	• Enables printing high-viscosity bioink. • Convenient to use	• Relative low resolution • High shear stress that causes cell damage
Coaxial printing	• Hollow fibers were made possible by coaxial printing, allowing for the direct bioprinting of blood arteries.	• Allows for contemporaneous and concentric deposition of several materials. • Enables printing low-viscosity bioink.	• Crosslinker solution needs to be removed • Requires rapid crosslinking to maintain the structure
Suspension bioprinting	It enables omnidirectional printing of complex structures by depositing bioink at discrete areas, overcoming the limitations of bottom-up and layer-by-layer printing methods.	• Enables printing of low-viscosity yet high-biocompatibility bioink • Allows comprehensive printing of sophisticated constructions.	• Suspension medium (should have suitable properties) must be carefully removed to avoid injuring fragile structures.
Laser Assisted- Laser-induced forward transfer (LIFT)	This method prevents direct contact between regulating devices and bioink, minimizing cell damage. Laser-induced forward transfer (LIFT) uses a laser to write on an energy-absorbing metal layer on top of a biomaterial layer, creating droplets of bioink.	• Resolution is high • Perforating • High Cell viability	• Requires fast-crosslinking bioink • Time-consuming
Stereolithography (SLA) and Digital light processing (DLP)	Unlike other conventional printing methods, SLA prints light-sensitive hydrogels layer by layer instead of in stripes or droplets, enabling the production of individual 3D structures in a matter of seconds.	• Perforating • Highly efficient • Fast speed • Resolution is high	• This technique could result in phototoxicity, which could impede the proliferation of cells. • Produce only 2D structure
2-PP	This is photosensitive hydrogel's 3-order nonlinear process is triggered by a pulse of a near-infrared laser (wave length: approximately 800 nm). Hydrogel polymerizes in regions that are exposed to dense photons and simultaneously absorb two or more photons.	• Produces bioink randomly and comprehensively. • Enables printing of complicated structures.	• Photosensitive bioink required • Printing speed is slow

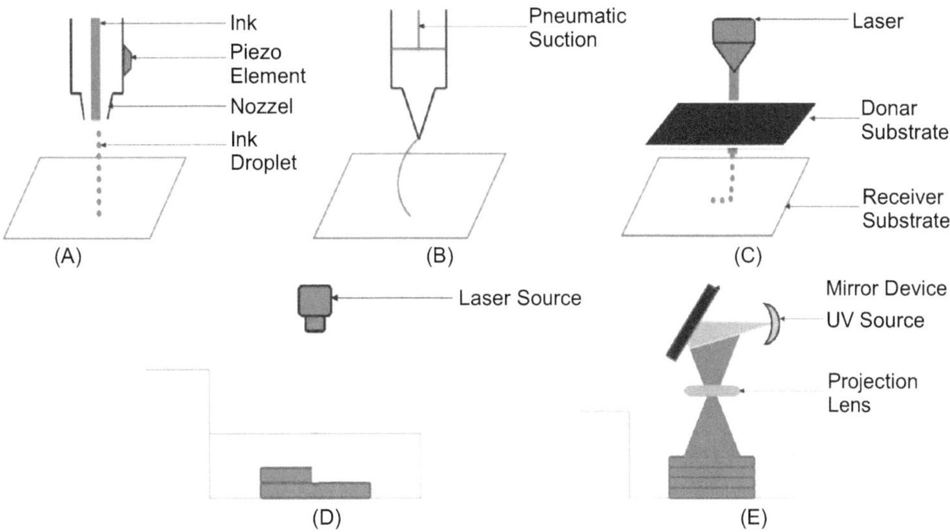

Fig. 3   Four main techniques of 3D Bioprinting. (A) Inkjet Bioprinting. (B) Extrusion Bioprinting. (C) LIFT. (D) SLA (E) DLP. (Kryou, C., et al. (2019)

5.   Bioprinted Liver Tissue Models

These days, 3D bioprinting is an interdisciplinary field that combines computer science, materials science, biology, medicine, and mechanics. It has enormous promise for precisely regulating the spatial distribution of cells and the surrounding milieu in tissue and organ engineering. Three distinct phases can be identified in the development of 3D bioprinting: non-biocompatible materials, biocompatible and biodegradable materials, and finally cells. Human organs including the hearts, kidneys, and lungs have been successfully constructed in vitro in this field thus far, offering fresh promise for human organ regeneration and repair as well as for the modeling of human disease. For most tissue engineers, creating fully functional hepatic networks is still a difficult task. As a result, many different kinds of 3D printing techniques are anticipated to get over present constraints. Because the liver is one of the most complex organs in the human body, liver tissue engineering has been a popular but difficult research area. Efforts to 3D print liver tissue have resulted in the creation of multicellular and multi-technology bioprinting. The liver's microscopic structure is complex, consisting of capillaries lined with specialized stellate macrophages (Kupffer cells) that continuously break down red blood cells, sinusoid ducts that pass through hepatocyte plates, and hexagonal hepatic lobules with hepatocytes irradiating from a central vein (Bismuth, H. (1982)).

Due to the organ's complexity, attempts to produce liver tissue have not been very successful, making liver transplants the only functional solution available as yet. However, the prospect of creating a three-dimensional liver construct is intriguing not only for disease modeling and regeneration but also for toxicological research (Nguyen, D. G., Funk, etal. (2016).

6.   Applications of 3D Bioprinting

The liver, the body's largest gland, is responsible for metabolism, bile generation, detoxification, and the management of water and electrolytes. Toxins or medications absorbed by the gastrointestinal tract are first transported to the liver before entering the blood stream. Liver disease is among the top causes of death worldwide. As a result, an in vitro liver tissue model that mimics the liver's primary functions can serve as a viable platform for studying liver illnesses and creating new therapeutics. Furthermore, the constraints of standard planar monolayer cell cultures and animal experiments for assessing drug candidate toxicity and efficacy can be addressed. Currently, the rapidly emerging 3D bioprinting technologies can generate in vitro liver tissue models in both static scaffolds (Ma, L., Wu, et al. (2020)). Figure 4 illustrates the various applications of 3D Bioprinting.

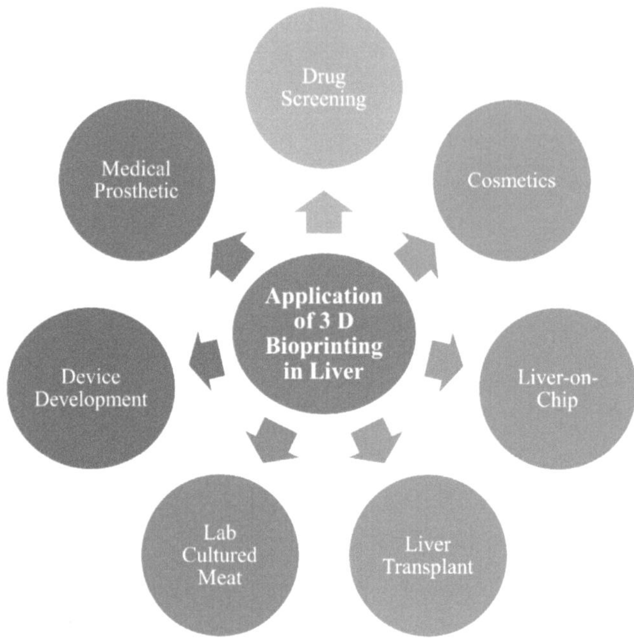

Fig. 4   Application of 3D Bioprinting

7.   Discussion and Future Directions

The absence of adequate animal and cell research models impedes the advancement of this field's study. Currently, organoids, 2D cells, and mice models are the most commonly used research models for liver regeneration. Patient-derived xenograft (PDX) models are among the most widely used three-dimensional (3D) disease models; yet, they have some disadvantages, such as ethical controversy, lengthy protocols, high expense, unsuitability for testing immunotherapies, and complicated operation. Another model, organoids, is likewise not an ideal representation of primary cells since it lacks the essential vascular network and immune system made up of several stromal cell types. Long-term in vitro cultivation of conventional cell lines causes an adaptive transformation that differs significantly from genuine cells in vivo. Numerous intrinsic properties of primary cells are lost in the three-dimensional in vivo environment. As a result, 2D cell culture models even give false positive results since they are unable to accurately replicate the milieu of a tissue or organ in life. Since 3D bioprinting involves the spatial organization of cells and their surroundings, it offers tremendous promise for use in the development of new tissues and organs. Tissue-like three-dimensional structures made of cells, biomaterial, and other components can encourage the expression of in vivo functions by the cells. Several techniques for creating biologically functional tissues have been made possible by 3D bioprinting in the last ten years. At the forefront of 3D printing technology is bioprinting of different cells, which has been used for in vitro rebuilding of tissues and organs like the heart, blood arteries, and lungs. This technology may help address the organ shortage dilemma. With the advent of 3D Bioprinting, designing complex structures has become easier. These intricate models, which were once challenging to create,can now be conveniently designed and modeled .

8.   Limitations

Vascularization and post-print sustainability are two major limitations of 3D bioprinting of tissues and organs. Another major challenge is to bioprint functional and living dense tissues. Even though the media enthusiastically promotes the timely development of organ bioprinting, and 3D bioprinting offers a novel alternative to traditional treatment, considerable work remains before it can be used in clinical settings. Before the bioprinted liver can be used in clinical settings, more study is needed to confirm its safety and effectiveness. It is now in the experimental stage. Furthermore, to confirm its efficacy in treating liver illnesses, clinical trials would be required. It is crucial to take into account any potential ethical ramifications of 3D-bioprinted livers, as these could include issues with ownership and consent related to the use of human tissue samples.

Conclusion

When compared to non-biological printing, 3D bioprinting entails additional complexities such as material selection, cell types, growth and differentiation factors, and technical challenges related to the sensitivities of living cells and tissue assembly and as a result of that 3D bioprinting has made significant progress towards functional tissue printing. Using biomaterials and living cells, 3D bioprinting techniques create biomimetic tissues in a predetermined pattern or on an already-existing 3D matrix. One promising tool for drug testing, regenerative medicine, and liver ailments is a bioartificial liver. High-resolution cell structures, the creation of 3D scaffolds for cell growth, inkjet printing, extrusion printing, LAB, and vat photopolymerization are frequently selected due to their adaptability to culture settings. More work is still needed to overcome the obstacles to accurately simulating the 3D liver tissue environment in drug development, regenerative medicine, and disease modeling. Despite obstacles, early research indicates that bioprinting is a promising area for further study. Although more time, effort, and diverse expertise are required to realize the clinical potential of this technology, the future looks promising.

References

Acun, A., Oganesyan, R. and Uygun, B.E. (2019). Liver bioengineering: promise, pitfalls, and hurdles to overcome. *Current transplantation reports, 6*, 119–126.

Andriotis, E.G., Eleftheriadis, G.K., Karavasili, C. and Fatouros, D.G. (2020). Development of bio-active patches based on pectin for the treatment of ulcers and wounds using 3D-bioprinting technology. *Pharmaceutics, 12*(1), 56.

Bishop, E.S., Mostafa, S., Pakvasa, M., Luu, H.H., Lee, M.J. et al. (2017). 3-D bioprinting technologies in tissue engineering and regenerative medicine: Current and future trends. *Genes & diseases, 4*(4), 185–195.

Bismuth, H. (1982). Surgical anatomy and anatomical surgery of the liver. *World journal of surgery, 6*, 3–9.

Deng, J.; Wei, W.; Chen, Z.; Lin, B.; Zhao, W. et al. Engineered liver-on-a-chip platform to mimic liver functions and its biomedical applications: A review. *Micromachines* 2019, *10*, 676.

Fetah, K.; Tebon, P.; Goudie, M.J.; Eichenbaum, J.; Ren, L. et al. The emergence of 3D bioprinting in organ-on-chip systems. *Prog. Biomed. Eng.* 2019, *1*, 012001.

Ge, Q. 3D printing of highly stretchable hydrogel with diverse UV curable polymers. Sci. Adv. 7, eaba4261 (2021).

Gu, Z., Fu, J., Lin, H. and He, Y. (2020). Development of 3D bioprinting: From printing methods to biomedical applications. *Asian Journal of Pharmaceutical Sciences, 15*(5), 529–557.

Janani, G., Priya, S., Dey, S. and Mandal, B.B. (2022). Mimicking native liver lobule microarchitecture in vitro with parenchymal and non-parenchymal cells using 3D bioprinting for drug toxicity and drug screening applications. *ACS Applied Materials & Interfaces, 14*(8), 10167-10186.

Jin, B., Liu, Y., Du, S., Sang, X., Yang, H. et al. (2022). Current trends and research topics regarding liver 3D bioprinting: A bibliometric analysis research. *Frontiers in Cell and Developmental Biology, 10*, 1047524.

Kryou, C., Leva, V., Chatzipetrou, M. and Zergioti, I. (2019). Bioprinting for liver transplantation. *Bioengineering, 6*(4), 95.

Li, C., Jiang, Z. and Yang, H. (2022). Advances in 3D bioprinting technology for liver regeneration. *Hepatobiliary Surg Nutr, 11*(6), 917–919.

Liu, F., Chen, Q., Liu, C., Ao, Q., Tian, X. et al. (2018). Natural polymers for organ 3D bioprinting. *Polymers, 10*(11), 1278.

Ma, L., Wu, Y., Li, Y., Aazmi, A., Zhou, H. et al. (2020). Current advances on 3D-bioprinted liver tissue models. *Advanced Healthcare Materials, 9*(24), 2001517.

Nguyen, D.G., Funk, J., Robbins, J.B., Crogan-Grundy, C., Presnell, S.C et al., (2016). Bioprinted 3D primary liver tissues allow assessment of organ-level response to clinical drug induced toxicity in vitro. *PloS one, 11*(7), e0158674.

Sun, L., Wang, Y., Zhang, S., Yang, H. and Mao, Y. et al. (2023). 3D bioprinted liver tissue and disease models: Current advances and future perspectives. *Biomaterials Advances*, 213499.

Sun, Y. 3D bioprinting dual-factor releasing and gradient-structured constructs ready to implant for anisotropic cartilage regeneration. Sci. Adv. 6, eaay1422 (2020).

3D Bioprinting Lung Tissue

Yofiel Wyle,[1] *Rahul Sayal*[1] and
Mereena George Ushakumary[2]*

1. Introduction

The human respiratory system is an incredible ensemble of specialized structures and organs responsible for the life-sustaining process of gas exchange. While the lung is the most crucial organ for gas exchange, our body depends on an intricate system of interconnected organs to facilitate efficient and resilient respiration. The larynx, situated in the neck and housing the vocal cords, contributes to respiration, voice production, and safeguarding the trachea from food inhalation. Similarly, although commonly associated with digestion, the pharynx also serves an essential function in the respiratory system by facilitating air passage. The lung sits in the thoracic cavity, which is physically manipulated by the diaphragm and intercostal muscles. When the diaphragm contracts, it moves downward, and the external intercostal muscles contract to lift the rib cage and sternum up and out. This combined action increases the volume of the thoracic cavity, which decreases the intrathoracic pressure below atmospheric pressure, causing air to flow into the lungs. When the diaphragm relaxes, it moves upward, and the internal intercostal muscles along with other muscles involved in forced expiration contract to bring the rib cage and sternum down and in. This action decreases the volume of the thoracic cavity, increasing the intrathoracic pressure above atmospheric pressure, pushing air out of the lungs. For the remainder of this chapter, we will focus on the structures which comprise the lung itself rather than the various other structures and organs necessary for proper respiratory function. The trachea, or windpipe, is a flexible tube located in the throat that connects the larynx to the bronchi and allows air to flow in and out of the lungs. It extends from the larynx and branches into the right and left bronchi, which further divide into smaller bronchi and bronchioles. The bronchi are the next level of branching, extending from the trachea into the lungs. They further divide into smaller bronchioles, which play a vital role in distributing air throughout the lungs. Finally, the smallest and most numerous structures in the respiratory system are the alveoli. The alveoli are the endpoint of the respiratory tree and are crucial for the gas exchange process. Each alveolus is enveloped by a network of around 2,000 capillaries,

[1] UC Davis Center for Surgical Bioengineering, University of California Davis, U.S.A.
[2] Biological Sciences Division, Pacific Northwest National Laboratory, Richland, U.S.A.
* Corresponding author: mereena.ushakumary@pnnl.gov

where the blood releases carbon dioxide and absorbs oxygen through the thin alveolar walls. In total, the human lungs contain approximately 300 to 500 million alveoli, creating a vast surface area to maximize the exchange of gasses. To maximize bidirectional diffusion each alveolus is extremely thin, around 200 nm across-about 500 times thinner than a single strand of hair (Stanton, Bruce and Koeppen, Bruce, 2008) The surface of each alveolus is coated with a surfactant, a substance that reduces surface tension and prevents the nanoscopic alveolar walls from collapsing during exhalation. The inherent intricacy and complexity of the lung has thus far prevented effective treatments for repairing the lung.

Furthermore, lung tissue has a relatively low regenerative capacity compared to other tissues like skin or liver. The lungs' stem and progenitor cells, which are essential for tissue repair and regeneration, are less abundant and have a more limited capacity for proliferation and differentiation. This is compounded by the lungs' constant exposure to environmental toxins, pathogens, and mechanical forces, which can lead to cumulative damage over time and further impair regenerative processes (Figure 1). The immune response also poses a challenge in lung tissue regeneration. Inflammation, a natural part of the healing process, can become a hindrance if it is chronic or excessive, leading to scarring (fibrosis) that disrupts normal tissue architecture and function. In many lung diseases, pulmonary fibrosis is irreversible and gradually reduces gas exchange, requiring mechanical ventilation until patients die of complete respiratory failure (Du Bois and M, 2010).

On the support new lung tissue is highly intricate. Establishing a blood supply to newly formed lung structures is critical for delivering nutrients and oxygen but is a significant hurdle in tissue engineering. There are currently no therapies which address lung cell death implicated in various lung diseases including chronic obstructive pulmonary disease (COPD), pulmonary fibrosis, and lung cancer. Depending on the condition, patients will progress from moderate stages of the disease, which may include chronic cough, to severe age stages of the disease which force hospitalizations. In end stage lung diseases, patients experience fatigue and weight loss as the body is no longer able to adequately supply organs with oxygen, due to respiratory failure(Du Bois and M, 2010). With an inability to adequately heal the lung after damage, physicians rely on whole lung transplantation after late-stage lung failure. With a growing elderly population, there is a growing demand for healthy lungs for transplantation, defined as lungs taken from patients between the ages of 20-45 that did not suffer from cardiovascular disease. In the United States, there are 4,117 patients on the lung transplant waiting list, an increase of over 27% compared to the last decade (Valapour et al., 2023). Due to the limited supply, currently only 1/6 to 1/7 patients suffering from complete lung failure will have the chance to receive a new lung, meaning over 85% of patients experiencing end-stage lung disease are left with no hope of improvement. (*NHS Blood and Transplant Annual Report and Accounts 2014/15*, 2015). After undergoing lung transplantation, patients often encounter a myriad of challenges that can impact their recovery and long-term health. The most pressing issue is the risk of chronic lung allograft dysfunction (CLAD), which affects approximately 50% of recipients within five years, significantly diminishing lung function and survival rate (Bos et al., 2020). Additionally, patients may face complications from immunosuppressive medications, including side effects and increased susceptibility to infections. Physical health status can also be compromised due to factors like age, the type of transplant received (single-lung vs. bilateral), and the underlying disease that necessitated the transplant (Diel et al., 2023). Pulmonary function, while initially improved, typically declines over time due to CLAD or other complications, and exercise tolerance often does not fully return to expected levels, possibly due to pre-existing skeletal muscle weakness (Thabut and Mal, 2017).

The advent of 3D lung bioprinting signifies a groundbreaking stride in regenerative medicine and transplant science. The critical shortage of donor lungs suitable for transplantation has fueled the need for alternative solutions to treat end-stage lung disease. With the high precision of 3D bioprinting, it is now possible to construct complex, three-dimensional tissues that mimic the intricate structures of the lung, including its fine network of airways and blood vessels (Grigoryan et al., 2019). This technology holds the promise of producing personalized lung tissue for repair or replacement,

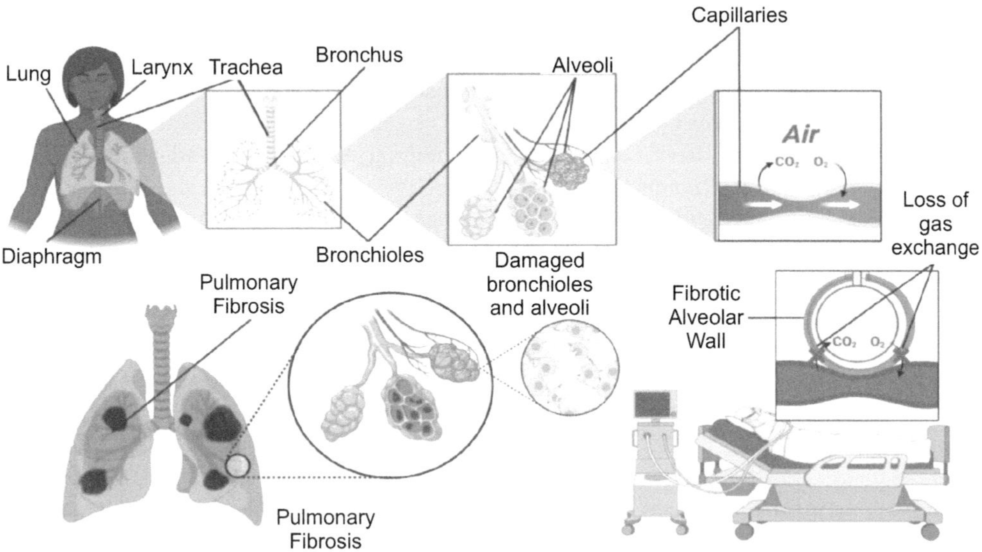

Fig. 1   Overview of human respiratory physiology including the larynx, diaphragm, and bronchus. The bronchus splits up into smaller regions called bronchioles which lead to gas-exchanging alveolar subunits. In diseases such as pulmonary fibrosis, alveoli become damaged, leading to a loss of gas exchange and eventually respiratory failure.

which could be tailored to the specific immunological and architectural requirements of the patient, thereby reducing the risk of rejection and the need for lifelong immunosuppression. Additionally, 3D bioprinted lung models serve as invaluable platforms for drug testing and disease modeling, allowing scientists to study lung pathologies and treatments in a controlled, patient-specific manner (James et al., 2020), (Hong et al., 2020). The potential to replicate the unique biomechanical and biochemical properties of the lung parenchyma paves the way for novel therapeutic strategies and a deeper understanding of pulmonary diseases, ultimately contributing to enhanced patient outcomes and longevity. The imperative to develop 3D bioprinting for the lung stems from a critical need to address the chronic shortage of donor organs and offer more effective treatment options for those suffering from severe lung diseases. This technology heralds a new era in personalized medicine, potentially circumventing the risks of immune rejection by utilizing a patient's own cells to create compatible lung structures. Moreover, 3D bioprinting has the unique capability to replicate the lung's complex architecture, encompassing its delicate alveoli and intricate vascular networks—a feat that has remained elusive with conventional tissue engineering techniques. This advancement not only promises to revolutionize organ transplantation but also provides an invaluable tool for research and drug testing, facilitating the development of new pharmaceuticals with greater accuracy and less reliance on animal models. Furthermore, by tailoring tissues to the specific anatomy of an individual patient, 3D bioprinting could significantly reduce post-transplant complications and improve the long-term success of lung transplants. It also spurs innovation in treating a variety of pulmonary conditions, including those previously deemed intractable, by harnessing the potential of regenerative medicine. Beyond the profound health benefits, the economic implications of reducing healthcare costs through durable treatments and decreasing the need for recurrent hospitalizations— estimated to cost the world economy over \$4.326 trillion for COPD treatment alone (Chen et al., 2023). Modern bioengineering approaches including 3D bioprinting offer some hope that clinically tractable treatments for lung replacement may be developed in the coming years.

2.   Current Methods for 3D Lung Bioprinting

Here, we describe various methods implicated in 3D bioprinting of lungs and their potential strategies and limitations.

2.1 *Stereolithography (SLA)*

Stereolithography (SLA) is a modern form of additive manufacturing that has significantly advanced the field of tissue engineering. This technique utilizes a laser to cure and solidify photo-reactive polymer resins layer by layer, creating high-resolution three-dimensional structures with intricate details and smooth surface finishes. In bioprinting, SLA has been adapted to work with bioinks—materials that are compatible with living cells—to fabricate complex tissue constructs with precise architectural control. The potential for high resolution (100 um) and precision of SLA is particularly beneficial for creating the vascular networks and micro-channels necessary for the survival and function of cells within larger tissue constructs. SLA has been leveraged to create "breathing models" of the lung, which simulate tidal breathing of the lung and blood flow around lung tissues. In this model, Grigoryan et al. could model pulmonary transport and measure blood oxygenation in and out of the mode (Grigoryan et al., 2019). Similarly, SLA has been used to generate lung-inspired flow fields to better understand the directionality and pressure of air as it enters and exits the lung (Muñoz-Perales et al., 2023). The ability to mimic airflow and the high resolution makes SLA desirable for printing alveolar sacs with complex geometry compared to the printing methods described below. although a pioneering technique in 3D printing, faces several challenges in the bioprinting of lung tissues. The photo-reactive resins typically used in SLA are not inherently biocompatible, posing a significant hurdle in creating an environment that supports cell adhesion, growth, and differentiation essential for lung tissue engineering. Furthermore, the UV light and heat involved in the curing process can compromise cell viability, a critical aspect for creating living tissues. Moreover, the complex assembly of different tissue types within the native lung is difficult to recapitulate through SLA, as researchers are generally limited to a single material type. For example, to model the interaction between alveoli and capillary beds, each structure would have to be printed separately before assembly. The sheer scale and hierarchical organization stretch the capabilities of current SLA systems due to limited speed and throughput. In addition, the limited bioinks compatible with SLA printing limits the mechanical properties of the materials that can be produced through this process. It has become clear that the biophysical properties of tissue impact cell fate and function-which is particularly important in the lung which requires elasticity and must withstand dynamic changes in airflow and pressure. Another obstacle is the development of suitable bioinks that can be broken down and replaced by the patient's own tissues over time after photo-crosslinking. For clinical application, sterilization of the printed structures is another critical issue. If printing occurs in an unsterile environment, the construct must be sterilized without damaging the construct or embedded cells. Lastly, the cost and printing speed of SLA do not currently align with the needs for mass production or rapid creation of large, clinically sized tissues, making it an impractical choice for widespread clinical use in its current state, thus highlighting the need for continued innovation and refinement in the technique for it to be viable for lung bioprinting in regenerative medicine.

2.2 *Fused Deposition Modeling (FDM)*

In contrast to SLA's approach to 3D printing, Fused Deposition Modeling (FDM) operates on a more mechanical basis, where thermoplastic filaments are heated and extruded through a precision nozzle, laying down material layer by layer to construct the 3D model. While FDM may not match the fine resolution of SLA, it compensates with its cost-effectiveness and the diversity of materials it can process. These advantages make FDM a popular choice in the initial stages of lung model prototyping, where the requirements for detail are balanced against the need for cost control and material properties. Although the fidelity in replicating the nuanced structures of the lung may be less than that achieved with SLA, FDM remains a valuable tool for creating larger, more macroscopic features of lung anatomy or for producing templates around which more detailed work can be performed. While FDM may not be suitable for printing the living tissue itself, it can aid in the development and testing of respiratory treatments and diagnostics. By producing patient-specific airway models with FDM, researchers can simulate the respiratory tract's anatomy to study the deposition patterns of inhaled medications, as seen in studies analyzing salbutamol sulfate delivery (Lim et al., 2021). Such models can be used to optimize inhaler design, adjust dosages, and improve the efficacy of treatments for conditions like asthma and COPD. Moreover, FDM is instrumental in creating highly detailed and accurate lung phantoms from patient CT datasets, which are then used for calibrating CT imaging intensity and validating image quantification software. These phantoms, complete with artificial lesions, enable the precise evaluation of imaging techniques and software, crucial for detecting and quantifying lung abnormalities (Hong et al., 2020). Lastly, FDM can be used in conjunction with other technologies, such as Particle Image Velocimetry (PIV), to visualize fluid flow using patient-specific models of respiratory tract geometry (Vermeulen et al., 2013). By leveraging the rapid prototyping potential of PIV, clinicians can determine optimal delivery strategies for lungs which have undergone extensive tissue remodeling. Through these applications, FDM contributes to personalized medicine by providing tools for a better understanding of drug delivery dynamics and enhancing the accuracy of diagnostic imaging, thereby supporting the development of targeted interventions for lung diseases.

2.3 *Selective Laser Sintering (SLS)*

Selective Laser Sintering (SLS) is a sophisticated 3D printing technique that stands as a promising tool for lung bioprinting applications, leveraging a high-powered laser to fuse polymer powder into complex structures after digital modeling. This method could revolutionize surgical planning and simulation by producing precise and detailed anatomical lung models that allow surgeons to practice and perfect their techniques before actual operations, with slightly better resolution than FDM. SLS has been used for over 20 years to produce detailed physical models of complex respiratory features such as hollow tracheobronchial airway models with features less than 2 mm in diameter (Clinkenbeard et al., 2002). In therapeutic realms, SLS has the potential to fabricate intricate scaffolds that emulate the lung's unique architecture, providing a framework for the growth of new lung tissue, with the added advantage of utilizing biocompatible materials conducive to cell attachment and integration. The ability of SLS to create highly porous and customizable structures is invaluable for ensuring tissue viability, supporting essential processes like vascularization and nutrient diffusion within cell-laden scaffolds. Research into lung bioprinting could harness SLS to construct complex, patient-specific geometries that address individual medical needs, such as custom prosthetics for lung repair. Notably, the SLS process inherently supports the creation of delicate internal structures without the need for additional supports due to the surrounding powder bed, facilitating the generation of the intricate networks reminiscent of lung tissue. Compared to FDM, SLS is better suited for bio-based polymeric powders like polybutylene succinate (PBS) that can support cell growth, while maintaining physiologically-relevant parameters of the microenvironment and tissue-level macrostructure (Colucci et al., 2024).

SLS excels in fabricating complex geometries with high geometric accuracy, such as intricate six-pointed stars and hexagonal structures, without the need for support structures, thus avoiding the post-processing required with FDM. The SLS process yields part with uniform thermal and viscoelastic properties, which are crucial for applications that FDM can struggle with due to the extrusion-based process's inherent material inconsistencies. Furthermore, SLS-produced samples demonstrate a good level of definition and porosity, desirable attributes for biomedical applications like scaffolds and drug carriers, without further modification after printing. The preliminary cytocompatibility results of PBS suggest that SLS technology can create biocompatible parts that do not release harmful substances, eliminating the need for additional treatments or post-processing. This positions SLS as a highly suitable technology for producing biodegradable, precise, and medically safe components, pushing the boundaries of applications well beyond what is typically achievable with FDM and other 3D printing methods. Although directly printing fully functional lung tissue is beyond current capabilities, SLS offers immense potential in advancing the development of scaffolds and models that could significantly impact the study and treatment of pulmonary disorders, positioning itself as a cornerstone technology in the evolution of personalized medicine and regenerative therapies for lung conditions. As SLS technology and bioinks continue to improve, SLS may emerge as a dominant bioprinting option for tissues with complex and intricate morphology such as the lung.

2.4　*Digital Light Processing (DLP)*

Digital Light Processing (DLP) represents a cutting-edge approach for the creation of complex tissue structures, such as lung tissue, which require high resolution and precision. DLP technology, which harnesses light to cure photo-sensitive resins layer by layer, can potentially provide the fine detail necessary to replicate the intricate alveolar structures and vascular networks of the lung. This is particularly advantageous when considering the lung's delicate air sacs and the need for precise vascularization to ensure tissue viability and function. The high resolution of DLP, often down to the single micron level, allows for the creation of the detailed and porous structures that are critical for gas exchange in lung tissue or creating lung-on-a-chip systems for improving throughput (Razavi Bazaz et al., 2019). In bioprinting, DLP can be used to solidify bioinks that contain living cells and biomaterials, enabling the construction of scaffolds that support the growth and organization of cells into functional lung tissue. The speed of the DLP process, compared to other 3D printing methods, is beneficial for maintaining cell viability during the printing process, as prolonged exposure to environmental stress can compromise cell health. Furthermore, the capability of DLP to swiftly cure materials minimizes the duration that cells spend in an artificial environment. This aspect is particularly crucial for the viability of sensitive lung cells. In the pursuit of creating functional lung tissue, researchers can utilize DLP to print patient-specific geometries derived from medical imaging data, leading to personalized tissue constructs that could be used for transplantations or therapeutic applications.

DLP has been used to create *in vitro* air-blood barrier interfaces to simulate gas exchange by printing human lung and umbilical vein cells together in culture (Horváth et al., 2015). The extraordinary potential of DLP was more recently demonstrated through a collaborative effort by Jordan Miller and Kelly Stevens by constructing an intricate vascular network surrounding alveolar-like structures—recapitulating the intricate and complex architecture of the native gas exchanging units in the human lung. In this study, bioprinted structures were seeded with cells and transplanted into live mice to demonstrate biocompatibility and potential therapeutic application of DLP-generated structures (Grigoryan et al., 2019). DLP has also been leveraged to generate models of non-small cell lung cancer, integrating human blood vessels with cancer cells. This model facilitates the screening of cancer treatments, providing a physiologically relevant 3D structure that closely mimics the interaction between lung cancer tissue and vasculature.

While direct printing of fully functional lung tissue is not yet a reality, DLP holds promise for the fabrication of complex tissue scaffolds and is a key technology in ongoing research into tissue engineering and regenerative medicine. Its high resolution and speed, combined with the potential for customization, make DLP a promising tool for advancing lung tissue bioprinting and bringing us closer to the goal of creating viable, transplantable lung tissue in the laboratory.

2.5　*Multi-Photon Polymerization (MPP)*

Multi-Photon Polymerization (MPP) operates on the principle of using two-photon absorption at the focal point of a laser, permitting the polymerization of photosensitive resins with an exceptional degree of spatial control: down to 100 nm lateral resolution and 1 um vertical resolution. In lung 3D printing, MPP offers sub-micron resolution enabling the construction of the fine branching structures of bronchioles, alveolar sacs, and capillary networks. The enhanced precision and resolution of

MPP enables the creation of vascular structures with the necessary porosity and interconnectivity to facilitate blood flow and nutrient transport, key factors for tissue viability and function. By using patient-specific imaging data, MPP can be used to print lung tissues that precisely match the anatomical features of individual patients, aiding in pre-surgical planning or in the development of personalized lung implants. Furthermore, the ability of MPP to fabricate scaffolds with a biomimetic environment is critical for studying lung cancer progression and for drug discovery, providing a more accurate in vitro model that can replicate tumor-stroma interactions and tissue mechanics. Additionally, MPP's use of biocompatible materials can lead to the printing of scaffolds that, once implanted, can support the body's own cells to repopulate and eventually integrate into the host tissue, potentially leading to breakthroughs in regenerative medicine for lung disease. To date, only a few groups have employed MPP for lung printing. One group has patterned lung carcinoma lines as a proof of principle towards generating an organ-on-a-chip. Others have used MPP to generate monolithic devices for delivering aqueous drugs into the airway (Last, 2022). Another group has used MPP to generate 500 nm scaffolds made from ECM derived from normal and fibrotic lung tissue to investigate the impact of remodeled ECM on cell behavior (James et al., 2020). While this technology has thus far been primarily used for basic biological investigation, the superior resolution endowed by MPP will allow researchers to generate intricate pulmonary structures on the nanometer scale.

2.6 Material Extrusion

Material extrusion (ME) is perhaps the most common and well understood method of 3D bioprinting. ME bioprinting involves the precise layer-by-layer deposition of bioinks, generally biocompatible materials, through a computer-controlled extrusion nozzle. Early in its development, the focus of ME bioprinting was primarily on creating simple tissue constructs, but the technology has since evolved to enable the fabrication of more intricate structures that more closely mimic the native lung architecture (Fu et al., 2021). With advancements in bioink formulations, researchers can tailor the mechanical properties and degradation rates to better suit lung tissue's unique requirements. These optimized bioinks can support the complex cellular environments necessary for lung function, including the presence of multiple cell types such as the lung epithelium, mesenchyme, and lung vascular cells (Horváth et al., 2015). Recent innovations have also seen the integration of decellularized extracellular matrix components into bioinks, enhancing the biomimetic nature of the printed construct (van Tienderen et al., 2022). Cutting-edge research is focusing on refining ME bioprinting to replicate the highly ordered alveolar structure, essential for gas exchange. Scientists are increasingly able to create porous scaffolds that facilitate cell infiltration and vascularization-key factors for tissue survival and integration post-implantation. Concurrently, the development of dynamic bioinks that can respond to environmental stimuli has opened new avenues for creating scaffolds that can actively participate in the maturation and functionalization of lung tissue.

The precision of ME bioprinting has also seen considerable improvement, with the advent of multi-nozzle printing systems allowing for the simultaneous deposition of different materials. This multi-material capability is crucial for building the complex gradients and interfaces seen between different tissue types within the lung. Work has already been done to modify gelation and de-gelation times, which holds the extruded material in place while it polymerizes. This increases the resolution and fidelity of existing bioink materials-which would ordinarily lack "printability" due to their fluidity at lower temperatures. For example, materials with desirable mechanical properties such as Poly(vinyl alcohol) (PVA) or Hyaluronic acid can now be used to print complex designs through the use of print baths or slurries. Despite these advancements, ME bioprinting for lung tissue faces several unmet challenges. The resolution of ME, while improving, still falls short of replicating the microscale features of lung tissue, such as the delicate alveolar sac (Grigoryan et al., 2019). The mechanical forces involved in the extrusion process can also be detrimental to the viability and function of the cells within the bioink. Moreover, ensuring the long-term stability and functionality of printed lung constructs remains a significant hurdle, as does replicating the lung's intricate vascular networks that are essential for tissue survival. Another pressing challenge is the scaling up of ME bioprinting processes for the production of tissues large enough for clinical applications while maintaining high cell viability and construct fidelity (Díaz Lantada et al., 2018). Additionally, the integration of printed lung tissues with the host's native tissue post-transplantation, to ensure proper integration and function, is an area that requires further research. In summary, ME bioprinting holds considerable promise for lung tissue engineering. Nevertheless , this is an area ripe for ongoing research aimed at overcoming the current limitations related to resolution, cell viability, vascularization, and the integration of engineered tissues with host systems. Addressing these challenges is crucial for advancing the field toward viable clinical solutions for lung disease and injury.

Each of these 3D printing technologies offer unique benefits and pose distinct challenges when applied to the task of lung replication. The choice often depends on the specific requirements of the project at hand, including necessary resolution, material properties, speed, and cost. As the field of 3D bioprinting evolves, these technologies continue to advance, expanding the possibilities for creating accurate and functional lung models for a range of applications in medicine and research.

3.   Biomaterials and Bioink

Biomaterials and bioinks are inevitable components of tissue engineering. Bioinks are often a combination of biocompatible materials with living cells. The biomaterial of choice would be an important aspect as it is meant to support the physical and mechanical properties of the tissue. In this session, we describe different biomaterials and bioinks used for the 3D bioprinting of lung tissue.

3.1   Hydrogels

Hydrogels have become an indispensable tool in 3D lung bioprinting, largely due to their capacity to emulate the extracellular matrix (ECM) of pulmonary tissues with high fidelity. These hydrated polymers, such as alginate, gelatin-methacryloyl (GelMA), and hyaluronic acid-based hydrogels, can be precisely formulated to match the complex biomechanical properties of lung tissue such as stiffness, porosity, and degradation rate (Wang et al., 2017) (Figure 2). Their application in lung bioprinting extends beyond mere structural support; hydrogels can be functionalized with lung-specific peptides, like fibronectin or elastin, to promote cellular activities essential for recreating functional alveolar sacs and bronchiolar structures. For example, the inclusion of integrin, laminin or collagen in hydrogel formulations has been shown to significantly enhance epithelial and endothelial cell interactions, which are critical for re-establishing the alveolar-capillary barrier necessary for gas exchange (Busch et al., 2021). Scientists are identifying precise peptide sequences that can selectively attract and maintain distinct cell populations such as RGD motifs, SILY, or LXW7. LXW7, for example, was able to selectively recruit endothelial cells and assist in blood vessel regeneration (Hao et al., 2017) Other hydrogels like PEGDA (polyethylene glycol diacrylate) have been used to create the fine, branching structures of the bronchial tree. Meanwhile, more elastic hydrogels are used to mimic the compliance of the alveolar regions (Galliger et al., 2019).

Additionally, the use of decellularized ECM (dECM) from lung tissue as a bioink has shown great potential. dECM hydrogels retain the complex composition of lung-specific ECM, providing a conducive environment for lung cells to remodel and mature into functional tissues (Figure 3). This approach has been integral in bioprinting efforts aimed at generating scaffolds for lung tissue repair or for modeling diseases such as pulmonary fibrosis or chronic obstructive pulmonary disease (COPD) (Du Bois and M, 2010), (James et al., 2020). The tunable degradation rates of hydrogels are also critical for in vivo applications. For instance, a hydrogel might be engineered to degrade at a rate that corresponds with the integration of the bioprinted tissue into the host's lung tissue, thereby ensuring that the scaffold supports the tissue only as long as needed (Khan and Tanaka, 2017).

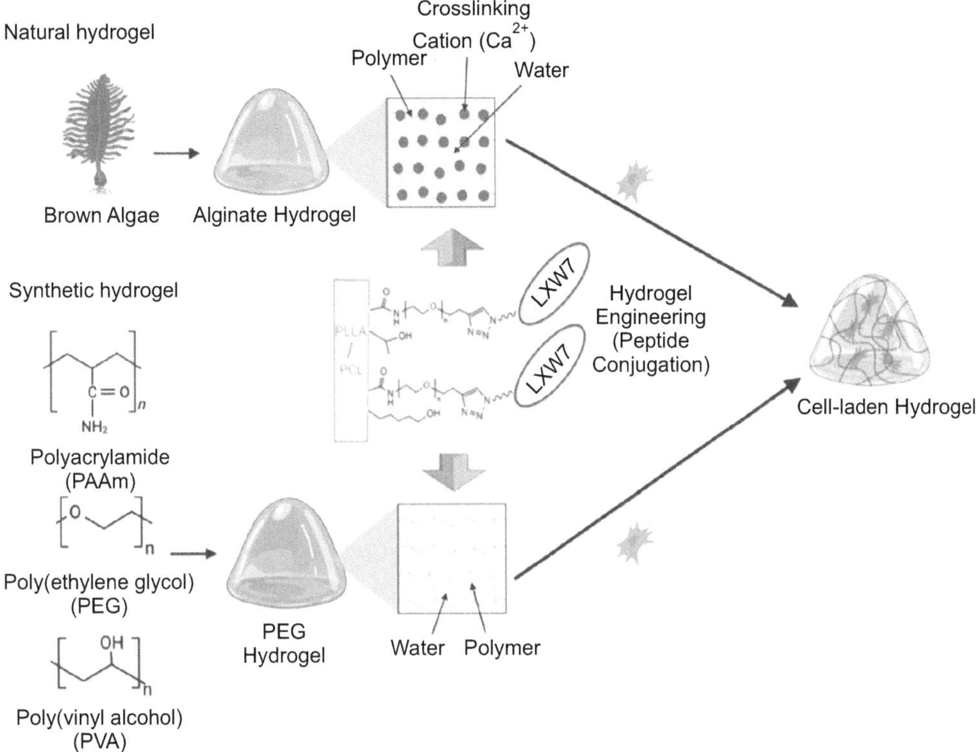

Fig. 2 Fabrication of natural or synthetic hydrogels for cell culture. In this example, brown algae is treated with acid to form alginic acid and then alkalized into sodium alginate solution. This solution is then diluted, filtered, and re-acidified to precipitate the alginic acid once more. In contrast, synthetic hydrogels are produced through either bulk polymerization or solution polymerization techniques. Bulk polymerization involves a radical initiator and a liquid monomer, while solution polymerization is characterized by the presence of an initiator, monomer, and a crosslinking agent within a single solution. These hydrogels can be custom-designed to incorporate various bioactive molecules that facilitate cell adhesion and integration.

Through ongoing research and development, hydrogels are becoming increasingly sophisticated, with the integration of smart hydrogels capable of responding to physiological stimuli, thus paving the way for dynamic tissue constructs that can react and adapt to their environment in a manner similar to native lung tissue. This innovation could lead to breakthroughs in personalized medicine, where bioprinted lung tissues are tailored not only to the general structural requirements but also to patient-specific conditions, potentially revolutionizing the treatment of a vast array of pulmonary diseases.

3.2 *Natural Polymers*

Natural polymers such as collagen, elastin, and hyaluronic acid play an integral role in replicating the lung's extracellular matrix due to their bioactivity and ability to communicate with cells. These polymers are key components of the lung's ECM and are employed for their exceptional ability to influence cellular behavior, including differentiation, proliferation, and migration. By incorporating these materials into 3D bioprinted lung models, scientists can create more biologically accurate scaffolds that not only support the physical structure of the lung but also actively participate in the formation of functional tissue by providing essential signals to the residing cells.

Hydrogels such as alginate, gelatin, and fibrin have gained prominence in the field of tissue engineering, especially for creating environments that foster cell growth and differentiation, making

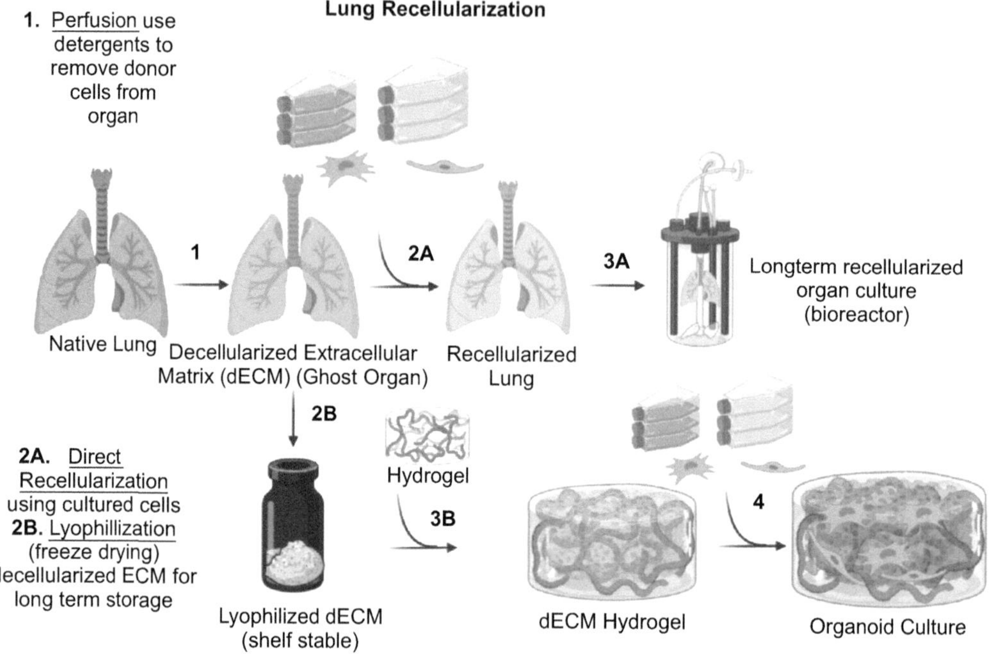

Fig. 3 Overview of lung recellularization process. 1. Native lung is perfused with detergents to remove all native cells, while retaining the extracellular matrix, creating a "ghost organ". Ghost organs can be directly recellularized to retain the architecture of the matrix or be lyophilized for later use. Recellularized organs can be cultured for long term maintenance in bioreactor culture. Lyophilized matrix material can be combined with hydrogel to improve the biocompatibility of synthetic or natural gel materials.

them ideal candidates for bioinks in 3D bioprinting. These substances possess viscoelastic properties that closely emulate the natural extracellular matrix (ECM) of the lung, providing a soft and moist environment that facilitates the proliferation and biological function of cells. Their inherent biocompatibility and ability to encapsulate cells uniformly make natural hydrogels indispensable in the creation of tissue constructs that not only resemble the physical architecture of the lung but also support its vital biological processes. Hydrogels can be tuned to create desired physical properties for printed cells. For example, alginate can be tuned to create stiffer materials by increasing the concentration of calcium ions by adding a greater proportion of calcium sulfate or calcium chloride to the gel solution, which increases the crosslinking density by providing a divalent cation to form a molecular bridge between two strands of the negatively charged backbone.

3.3 *Synthetic Polymers*

Synthetic polymers have emerged as versatile materials for use in 3D bioprinting applications, especially for replicating the intricate structures of lung tissue. Polymers such as polycaprolactone (PCL), poly(lactic-co-glycolic acid) (PLGA), and polyethylene glycol (PEG) have been extensively investigated due to their tunable mechanical properties, biocompatibility, and controllable degradation rates. These synthetic polymers can be engineered to achieve the desired tensile strength, elasticity, and porosity needed to mimic the lung's complex architecture, from the sturdy bronchial passages to the delicate alveolar sacs. For instance, PCL has been utilized for its slow degradation rate and mechanical robustness, making it a suitable candidate for creating the supportive framework of the bronchial tree within lung constructs (Li et al., 2006). PLGA, on the other hand, offers a faster degradation rate, which can be precisely adjusted by varying the ratio of its copolymers, allowing the bioprinted constructs to integrate seamlessly with the host tissue over time. Polylactic acid (PLA) is another synthetic gel that offers biocompatibility and superior mechanical strength (Ranakoti et al., 2023). These materials can be precisely manipulated to form the intricate scaffold of the lung's airways, providing the necessary support for the complex structures within. The degradation rate of these polymers can be tuned to match the tissue remodeling process, ensuring that the scaffold provides temporary support while native tissue regenerates. The use of PCL and PLA allows researchers to create stable structures that can withstand manipulation during the maturation and integration of the engineered lung tissue.

3.4 Composite Materials

Synthetic polymers can be functionalized with bioactive molecules to support cellular adhesion, proliferation, and differentiation. Bioactive signals can be incorporated into the polymer matrix, either by blending with natural polymers or by surface modifications, to provide cues for lung-specific cell functions. This is crucial for establishing a functional air-blood barrier and facilitating the complex interactions between epithelial and endothelial cells in the recreated lung tissue. The versatility of synthetic polymers also enables the creation of composite materials, where the polymer can be blended with natural ECM components or nanoparticles to enhance the bioactivity of the printed structure. Such composites can effectively bridge the gap between the mechanical robustness of synthetic materials and the bioactivity of natural substances. Moreover, advancements in the field have led to the development of smart polymers that respond to environmental stimuli, such as temperature or pH, allowing for dynamic changes in the bioprinted constructs post-fabrication (Khan and Tanaka, 2017). These stimuli-responsive materials can be engineered to undergo changes in their properties in response to the biological milieu, thereby providing temporal control over the scaffold's function and facilitating tissue development and maturation. The integration of such polymers in lung bioprinting holds significant promise for creating scaffolds that not only support initial cell growth but also evolve alongside the developing tissue, ultimately leading to more sophisticated and biomimetic lung models. As research progresses, the potential of synthetic polymers in 3D bioprinting continues to expand, offering new possibilities for creating functional lung tissues for transplantation, disease modeling, and drug screening applications.

The development of composite materials in lung tissue engineering represents a strategic approach to optimizing the mechanical and biological properties of the printed structures. By combining various biomaterials, such as hydrogels with synthetic or natural polymers, it is possible to create constructs that better mimic the lung's physical and biochemical environment. Composite materials can be engineered to have the strength required to maintain the airways' patency while providing a biologically active matrix that promotes cell attachment, proliferation, and differentiation, which are critical for replicating the intricate functionality of lung tissue. Additionally, composite materials offer the advantage of tailoring the properties of the scaffold to meet specific requirements. For example, the mechanical properties can be adjusted by varying the ratio of different materials, while the addition of bioactive components can enhance cell signaling and tissue integration. Some examples of composite hydrogels are alginate-polyethylene glycol blends, gelatin-methacryloyl combined with hyaluronic acid, and collagen-based hydrogels reinforced with synthetic polymers like poly (caprolactone) or poly (lactic acid).

4. Advances in Lung Bioprinting: Current Models and Future Directions

4.1 Primary Cell Lines and Their Functional Roles

Primary cell lines, when sourced directly from donor lung tissues, retain many of the functional characteristics required for creating a physiologically relevant lung model. In bioprinting applications, these cells are often isolated, cultured, and then used in combination with biomaterials to create tissue constructs that replicate the complex architecture and function of the lung environment. Lung epithelial cells, specifically, are crucial for replicating the air-liquid interface found in the pulmonary system. They form the lining of the airway and alveoli and are responsible for crucial functions such as mucociliary clearance and the secretion of pulmonary surfactant, which reduces surface tension to prevent alveolar collapse during respiration. Human airway epithelium cells have been printed that could support the growth of various epithelial cell types and allow for the study of diseases like asthma and COPD (Doryab et al., 2022). Endothelial cells are another primary cell line used in lung bioprinting. They form the interior surface of blood vessels and are key regulators of vascular function, contributing to hemostasis, permeability, and angiogenesis. The incorporation of endothelial cells into bioprinted lung constructs is essential for developing perfusable vasculature within the tissues. Endothelial cells have recently been bioprinted alongside other lung cells to create vascularized lung constructs that demonstrate barrier function and mechanical properties similar to native tissue (Ng et al., 2021).

Researchers from the University of Minnesota generated and printed vascularized lung cancer tissue to better understand molecular mechanisms which underlie lung cancer growth and metastasis (Meng et al., 2019). Lung fibroblasts are responsible for producing and organizing the extracellular matrix (ECM), which provides structural support to the lung tissue and plays a significant role in wound healing and tissue repair (Ushakumary et al., 2021). Their inclusion in bioprinted constructs is vital for recreating the supportive scaffold needed for other cell types. Integrated lung fibroblasts within a bioprinted construct that exhibited organized ECM deposition and mechanical properties were conducive to cell attachment and proliferation (Galliger et al., 2019). Combining these primary cell lines in a bioprinted model requires precise control over the spatial deposition of cells to mimic the lung's native architecture. Coaxial bioprinting techniques, for instance, have been explored to create hollow, tube-like structures that replicate the airways and vasculature, with the potential to seed different cell types in concentric layers to mimic native tissue structures (Grigoryan et al., 2019). Furthermore, the functional roles of these cell types have been demonstrated in several in vitro studies, where bioprinted lung constructs have been used to model pulmonary diseases, test drug responses, and study the lung's response to environmental toxins. For instance, Horváth and team used a bioprinted 3D lung model with primary human bronchial epithelial cells to assess the toxicological response to nanoparticle exposure, highlighting the model's potential for inhalation toxicology research (Horváth et al., 2015).

4.2   Stem Cells and Induced Pluripotent Stem Cells (iPSCs)

Stem cells, and particularly induced pluripotent stem cells (iPSCs), have revolutionized the field of tissue engineering due to their ability to differentiate into a wide variety of cell types, including those required for lung tissue construction. iPSCs are derived from adult cells that have been genetically reprogrammed to an embryonic stem cell-like state, allowing them to proliferate indefinitely and differentiate into cells of all three germ layers. Researchers have leveraged these cells to generate complex, multicellular constructs that more accurately recapitulate the cellular diversity and function of lung tissues (Figure 4 and 5). For lung bioprinting, iPSCs can be differentiated into alveolar epithelial cells, endothelial cells, and lung fibroblasts, which are the primary cell types found in the lung parenchyma. This differentiation process often involves the use of specific growth factors and signaling molecules that guide the iPSCs through stages that resemble embryonic lung development. Hawkins and others from Boston University demonstrated the differentiation of human iPSCs into functional alveolar epithelial cells, which could be further used in tissue-engineered lung models for disease studies and drug screening (Hawkins et al., 2017). The ability of iPSCs to generate patient-specific cells is particularly promising for personalized medicine. For example, iPSCs derived from patients with cystic fibrosis have been used to produce lung epithelial cells that exhibit disease-specific characteristics (Calvert and Ryan Firth, 2020).

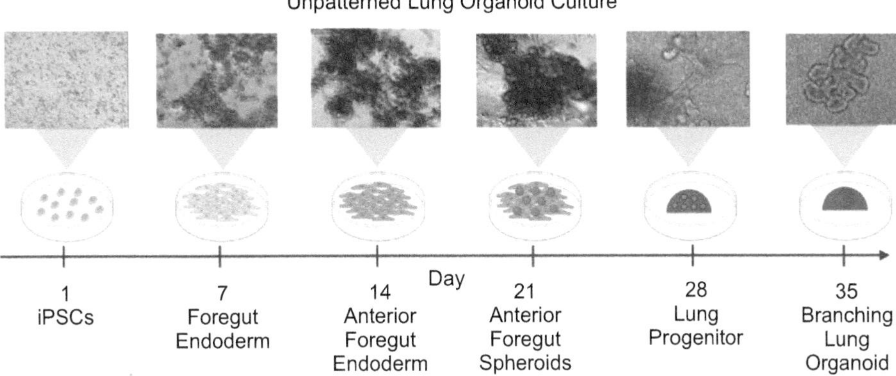

Fig. 4   Overview of a as 5 week differentiation protocol for unpatterned lung organoids. iPSCs are seeded as 2D monolayer on Matrigel-coated culture plates. iPSCs are biochemically differentiated into foregut endoderms, and then anterior foregut endoderms. Cells are then encapsulated into a 3D matrix such as Matrigel to form spheroids. By day 28, the spheroids further differentiate into lung progenitor cells, marked by NXK2.1. By day 35 lung progenitor cells have fully differentiated into branching lung organoids which begin to express mature lung markers such as SFTPC.

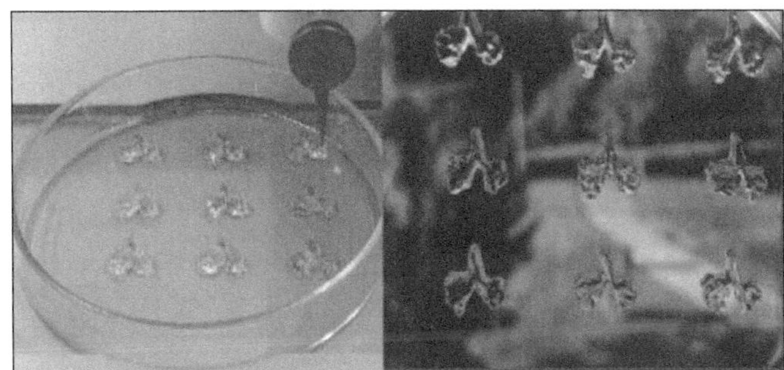

Fig. 5   Using fetal lung scans, a whole lung organoid was printed to recapitulate the 3D architecture of the native embryonic lung at Carnegie Stage 18. These organoids can be printed using biocompatible materials to generate physiologically relevant lung shapes for disease modeling and drug evaluation. In the future, these methods may be used to generate transplantable tissue for regenerative medicine (Wyle 2023).

These patient-derived cells can be used within bioprinted models to study disease mechanisms, evaluate new drugs, and potentially screen for personalized therapies. 3D bioprinting has been instrumental in advancing the development of lung organoids, which are self-organizing, three-dimensional cell cultures that replicate much of the complexity of actual lung tissue. Lung organoids offer an exciting platform for studying lung development, modeling diseases, and screening potential therapeutics. In recent years, researchers have begun to combine the organoid technology with bioprinting, embedding lung organoids within biocompatible scaffolds to enhance their structure and functionality. Encapsulating lung organoids derived from human iPSCs within a hydrogel matrix and printing into lung structures can now be used to screen drugs and study infection (Choi et al., 2023).

Summary

Within the realm of regenerative medicine, lung organoids have emerged as a revolutionary asset, offering researchers miniature, three-dimensional models of the lung fabricated from pluripotent stem cells or organ-specific progenitor cells. These lung organoids are not mere cell clusters; they are complex, self-organizing structures that replicate the cellular and molecular intricacies of the lung, to an extent. They provide invaluable insights into pulmonary development, disease pathogenesis, and the potential efficacy of pharmacological interventions, in a controlled and reproducible laboratory setting. The synergy between organoid biology and 3D bioprinting technologies has been particularly transformative. By employing 3D printed scaffolds, scientists can guide the growth and spatial organization of lung organoids, allowing them to shape these structures in ways that more closely resemble the actual organ. This approach not only aids in studying disease within a relevant three-dimensional context but also holds the key to future applications such as high-throughput drug screening and the creation of organoid-based tissue constructs for therapeutic purposes. The goal of this synergy is ambitious yet profoundly impactful: to cultivate fully functional, transplantable tissues or even whole organs tailored to individual patients, effectively bypassing many challenges associated with traditional organ transplantation. Lung organoids have also been used to study infectious diseases, such as COVID-19, as these stem cell derived tissues can accurately model infection and transmission of the virus (Han et al., 2022). In the future, printed models of lung organoids will endow a deeper understanding of the spread of disease within a physiologically relevant tissue architecture.

By integrating the sophistication of organoid biology with the precision of 3D bioprinting, these studies underscore the potential to create even more refined lung models. Not only do these models hold promise for enhancing our understanding of lung function and disease but they also serve as test beds for pharmacological studies and the development of personalized therapeutic interventions. As bioprinting technology continues to evolve, the fidelity of lung organoids as in vitro models of the human lung is expected to increase, further bridging the gap between preclinical studies and clinical applications.

References

Bos, S., Vos, R., Van Raemdonck, D.E. and Verleden, G.M. (2020). Survival in adult lung transplantation: Where are we in 2020? *Current Opinion in Organ Transplantation*, *25*(3), 268–273. https://doi.org/10.1097/MOT.0000000000000753

Busch, S.M., Lorenzana, Z. and Ryan, A.L. (2021). Implications for Extracellular Matrix Interactions With Human Lung Basal Stem Cells in Lung Development, Disease, and Airway Modeling. *Frontiers in Pharmacology*, *12*, 645858. https://doi.org/10.3389/fphar.2021.645858

Calvert, B.A. and Ryan Firth, A.L. (2020). Application of iPSC to Modelling of Respiratory Diseases. *Advances in Experimental Medicine and Biology*, *1237*, 1–16. https://doi.org/10.1007/5584_2019_430

Chen, S., Kuhn, M., Prettner, K., Yu, F., Yang, T. et al. (2023). The global economic burden of chronic obstructive pulmonary disease for 204 countries and territories in 2020-50: A health-augmented macroeconomic modelling study. *The Lancet. Global Health*, *11*(8), e1183–e1193. https://doi.org/10.1016/S2214-109X(23)00217-6

Choi, Y., Lee, H., Ann, M., Song, M., Rheey, J. et al. (2023). 3D bioprinted vascularized lung cancer organoid models with underlying disease capable of more precise drug evaluation. *Biofabrication*, *15*(3), 034104. https://doi.org/10.1088/1758-5090/acd95f

Clinkenbeard, R.E., England, E.C., Johnson, D.L., Esmen, N.A. and Hall, T.A. et al. (2002). A field comparison of the IOM inhalable aerosol sampler and a modified 37-mm cassette. *Applied Occupational and Environmental Hygiene*, *17*(9), 622–627. https://doi.org/10.1080/10473220290095943

Colucci, G., Piano, M., Lupone, F., Baruffaldi, D., Frascella, F. et al. (2024). Printability study by selective laser sintering of bio-based samples obtained by using PBS as polymeric matrix. *Polymer Testing*, *131*, 108327. https://doi.org/10.1016/j.polymertesting.2024.108327

Díaz Lantada, A., Pfleging, W., Besser, H., Guttmann, M., Wissmann, M. et al. (2018). Research on the Methods for the Mass Production of Multi-Scale Organs-On-Chips. *Polymers*, *10*(11), 1238. https://doi.org/10.3390/polym10111238

Diel, R., Simon, S. and Gottlieb, J. (2023). Chronic Lung Allograft Dysfunction Is Associated with Significant Disability after Lung Transplantation—A Burden of Disease Analysis in 1025 Cases. *Advances in Respiratory Medicine*, *91*(5), 432–444. https://doi.org/10.3390/arm91050033

Doryab, A., Taskin, M.B., Stahlhut, P., Groll, J. and Schmid, O. et al. (2022). Real-Time Measurement of Cell Mechanics as a Clinically Relevant Readout of an In Vitro Lung Fibrosis Model Established on a Bioinspired Basement Membrane. *Advanced Materials*, *34*(41), 2205083. https://doi.org/10.1002/adma.202205083

Du Bois and M, R. (2010). Strategies for treating idiopathic pulmonary fibrosis. *Nature Reviews Drug Discovery*, *9*(2), Article 2. https://doi.org/10.1038/nrd2958

Fu, Z., Naghieh, S., Xu, C., Wang, C., Sun, W. et al. (2021). Printability in extrusion bioprinting. *Biofabrication*, *13*(3). https://doi.org/10.1088/1758-5090/abe7ab

Galliger, Z., Vogt, C.D. and Panoskaltsis-Mortari, A. (2019). 3D Bioprinting for Lungs and Hollow Organs. *Translational Research: The Journal of Laboratory and Clinical Medicine*, *211*, 19–34. https://doi.org/10.1016/j.trsl.2019.05.001

Grigoryan, B., Paulsen, S.J., Corbett, D.C., Sazer, D.W., Fortin, C.L. et al. (2019). Multivascular networks and functional intravascular topologies within biocompatible hydrogels. *Science (New York, N.Y.)*, *364*(6439), 458–464. https://doi.org/10.1126/science.aav9750

Han, Y., Yang, L., Lacko, L.A. and Chen, S. (2022). Human organoid models to study SARS-CoV-2 infection. *Nature Methods*, *19*(4), Article 4. https://doi.org/10.1038/s41592-022-01453-y

Hao, D., Xiao, W., Liu, R., Kumar, P., Li, Y. et al. (2017). Discovery and Characterization of a Potent and Specific Peptide Ligand Targeting Endothelial Progenitor Cells and Endothelial Cells for Tissue Regeneration. *ACS Chemical Biology*, *12*(4), 1075–1086. https://doi.org/10.1021/acschembio.7b00118

Hawkins, F., Kramer, P., Jacob, A., Driver, I., Thomas, D.C. et al. (2017). Prospective isolation of NKX2-1-expressing human lung progenitors derived from pluripotent stem cells. *The Journal of Clinical Investigation*, *127*(6), 2277–2294. https://doi.org/10.1172/JCI89950

Hong, D., Lee, S., Kim, G.B., Lee, S.M., Kim, N. et al. (2020). Development of a CT imaging phantom of anthromorphic lung using fused deposition modeling 3D printing. *Medicine*, *99*(1), e18617. https://doi.org/10.1097/MD.0000000000018617

Horváth, L., Umehara, Y., Jud, C., Blank, F., Petri-Fink, A. et al. (2015). Engineering an in vitro air-blood barrier by 3D bioprinting. *Scientific Reports*, *5*, 7974. https://doi.org/10.1038/srep07974

James, D.S., Jambor, A.N., Chang, H.-Y., Alden, Z., Tilbury, K.B. et al. (2020). Probing ECM remodeling in idiopathic pulmonary fibrosis via second harmonic generation microscopy analysis of macro/supramolecular collagen structure. *Journal of Biomedical Optics*, *25*(1), 014505. https://doi.org/10.1117/1.JBO.25.1.014505

Khan, F. and Tanaka, M. (2017). Designing Smart Biomaterials for Tissue Engineering. *International Journal of Molecular Sciences*, *19*(1), 17. https://doi.org/10.3390/ijms19010017

Last, T. (2022). *Advancing portable, aqueous drug delivery to the human lung*. https://urn.kb.se/resolve?urn=urn:nbn:se:kth:diva-320164

Lim, S.H., Park, S., Lee, C.C., Ho, P.C.L., Kwok, P.C.L. et al. (2021). A 3D printed human upper respiratory tract model for particulate deposition profiling. *International Journal of Pharmaceutics*, *597*, 120307. https://doi.org/10.1016/j.ijpharm.2021.120307

Meng, F., Meyer, C.M., Joung, D., Vallera, D.A., McAlpine, M.C. et al. (2019). 3D Bioprinted In Vitro Metastatic Models via Reconstruction of Tumor Microenvironments. *Advanced Materials*, *31*(10), 1806899. https://doi.org/10.1002/adma.201806899

Muñoz-Perales, V., van der Heijden, M., García-Salaberri, P.A., Vera, M. and Forner-Cuenca, A. et al. (2023). Engineering Lung-Inspired Flow Field Geometries for Electrochemical Flow Cells with Stereolithography 3D Printing. *ACS Sustainable Chemistry and Engineering*, *11*(33), 12243–12255. https://doi.org/10.1021/acssuschemeng.3c00848

Ng, W.L., Ayi, T.C., Liu, Y.-C., Sing, S.L., Yeong, W.Y. et al. (2021). Fabrication and Characterization of 3D Bioprinted Triple-layered Human Alveolar Lung Models. *International Journal of Bioprinting*, *7*(2), 332. https://doi.org/10.18063/ijb.v7i2.332

NHS Blood and Transplant Annual Report and Accounts 2014/15. (2015).

Ranakoti, L., Gangil, B., Bhandari, P., Singh, T., Sharma, S. et al. (2023). Promising Role of Polylactic Acid as an Ingenious Biomaterial in Scaffolds, Drug Delivery, Tissue Engineering, and Medical Implants: Research Developments, and Prospective Applications. *Molecules*, *28*(2), 485. https://doi.org/10.3390/molecules28020485

Razavi Bazaz, S., Kashaninejad, N., Azadi, S., Patel, K., Asadnia, M. et al. (2019). Rapid Softlithography Using 3D-Printed Molds. *Advanced Materials Technologies*, *4*(10), 1900425. https://doi.org/10.1002/admt.201900425

Stanton, Bruce and Koeppen, Bruce. (2008). *Berne and Levy Physiology* (6th ed.). Mosby/Elsevier.

Thabut, G. and Mal, H. (2017). Outcomes after lung transplantation. *Journal of Thoracic Disease*, *9*(8), 2684–2691. https://doi.org/10.21037/jtd.2017.07.85

Ushakumary, M.G., Riccetti, M. and Perl, A.-K.T. (2021). Resident Interstitial Lung Fibroblasts and their Role in Alveolar Stem Cell Niche Development, Homeostasis, Injury, and Regeneration. *Stem Cells Translational Medicine*, *10*(7), 1021–1032. https://doi.org/10.1002/sctm.20-0526

Valapour, M., Lehr, C.J., Schladt, D.P., Smith, J.M., Goff, R. et al. (2023). OPTN/SRTR 2021 Annual Data Report: Lung. *American Journal of Transplantation*, *23*(2), S379–S442. https://doi.org/10.1016/j.ajt.2023.02.009

van Tienderen, G.S., van Beek, M.E.A., Schurink, I.J., Rosmark, O., Roest, H.P. et al. (2022). Modelling metastatic colonization of cholangiocarcinoma organoids in decellularized lung and lymph nodes. *Frontiers in Oncology*, *12*, 1101901. https://doi.org/10.3389/fonc.2022.1101901

Vermeulen, M., Claessens, T., Van Der Smissen, B., Van Holsbeke, C.S., De Backer, J.W. et al. (2013). Manufacturing of patient-specific optically accessible airway models by fused deposition modeling. *Rapid Prototyping Journal*, *19*(5), 312–318. https://doi.org/10.1108/RPJ-11-2011-0118

Wang, X., Ao, Q., Tian, X., Fan, J., Tong, H. et al. (2017). Gelatin-Based Hydrogels for Organ 3D Bioprinting. *Polymers*, *9*(9), Article 9. https://doi.org/10.3390/polym9090401

Wyle, Y., Haczku, A. and Wang, A. (2023). Rescue potential of placenta- and amniotic fluid-derived mesenchymal stem cell extracellular vesicles (EVs) in human lung models of oxidative stress and apoptosis [Abstract]. Lung Development, Injury and Repair, Gordon Research Conference, Waterville Valley Resort, 56 Packard's Road, Waterville Valley, NH, United States.

3D Bioprinting Skin Tissue

Manisha Sonthalia[1,2] and *Amit Kumar Jaiswal*[2*]

1. Introduction

Our skin is the most extensive sensory organ, performing various biological functions. It serves as the primary line of defence between the body and the outside environment, aids in, thermoregulation, excretion, and is capable of performing versatile functions (Ibrahim et al., 2021). The skin is part of the integumentary system, weighing close to 15% of the body weight, which defends the body from the external environment (Richardson M, 2003). The skin is a complex, heterogeneous, multi-layered tissue comprising fibres, cells, and extracellular matrix (ECM) that have specific functions based on location (Watt FM et al., 2011). The skin is prone to various complications like wounds, burn injuries, skin cancer, etc. In accordance with these challenges, technological advancements have led to the development of tissue-engineered skin and its subsequent application (Zhang M et al., 2023). An increasing number of additive manufacturing techniques, such as three-dimensional (3D) bioprinting, are becoming increasingly popular among the various approaches to the development of artificial skin. These techniques are useful for the production of artificial skin for use in pre-clinical, medical, and cosmetic applications (Olejnik A et al., 2021). A microenvironment that is similar to that of the human skin can be created using these. A comprehensive explanation of the skin, as well as the various methods that are utilised in the process of 3D bioprinting in the growth of skin tissue, as well as the practical applications of 3D bioprinted skin, will be presented in this chapter.

1.1 Skin Anatomy and Function

Figure 1 illustrates that the epidermis, dermis, and hypodermis are the three layers that make up the skin, arranged from the outermost layer to the innermost layer. The skin is a complex structure consisting of these three layers (Pereira R.F. et al., 2017).

[1] School of Bio-Sciences and Technology (SBST).

[2] Centre for Biomaterials Cellular and Molecular Theranostics (CBCMT), Vellore Institute of Technology (VIT) Vellore, Vellore, India.

[*] Corresponding author: amitj@vit.ac.in

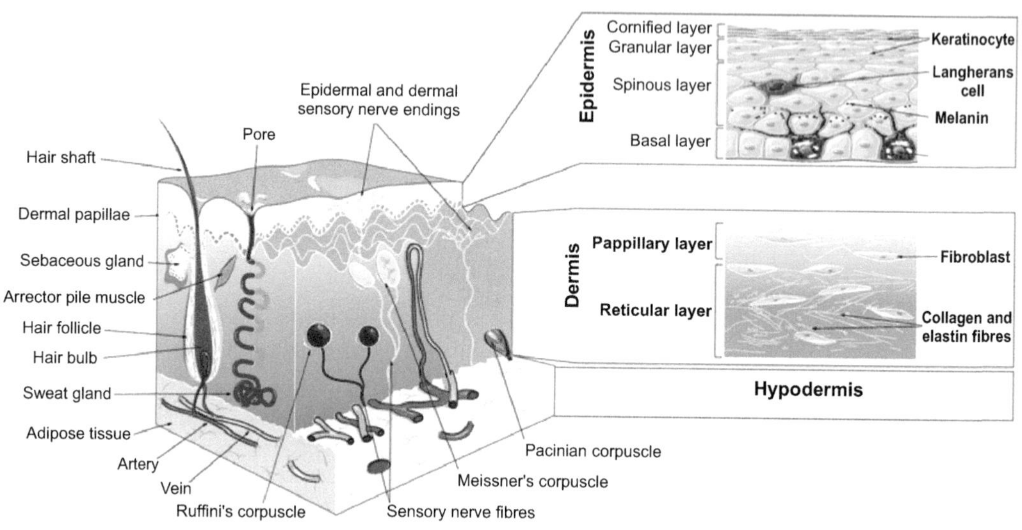

Fig. 1 The stratified structure of human skin is depicted in this illustration. The four primary layers of the skin, as well as the cellular components of the epidermis, such as melanocytes, keratinocytes, and Langerhans cells, are the primary focus of this discussion. The image reveals distinct regions within the dermis, specifically fibroblasts and a zonal pattern of collagen and elastin fibres. These regions are visible in the image. Blood vessels, lymph vessels, sweat glands, hair follicles, and sensory cells are some of the specialized components that can be found in the skin in large quantities. Reproduced from (Pereira RF et al., 2017) with permission from © SNCSC

The epidermis, which is the outermost layer of the skin, is composed of numerous cells, including keratinocytes (KCs), melanocytes, Merkel cells, and Langerhans cells. After the basal layer, the epidermis is further divided into five layers: the stratum basale, the stratum spinosum, the stratum granulosum, the stratum lucidum, and the stratum corneum. These layers are located from the basal layer to the uppermost layer (Rousselle P et al., 2015). Because the epidermis does not contain an ECM, the epidermis acts as a barrier that protects the skin from environmental factors such as dehydration, high temperatures, pathogens, and ultraviolet (UV) radiation. A basal membrane functions as a connection between the inner layer of the epidermis and the layer that is adjacent to it (Hofmann E et al., 2023).

When compared to the topmost layer, the dermis, which is the middle layer, is significantly thicker. The papillary dermis and the reticular dermis are the two components that make up the total structure. Follicles for hair and sweat glands are examples of skin appendages that are found in the dermis. These appendages contribute to the functions of protection and thermoregulation in the skin (Hofmann E et al., 2023). Specific nerves facilitate the perception of external stimuli such as tactile sensations, pressure, and temperature. The circulatory vessels are the source of both oxygen and nutrients that are supplied to the body. A dermis layer is a form of connective tissue that has a higher concentration of ECM. It helps to strengthen the tissue's mechanical integrity (Brown TM et al., 2024). Collagen forms the main structure of the extracellular matrix (ECM), providing a supportive and protective network for the skin. The skin gains its elasticity from the presence of elastin fibres (Pfisterer K et al., 2021). Hypodermis, also referred to as the subcutaneous layer, is the layer that is located deepest within the skin. It predominantly comprises adipocytes that help cushion and insulate the body during violent trauma and cold temperatures. This layer provides buoyancy to the tissue and stores energy. It attaches the skin to the underlying muscles and bones (Driskell RR et al., 2014). The different layers of the skin perform specific functions supporting the skin's physiology. Many technological advancements are required to mimic the skin's microenvironment and, hence, the skin tissue. The cell pattern and ECM distribution, the porous structure, and many other factors play an essential role in forming human skin equivalents (Weng T et al., 2021).

2.   Importance of Skin Tissue Engineering

The skin, as the outer covering, is susceptible to injuries and diseases. The development of in vitro models for diseases, drug testing, and cosmetic testing, as well as the requirement for skin grafts for surgical procedures, paved the way for the development of skin tissue engineering strategies (Przekora A, 2022). In terms of statistics, it is anticipated that the value of the global market for tissue-engineered skin substitutes will increase from 2.2 billion dollars in 2022 to 4.1 billion dollars in 2029 (Ghosh S, 2029). Tissue engineering takes two primary approaches: the top-down approach and the bottom-up approach. Both approaches are described below. One method involves seeding cells onto a porous scaffold. This is the first approach. Over the course of time, cells multiply, and ECM is deposited, all while the scaffold is degrading simultaneously. This process ultimately results in the formation of established tissue. In the latter method, the building blocks that are assembled to produce a mature engineered tissue are cell sheets, cell aggregates, or hydrogels that are loaded with cells (Schmidt T et al., 2021). Regarding wounds where the underlying tissue has lost its regenerative ability, a tissue-engineered skin construct helps in wound healing while restoring the functionality of the original skin. Burn wounds, deep cut wounds, or diabetic wounds take longer to heal, which can lead to infection during the healing process (Tottoli EM et al., 2020). The skin grafts are developed using the cells from the patient's skin biopsies, thus avoiding the complications of graft rejection. In addition to medical applications, it is crucial to have an in vitro model that can replicate the 3D microenvironment of native tissue for drug testing in preclinical trials and toxicology testing of skin care products (Przekora A., 2020).

Based on the application, different types of artificial skin tissue have been developed **(Table 1)**. Single-layered epidermal and dermal substitutes are used for grafting purposes, such as autografts and allografts, while bilayered skin substitutes are used for in vitro testing and for the treatment of slow-healing wounds. The skin substitutes can be cellular or acellular. They mostly consist of an ECM-like matrix composed of either natural, synthetic, or hybrid biopolymeric materials based on the duration of usage, mechanical strength, and several other factors that align with the properties of the native tissue. The skin construct is considered ideal when it can biomimic the mechanical and physiological characteristics of the natural tissue (Oualla-Bachiri W et al., 2020).

Ongoing research is being conducted with the aim of developing a highly desirable skin substitute in the upcoming period. Currently, there are several tissue engineered skin substitutes commercially available for application in burn injuries, wounds, diabetic ulcers, chronic ulcers and a few other skin diseases. These substitutes are of varying thickness and consist of different cell types based on aptness (Vecin NM, Kirsner RS, 2023). The major issue with the existing tissue models is that they need cell distribution throughout the many strata of skin tissue and its ECM. These substitutes are primarily composed of two types of cells: keratinocytes, which make up the epidermis, and fibroblasts, which make up the dermis. The existence of pigmentation, vascularization , and invagination within the epidermal and dermal layers will contribute to the formation of fully operational skin tissue. These can serve as disease models for toxicology assays and in other diverse investigations (Díaz-García D et al., 2021; Urciuolo F et al., 2019).

3.   3D Bioprinting

In order to overcome the constraints above, 3D bioprinting became popular in the early 2000s after skin tissue was successfully bioprinted using KCs and FBs in a collagen hydrogel for the first time (Lee W et al., 2009). Bioprinting is the most favoured technique in tissue engineering for its precision and time-saving process. Individual layers can be bioprinted and assembled for the skin bioprinting to get a full-thickness functional skin substitute (Weng T et al., 2014). Leading cosmetic companies are currently working on a cutting-edge 3D bioprinted skin model to conduct in vitro testing of their cosmetic products. This innovative approach comes in response to the recent ban by PETA on cosmetic testing on animals. Although there is no ban on the testing of pharmaceutical

Table 1   Commercially available cellular skin substitutes reprinted from an open-access source (Oualla-Bachiri W et al., 2020) under Creative Commons Attribution License (CC BY)

Commercial brand	Source	Conformation	Anatomical structure	Type of biomaterial	Description	Clinical use
Apligraf® (Zaulyanov L, Kirsner RS, 2007)	Allogenic	Bi-layered	Composite	Biological	nHEK and hFbs cultured in a type I collagen matrix derived from bovine sources	Exclusively authorized to treat diabetic foot ulcers (DFUs) and venous leg ulcers (VLUs).
Bioseed-S (Johnsen et al., 2005)	Autologous	Single-layered	Epidermal	Biological	Autologous KCs are suspended in a fibrin sealant	Therapy-resistant chronic VLUs
CryoSkin (Hilmi ABM, 2015)	Allogeneic	Spray	Epidermal	Biological	A KC cell spray originating from newborn foreskin and cultured on silicone	Minor wounds
Dermagraft® (Hart CE et al., 2012)	Allogeneic	Single-layered	Dermal	Biological	HFFs, which secrete growth factors and extracellular matrix, are placed on a bioabsorbable polyglactin mesh scaffold	Delayed healing of DFUs and other medical conditions
EPIBASE® (Acher-Chenebaux A et al., 2006; Carsin H et al., 2000)	Autologous	Single-layered	Epidermal	Biological	KCs obtained from a small biopsy were cultured and then applied to the wound as a CEA spray	Cutaneous calciphylaxis and burns
Epicel® (Vacher D, 2003)	Autologous	Single-layered	Epidermal	Biological	KCs adhered to a petrolatum gauze substrate	Full-thickness burns
Epidex TM® (Tausche AK et al., 2003)	Autologous	Single-layered	Epidermal	Biological	Epidermal KC precursor cells from the outer root sheath (ORS) of hair follicles were expanded by plucking hair onto a silicone membrane disc	Chronic leg ulcers
Hyalograft 3D® (Uccioli L, 2016)	Autologous	Single-layered	Dermal	Biological	Hyaluronic acid scaffold seeded with autologous fibroblasts	Full-thickness and deep partial wound

Contd.

Table 1 *Contd.*

Commercial brand	Source	Conformation	Anatomical structure	Type of biomaterial	Description	Clinical use
Laserkin® (Uccioli L, 2016)	Autologous	Single-layered	Epidermal	Biosynthetic	KCs cultured on a hyaluronic acid microperforated membrane	Wound resurfacing
Orcel® (Still J et al., 2023)	Allogeneic	Bi-layered	Composite	Biological	KCs from the epidermis and fibroblasts from the dermis were co-cultured in distinct layers within the collagen sponge matrix	Patients with severe burns
PolyActive® (van Dorp AGM et al., 1999)	Autologous	Bi-layered	Composite	Biological	With keratinocytes and fibroblasts, there are two types of terephthalates : a soft polyethylene oxide component and a hard polybutylene component	Not mentioned
Recell® (Holmes JH et al., 2019)	Autologous	Single-layered	Epidermal	Biological	KCs and melanocytes disperse	Depth burns

products, the in vitro skin model exhibits a closer resemblance to native tissue compared to animal models (D S, N M et al., 2020). Utilising 3D bioprinting techniques, the skin tissue can be created through a series of steps, including bioink preparation, printing, and allowing the printed construct to mature at the air-liquid interface (ALI) (Akh LA et al., 2020). The bioink is composed of material that provides viscosity and mechanical strength to the tissue and supports cells to adhere, proliferate, differentiate and secret its ECM, which leads to the formation of mature tissue (Olejnik A et al., 2021).

3.1 *Materials/Bioink Selection*

Material selection is a crucial step for bioprinting. The materials used in 3D bioprinting are often biodegradable in nature. These materials are referred to as biomaterials and can be of either natural or synthetic origin based on their production method. For bioprinting, the biomaterials should exhibit good printability, biocompatibility, excellent mechanical properties, and shape fidelity post-printing. Biomaterials for bioprinting of skin tissue should demonstrate good shear thinning properties and be non-toxic and non-immunogenic to encourage cells to adhere and proliferate within the printed structure. Another important biomaterial feature is to support secretion of the ECM by the cells present within, corresponding to the simultaneous degradation of the biomaterial to nullify the negative effect of the biomaterial on ECM production (Ishack S, Lipner SR, 2020; Javaid M, Haleem A, 2021; Manita PG et al., 2021).

Collagen is a naturally occurring biopolymer that is most frequently employed to fabricate artificial skin because it is widely distributed in the extracellular matrix of skin tissue. **Table 2**

Table 2 Features, benefits, and 3D printing methods employed with bioinks based on collagen, chitosan, cellulose, hyaluronic acid, and alginate. Readapted from open access source (Antezana PE et al., 2022) under Creative Commons Attribution License (CC BY)

Natural Polymer Bioink	*Characteristics*	*Benefits*	*3D bioprinting technologies*	*Cells used in bioprinting*
Collagen-based bioink	Good biocompatibility, natural polymer material that encourages migration, proliferation, and adhesion of cells. It does not result in significant inflammation and is safe for the host. It is capable of being broken down by enzymes. (Weng T et al., 2021)	High porosity, absorbency, and low immunogenicity. Strong cellular adhesion. (Fayyazbakhsh F, Leu MC, 2020; Pugliese R et al., 2021)	Low temperatures can be used for printing, and at body temperature, it solidifies into a gel. Collagen with a low concentration of 0.1 wt% is suitable for the processes of droplet ejection, inkjet printing, and laser-assisted 3D bioprinting. When the concentration of the substance exceeds 1.25 wt%, it reaches a viscosity that is suitable for extrusion. (Weng T, et al., 2021; Valot L et al., 2019)	Primary HFFs (Teoh JH et al., 2019)
Chitosan-based bioink	Chitosan is derived from chitin, a polysaccharide present in the exoskeleton of crustaceans and various other marine arthropods. The linear structure facilitates the swift creation of a gel matrix through the utilization of NaOH. (Weng T et al., 2021)	Chitosan demonstrates exceptional compatibility with living organisms and the ability to break down naturally over time. Mild gelation conditions and antimicrobial properties. (Weng T et al., 2021; Fayyazbakhsh F, Leu MC. 2020)	Chitosan hydrogels are commonly utilized with an extrusion bioprinter, and there is limited research on chitosan printing using jet-based bioprinting techniques. (Zhou D et al., 2019)	Keratinocytes and human dermal fibroblasts (Hafezi F et al., 2020)
Cellulose-based bioink	Cellulose is a common linear polysaccharide and a widely occurring natural polymer. It is both biocompatible and nontoxic. (Badhe RV et al., 2020)	Cellulose hydroxyl groups have the potential for chemical modification through various processes, including esterification, graft copolymerization, etherification, selective oxidation, or intermolecular crosslinking reactions. These processes offer a wide range of possibilities for bioink formulation. (Pradhan RA et al., 2021)	It is commonly used in bioinks for its excellent bio-adhesion and mechanical properties. (Badhe RV et al., 2020)	Fibroblasts (Rastin H et al., 2021)

Contd.

Table 2 *Contd.*

Natural Polymer Bioink	Characteristics	Benefits	3D bioprinting technologies	Cells used in bioprinting
Hyaluronic acid-based bioink	Hyaluronic acid is a negatively charged complex carbohydrate that stimulates the regrowth of tissues. Hyaluronic acid with low molecular weight can stimulate cell differentiation and the formation of new blood vessels. (Weng T et al., 2021)	Outstanding moisture retention and stimulates cell growth. (Si, Xing et al., 2019)	It is commonly used alongside various biomaterials to improve the physical properties of the bioink mixture, although it can also be utilized independently. (Valot L et al., 2019)	Human dermal fibroblasts (Fayyazbakhsh F et al., 2020)
Alginic acid-based bioink	Diminished cellular adhesion. Alginate is a naturally occurring linear polymer that is derived from the cell walls of brown algae. Alginate is a polysaccharide with a negative charge. This soluble biopolymer promotes cell growth and demonstrates excellent biocompatibility. (Pugliese R et al., 2021; Axpe E, Oyen Mn, 2016)	Effortless, rapid gelation at a minimal cost. (Fayyazbakhsh F, Leu MC, 2020)	Multiple bioinks described in scientific literature comprise alginate, either as an individual material or in combination with various other biopolymers. The ionotropic gelation process's ease of use and sodium alginate, a readily available and reasonably priced network precursor, both contribute to its popularity. (Valot L et al., 2019)	Human amniotic epithelial cells and Wharton's jelly-derived MSCs (Liu P et al., 2019)

highlights the major natural bioinks that are used (Antezana PE et al., 2022). There are advantages and disadvantages associated with both natural and synthetic polymers. In contrast to synthetic polymers, natural polymers are known to exhibit superior biocompatibility when compared to synthetic polymers, but they have a lower mechanical strength. The need for an optimised material that has good printability and rheology and exhibits good shape fidelity has led to the fabrication of composite biomaterials. These show excellent printability and shape fidelity (Puertas-Bartolomé M et al., 2021). Different skin substitutes made of natural polymers and synthetic materials are presented in **Table 3** below (Wei C et al., 2021).

Table 3 A combination of natural and synthetic materials used in the process of tissue engineering to create skin substitutes. Reproduced from (Wei C et al., 2021) with permission of the publisher (Taylor and Francis Ltd, http://www.tandfonline.com)

Biomaterial composition	Structural type of substitute	Cellular content	Demonstrated effect in vitro or in vivo
Poly(globalide), cellulose	Epidermal	Acellular	Stimulation of KC proliferation and increased cellular metabolic function in laboratory conditions (Homaeigohar S, Boccaccini AR, 2020)
PLA, PCL, gelatin	Dermal	Acellular	Stimulated fibroblast growth and elevated collagen accumulation in a laboratory setting (Chandrasekaran AR et al., 2011)

Contd.

Table 3 *Contd.*

Biomaterial composition	Structural type of substitute	Cellular content	Demonstrated effect in vitro or in vivo
Collagen, elastin, PCL	Dermal	Acellular	Enhanced growth of keratinocytes and fibroblasts, enhanced tissue integration, and accelerated early-stage angiogenesis in a mouse model (Chong C et al., 2019)
PVP, PGS	Dermal	Acellular	Human dermal fibroblast cells exhibit strong viability and proliferation in an in vitro environment (Keirouz A et al., 2019)
Human-like collagen, carboxymethylated chitosan	Dermal	Acellular	Complete restoration of skin structure and tissue regeneration in a full-thickness skin defect
Fish collagen, chitosan, chondroitin sulfate, basic fibroblast growth factor(bFGF)-loaded PLGA microspheres	Dermal	Acellular	Enhancing fibroblast cell growth and promoting skin tissue regeneration in a rat model with full-thickness skin defects (Cao H et al., 2019)
Chitosan, collagen	Dermal	Cellular (fibroblasts)	In a rat model with a full-thickness skin defect, improved wound healing and re-epithelialization (Chen K-Y et al., 2009)
Collagen, silk fibroin	Dermal	Cellular (BMSCs)	Improved wound healing and decreased scar formation in a full-thickness skin defect rat model (Cui B et al., 2020)
Fibrin-coated PLA, collagen	Dermo-epidermal	Cellular (keratinocytes, fibroblasts)	Enhancement of a uniform basal layer and increased migration of fibroblasts in a laboratory setting (Bacakova M, Pajorova J et al., 2019)

3.2 *Cells-keratinocytes, Fibroblasts, Melanocytes/Cell Sources*

The vital component of a bioink is the cells that are required to make up the tissue. The deposition of cells layer by layer mimics the architecture of natural human skin. The selection of cells is based on the functional properties that help in the regeneration of the tissue construct (Ashammakhi N et al., 2019; Gungor-Ozkerim PS et al., 2018). The cell types used majorly are keratinocytes, fibroblasts, melanocytes, and endothelial cells. The epidermis is primarily composed of KCs and melanocytes. KCs proliferate, differentiate, and keratinise, which is the unique property of this cell type, in order to create a protective barrier separating the external environment from the body (Lee J-S et al., 2013). These cells have good regenerative properties which makes them an important component in wound healing. The skin colour is due to the pigment-containing cells known as melanocytes. It helps in protection against harmful UV radiation (Lee J-S et al., 2013). Adding melanocytes to a tissue construct can assist in attaining the patient's skin tone more accurately. These cells are the prime target of skin cancers such as melanoma (Helgadottir H et al. 2018). In addition to the epidermal layer, fibroblasts are responsible for the growth that occurs within the dermal layer. This growth leads to the development of full-thickness skin tissue, which can be utilized as an in vitro skin model for the testing of cosmetics and pharmaceuticals. The fibroblasts secrete collagen, which is a significant part of the ECM (Reijnders CMA et al., 2015). The vascularization of the tissue contributes to the fabrication of a more human skin-like equivalent, and the incorporation of endothelial cells into the bioink in order to stimulate angiogenesis can be beneficial. However, to increase the similarity between native skin and bioprinted skin, efforts have been made to culture specialized structures like hair follicles and sweat glands. (Zhang Y, et al., 2021).

3.3 3D Printing Techniques

Skin tissue formation and development through bioprinting is the upcoming technology for fabrication as it gives more precision and time. The spatial arrangement of the skin cells across the scaffold helps in the development of layered skin tissue, which is closely like human skin tissue (Pasierb A et al., 2022; Weng T et al., 2021). The process of producing biomedical components that most closely resemble natural tissue/organ characteristics is known as 3D bioprinting. It involves printing cells, biomaterials and growth factors layer by layer using rapid prototyping technologies (Tripathi S et al., 2022). Bioprinting is a sophisticated, rapid prototype creation and printing method via additive manufacturing. This method creates intricate 3D biocompatible structures by automatically depositing biological materials onto a surface with the help of computer-aided technology (Gu BK et al., 2018). **Table 4** highlights the key features of different bioprinting technologies.

Table 4   An illustration of the key features of bioprinting technologies. Readapted (Pereira RF et al., 2017) with permission from © SNCSC

Technology	*Characteristics*
Inkjet bioprinting	
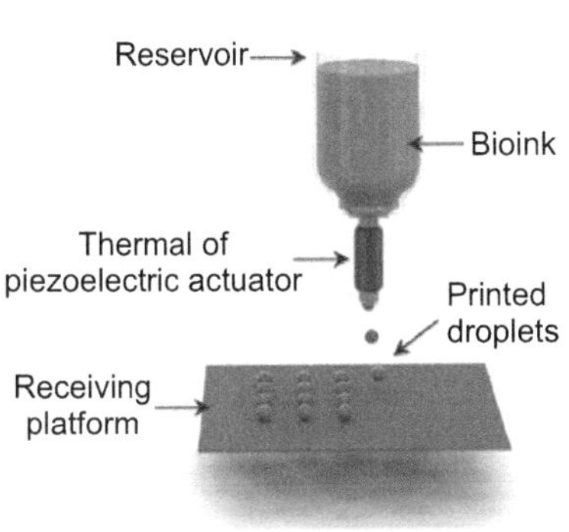	Benefits: Non-contact printing using multiple printheads for high throughput at a medium printing speed and low cost. Limitations: Low bioink viscosity, clogging problems, potential for cell clumping and settling
Laser-assisted bioprinting	
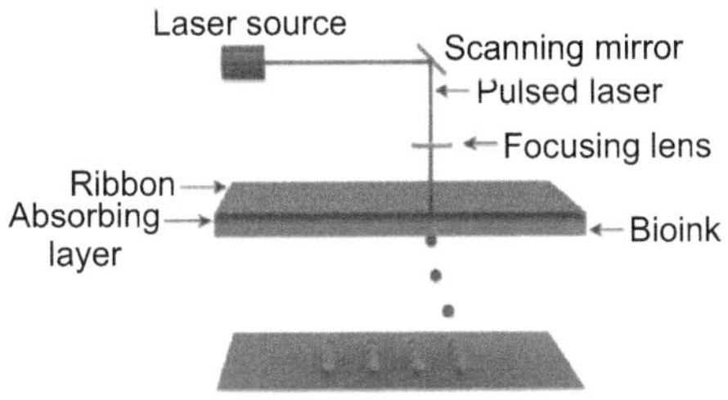	Benefits: Features include a high cell count, thick inks, superior resolution, consistent repeatability, and fast printing speed. It has a moderate throughput, operates without nozzles, and is non-contact Limitations: Interactions between cells and lasers, extended printing durations, challenges in constructing objects on the millimetre scale, and high expenses and time constraints.
Extrusion-based bioprinting	
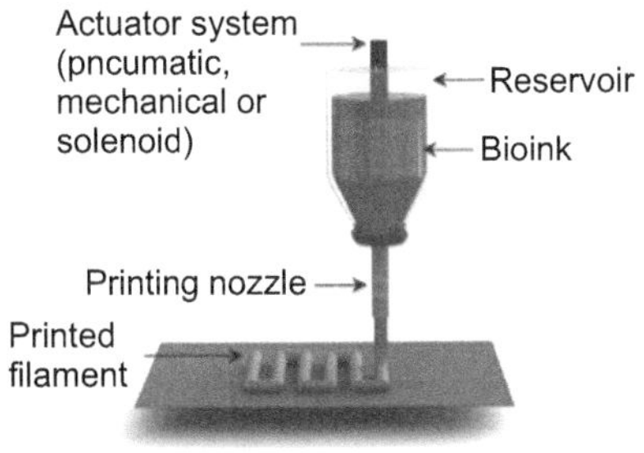	Benefits: Uninterrupted printing of thick bioinks and elevated cell concentrations; the ability to produce 3D structures at sizes important for medical treatment; simple combination with other biofabrication methods; Moderate throughput, resolution, and expenditures Limitations: Mechanical tensions produced throughout the bioink deposition process; challenging to create complex geometrized 3D structures arranged in a hierarchical manner

3.4 Inkjet Bioprinting

Inkjet bioprinting, also referred to as drop-on-demand (DOD) printing, is favoured over continuous droplet expulsion systems because of the precise patterning capability of DOD systems in replicating the cell structure of native tissue (Jamee R et al., 2021). Currently, research on acoustic-based bioprinting is restricted because of the lack of control over the printing system. The two types of inkjet printing techniques that are most frequently used for bioprinting are thermal and piezoelectric DOD techniques (Kumar P et al., 2021). Thermal bioprinting utilizes a brief pulse of voltage that heats the bioink, forming a vapour bubble that quickly expands and breaks down, causing pressure to build up within the bioink reservoir. Applying pressure aids the bioink in overcoming the surface tension surrounding the nozzle's tip, resulting in the expulsion of a droplet (Bhushan S et al., 2022). The piezoelectric bioprinting technology utilises a voltage pulse to induce expansion in a piezoelectric crystal, resulting in the generation of pressure waves in the bioink reservoir. This wave facilitates the bioink in surmounting surface tension in the vicinity of the nozzle tip, resulting in the ejection of a droplet. The critical factors in a piezoelectric bioprinting method include the viscosity and rheological characteristics of the bioink, the amplitude, frequency range, and duration of the voltage pulse, as well as the activation patterns of the piezoelectric crystal, which involve both pull-push and push-pull actions (Gu Z et al., 2020). The microvalve bioprinting system uses pneumatic pressure to extrude the cell-containing bioink through the nozzle. A solenoid-operated electromechanical valve regulates the nozzle's aperture. The bioink's viscosity, surface tension, as well as additional rheological properties, along with the pneumatic pressure, frequency and duration of valve openings, and the nozzle diameter, are the factors that define the droplet characteristics (Ng WL et al., 2017).

Using a hybrid technique combining inkjet and microextrusion, a study by Lee et al. aimed to create a repeatable process for printing skin layers. They enhanced bioinks for optimal cell viability in both dermal and epidermal layers. The inkjet printing technique produced an equivalent of human skin with structure, which improved accuracy and uniformly distributed epidermal keratinocytes on the dermal layer. The printed skin model included a dermis, basement membrane, and an epidermal layer expressing skin-specific markers. The study showed that it is possible to create a complex skin equivalent using printing methods, emphasizing the potential of bioprinting in generating skin tissue and proposing directions for future research. The study contrasted manual pipetting techniques with inkjet printing for the deposition of epidermal keratinocytes. In the skin model, inkjet printing produced a more even dispersion of keratinocytes on the dermal layer, resulting in a broad and well-organized epidermal layer. Manual pipetting resulted in uneven layers with cell aggregations, suggesting a less precise and consistent deposition technique (Lee H-R et al., 2021).

Yanez et al. developed artificial skin by utilizing inkjet printing technology and a combination of different biological components. They used various types of cells, including nHDFs, KCs and human umbilical vascular endothelial cells (HUVECs), to enhance the vascularization of the printed skin tissues. An engineered skin graft was inserted into a wound on the backs of mice that lacked a functioning thymus. It showed that 3D-printed skin grafts have the potential to speed up wound healing, as new blood vessels were observed in the grafts just 2 weeks after the surgery. HUVECs are well-known among the indicated cell types (Yanez M et al., 2015). For instance, Rimann et al. used inkjet bioprinting to create the dermal section of a bilayer skin structure by alternating layers composed of primary dermal fibroblasts with cell-free layers using PEG-based bioink. Next, the bioprinted dermal equivalent was covered with seeded primary epidermal keratinocyte cultures to form the skin bilayer structure (Rimann M et al., 2016). Conversely, Kim et al. made use of inkjet printing to create the epidermal compartment for the vascularized skin model using epidermal cells that were suspended in a cell culture medium (Kim BS et al., 2017). Using a combination of wound scanning imaging technology and inkjet bioprinting technology, Albanna et al. were able to deliver HDFs and KCs directly to a full-thickness wound. The cells were supported by a fibrin/collagen hydrogel and applied layer-by-layer, integrating along the topography and depth of the wound.

The data showed accelerated healing with improved re-epithelialization, reduced contraction, and notable collagen fibre deposition, indicating comparable effectiveness to current clinical cell spraying techniques (Albanna M et al., 2019).

3.5 *Laser-assisted Bioprinting*

The upside of laser-assisted bioprinting (LAB) is the precise deposition of bioink to fabricate a 2D biomaterials' layer-by-layer stacked 3D scaffold. The critical components of laser-assisted bioprinting are a pulsed laser source, a ribbon, and a substrate at the receiving end. The basic principle of working has been described in detail in previous chapters. The ribbon containing the bioink, which is made up of cells, hydrogels, and bioactive components, is vaporised by a pulsed laser source, which typically uses nanosecond lasers using UV or close to UV wavelengths. By concentrating the laser beam on the ribbon for a precise period, the metal layer on the hydrogel is dissolved. The high-pressure bubble propels the bioink onto the receptive substrate (Ventura RD, 2010). This method significantly contributes to the field of tissue engineering applications. LAB addresses the limitations of conventional bioprinting methods, including issues like print head blockage, cell clumping, and ink evaporation, by providing a non-contact, nozzle-free bioprinting technology. Because of LAB's exceptional resolution and precision, very viscous bioinks that closely resemble natural tissues and organs may be printed with excellent cell viability and accuracy (Gu Z et al., 2020).

Laser-assisted bioprinting (LAB) is a printing technique that utilizes laser energy to place cell-laden bioink droplets onto a substrate without physical contact, eliminating the need for a nozzle. Several laser-based bioprinting methods exist, all based on a fundamental concept but varying in their experimental setups. There are several commonly used techniques in the field, such as biological laser processing (BioLP), matrix-assisted pulsed laser evaporation direct writing (MAPLE DW), laser-guided direct writing (LG DW), laser-induced forward transfer (LIFT), and absorbing film-assisted laser-induced forward transfer (AFA-LIFT) (Schiele NR et al., 2010).

Micheal et al. created a novel technique for producing tissue-engineered skin replacements using laser-assisted bioprinting. They utilized the LAB method to develop skin substitutes. They placed fibroblasts on a stabilizing matrix called Matriderm. The skin wounds in the nude mice were then filled with the grafts. The grafts successfully bonded to the surrounding tissue of the skin wound within 11 days. It was observed that certain blood vessels extended towards the printed cells from the injured area's bottom and wound margins. The normal skin integrated with the printed dermis collagen layer, exhibiting sparse collagen in the bottom layer and rich collagen in the top layer, mirroring the typical dermal structure of the human body (Slominski AT et al., 2013).

In a study by Koch et al., NIH3T3 and HaCaTs bioprinted using the LIFT technique were examined for cell viability, proliferation, apoptosis and DNA disintegration. The post-printing vitality of these cells was remarkable, while their proliferation rate was comparable to that of a manually produced control. When evaluating post-printed apoptosis activity, there were consistent levels of caspase 3/7 activity, indicating cell death, between 12 and 48 hours following laser transfer. The comet assay showed that the LIFT process did not cause any DNA damage or fragmentation in the post-printed cells. This work is not a stratified skin model but a cell viability post-printing evaluation employing the LAB method (Koch L et al., 2010). Utilizing the LIFT technique, they also sought to create a stratified three-dimensional model of skin. The layer that absorbed laser energy was made of a thin 60 nm layer of gold. NIH3T3 and HaCaT cells were incorporated into collagen and placed on the donor slide. The Matriderm™ sheet was used as the base for printing the bioink-containing cells. Twenty layers of collagen were 3D printed using NIH3T3 fibroblasts, and subsequently, additional twenty levels using HaCaT keratinocytes. Different staining methods were utilized to assess the cell viability and cell proliferation in the printed construct over time, confirming that the cells were alive and continued to grow post-printing. Gap and adherens junctions among keratinocytes in normal skin tissue show intercellular adhesion. This study represents the initial attempt to utilize bioprinting technology to create a multi-layered skin tissue. The subsequent biological analysis was conducted within a short span of 10 days. This study lacks long-term culture and additional biological characterization, such as examining extracellular matrix production of cells after printing (Koch L et al., 2012).

Researchers utilised a 4D bioprinting technique to develop a new model capable of mimicking the dynamic restructuring of fibroblasts in a laboratory setting. Fibroblasts were arranged on collagen gels using laboratory techniques to investigate the resulting alterations in the matrix structure. This technique was employed to arrange both sets of collagen gels in uniform isotropic patterns with exceptional precision, density, and viability. The fibroblasts and myofibroblasts that were created using bioprinting techniques were arranged and rearranged into either scattered or grouped cells during their growth and development. 4D bioprinting was utilized to stimulate and align the dynamic matrix remodelling processes of different fibroblastic groups and structures on collagen through LAB patterning. This approach offers a versatile tool for examining the structures, properties, and healing mechanisms of the skin, as well as exploring potential therapeutic opportunities in future studies (Douillet C et al., 2022).

3.6 Extrusion-based Bioprinting

Extrusion-based bioprinting (EBB) uses pneumatic force to extrude the bioink through a narrow diameter, which aligns with the CAD model. Through automated machine systems and fluid distribution systems, extrusion-based bioprinting technology produces extremely controllable printing (Malekpour A et al., 2022). The bioink containing cells is driven by a computer and is pushed through a micro-nozzle in continuous strands using a screwdriver, piston, or even pneumatic methods. An entire three-dimensional structure is formed by printing one layer at a time (Potere F et al., 2022). Pneumatic-based extrusion bioprinting works best with hydrogels that have shear-thinning properties since they help maintain the filament's condition post-extrusion. The utilization of a screw-driven mechanism enables the printing of bioink with high viscosity, resulting in the creation of more durable 3D-bioprinted tissue (Hospodiuk M et al., 2018). Modern extrusion bioprinters are equipped with multiple printer heads to concurrently apply various bioinks, thereby reducing the likelihood of cross-contamination (Munaz A et al., 2016). Furthermore, they enable enhanced control over the printed structure's porosity, form, and distribution of cells. Extrusion bioprinting offers faster printing speed, a more comprehensive range of printable bioink types, and enhanced mechanical strength in printed products compared to droplet-based bioprinting and laser-assisted bioprinting (Chen XB et al., 2023). More significantly, this can produce bionic effects, encourage the flow of nutrients and metabolites, and print a porous grid structure. This technique is very adaptable and ideal for creating scaffolds or prosthetic implants for tissue engineering. But the resolution of EBB is lower. The minimum resolution typically surpasses 100 μm (Loh QL et al., 2013).

Lee et al. employed the pneumatic microextrusion method to create a durable dermal layer consisting of collagen and primary HDFs. Later on, piezoelectric inkjet printing was used to apply a layer of primary HEKs, creating a uniform and highly viable epidermal layer. Viscosity was measured in the presence of dermal fibroblasts to enhance the printability of collagen ink. A study was performed on the epidermal bioink, which consists of media and epidermal keratinocytes, under different conditions in order to enhance the inkjet printing procedure. The culture conditions, including the bioink and culture media, were validated to ensure the survival of cells. After immersing the dermal culture for about 2 weeks and then exposing it to air for another 2 weeks, histological staining and immunostaining was conducted to evaluate the quality of our printed skin models. This hybrid process can establish an uncomplicated and dependable printing technique for fabricating skin models with multiple layers. Moreover, it enables the modification of the outermost epidermal layer by altering the parameters of inkjet printing (Lee H-R et al., 2021).

Cho's group presented a 3D bioprinted skin tissue using a skin-derived extracellular matrix (S-dECM). Decellularized porcine skin, due to its similarity to human skin, was utilized as a bioink. This bioink contains essential factors for cell growth and demonstrated exceptional stability for two weeks. In vivo experiments showed impressive wound healing capabilities of this new construct. However, the discrepancy between the excellent biocompatibility and the limited ability to be shaped by dECMs has limited their widespread application (Kim BS et al., 2017). A cryogenic free-form extrusion bioprinter was explicitly developed for printing decellularized small intestinal submucosal (dSIS) material obtained from porcine skin. By utilizing this method, dSIS scaffolds were created with outstanding physical and chemical properties and improved compatibility with living tissues (Shi L et al., 2019). This approach may pave the way for new research in the future because of the chemical similarities between dSIS and the components of dECM, which primarily consist of collagens and polysaccharides.

By layering hFBs and hKCs into a collagen hydrogel to create multi-layered engineered tissue composites with an external layer of hKCs and an internal layer of hFBs, the viability of employing bioprinting to create in vitro skin tissue constructs was first demonstrated. More precisely, a microvalve-controlled pneumatic extrusion bioprinter with four nozzles was created. By employing ten distinct tiers of the protein collagen hydrogel precursors, fibroblasts were deposited in the following layer with hKCs in the eighth layer, resulting in the development of intricate engineered composite tissues that imitate the layers of natural skin (Lee W et al., 2009). An eight-nozzle bioprinting device was utilized to fabricate several layers comprising crosslinked collagen, incorporating either human fibroblasts or human keratinocytes, in order to mimic the epidermal layer, dermis layer, and extracellular matrix of native skin tissue. The bioprinted skin constructs closely resemble human skin tissue biology and structure and demonstrates superior shape and structure preservation during in vitro cultures (Lee V et al., 2014).

The cellular behaviour of a collagen scaffold developed by Kim and colleagues was impressive. However, the scaffold's mechanical stability was compromised due to the high porosity (>95%) and the inadequate mechanical attributes of collagen (Kim G et al. 2009). In order to address this limitation, a scaffold was developed that comprised a collagen core and an outer layer made of alginate. This scaffold exhibited remarkable structural stability and allowed for accurate measurement of the growth and proliferation of healthy hFB and hKC cells after 7 days of both in vitro and in vivo culture. The constructed framework exhibited a Young's modulus, which was approximately 6.7 times greater than that observed in pristine collagen, resembling the modulus of the skin (Kim G et al., 2011). In a separate study, the same scientists employed this technique to create collagen-based scaffolds that formed the dermal part of a skin substitute using a poly(ε-caprolactone) PCL mesh. The inclusion of PCL mesh stabilized the dermal matrix and prevented collagen shrinkage during maturation. A recent study presented a thermosensitive hydrogel composed of p(NIPAAm-AA) for application in various 3D printing methods, including single nozzle and single syringe, coaxial needles with double syringes, and single nozzle with double syringes (Kim BS et al., 2017). The hybrid bioink, composed of p(NIPAAm-AA) and fibrin, was utilized in 3D printing to generate keratinocytes, fibroblasts, and endothelial cells, exhibiting notably high cell viability. In addition, the analysis included studying the growth and division of the cells beneath the skin and the outer layer's process of becoming cornified (Zhang J et al., 2020).

4. Application of 3D Bioprinted Skin Tissues

Bioengineered human skin substitutes can be utilized for various clinical and research purposes. The world is becoming more concerned with the repair of lost or damaged tissue, and there is an increasing need for skin biofabrication due to the growing interest in cosmetic/aesthetic procedures, obesity, diabetes, and ageing populations (Sarkiri M et al., 2019). Skin bioprints are proposed as an alternative method for the following: (a) Clinical applications of regenerative medicine include ulcerations, burns, chronic wounds, and reconstructive surgery following extensive oncological

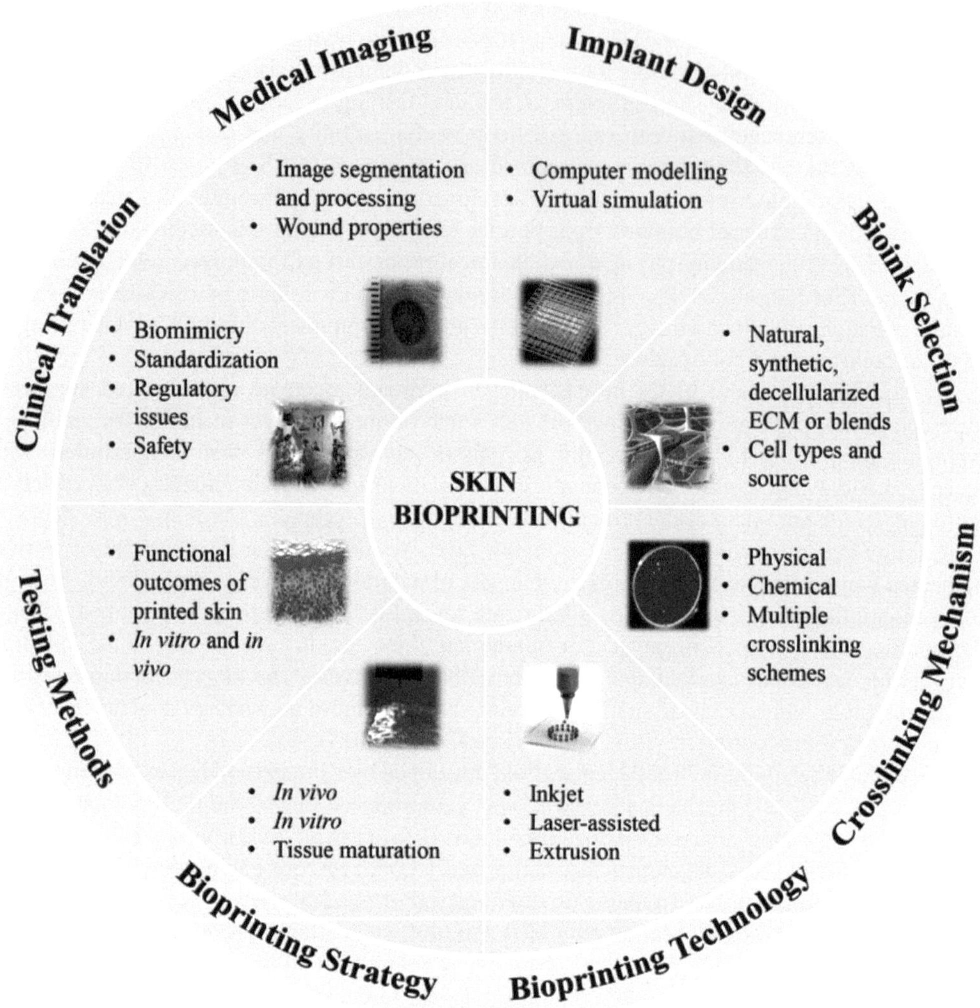

Fig. 2   An illustration of the various interdisciplinary tasks required for designing 3D structures for skin rejuvenation and repair using bioprinting technologies. Images are reprinted from (Pereira RF et al., 2017) with permission © SNCSC

resections , (b) modelling pathological and physiological conditions such as ageing, genodermatoses, wound repair, UV response, drug reaction, photoirradiation, penetration of the skin barrier, and inflammatory conditions and (c) concerns in the cosmetic and pharma industry including the safety and effectiveness of active ingredients, drug absorption, drug metabolism, and personalised therapies (Prescott SL et al., 2017; Tavakoli S et al., 2021; Smandri A et al., 2020; Velasquillo C et al., 2013). **Figure 2** shows the various applications of 3D bioprinted skin.

Since testing on animals for cosmetic purposes is now entirely prohibited by the European Union Cosmetic Regulation (EU/1223/2009), there is a great need to find skin equivalents that could be used in place of animal trials. In addition to ethical concerns, the limited resemblance of animal skin to human skin further limits the use of animal models (Silva RJ, Tamburic S, 2022). Hence, the research findings sometimes need to be clarified. Comparatively speaking, the animal and human physiological systems are distinct. As a result, about 50% of medications that did well in animal testing turned out to be harmful to people, and vice versa (Van Norman GA, 2019). Global cosmetics and pharmaceutical industries focus on finding skin models that can effectively test new topical formulations and substances. Thus, skincare companies have shown a growing interest in 3D bioprinting. This new technology is predicted to change topical and cosmetic product testing completely. The skin is composed of numerous layers and comprises various types of cells (Olejnik A et al., 2021). 3D bioprinting enables the accurate positioning of cells in a predetermined arrangement. 3D bioprinted skin offers numerous benefits for the cosmetic and pharmaceutical sectors. Prior to conducting clinical trials on any novel substance or medication, it is imperative to assess its safety through in vitro testing (Weng T et al., 2021). Pharma and chemical companies have the ability to conduct product testing using skin models generated by 3D bioprinters. On the other hand, cosmetic formulations must undergo testing to assess potential allergic reactions and toxicity prior to being made available for purchase. Thus, 3D bioprinted skin can serve as a suitable platform for evaluating and testing cosmetic and pharmaceutical products. This technology has the ability to accelerate, decrease expenses, and improve the effectiveness of drug and product testing. It is possible for it to be ethical as well. Production costs can be reduced by implementing a fully standardized and automated method. It is necessary to create fake versions of various skin types, including normal, oily, dry, and sensitive, for cosmetic testing (Ng WL et al., 2019). In addition, 3D skin bioprinting can be employed to examine the permeation and assimilation of pharmaceuticals or active substances into the skin. Esteemed multinational cosmetic corporations such as L'Oreal and Proctor and Gamble were attracted to this technology and allocated funds to research and develop 3D bioprinted skin models (Millás A et al., 2019).

3D tumour models can aid in analyzing the mechanisms involved in cancer growth and spread, as well as the response to specific drugs. Tumor cells can be added to bioprinted tissues to create a new disease model. Therefore, melanoma was introduced to the in vitro model of human skin (Germain N et al., 2022). Liu et al. generated skin tissues in order to establish disease models for Atopic Dermatitis (AD). The models have identified several characteristic features of Alzheimer's disease, such as hyperplasia and spongiosis, elevated levels of pro-inflammatory cytokines, along the initial and final levels of differentiated proteins. Bioprinting can be utilized to create human skin substitutes of different cellular complexity, which can accurately simulate specific diseases, as indicated by this study (Liu X et al., 2020). This method provides a chance to comprehend the mechanisms of different pathologies.

Many individuals experience nonhealing skin wounds. Typically, skin injuries are treated with transplants taken from patients' bodies or donors. 3D bioprinting could serve as a substitute for the previously mentioned technique. This innovative technology's primary benefit is the efficient and cost-effective creation of skin equivalents in a shorter time frame (Manita PG et al., 2021). 3D bioprinting has the capacity to revolutionize the methodical approach to injury and surgery treatment. It can be especially advantageous for treating damaged skin caused by burns. Researchers have created 3D bioprinters specifically designed to facilitate the production of skin for individuals who have sustained injuries. Two techniques are employed to fabricate skin for wound healing therapies: Bioprinting techniques include ex vivo and in situ methods (Varkey M et al., 2019). Ex vivo techniques, including inkjet, extrusion, and laser-based bioprinting, are employed to fabricate a skin structure composed of dermis and epidermis. If necessary, this construct is subsequently cultured in vitro to promote maturation. Afterwards, it is affixed to the patient's wound via grafting. Extrusion-based bioprinting is the most direct and efficient ex vivo technique. This method allows for the simultaneous deposition of all the necessary elements, including calcium chloride, human plasma, and fibroblasts, to form the dermis. An epidermis is formed by placing a layer of human keratinocytes on top. An inherent limitation of 3D bioprinting technology for wound recovery treatments is the time-consuming process of acquiring a sufficient number of autologous cells to generate a substantial skin surface. Patients suffering from severe burns require immediate medical intervention. Therefore, it is crucial to promptly utilize bioprinted skin equivalents in order to expedite wound healing and minimize the formation of hypertrophic scar tissue (Gu Z et al., 2020; Olejnik A et al., 2021).

5. Conclusion and Future Prospects

Skin bioprinting is showing promise as it moves from the bench to the bedside. Regenerative medicine has uncovered various potential clinical applications, such as tissue engineering and cell therapy (including the use of stem cell therapeutics as well as cell-based immunotherapy), with 3D bioprinting for the rejuvenation of skin and appendages. Given this, skin grafts are among the most crucial clinical requirements. The replication of a skin biological scaffold could be used as a substitute for conventional skin grafts to reduce the need for donors and improve the effectiveness of skin grafting treatment. Furthermore, burns, venous, diabetic, and pressure ulcers are among persistent and nonhealing wounds that can be treated with this technology (Jarrige M et al., 2021). Günther et al. created portable 3D bioprinting devices that improved the healing process in pigs with third-degree burns. The system improves the process of skin regeneration and reduces the appearance of scars, indicating potential for future use in medical settings (Hakimi N et al., 2018).

Furthermore, skin bioprinting can revolutionize cosmetic medical procedures. 3D skin bioprinting has the potential to replicate the cancer microenvironment. It can be employed to create cancer models by using cancer cells from patients, assisting in the personalization of anti-cancer drugs. This procedure can be a potent tool for investigating the roles of different biochemical pathways in the initiation and progression of carcinoma (Wu B-X et al., 2023). 3D skin bioprinting has another clinical application in precision medicine. Because of that, it can be utilized to provide patients with customized medication based on their genetic profile and overall health. Furthermore, one of the tissue engineering techniques that holds promise for astronauts on long-term space missions in the future is personalised skin bioprinting (Ghidini T, 2018). We must keep in mind that human skin bioprinting remains in its early stages of clinical development despite these excellent viewpoints. Automated procedures must be implemented to translate bioprinted skin into clinical settings effectively. Its quick clinical application is hampered by a number of ethical, financial, regulatory, and experimental issues.

Acknowledgments

This book chapter was written while executing an Indo-Austria project (DST/IC/Austria/P-14/2021 (G)). We extend our heartfelt appreciation to the Department of Science and Technology (DST) for funding the project. This project has provided a range of viewpoints and insights which were helpful in writing this book chapter.

References

Acher-Chenebaux, A., Maillard, H., Potier, A., Nzeyimana, H., Cazals, F. and Celerier, P. (2006, March). Nécrose cutanée par calciphylaxie traitée par greffe de kératinocytes autologues et parathyroïdectomie partielle. In Annales de dermatologie et de vénéréologie (Vol. 133, No. 3, pp. 260–263).

Akh L.A., Ishak M.O., Harris J.F., Glaros T.G., Sasiene Z.J. et al. Omics potential of in vitro skin models for radiation exposure. Cellular and Molecular Life Sciences. 2022; 79(7).

Albanna M., Binder K.W., Murphy S.V., Kim J., Qasem S.A. et al. In Situ Bioprinting of Autologous Skin Cells Accelerates Wound Healing of Extensive Excisional Full-Thickness Wounds. Scientific Reports. 2019; 9(1).

Antezana P.E., Municoy S., Álvarez-Echazú M.I., Santo-Orihuela P.L., Catalano P.N., et al. The 3D Bioprinted Scaffolds for Wound Healing. Pharmaceutics. 2022; 14(2).

Ashammakhi N., Ahadian S., Xu C., Montazerian H., Ko H. et al. Bioinks and bioprinting technologies to make heterogeneous and biomimetic tissue constructs. Materials Today Bio. 2019; 1.

Axpe E., Oyen M. Applications of Alginate-Based Bioinks in 3D Bioprinting. International Journal of Molecular Sciences. 2016; 17(12).

Bacakova M., Pajorova J., Broz A., Hadraba D., Lopot F. et al. A two-layer skin construct consisting of a collagen hydrogel reinforced by a fibrin-coated polylactide nanofibrous membrane. International Journal of Nanomedicine. 2019; Volume 14: 5033–50.

Badhe R.V., Nipate S.S. Cellulosic materials as bioinks for 3D printing applications. Advanced 3D-Printed Systems and Nanosystems for Drug Delivery and Tissue Engineering 2020. p. 109–37.

Bhushan S., Singh S., Maiti T.K., Sharma C., Dutt D. et al. Scaffold Fabrication Techniques of Biomaterials for Bone Tissue Engineering: A Critical Review. Bioengineering. 2022; 9(12).

Brown T.M., Krishnamurthy K. Histology, Dermis. StatPearls. Treasure Island (FL) ineligible companies. Disclosure: Karthik Krishnamurthy declares no relevant financial relationships with ineligible companies. 2024.

Cao H., Chen M-M., Liu Y., Liu Y-Y., Huang Y-Q. et al. Fish collagen-based scaffold containing PLGA microspheres for controlled growth factor delivery in skin tissue engineering. Colloids and Surfaces B: Biointerfaces. 2015; 136: 1098–106.

Carsin H., Ainaud P., Le Bever H., Rives J-M., Lakhel A. et al. Cultured epithelial autografts in extensive burn coverage of severely traumatized patients: a five year single-center experience with 30 patients. Burns. 2000; 26(4): 379–87.

Catros S., Fricain J-C, Guillotin B., Pippenger B., Bareille R. et al. Laser-assisted bioprinting for creating on-demand patterns of human osteoprogenitor cells and nano-hydroxyapatite. Biofabrication. 2011; 3(2).

Chandrasekaran A.R., Venugopal J., Sundarrajan S., Ramakrishna S. Fabrication of a nanofibrous scaffold with improved bioactivity for culture of human dermal fibroblasts for skin regeneration. Biomedical Materials. 2011; 6(1).

Chen K-Y., Liao W-J., Kuo S-M., Tsai F-J, Chen Y-S. et al. Asymmetric Chitosan Membrane Containing Collagen I Nanospheres for Skin Tissue Engineering. Biomacromolecules. 2009; 10(6): 1642–9.

Chen X.B., Fazel Anvari-Yazdi A., Duan X., Zimmerling A., Gharraei R. et al. Biomaterials / bioinks and extrusion bioprinting. Bioactive Materials. 2023; 28: 511–36.

Chong C., Wang Y., Fathi A., Parungao R., Maitz P.K. et al. Skin wound repair: Results of a pre-clinical study to evaluate electropsun collagen–elastin–PCL scaffolds as dermal substitutes. Burns. 2019; 45(7): 1639–48.

Cui B., Zhang C., Gan B., Liu W., Liang J. et al. Collagen-tussah silk fibroin hybrid scaffolds loaded with bone mesenchymal stem cells promote skin wound repair in rats. Materials Science and Engineering: C. 2020; 109.

D S, N.M., Pise A., Pise S., Vs L. et al. Ban of Cosmetic Testing on Animals: A Brief Overview. International Journal of Current Research and Review. 2020; 12(14): 113–116.

Díaz-García D., Filipová A., Garza-Veloz I., Martinez-Fierro M.L. A Beginner's Introduction to Skin Stem Cells and Wound Healing. International Journal of Molecular Sciences. 2021; 22(20).

Douillet C., Nicodeme M., Hermant L., Bergeron V., Guillemot F., Fricain J-C, et al. From local to global matrix organization by fibroblasts: a 4D laser-assisted bioprinting approach. Biofabrication. 2022; 14(2).

Driskell R.R., Jahoda CAB, Chuong C.M., Watt F.M., Horsley V. et al. Defining dermal adipose tissue. Experimental Dermatology. 2014; 23(9): 629–31.

Fayyazbakhsh F., Leu M.C. A Brief Review on 3D Bioprinted Skin Substitutes. Procedia Manufacturing. 2020; 48: 790–796.

Germain N., Dhayer M., Dekiouk S., Marchetti P. Current Advances in 3D Bioprinting for Cancer Modeling and Personalized Medicine. International Journal of Molecular Sciences. 2022; 23(7).

Ghidini T. Regenerative medicine and 3D bioprinting for human space exploration and planet colonisation. Journal of Thoracic Disease. 2018; 10(S20): S2363–S75.

Ghosh S. Tissue Engineered Skin Substitute Market Snapshot (2022 to 2029) [Available from: https://www.futuremarketinsights.com/reports/tissue-engineered-skin-substitute-market#:~:text=What%20will%20be%20demand%20outlook,9.6%25%20over%20the%20forecast%20period.

Gu B.K., Choi D.J., Park S.J., Kim Y-J, Kim C-H et al. 3D Bioprinting Technologies for Tissue Engineering Applications. Cutting-Edge Enabling Technologies for Regenerative Medicine. Advances in Experimental Medicine and Biology 2018. p. 15–28.

Gu Z., Fu J., Lin H., He Y. Development of 3D bioprinting: From printing methods to biomedical applications. Asian Journal of Pharmaceutical Sciences. 2020; 15(5): 529–57.

Gungor-Ozkerim P.S., Inci I., Zhang Y.S., Khademhosseini A., Dokmeci M.R. et al. Bioinks for 3D bioprinting: an overview. Biomaterials Science. 2018; 6(5): 915–46.

Hafezi F., Shorter S., Tabriz A.G., Hurt A., Elmes V. et al. Bioprinting and Preliminary Testing of Highly Reproducible Novel Bioink for Potential Skin Regeneration. Pharmaceutics. 2020; 12(6).

Hakimi N., Cheng R., Leng L., Sotoudehfar M., Ba P.Q. et al. Handheld skin printer: in situ formation of planar biomaterials and tissues. Lab on a Chip. 2018; 18(10): 1440–51.

Hart C.E., Loewen-Rodriguez A., Lessem J. Dermagraft: Use in the Treatment of Chronic Wounds. Advances in Wound Care. 2012; 1(3): 138–41.

Helgadottir H., Rocha Trocoli, Drakensjö I., Girnita A. Personalized Medicine in Malignant Melanoma: Towards Patient Tailored Treatment. Frontiers in Oncology. 2018; 8.

Hilmi A.B.M. Vital roles of stem cells and biomaterials in skin tissue engineering. World Journal of Stem Cells. 2015; 7(2).

Hofmann E., Schwarz A., Fink J., Kamolz L-P., Kotzbeck P. et al. Modelling the Complexity of Human Skin In Vitro. Biomedicines. 2023; 11(3).

Holmes J.H., Molnar J.A., Shupp J.W., Hickerson W.L., King B.T. et al. Demonstration of the safety and effectiveness of the RECELL® System combined with split-thickness meshed autografts for the reduction of donor skin to treat mixed-depth burn injuries. Burns. 2019; 45(4): 772–82.

Homaeigohar S., Boccaccini A.R. Antibacterial biohybrid nanofibers for wound dressings. Acta Biomaterialia. 2020; 107: 25–49.

Hospodiuk M., Moncal K.K., Dey M., Ozbolat I.T. Extrusion-Based Biofabrication in Tissue Engineering and Regenerative Medicine. 3D Printing and Biofabrication 2018. p. 255–81.

Ibrahim A.A.E., Bagherani N., Smoller B.R., Reyes-Baron C., Bagherani N. et al. Functions of the Skin. Atlas of Dermatology, Dermatopathology and Venereology 2021. p. 1–11.

Ishack S., Lipner S.R. A Review of 3-Dimensional Skin Bioprinting Techniques: Applications, Approaches, and Trends. Dermatologic Surgery. 2020; 46(12): 1500–1505.

Jamee R., Araf Y., Naser I.B., Promon S.K. The promising rise of bioprinting in revolutionalizing medical science: Advances and possibilities. Regenerative Therapy. 2021; 18: 133–45.

Jarrige M., Frank E., Herardot E., Martineau S., Darle A. et al. The Future of Regenerative Medicine: Cell Therapy Using Pluripotent Stem Cells and Acellular Therapies Based on Extracellular Vesicles. Cells. 2021; 10(2).

Javaid M., Haleem A. 3D bioprinting applications for the printing of skin: A brief study. Sensors International. 2021; 2.

Johnsen, Ermuth, Tanczos, Bannasch, Horch et al. Treatment of therapy-refractive ulcera cruris of various origins with autologous keratinocytes in fibrin sealant. Vasa. 2005; 34(1): 25–29.

Keirouz A., Fortunato G., Zhang M., Callanan A., Radacsi N. et al. Nozzle-free electrospinning of Polyvinylpyrrolidone/ Poly(glycerol sebacate) fibrous scaffolds for skin tissue engineering applications. Medical Engineering & Physics. 2019; 71: 56–67.

Kim B.S., Kim H., Gao G., Jang J., Cho D-W et al. Decellularized extracellular matrix: a step towards the next generation source for bioink manufacturing. Biofabrication. 2017; 9(3).

Kim B.S., Lee J-S, Gao G., Cho D-W. Direct 3D cell-printing of human skin with functional transwell system. Biofabrication. 2017; 9(2).

Kim G., Ahn S., Kim Y., Cho Y., Chun W. et al. Coaxial structured collagen–alginate scaffolds: fabrication, physical properties, and biomedical application for skin tissue regeneration. Journal of Materials Chemistry. 2011; 21(17).

Kim G., Ahn S., Yoon H., Kim Y., Chun W. et al. A cryogenic direct-plotting system for fabrication of 3D collagen scaffolds for tissue engineering. Journal of Materials Chemistry. 2009; 19(46).

Koch L., Deiwick A., Schlie S., Michael S, Gruene M. et al. Skin tissue generation by laser cell printing. Biotechnology and Bioengineering. 2012; 109(7): 1855–63.

Koch L., Kuhn S., Sorg H., Gruene M., Schlie S., et al. Laser Printing of Skin Cells and Human Stem Cells. Tissue Engineering Part C: Methods. 2010; 16(5): 847–54.

Kumar P., Ebbens S., Zhao X.. Inkjet printing of mammalian cells – Theory and applications. Bioprinting. 2021; 23.

Lee H-R, Park J.A., Kim S., Jo Y., Kang D. et al. 3D microextrusion-inkjet hybrid printing of structured human skin equivalents. Bioprinting. 2021; 22.

Lee J-S, Kim D-H, Choi D-K, Kim C.D., Ahn G-B et al. Comparison of Gene Expression Profiles between Keratinocytes, Melanocytes and Fibroblasts. Annals of Dermatology. 2013; 25(1).

Lee V., Singh G., Trasatti J.P., Bjornsson C., Xu X. et al. Design and Fabrication of Human Skin by Three-Dimensional Bioprinting. Tissue Engineering Part C: Methods. 2014; 20(6): 473–84.

Lee W., Debasitis J.C., Lee V.K., Lee J-H, Fischer K. et al. Multi-layered culture of human skin fibroblasts and keratinocytes through three-dimensional freeform fabrication. Biomaterials. 2009; 30(8): 1587–95.

Liu J., Zhou Z., Zhang M., Song F., Feng C. et al. Simple and robust 3D bioprinting of full-thickness human skin tissue. Bioengineered. 2022; 13(4): 10090–100.

Liu P., Shen H., Zhi Y., Si J., Shi J. et al. 3D bioprinting and in vitro study of bilayered membranous construct with human cells-laden alginate/gelatin composite hydrogels. Colloids and Surfaces B: Biointerfaces. 2019; 181: 1026–34.

Liu X., Michael S., Bharti K., Ferrer M., Song M.J. et al. A biofabricated vascularized skin model of atopic dermatitis for preclinical studies. Biofabrication. 2020; 12(3).

Loh Q.L., Choong C. Three-Dimensional Scaffolds for Tissue Engineering Applications: Role of Porosity and Pore Size. Tissue Engineering Part B: Reviews. 2013; 19(6): 485–502.

Malekpour A., Chen X. Printability and Cell Viability in Extrusion-Based Bioprinting from Experimental, Computational, and Machine Learning Views. Journal of Functional Biomaterials. 2022; 13(2).

Manita P.G., Garcia-Orue I., Santos-Vizcaino E., Hernandez R.M., Igartua M. et al. 3D Bioprinting of Functional Skin Substitutes: From Current Achievements to Future Goals. Pharmaceuticals. 2021; 14(4).

Millás A., Lago J., Vasquez-Pinto L., Massaguer P., Maria-Engler S.S. et al. Approaches to the development of 3d bioprinted skin models: the case of natura cosmetics. International Journal of Advances in Medical Biotechnology - IJAMB. 2019; 2(1).

Munaz A., Vadivelu R.K., St. John J., Barton M., Kamble H. et al. Three-dimensional printing of biological matters. Journal of Science: Advanced Materials and Devices. 2016; 1(1): 1–17.

Ng W.L., Lee J.M., Yeong W.Y., Win Naing M. Microvalve-based bioprinting – process, bio-inks and applications. Biomaterials Science. 2017; 5(4): 632–47.

Ng W.L., Yeong W.Y. The future of skin toxicology testing – Three-dimensional bioprinting meets microfluidics. International Journal of Bioprinting. 2019; 5(1).

Olejnik A., Semba J.A., Kulpa A., Dańczak-Pazdrowska A., Rybka J.D. et al. 3D Bioprinting in Skin Related Research: Recent Achievements and Application Perspectives. ACS Synthetic Biology. 2021; 11(1): 26–38.

Oualla-Bachiri W., Fernández-González A., Quiñones-Vico M.I., Arias-Santiago S. From Grafts to Human Bioengineered Vascularized Skin Substitutes. International Journal of Molecular Sciences. 2020; 21(21).

Pasierb A., Jezierska M., Karpuk A., Czuwara J., Rudnicka L. et al. 3D skin bioprinting: future potential for skin regeneration. Advances in Dermatology and Allergology. 2022; 39(5): 845–51.

Pereira R.F., Sousa A., Barrias C.C., Bayat A., Granja P.L. et al. Advances in bioprinted cell-laden hydrogels for skin tissue engineering. Biomanufacturing Reviews. 2017; 2(1).

Pfisterer K., Shaw L.E., Symmank D., Weninger W. The Extracellular Matrix in Skin Inflammation and Infection. Frontiers in Cell and Developmental Biology. 2021; 9.

Potere F., Belgio B., Croci G.A., Tabano S., Petrini P. et al. 3D bioprinting of multi-layered segments of a vessel-like structure with ECM and novel derived bioink. Frontiers in Bioengineering and Biotechnology. 2022; 10.

Pradhan R.A., Rahman S.S., Qureshi A., Ullah A. Biopolymers. Biopolymers and their Industrial Applications2021. p. 281–303.

Prescott S.L., Larcombe D-L., Logan A.C., West C., Burks W. et al. The skin microbiome: impact of modern environments on skin ecology, barrier integrity, and systemic immune programming. World Allergy Organization Journal. 2017; 10.

Przekora A. A Concise Review on Tissue Engineered Artificial Skin Grafts for Chronic Wound Treatment: Can We Reconstruct Functional Skin Tissue In Vitro? Cells. 2020; 9(7).

Puertas-Bartolomé M., Mora-Boza A., García-Fernández L. Emerging Biofabrication Techniques: A Review on Natural Polymers for Biomedical Applications. Polymers. 2021; 13(8).

Pugliese R., Beltrami B., Regondi S., Lunetta C. Polymeric biomaterials for 3D printing in medicine: An overview. Annals of 3D Printed Medicine. 2021; 2.

Rastin H., Ramezanpour M., Hassan K., Mazinani A., Tung T.T. et al. 3D bioprinting of a cell-laden antibacterial polysaccharide hydrogel composite. Carbohydrate Polymers. 2021; 264.

Reijnders C.M.A., van Lier A., Roffel S., Kramer D., Scheper R.J., Gibbs S. et al. Development of a Full-Thickness Human Skin Equivalent In Vitro Model Derived from TERT-Immortalized Keratinocytes and Fibroblasts. Tissue Engineering Part A. 2015; 21(17–18): 2448–59.

Richardson M. Understanding the structure and function of the skin. Nurs Times. 2003; 99(31): 46–48.

Rimann M., Bono E., Annaheim H., Bleisch M., Graf-Hausner U. et al. Standardized 3D Bioprinting of Soft Tissue Models with Human Primary Cells. SLAS Technology. 2016; 21(4): 496–509.

Rousselle P., Gentilhomme E., Neveux Y. Epidermal Physiology. Agache's Measuring the Skin 2015. p. 1–9.

Sarkiri M., Fox S., Fratila-Apachitei L., Zadpoor A. Bioengineered Skin Intended for Skin Disease Modeling. International Journal of Molecular Sciences. 2019; 20(6).

Schiele N.R., Corr D.T., Huang Y., Raof N.A., Xie Y. et al. Laser-based direct-write techniques for cell printing. Biofabrication. 2010; 2(3).

Schmidt T., Xiang Y., Bao X., Sun T. A Paradigm Shift in Tissue Engineering: From a Top–Down to a Bottom–Up Strategy. Processes. 2021; 9(6).

Shi L., Hu Y., Ullah M.W., ullah I., Ou H. et al. Cryogenic free-form extrusion bioprinting of decellularized small intestinal submucosa for potential applications in skin tissue engineering. Biofabrication. 2019; 11(3).

Si, Xing, Ding, Zhang, Yin, Zhang. 3D Bioprinting of the Sustained Drug Release Wound Dressing with Double-Crosslinked Hyaluronic-Acid-Based Hydrogels. Polymers. 2019; 11(10).

Silva R.J., Tamburic S. A State-of-the-Art Review on the Alternatives to Animal Testing for the Safety Assessment of Cosmetics. Cosmetics. 2022; 9(5).

Slominski A.T., Michael S., Sorg H., Peck C-T., Koch L. et al. Tissue Engineered Skin Substitutes Created by Laser-Assisted Bioprinting Form Skin-Like Structures in the Dorsal Skin Fold Chamber in Mice. PLoS ONE. 2013; 8(3).

Smandri A., Nordin A., Hwei N.M., Chin K-Y, Abd Aziz I. et al. Natural 3D-Printed Bioinks for Skin Regeneration and Wound Healing: A Systematic Review. Polymers. 2020; 12(8).

Still J., Glat P., Silverstein P., Griswold J., Mozingo D. et al. The use of a collagen sponge/living cell composite material to treat donor sites in burn patients. Burns. 2003; 29(8): 837–41.

Tausche A.K., Skaria M., Böhlen L., Liebold K., Hafner J. et al. An autologous epidermal equivalent tissue-engineered from follicular outer root sheath keratinocytes is as effective as split-thickness skin autograft in recalcitrant vascular leg ulcers. Wound Repair and Regeneration. 2003;11(4): 248–52.

Tavakoli S., Klar A.S. Bioengineered Skin Substitutes: Advances and Future Trends. Applied Sciences. 2021; 11(4).

Teoh J.H., Thamizhchelvan A.M., Davoodi P., Ramasamy S., Vijayavenkataraman S. et al. Investigation of the application of a Taylor-Couette bioreactor in the post-processing of bioprinted human dermal tissue. Biochemical Engineering Journal. 2019; 151.

Tottoli E.M., Dorati R., Genta I., Chiesa E., Pisani S. et al. Skin Wound Healing Process and New Emerging Technologies for Skin Wound Care and Regeneration. Pharmaceutics. 2020; 12(8).

Tripathi S., Mandal S.S., Bauri S., Maiti P. 3D bioprinting and its innovative approach for biomedical applications. MedComm. 2022; 4(1).

Uccioli L. A Clinical Investigation on the Characteristics and Outcomes of Treating Chronic Lower Extremity Wounds using the TissueTech Autograft System. The International Journal of Lower Extremity Wounds. 2016; 2(3): 140–51.

Urciuolo F., Casale C., Imparato G., Netti P.A. Bioengineered Skin Substitutes: The Role of Extracellular Matrix and Vascularization in the Healing of Deep Wounds. Journal of Clinical Medicine. 2019; 8(12).

Vacher D. [Autologous epidermal sheets production for skin cellular therapy]. Ann Pharm Fr. 2003; 61(3): 203–6.

Valot L., Martinez J., Mehdi A., Subra G. Chemical insights into bioinks for 3D printing. Chemical Society Reviews. 2019; 48(15): 4049–86.

van Dorp A.G.M., Verhoeven M.C.H., Koerten H.K., van Blitterswijk C.A., Ponec M. et al. Bilayered biodegradable poly(ethylene glycol)/poly(butylene terephthalate) copolymer (Polyactive?) as substrate for human fibroblasts and keratinocytes. Journal of Biomedical Materials Research. 1999; 47(3): 292–300.

Van Norman G.A. Limitations of Animal Studies for Predicting Toxicity in Clinical Trials. JACC: Basic to Translational Science. 2019; 4(7): 845–54.

Varkey M., Visscher D.O., van Zuijlen P.P.M, Atala A., Yoo J.J. et al. Skin bioprinting: the future of burn wound reconstruction? Burns and Trauma. 2019; 7.

Vecin N.M., Kirsner R.S. Skin substitutes as treatment for chronic wounds: current and future directions. Frontiers in Medicine. 2023; 10.

Velasquillo C., Galue E.A., Rodriquez L., Ibarra C., Ibarra-Ibarra L.G. et al. Skin 3D Bioprinting. Applications in Cosmetology. Journal of Cosmetics, Dermatological Sciences and Applications. 2013; 03(01): 85–89.

Ventura R.D. An Overview of Laser-assisted Bioprinting (LAB) in Tissue Engineering Applications. Medical Lasers. 2021; 10(2): 76–81.

Watt F.M., Fujiwara H. Cell-Extracellular Matrix Interactions in Normal and Diseased Skin. Cold Spring Harbor Perspectives in Biology. 2011; 3(4): a005124-a.

Wei C., Feng Y., Che D., Zhang J., Zhou X. et al. Biomaterials in skin tissue engineering. International Journal of Polymeric Materials and Polymeric Biomaterials. 2021; 71(13): 993–1011.

Weng T., Zhang W., Xia Y., Wu P., Yang M. et al. 3D bioprinting for skin tissue engineering: Current status and perspectives. Journal of Tissue Engineering. 2021; 12.

Wu B-X., Wu Z., Hou Y-Y., Fang Z-X., Deng Y. et al. Application of three-dimensional (3D) bioprinting in anti-cancer therapy. Heliyon. 2023; 9(10).

Yanez M., Rincon J., Dones A., De Maria C., Gonzales R. et al. In Vivo Assessment of Printed Microvasculature in a Bilayer Skin Graft to Treat Full-Thickness Wounds. Tissue Engineering Part A. 2015; 21(1–2): 224–33.

Zaulyanov L., Kirsner R.S. A review of a bi-layered living cell treatment (Apligraf) in the treatment of venous leg ulcers and diabetic foot ulcers. Clinical Interventions in Aging. 2007; 2(1): 93–98.

Zhang J., Yun S., Karami A., Jing B., Zannettino A. et al. 3D printing of a thermosensitive hydrogel for skin tissue engineering: A proof of concept study. Bioprinting. 2020; 19.

Zhang M., Zhang C., Li Z., Fu X., Huang S et al. Advances in 3D skin bioprinting for wound healing and disease modelling. Regenerative Biomaterials. 2023; 10.

Zhang Y., Kumar P., Lv S., Xiong D., Zhao H. et al. Recent advances in 3D bioprinting of vascularized tissues. Materials & Design. 2021; 199.

Zhou D., Chen J., Liu B., Zhang X., Li X. et al. Bioinks for jet-based bioprinting. Bioprinting. 2019; 16.

Building Better Faces: The 3D Bioprinting Breakthrough in Maxillofacial Surgery

Namratha B,[1] *Dheeraj D*[2] and *Santosh LG*[2]*

1. Introduction

The craniofacial tissues possess a sophisticated three-dimensional structure composed of fourteen facial bones and eight cranial bones. These structures support and shape the soft tissues of the face (Zhang and Yelick, 2018). The bones undergo either intramembranous or endochondral ossification processes, leading to the creation of a composite structure comprising both inorganic and organic elements. Developed bone displays an osteonal structure, characterized by haversian systems containing concentric lamellae that enclose osteocytic lacunae (Kim et al., 2015). Conversely, the cartilaginous component is constructed by chondroblasts and encompasses chondrocytes. Recreating the intricate three-dimensional structure and cellular interactions of craniofacial tissues poses a noteworthy challenge, particularly in the context of functionally reconstructing defects. Lack of availability of autogenous grafts limits their application and paves the way for new discoveries. The emerging field of biofabrication offers a hopeful alternative by leveraging living cells and extracellular matrices to fabricate tissues and organs using bioprinting technology (Mir et al., 2018). This innovative approach holds great potential in surmounting the limitations associated with autogenous grafts in the realm of craniofacial reconstruction.

Bioprinting, a state-of-the-art technology, entails the step-by-step deposition of living cells and biomaterials under the guidance of computer-aided design. While it boasts significant promise in regenerative medicine, the practical application of bioprinting in clinical settings remains largely limited to research. This is mainly because current bioprinting capabilities are primarily capable of producing simple and uniform tissues (Dey and Ozbolat, 2020). Nonetheless, on-going advancements

[1] Department of Chemistry, The Yenepoya Institute of Arts, Science, Commerce and Management, Yenepoya (Deemed to be University), Mangaluru, India.
[2] Department of Oral surgery, Century Dental College, Poinachi, India.
[3] Department of Chemistry, Manipal Institute of Technology, Manipal Academy of Higher Education, Manipal, India
* Corresponding author: sl.gaonkar@manipal.edu

indicate the possibility of its future capacity to fabricate more intricate and diverse tissues, which would considerably expand its clinical applications. Craniofacial anomalies, whether congenital or acquired, can exert profound negative psychological consequences on affected individuals. These abnormalities impact the craniofacial complex's soft and hard tissues to varying extents. The optimal management of such patients necessitates a multidisciplinary approach involving a team of experts. This interdisciplinary team typically comprises cranio-maxillofacial surgeons, plastic and reconstructive surgeons, otorhinolaryngologists, neurosurgeons, pediatricians, orthodontists, psychologists, as well as speech and language therapists. A collaborative effort among these professionals is indispensable in order to address both functional and aesthetic concerns, thereby delivering comprehensive care for patients afflicted with craniofacial deformities (Mahon et al., 2015).

The advancement in the field of manufacturing technology is due to the significant efforts shown by research scientists and engineers. During the 1970s, the CAD/CAM system was introduced, primarily utilized in the automotive and aerospace sectors, and subsequently embraced in dentistry for numerous tooth restorations (Suganna et al., 2022). This particular system allows for the creation of digital designs through software, followed by the manufacturing of prototypes with computer assistance. In the initial stages, prototypes were fashioned by carving ingots or blocks using the CAM system. However, progress in the field led to the emergence of 3D bioprinting involved in customized biomedical treatment. Additive manufacturing (AM) technology deposits bioink layer by layer to fabricate prototypes or scaffolds, thereby facilitating precise control and replication of the intricate architecture found in human tissue. Recent advancements have made it possible to deposit multicomponent bioinks with great accuracy, thereby augmenting the potential for tissue engineering applications (Rijal, 2023).

3D bioprinting stands as a notable leap forward in comparison to conventional 3D printers because of its ability to accurately place cells in specific arrangements and fabricate tissues originating from various sources that closely mimic native tissues (Swarnima et al., 2020). Despite demonstrating successful insertion of 3D bioprinted tissues in different *in vivo* scenarios, approval for human transplantation trials is still pending. The transition of 3D bioprinting from laboratory research to practical clinical application is followed by the evolution in the fields of cytology, transplantation technology and biomaterials. Nevertheless, the complete integration of 3D bioprinting into clinical practice is currently pending further advancements and regulatory approvals (Tripathi et al., 2020). 3D bioprinting caters to several applications. It allows for the precise modulation of both the internal and external 3D structure of scaffold systems, which facilitates the creation of intricate tissue formations. The process itself is relatively straightforward, providing a level of ease in the fabrication process. Additionally, it grants the ability to produce scaffolds that are tailored to the individual needs of patients, with a high level of precision. Moreover, this technique allows for the printing of multiple materials, thereby increasing the versatility of scaffold fabrication. 3D bioprinting holds well defined control over behaviour of the cells and the mechanical properties of the construct by predefining the scaffold's architecture. This can lead to various applications in regenerative medicine (Kačarević et al., 2018).

The exact transfer of biofabricated tissue scaffolds to the operating room for implantation presents notable healing and logistical benefits in craniofacial regeneration (Murphy and Atala, 2014). Furthermore, the development of bioinks with properties such as viscoelasticity and nonlinear performance, akin to innate cartilage in structures like the temporo-mandibular joint disc, the auricular cartilage, or nasal cartilage, holds potential for fabricating such tissues through bioprinting (Hyun-Wook et al., 2016).

2.   3D Bioprinting Tools

While the terms 3D printing, additive manufacturing, and rapid prototyping are frequently utilized interchangeably, they diverge from 3D bioprinting in terms of the substances employed and the printing abilities. In the realm of 3D printing, inert or bioactive frameworks are generated devoid of living cells, which are designated as acellular frameworks. Conversely, 3D bioprinting encompasses the utilization of cell-laden biomaterial that enables the printing of both cells and frameworks without the need for scaffolds. This pivotal differentiation underlines the potential of 3D bioprinting to fabricate intricate tissue structures featuring living cellular components, thus distinguishing it from conventional 3D printing techniques. The process of 3D bioprinting entails the utilization of bioink, which denotes a solution or amalgamation of biomaterial, generally hydrogel, enclosing desired cell types in order to fabricate tissue constructs. In order to achieve precise physical configuration and architecture, bioink is either stabilized or crosslinked during the bioprinting process or immediately after printing. The perfect bioink ought to exhibit suitable chemical, biological, mechanical, and rheological characteristics to guarantee operative and structural precision in bioprinted organs (Dwivedi et al., 2020). These biomaterials, which can be of natural, artificial, or hybrid origin, propose possible alternatives to typical autologous or allogeneic grafts for attaining therapeutically effective bone regeneration.

Embryonic, mesenchymal, and induced pluripotent stem cells are the chief sources of stem cells consumed in bioinks of tissue engineering applications (Gao et al., 2016). Embryonic stem cells offer the highest level of multipotency, their acquisition posing challenges, along with moral concerns and potential immunogenicity issues. The effectiveness of mesenchymal stem cells (MSC) is relatively less than that of embryonic stem cells (ESCs), despite their ease of access and ability to promote immunotolerance in specific tissues. Induced pluripotent stem cells (iPSC) exhibit an amplified degree of multipotency, but apprehensions exist about their potential involvement in tumorigenesis (Dwivedi and Mehrotra, 2020). Another technique employed in tissue engineering is the use of cell aggregates devoid of scaffolds, such as cellular spheroids. Such aggregates are organized into tubular or ring-like structures without the requirement of a scaffold, thereby reducing the chances of toxicity or immunogenicity (Miura et al., 2009). The incorporation of cells within a biocompatible hydrogel facilitates cell survival and provides mechanical support. Nevertheless, challenges arise in terms of the time needed for spheroids to form larger tissue structures and the potential lack of uniformity. Advancements in this area encompass the development of multicellular cylinders, which offer greater control over shape. While the majority of research is conducted in vitro, further investigations are essential to evaluate the safety and integrity of scaffold-free constructs *in vivo* (Safhi, 2022).

3. Techniques in 3D Bioprinting

Contemporarily, there has been a significant increase in the accessibility of bioprinting methodologies. Among these methodologies, the most prevalent and established modalities of 3D bioprinting encompass laser-assisted, inkjet bioprinting, and extrusion-based bioprinting. Furthermore, other techniques such as multi-head deposition systems, 4D bioprinting technology, and custom-made bioprinting systems are in existence. These methodologies entail the utilization of a computer-aided design/computer-aided manufacturing (CAD/CAM) system for the determination of designing the 3D structure (Khalil and Sun, 2009; Wu et al., 2016).

3.1 Laser Bioprinting Technology

Laser Induced Forward Transfer (LIFT) serves as the fundamental source of laser bioprinting technology, playing an essential and influential role within the arena of tissue engineering. This method employs a pulsed laser source that is directed towards a transparent support. Upon stimulation, the support generates droplets of bioink which are subsequently collected on a substrate for cross-linking purposes (Figure 1). Unlike inkjet bioprinters, laser-assisted bioprinters do not possess nozzles, thereby reducing the risk of material or cell blockage. Moreover, this allows for the creation of high-resolution outcomes that are attuned with various viscosity materials, while maintaining the viability of cells. Selective Laser Sintering (SLS), Stereolithography (SLA), and Laser Induced Forward Transfer represent popular variants of laser-assisted 3D bioprinting (Tan et al., 2005).

Selective Laser Sintering utilizes high-powered lasers to merge powder materials in a step-by-step manner. This method presents noteworthy adaptability in the creation of scaffolds for intricate tissue regeneration. Despite its high efficiency in fabricating intricate 3D constructs, Selective Laser Sintering does face certain challenges, including complexities in laser control and potential side effects arising from exposure to the laser. Nevertheless, when compared to other bioprinting technologies, Selective Laser Sintering remains unparalleled in terms of efficiency, flexibility, and the complexity of 3D construct fabrication. The progress in this particular domain is impeded due to the complex regulation of laser systems and the potential adverse consequences linked to laser exposure (Roskies et al., 2016).

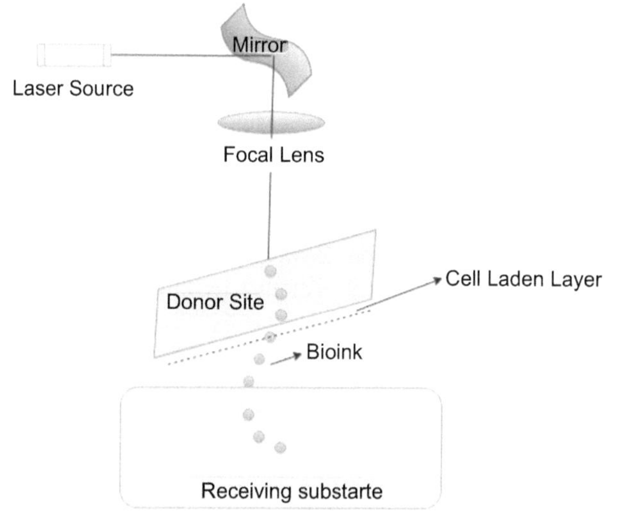

Fig. 1   Schematic representation of laser bioprinting.

3.2   *Inkjet Bioprinting*

Inkjet (droplet) bioprinting is characterized by a sequential process of droplet ejection in the downstream direction, which is initiated by a pressure alteration caused by a minor modification in volume introduced in the upstream region of the nozzle. This ejection is made possible by either piezoelectrically induced inkjet head systems or thermally induced systems. Piezoelectric heads induce changes in the volume of a biomaterial by applying voltage pulses, whereas thermal-induced heads employ the vaporization of a fluid to create bubbles which subsequently expand and propel droplets through the nozzle (Rémi et al., 2005). This particular technology demonstrates versatility by accommodating various biomaterials such as polymers, ceramics, proteins, and cells, with a viscosity range limited to 5–20 Pa in order to prevent continuous flow or high ejection pressures (Figure 2). This method possesses an advantage over its counterparts due to its cost-effectiveness, rapid printing speed, and ability to encapsulate cells within biomaterials (Shirazi et al., 2015).

3.3   *Extrusion-based Bioprinting*

Frequently recognized as one of the primary techniques for bioprinting, fused deposition modelling (FDM) printers/extrusion-based printers exhibit a wide range of capabilities. These printers operate by melting a continuous thermoplastic polymer filament at the nozzle, which then extrudes onto previously deposited layers in a partially solidified state. Once the material solidifies at room

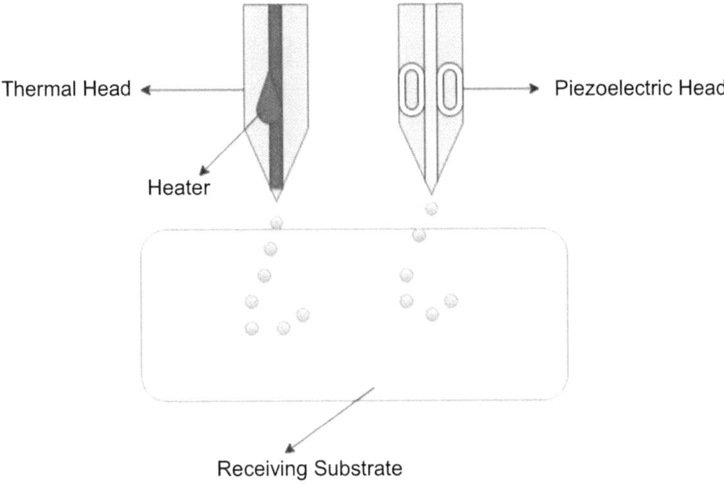

Fig. 2 Diagrammatic representation of inkjet Bioprinting.

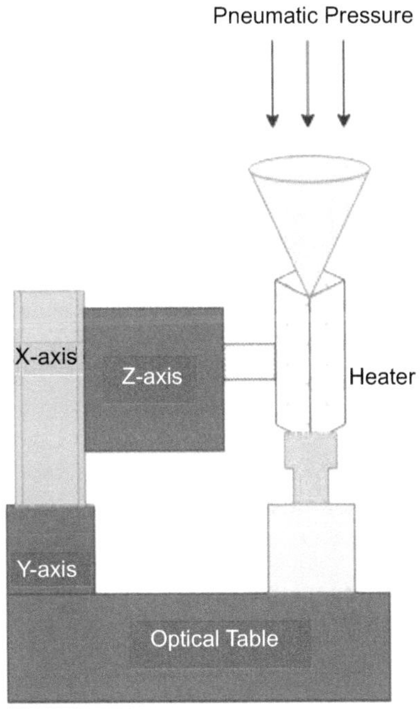

Fig. 3 A diagrammatic depiction of bioprinting based on the extrusion technique.

temperature, it merges together to form a constant structure (Figure 3). The value of the tissue construct produced by these printers relies heavily on the bioprinting speed, the alignment of the construct, and the thickness of each layer (Xin et al., 2017). Judging against other bioprinters, extrusion-based 3D bioprinters excel in speedily fabricating significant designs and have the capability to dispense various materials that possess osteo-inductive properties. Furthermore, these printers possess the ability to simultaneously print multiple materials by utilizing multi-nozzle systems, resulting in a more cost-effective approach. However, it is important to note that the biomaterials used in Fused deposition modelling printing must have low melting points (Li et al., 2017).

3.4 Multi-head Deposition Systems (MHDS)

The Multi-head deposition system (MHDS), a 3D plotting technique, bears a strong resemblance to Fused Deposition Modelling. The arrangement of various cartridges on an XYZ stage enables the precise control of location, pressure, and temperature for each cartridge within this system. Viscous material is extruded from the nozzles onto a platform under either pneumatic or mechanical pressure. Like Fused deposition modelling, the Multi-head deposition system enables the printing of heterogeneous configurations using multiple materials. To facilitate bioprinting and material curing, reactive components are extruded through mixing nozzles and then exposed to either UV light or heat, resulting in the desired heterogeneous construct (Figure 4). The utilization of a diverse range of substances, including hydrogels, plastics, pastes, and solutions, is a notable advantage of the Multi-head deposition system due to its inherent flexibility. These materials are all biocompatible and allow for cell encapsulation prior to bioprinting. However, it is worth noting that this method tends to have lower resolution and speed when compared to Fused deposition modelling (Wenz et al., 2017).

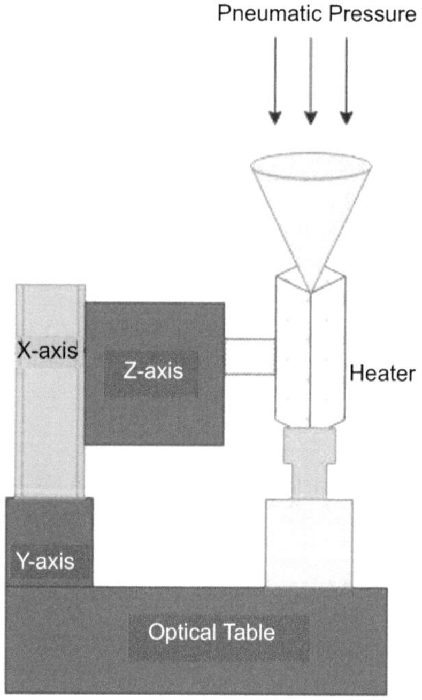

Fig. 4 Schematic representation of multi-head deposition systems

4. 4D Bioprinting

The emergence of a novel technological advancement, known as "four-dimensional (4D) bioprinting," is currently underway. This ground-breaking technology allows for the alteration of both form and function of bioprinted constructs after the printing process, in response to external stimuli. This unique capability opens up new possibilities for performance-driven applications, which rely on the utilization of innovative biomaterials that cooperate with environmental aspects, such as humidity, temperature, or chemicals. Consequently, these interactions induce modifications in the form and function of the constructs subsequent to their fabrication (Scheithauer et al., 2017). Presently, the application of 4D bioprinting in scaffold fabrication predominantly revolves around the use of polymers, with only limited efforts made in exploring ceramic-based functionally graded materials. The availability of scaffolds required for the tissue engineering of bones is somewhat restricted.

Nevertheless, the outlook for 4D bioprinting seems optimistic, given its considerable capacity to create implantable scaffolds that can be programmatically designed to foster bone regeneration (Li et al., 2016).

5.   3D Bioprinting Process

The fundamental procedure underlying the phenomenon of 3D bioprinting can be categorized as prebioprinting, bioprinting, and postbioprinting stages (Ashkan and Anthony, 2016).

5.1   Prebioprinting

The initiation of the prebioprinting process necessitates the development of an intricate computer-aided design (CAD) representation that accurately represents the desired structure of the tissue. This particular stage is of utmost importance as it serves as a critical guide for the subsequent bioprinting process. Moreover, the selection of suitable biomaterials ensures compatibility with both the target tissue and the employed bioprinting technique (Phillippi et al., 2018).

Computed tomography (CT) and magnetic resonance imaging (MRI) are widely recognized imaging methods that play a crucial role in detailed visualizations of the tissue in the Digital Imaging and Communications in Medicine (DICOM) format. These imaging datasets are subsequently converted into the Standard Triangle Language (STL) format, which can be interpreted by the bioprinter, thus facilitating the accurate reproduction of the tissue design. However, prior to the initiation of the actual bioprinting process, there are essential preparatory steps that need to be carried out. These steps involve the isolation and proliferation of the desired cells, which are the fundamental components for the construction of the tissue. The separated cells are subsequently combined with a culture medium that is enriched with vital growth factors such as Transforming Growth Factor Beta (TGFb), Fibroblast Growth Factor (FGF), Platelet-derived Growth Factor (PDGF), Bone Morphogenetic Proteins (BMP), Vascular Endothelial Growth Factor (VEGF), and Insulin-like Growth Factor (IGF). This culture medium enhances the viability and functionality of cells by providing nourishment and supporting their functionality (Mironov et al., 2003).

Alongside the growth factors, the growth medium may also contain other substances such as antioxidants, ascorbic acid, rosiglitazone, and dexamethasone, which further contribute to the maintenance and enhancement of cell viability. These components play crucial roles in cellular function, stress reduction, and overall tissue health. Alternatively, cell aggregates without scaffolds can be employed, where the cells are enclosed within cellular spheroids with an approximate diameter of 500 μm. This approach presents a method devoid of scaffolds for organizing and structuring the cells, thereby enhancing their cohesion and functionality within the printed tissue construct (Phillippi et al., 2018).

5.2   Bioprinting

The procedure for bioprinting entails the placement of a bioink, typically composed of cells, extracellular matrix components, and nutrients, into a printer cartridge. This bioink is subsequently utilized by the bioprinter to construct tissue structures in accordance with a layer-by-layer methodology. Each layer is precisely deposited based on the CAD model, progressively constructing the sought-after tissue architecture. After the completion of bioprinting, the pre-tissue is moved to an incubator to undergo maturation. This period of incubation allows the cells to further develop and interact with their surrounding environment, thereby facilitating tissue maturation and functional integration. Cells are distributed throughout or within a biocompatible framework through a methodical layer-by-layer procedure. This technique enables the production of three-dimensional biological constructs resembling natural tissues in terms of their intricate structural integrity and functionality (Harmon, 2013; Thomas, 2016).

5.3 Postbioprinting

To guarantee the stability and mechanical soundness of a three-dimensional structure produced through the process of bioprinting, it is imperative to implement appropriate post-bioprinting procedures. The regulation of tissue remodeling and growth involves the transmission of signals to cells through both mechanical and chemical stimuli. These signals play a crucial role in maintaining the structure of the tissue. In recent times, the field of tissue engineering has witnessed notable progress with the introduction of bioreactors. These bioreactors have become essential in enhancing the survival, maturation, and vascularization of transplanted tissues. Bioreactors are furnished with various modules that are specifically designed to create the most favourable conditions for tissue development. These modules include convective nutrient transport, the establishment of microgravity environments, alterations in pressure to facilitate the flow of solutions through cells, and the application of compression to induce vibrant or stationary loading. Compression bioreactors offer considerable benefits for tissues like cartilage. These bioreactors subject the tissue to controlled compression, thereby emulating physiological conditions and fostering the growth of functional cartilaginous tissue (Singh and Thomas, 2018).

6.   Biomaterials Utilized for Craniofacial Reconstruction

The utilization of 3D bioprinters involves the creation of bony and cartilaginous scaffolds that are meticulously customized to correspond to specific defects with a remarkable level of precision. The significance of bone transplantation is emphasized by the prevalence of bone loss resulting from a variety of factors, such as trauma, osteoporosis, and tumours. As a result, bone ranks are among the most commonly transplanted tissues, alongside cartilage. Yet, for these transplants to be successful, the biomaterials used must meet various criteria. Specifically, they must be biocompatible, thereby not inciting an adverse immune response. Additionally, they must possess the ability to be printed, thereby enabling the accurate fabrication of intricate structures. Furthermore, the biomaterials must be osteo-conductive, thus promoting bone growth, as well as osteo-inductive, thereby stimulating bone formation. Ultimately, they have the ability to offer substantial reinforcement and steadfastness due to their mechanical attributes that imitate those of the natural bone (Seyednejad et al., 2012).

Multiple classifications of biomaterials are required for the advancement of bone and cartilage tissue engineering. These encompass bioceramics, which offer exceptional biocompatibility and osteoconductivity, as well as polymers renowned for their versatility and adjustable properties. Furthermore, composites, which amalgamate the advantages of multiple materials, are also employed. Hydrogels are additionally prevalent due to their capacity to effectively replicate the extracellular matrix and facilitate cell growth (Tao et al., 2019).

6.1 Bioceramics

Bioceramics composed of mineral phases consisting of calcium and phosphate, such as hydroxyapatite (HA), β-tricalcium phosphate (TCP), and bioactive glasses (BGs), are frequently selected biomaterials for applications in tissue engineering. These bio-ceramics have demonstrated their ability to stimulate bone formation by creating a microenvironment rich in bioactive ions and facilitating cell growth through close cell-cell interactions. However, the use of bioceramic scaffolds poses challenges, especially in load-bearing regions of the craniofacial area, such as maxilla-mandibular defects. Research findings indicate that HA/αTCP composite scaffolds are not suitable for these applications due to their insufficient strength and dimensional stability. Scientists have proposed various methods to enhance the biological functionality and mechanical strength of bioceramics. For instance, the substitution of magnesium ions into wollastonite has significantly improved the flexural strength in comparison to βTCP and other calcium-silicate bioceramics (Kargozar et al., 2018).

Moreover, the inclusion of metallic ions such as cupric ions and cobaltous ions into bioactive glasses has been demonstrated to stimulate angiogenic activity *in vivo*, thereby facilitating expeditious wound healing. The efficacy of tissue-engineered constructs can be enhanced by incorporating bioceramics into composite materials, which enriches their bone-inducing properties. These advancements underscore the continuous efforts being made to optimize bioceramic-based scaffolds for bone tissue engineering applications (Lobo et al., 2015).

6.2 Polymers

Polymers are highly favoured materials for the bioprinting of craniofacial tissues due to their exceptional printability and capacity to efficiently promote osteogenesis. However, traditional polymers such as Polyglycolic acid (PGA) and Polylactic acid (PLA) are less frequently employed for bone scaffolds due to their inadequate compressive strength and osteoconductivity. In contrast, the copolymer Poly lactic-co-glycolic acid (PLGA) has exhibited breakneck osteoconductivity and improved mechanical properties. Another polymer, known as Polycaprolactone (PCL), is highly regarded for its utility in bone tissue engineering applications due to its ready availability, cost-effectiveness, and modifiability to cater to specific requirements. Polycaprolactone's capability to endure physical, chemical, and mechanical strains without substantial property deterioration, along with its slow degradation rate, enables the creation of denser tissues (Liu et al., 2018). Furthermore, the low melting point of Polycaprolactone renders it appropriate for extrusion-based bioprinting techniques such as Fused deposition modelling (FDM).

More recent bioprinters utilizing Selective Laser Sintering (SLS) offer improved precision, enabling control over scaffold porosity for optimal cell growth and proliferation. Polycaprolactone scaffolds produced through Selective Laser Sintering demonstrate higher stiffness in comparison to traditional 3D polymers, although it remains below the stiffness level of human trabecular bone. Nevertheless, a key drawback of Polycaprolactone is its comparative lack of bioactivity. To overcome this limitation, the proposal suggests the use of composite scaffolds that integrate bio-inert polycaprolactone frameworks with growth factors and biologically active constituents such as β-tricalcium phosphate (βTCP), hydroxyapatite (HA), and de-cellularized trabecular bone. This approach enhances the bioactivity and biological functionality of Polycaprolactone scaffolds, thereby rendering them more suitable for tissue regeneration applications. Polyaryletherketones (PEAKs), which are high-performance polymers, serve as favorable substitutes for craniofacial tissues owing to their mechanical properties that closely resemble those of natural bone (Ben et al., 2016).

6.3 Hydrogels

Hydrogels are renowned for their capacity to produce extracellular matrices, rendering them highly valuable in the field of tissue engineering. Hydrogels encapsulating chondrocytes or mesenchymal stem cells (MSCs) involve the utilization of micro-extrusion techniques. These hydrogel formulations that contain cells encompass a diverse range of materials, including alginate, collagen, and other natural polymers, as well as synthetic alternatives like Gel MA and polyethylene glycol dimethacrylate (PEGDMA). Nevertheless, a primary challenge in the use of hydrogels lies in determining the appropriate concentration of polymers. Higher concentrations of polymers are desirable in order to enhance mechanical properties and construct viscosity, while lower concentrations are more effective for promoting cell proliferation and chondrogenic differentiation. Documentation exists regarding the creation of hydrogel scaffolds with soft characteristics, incorporating both robust polymers and stem cells through a tissue-organ bioprinter. The selection of material for bone bioprinting is bioink composed of gelatin, hyaluronic acid, and Tricalcium phosphate (TCP) (Lee et al., 2014; Mantha et al., 2019).

7.   Conclusion and Forward Trajectory

By incorporating composite biomaterials with stem cells in the bioink, the generation of various tissues and organs in the craniofacial region can be achieved through the application of 3D bioprinting. This advanced technology holds great potential in meeting the increasing demand for effective tissue regeneration therapies, providing tailored solutions for patients with diverse requirements. It is highly likely that 3D printing technology will become an indispensable tool for plastic, maxillofacial, and reconstructive surgeons in the near future, potentially enhancing the outcomes of facial reconstruction surgeries as well as patient gratification and overall value of life. While there have been numerous studies reporting successful outcomes of 3D bioprinting, the future applications of tissue engineering for craniofacial bones and cartilages should be supported by a more substantial body of evidence. The primary obstacle to the widespread adoption of this methodology is the initial investment required. However, once a bioprinter is acquired, the production of scaffolds through 3D printing becomes relatively cost-effective, as it minimizes wastage by utilizing only the necessary materials.

The careful selection of prerequisite biomaterials is crucial for the successful clinical construction of tissues using 3D bioprinting. Traditionally employed biomaterials with sufficient biological activity may lead to unfavorable cell-to-cell communications, resulting in undesired and spontaneous differentiation of stem cells. While innovative biopolymers and hydrogels have a similar nanostructural resemblance to native tissue, they lack the necessary structural integrity required for conventional 3D bioprinting. Combining two different biomaterials can be chosen as a solution to create a strong scaffold with multifarious mechanical strength and harness respective benefits (Salah et al., 2020). Furthermore, there are additional drawbacks such as the significant time investment needed for bioprinting, challenges in consistently delivering the required number of cells for tissue regeneration, and potential changes in cellular shape that may lead to cell death. Therefore, there is a need to improve the overall effectiveness of the bioprinting procedure.

Another significant hurdle in bioprinting functional tissues involves creating a sufficient vascular system crucial for tissue survival. The presence of a vasculature during the early stages is of utmost importance in order to prevent tissue death and promote the fixation and growth of endothelial cells. Insufficient development of vasculature can result in inadequate tissue formation and necrosis due to a lack of essential nutrients in the newly formed tissue constructs. *In vivo* tissue growth beyond the limited range of oxygen diffusion (100-200 µm) necessitates the presence of a vascular network. Additionally, the vasculature plays various roles in waste filtration, inflammation, coagulation, and other homeostatic processes, as observed during normal development (Carmeliet and Jain, 2000). The bioprinting of vasculature presents a challenge due to the current limitations in the printing resolution of bioprinters. Capillaries ideally require a diameter resolution of 3 µm, but current laser-based bioprinters can only achieve a resolution of 20 µm. To address these obstacles, it is proposed to include angiogenic growth factors in the bioink to encourage the regeneration of host vasculature post *in-vivo* implantation. Alternatively, synthetic vasculature can be utilized.

Another area of focus should be the advancement of intelligent polymers that can adapt at the molecular level in response to environmental stimuli (Jingcheng et al., 2021). These advancements are critical for the production of next-generation smart tissue constructs. Moreover, the incorporation of microRNAs into 3D bioprinted constructs shows promise in initiating vascularization and bone formation in these tissue constructs.

References

Ashkan, S. and Anthony A. (2016) Printing technologies for medical applications. *Trends in Molecular Medicine*, 22(3): 254–265. doi: 10.1016/j.molmed.2016.01.003.

Ben, P.H., Bilal, A.N., Ethan, L.N., Miguel, D., Christina A.H et al. (2016) Three-dimensional printing of bone extracellular matrix for craniofacial regeneration. *ACS Biomaterials and Engineering, 2*: 1806–1816. doi:10.1021/acsbiomaterials.6b00101.

Carmeliet, P. and Jain, R.K. (2000) Angiogenesis in cancer and other diseases. *Nature, 407*(6801): 249–57. doi: 10.1038/35025220.

Dey, M. and Ozbolat, I.T. (2020) 3D bioprinting of cells, tissues and organs. *Scientific Reports, 10*, 14023 doi:10.1038/s41598-020-70086-y.

Dwivedi, R., Kumar, S., Pandey, R., Mahajan, A., Nandana, D. et al. (2020) Polycaprolactone as biomaterial for bone scaffolds: Review of literature. *Journal of Oral Biology and Craniofacial Research, 10*(1): 381–388. doi: 10.1016/j.jobcr.2019.10.003.

Dwivedi, R. and Mehrotra, D. (2020) 3D bioprinting and craniofacial regeneration. *Journal of Oral Biology and Cranofacial Research, 10*(4): 650–659. doi: 10.1016/j.jobcr.2020.08.011.

Gao, F., Chiu, S.M., Motan, D.A., Zhang, Z., Chen, L. et al. (2016) Mesenchymal stem cells and immunomodulation: current status and future prospects. *Cell Death and Disease, 7*(1): e2062. doi: 10.1038/cddis.2015.327.

Harmon, K. (2013) A sweet solution for replacing organs. *Scientific American, 308*(4): 54–55. doi: 10.1038/scientificamerican0413-54.

Hyun-Wook, K., Sang, J.L., In, K.K., Carlos, K., James, J.Y. et al. (2016) A 3D bioprinting system to produce human-scale tissue constructs with structural integrity. *Nature Biotechnology, 34*: 312–319. doi:10.1038/nbt.3413.

Jingcheng, L., Reddy, V.S., Jayathilaka, W.A.D.M., Chinnappan, A., Ramakrishna, S. et al. (2021) Intelligent Polymers, Fibers and Applications. *Polymers (Basel), 13*(9): 1427. doi: 10.3390/polym13091427.

Kačarević, Ž.P., Rider, P.M., Alkildani, S., Retnasingh, S., Smeets, R. et al. (2018) An Introduction to 3D Bioprinting: Possibilities, Challenges and Future Aspects. *Materials (Basel), 11*(11): 2199. doi: 10.3390/ma11112199.

Kargozar, S., Baino, F., Hamzehlou, S., Hill, R.G. and Mozafari, M. et al. (2018) Bioactive Glasses: Sprouting Angiogenesis in Tissue Engineering. *Trends in Biotechnology. 36*(4): 430–444. doi: 10.1016/j.tibtech.2017.12.003.

Khalil, S. and Sun, W. (2009) Bioprinting endothelial cells with alginate for 3D tissue constructs. *Journal of Biomechanical Science and Engineering, 131*(11): 111002. doi: 10.1115/1.3128729.

Kim, J.N., Lee, J.Y., Shin, K.J., Gil, Y.C., Koh, K.S. et al. (2015) Haversian system of compact bone and comparison between endosteal and periosteal sides using three-dimensional reconstruction in rat. *Anatomy and Cell Biology, 48*(4): 258–61. doi: 10.5115/acb.2015.48.4.258.

Lee, J.S., Hong, J.M., Jung, J.W., Shim, J.H., Oh, J.H. et al. (2014) 3D printing of composite tissue with complex shape applied to ear regeneration. *Biofabrication, 6*: 024103. doi: 10.1088/1758-5082/6/2/024103.

Li, J., Chen, M., We,i X., Hao, Y. and Wan,g J. et al. (2017) Evaluation of 3D-Printed Polycaprolactone Scaffolds Coated with Freeze-Dried Platelet-Rich Plasma for Bone Regeneration. *Materials (Basel), 10*(7): 831. doi: 10.3390/ma10070831.

Li, Y.C., Zhang, Y.S., Akpek, A., Shin, S.R. and Khademhosseini, A. et al. (2016) 4D bioprinting: the next generation technology for biofabrication enabled by stimuli-responsive materials. *Biofabrication, 9*(1): 012001. doi: 10.1088/1758-5090/9/1/01200.

Liu, F., Chen, Q., Liu, C., Ao, Q., Tian, X. et al. (2018) Natural Polymers for Organ 3D Bioprinting. *Polymers (Basel), 10*(11): 1278. doi: 10.3390/polym10111278.

Lobo S.E., Glickman R., da Silva W.N., Arinzeh T.L. and Kerkis I. et al. (2015) Response of stem cells from different origins to biphasic calcium phosphate bioceramics. *Cell and Tissue Research, 361*(2): 477–95. doi: 10.1007/s00441-015-2116-9.

Mahon, N.A., Joyce, C.W., Thomas, S., Concannon, E. and Murray, D. et al. (2015) The 50 Most Cited Papers in Craniofacial Anomalies and Craniofacial Surgery. *Archives of Plastic Surgery, 42*(5): 559–66. doi: 10.5999/aps.2015.42.5.559.

Mantha, S., Pillai, S., Khayambashi, P., Upadhyay, A., Zhang, Y. et al. (2019) Smart Hydrogels in Tissue Engineering and Regenerative Medicine. *Materials (Basel), 12*(20): 3323. doi: 10.3390/ma12203323.

Mir, T.A., Iwanaga, S., Kurooka, T., Toda, H., Sakai, S. et al. (2018) Biofabrication offers future hope for tackling various obstacles and challenges in tissue engineering and regenerative medicine: A Perspective. *International Journal of Bioprinting, 5*(1): 153. doi: 10.18063/ijb.v5i1.153.

Mironov, V., Boland, T. and Trusk, T. (2003) Organ printing: computer-aided jet-based 3D tissue engineering. *Trends in Biotechnology, 21*(4): 157–161.

Miura, K., Okada, Y., Aoi, T., Okada, A., Takahashi, K. et al. (2009) Variation in the safety of induced pluripotent stem cell lines. *Nature Biotechnology, 27*(8): 743–5. doi: 10.1038/nbt.1554.

Murphy, S. and Atala, A. (2014) 3D Bioprinting of Tissues and Organs. *Nature biotechnology, 32*(8): 773–785. doi:10.1038/nbt.2958.

Phillippi, J.A., Miller, E., Weiss, L., Huard, J., Waggoner, A. et al. (2008) Microenvironments engineered by inkjet bioprinting spatially direct adult stem cells toward muscle-and bone-like subpopulations. *Stem Cell, 26*(1): 127–134. doi: 10.1634/stemcells.2007-0520.

Rémi, N., Martine, L. and Thierry, C. (2005) 3D fine scale ceramic components formed by ink-jet prototyping process, *Journal of the European Ceramic Society, 25*(12): 2055–2059. doi:10.1016/j.jeurceramsoc.2005.03.223.

Rijal, G. (2023) Bioinks of Natural Biomaterials for Printing Tissues. *Bioengineering, 10*(6): 705. doi:10.3390/bioengineering10060705.

Roskies, M., Jordan, J.O., Fang, D., Abdallah, M.N., Hier, M.P. et al. (2016) Improving PEEK bioactivity for craniofacial reconstruction using a 3D printed scaffold embedded with mesenchymal stem cells. *Journal of Biomaterial Applications, 31*(1): 132–9. doi: 10.1177/0885328216638636.

Safhi, A.Y. (2022) Three-Dimensional (3D) Printing in Cancer Therapy and Diagnostics: Current Status and Future Perspectives. *Pharmaceuticals (Basel), 15*(6): 678. doi: 10.3390/ph15060678.

Salah, M., Tayebi, L., Moharamzadeh, K. and Naini, F.B. (2020) Three-dimensional bio-printing and bone tissue engineering: technical innovations and potential applications in maxillofacial reconstructive surgery. *Maxillofacial Plastic and Reconstructive Surgery, 42*(1): 1–9. doi: 10.1186/s40902-020-00263-6.

Scheithauer, U., Weingarten, S., Johne, R., Schwarzer, E., Abel, J. et al. (2017) Ceramic-Based 4D Components: Additive Manufacturing (AM) of Ceramic-Based Functionally Graded Materials (FGM) by Thermoplastic 3D Printing (T3DP). *Materials (Basel), 10*(12): 1368. doi: 10.3390/ma10121368.

Seyednejad, H., Gawlitta, D., Kuiper, R.V., de Bruin, A., van Nostrum, C.F et al. (2012) *In vivo* biocompatibility and biodegradation of 3D-printed porous scaffolds based on a hydroxyl-functionalized poly(ε-caprolactone). *Biomaterials, 33*(17): 4309–18. doi: 10.1016/j.biomaterials.2012.03.002.

Shirazi, S.F., Gharehkhani, S., Mehrali, M., Yarmand, H., Metselaar, H.S. et al. (2015). A review on powder-based additive manufacturing for tissue engineering: selective laser sintering and inkjet 3D printing. Science and Technology of Advanced Materials, *16*: 033502. doi:10.1088/1468-6996/16/3/033502.

Singh, D. and Thomas, D. (2018) Advances in medical polymer technology towards the panacea of complex 3D tissue and organ manufacture. *The American Journal of Surgery, 217*(4): 807–808. doi: 10.1016/j.amjsurg.2018.05.012.

Suganna, M., Kausher, H., Tarek, A.S., Sultan, A.H., Faraj, A.B. et al. (2022) Contemporary Evidence of CAD-CAM in Dentistry: A Systematic Review. *Cureus, 14*(11): e31687. doi: 10.7759/cureus.31687.

Swarnima, A., Shreya, S., Vamsi, K.B., Aniruddha, P., Ananya, B. and Subhadip, B. (2020) Current Developments in 3D Bioprinting for Tissue and Organ Regeneration–A Review. *Frontiers in Mechanical Engineering, 6,* 589171. doi:10.3389/fmech.2020.589171.

Tan, K.H., Chua, C.K., Leong, K.F., Cheah, C.M., Gui, W.S. et al. (2005) Selective laser sintering of biocompatible polymers for applications in tissue engineering. *Biomedical Material and Engineering, 15*(1-2): 113–24. PMID: 15623935.

Tao, O., Kort-Mascort, J., Lin, Y., Pham, H.M., Charbonneau, A.M. et al. (2019) The Applications of 3D Printing for Craniofacial Tissue Engineering. *Micromachines (Basel), 10*(7): 480. doi: 10.3390/mi10070480.

Thomas, D.J. (2016) Could 3D bioprinted tissues offer future hope for microtia treatment? *International Journal of Surgery, 32*: 43–44. doi: 10.1016/j.ijsu.2016.06.036.

Tripathi, S., Mandal, S.S., Bauri, S. and Maiti, P. (2020) 3D bioprinting and its innovative approach for biomedical applications. *MedComm, 4*(1): e194. doi: 10.1002/mco2.194.

Wenz, A., Borchers, K., Tovar, G.E.M. and Kluger, P.J. (2017) Bone matrix production in hydroxyapatite-modified hydrogels suitable for bone bioprinting. *Biofabrication, 9*(4): 044103. doi: 10.1088/1758-5090/aa91ec.

Wu, Z., Su, X., Xu, Y., Kong, B., Sun, W. et al. (2016) Bioprinting three-dimensional cell-laden tissue constructs with controllable degradation. *Scientific Reports, 6*: 24474. doi: 10.1038/srep24474.

Xin, W., Man, J., Zuowan, Z., Jihua, G. and David, H. et al. (2017) 3D printing of polymer matrix composites: A review and prospective. *Composites Part B: Engineering, 110*: 442–458. doi:10.1016/j.compositesb.2016.11.034.

Zhang, W. and Yelick, P.C. (2018) Craniofacial Tissue Engineering. *Spring Harbour Perspectives in Medicine, 8*(1): a025775. doi: 10.1101/cshperspect.a025775.

3D Bioprinting of Cartilage

Jesús Manuel Rodríguez Rego,[1*]
Ana Isabel Rodríguez Cendal,[3]
Silvia María Díaz Prado,[3] *Antonio Macías García,*[2]
Alfonso Carlos Marcos Romero[1] *and*
Laura Mendoza Cerezo[1]

1. Introduction

Articular cartilage is an elastic, connective tissue that lines joints and has the primary function of reducing friction between bone surfaces to allow smooth, uninterrupted movement. Unlike most body tissues, articular cartilage has no blood vessels, nerves or lymphatic system (Z. Ouyang et al., 2023). The main mechanism for the nutrition of articular cartilage is diffusion from the synovial fluid. This process transports nutrients and other vital elements needed by the tissue cells. Articular cartilage consists of the extracellular matrix, which consists mainly of collagen fibers, proteoglycans and water. The mechanical characteristics of this tissue depend on the interaction of these components with one another (A.J. Sophia Fox et al., 2009). The articular cartilage consists of three different zones: the superficial zone, the transition/middle zone and the radial/deep zone. After these regions is the "tidemark" and the calcified cartilage layer. Depending on the zone, the density of chondrocytes, the orientation of collagen fibers and the water content vary. The superficial region is the outermost layer of articular cartilage and contains the greatest amount of water. It contains the highest density of chondrocytes and the collagen fibrils are aligned to the articular surface. In the transition zone there is a lower cell density and the collagen fibers are thicker and have an oblique orientation. The deep zone, which has a lower water content, has the highest levels of proteoglycans, molecules that help improve the ability to absorb shock. The chondrocytes in this zone are aligned perpendicularly in a columnar fashion and the collagen fibers are oriented parallel to these chondrocytes. Finally,

[1] Department of Graphic Expression, University of Extremadura, Spain.
[2] Department of Mechanical, Energy and Materials Engineering. School of Industrial Engineering. University of Extremadura. Avenida de Elvas, Badajoz. Spain.
[3] Biomedical Research Institute of A Coruña (INIBIC). Building attached to the Hospital Materno Infantil Teresa Herrera, 1st floor. Carretera As Xubias, A Coruña, Spain.
* Corresponding author: jesusrodriguezrego@unex.es

the calcified cartilage layer interacts with the subchondral bone. This area has a low cell density and characteristics of both cartilage and bone (M. Oliveira Silva et al., 2020).

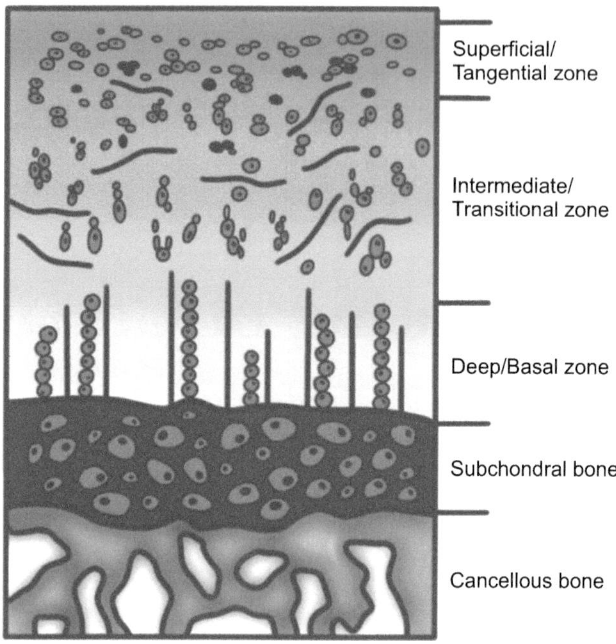

Fig. 1   Composition of articular cartilage.

The balance of articular cartilage depends on anabolic and catabolic mechanisms, along with anti-inflammatory and pro-inflammatory factors. Articular chondrocytes, which represent less than 10% of the tissue volume, are the unique cell type of cartilage. They play a crucial role in maintaining this balance and in reacting to mechanical and biochemical signals. Injury to cartilage can cause irreversible loss due to the inability of differentiated chondrocytes to compensate for the deterioration that has occurred (G. Schulze-Tanzil et al., 2009).

2. Osteoarthritis

Osteoarthritis is a complex disorder affecting mobile joints and is characterized by degeneration of the extracellular matrix of cartilage and cellular stress. The onset and development of the disease is marked by the production of catabolic proteins, such as interleukin IL1, IL6 and tumor necrosis factor (TNFα), which cause inflammation and the release of tissue-damaging proteolytic enzymes (C. Manferdini et al., 2022). Arthritic cartilage has a higher proportion of chondroprogenitor cells (chondrocyte precursor cells) compared to normal cartilage. However, in osteoarthritic cartilage, these have low proliferation rates, so they do not divide and multiply as fast as they should. In addition, their telomeres, which are protective layers at the ends of chromosomes that shorten with each cell division, show increased erosion in diseased tissue (M. Piñeiro-Ramil, 2023). The disease begins as a molecular alteration, followed by anatomical and physiological changes, such as cartilage degradation, bone remodeling, osteophyte formation, inflammation and loss of normal joint function, which can ultimately lead to the onset of symptoms (V.B. Kraus, 2015). The physical manifestations and signs of the disease are usually joint pain, limitation of movement, crunching and occasionally varying degrees of swelling or even synovial effusion. Osteoarthritis can develop in any synovial joint in the body, although it is most common in the hip, knee, and hand joints (F. J. Blanco, 2021).

The main risk factors for the disease are genetic predisposition, gender, age, tobacco use, pathogens, hormonal influences, dietary habits, socio-economic status and ethnic characteristics (Y. Alamanos and A.A. Drosos, 2005). Due to an increasingly aging population and rising obesity rates, the prevalence of the disease is increasing. The number of people with osteoarthritis is expected to increase by 50% in the next 20 years and already affects a significant percentage of the population (303 million people worldwide), especially women aged 60 years and older. Osteoarthritis also incurs substantial medical costs in high-income countries (T. Chen, 2021; W. Wei, 2021).

2.1   *Current Therapies for Osteoarthritis*

Current therapies for osteoarthritis, such as education, physical activity, weight control, pain relief medications and injections into the affected joint, do not effectively stop the gradual deterioration of cartilage associated with the disease (T. Chen, 2021). Tissue engineering is now being used to improve and find new ways to treat osteoarthritis. This field, which combines principles of engineering and life sciences, aims to create biological alternatives that can repair, maintain or improve the functionality of damaged tissues that have a limited capacity for self-renewal (C. Sanjurjo-Rodríguez, 2017). To achieve tissue repair, three strategies are being investigated independently or together: cell-based therapy (C. Sanjurjo-Rodríguez 2017; E. Muiños-López et al., 2016; C. Sanjurjo-Rodríguez et al., 2016 and A.I. Rodríguez-Cendal et al., 2023). (C. Sanjurjo-Rodríguez 2017; E. Muiños-López et al., 2017) growth factors and scaffolds (C. Sanjurjo-Rodríguez et al., 2016) and biomaterials (A I. Rodríguez-Cendal et al., 2023).

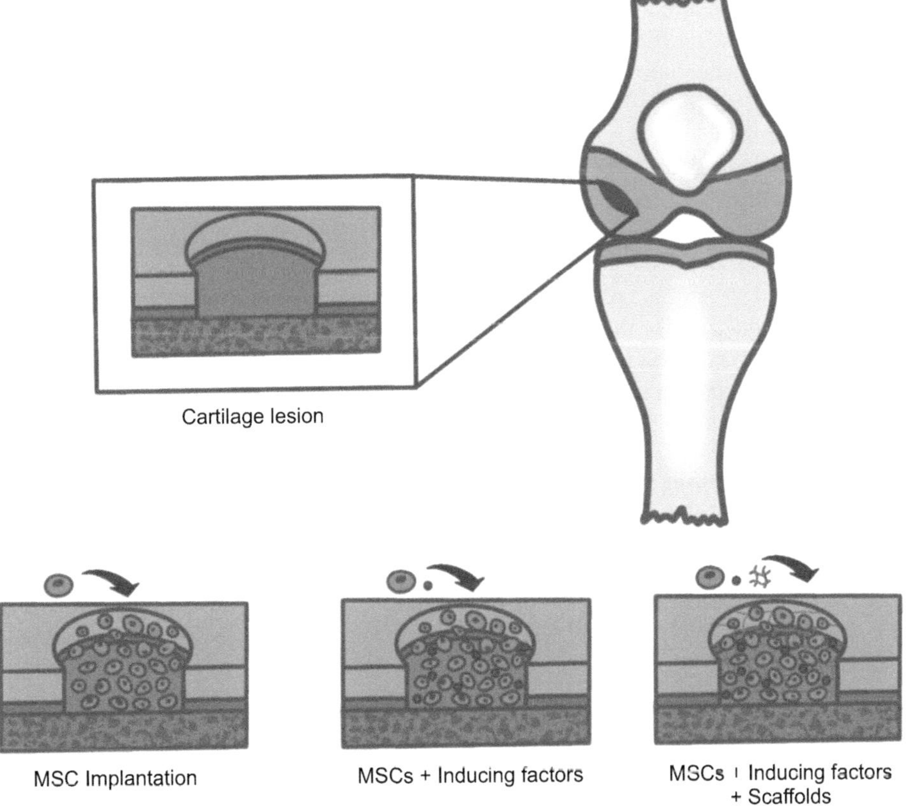

Fig. 2   Strategies studied to repair damaged articular cartilage.

Suitable cell sources for cartilage tissue engineering include mesenchymal stem cells and chondrocytes (S. McGivern et al., 2021). Mesenchymal stem cells are characterized by their ability to proliferate in culture and mesodermal differentiation. This cell type has been found in all joint tissues, including the cartilage surface, and are an attractive cell source for focal repair of osteochondral defects and potentially cartilage regeneration in osteoarthritis (Zhang et al., 2016).

Various surgical approaches using cells to treat cartilage defects have been used in clinical practice for many decades. These methods include the microfracture technique, where a perforation is made in the subchondral bone to facilitate the migration of mesenchymal stem cells from the bone marrow into the cartilage defect; autologous chondrocyte insertion (ACI), which involves filling the cartilage defect with laboratory-grown chondrocytes and covering them with a periosteal flap; and matrix-induced ACI, where chondrocytes previously grown in the laboratory are placed in a collagen or hyaluronic acid matrix prior to implantation. However, these surgical interventions have disadvantages, such as potential mechanical instability and unwanted fibrocartilaginous tissue formation (S. McGivern et al., 2021).

The limitations associated with the above techniques have led to the development of new therapeutic strategies. A wide range of natural and synthetic materials, such as alginate and collagen, have been investigated as scaffolds for cartilage repair (S. Wang et al., 2022). Within biomaterials, hydrogels in the form of three-dimensional polymeric matrices are proving to be good candidates for this task due to their structure and physicochemical properties (E. Merotto, 2023). In addition, because their properties can be modified as desired, hydrogels can bring benefits to the disease at different stages of the pathology. In the early stages of osteoarthritis, cartilage begins to break down, resulting in symptoms such as joint pain, stiffness and limited range of motion. Hydrogels due to their ability to absorb and retain water or biological fluids can help to lubricate and cushion the affected joint, reducing friction and relieving pain (E. Merotto, 2023). In turn, hydrogels can be designed to release therapeutic agents, such as anti-inflammatory drugs or growth factors, to further enhance the healing process of the joint (R. Nicu, 2023). Most of the drugs used for this purpose have formulations that dissolve rapidly after intra-articular injection, resulting in a shorter time for action and therapeutic efficacy. To overcome this limitation, the use of biomaterials is proposed, which may be an ideal support to encapsulate and control the release of these drugs, thus offering a solution to prolong their permanence at the site of action and optimize their clinical effectiveness (M.C. Bruno, 2022).

In an advanced stage of the pathology, the cartilage may have thickness defects on the cartilage surface, making it difficult for the body's own stem cells, called mesenchymal stem cells from the bone marrow, to migrate or be recruited to the damaged area. The structure of the hydrogel allows cells to be loaded, which can strengthen the body's natural repair mechanism of damaged articular cartilage. (S. Wang et al., 2022).

2.2   *Alternative Therapies to Treat Cartilage Defects*

The use of 3D printing in the manufacture of hydrogel scaffolds offers several advantages, such as the ability to create complex and customized architectures, cost-effectiveness and precise control of the spatial and temporal distribution of cells within the scaffold. (E. Merotto et al., 2023). To improve the control of cell growth and differentiation within the hydrogel scaffold, cells can be encapsulated prior to the 3D printing process (W. Fang, 2023). This means that the cells are embedded in the hydrogel material and distributed throughout the scaffold during the printing process. This encapsulation technique not only allows improved spatial and temporal control over cell distribution within the scaffold, ensuring their placement in specific areas and densities, but can also protect the cells against external stress and provide them with a microscopic environment suitable for their development and function (H. Chen et al., 2023). In the field of bioprinting for cartilage tissue engineering, hydrogels are considered an ideal choice as bioink materials, due to their hydrophilic nature, structural similarities to native cartilage and ability to retain a large amount of water (S. McGivern et al., 2021).

3. Bioprinting

3D bioprinting represents a developing additive manufacturing technology that enables the controlled dispensing of biological materials, bioactive factors and living cells in a precise and sequential manner, allowing the progressive construction of three-dimensional structures that can serve as replacements for natural tissues or organs (J. Malda, 2013). It emerges as a pioneering field at the intersection of tissue engineering and regenerative medicine, challenging the conventional boundaries of tissue and organ manufacturing. This innovative discipline fuses the principles of 3D printing with cell biology. Their ability to replicate both the microscopic and macroscopic architecture of biological tissues opens up a range of possibilities in the field of medicine and research, offering possibilities as important as the regeneration of damaged tissues to the creation of disease models for pharmacological studies. Among these applications is the regeneration of cartilage, through the controlled deposition of materials suitable for the proliferation and development of progenitor cells. There are different types of bioprinting, in which different techniques are used to achieve layer-by-layer material deposition:

3.1 Inkjet-based Bioprinting

Inkjet-based printing is an evolution of traditional 2D printers, where picolitre-sized droplets of bio-ink are precisely placed on a substrate by computer control, without direct contact (G. Huang, 2024). This technology uses two main methods: continuous inkjet printing (CIJ) and droplets on demand (DOD). CIJ produces continuous drops while DOD produces drops on demand. Although CIJ is faster, its medical application is limited by conductivity and contamination issues. DOD, which is more accurate and less wasteful, uses different technologies to control droplet deposition:

- **Thermal inkjet bioprinting:** It uses a thermal actuator to heat the fluid, creating a vapor bubble that precisely ejects a droplet of bio-ink (X. Cui, n.d). Although the temperature reached is high, its short duration limits the temperature rise of the liquid. It is speculated that this process could induce temporary cellular reprogramming due to the stretching and compression of cell membranes, activating the expression of primitive genes.
- **Piezoelectric inkjet bioprinting:** It employs piezoelectric actuators that convert electrical energy into mechanical energy efficiently and precisely. In piezoelectric inkjet bioprinting, a voltage pulse applied to a piezoelectric actuator causes a deformation in the wall of the bio-ink chamber, ejecting a droplet with precision (X. Gao, 2020). Optimization is achieved by adjusting the actuation mode and the characteristics of the voltage pulse. Although this process can cause the death of some cells, cell viability is usually above 85%, even better than extrusion printing.
- **Electrostatic inkjet bioprinting:** In this technique droplets are generated by electrostatic manipulation of the fluid chamber volume. The application of an electrical charge between the pressure plate and the electrode creates a curvature in the plate, increasing the volume of the chamber and ejecting the droplets when the charge is deactivated (D. Zhou et al., 2019). This method is notable for its energy efficiency, gentle handling of the bioink and absence of heat generation, protecting cell integrity. However, the fixed nozzle size may present limitations and be susceptible to clogging.
- **Microvalve inkjet bioprinting:** It uses a three-axis mobile robotic platform, multiple microvalve print heads and an individual gas regulation system to control the pressure and valve opening time. The microvalves, consisting of a solenoid coil and plunger, control the flow of bioink stored in a pressurized chamber. When a voltage pulse is applied to the coil, a magnetic field is generated that opens the valve, releasing a drop of bio-ink with millimeter precision (W. Long Ng e al., 2017). During bioprinting, factors such as pneumatic pressure, nozzle geometry and bioink composition affect droplet size and cell viability.

3.2 Extrusion-based Bioprinting

It employs technology very similar to that of conventional 3D printers, using pneumatic pressure forces or mechanical tools for material deposition. The process begins with the loading of the biomaterial into a cartridge or syringe, which is placed into a controlled extrusion device to regulate the flow through the nozzle (J. Yu, 2020). This nozzle moves precisely over a printing platform depositing the biomaterial layer by layer to form the desired structure, while controlling the temperature to avoid damage to the biomaterial and cells. Some bioprinters also have humidification systems to prevent drying of the biomaterial. The control software allows parameters such as speed, pressure and temperature to be adjusted to suit the material being printed.

3.3 Laser-assisted Bioprinting

Laser-assisted bioprinters consist of a donor slide composed of glass, laser-absorbing metal and bio-ink, together with a pulsed laser beam and a receiver slide. The LAB technique works by vaporizing the metal film underneath the hydrogel with a laser pulse, creating a cavitation bubble that drives microdroplets of bio-ink onto the substrate. This technology offers picolitre-level resolution, allowing cell density and three-dimensional spatial organization to be precisely controlled, even at the individual cell level, representing a major advance in tissue engineering (V. Keriquel, 2017).

3.4 Bioprinting Based on in-tray Polymerisation

This method employs a light source, either ultraviolet or visible, which selectively solidifies a photosensitive liquid resin layer by layer within a cuvette, forming a pre-designed three-dimensional structure. The photosensitive liquid resin, together with cells and growth factors, forms the bioink. This technology allows the fabrication of complex structures with high resolution and precision, ideal for the creation of customized tissues and organs for medical applications. There are two types of bioprinting based on vat polymerization:

- **Stereolithography-based bioprinting (SLA):** This builds 3D tissue structures layer by layer by converting a 3D model into superimposed 2D images, similar to biomedical image processing. The biomaterials used must be photosensitive for cross-linking with the appropriate light source, on whose characteristics the quality of the bioprinted structures depends. The process begins by mixing a biocompatible photosensitive polymer with cells to create the bioink, which is added to the SLA bioprinter tray. The manufacturing platform is then irradiated point-by-point with the light source to solidify each layer. Once solidified, the platform is lowered to a defined height and the process is repeated layer by layer until the three-dimensional structure is completed (Stereolithography 3D Bioprinting | Springer Nature Experiments, n.d).
- **Light processing-based bioprinting (DLP):** This uses a process similar to SLA bioprinting to create three-dimensional structures. Instead of irradiating the bioink dot by dot with a light source, it uses a projector to photocure the image of each layer at once. The projector is located underneath the tray, and the manufacturing platform is raised to solidify successive layers. This method allows complex and fast printing, but has a reduced printable area due to the resolution requirements of the digital light mirrors and the size of the projection area (Z. Zheng et al., 2020).

4. Cartilage Bioprinting

The bioprinting process for the generation of different types of tissue is broken down into three phases: First, computed tomography (CT) and magnetic resonance imaging (MRI) technologies are used to collect data on the properties of biological tissues or organs to generate three-dimensional models; then the bioink required for the regeneration of the tissues or organs is formulated. Finally, the bioprinter is used to assemble three-dimensional structures corresponding to the natural tissues or organs (M.A. Heinrich, 2019).

The three-dimensional construction of cartilage by bioprinting depends on three essential elements: a sufficient number of stem cells with normal functionality, the selection of suitable support materials (bioinks) and the incorporation of relevant growth factors (N. Bhardwaj et al., 2015). Bioinks need to have optimal printability and be highly compatible with the organism, as well as creating a microscopic environment conducive for cell development (M. Hospodiuk et al., 2016). Moreover, the generation of scaffolds with gradients of pore size and hole geometry can mimic the zonal organization of articular cartilage and provide similar mechanical strength characteristics to some extent. Thus, 3D printed cartilage scaffolds with tissue gradients, loaded with MSCs, can further simulate the zonal structure of articular cartilage, promoting increased cell viability, cell proliferation, type II collagen deposition and cartilage-related gene expression (J. Huang, 2021).

Numerous studies have been conducted on various natural (such as sodium alginate, hyaluronic acid, collagen, fibrin, gelatin, etc.) and synthetic (including polyvinyl alcohol (PVA), polyethylene glycol (PEG), polycaprolactone (PCL), etc.) biomaterials that have been used in cartilage regeneration (M. Li et al., 2022). Occasionally, inorganic materials are integrated into the scaffold, such as nanohydroxyapatite, tricalcium phosphate, graphene oxide, carbon nanotubes, nanocellulose, iron oxide nanoparticles and silver nanoparticles. Similarly, nanotechnology can offer a solution to mimic the highly complex structure of cartilage, which has exceptional mechanical properties that are difficult to replicate artificially. For example, carbon nanotubes have been shown to improve the physical characteristics of cartilage scaffolds (T. Szymański, 2020). Moreover, carboxylated cellulose nanocrystals enable the development of cell-stable and cell-free inks, with excellent physicochemical properties and biocompatibility (A. Kumar et al., 2020), and magnetic nanoparticles are suitable for use as a bioink to generate a magnetic nanocomposite hydrogel for cartilage tissue engineering (J. Huang, 2020).

Some of the most commonly used materials are hydrogels, three-dimensional networks composed of cross-linked polymer chains with a high water absorption capacity. Due to their hydrophilic nature and high water content, hydrogels are often considered the best choice for encapsulating the cells to be bioprinted. Hydrogels also bear a strong resemblance to the extracellular matrix (ECM) of natural cartilage and are considered a promising option in tissue engineering (A. Dhawan et al., 2019). Furthermore, cells and growth factors can be incorporated into the hydrogel solution before it solidifies, using curing agents and varying pH, ion concentration and temperature (A. Blaeser et al., 2017). Hydrogels can be composed of both natural and synthetic materials. The excellent cell affinity of implants made from natural materials leads to their degradation in biological environments in vivo, which can result in a loss of adequate mechanical support at the defect site. In contrast, synthetic materials, being artificially manufactured, offer implants with superior mechanical properties and controlled performance, and tend to be bioinert due to the lack of cell attachment sites, allowing them to maintain structural stability in the implantation environment (M. Li et al., 2022). For cartilage regeneration by bioprinting, it is common to use composite bioinks that combine natural and synthetic materials for cartilage regeneration.

4.1 *Cartilage Bioprinting Materials*

In cartilage bioprinting, the selection of suitable materials for the generation of appropriate bioinks is of vital importance. Optimal bioinks for 3D printing of articular cartilage are sought to possess adequate mechanical strength, controlled degradation, robust interfacial strength, favorable biocompatibility and optimal printability (Y. Huang et al., 2022). Both natural and synthetic materials offer unique advantages and disadvantages in terms of biocompatibility, structural stability and cell support capability. There is a wide variety of materials used in the manufacture of bioinks for cartilage bioprinting, ranging from biomaterials derived from natural sources to synthetic polymers. Understanding these materials will advance the development of effective cartilage tissue engineering strategies.

4.2   Natural Materials Most Commonly used in Cartilage Bioprinting

Natural polymers are considered good choices for bioinks due to their high water content, excellent biocompatibility, superior degradability and low immunological response, although they have shortcomings in terms of their mechanical properties and their ability to maintain the desired shape during and after the printing process reducing their application in tissues that experience loading, such as articular cartilage (F. You et al., 2017). Some studies suggest that collagen together with heparan sulphate are suitable for use as a scaffold for cartilage repair (C. Sanjurjo-Rodríguez et al., 2016), and even new strategies such as the use of human amniotic membrane as a scaffold for articular cartilage repair are being proposed with good results (S. Díaz-Prado 2010). The natural materials commonly used in the study of cartilage tissue regeneration are divided into polysaccharides and proteins:

4.2.1   Polysaccharides

- **Alginate:**   This is a biopolymer extracted from calcium, magnesium and sodium alginate salts present in brown algae consisting of β-D-mannuronic acid (M-block) and α-L-guluronic acid (G-block) units bonded in a (1-4) structure, forming a linear polyanionic block copolymer. Being negatively charged, alginate is considered biocompatible and can promote cell growth. G-blocks facilitate gel formation, while MG- and M-blocks increase flexibility. Their structure allows water and other molecules to be trapped in a matrix, but allows them to diffuse, making alginate hydrogels ideal for bioink formulations (E. Axpe and M.L. Oyen, 2016).

- **Chitosan:**   This is a biocompatible natural polymer of polycationic nature that is stable under physiological conditions and has a suitable viscosity for use in bioprinting processes. Studies have shown that chitosan-based bioinks promote appropriate cell proliferation and differentiation. Furthermore, they can be tuned to effectively mimic the native extracellular matrix of tissues. Despite these advantages, it has a slow gelation rate and weak mechanical strength (M. Taghizadeh, 2022).

- **Agarose:**   This is a natural linear polysaccharide extracted from marine or red algae, consisting of repeating polymeric chains of d-galactose and 3,6-anhydro-l-galactopyranose linked by α-1,3 and β-1,4 glycosidic bonds. It gels rapidly at low temperature, making it ideal as a bioink material for 3D printing, and its mechanical and swelling properties can be adjusted by varying the hydrogel concentration. However, its usefulness as a matrix for encapsulating cells is limited due to the lack of extracellular adhesion motifs that promote cell adhesion (A. Dravid et al., 2022).

4.2.2   Proteins

- **Hyaluronic acid:**   This is a natural, non-immunogenic polymer present in the extracellular matrix of various tissues with excellent biocompatibility and hydrophilicity and the ability to regulate many cellular behaviors and tissue functions. Despite its good biological properties, due to its low mechanical strength and fast degradation rate it cannot be used as a bioink on its own, so it has to be modified and/or blended to improve its properties (Y.-W. Ding et al., 2023).

- **Collagen:**   This is the main structural protein of the extracellular matrix, with a high affinity for adherent cells. Most collagen hydrogels are derived from type I collagen, which constitutes approximately 90% of the protein mass in mammalian connective tissues. The collagen types that produce the best chondrogenic phenotypes of bone marrow mesenchymal stromal cells are collagen type I (Col I), Col I and heparan sulphate (Col I+HS), Col I and collagen type II (Col II) and HS (Col I+Col II+HS) and Col I and Col II and chondroitin sulphate (Col I+Col II+CHS). (C. Sanjurjo-Rodríguez 2017). This type of collagen belongs to the group of fibril-forming collagens and is composed of three alpha helices that intertwine to form a triple helical structure. Under normal physiological conditions, such as neutral pH and a temperature of 37°C, collagen molecules tend to self-assemble into fibrils, resulting in the formation of a hydrogel from the collagen solution. The ability of the collagen bioink to be printed depends on the speed of this process: the faster it is, the higher the precision of the print achieved (E. O. Osidak et al., 2020).

- **Silk fibroin:** Silk fibroin is a protein obtained from the silkworm *Bombyx mori*, which has solid-forming, spinning, biodegradable and biocompatible properties. It has characteristics that make it highly suitable as a support matrix, as has been demonstrated for many cell types, including chondrocytes (R. Seda Tığlı, 2009).
- **Gelatine:** This is a water-soluble protein derived from the partial hydrolysis of collagen, an important function of which is to maintain the integrity of connective tissues such as bones, cartilage, corneas, tendons, ligaments, blood vessels and dentine. Gelatine-based hydrogels possess unique characteristics such as excellent biocompatibility, rapid biodegradability and non-immunogenicity in clinical applications (X. Wang et al., 2017).

4.3 Synthetic Materials Most Commonly used in Cartilage Bioprinting

Synthetic polymers generally offer superior mechanical strength and printing precision compared to natural polymers, although they have a fixed covalent network structure, which makes them difficult to resist mechanical stress (Y. Huang et al., 2022).

- **PVA:** It is a water-soluble synthetic polymer with good hydrophilicity, biocompatibility and toughness properties, helping to improve the toughness of other hydrogels. It has physical cross-linking properties by repeated freezing and thawing without the addition of any cross-linking compounds, allowing porous scaffolds to be developed when used in conjunction with other hydrogels (Q. Wei, 2021).
- **PEG:** It is a highly biocompatible synthetic poly(ether) that dissolves in both organic solvents and aqueous solutions. Its use does not adversely affect cell adhesion or proliferation, and allows the addition of cell binding motifs, such as Arg-Gly-Asp peptides, to the hydrogel network to improve cell adhesion (R. Khoeini et al., 2021).
- **PCL:** This is a biodegradable, high molecular weight, semi-crystalline, biodegradable polymer with thermoplastic behavior, high mechanical strength and low melting point (60°C). However, the melting temperature is too high to be supported by the cells, so they have to be added to the structure after printing (J.K. Carrow et al., 2015).

4.4 Growth Factors

Growth factors have the ability to regulate cell behavior, increase activity and cause functional differentiation, remodeling tissue in the affected area. Several growth factors have been tested in clinical trials, including TGF-β, BMP, IGF-1, FGF, HGF and PDGF (M. Li et al., 2022) that can direct chondrocyte and stem cell differentiation. These factors, either individually or in combination, enhance cartilage regeneration:

- TGF-β1 enhances chondrocyte differentiation.
- TGF-β2 and TGF-β3 promote extracellular matrix production in cartilage tissue. (A.S. Patil et al., 2011).
- bFGF and TGF-β can work together to regulate gene expression and repair cartilage.

Although studies indicate that these factors work with chondrogenic cells, their mechanism of action is not fully understood, so the control of these dynamic cellular processes is not yet precise, and more research is needed to make this a reality for clinical application (M. Li et al., 2022).

5. Bio-ink Reinforcement for Cartilage Generation

It is difficult to replicate the mechanical properties of articular cartilage using biotites composed only of natural polymers or synthetic polymers, as cartilage has high strength and excellent elastic and shock-absorbing properties (Z. Wang, 2022). Therefore, various reinforcement strategies are proposed to develop printable bioinks with desirable characteristics that meet the mechanical requirements of articular cartilage, including methods to achieve strength, elasticity and self-healing properties:

5.1 Functionalization of Polymers

Hydrogels are typically formed by physical (weaker, reversible and susceptible to environmental influences) or covalent (stronger) cross-linking. One strategy to follow is functionalization, which involves modifying the methacrylate groups in the main polymer chain to produce covalent cross-linking. Methacrylation is applied to polysaccharides such as alginate and hyaluronic acid, and UV curing techniques are used to print low-viscosity hydrogels (Y. Zhang, 2019).

5.2 Formation of an Interpenetrating Network (IPN)

IPNs are structures composed of two polymeric networks, one primary (flexible and elastic polymers) and one secondary (rigid and brittle polymers), linked by covalent or ionic cross-linking, or both. They offer higher toughness and fracture resistance compared to a single polymeric network. Currently, IPNs are divided into ionic-covalent cross-linked (ICE) and dual networks. ICE networks, which can be physically or chemically cross-linked, undergo fast cross-linking and are less sensitive to external factors such as temperature and pH, making them ideal for 3D bioprinting. On the other hand, dual networks consist of covalently cross-linking polymer chains to form a primary network, followed by dispersion and cross-linking of secondary polymer monomers to form the secondary network. However, this process is too slow for 3D bioprinting applications (Y. Huang et al., 2022).

5.3 Use of Polymer Support Scaffolding

Synthetic polymers, with good mechanical properties but poor adhesion and cell survival properties, can be used as a structural material for cell-loaded natural bioinks that have good cell viability but low mechanical stability. Thus, synthetic polymers can be combined with natural polymers to achieve adequate mechanical properties (Y. Huang et al., 2022).

5.4 Incorporation of Nanomaterials

Nanocomposites, having a higher surface area to volume ratio, improve the mechanical properties and bioavailability of hydrogels. Nanomaterials are added to bioinks to reinforce them, thus improving their mechanical properties through physical and chemical interactions ('Hydrogel Bioink Reinforcement for Additive Manufacturing: A Focused Review of Emerging Strategies - Chimene-2020). These nanoparticles can also introduce new biological functions and affect cell-material interactions. For example, the incorporation of carbon nanotubes increases toughness and electrical conductivity, while some nanoparticles, such as silicate nanoclay, can enhance osteogenic differentiation of mesenchymal stem cells.

Conclusions

Bioprinting technology applied to cartilage regeneration represents a revolutionary advance in regenerative medicine with the potential to transform the way cartilage-related injuries and diseases are treated. Through the ability to precisely print complex three-dimensional structures that mimic the architecture and function of native cartilage, this technology offers the potential for new, more effective and personalized therapies for patients suffering from osteoarthritis, traumatic joint injuries and other degenerative conditions. One of the main benefits of cartilage bioprinting is its ability to provide an adaptable scaffold for tissue engineering by combining biomaterials, cells and growth factors, designing cartilage constructs that can be tailored to the specific needs of each patient.

However, there are still significant challenges to overcome, as accurately reproducing the complex microarchitecture of cartilage, promoting proper integration with surrounding tissue and improving the long-term viability of bioprinted tissues are barriers that still need to be overcome.

As we move into the future, it is critical to continue research and develop new strategies and technologies to improve the efficacy and feasibility of cartilage bioprinting, and interdisciplinary collaboration between scientists, engineers, clinicians and other healthcare professionals is key to addressing these challenges and bringing this technology to clinical applications, with the potential to vastly improve patients' quality of life.

References

A. Blaeser, D.F. Duarte Campos and H. Fischer, '3D bioprinting of cell-laden hydrogels for advanced tissue engineering', *Curr. Opin. Biomed. Eng.*, vol. 2, pp. 58–66, Jun. 2017, doi: 10.1016/j.cobme.2017.04.003.

A. Dhawan, P.M. Kennedy, E.B. Rizk and I.T. Ozbolat, 'Three-dimensional Bioprinting for Bone and Cartilage Restoration in Orthopaedic Surgery', *JAAOS - J. Am. Acad. Orthop. Surg.*, vol. 27, no. 5, p. e215, Mar. 2019, doi: 10.5435/JAAOS-D-17-00632.

A. Dravid, A. McCaughey-Chapman, B. Raos, S.J. O'Carroll, B. Connor et al., 'Development of agarose-gelatin bioinks for extrusion-based bioprinting and cell encapsulation', *Biomed. Mater.*, vol. 17, no. 5, p. 055001, Jun. 2022, doi: 10.1088/1748-605X/ac759f.

A.I. Rodríguez-Cendal, I. Gómez-Seoane, F.J. de Toro-Santos, I.M. Fuentes-Boquete, J. Señarís-Rodríguez et al., 'Biomedical Applications of the Biopolymer Poly(3-hydroxybutyrate-co-3-hydroxyvalerate) (PHBV): Drug Encapsulation and Scaffold Fabrication', *Int. J. Mol. Sci.*, vol. 24, no. 14, Art. no. 14, Jan. 2023, doi: 10.3390/ijms241411674.

A.J. Sophia Fox, A. Bedi and S.A. Rodeo, 'The Basic Science of Articular Cartilage', *Sports Health*, vol. 1, no. 6, pp. 461–468, Nov. 2009, doi: 10.1177/1941738109350438.

A. Kumar, I.A. A.I. Matari and S.S. Han, '3D printable carboxylated cellulose nanocrystal-reinforced hydrogel inks for tissue engineering', *Biofabrication*, vol. 12, no. 2, p. 025029, Mar. 2020, doi: 10.1088/1758-5090/ab736e.

A.S. Patil, R.B. Sable and R.M. Kothari, 'An update on transforming growth factor-β (TGF-β): sources, types, functions and clinical applicability for cartilage/bone healing', *J. Cell. Physiol.* vol. 226, no. 12, pp. 3094–3103, Dec. 2011, doi: 10.1002/jcp.22698.

C. Manferdini, 'Mesenchymal Stromal Cells Laden in Hydrogels for Osteoarthritis Cartilage Regeneration: A Systematic Review from In Vitro Studies to Clinical Applications', *Cells*, vol. 11, no. 24, p. 3969, Dec. 2022, doi: 10.3390/cells11243969.

C. Sanjurjo-Rodríguez, 'Human Cartilage Engineering in an In Vitro Repair Model Using Collagen Scaffolds and Mesenchymal Stromal Cells', *Int. J Med. Sci.* vol. 14, no. 12, pp. 1257–1262, Sep. 2017, doi: 10.7150/ijms.19835.

C. Sanjurjo-Rodríguez, 'Ovine Mesenchymal Stromal Cells: Morphologic, Phenotypic and Functional Characterization for Osteochondral Tissue Engineering', *PLOS ONE*, vol. 12, no. 1, p. e0171231, Jan. 2017, doi: 10.1371/journal.pone.0171231.

C. Sanjurjo-Rodríguez, A.H. Martínez-Sánchez, T. Hermida-Gómez, I. Fuentes-Boquete, S. Díaz-Prado et al. 'Differentiation of human mesenchymal stromal cells cultured on collagen sponges for cartilage repair', *Histol. Histopathol.*, vol. 31, no. 11, pp. 1221–1239, Nov. 2016, doi: 10.14670/HH-11-754.

C. Sanjurjo-Rodríguez, A.H. Martínez-Sánchez, T. Hermida-Gómez, I. Fuentes-Boquete, S.D. Prado et al., 'Human Cartilage Tissue Engineering Using Type I Collagen/Heparan Sulfate Scaffolds', *J. Regen. Med.*, vol. 2014, Mar. 2016, doi: 10.4172/2325-9620.1000116.

D. Zhou, J. Chen, B. Liu, X. Zhang, X. Li et al., 'Bioinks for jet-based bioprinting', *Bioprinting*, vol. 16, p. e00060, Dec. 2019, doi: 10.1016/j.bprint.2019.e00060.

E. Axpe and M.L. Oyen, 'Applications of Alginate-Based Bioinks in 3D Bioprinting', *Int. J. Mol. Sci.*, vol. 17, no. 12, Art. no. 12, Dec. 2016, doi: 10.3390/ijms17121976.

E. Merotto, P.G. Pavan and M. Piccoli, 'Three-Dimensional Bioprinting of Naturally Derived Hydrogels for the Production of Biomimetic Living Tissues: Benefits and Challenges', *Biomedicines*, vol. 11, no. 6, Art. no. 6, Jun. 2023, doi: 10.3390/biomedicines11061742.

E. Muiños-López, T. Hermida-Gómez, I. Fuentes-Boquete, J. de Toro-Santos, F.J. Blanco et al., 'Human Amniotic Mesenchymal Stromal Cells as Favorable Source for Cartilage Repair', *Tissue Eng. Part A*, vol. 23, no. 17–18, pp. 901–912, Sep. 2017, doi: 10.1089/ten.TEA.2016.0422.

E.O. Osidak, V.I. Kozhukhov, M.S. Osidak and S.P. Domogatsky, 'Collagen as Bioink for Bioprinting: A Comprehensive Review', *Int. J. Bioprinting*, vol. 6, no. 3, p. 270, Apr. 2020, doi: 10.18063/ijb.v6i3.270.

F.J. Blanco, 'Prevalence of symptomatic osteoarthritis in Spain: EPISER2016 study', *Rheumatol. Clinica*, vol. 17, no. 8, pp. 461–470, Oct. 2021, doi: 10.1016/j.reuma.2020.01.008.

F. You, B.F. Eames and X. Chen, 'Application of Extrusion-Based Hydrogel Bioprinting for Cartilage Tissue Engineering', *Int. J. Mol. Sci.*, vol. 18, no. 7, Art. no. 7, Jul. 2017, doi: 10.3390/ijms18071597.

G. Huang, 'Applications, advancements and challenges of 3D bioprinting in organ transplantation', *Biomater. Sci.*, vol. 12, no. 6, pp. 1425–1448, 2024, doi: 10.1039/D3BM01934A.

G. Schulze-Tanzil, 'Activation and dedifferentiation of chondrocytes: implications in cartilage injury and repair', *Ann. Anat. Anat. Anz. Off. Organ Anat. Ges.*, vol. 191, no. 4, pp. 325–338, Oct. 2009, doi: 10.1016/j.aanat.2009.05.003.

H. Chen, G. Gonnella, J. Huang and L. Di-Silvio, 'Fabrication of 3D Bioprinted Bi-Phasic Scaffold for Bone-Cartilage Interface Regeneration', *Biomimetics*, vol. 8, no. 1, Art. no. 1, Mar. 2023, doi: 10.3390/biomimetics8010087.

'Hydrogel Bioink Reinforcement for Additive Manufacturing: A Focused Review of Emerging Strategies - Chimene - 2020 - Advanced Materials - Wiley Online Library'. Accessed: Mar. 27, 2024. [Online]. Available: https://onlinelibrary.wiley.com/doi/full/10.1002/adma.201902026?casa_token=X6USfzB1VqgAAAAA%3AiHWDQxpoLsUWUBOR8v_DAmytmXDA_wkESl8DTbccNG1_zu0ZEtthg3_HQv7esnKOVXkP3ALd1wDm

J. Huang, '3D Bioprinting of Hydrogels for Cartilage Tissue Engineering', *Gels*, vol. 7, no. 3, Art. no. 3, Sep. 2021, doi: 10.3390/gels7030144.

J. Huang, 'Pulse electromagnetic fields enhance the repair of rabbit articular cartilage defects with magnetic nano-hydrogel', *RSC Adv.*, vol. 10, no. 1, pp. 541–550, 2020, doi: 10.1039/C9RA07874F.

J.K. Carrow, P. Kerativitayanan, M.K. Jaiswal, G. Lokhande and A.K. Gaharwar et al, 'Polymers for Bioprinting', in *Essentials of 3D Biofabrication and Translation*, A. Atala and J.J. Yoo, Eds., Boston: Academic Press, 2015, pp. 229–248. doi: 10.1016/B978-0-12-800972-7.00013-X.

J. Malda, '25th anniversary article: Engineering hydrogels for biofabrication', *Adv. Mater. Deerfield Beach Fla*, vol. 25, no. 36, pp. 5011–5028, Sep. 2013, doi: 10.1002/adma.201302042.

J. Yu, 'Current Advances in 3D Bioprinting Technology and Its Applications for Tissue Engineering', *Polymers*, vol. 12, no. 12, Art. no. 12, Dec. 2020, doi: 10.3390/polym12122958.

M.A. Heinrich, '3D Bioprinting: from Benches to Translational Applications', *Small Weinh. Bergstr. Ger.*, vol. 15, no. 23, p. e1805510, Jun. 2019, doi: 10.1002/smll.201805510.

M.C. Bruno, 'Injectable Drug Delivery Systems for Osteoarthritis and Rheumatoid Arthritis', *ACS Nano*, vol. 16, no. 12, pp. 19665–19690, Dec. 2022, doi: 10.1021/acsnano.2c06393.

M. Hospodiuk, M. Dey, D. Sosnoski and I.T. Ozbolat, 'The bioink: A comprehensive review on bioprintable materials', *Biotechnol. Adv.*, vol. 35, no. 2, pp. 217–239, Mar. 2017, doi: 10.1016/j.biotechadv.2016.12.006.

M. Li, D. Sun, J. Zhang, Y. Wang, Q. Wei et al., 'Application and development of 3D bioprinting in cartilage tissue engineering', *Biomater. Sci.*, vol. 10, no. 19, pp. 5430–5458, Sep. 2022, doi: 10.1039/D2BM00709F.

M. Oliveira Silva, J.L. Gregory, N. Ansari and K.S. Stok, 'Molecular Signaling Interactions and Transport at the Osteochondral Interface: A Review', *Front. Cell Dev. Biol.*, vol. 8, Aug. 2020, doi: 10.3389/fcell.2020.00750.

M. Piñeiro-Ramil, 'Generation of human immortalized chondrocytes from osteoarthritic and healthy cartilage', *Bone Jt. Res.*, vol. 12, no. 1, pp. 46–57, Jan. 2023, doi: 10.1302/2046-3758.121.BJR-2022-0207.R1.

M. Taghizadeh, 'Chitosan-based inks for 3D printing and bioprinting', *Green Chem.*, vol. 24, no. 1, pp. 62–101, 2022, doi: 10.1039/D1GC01799C.

N. Bhardwaj, D. Devi and B.B. Mandal, 'Tissue-Engineered Cartilage: The Crossroads of Biomaterials, Cells and Stimulating Factors', *Macromol. Biosci.* vol. 15, no. 2, pp. 153–182, 2015, doi: 10.1002/mabi.201400335.

Q. Wei, 'Design and evaluation of sodium alginate/polyvinyl alcohol blend hydrogel for 3D bioprinting cartilage scaffold: molecular dynamics simulation and experimental method', *J. Mater. Res. Technol.*, vol. 17, pp. 66–78, Mar. 2022, doi: 10.1016/j.jmrt.2021.12.130.

R. Khoeini, 'Natural and Synthetic Bioinks for 3D Bioprinting', *Adv. NanoBiomed Res.*, vol. 1, no. 8, p. 2000097, 2021, doi: 10.1002/anbr.202000097.

R. Nicu, '3D Matrices for Enhanced Encapsulation and Controlled Release of Anti-Inflammatory Bioactive Compounds in Wound Healing', *Int. J. Mol. Sci.*, vol. 24, no. 4, Art. no. 4, Jan. 2023, doi: 10.3390/ijms24044213.

R. Seda Tığlı, 'Comparative chondrogenesis of human cell sources in 3D scaffolds', *J. Tissue Eng. Regen. Med.*, vol. 3, no. 5, pp. 348-360, 2009, doi: 10.1002/term.169.

S. Díaz-Prado, 'Potential use of the human amniotic membrane as a scaffold in human articular cartilage repair', *Cell Tissue Bank.*, vol. 11, no. 2, pp. 183–195, May 2010, doi: 10.1007/s10561-009-9144-1.

S. McGivern, H. Boutouil, G. Al-Kharusi, S. Little, N.J. Dunne et al., 'Translational Application of 3D Bioprinting for Cartilage Tissue Engineering', *Bioengineering*, vol. 8, no. 10, Art. no. 10, Oct. 2021, doi: 10.3390/bioengineering8100144.

S. Wang, Y. Qiu, L. Qu, Q. Wang and Q. Zhou et al., 'Hydrogels for Treatment of Different Degrees of Osteoarthritis', *Front. Bioeng. Biotechnol.*, vol. 10, Jun. 2022, doi: 10.3389/fbioe.2022.858656.

Stereolithography 3D Bioprinting | Springer Nature Experiments. Accessed: Mar. 03, 2024. [Online]. Available: https://experiments.springernature.com/articles/10.1007/978-1-0716-0520-2_6

T. Chen, W. Weng, Y. Liu, R.H. Aspera-Werz, A.K. Nüssler et al. 'Update on Novel Non-Operative Treatment for Osteoarthritis: Current Status and Future Trends', *Front. Pharmacol.*, vol. 12, p. 755230, Sep. 2021, doi: 10.3389/fphar.2021.755230.

T. Szymański, 'Utilization of Carbon Nanotubes in Manufacturing of 3D Cartilage and Bone Scaffolds', *Materials*, vol. 13, no. 18, Art. no. 18, Jan. 2020, doi: 10.3390/ma13184039.

V.B. Kraus, F.J. Blanco, M. Englund, M.A. Karsdal and L.S. Lohmander et al., 'Call for standardized definitions of osteoarthritis and risk stratification for clinical trials and clinical use', *Osteoarthritis Cartilage*, vol. 23, no. 8, pp. 1233–1241, Aug. 2015, doi: 10.1016/j.joca.2015.03.036.

V. Keriquel, 'In situ printing of mesenchymal stromal cells, by laser-assisted bioprinting, for in vivo bone regeneration applications', *Sci. Rep.*, vol. 7, Dec. 2017, doi: 10.1038/s41598-017-01914-x.

W. Fang, 'Hydrogels for 3D bioprinting in tissue engineering and regenerative medicine: Current progress and challenges', *Int. J. Bioprinting*, vol. 9, no. 5, p. 759, 2023, doi: 10.18063/ijb.759.

W. Long Ng, J. Min Lee, W. Yee Yeong and M.W. Naing, 'Microvalve-based bioprinting - process, bio-inks and applications', *Biomater. Sci.*, vol. 5, no. 4, pp. 632–647, 2017, doi: 10.1039/C6BM00861E.

W. Wei, 'Advanced hydrogels for the repair of cartilage defects and regeneration', *Bioact. Mater.*, vol. 6, no. 4, pp. 998–1011, Apr. 2021, doi: 10.1016/j.bioactmat.2020.09.030.

W. Zhang, H. Ouyang, C.R. Dass and J. Xu, 'Current research on pharmacologic and regenerative therapies for osteoarthritis', *Bone Res.*, vol. 4, no. 1, pp. 1–14, Mar. 2016, doi: 10.1038/boneres.2015.40.

X. Cui, T. Boland, D.D. D'Lima and M.K. Lotz, 'Thermal Inkjet Printing in Tissue Engineering and Regenerative Medicine', *Recent Pat. Drug Deliv. Formul.*, vol. 6, no. 2, pp. 149–155.

X. Gao, 'Piezoelectric Actuators and Motors: Materials, Designs, and Applications', *Adv. Mater. Technol.*, vol. 5, no. 1, p. 1900716, 2020, doi: 10.1002/admt.201900716.

X. Wang, 'Gelatin-Based Hydrogels for Organ 3D Bioprinting', *Polymers*, vol. 9, no. 9, Art. no. 9, Sep. 2017, doi: 10.3390/polym9090401.

Y. Alamanos and A.A. Drosos, 'Epidemiology of adult rheumatoid arthritis', *Autoimmun. Rev.*, vol. 4, no. 3, pp. 130–136, Mar. 2005, doi: 10.1016/j.autrev.2004.09.002.

Y. Huang, X. Li, A.J. Poudel, W. Zhang and L. Xiao et al., 'Hydrogel-based bioinks for 3D articular cartilage bioprinting: A comprehensive review with focus on mechanical reinforcement', *Appl. Mater. Today*, vol. 29, p. 101668, Dec. 2022, doi: 10.1016/j.apmt.2022.101668.

Y.S. Kim and F. Guilak, 'Engineering Hyaluronic Acid for the Development of New Treatment Strategies for Osteoarthritis', *Int. J. Mol. Sci.*, vol. 23, no. 15, p. 8662, Aug. 2022, doi: 10.3390/ijms23158662.

Y. Zhang, 'In situ bone regeneration enabled by a biodegradable hybrid double-network hydrogel', *Biomater. Sci.*, vol. 7, no. 8, pp. 3266–3276, 2019, doi: 10.1039/C9BM00561G.

Y.-W. Ding, X.-W. Zhang, C.-H. Mi, X.-Y. Qi, J. Zhou et al 'Recent advances in hyaluronic acid-based hydrogels for 3D bioprinting in tissue engineering applications', *Smart Mater. Med.*, vol. 4, pp. 59-68, Jan. 2023, doi: 10.1016/j.smaim.2022.07.003.

Z. Ouyang, 'Cartilage-Related Collagens in Osteoarthritis and Rheumatoid Arthritis: From Pathogenesis to Therapeutics', *Int. J. Mol. Sci.*, vol. 24, no. 12, Art. no. 12, Jan. 2023, doi: 10.3390/ijms24129841.

Z. Wang, 'High-Strength and Injectable Supramolecular Hydrogel Self-Assembled by Monomeric Nucleoside for Tooth-Extraction Wound Healing', *Adv. Mater.*, vol. 34, no. 13, p. 2108300, 2022, doi: 10.1002/adma.202108300.

Z. Zheng, D. Eglin, M. Alini, R. Richards, L. Qin et al., 'Visible Light-Induced 3D Bioprinting Technologies and Corresponding Bioink Materials for Tissue Engineering: A Review', *Engineering*, vol. 7, Sep. 2020, doi: 10.1016/j.eng.2020.05.021.

26

3D-Bioprinting of Eye

Sule Ilgar,[1,2] *Musa Ayran,*[1,3] *Dilruba Baykara,*[1,3]
Songul Ulag[1,4,5]* and *Oguzhan Gunduz*[1,4]*

1. Introduction

The most common eye diseases such as cataracts, diabetic retinopathy, macular degeneration, glaucoma, and corneal diseases are becoming increasingly common and affect people worldwide. Some pathological eye diseases have the potential to cause severe visual impairment. It is estimated that there are around 385 million people with visual impairment (Akter, 2016). More than 10 million people worldwide suffer from vision loss due to corneal defects, which have a complex anatomy. Corneal blindness, which plays an important role in the optical system, requires corneal transplantation. According to research, 40,000 corneal transplants are performed every year in the United States of America (Ghezzi et al., 2015). The eye has a static or dynamic protective mechanism and the successful administration of medication is a challenge (Zamboulis, 2020). However, this treatment has some limitations. To overcome these limitations, it has been found that there is an increasing need in the clinic for graft materials produced as corneal grafts using 3D printing techniques. Conventional treatment of corneal damage has some limitations. Rejection of the graft material used for treatment and lack of donors are the main limitations (Fagerholm et al, 2009). In addition, the complex anatomy of the eye limits the effective use of drugs to treat disease. Topical eye drops or intravitreal injections used for treatment cause poor bioavailability, resulting in more frequent dosages. They require more effective treatment due to their shorter duration of stay in the eye (Wu et al., 2023).

The difficulties experienced in traditional treatment methods have led researchers to find innovative treatment methods. Regenerative medicine and tissue engineering play an important role in the development of materials and products that can be used in the treatment of patients with treatment techniques developed on the premise of the fields. Scaffolds produced using 3D

[1] Center for Nanotechnology & Biomaterials Application and Research (NBUAM), Marmara University, Istanbul, Turkey.
[2] Department of Bioengineering, Faculty of Chemistry and Metallurgy, Yildiz Technical University, Turkey.
[3] Institute of Pure and Applied Sciences, Marmara University, Department of Metallurgical and Materials Engineering, Istanbul.
[4] Department of Metallurgical and Materials Engineering, Faculty of Technology, Marmara University, Istanbul, Turkey
[5] Health Institutes of Turkey (TUSEB), Istanbul, Turkey.
* Corresponding author: songul.ulag@marmara.edu.tr; ucemogu@ucl.ac.uk

printing techniques can replace donor tissue or contribute to wound healing (Aghamirs, 2022). This technology, which aims to mimic the real environment of the tissue, enables the production of 3D tissues and organs consisting of scaffolds, cells and the microenvironment. It is important to ensure that cells transplanted into scaffolds, created via 3D printing techniques, receive the necessary physical support to maintain physiological functions. Due to the fact that the shape, size and porosity of the scaffolds produced can be easily designed, the 3D printing technique is one of the most recent preferred methods. The structures produced with high precision have the potential to be an effective method for understanding the mechanism of the drug in treatment methods or organ transplants (Fakhoury et al., 2022).

1.1   Overview of Three-dimensional (3D) Printing

Personalization is becoming an increasingly adopted approach in modern medicine. Every day, advances and revolutions in technological, biological, and soft matter fields enable the development of new devices for biological and medical research. These advances contribute to a deeper understanding of each patient's unique pathophysiology and physiology (Garg, 2022). 3D Printing technology, which allows complex structures to be printed with high precision, has the potential to enable the production of personalized medical products that are not possible with conventional manufacturing processes (Tan et al., 2022). The emergence of breakthrough technologies such as 3D printing has raised high hopes in the scientific community. It is expected that these advances will not only improve the well-being of patients with serious diseases but also make more efficient use of healthcare resources (Ruiz-Alonso, 2021). These advancements in 3D printing technologies have made the technology broadly applicable as a game-changing instrument in biomedical applications, tissue engineering, and regenerative medicine (Zhu et al., 2016). There are different areas where 3D printers are used in ophthalmology. People suffering from various eye diseases can benefit from the advantages and applications of 3D printing. Advances in 3D printing are paving the way for new possibilities in the management of ocular conditions in the field of ophthalmology (Tan et al., 2022). Examples of areas where this technology is used include contact lenses, drug delivery systems, iris rings, implants, artificial corneas, customized surgical instruments, and anatomical models (Ali, 2023).

1.2   History of 3D Printing

SLA (Stereolithography), which aims to create 3D objects using light-curable polymers and ultraviolet light, is among the oldest types of additive manufacturing (I.K. Cingesar et al., 2022). It was developed in 1981 by Hideo Kodama at the Nagoya Municipal Industrial Research Institute of Japan, but he applied for a patent and used it for the automatic production of three-dimensional plastic. He detailed it in his article titled Method. However, it did not become a full patent because it was not filed before the one-year deadline. It can be seen that his published article contributed to history and marked the beginning of rapid growth in this field. Charles W. Hull, who was the first to commercialize 3D printing techniques, invented the stereolithography apparatus (SLA) in 1984. After patenting his invention, he contributed to the development of 3D printer technology by producing the SLA printer, the first printer in the medical field, in 1988 (Ali, 2023). In 1989, new printing techniques were developed. After the "Fused Deposition Modelling" (FDM) and "Selective Laser Sintering" (SLS) printing techniques were patented in 1989, 3D printing techniques began to become more popular in different sectors (Tsui et al., 2022). This technology, which enables customized and faster production, was first called "3D printing" by Professor Emanuel Sachs, who is associated with the Massachusetts Institute of Technology (MIT) (Sommer, Blumenthal, 2019). Some of the areas where 3D printers are used are jewellery collections, PGA rocket engine, artificial heart pump, aerospace industry and 3D printed cornea (Cingesar et al., 2022). When we look at the studies carried out in the field of health, it was used in surgical planning for the treatment of skull defects in 1994. The use of 3D printing techniques in the field of eye (ophthalmology) has been slower than other fields. In 2015, a personalized eye prosthesis was one of the remarkable studies (Tsui et al., 2022).

1.3 Materials and Techniques in 3D Printing Eyes

Nowadays, selecting the appropriate method and the right material to print complex shapes that match the patient's anatomy is crucial. To fulfil the required performances of the complex anatomical structure, it is necessary to choose materials with suitable mechanical properties (Aimar et al., 2019). For example, the fulfilment of critical functions of the natural corneal structure is an important factor. Examples of critical properties of the corneal structure are protection, conductivity, and refraction. In tissue engineering studies, the design should take into account the basic properties to fulfil these characteristics. To produce a corneal structure with a functional one, it should be able to promote epithelial cell migration. It should also be a viscoelastic structure with adequate tensile strength and resistance to intraocular pressure. It should be transparent enough to provide the refractive index. It is also necessary to maintain the functional keratocytes for the production of collagen tissue in the cornea. To minimize the risk of optical blurring in the designed structure, it is important to select materials with suitable swelling properties that can ensure the circulation and distribution of the water content (Tsui et al., 2022). Various natural or synthetic materials are used to develop corneal tissue scaffolds for 3D printing. Chitosan, collagen, gelatin, methacrylated gelatin (GelMA), alginate, and silk fibroin are the preferred natural biomaterials in this field due to their similarity to their suitability for cell proliferation. They have superior properties such as good biocompatibility and biodegradability. These natural materials are biomaterials used in cellular bioprinting (Balters, Reichl, 2023).

Collagen occurs in various structural and hierarchical arrangements in the human body. Type 1 collagen is the most abundant protein in the skin, tendons, and cornea, while types ii and iv are abundant in cartilage and the basal metabolic rate. The triple helix with the RGD (arginine-glycine-aspartic acid) motif in its structure makes it a biocompatible protein. It therefore enables cell adhesion, growth, and attachment. Since it has low mechanical strength, the collagen protein can be made more functional by increasing its mechanical strength through a chemical methacrylation process. Furthermore, by using it with different biomaterials, structures with the desired strength can be produced (Ahearne et al., 2020). Gingras et al. aimed to produce a stromal structure for the cornea using alginate to increase the mechanical strength of collagen. The dome-shaped scaffold produced using the extrusion printing technique exhibited high transparency (Gingras, 2023).

Gelatine is a polymer with the same amino acid sequences that is obtained by partial hydrolysis of collagen. Derived from animals such as pigs, fish and cattle, the polymer is often favoured in tissue engineering studies as it protects the connective tissue integrity of cornea, tendon cartilage and blood vessels (Aghamirsalim, 2022; Gingras, 2023). It is a polymer used in corneal tissue engineering, mainly because of its low cost, excellent biocompatibility and good transparency. Methacrylated gelatin (GelMA), which is obtained by chemical modification of gelatin, enhances the heat resistance of the gelatin and protects the cell binding sites. The RGD patterns (arginine, glycine and aspartate) in GelMA hydrogel make the material advantageous in terms of biocompatibility (Sang et al., 2022). For example, in 2021, Farasatkia et al. created a design using silk fibroin and GelMA polymers for use in corneal tissue engineering studies. In this study, which was designed to make the complex structure and mechanical properties of the cornea structure similar, they achieved high transparency and high mechanical strength (over 85%). (Farasatkia et al., 2021).

Silk fibroin, which is extracted from the cocoon of the silkworm Bombyx mori, is a preferred protein in regenerative medicine and tissue engineering studies due to its robust mechanical properties and controllable degradation rate. Silk cocoons consist of silk fibroin and the protein sericin, which holds these proteins together. It is a protein that is characterized by its affinity for water and has a molecular weight of around 350 kilodaltons (Wani et al., 2022). Studies have shown that it plays a role in the proliferation and adhesion of epithelia and fibroblasts. The efficacy of silk fibroin in this regeneration is of interest for ocular tissue engineering studies, e.g. in wound healing. The silk fibroin protein may serve as a therapeutic agent to bring healthy epithelial cells closer to the injured site (Lawrence et al., 2008). Sahi et al. developed scaffolds using silk fibroin and gelatin polymers to create a structure equivalent to the corneal stromal structure. The mechanical and transparency properties of the fabricated samples were found to be similar to the natural cornea. Viability analysis using fibroblast cells showed high cellular biocompatibility (Sahi et al., 2021).

Chitosan, the second most abundant polysaccharide in the world, is one of the suitable candidates for ophthalmic applications due to its biocompatibility, antibacterial and antifungal activity, and biodegradability. It is produced using chemical and biological methods. In biological methods, enzymes or bacteria are used for production. Chemical methods require the necessary chemicals. The synthesis stage takes place in 3 steps. These steps are demineralization, deproteinization, and deacetylation. Chitosan, which is obtained from the exoskeletons of crustaceans and insects, increases the permeability of the mucosal barriers in the eye. It plays an important role in wound healing by promoting the migration of keratinocytes (Irimia et al., 2018). CH et al. developed an Antimicrobial peptide loaded Gelatin Methacryloyl (GelMA)/Chitosan Methacryloyl (ChiMA) lens to treat Bacterial Keratitis. They prevented frequent dosing along with controlled drug release. In the animal experiment applied, bacteria had a significant effect on reducing bacteria.

3D printing techniques are used to create structures from designed 3D model data using these biomaterials, which are widely used in ocular tissue engineering. The underlying mechanism of operation for 3D printing techniques is to combine materials layer by layer to create the designed 3D structure. 3D printing technology covers 4 basic stages (Figure 1). (1) A CAD file is converted into a format that 3D printers can read. This is a commonly used Standard Triangle Language (STL) file. (2) It is the process of 3D printing using a 3D printing system with the desired feature. (3) After the printing process is completed, the structure is removed from the printer. This structure can be easily separated from the platform or it can be more complex. (4) After printing, other processes can be applied for functional or aesthetic requirements (Fakhoury et al., 2022). Because of the diverse range of materials accessible, extrusion, Stereolithography (SLA) and inkjet bioprinting methods are extensively implemented in the realm of ocular tissue engineering (Zhang, 2023). Recent studies in the field of ocular tissue engineering using biomaterials and different printing techniques are summarized in Table 1.

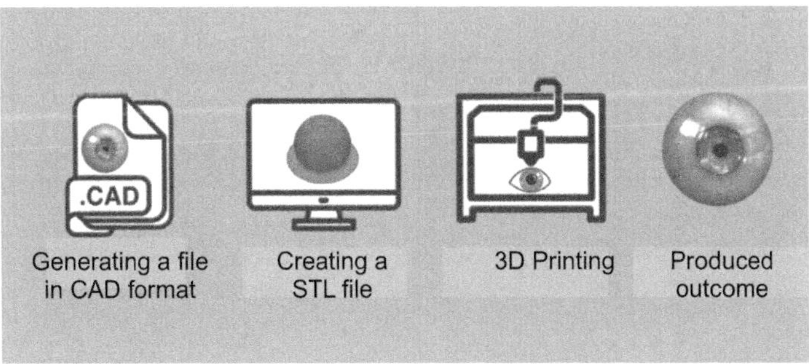

Fig. 1   Manufacturing procedure utilizing a 3D printer.

The extrusion printing technique applied to polymer blends with other elements is a widely used technology because it is an inexpensive technique. (Jiang et al., 2020). The device has a printhead that semi-fluidizes the thermoplastic to create the designed model (Fakhoury et al., 2022). The printing resolution depends on the diameter of the nozzle as well as the precision of the nozzle movement (Miri, 2019). By applying pressure, mechanical or pneumatic force, even polymers with high viscosity can be easily printed. The most important advantage is high throughput. For example, for cornea printing, a production time of less than 10 minutes was easily realized (Balters, Reichl,

2023). With this technique, cell-dense bioprinting can be realized. This is an innovative method for medical applications. However, the existing shear stresses carry the risk of decreasing cell viability (Aghamirsalim, 2022).

Stereolithography (SLA) is one of the oldest techniques for printing a wide variety of materials in which a photopolymer is exposed to curing radiation. To print the designed structure, the height of the building platform is varied, allowing additional layers to be built on top of each other (Fakhoury et al., 2022). The three main components of this technique are a photopolymer layer capable of absorbing laser energy, a donor slide, and a laser beam source. This method allows the formation of high-resolution structures but is slightly more expensive than other techniques (O'Brien et al., 2015). It is highly advantageous for co-printing many biological materials such as living cells, peptides, and DNA with the polymer (Hou et al., 2018). In the inkjet technique, a heating unit at the nozzle allows the formation of bubbles. After bubble formation, a driving force is generated that can eject the droplets one by one. In this technique, which uses thermal heaters or piezoelectric actuators, the material is deposited in droplets (Zhang, 2019). It allows the printing of peptides or growth factors from different living cells. It is not a fast technique for printing complex structures. Also, the mechanical properties of the scaffolds formed may be low.

Table 1   Recent studies in the field of ocular tissue engineering

Year	*Natural Base Materials*	*Method*	*Targeted tissue of eye*	*Cells for In vitro evaluation*	*Ref.*
2024	Polylactic acid (PLA)-amniotic fornical ring (AFR)	Extrusion 3D printing	Ocular surface reconstruction	–	(Zhang, 2023)
2023	GelMA/collagen	Extrusion 3D printing	Cornea	Corneal epithelial cells (RCECs)	
2023	Cellulose acetate (CA), and chloramphenicol (CAM)	Electrohydrodynamic (EHD) printing	Cornea	L929 cells	(Sun et al., 2023)
2023	Collagen, alginate, and alginate-gelatin	Extrusion 3D printing	Cornea	–	(Gingras, 2023)
2023	Decellularized extracellular matrix/ gelatin methacryloyl (CECM-GelMA)	Digital light processing (DLP) 3D bioprinting	Cornea	Human corneal fibroblasts (hCFs)	(Zhang, 2023)
2022	Gelatin methacrylate (GelMA) and long-chain poly (ethylene glycol) diacrylate (PEGDA)	Digital light processing (DLP) 3D bioprinting	Epithelium/stroma bilayer	Rabbit corneal epithelial cells (rCECs)-laden epithel-rabbit adipose-derived mesenchymal stem cells (rASCs)	(He, 2022)

1.4   Eye Anatomy

Although the eye is often described as spherical, it is a structure surrounded by three layers in which two spheres of different radii are arranged side by side. The anatomy of the eye is as shown in Figure 2. The posterior part, which has a white and opaque structure, is called the sclera. The more curved anterior part is the cornea (Brooks, 2007). The cornea and sclera, which have a relatively inflexible structure, surround the entire eye structure and serve as a protective layer for the internal structures. The cornea of the eye has a three-layered structure and serves as a transparent barrier that protects the eye. Its three basic layers, from the outside in, are defined as squamous epithelium, stroma, and a monolayer of specialized endothelial cells (Sridhar, 2018). The middle tissue layer of the eye consists of the iris, the ciliary body, and the choroid. The iris forms the colored part of the eye and has a circular opening in the middle. This opening is called the pupil and there are two muscle groups with opposing movements to regulate the size of the pupil (Purves, 2024). The iris controls the amount of light that reaches the retina by adjusting the diameter of the pupil (Bloom, 2005). The ciliary body is the ring of tissue that surrounds the lens as an extension of the iris. It contains a muscular component that is important in changing the shape of the lens to focus on objects at different distances (Delamere, 2005). Another important function of the lens is the production of a fluid called aqueous humor. This fluid plays an important role in maintaining the shape of the eye by maintaining eye pressure (Janssen, 2012). The choroid is composed of blood vessels and supplies the outer retina as the main blood supply to the photoreceptors of the retina (Nickla, 2009).

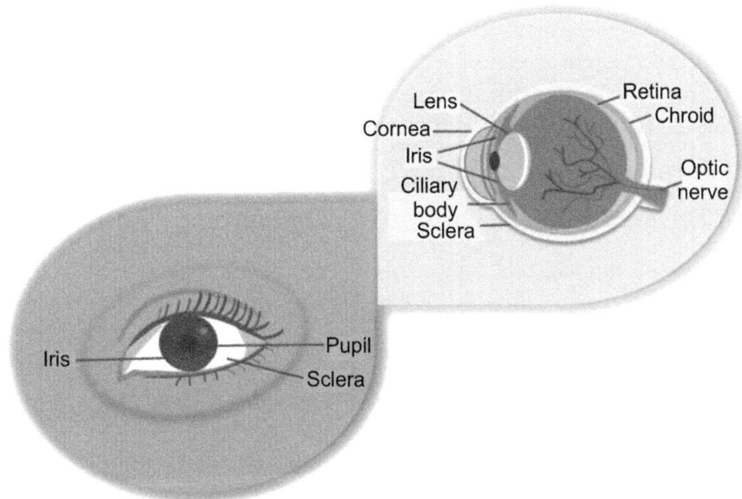

Fig. 2   Anatomy of eye

2. Applications of 3D Printing in Ophthalmology

2.1 *Diagnosis*

According to the World Health Organization, at least 2.2 billion people worldwide are affected by vision impairment, with almost 50% of these cases being potentially preventable (Onugwu, 2023). Notable eye diseases, such as cataracts, keratoconus, glaucoma, diabetic retinopathy, and age-related macular degeneration, result in significant vision impairment. These conditions can substantially diminish the quality of life, and if not treated correctly, may lead to total blindness. The economic and social impact of blindness is substantial (Chakravarthy et al., 2017). The advancements in eye surgery progress in tandem with scientific developments. Emerging technologies such as 3D bio-printing, mathematical modeling, and advancements in lab-on-a-chip prototyping are utilized in procedures like eye enucleation. These innovations extend to the detection of eye biomarkers at the cellular level, biosensors, and new diagnostic tests, all aimed at improving the post-surgical quality of life for patients (Ospina et al., 2016).

The potential of 3D printing in the field of precision medicine within ophthalmology holds considerable significance. Specifically, advancements in technologies capable of printing at the nanometer-micrometer scale have heightened the application of 3D printing in areas such as ophthalmic devices, intraocular implants, ocular prosthetics, and surgical tools, all of which demand intricate details. 3D-printed anatomical models, utilized for medical education, prove effective in educating students and medical professionals on the intricate structure of the eye (Ye, 2018). Likewise, 3D-printed surgical guides provide precise solutions in surgery, aiding ophthalmologists in reducing surgical durations and improving patient outcomes (Lichtenberger et al., 2018; Jones et al., 2016). Furthermore, the evolving field of bioprinting opens avenues for novel research in ophthalmology, facilitating the creation of artificial corneal, retinal, and conjunctival tissue models. This presents promising prospects for future regenerative medicine interventions to address vision loss (Wang, 2022). The conceptual framework of 3D printing applications in ophthalmology closely aligns with that of other medical fields. However, the unique characteristics of the eye, including the accessibility to the inner eye and particularly the anterior segment, the immune privileged status, and the array of diagnostic tools for identifying ocular conditions, make the eye an ideal terrain for the integration of innovative 3D printing solutions. Progress in biocompatible materials and the utilization of autologous stem cells not only improve implant adaptability but also mitigate the risks of rejection and irritation associated with implanted materials (Sommer, Blumenthal, 2019). Personalized diagnostic or treatment devices, 3D-printed contact lenses, and intraocular implants that aid in the early detection of common ocular conditions can be manufactured using 3D printing technology. Furthermore, various applications encompass models that assist in surgical planning and products that contribute to the education of both patients and healthcare personnel (Ruiz-Alonso, 2021).

2.2 *Medical Devices in 3D Printing of Ophthalmology and Eye Care*

Production of prostheses, models, and devices used in ophthalmology with 3D printing technology offers significant advantages in terms of pressure resistance, cost, and customization compared to traditional production methods. Ophthalmological medical devices and implants which are typically small and delicate, can be manufactured to suit individual needs thanks to 3D printing, despite individual differences. Additionally, 3D printing has advantages such as short design and production times, durability, low cost, and customization (Canabrava et al., 2015). Glasses produced with specially designed 3D printers can be applied to patients with facial deformities. Since many children with facial deformities need to wear glasses, it is important to provide appropriate frames for this patient group. The mentioned 3D printing technique may offer a new and accurate alternative. For special occasions, it is also possible to produce personalized glasses with this technique to maximize optical alignment and comfort (Ayyildiz, 2018). In another study, personalized eyeglass frames using 3D printing technology were produced for the optical rehabilitation of patients with dysmorphic features (Altinkurt et al., 2020). It enabled the development of Cana's Ring (CR), a 3D pupil dilation device; This was the first intraocular model designed and manufactured using 3D printing technology. CR is an iris expansion ring that expands the pupil to a diameter of 6.5 millimeters (Canabrava et al., 2015).

Devices related to vision, such as fundus cameras and slit lamps, are often expensive and come with a price tag that is hard for most general practitioners or primary care providers to afford. In 2015, Hong unveiled a slit-lamp microscope adapter for smartphones that was made using 3D printing and had a manufacturing cost much lower than traditional equipment. This adapter can capture images and document pathologies in the front part of the eye. Additionally, a portable adapter for retina imaging, also 3D printed, was introduced for mobile phones. These kinds of devices can send data electronically to eye specialists worldwide and are easily accessible in rural or underdeveloped regions, aiding local medical personnel in promptly and accurately diagnosing and treating common eye conditions (Hong et al., 2015). Additive manufacturing emerges as a viable approach for producing ophthalmic models, devices, and instruments at a relatively low cost using biocompatible materials. This pioneering method holds the potential to introduce novel perspectives for the utilization of 3D printing, an innovative technology with significant applicability in the domain of ophthalmology.

2.2.1 Artificial corneas

The cornea, with its transparent and avascular structure, plays vital protective and refractive roles. Its anterior position allows it to transmit and refract incoming light, while also serving the function of protecting the eye from mechanical damage, infections, and ultraviolet (UV) radiation (Tan et al, 2012). The cornea, a significant component of the optical system, is a highly organized, dense, avascular, transparent connective tissue that protects the eye from external factors. The average diameter of the adult cornea falls within the range of 11.04 to 12.50 mm for males and 10.70 to 12.58 mm for females (Rüfer et al., 2005). The cornea is composed of three main cellular layers, progressing from the outermost to the innermost: the outermost epithelium, the middle layer known as stroma, and the innermost endothelium. Additionally, it features two acellular interfaces named Bowman's layer and Descemet's membrane (Ulag, 2020).

The advent of contemporary surgical techniques and the proficiency of surgeons have propelled keratoplasty, commonly recognized as whole cornea transplantation, to the forefront of solid tissue transplantation globally. It is acknowledged as the preeminent procedure, widely accepted as the sole treatment modality for corneal blindness (Saverymuttu et al., 2009; Niederkorn, 2002). The trend toward personalized treatment for patients is swiftly gaining prominence in modern medicine. In this context, the conventional production methods of artificial corneas are under scrutiny, evaluating their cost-effectiveness and direct recoverability tailored to the individual needs of integrated corneal functions. The cornea, one of the intricate tissues with refractive power, poses a challenge in achieving individual functional restoration for many tissues and organs due to its structure and materials' specific functions and characteristics. To realize this objective, additive manufacturing, especially the potential of 3D printing, is currently a subject of active investigation (Zhang, 2019). The designed three-dimensional scaffold not only replaces the damaged cornea to provide mechanical and structural stability but also creates a suitable microenvironment for cell regeneration. In essence, the scaffold is a designed template that mimics the extracellular matrix (ECM) of natural tissue, supporting cell proliferation, migration, and the establishment of their microenvironments, thus mimicking the in vivo environment (Chan, Leong, 2008). The corneal substitute should mimic the structural, functional, and morphological properties of the natural cornea, while also ensuring high repeatability, low cost, and high quality. It must demonstrate biocompatibility to prevent autoimmune reactions and resist surgical procedures, and its materials should facilitate the diffusion of oxygen, carbon dioxide, and nutrients. Shape and structure significantly affect the cornea's optical properties, thus current research focuses on advancements in production methods to meet various requirements of corneal substitutes (Wang et al, 2016).

The scaffolds investigated for corneal replacement in ophthalmology can be classified into three categories: synthetic, naturally derived, and hybrid materials. Polyethylene glycol, polyamides, polydimethylsiloxane, acrylic-established polymers, polyvinyl alcohol-established polymers, and polyesters are the primary synthetic materials scrutinized for corneal substitutions (Rafat, 2008; Aldave et al., 2008; Zorlutuna et al., 2006; Liu, Sheardown, 2004; Deng et al., 2004; "Effects of Ultra High Molecular Weight, 2024). Despite the possession of these synthetic polymer adjustable chemical and mechanical properties compatible, it has been found essential to significantly enhance the biomimetic properties necessary for effective cell adhesion, proliferation, and integration with host tissue in clinical settings before their use (Sharma, 2019). Natural biopolymers offer notable biomimetic properties and biological functions, along with biocompatibility and biological degradability. The majority of studies on naturally derived corneal scaffolds focus on scaffolds made from proteins or polysaccharides. Collagen stands out as one of the most extensively researched protein-based scaffolds for artificial corneas. This is attributed to collagen's compatibility with living tissues, minimal harmful effects, and the retention of sequences like arginine-glycine-aspartic acid, which promote the attachment of cells to the scaffold (Li, 2005). Although collagen-based scaffolds exhibit promising characteristics (McLaughlin, 2009; Liu, 2008), further development is still required to fully match their biomimetic properties with those found in specific natural tissues

(Duan et al., 2006). In addition, gelatin, fibrin, and silk are potential candidates being investigated among other protein-based biopolymers as corneal substitutes (Lawrence et al., 2008; Lai, Li, 2019; Alaminos, 2006).

With its potential in artificial cornea production, 3D bioprinting provides progress in important areas such as precise control of shape and properties, surface quality, and mechanical strength control in corneal tissue engineering. In addition, this technology enables the production of full-layer multicellular cornea models in vitro and contributes to ensuring surface quality as well as biomechanical durability in artificial cornea production (Zhang, 2019). He et al. propose 3D printing of a biomimetic epithelial/stroma bilayer implant due to difficulties in corneal regeneration and undesirable transformations. This method is based on a corneal scaffold using Digital Light Processing (DLP) technology with different mechanical strengths such as GelMA and PEGDA, which supports cell durability, proliferation, and migration and provides a suitable microenvironment (He, 2022). In their study, Sorkio et al. conducted a three-dimensional bioprinting of a stromal structure containing human adipose tissue-derived stem cells (hASCs), successfully mimicking the properties of the natural corneal stroma with high cell survival rates (Sorkio, 2018). Isaacson et al. utilized a computer-aided design tool based on the standard commercial contact lens size to perform three-dimensional (3D) modeling, followed by the selection of suitable materials and the 3D printing of contact lenses (Isaacson et al, 2018).

Kim et al. achieved the alignment of a collagen structure derived from corneal stroma through the induction of shear stress in cell-depleted ECM bioink using a 3D cell printing technique. Cutting-related 3D printing parameters can be utilized to spatially control the orientation of collagen fibrils within structures, and it has been demonstrated that shear stresses associated with various nozzle diameters lead to different distributions of collagen fibril orientation (Kim, 2019). Three-dimensional corneal in vitro models represent valuable techniques for examining interactions between cells, as well as the processes of development and disease pathophysiology in corneal research. Such progressions are expected to diminish the dependence on live animal models in corneal research and potentially offer new avenues for treating corneal disorders and diseases in the future (Shiju et al., 2020). Kutlehria et al. employed a combination of stereolithography, extrusion-based printing, and micro-transfer molding methodologies, yielding the effective fabrication of 3D-printed corneal stromal equivalents (Kutlehria et al., 2020).

2.2.2 Intraocular lenses

Our ability to perceive sight significantly depends on the transparency and refractive characteristics of the tissues comprising the optical pathway responsible for focusing light onto the retina, in conjunction with the ocular environment (Herranz, Herran, 2012). Typically, the eye is simplified as a basic system composed of two refractive components (the cornea and the lens). The cornea, coupled with the tear film overlaying it, contributes roughly two-thirds of the eye's overall optical power, with the lens providing the remainder of the focusing power (Atchison, 2023; Lovicu et al., 2011). Over 95 million people worldwide suffer from cataracts, the primary cause of blindness (Liu et al., 2017). Intraocular lens (IOL) implantation remains the most effective method of combating cataracts (Allen, Vasavada, 2006). Three-dimensional printing presents significant promise within biomedical engineering research and ophthalmological applications, facilitating the creation of cost-effective tools and products tailored for individual cataract patients, notably intraocular lenses designed for therapeutic purposes (Sommer, Blumenthal, 2019). An IOL implanted during cataract surgery must meet certain basic criteria, such as being biocompatible, not causing any surgery or tissue disease, and having excellent optical data for recovery. Although clinical and material degradation of IOLs is rare, replacements such as lens removal have been reported to cause significant degradation. Various types of degradation have been described, including photochemical material degradation, surface degradation, deposition with the IOL material itself, breakage, surface coatings, and color changes. These typically appear to be related to the type of IOL material used or the manufacturing process used to create such implants (Stanojcic et al., 2020).

Advancements in three-dimensional printing of IOLs should focus on processing the ultrafine roughness of the IOL surface at the micro/nano level, ensuring high transparency and UV protection, achieving optimal flexibility, water retention, and micromechanical properties, and guaranteeing the biosafety of the materials (Fang et al., 2023). For ophthalmic usage, PNIPAM has been utilized as a platform for controlled delivery of drugs and has been noted to decrease intraocular pressure following topical or intravitreal administration in vivo. Additionally, employing linear PNIPAAm crosslinked with nanoparticles as a combination has shown a greater reduction in intraocular pressure compared to a linear PNIPAAm system (Zou et al., 2011). Li et al. rapidly fabricated a GAT-loaded IOL based on a bulk synthesized poly (urethane acrylate) (PUA) prepolymer, isobornyl methacrylate (IBOMA), N-vinyl-2-pyrrolidone (NVP), and adjuvants using light-induced curing in a 3D printed mold (Li, 2023). Li et al. assessed the biocompatibility of poly(acrylamide-co-sodium acrylate) hydrogel (PAH) as a material for 3D-printed intraocular lenses (IOLs) and concluded that PAH is a safe material for the 3D printing of personalized IOLs with great potential for future clinical applications (Li, 2020). Zhang et al. reported the success of smooth sidewall contact lens structures using a continuous liquid film-confined 3D printing strategy. By modifying the characteristics of the ink and adjusting the printing settings, it is possible to effectively manage the thickness of the liquid film and the smoothness of the surface in the 3D-printed contact lens structure. Additionally, prolonged continuous printing can be facilitated without excessive heat build-up or poor thermal dissipation, ensuring the stable production of contact lens structures characterized by smooth sidewalls, superior optical properties, uniform material properties, and compatibility with biological systems (Zhang et al., 2022). Alam et al. 3D printed intraocular lenses made of poly-2-hydroxyethyl methacrylate (pHEMA) and polyethylene glycol diacrylate (PEGDA) resin, which provide high transparency, enriched with Atto 565 dye, using a digital light processing (DLP) 3D printer. The lenses were created three-dimensionally by adding the dye to this transparent resin (Alam et al., 2023).

3D printing technology has the potential to overcome complex challenges and play a significant role in sourcing corneal tissues and supply chains. This technology can facilitate the creation of human anterior segment models, leading to a deeper understanding of aqueous physiology and fluid dynamics. Bio-printed ocular anatomy models are being investigated for surgical education and can facilitate problem-based learning. Drug-loaded copolymer intraocular lenses offer a promising alternative approach to prevent postoperative endophthalmitis. Moreover, it is believed that the cost of customized adjustable lenses can be significantly reduced through 3D printing. The benefit of remote printing appears on the horizon; this means that medical personnel can leverage each other's expertise and produce the required 3D materials in their respective fields (Ali, 2023).

2.2.3 Retina

The retina is a complex and light-sensitive layer that plays a critical role in maintaining vision, covers the inner surface of the eyeball and is part of the central nervous system (Singh et al., 2018). The vertebrate retina consists of distinct cellular layers: inner neuroepithelial and outer pigmented epithelial. Between these layers, light-sensitive photoreceptors such as cones and rods carry out visual phototransduction. The light entering the eye reaches the outer parts of the photoreceptors through the passage of the retinal layers, where the photon energy is converted into electrical signals and the vision process is initiated. The retinal pigment epithelium (RPE) is located between the photoreceptors and the choroid and helps increase visual resolution by supporting and insulating the photoreceptors (Strauss, 2005). Photoreceptor cells (PRs) situated in the intermediate strata of the retina are accountable for light perception. Their deterioration can result in blindness in different ailments, such as retinitis pigmentosa and age-related macular degeneration (AMD) (Ballios, 2015).

The utilization of 3D printing technology to reproduce optical coherence tomography angiography (OCTA) scans represents a breakthrough geared towards achieving thorough and dye-free depiction of the retinal, choroidal vasculature and choroidal tumors. In a recent study conducted by Maloca and colleagues, the original OCTA data underwent processing to generate a printable 3D rendition, illustrating the spatial arrangement of vasculature across the inner retinal surface and vertical branches linking to deeper retinal vascular networks (Maloca, 2019; Kador, 2016). 3D printing has the potential to determine cell identities in conjunction with specifically designed radial electrospun scaffolds to detect RGC placement and regulate axon guidance. The effects of thermal inkjet printing using different buffers, ejection energies, and cell distributions on the survival and neurite distribution of polymers RGCs in vitro were examined (Kador, 2016). The inkjet printing technology was explored to investigate whether it could be expanded to print adult rat central nervous systems, retinal ganglion cells (RGC), and glial cells, and its effects on the survival and growth of these cells in culture. It could be a step in developing tissue grafts for regenerative medicine and may aid in the treatment of blindness (Lorber et al., 2013). Clinical management of retinal vascular diseases often requires repeated intravitreal medication due to short effectiveness, resulting in healthcare costs and patient inconvenience. Thus, there is a pressing need for the development of an advanced drug delivery system capable of extending drug activity while minimizing adverse effects. The coaxial printing method enabled the simultaneous release of two distinct drugs within the same area, each exhibiting different release kinetics, achieved by employing a polymeric shell and a hydrogel core, respectively. This innovative printing approach facilitates the production of drug sticks of varying sizes and concentrations, and the multilayer configuration allows for precise modulation of the release profile of the binary drug delivery system (Won et al., 2020).

Recent progress in generating cellular three-dimensional structures has resulted in promising advancements in the fabrication of a three-dimensional printed retina. Furthermore, recent studies have demonstrated that specific types of mammalian retinal cells, including adult rat retinal ganglion cells and glia can be effectively printed without compromising their viability and certain phenotypic characteristics. Additionally, overcoming challenges associated with the creation of a functional three-dimensional printed retina involves addressing issues such as cell density, spatial and functional integration of diverse cell types, and ensuring long-term cell survival within the complex tissue construct. Ultimately, realizing the potential for research and creating implantable 3D printed retinas necessitates substantial engineering refinement, regulatory endeavors, and significant capital investment (Abedin Zadeh et al., 2019).

2.2.4 Orbital bone

Orbital blowout fractures frequently occur as a result of maxillofacial trauma, with the abrupt rise in pressure within the eye socket recognized for causing harm to the thin and fragile walls surrounding it (Al-Sukhun et al., 2005). The primary reasons behind orbital blowout fractures often stem from assaults, motor vehicle accidents, injuries sustained during sports activities, and falls. Complications linked with these fractures encompass double vision, sunken appearance of the eye, and reduced sensation along the infraorbital nerve (Brucoli et al., 2011). The main objective of surgery for orbital fractures is to repair the injured orbital wall and return the orbital volume to normal, thus relieving restricted eye movements (Kochhar, Byrne, 2013). Because of the intricate structure of the orbit, one of the difficulties in conventional reconstructive surgery involves molding and carving accurate implant shapes during the procedure. Furthermore, because of the restricted surgical area, positioning and sculpting implants in orbit can be time-consuming and rely heavily on the expertise and proficiency of the surgeon (Scawn, 2015).

Three-dimensional printing enables the production of physical objects from digital 3D models and allows for customization for medical treatment. In orbital surgery, 3D printing can be employed to produce a replica of the fractured orbit or to generate a mirrored representation of the uninjured orbit on the opposite side (Tack et al., 2016). These models can assist in shaping an orbital implant before surgery to ensure a perfect fit with the patient's anatomy. Furthermore, they can be used to directly fabricate an orbital implant designed on a computer. Although the impact of 3D printing in craniofacial surgery has been studied, there is a lack of comprehensive evidence regarding its role specifically in orbital reconstruction (Park et al., 2015). Some research endeavours propose that 3D printing in orbital reconstruction could address certain constraints associated with conventional surgical methods. Models created via printing, devoid of soft tissue, provide a wider perspective of the fracture area, enabling precise preoperative customization of an implant. Moreover, this customization is no longer part of the intraoperative process, which could potentially decrease the duration of surgery and minimize the necessity for multiple insertions of the implant through delicate soft tissues (Jacobs, Lin, 2017). Vehmeijer et al. devised an uncomplicated and economical technique for manufacturing customized orbital implants. This method involves utilizing computed tomography (CT) imaging and virtual planning, along with 3D-printed molds and autologous bone grafts (Vehmeijer et al., 2016). Manmadhachary et al. reconstructed damaged orbital floor defects via 3D printed implants and transformed the orbital floor to its original shape. Additionally, the designed implants were produced using a biocompatible material 3D printer. Application of the implant with biocompatible material resulted in the production of implants at the minimum cost (Mohan, ve Reddy, 2021).

3D printers offer tailored solutions specific to individual patients' needs in addressing surgical difficulties. The repair of orbital floor damage in two patients with intricate fractures was directed by a customized three-dimensional printed model of the orbital floor defect. Preoperative preparation for orbital floor reconstruction using porous polyethylene was facilitated through the utilization of 3D printing technology readily accessible in the local area (Pang et al., 2018). A novel, individually crafted, 3D-printed supportive implant can be manufactured for the reconstruction of cranial or orbital areas utilizing PMMA. By utilizing data from computed tomography scans processed in Medical Imaging and Communications in Medicine format and transferred to treatment planning software, a three-dimensional master model for the prosthesis was designed and digitally printed. This method was applied to treat five patients with defects in the cranial or orbital regions caused by tumors or trauma. Over a follow-up period of 5-7 years, no complications arose that required removal of the prostheses (Martinez-Seijas et al., 2018). Mourits et al. employed 3D imaging and printing techniques to precisely analyze and calculate the shape of the cysts and the defects they create in the orbital wall. They also successfully used 3D methods to support cystectomy and orbital reconstruction (Mourits et al., 2016). The advent of 3D printing technology allows surgeons to develop an in-depth and objective understanding of the injury situation before surgery, allowing them to plan surgery. Manufacturing prosthetic materials with 3D printers can reduce orbital repair operation time, minimize surgical risk, and increase the accuracy of repairing fracture defects (Chai et al., 2021).

2.2.5 Ocular prostheses

The loss of an eye or a deformed eye has a significant impact on the psychology of the individual. In addition, this situation also affects the person's social and professional life. Aesthetic rehabilitation with personalized prostheses alleviates the problems by giving these people professional and social acceptance (Raizada ve Rani, 2007). Ocular prosthesis treatment aims to correct deformities in the eye socket, provide facial aesthetics, preserve the anophthalmic cavity, correct the direction of tears, and prevent the accumulation of tear fluid in the eye socket (Goiato et al., 2014). Eye prostheses can be found in two different types: stock and custom. Stock ocular prostheses generally come in a variety of standard sizes, lengths, and variations (Choubisa, 2017). They can be used almost anywhere, temporarily or after surgery. Ocular prostheses can be classified in different ways, such as artificial eyes, specially shaped eyes, cosmetic contact shells, cosmetic contact lenses, or spectacle prostheses (Hallikerimath et al., 2009).

3D printing has the potential to assist in creating and manufacturing ocular prostheses for cases of enucleation resulting from ocular cancer and serious traumatic eye injuries. This technology may also be beneficial in the subsequent reconstruction phase. Ruiters et al. have developed a novel approach for producing personalized ocular prostheses using computer-aided design and computer-aided manufacturing techniques. An ocular prosthesis based on three-dimensional (3D) molds of an ophthalmic space has been successfully applied to a 68-dimensional male. To our knowledge, this is the first case of a personalized ocular prosthesis prepared using three-dimensional printing (Ruiters et al., 2016). Sedlak et al. designed and manufactured an aesthetic eye prosthesis prototype based on the 3D model obtained by scanning the acrylic prosthesis and its additive using PolyJet technology (Sedlak et al., 2020). In a clinical study consisting of ten patients, 3D-printed sphere implantation was performed after evisceration. None of the patients encountered issues such as systemic or local toxicity, infection, inflammation, extrusion, or exposure (Kormann et al., 2019).

2.2.6 Punctal plug

Vision is considered one of the most basic sensory experiences of humans (Awwad, 2017). Dry eye syndrome is a prevalent, persistent condition impacting millions globally and poses an escalating public health concern (Uchino A. Schaumberg, 2013). This ailment, stemming from causes like insufficient tear production or heightened evaporation of tear film, may cause inflammation in the cornea and conjunctiva if not addressed. The static and dynamic defences guarding against external substances like pathogens and therapeutic compounds reaching the eye have continually presented hurdles for delivering drugs to the eye. Topical methods, like eye drops, remain the favored approach for delivering therapeutic substances to the front part of the eye, as they reduce systemic side effects, are non-invasive, and are simple to apply. However, the effectiveness of topical applications in the eye is generally low (less than 5%), which results from several factors such as the lack of drug retention in the eye, blinking, high tear flow rate, and nasolacrimal drainage (Gote et al., 2019; A. Patel et al., 2013).

Punctal plugs are a commonly preferred treatment strategy for alleviating dry eye syndromes. These plugs block tear drainage channels connecting the eyes to the nose. Research has shown that occlusion of the punctum improves tear film stability, tear osmolarity, and functional visual acuity in patients with dry eyes. Punctual plugs can generally be easily inserted and removed, while canalicular plugs are less visible and can be more challenging to remove (Ervin et al., 2017; Xie, 2017). Xu et al's. digital light processing (DLP) 3D printing was employed to fabricate dexamethasone-loaded punctal plugs. This research outlines the potential of utilizing DLP 3D printing for directly creating drug-loaded punctal plugs, marking a novel approach with extensive potential in enhancing the delivery of ocular therapies. The manufacturing process is straightforward and accomplished in a single step under mild conditions, contrasting with earlier methods for drug-loaded punctal plugs. In comparison to conventional molding techniques for preparing punctal plugs, DLP 3D printing provides significant flexibility in tailoring the size, shape, and material of the plug to meet the requirements of individual patients (Xu et al., 2021). Effective 3D printed punctal plugs are produced for personalized punctal occlusion and long-term ocular drug delivery for dry eye disease (Khanna et al., 2023). One key benefit of utilizing 3D printed personalized punctal plugs is the customized design and dimensions of the device tailored to the patient's unique punctal size. Another significant advantage of these customized plugs is that, apart from being tailored to individuals, they have a brief printing duration and are cost-efficient (Best et al., 2018). A variety of punctal plugs are available in the market and are not limited to the non-pharmacological treatment of dry eyes but are also preferred in many other ophthalmic diseases. However, there are some limitations in the use of these plugs and regular monitoring is required after placement. Future studies will be important to compare the effectiveness of different types of plugs and evaluate long-term outcomes. New technologies and ongoing research are expected to contribute to the fact that punctal plugs will continue to play an important role in the treatment of various eye diseases (Jehangir et al., 2016).

2.3 Surgical Planning

The utilization of 3D printing technology has supplied an efficient instrument for presurgical modeling, illustrating an entirely distinct viewpoint from conventional fracture mending. Data on anatomy concerning fracture sites are acquired from computed tomography scans and transformed into virtual three-dimensional models employing computer-aided design software. It is then possible to produce appropriate fracture models using special 3D printing techniques, allowing suitable implants to be easily prepared. Additionally, alongside the reduction of implant preparation duration, the precision of shaped implants experiences a notable augmentation. Surgical interventions aided by 3D printing have been extensively employed in clinical investigations to execute orbital reconstruction with greater dependability (Callahan et al., 2017; Oh et al., 2016).

For intricate orbital and periorbital fractures, instances with bone deficiencies and tumors, the three-dimensional printed skull permits the surgeons to acquaint themselves with particular anatomy prior to surgery and empowers them to observe the defect from varying perspectives with tactile feedback (Engel et al., 2015). In this manner, the desired positioning and configuration of surgical incisions, as well as the complexities of orbital bone surgical procedures, can be premeditated and simulated. Moreover, the selection of implants and instrumentation, along with the positioning of screws, can be appraised using the pre-structured and three-dimensionally printed orbit as a navigational tool prior to surgical intervention (Xue, 2019). The principal advantage of 3D printing resides in its capability to fabricate medical structures characterized by considerable diversity in size and morphology. These models offer invaluable assistance in strategizing complex surgical interventions, thereby contributing to enhanced surgical outcomes and a reduction in operative duration. (Mourits et al., 2016). In a study involving six patients who had previously undergone orbital surgery, the use of 3D printing to discuss how customized implants can be tailored to manage the migration (movement away from the center and displacement) of inferotemporal globe orbit implants was discussed (Dave, 2018). Preoperative fabrication of customized titanium mesh based on the production of 3D printed designs reduces surgical time and lowers the risk of surgery. Post-operative CT scans showed that the personalized titanium mesh placed could more accurately repair orbital wall fractures. No patient experienced infection, titanium mesh loosening, prolapse, or rejection (Li-bo et al., 2017). Furdová et al. described a new method for imaging intraocular tumors before stereotactic radiosurgery. Using CT and MRI data, five color eye models were created, each with an estimated suppression time of 15 to 30 minutes. These models included the sclera, cornea, lens, optic nerve, and tumor mass. These 3D models helped doctors better define tumor boundaries, thus contributing to increasing surgical experience and skills to improve clinical outcomes. They can be used before surgery on a real patient (Furdová et al., 2017). In their study Han et al., demonstrated that 3D printing technology allows the rapid preparation of PCL-β-TCP fibrous membranes and customized production is possible according to the shape of the bone defect obtained from CT scan data (Ho Han, 2018). A digital model of the trocar-cannula system for vitreoretinal surgery was generated utilizing computer-aided design (CAD) software and fabricated using a laser sintered 3D printer with modified ABS thermoplastic material. Subsequently, prototypes of the trocar cannula underwent testing in porcine eyes (Navajas et al., 2017).

3. Drug Delivery Systems in 3D printing

A drug product refers to a fully formulated dosage form, exemplified by tablets, capsules, or solutions, containing an active drug ingredient often in combination with inert components. The utilization of three-dimensional (3D) printing in the domain of drug products deals with the production of finalized pharmaceutical entities using active pharmaceutical ingredients and excipients. This departure from the conventional synthesis of drug substances involves a 3D printing methodology that is both computer-controlled and circumvents stepwise processes (Norman et al., 2017). In contrast to conventional pharmaceutical procedures, 3D printing distinguishes itself in terms of product intricacy, adaptability, and performance. The substantial disparities between 3D printing and established pharmaceutical methods present promising prospects for the advancement of drug delivery. A contemporary trend within the domain of 3D printing relates to the utilization of novel materials and the deliberate incorporation of varying material intensities throughout the printing technique. As an example of a 3D printing technique, Material Jetting has been utilized by researchers to successfully produce microparticles for drug delivery purposes (Kim et al., 2011). Recent advancements in this area include the application of 3D printing techniques to silicones (Plott et al., 2018) and stimuli-responsive polymers (Zhang, 2015), highlighting potential implications in the field of drug delivery.

Additive manufacturing, commonly referred to as 3D printing, holds the potential for the fabrication of delivery devices or the corresponding molds employed in their casting processes. Lee et al. direct their attention towards the design, simulation, and fabrication of an implantable ocular drug delivery device (Lee et al., 2012). This device incorporates micro-/nanochannels situated between upper and lower covers, and the drug reservoir is crafted from polydimethylsiloxane (PDMS), a silicone-based organic and biodegradable polymer, utilizing stereolithography (SLA) printing. Their innovative approach extends to the creation of an intravitreal, transscleral-sutured delivery device, incorporating micro- and nanochannels, with the constituent components manufactured through the utilization of 3D-printed molds. In another study, researchers developed a semi-transparent mold using SLA-based 3D printing for the fabrication of a microfluidic device (Kulkarni et al., 2023). This device was seamlessly integrated with a portable and automated thermal management platform, employing soft lithography techniques for nanomicelles. These nanomicelles are recognized as exceptional pharmaceutical carriers due to their small size, effectiveness in minimizing side effects and drug degradation, and improved ability to penetrate the cornea. This innovation holds promise for applications in ocular drug delivery.

With regard to other devices, Kojima et al. explicated their innovative initiatives in formulating a periocular, transscleral, 3D-printed delivery system featuring human retinal pigment epithelium (RPE) cells, ensuring protracted delivery of brain-derived neurotrophic factor to the retinal milieu (Kojima et al., 2020). Leveraging advancements in cell sheet engineering and 3D printing technologies, our research initiatives culminated in the development of a self-sustainable cell-encapsulation device, poised to function as a minimally invasive periocular conduit for the targeted therapeutic intervention in retinal diseases. Another study focused on the formulation of an open-source design and the application of 3D printing to create a proficient model of a punctal plug endowed with an integrated drug delivery system (Khanna et al., 2023). This technological advancement shows potential in addressing diverse ocular conditions requiring recurrent drug administration or necessitating the obstruction of the nasolacrimal pathway. The investigation underscored the prospective advantages associated with 3D printing of punctal plugs incorporating built-in drug delivery systems, especially when customized to individual patients based on their punctum size. This individualized therapeutic strategy holds substantial promise for enhancing therapeutic outcomes in ocular healthcare. It is worth noting that another study identified a 3D-printed refillable drug delivery system (DDS) designed to conform to the curvature of the eyeball (Hori, 2023). This DDS comprises three components: a drug injection port for reloading, a drug release port featuring an aperture for unidirectional release into the sclera, and a drug tank for retention. In vitro evaluations were conducted to assess the sustained release of fluorescein isothiocyanate conjugate (FITC)-albumin, employed as a model drug, from a 20 wt% poly (vinyl alcohol) (PVA) hydrogel positioned at the release port, spanning a period of 200 days. A significant feature of this drug delivery system (DDS) is its ability to be reloaded with drugs without requiring extraction from its implantation site. The assessment also investigated the viability of achieving sustained drug release from the device and examined the feasibility of reloading drugs into the device, along with their stable re-release.

In relation to the surgical devices, Fan et al. conducted a comparative assessment between the clinical outcomes of 3D-assisted orbital reconstructions and conventional surgical approaches (Fan, 2017). Their study highlights the significant utility of the 3D printing technique in accurately predicting fracture zones both before and during personalized surgery. This technological approach proves valuable in enabling surgeons to achieve precise anatomical reconstruction for the repair of blowout orbital fractures. The application of a simulated bone template generated through 3D printing models ensures an authentic orbital reconstruction, leading to reduced surgical duration and improved precision and safety. Moreover, the incorporation of 3D printing techniques facilitates the production of a precisely customized implant based on the size and contour of the artificial bone template, thereby refining the surgical procedure. In addition, Annuryanti et al. aimed to develop an improved delivery system for Triamcinolone acetonide (TA) that extends its release duration while minimizing potential side effects (Annuryanti et al., 2023). The envisioned outcome of this strategy has broader implications, particularly in the context of precision 3D printing of ocular implants. The experimental approach employed a 3D bioprinter to fabricate implants using polycaprolactone (PCL) loaded with TA. Examination of the drug release data revealed that filament-shaped implants demonstrated the highest cumulative drug release among all shapes, showcasing their effectiveness over a 180-day period.

Within the recent landscape of 3D printing technologies, a discernible trend emerges towards the advancement of drug-eluting Implants, with microneedles standing out as an exceptional example for sophisticated drug delivery systems. A recent report indicates that the global market size for microneedle drug delivery systems reached approximately $2.65 billion in 2021, experiencing a subsequent increase to about $2.83 billion in 2022 (Global Microneedle Drug Delivery Systems, 2024). Projections anticipate a substantial expansion in the microneedle market, estimating a value of approximately $7.8 billion by 2027 (Aldawood et al., 2024; Microneedle Drug Delivery Systems, 2024). In this context, 3D-printed hydrogel-based microneedles are gaining considerable attention as a responsive drug-delivery system, particularly attuned to environmental stimuli (Willemen et al., 2021). Microneedles present a straightforward and minimally invasive approach to drug delivery, characterized by a minimal pain sensation. The malleability of microneedle shapes during the 3D printing process, enabling modifications through dissolution, pressure, or UV curing, significantly enhances the precision of drug-eluting implants. Particularly noteworthy are implants integrating biomaterials responsive to intraocular pressure, thereby facilitating the controlled release of drugs aimed at lowering intraocular pressure (IOP). This targeted therapeutic strategy holds considerable promise for the effective treatment of glaucoma (Tan et al., 2022; Lin et al., 2024).

Microneedles find application in drug and vaccine delivery, as well as in diagnostics, and their categorization involves multiple criteria. Predominant classifications consider factors such as geometry, the material employed in system development, fabrication methods, drug loading techniques, and modes of drug delivery (Bhatnagar et al., 2019). In eye drug delivery, four types of microneedles are distinguished based on construction and action: (i) Solid microneedles puncture and form drug channels. Post-penetration, they are removed, and pores are filled with the drug-loaded formulation. (ii) Drug-coated microneedles dissolve on administration, allowing drug diffusion into deeper regions. (iii) Dissolving microneedles release drugs as the matrix dissolves or undergoes hydrolysis. (iv) Hollow microneedles, linked to a pressure-driven unit, propel drug-loaded liquid into the targeted site (Huang et al., 2018; Gadziński, 2022).

The investigation scrutinized the drug release kinetics of microneedle arrays with varying needle quantities (8, 12, and 16) over a four-week period. Results indicated that the microneedle arrays demonstrated a significantly more uniform drug release profile in comparison to singular injections. Specifically, only the 16-needle microneedle array achieved complete release of the loaded drug by the conclusion of the four-week period (Amer, 2020). Building upon prior research, the researchers devised stimuli-sensitive bifunctional hydrogel microneedle arrays. Following application to the ocular region and membrane penetration, the needles underwent swelling, generating a wedging effect. Subsequent to drug release, exposure to UV light (365 nm, 10 mW/m2) for 14 minutes induced a 20% reduction in needle size, facilitating safe removal without causing damage to the eye. The microneedle matrix comprised a blend of polyvinyl alcohol (PVA) and spiropyran-conjugated N-isopropylacrylamide (NIPPAM) (Amer, 2022). In an alternative research endeavor, the objective is to formulate bilayer dissolving microneedle (MN) arrays incorporating nanoparticles (NPs) to achieve sustained and minimally invasive delivery of protein drugs. Poly(lactic-co-glycolic acid) (PLGA) NPs, encapsulating ovalbumin (OVA) and prepared through a water-in-oil-in-water (W/O/W) double emulsion method, were subject to optimization. The investigation systematically assessed the influence of stabilizers and the duration of primary sonication on the stability of encapsulated OVA, employing an enzyme-linked immunosorbent assay (ELISA). The outcomes revealed that a reduction in primary sonication time effectively prolonged the release, extending it to 77 days with a 28.5% OVA loading. (Wu, 2021). As elucidated in this chapter, the adoption of 3D printing technology for the development of specific drug delivery systems within the field of ophthalmology emerges as a promising avenue. Furthermore, leveraging this technology to fabricate artificial tissues closely mirroring native structures proves instrumental in the screening of novel drugs targeting ocular diseases. Nevertheless, for the widespread integration of this technology into clinical settings, various regulatory considerations must be thoroughly addressed.

4. Challenges Encountered in 3D Printing Applications

Dealing with ocular diseases, particularly those impacting deeper ocular tissues, presents challenges stemming from restricted accessibility and inherent anatomical and physiological barriers within the eye. Conventional therapeutic modalities, including topical formulations such as eye drops and gels, as well as systemic interventions, frequently confront issues of limited drug bioavailability, leading to inefficacy in treatment outcomes. The integration of 3D printing has emerged as a transformative tool, offering potential solutions to overcome these challenges in ocular disease treatment. In navigating the intersection of health and financial resources, ethical challenges arise. The technological capacity to bioprint and transplant organs or tissues as an alternative treatment for advanced diseases introduces the possibility of societal stratification. While components such as bioinks and 3D bioprinting may not individually incur exorbidant expenses, the overall high costs are influenced by the multidisciplinary nature of the process. This approach may be economically unfeasible for the entire spectrum of society, limiting access to a subgroup with financial means. Bio-impression for organ creation may only be accessible to those financing such procedures, potentially affording them an extended and enhanced quality of life. This could reduce dependence on immune-suppressant drugs for organ rejections. The prospect of implanting engineered organs or tissues with superior biological properties extends beyond disease treatment, offering enhanced physiological performance. This could lead to the development of "super" bio-items aligned with eugenic objectives, such as exceptionally high-performing eyes or retinas (Arslan-Yildiz, 2016; Ruiz-alonso, 2021).

In the field of ocular applications, the improvement of 3D printing material properties is crucial. Initial research is needed to develop biocompatible materials for ocular devices, requiring comprehensive safety studies before clinical implementation. Optimal materials for ocular prostheses are anticipated to exhibit qualities such as non-immunogenicity, customizable transparency, flexibility, and mechanical resilience. Subsequent investigations should focus on assessing long-term complications and the impact on patients' quality of life. Conventional polymeric materials frequently employed in 3D printing are frequently characterized by insufficient softness and flexibility, resulting in challenges when attempting to faithfully reproduce the dynamic and fluidic properties inherent to ocular tissues. To facilitate precise training in surgical simulation and dissection models, biomimetic materials with customizable directional strength are necessary. For cases requiring structural implants with uniformity, consideration of anisotropy associated with techniques like FDM printing is vital. Alternatively, isotropic printing techniques such as SLA may be preferable for consistent directional properties. Concurrent development of composite scaffolds and stimuli-responsive biomaterials, facilitating tissue remodelling, holds promise for future advancements in ocular bioprinting (Lin et al., 2024; Kador, 2016; Mao, 2020; Wang, 2018).

Another challenge associated with the utilization of 3D bioprinting in the pharmaceutical sector stem from various technique printing parameters. These include factors such as slow printing speed, which can impede efficiency, as well as issues related to clogging and lower resolution, which may compromise the precision and quality of printed structures. Furthermore, challenges arise from the rheological properties of biomaterials, which can affect the printability and structural integrity of the final product. Moreover, the requirement for high temperatures in certain 3D printing processes or biomaterial sterilization methods may not be conducive to maintaining the stability and efficacy of drug formulations embedded within the biomaterial matrix. Thus, these considerations underscore the need for careful optimization and innovation to address the technical challenges associated with 3D bioprinting in pharmaceutical applications.

Beyond the difficulties associated with attaining a sophisticated bio-printed construct comparable to native tissues, a crucial aspect for clinical application revolves around the establishment of vascularization and innervation in tissue-engineered constructs subsequent to transplantation. Currently, the majority of 3D-printed tissues exhibit a deficiency in a functional vascular network, impeding the supply of oxygen and nutrients post-implantation. Approaches aimed at mitigating this challenge encompass the incorporation of angiogenic growth factors, integration of microchannels to enhance diffusion, and the direct fabrication of vasculature. (Murphy et al., 2020). Nevertheless, the replication of the intricate vascular network essential for clinical applicability poses a formidable challenge. In the context of ocular tissues, the successful bioprinting of a comprehensive ocular structure precedes the consideration of vascularization and innervation. Particularly in the retina, a pivotal component responsible for converting light signals into electrical impulses, the attainment of functional electrophysiological properties in bio-printed retinal ganglion cells represents a significant step forward in the development of prospective retinal constructs. (Kador et al., 2016). The fundamental goal of these constructs is to foster pertinent cellular connections across various retinal layers, thereby supporting the intricate process of visual phototransduction.

5.   Conclusion and Future Prospects

Over the last decade, 3D printing has exhibited a diverse array of applications in eye treatment. This technology enables the precise modelling of eye anatomy, facilitating surgical planning and the creation of custom-fit implants or devices within the field of oculoplastic surgery. Additionally, 3D printing has found utility in the design of surgical instruments, diagnostic tools, drug delivery devices, and elements constituting personal protective equipment. The rapid advancement of 3D printing technology has resulted in widespread accessibility, albeit with significant variations in equipment design and quality. Even in instances where equipment may be unavailable or lacks adequate quality, designers can overcome these limitations by uploading their three-dimensional files to third-party services for outsourced printing. This chapter underscores the pivotal role of 3D printing in democratizing access to manufacturing capabilities and ensuring the broader applicability of this technology in various fields, including eye treatment. The versatility of 3D printing not only facilitates innovation but also promotes inclusivity by allowing diverse users to harness its potential, transcending limitations posed by equipment availability or quality constraints.

While the application of 3D printing technology in eye treatment holds the promise of diminishing the need for animal testing, the transformative concept of printing ocular tissues and potentially entire organs introduces ethical and regulatory concerns that require thorough examination. The profound implications of utilizing 3D printing for eye-related tissues and organ fabrication underscore the necessity for indepth assessments within ethical and regulatory frameworks. This ensures that advancements in ocular treatment align with responsibly and ethically sound practices. Recent advancements in 3D printing, especially within ocular tissue engineering, exhibit potential for prospective biomedical applications. Nevertheless, several formidable challenges must be surmounted before clinical translation becomes viable. The intricate task of replicating organ complexity and heterogeneity, encompassing diverse functional and supporting cell types, alongside the integration of vital components such as vasculature and innervation, presents formidable obstacles. The recent ability to recreate intricate ocular structures using advanced techniques like bioprinting has revolutionized training, pre-operative planning, and surgical efficiency in ophthalmology. Bioprinting allows for the fabrication of 3D-printed ocular tissues, holding significant potential for regenerative treatments of corneal, retinal, and conjunctival diseases. However, achieving greater complexity, ensuring biocompatibility of materials, and standardizing protocols at cost-effective levels remain key challenges to fully unlock the potential of this technology. Anticipated advancements in 3D printing technology offer promising solutions to overcome these hurdles and benefit patients further. Continuous collaboration between clinicians, scientists, engineers, and industry partners is crucial for addressing these challenges and seamlessly integrating 3D printing into routine clinical practice. The synergy between 3D printing and ophthalmology presents exciting opportunities for improved patient care, enhanced surgical precision, and advancements in medical education. As this field rapidly evolves, the adoption of 3D printing technologies is poised to significantly shape the future of ophthalmic innovation and progress in ocular health.

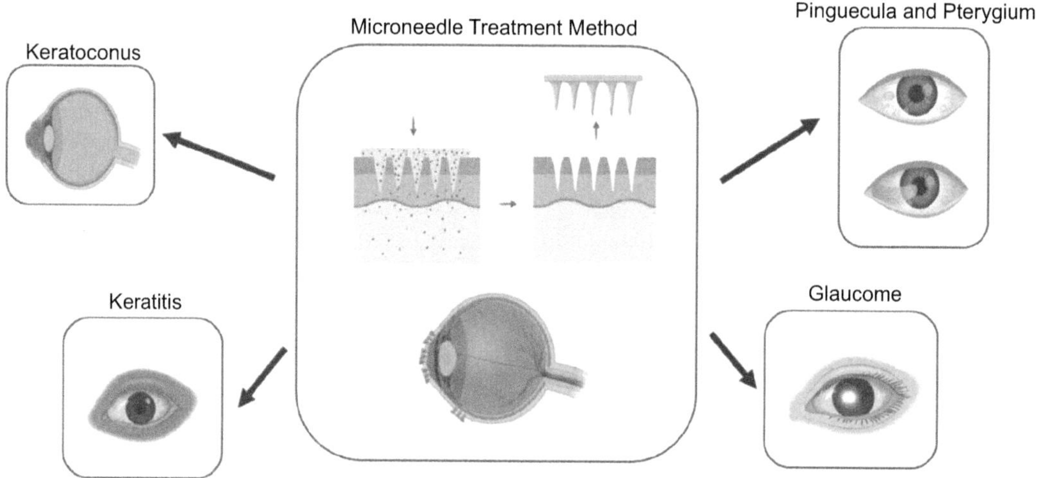

Fig. 3   Microneedle drug-eluting implants designed for the treatment of Keratoconus, Keratitis, Glaucoma, Pinguecula, and Pterygium.

In summary, 3D printing stands as a vital manufacturing method for personalized items like orbital implants, ocular prostheses, surgical instruments, and optical devices. Its evolution has significantly enhanced surgical planning, simulation, training, and educational practices in ophthalmology. The increasing adoption of this technology among ophthalmologists and other clinicians in the near future (Fakhoury et al., 2022). 3D printing advancements hold promise for printing viable ocular tissues, offering potential solutions for corneas, retinas, and surgical devices. The prospect of creating a functional retina for treating blindness appears attainable, emphasizing the need for continuous improvement in technologies, materials, and new printing equipment. Additionally, the potential approach of 4D printing and tissue regeneration holds exciting prospects, including applications in implants, medical devices, artificial corneas, and intricate surgeries. 4D printing involves using hydrogel, responsive to environmental stimuli, to create drug delivery systems such as microneedles (Willemen, 2021). These 4D printed microneedles can dynamically alter their shapes through dissolving, bending, and UV curing, enhancing cell adhesion. Such alterations hold potential for the development of drug-eluting implants. In future, these innovative designs utilizing 4D printing technologies can particularly advance ophthalmic applications, specifically drug-eluting implants for the treatment of Keratoconus, Keratitis, Glaucoma, Pinguecula, and Pterygium (Figure 3).

References

A.A. Gingras *vd.*, "3D Bioprinting of Acellular Corneal Stromal Scaffolds with a Low Cost Modified 3D Printer: A Feasibility Study", *Current Eye Research*, c. 48, sy 12, ss. 1112–1121, Ara. 2023, doi: 10.1080/02713683.2023.2251172.

A. Aimar, A. Palermo, ve B. Innocenti, "The Role of 3D Printing in Medical Applications: A State of the Art", *Journal of Healthcare Engineering*, c. 2019, s. e5340616, Mar. 2019, doi: 10.1155/2019/5340616.

A. Arslan-Yildiz *vd.*, "Accessible bioprinting: adaptation of a low-cost 3D-printer for precise cell placement and stem cell differentiation", *Biofabrication*, c. 8, sy 2, s. 025017, Haz. 2016, doi: 10.1088/1758-5090/8/2/025017.

A.B. Callahan, A.A. Campbell, C. Petris, ve M. Kazim, "Low-Cost 3D Printing Orbital Implant Templates in Secondary Orbital Reconstructions", *Ophthalmic Plastic and Reconstructive Surgery*, c. 33, sy 5, ss. 376-380, Eyl. 2017, doi: 10.1097/IOP.0000000000000884.

A.C. Sommer ve E.Z. Blumenthal, "Implementations of 3D printing in ophthalmology", *Graefes Arch Clin Exp Ophthalmol*, c. 257, sy 9, ss. 1815–1822, Eyl. 2019, doi: 10.1007/s00417-019-04312-3.

A. Farasatkia, M. Kharaziha, F. Ashrafizadeh, ve S. Salehi, "Transparent silk/gelatin methacrylate (GelMA) fibrillar film for corneal regeneration", *Materials Science and Engineering: C*, c. 120, s. 111744, Oca. 2021, doi: 10.1016/j.msec.2020.111744.

A. Furdová, M. Sramka, A. Thurzo, ve A. Furdová, "Early experiences of planning stereotactic radiosurgery using 3D printed models of eyes with uveal melanomas", *Clinical Ophthalmology*, c. 11, ss. 267–271, Oca. 2017, doi: 10.2147/OPTH.S123640.

A. Isaacson, S. Swioklo, ve C.J. Connon, "3D bioprinting of a corneal stroma equivalent", *Experimental Eye Research*, c. 173, ss. 188–193, Ağu. 2018, doi: 10.1016/j.exer.2018.05.010.

A.J. Aldave, K.M. Kamal, R.C. Vo, ve F. Yu, "The Boston Type I Keratoprosthesis: Improving Outcomes and Expanding Indications", *Ophthalmology*, c. 116, sy 4, ss. 640–651, Nis. 2009, doi: 10.1016/j.ophtha.2008.12.058.

A.K. Miri *vd.*, "Effective bioprinting resolution in tissue model fabrication", *Lab Chip*, c. 19, sy 11, ss. 2019–2037, May. 2019, doi: 10.1039/C8LC01037D.

A.K. Sahi, N. Varshney, S. Poddar, S. Gundu, ve S.K. Mahto et al, "Fabrication and Characterization of Silk Fibroin-Based Nanofibrous Scaffolds Supplemented with Gelatin for Corneal Tissue Engineering", *Cells Tissues Organs*, c. 210, sy 3, ss. 173–194, Tem. 2021, doi: 10.1159/000515946.

A. Kochhar ve P.J. Byrne, "Surgical Management of Complex Midfacial Fractures", *Otolaryngologic Clinics of North America*, c. 46, sy 5, ss. 759–778, Eki. 2013, doi: 10.1016/j.otc.2013.06.002.

A.L. Onugwu *vd.*, "Nanotechnology based drug delivery systems for the treatment of anterior segment eye diseases", *Journal of Controlled Release*, c. 354, ss. 465–488, Şub. 2023, doi: 10.1016/j.jconrel.2023.01.018.

A. Patel, K. Cholkar, V. Agrahari, ve A.K. Mitra, "Ocular drug delivery systems: An overview", *World J Pharmacol*, c. 2, sy 2, ss. 47–64, 2013, doi: 10.5497/wjp.v2.i2.47.

A. Sorkio *vd.*, "Human stem cell based corneal tissue mimicking structures using laser-assisted 3D bioprinting and functional bioinks", *Biomaterials*, c. 171, ss. 57–71, Tem. 2018, doi: 10.1016/j.biomaterials.2018.04.034.

A. Zamboulis *vd.*, "Chitosan and its Derivatives for Ocular Delivery Formulations: Recent Advances and Developments", *Polymers*, c. 12, sy 7, Art. sy 7, Tem. 2020, doi: 10.3390/polym12071519.

A.-L. Best, M. Labctoulle, M. Legrand, M. M'garrech, E. Barreau, ve A. Rousseau, "[Punctal and canalicular plugs: Indications, efficacy and safety (French translation of the article)]", *J Fr Ophtalmol*, c. 42, sy 4, ss. 404–414, Nis. 2019, doi: 10.1016/j.jfo.2018.10.003.

A.-M. Ervin, A. Law, ve A. D. Pucker, "Punctal occlusion for dry eye syndrome", *Cochrane Database of Systematic Reviews*, sy 6, 2017, doi: 10.1002/14651858.CD006775.pub3.

B.D. Lawrence, J.K. Marchant, M.A. Pindrus, F.G. Omenetto, ve D.L. Kaplan et al., "Silk film biomaterials for cornea tissue engineering", *Biomaterials*, c. 30, sy 7, ss. 1299–1308, Mar. 2009, doi: 10.1016/j.biomaterials.2008.11.018.

B. Fan *vd.*, "Clinical effects of 3-D printing-assisted personalized reconstructive surgery for blowout orbital fractures", *Graefe's Archive for Clinical and Experimental Ophthalmology*, c. 255, sy 10, ss. 2051–2057, Eki. 2017, doi: 10.1007/S00417-017-3766-Y/FIGURES/6.

B.G. Ballios *vd.*, "A Hyaluronan-Based Injectable Hydrogel Improves the Survival and Integration of Stem Cell Progeny following Transplantation", *Stem Cell Reports*, c. 4, sy 6, ss. 1031–1045, Haz. 2015, doi: 10.1016/j.stemcr.2015.04.008.

B.H. Kim, S. Il Kim, J.C. Lee, S.J. Shin, ve S.J. Kim et al., "Dynamic characteristics of a piezoelectric driven inkjet printhead fabricated using MEMS technology", *Sensors and Actuators, A: Physical*, c. 173, sy 1, ss. 244–253, Oca. 2012, doi: 10.1016/J.SNA.2011.10.010.

B. He *vd.*, "3D printed biomimetic epithelium/stroma bilayer hydrogel implant for corneal regeneration", *Bioactive Materials*, c. 17, ss. 234–247, Kas. 2022, doi: 10.1016/j.bioactmat.2022.01.034.

B. Lorber, W.-K. Hsiao, I.M. Hutchings, ve K.R. Martin, "Adult rat retinal ganglion cells and glia can be printed by piezoelectric inkjet printing", *Biofabrication*, c. 6, sy 1, s. 015001, Ara. 2013, doi: 10.1088/1758-5082/6/1/015001.

B.P. Chan ve K.W. Leong, "Scaffolding in tissue engineering: general approaches and tissue-specific considerations", *Eur Spine J*, c. 17, sy 4, ss. 467–479, Ara. 2008, doi: 10.1007/s00586-008-0745-3.

B. Zhang *vd.*, "3D bioprinting for artificial cornea: Challenges and perspectives", *Medical Engineering & Physics*, c. 71, ss. 68–78, Eyl. 2019, doi: 10.1016/j.medengphy.2019.05.002.

Bloom J., "Anatomy, Head and Neck: Eye Iris Sphincter Muscle", *StatPearls*, 2023.

C.A. Jacobs ve A.Y. Lin, "A New Classification of Three-Dimensional Printing Technologies: Systematic Review of Three-Dimensional Printing for Patient-Specific Craniomaxillofacial Surgery", *Plastic and Reconstructive Surgery*, c. 139, sy 5, ss. 1211–1220, May. 2017, doi: 10.1097/PRS.0000000000003232.

C.E. Ghezzi, J. Rnjak-Kovacina, ve D.L. Kaplan, "Corneal Tissue Engineering: Recent Advances and Future Perspectives", *Tissue Engineering Part B: Reviews*, c. 21, sy 3, ss. 278–287, Haz. 2015, doi: 10.1089/ten.teb.2014.0397.

C.M. O'Brien, B. Holmes, S. Faucett, ve L.G. Zhang, "Three-Dimensional Printing of Nanomaterial Scaffolds for Complex Tissue Regeneration", *Tissue Engineering Part B: Reviews*, c. 21, sy 1, ss. 103–114, Şub. 2015, doi: 10.1089/ten.teb.2014.0168.

C.P. Sharma, *Biointegration of Medical Implant Materials*. Woodhead Publishing, 2019.

C.R. McLaughlin *vd.*, "Regeneration of functional nerves within full thickness collagen–phosphorylcholine corneal substitute implants in guinea pigs", *Biomaterials*, c. 31, sy 10, ss. 2770–2778, Nis. 2010, doi: 10.1016/j.biomaterials.2009.12.031.

C.W. Brooks, "The Ophthalmic Assistant: A Text for Allied and Associated Ophthalmic Personnel, 8th ed.", *Optometry and Vision Science*, c. 84, sy 3, s. 162, Mar. 2007, doi: 10.1097/01.opx.0000258437.13457.32.

D. Allen ve A. Vasavada, "Cataract and surgery for cataract", *BMJ*, c. 333, sy 7559, ss. 128–132, Tem. 2006, doi: 10.1136/bmj.333.7559.128.

D. Atchison, *Optics of the Human Eye*, 2. bs. Boca Raton: CRC Press, 2023. doi: 10.1201/9781003128601.

D.B. Jones, R. Sung, C. Weinberg, T. Korelitz, ve R. Andrews et al., "Three-Dimensional Modeling May Improve Surgical Education and Clinical Practice", *Surg Innov*, c. 23, sy 2, ss. 189–195, Nis. 2016, doi: 10.1177/1553350615607641.

D. Choubisa, "A simplified approach to rehabilitate an ocular defect: Ocular prosthesis", *J Indian Prosthodont Soc*, c. 17, sy 1, ss. 89–94, 2017, doi: 10.4103/0972-4052.179260.

D. Huang, Y.S. Chen, ve I.D. Rupenthal, "Overcoming ocular drug delivery barriers through the use of physical forces", *Advanced Drug Delivery Reviews*, c. 126, ss. 96–112, Şub. 2018, doi: 10.1016/J.ADDR.2017.09.008.

D.L. Mourits *vd.*, "3D Orbital Reconstruction in a Patient with Microphthalmos and a Large Orbital Cyst—A Case Report", *Ophthalmic Genetics*, c. 37, sy 2, ss. 233–237, Nis. 2016, doi: 10.3109/13816810.2015.1033558.

D.L. Nickla ve J. Wallman, "The multifunctional choroid", *Progress in Retinal and Eye Research*, c. 29, sy 2, ss. 144–168, Mar. 2010, doi: 10.1016/j.preteyeres.2009.12.002.

D. Purves *vd.*, "Neurotransmission in the Visceral Motor System", içinde *Neuroscience. 2nd edition*, Sinauer Associates, 2001. Erişim: 18 Şubat 2024. [Çevrimiçi]. Erişim adresi: https://www.ncbi.nlm.nih.gov/books/NBK10854/

D.T. Tan, J.K. Dart, E.J. Holland, ve S. Kinoshita, "Corneal transplantation", *The Lancet*, c. 379, sy 9827, ss. 1749–1761, May. 2012, doi: 10.1016/S0140-6736(12)60437-1.

E. Altinkurt, N.A. Ceylan, U. Altunoglu, ve G.T. Turgut, "Manufacture of custom-made spectacles using three-dimensional printing technology", *Clinical and Experimental Optometry*, c. 103, sy 6, ss. 902–904, Kas. 2020, doi: 10.1111/cxo.13038.

E.V. Navajas ve M. ten Hove, "Three-Dimensional Printing of a Transconjunctival Vitrectomy Trocar-Cannula System", *Ophthalmologica*, c. 237, sy 2, ss. 119–122, Mar. 2017, doi: 10.1159/000457807.

"Effects of Ultra High Molecular Weight Poly-γ-glutamic Acid from Bacillus subtilis (chungkookjang) on Corneal Wound Healing -Journal of Microbiology and Biotechnology | Korea Science". Erişim: 07 Şubat 2024. [Çevrimiçi]. Erişim adresi: https://koreascience.kr/article/JAKO201018860404901.page

F. Akter, "Chapter 5 - Ophthalmic Tissue Engineering", içinde *Tissue Engineering Made Easy*, F. Akter, Ed., Academic Press, 2016, ss. 43-54. doi: 10.1016/B978-0-12-805361-4.00005-9.

F. Alam, M. Ali, M. Elsherif, A.E. Salih, N. El-Atab et al., "3D printed intraocular lens for managing the color blindness", *Additive Manufacturing Letters*, c. 5, s. 100129, Nis. 2023, doi: 10.1016/j.addlet.2023.100129.

F. Annuryanti, J. Domínguez-Robles, Q.K. Anjani, M.F. Adrianto, E. Larrañeta et al., "Fabrication and Characterisation of 3D-Printed Triamcinolone Acetonide-Loaded Polycaprolactone-Based Ocular Implants", *Pharmaceutics*, c. 15, sy 1, s. 243, Oca. 2023, doi: 10.3390/PHARMACEUTICS15010243/S1.

F.J. Lovicu, J. W. McAvoy, ve R.U. de Iongh, "Understanding the role of growth factors in embryonic development: insights from the lens", *Philosophical Transactions of the Royal Society B: Biological Sciences*, c. 366, sy 1568, ss. 1204–1218, Nis. 2011, doi: 10.1098/rstb.2010.0339.

F.K. Aldawood, S.K. Parupelli, A. Andar, ve S. Desai, "3D Printing of Biodegradable Polymeric Microneedles for Transdermal Drug Delivery Applications", *Pharmaceutics 2024, Vol. 16, Page 237*, c. 16, sy 2, s. 237, Şub. 2024, doi: 10.3390/PHARMACEUTICS16020237.

F. Li vd., "Recruitment of multiple cell lines by collagen-synthetic copolymer matrices in corneal regeneration", *Biomaterials*, c. 26, sy 16, ss. 3093–3104, Haz. 2005, doi: 10.1016/j.biomaterials.2004.07.063.

F. Rüfer, A. Schröder, ve C. Erb, "White-to-White Corneal Diameter: Normal Values in Healthy Humans Obtained With the Orbscan II Topography System", *Cornea*, c. 24, sy 3, s. 259, Nis. 2005, doi: 10.1097/01.ico.0000148312.01805.53.

G. Chai, D. Zhang, W. Hua, J. Yin, Y. Jin et al., "Theoretical model of pediatric orbital trapdoor fractures and provisional personalized 3D printing-assisted surgical solution", *Bioactive Materials*, c. 6, sy 2, ss. 559–567, Şub. 2021, doi: 10.1016/j.bioactmat.2020.08.029.

"Global Microneedle Drug Delivery Systems Market Size and Forecast to 2030". Erişim: 09 Şubat 2024. [Çevrimiçi]. Erişim adresi: https://www.skyquestt.com/report/microneedle-drug-delivery-systems-market

G. Tan, N. Ioannou, E. Mathew, A.D. Tagalakis, D.A. Lamprou et al., "3D printing in Ophthalmology: From medical implants to personalised medicine", *International Journal of Pharmaceutics*, c. 625, s. 122094, Eyl. 2022, doi: 10.1016/J.IJPHARM.2022.122094.

H. Ho Han vd., "Orbital wall reconstruction in rabbits using 3D printed polycaprolactone-β-tricalcium phosphate thin membrane", *Materials Letters*, c. 218, ss. 280–284, May. 2018, doi: 10.1016/j.matlet.2018.01.121.

H. Kim vd., "Shear-induced alignment of collagen fibrils using 3D cell printing for corneal stroma tissue engineering", *Biofabrication*, c. 11, sy 3, s. 035017, May. 2019, doi: 10.1088/1758-5090/ab1a8b.

H. Kojima, B. Raut, L.J. Chen, N. Nagai, T. Abe et al., "A 3D Printed Self-Sustainable Cell-Encapsulation Drug Delivery Device for Periocular Transplant-Based Treatment of Retinal Degenerative Diseases", *Micromachines 2020, Vol. 11, Page 436*, c. 11, sy 4, s. 436, Nis. 2020, doi: 10.3390/MI11040436.

H. Mao vd., "Recent advances and challenges in materials for 3D bioprinting", *Progress in Natural Science: Materials International*, c. 30, sy 5, ss. 618–634, Eki. 2020, doi: 10.1016/J.PNSC.2020.09.015.

I.K. Cingesar, M.-P. Marković, ve D. Vrsaljko, "Effect of post-processing conditions on polyacrylate materials used in stereolithography", *Additive Manufacturing*, c. 55, s. 102813, Tem. 2022, doi: 10.1016/j.addma.2022.102813.

J. Al-Sukhun, C. Lindqvist, ve R. Kontio, "Modelling of orbital deformation using finite-element analysis", *Journal of The Royal Society Interface*, c. 3, sy 7, ss. 255–262, Eyl. 2005, doi: 10.1098/rsif.2005.0084.

J.K.S. Tsui, S. Bell, L. da Cruz, A.D. Dick, ve M.S. Sagoo et al., "Applications of three-dimensional printing in ophthalmology", *Survey of Ophthalmology*, c. 67, sy 4, ss. 1287–1310, Tem. 2022, doi: 10.1016/j.survophthal.2022.01.004.

J. Norman, R.D. Madurawe, C.M.V. Moore, M.A. Khan, ve A. Khairuzzaman, "A new chapter in pharmaceutical manufacturing: 3D-printed drug products", *Advanced Drug Delivery Reviews*, c. 108, ss. 39–50, Oca. 2017, doi: 10.1016/J.ADDR.2016.03.001.

J.P. Lichtenberger, P.S. Tatum, S. Gada, M. Wyn, V.B. Ho et al., "Using 3D Printing (Additive Manufacturing) to Produce Low Cost Simulation Models for Medical Training", *Military Medicine*, c. 183, sy suppl_1, ss. 73–77, Mar. 2018, doi: 10.1093/milmed/usx142.

J. Plott, X. Tian, ve A.J. Shih, "Voids and tensile properties in extrusion-based additive manufacturing of moisture-cured silicone elastomer", *Additive Manufacturing*, c. 22, ss. 606–617, Ağu. 2018, doi: 10.1016/J.ADDMA.2018.06.010.

J. Sedlak, O. Vocilka, M. Slany, J. Chladil, A. Polzer et al., "Design and Production of Eye Prosthesis Using 3d Printing", *MM Science Journal*, ss. 3806-3812, Mar. 2020, doi: 10.17973/MMSJ.2020_03_2019127.

J. Xie vd., "A new strategy to sustained release of ocular drugs by one-step drug-loaded microcapsule manufacturing in hydrogel punctal plugs", *Graefes Arch Clin Exp Ophthalmol*, c. 255, sy 11, ss. 2173–2184, Kas. 2017, doi: 10.1007/s00417-017-3755-1.

J.Y. NIEDERKORN, "Immunology and Immunomodulation of Corneal Transplantation", *International Reviews of Immunology*, c. 21, sy 2-3, ss. 173–196, Oca. 2002, doi: 10.1080/08830180212064.

J.Y. Won vd., "3D printing of drug-loaded multi-shell rods for local delivery of bevacizumab and dexamethasone: A synergetic therapy for retinal vascular diseases", *Acta Biomaterialia*, c. 116, ss. 174–185, Eki. 2020, doi: 10.1016/j.actbio.2020.09.015.

J.-H. Lee, R.M. Pidaparti, G.M. Atkinson, ve R.S. Moorthy, "Design of an Implantable Device for Ocular Drug Delivery", *Journal of Drug Delivery*, c. 2012, 2012, doi: 10.1155/2012/527516.

J.-W. Li vd., "Biosafety of a 3D-printed intraocular lens made of a poly(acrylamide-co-sodium acrylate) hydrogel in vitro and in vivo", *Int J Ophthalmol*, c. 13, sy 10, ss. 1521–1530, Eki. 2020, doi: 10.18240/ijo.2020.10.03.

J.-Y. Lai ve Y.-T. Li, "Functional Assessment of Cross-Linked Porous Gelatin Hydrogels for Bioengineered Cell Sheet Carriers", *Biomacromolecules*, c. 11, sy 5, ss. 1387–1397, May. 2010, doi: 10.1021/bm100213f.

K.E. Kador *vd.*, "Control of Retinal Ganglion Cell Positioning and Neurite Growth: Combining 3D Printing with Radial Electrospun Scaffolds", *Tissue Engineering Part A*, c. 22, sy 3-4, ss. 286–294, Şub. 2016, doi: 10.1089/ten.tea.2015.0373.

K.E. Kador *vd.*, "Control of Retinal Ganglion Cell Positioning and Neurite Growth: Combining 3D Printing with Radial Electrospun Scaffolds", *Tissue Engineering - Part A*, c. 22, sy 3-4, ss. 286–294, Şub. 2016, doi: 10.1089/TEN.TEA.2015.0373.

K. Raizada ve D. Rani, "Ocular prosthesis", *Contact Lens and Anterior Eye*, c. 30, sy 3, ss. 152–162, Tem. 2007, doi: 10.1016/j.clae.2007.01.002.

K.Y. Wu, M. Joly-Chevrier, D. Akbar, ve S.D. Tran, "Overcoming Treatment Challenges in Posterior Segment Diseases with Biodegradable Nano-Based Drug Delivery Systems", *Pharmaceutics*, c. 15, sy 4, Art. sy 4, Nis. 2023, doi: 10.3390/pharmaceutics15041094.

L. Balters ve S. Reichl, "3D bioprinting of corneal models: A review of the current state and future outlook", *J Tissue Eng*, c. 14, s. 20417314231197793, Oca. 2023, doi: 10.1177/20417314231197793.

L. Liu ve H. Sheardown, "Glucose permeable poly (dimethyl siloxane) poly (N-isopropyl acrylamide) interpenetrating networks as ophthalmic biomaterials", *Biomaterials*, c. 26, sy 3, ss. 233–244, Oca. 2005, doi: 10.1016/j.biomaterials.2004.02.025.

L. Zou, A. Nair, H. Weng, Y.-T. Tsai, Z. Hu et al., "Intraocular Pressure Changes: An Important Determinant of the Biocompatibility of Intravitreous Implants", *PLOS ONE*, c. 6, sy 12, s. e28720, Ara. 2011, doi: 10.1371/journal.pone.0028720.

M.A, A. Mohan A, ve H. Reddy M, "Manufacturing of customized implants for orbital fractures using 3D printing", *Bioprinting*, c. 21, s. e00118, Mar. 2021, doi: 10.1016/j.bprint.2020.e00118.

M. Abedin Zadeh, M. Khoder, A.A. Al-Kinani, H.M. Younes, ve R.G. Alany et al., "Retinal cell regeneration using tissue engineered polymeric scaffolds", *Drug Discovery Today*, c. 24, sy 8, ss. 1669–1678, Ağu. 2019, doi: 10.1016/j.drudis.2019.04.009.

M. Aghamirsalim *vd.*, "3D Printed Hydrogels for Ocular Wound Healing", *Biomedicines*, c. 10, sy 7, Art. sy 7, Tem. 2022, doi: 10.3390/biomedicines10071562.

M. Ahearne, J. Fernández-Pérez, S. Masterton, P.W. Madden, ve P. Bhattacharjee et al., "Designing Scaffolds for Corneal Regeneration", *Advanced Functional Materials*, c. 30, sy 44, s. 1908996, 2020, doi: 10.1002/adfm.201908996.

M. Alaminos *vd.*, "Construction of a Complete Rabbit Cornea Substitute Using a Fibrin-Agarose Scaffold", *Investigative Ophthalmology & Visual Science*, c. 47, sy 8, ss. 3311-3317, Ağu. 2006, doi: 10.1167/iovs.05-1647.

M. Amer ve R.K. Chen, "Hydrogel-Forming Microneedle Arrays for Sustained and Controlled Ocular Drug Delivery", *Journal of Engineering and Science in Medical Diagnostics and Therapy*, c. 3, sy 4, Kas. 2020, doi: 10.1115/1.4048481.

M. Amer, X. Ni, M. Xian, ve R.K. Chen, "Photo-Responsive Hydrogel Microneedles With Interlocking Control for Easy Extraction in Sustained Ocular Drug Delivery", *Journal of Engineering and Science in Medical Diagnostics and Therapy*, c. 5, sy 1, Şub. 2022, doi: 10.1115/1.4052627.

M.B. Kulkarni, K. Velmurugan, J. Nirmal, ve S. Goel, "Development of dexamethasone loaded nanomicelles using a 3D printed microfluidic device for ocular drug delivery applications", *Sensors and Actuators A: Physical*, c. 357, s. 114385, Ağu. 2023, doi: 10.1016/J.SNA.2023.114385.

M. Brucoli, F. Arcuri, R. Cavenaghi, ve A. Benech, "Analysis of Complications After Surgical Repair of Orbital Fractures", *Journal of Craniofacial Surgery*, c. 22, sy 4, s. 1387, Tem. 2011, doi: 10.1097/SCS.0b013e31821cc317.

M.C. Goiato, L.C. Bannwart, M.F. Haddad, D.M. dos Santos, A.A. Pesqueira et al., "Fabrication Techniques for Ocular Prostheses – An Overview", *Orbit*, c. 33, sy 3, ss. 229-233, Haz. 2014, doi: 10.3109/01676830.2014.881395.

M. Engel, J. Hoffmann, G. Castrillon-Oberndorfer, ve C. Freudlsperger, "The value of three-dimensional printing modelling for surgical correction of orbital hypertelorism", *Oral Maxillofac Surg*, c. 19, sy 1, ss. 91–95, Mar. 2015, doi: 10.1007/s10006-014-0466-1.

"Microneedle Drug Delivery Systems Market Size, Share, Trends And Forecast To 2033". Erişim: 09 Şubat 2024. [Çevrimiçi]. Erişim adresi: https://www.thebusinessresearchcompany.com/report/microneedle-drug-delivery-systems-global-market-report

M.J. Ali, "Progress in the application of 3D printing technology in ophthalmology", *Graefes Arch Clin Exp Ophthalmol*, c. 261, sy 4, ss. 901–902, Nis. 2023, doi: 10.1007/s00417-022-05907-z.

M. Li *vd.*, "A novel gatifloxacin-loaded intraocular lens for prophylaxis of postoperative endophthalmitis", *Bioactive Materials*, c. 20, ss. 271–285, Şub. 2023, doi: 10.1016/j.bioactmat.2022.05.032.

M. Rafat *vd.*, "PEG-stabilized carbodiimide crosslinked collagen–chitosan hydrogels for corneal tissue engineering", *Biomaterials*, c. 29, sy 29, ss. 3960–3972, Eki. 2008, doi: 10.1016/j.biomaterials.2008.06.017.

M. S. Sridhar, "Anatomy of cornea and ocular surface", *Indian J Ophthalmol*, c. 66, sy 2, ss. 190-194, Şub. 2018, doi: 10.4103/ijo.IJO_646_17.

M. Uchino ve D.A. Schaumberg, "Dry Eye Disease: Impact on Quality of Life and Vision", *Curr Ophthalmol Rep*, c. 1, sy 2, ss. 51–57, Haz. 2013, doi: 10.1007/s40135-013-0009-1.

M. Vehmeijer, M. Van Eijnatten, N. Liberton, ve J. Wolff, "A Novel Method of Orbital Floor Reconstruction Using Virtual Planning, 3-Dimensional Printing, and Autologous Bone", *Journal of Oral and Maxillofacial Surgery*, c. 74, sy 8, ss. 1608–1612, Ağu. 2016, doi: 10.1016/j.joms.2016.03.044.

M. Zhang *vd.*, "3D bioprinting of corneal decellularized extracellular matrix: GelMA composite hydrogel for corneal stroma engineering", *Int J Bioprint*, c. 9, sy 5, s. 774, Haz. 2023, doi: 10.18063/ijb.774.

N.A. Delamere, "Ciliary Body and Ciliary Epithelium", içinde *Advances in Organ Biology*, c. 10, J. Fischbarg, Ed., içinde The Biology of the Eye, vol. 10. , Elsevier, 2005, ss. 127–148. doi: 10.1016/S1569-2590(05)10005-6.

N.G.A. Willemen *vd.*, "From oral formulations to drug-eluting implants: using 3D and 4D printing to develop drug delivery systems and personalized medicine", *Bio-Design and Manufacturing 2021 5:1*, c. 5, sy 1, ss. 85–106, Eyl. 2021, doi: 10.1007/S42242-021-00157-0.

N. Jehangir, G. Bever, S.M.J. Mahmood, ve M. Moshirfar, "Comprehensive Review of the Literature on Existing Punctal Plugs for the Management of Dry Eye Disease", *Journal of Ophthalmology*, c. 2016, s. e9312340, Mar. 2016, doi: 10.1155/2016/9312340.

N. Lin, M. Gagnon, ve K.Y. Wu, "The Third Dimension of Eye Care: A Comprehensive Review of 3D Printing in Ophthalmology", *Hardware 2024, Vol. 2, Pages 1-32*, c. 2, sy 1, ss. 1–32, Oca. 2024, doi: 10.3390/ HARDWARE2010001.

N. Stanojcic, C. Hull, ve D.P. O'Brart, "Clinical and material degradations of intraocular lenses: A review", *European Journal of Ophthalmology*, c. 30, sy 5, ss. 823–839, Eyl. 2020, doi: 10.1177/1120672119867818.

N. Zhang *vd.*, "Personalized 3D-printed amniotic fornical ring for ocular surface reconstruction", *Int J Bioprint*, c. 9, sy 3, s. 713, Mar. 2023, doi: 10.18063/ijb.713.

O. Ayyildiz, "Customised spectacles using 3-D printing technology", *Clinical and Experimental Optometry*, c. 101, sy 6, ss. 747–751, Kas. 2018, doi: 10.1111/cxo.12795.

O. Strauss, "The Retinal Pigment Epithelium in Visual Function", *Physiological Reviews*, c. 85, sy 3, ss. 845–881, Tem. 2005, doi: 10.1152/physrev.00021.2004.

P.D. Ospina, M.C.C. Díaz, S. Lara, P.D. Ospina, M.C.C. Díaz et al. , "New Technologies in Eye Surgery — A Challenge for Clinical, Therapeutic, and Eye Surgeons", içinde *Advances in Eye Surgery*, IntechOpen, 2016. doi: 10.5772/61072.

P. Fagerholm, N.S. Lagali, D.J. Carlsson, K. Merrett, ve M. Griffith et al, "Corneal Regeneration Following Implantation of a Biomimetic Tissue-Engineered Substitute", *Clin Transl Sci*, c. 2, sy 2, ss. 162–164, Nis. 2009, doi: 10.1111/j.1752-8062.2008.00083.x.

P. Gadziński, A. Froelich, M. Wojtyłko, A. Białek, J. Krysztofiak et al., "Microneedle-based ocular drug delivery systems – recent advances and challenges", *Beilstein Journal of Nanotechnology 13:98*, c. 13, sy 1, ss. 1167–1184, Eki. 2022, doi: 10.3762/BJNANO.13.98.

P.M. Maloca *vd.*, "3D printing of the choroidal vessels and tumours based on optical coherence tomography", *Acta Ophthalmologica*, c. 97, sy 2, ss. e313-e316, 2019, doi: 10.1111/aos.13637.

P.M. Maloca *vd.*, "Enhanced resolution and speckle-free three-dimensional printing of macular optical coherence tomography angiography", *Acta Ophthalmologica*, c. 97, sy 2, Mar. 2019, doi: 10.1111/aos.13567.

P. Martinez-Seijas, L.A. Díaz-Galvis, J. Hernando, I.O. Leizaola-Cardesa, A. Aguilar-Salvatierra et al., "Polymethyl Methacrylate Custom-Made Prosthesis: A Novel Three-Dimension Printing-Aided Fabrication Technique for Cranial and/or Orbital Reconstruction", *Journal of Craniofacial Surgery*, c. 29, sy 5, s. e438, Tem. 2018, doi: 10.1097/SCS.0000000000004451.

P. Tack, J. Victor, P. Gemmel, ve L. Annemans, "3D-printing techniques in a medical setting: a systematic literature review", *BioMed Eng OnLine*, c. 15, sy 1, s. 115, Eki. 2016, doi: 10.1186/s12938-016-0236-4.

P. Wang *vd.*, "3D bioprinting of hydrogels for retina cell culturing", *Bioprinting*, c. 12, Ara. 2018, doi: 10.1016/J. BPRINT.2018.E00029.

P. Zorlutuna, A. Tezcaner, I. Kıyat, A. Aydınlı, ve V. Hasırcı et al., "Cornea engineering on polyester carriers", *Journal of Biomedical Materials Research Part A*, c. 79A, sy 1, ss. 104–113, 2006, doi: 10.1002/jbm.a.30772.

Q. Zhang, D. Yan, K. Zhang, G.H.-S. reports, ve undefined 2015, "Pattern transformation of heat-shrinkable polymer by three-dimensional (3D) printing technique", *nature.com Q Zhang, D Yan, K Zhang, G HuScientific reports, 2015•nature.com*, 2015, doi: 10.1038/srep08936.

R.B. Hallikerimath, K. Preethi, ve S. Dhaded, "Simplified technique for fabrication of custom ocular tray and making ocular impression", *The Journal of Indian Prosthodontic Society*, c. 9, sy 3, s. 171, Eyl. 2009, doi: 10.4103/0972-4052.57090.

R.B. Kormann, R. Mörschbächer, H. Moreira, ve P. Akaishi, "A three-dimensional printed photopolymer resin implant for orbital rehabilitation for evisceration", *Arq. Bras. Oftalmol.*, c. 82, ss. 471–475, Ağu. 2019, doi: 10.5935/0004-2749.20190090.

R.L. Scawn, A. Foster, B.W. Lee, D.O. Kikkawa, ve B.S. Korn et al, "Customised 3D Printing: An Innovative Training Tool for the Next Generation of Orbital Surgeons", *Orbit*, c. 34, sy 4, ss. 216–219, Tem. 2015, doi: 10.3109/01676830.2015.1049367.

R.M. Herranz ve R.M.C. Herran, *Ocular Surface: Anatomy and Physiology, Disorders and Therapeutic Care*. CRC Press, 2012.

R. Singh, O. Cuzzani, F. Binette, H. Sternberg, M.D. West et al., "Pluripotent Stem Cells for Retinal Tissue Engineering: Current Status and Future Prospects", *Stem Cell Rev and Rep*, c. 14, sy 4, ss. 463–483, Ağu. 2018, doi: 10.1007/s12015-018-9802-4.

R. Sun, B. Wang, X. Li, M.-W. Chang, X. Yan et al., "3D Electrohydrodynamic Printing of Contact Lens-Like Chloramphenicol-Loaded Patches for Corneal Abrasions Treatment", *Advanced Engineering Materials*, c. 25, sy 2, s. 2200970, 2023, doi: 10.1002/adem.202200970.

R. Xue *vd.*, "Application of Three-Dimensional Printing Technology for Improved Orbital-Maxillary-Zygomatic Reconstruction", *Journal of Craniofacial Surgery*, c. 30, sy 2, s. e127, Nis. 2019, doi: 10.1097/SCS.0000000000005031.

S. Awwad *vd.*, "Principles of pharmacology in the eye", *British Journal of Pharmacology*, c. 174, sy 23, ss. 4205–4223, 2017, doi: 10.1111/bph.14024.

S. Bhatnagar, P.R. Gadeela, P. Thathireddy, ve V.V.K. Venuganti, "Microneedle-based drug delivery: materials of construction", *Journal of Chemical Sciences*, c. 131, sy 9, ss. 1–28, Eyl. 2019, doi: 10.1007/S12039-019-1666-X/FIGURES/9.

S.C. Hong, "3D printable retinal imaging adapter for smartphones could go global", *Graefes Arch Clin Exp Ophthalmol*, c. 253, sy 10, ss. 1831–1833, Eki. 2015, doi: 10.1007/s00417-015-3017-z.

S. Canabrava, A. Diniz-Filho, P. Schor, D.F. Fagundes, A. Lopes et al., Batista, "Production of an intraocular device using 3D printing: an innovative technology for ophthalmology", *Arq. Bras. Oftalmol.*, c. 78, ss. 393–394, Ara. 2015, doi: 10.5935/0004-2749.20150105.

S.F. Janssen *vd.*, "Gene Expression and Functional Annotation of the Human Ciliary Body Epithelia", *PLOS ONE*, c. 7, sy 9, s. e44973, Eyl. 2012, doi: 10.1371/journal.pone.0044973.

S.H. Saverymuttu, S. Gupta, A. Keshavarzian, B. Donovan, ve H.J.F. Hodgson et al., "Effect of a Slow-Release 5′-Aminosalicylic Acid Preparation on Disease Activity in Crohn's Disease", *Digestion*, c. 33, sy 2, ss. 89–91, Oca. 2009, doi: 10.1159/000199279.

S. Kutlehria, T.C. Dinh, A. Bagde, N. Patel, A. Gebeyehu et al., "High-throughput 3D bioprinting of corneal stromal equivalents", *Journal of Biomedical Materials Research Part B: Applied Biomaterials*, c. 108, sy 7, ss. 2981–2994, 2020, doi: 10.1002/jbm.b.34628.

S. Li-bo, L. Yu-yan, Z. Li, ve Z. Hang-yu, "Application of an individualized titanium mesh based on digital model in the repair of orbital fracture", *Chinese Journal of Tissue Engineering Research*, c. 21, sy 14, s. 2158, May. 2017, doi: 10.3969/j.issn.2095-4344.2017.14.005.

S. Ruiters, Y. Sun, S. De Jong, C. Politis, ve I. Mombaerts et al., "Computer-aided design and three-dimensional printing in the manufacturing of an ocular prosthesis", *Br J Ophthalmol*, c. 100, sy 7, ss. 879–881, Tem. 2016, doi: 10.1136/bjophthalmol-2016-308399.

S. Ruiz-Alonso *vd.*, "Current Insights Into 3D Bioprinting: An Advanced Approach for Eye Tissue Regeneration", *Pharmaceutics*, c. 13, sy 3, s. 308, Şub. 2021, doi: 10.3390/pharmaceutics13030308.

S. Ruiz-alonso *vd.*, "Current Insights into 3D Bioprinting: An Advanced Approach for Eye Tissue Regeneration", *Pharmaceutics 2021, Vol. 13, Page 308*, c. 13, sy 3, s. 308, Şub. 2021, doi: 10.3390/PHARMACEUTICS13030308.

S.S.Y. Pang, C. Fang, ve J.Y.W. Chan, "Application of three-dimensional printing technology in orbital floor fracture reconstruction", *Trauma Case Reports*, c. 17, ss. 23–28, Eki. 2018, doi: 10.1016/j.tcr.2018.09.006.

S. Sang *vd.*, "Photo-crosslinked hydrogels for tissue engineering of corneal epithelium", *Experimental Eye Research*, c. 218, s. 109027, May. 2022, doi: 10.1016/j.exer.2022.109027.

S.U.D. Wani *vd.*, "Promising Role of Silk-Based Biomaterials for Ocular-Based Drug Delivery and Tissue Engineering", *Polymers*, c. 14, sy 24, Art. sy 24, Oca. 2022, doi: 10.3390/polym14245475.

S. Ulag *vd.*, "3D printed artificial cornea for corneal stromal transplantation", *European Polymer Journal*, c. 133, s. 109744, Haz. 2020, doi: 10.1016/j.eurpolymj.2020.109744.

S.V. Murphy, P. De Coppi, ve A. Atala, "Opportunities and challenges of translational 3D bioprinting", *Nature Biomedical Engineering*, c. 4, sy 4, ss. 370–380, Nis. 2020, doi: 10.1038/S41551-019-0471-7.

S.W. Park, J.W. Choi, K.S. Koh, ve T.S. Oh, "Mirror-Imaged Rapid Prototype Skull Model and Pre-Molded Synthetic Scaffold to Achieve Optimal Orbital Cavity Reconstruction", *Journal of Oral and Maxillofacial Surgery*, c. 73, sy 8, ss. 1540–1553, Ağu. 2015, doi: 10.1016/j.joms.2015.03.025.

S. Wang, C.E. Ghezzi, R. Gomes, R.E. Pollard, J.L. Funderburgh et al., "In vitro 3D corneal tissue model with epithelium, stroma, and innervation", *Biomaterials*, c. 112, ss. 1–9, Oca. 2017, doi: 10.1016/j.biomaterials.2016.09.030.

T. Hori *vd.*, "Three-dimensional-printed Refillable Drug Delivery Device for Long-term Sustained Drug Delivery to Retina", *Sensors and Materials*, c. 35, sy 4, ss. 1301–1313, 2023, doi: 10.18494/SAM4167.

T. Irimia, M.V. Ghica, L. Popa, V. Anuța, A.-L. Arsene et al., "Strategies for Improving Ocular Drug Bioavailability and Corneal Wound Healing with Chitosan-Based Delivery Systems", *Polymers*, c. 10, sy 11, Art. sy 11, Kas. 2018, doi: 10.3390/polym10111221.

T. Khanna, J.D. Akkara, V. Bawa, ve E.A. Sargunam, "Designing and making an open source, 3D-printed, punctal plug with drug delivery system", *Indian J Ophthalmol*, c. 71, sy 1, ss. 297–299, Oca. 2023, doi: 10.4103/ijo. IJO_997_22.

T. Khanna, J.D. Akkara, V. Bawa, ve E.A. Sargunam, "Designing and making an open source, 3D-printed, punctal plug with drug delivery system", *Indian Journal of Ophthalmology*, c. 71, sy 1, s. 297, Oca. 2023, doi: 10.4103/ IJO.IJO_997_22.

T.M. Shiju, R. Carlos de Oliveira, ve S.E. Wilson, "3D in vitro corneal models: A review of current technologies", *Experimental Eye Research*, c. 200, s. 108213, Kas. 2020, doi: 10.1016/j.exer.2020.108213.

T.S. Oh, W.S. Jeong, T.J. Chang, K.S. Koh, ve J.-W. Choi et al., "Customized Orbital Wall Reconstruction Using Three-Dimensionally Printed Rapid Prototype Model in Patients With Orbital Wall Fracture", *Journal of Craniofacial Surgery*, c. 27, sy 8, s. 2020, Kas. 2016, doi: 10.1097/SCS.0000000000003195.

T.V. Dave *vd.*, "Low-cost three-dimensional printed orbital template-assisted patient-specific implants for the correction of spherical orbital implant migration", *Indian J Ophthalmol*, c. 66, sy 11, ss. 1600–1607, Kas. 2018, doi: 10.4103/ijo.IJO_472_18.

U. Chakravarthy, E. Biundo, R.O. Saka, C. Fasser, R. Bourne et al., "The Economic Impact of Blindness in Europe", *Ophthalmic Epidemiology*, c. 24, sy 4, ss. 239–247, Tem. 2017, doi: 10.1080/09286586.2017.1281426.

U. Garg *vd.*, "The emerging role of 3D-printing in ocular drug delivery: Challenges, current status, and future prospects", *Journal of Drug Delivery Science and Technology*, c. 76, s. 103798, Eki. 2022, doi: 10.1016/j. jddst.2022.103798.

V. Gote, S. Sikder, J. Sicotte, ve D. Pal, "Ocular Drug Delivery: Present Innovations and Future Challenges", *J Pharmacol Exp Ther*, c. 370, sy 3, ss. 602–624, Eyl. 2019, doi: 10.1124/jpet.119.256933.

W. Liu *vd.*, "Collagen–phosphorylcholine interpenetrating network hydrogels as corneal substitutes", *Biomaterials*, c. 30, sy 8, ss. 1551-1559, Mar. 2009, doi: 10.1016/j.biomaterials.2008.11.022.

W. Zhu, X. Ma, M. Gou, D. Mei, K. Zhang et al., "3D printing of functional biomaterials for tissue engineering", *Current Opinion in Biotechnology*, c. 40, ss. 103-112, Ağu. 2016, doi: 10.1016/j.copbio.2016.03.014.

X. Duan, C. McLaughlin, M. Griffith, ve H. Sheardown, "Biofunctionalization of collagen for improved biological response: Scaffolds for corneal tissue engineering", *Biomaterials*, c. 28, sy 1, ss. 78–88, Oca. 2007, doi: 10.1016/j.biomaterials.2006.08.034.

X. Xu *vd.*, "3D Printed Punctal Plugs for Controlled Ocular Drug Delivery", *Pharmaceutics*, c. 13, sy 9, Art. sy 9, Eyl. 2021, doi: 10.3390/pharmaceutics13091421.

Y. Fakhoury, A. Ellabban, U. Attia, A. Sallam, ve S. Elsherbiny et al., "Three-dimensional printing in ophthalmology and eye care: current applications and future developments", *Therapeutic Advances in Ophthalmology*, c. 14, Oca. 2022, doi: 10.1177/25158414221106682/ASSET/IMAGES/LARGE/10.1177_25158414221106682- FIG3.JPEG.

Y. Fang, F. Chen, H. Wu, ve B. Chen, "Progress in the application of 3D printing technology in ophthalmology", *Graefes Arch Clin Exp Ophthalmol*, c. 261, sy 4, ss. 903–912, Nis. 2023, doi: 10.1007/s00417-022-05908-y.

Y. Wang *vd.*, "Application of Bioprinting in Ophthalmology", *Int J Bioprint*, c. 8, sy 2, s. 552, Şub. 2022, doi: 10.18063/ijb.v8i2.552.

Y. Wu *vd.*, "Long-acting nanoparticle-loaded bilayer microneedles for protein delivery to the posterior segment of the eye", *European Journal of Pharmaceutics and Biopharmaceutics*, c. 165, ss. 306-318, Ağu. 2021, doi: 10.1016/J.EJPB.2021.05.022.

Y. Zhang, L. Wu, M. Zou, L. Zhang, ve Y. Song et al., "Suppressing the Step Effect of 3D Printing for Constructing Contact Lenses", *Advanced Materials*, c. 34, sy 4, s. 2107249, 2022, doi: 10.1002/adma.202107249.

Y.-C. Liu, M. Wilkins, T. Kim, B. Malyugin, ve J.S. Mehta et al., "Cataracts", *The Lancet*, c. 390, sy 10094, ss. 600–612, Ağu. 2017, doi: 10.1016/S0140-6736(17)30544-5.

Z. Deng, Z. Zhang, L. Li, ve C. Zhou, "[Biocompatibility evaluation of chitosan-g-polyvinylpyrrolidone]", *Di Yi Jun Yi Da Xue Xue Bao*, c. 24, sy 6, ss. 639–41, 645, Haz. 2004.

Z. Hou, X. Tian, J. Zhang, ve D. Li, "3D printed continuous fibre reinforced composite corrugated structure", *Composite Structures*, c. 184, ss. 1005-1010, Oca. 2018, doi: 10.1016/j.compstruct.2017.10.080.

Z. Jiang, B. Diggle, M.L. Tan, J. Viktorova, C.W. Bennett et al., "Extrusion 3D Printing of Polymeric Materials with Advanced Properties", *Advanced Science*, c. 7, sy 17, s. 2001379, 2020, doi: 10.1002/advs.202001379.

Z. Ye *vd.*, "The role of 3D printed models in the teaching of human anatomy: a systematic review and meta-analysis", *BMC Medical Education*, c. 20, sy 1, s. 335, Eyl. 2020, doi: 10.1186/s12909-020-02242-x.

Towards 3D-Bioprinting the Artificial Ovary

Anastasia Kirillova[1]*

1. Introduction

Cancer is touching the fates of more and more women of reproductive age. Over the last 40 years, the incidence of cancer annually increased by 1.15% in the group of 25-39-year-old women (Kehm et al., 2019). Due to the fact that gonadotoxic oncological treatment leads to infertility, premature ovarian failure or even sterility (Letourneau et al., 2012; Morgan et al., 2012; Donnez and Dolmans, 2013), a lot of effort has been directed towards establishing oncofertility programs worldwide (Letourneau et al., 2011; Muñoz et al., 2016; Martinez et al., 2017; Oktay et al., 2018). Embryo and oocyte freezing after controlled ovarian stimulation is the golden standard of fertility preservation (Medrano et al., 2018). Yet ovarian tissue cryopreservation is the only option for prepubertal girls and can restore endocrine function (Wallace et al., 2016; Pacheco and Oktay, 2017; Poirot et al., 2019). This technology finally shed its experimental status with more than 130 children born worldwide (The Practice Committee of the American Society for Reproductive Medicine, 2019).

With all the progress in oncofertility made over the last decades, there are currently no established clinical approaches for fertility preservation for women with ovarian cancer and types of cancer metastasizing into ovaries. These patients undergo radical ovariectomy and irrevocably lose the ability to have biological children, which might lead to depression and decrease of life quality (Penrose et al., 2013; Lawson et al., 2014; Logan et al., 2019;). The technology of artificial ovary biofabrication would benefit this group of patients by restoring their reproductive and endocrine function and giving the opportunity for natural conception. Since the follicles are surrounded by the basal membrane, malignant cells cannot invade them. (Amorim and Shikanov, 2016). With the help of 3-d bioprinting technology, it is possible to bioengineer a functional artificial ovary free of malignant cells.

[1]   The Royal Women's Hospital, Locked Bag 300, Grattan St and Flemington Rd, Parkville.
*   Corresponding author: anastasia.kirillova@zoho.com

1.1 *The Principal of an Artificial Ovary Biofabrication*

The biofabricated artificial ovary should mimic the natural organ in terms of structure and function. Ideally, it should include all structural units present in the natural organ: follicles and different types of stromal cells. Follicles consist of oocytes surrounded by granulosa and theca cells. They can be successfully isolated using the tailored protocol with the application of the Liberase enzyme (Chiti, Dolmans, Hobeika, et al., 2017). Enzymatic digestion of ovarian tissue might be combined with mechanical isolation (Xu et al., 2006), sedimentation (Kniazeva et al., 2016) or microfluidics (Lai et al., 2013). For example, pseudo-grayscale photomasks in combination with backside diffused light lithography can form multi-level weir-type cell traps which can isolate the large ovarian follicles from the smaller cancer cells with 88% efficiency (Lai et al., 2013). We believe that all stages of preantral follicles should be included in the ovarian construct. The secondary follicles survive better than primordial–primary follicles after grafting and can promote angiogenesis (Chiti, Dolmans, Lucci, et al., 2017). However, as in a natural organ, primary follicles should be in majority. In the biofabricated ovary, the main pool of primordial follicles has to be maintained in dormancy as the burst activation of follicles would lead to the ovarian reserve depletion and premature artificial organ failure. Thus, there should be a direct communication between the follicles within the ovarian construct in order to provide selective follicle activation. The primordial follicles most likely secrete a diffusible inhibitor that prevents neighboring primordial follicles from growing (Da Silva-Buttkus et al., 2009). Studies on mice demonstrated that follicles were more likely to remain dormant if they had at least one primordial follicle within a 10 μm distance (Da Silva-Buttkus et al., 2009). Therefore, it is of great importance to arrange follicles at an adjusted distance from each other in a biofabricated ovary. The mesenchymal-derived stromal cells contain theca cells, neurons, endothelial cells and immune cells (Tagler et al., 2011). Stromal cells play an essential role in folliculogenesis by primordial follicles activation. These cells express bone morphogenetic proteins (BMP-4 and BMP-7) which promote primordial-primary follicle transition (W.-S. Lee et al., 2001, 2004; Nilsson, 2003; Tagler et al., 2011).

Theca cells are essential for physiological steroidogenesis and oogenesis. The majority of primordial follicles undergo apoptosis most likely due to the lack of theca cell protection and the onset of folliculogenesis is associated with the differentiation of theca cells around granulosa cells (Tajima et al., 2007). Theca cells synthesize precursor androgens which are aromatized by granulosa cells for estrogen production (Hillier et al., 1994). Androgens can regulate follicle growth and ovulation (Walters et al., 2008; Yang et al., 2020) and promote granulosa proliferation (Hickey et al., 2005). Thus, theca cells should be part of the biofabricated ovary as they are essential for appropriate organ function. Theca cells can be isolated from an ovary or cortical stromal cells can differentiate into theca cells in the presence of granulosa (Orisaka et al., 2006).

Human ovaries contain an intrinsic network of ovarian neurons which most likely play a role in ovarian steroidogenesis (Dees et al., 2006). It has been demonstrated on a rhesus monkey model that the number of neurons in an ovary changes throughout its lifetime: its number increases significantly at puberty, remains high during the reproductive stage and dramatically declines during the postreproductive life period (Dees et al., 2006). Thus, ovarian neurons might contribute to maintaining ovarian reproductive and endocrine function.

Natural ovaries also include the population of immune cells (adaptive T lymphocytes, Natural Killer cells, B lymphocytes), and innate immune system (monocytes and macrophages) which play a role in ovulation by a cytokine-mediated inflammatory response (Fan et al., 2019). Endothelial cells make up around 3% of all ovarian cells (Shahri et al., 2019). These cells are essential in the artificial ovary as they can improve the revascularization of the transplanted construct and decrease follicle degeneration due to ischemia. Dath and co-authors demonstrated that isolated endothelial cells can reorganize into vessel-like vascular tubular structures and provide good survival of co-transplanted cells (Dath et al., 2011). The best source of isolated stromal cells is the fresh medullary tissue as it provides higher cell yield and viability (Soares et al., 2017). The stromal cells can improve the vascularization of an ovarian construct by reorganizing into a rich vascular network. Furthermore, isolated ovarian cells can synthesize extracellular matrices and therefore provide support for the follicles (Soares et al., 2017) making it possible to apply scaffold-free biofabrication. The architecture of an ovary should be taken into consideration for ovarian construct biofabrication. The outer cortical layer is more rigid with parallel organized stromal cells and a rounded structure, while the medulla is looser with the random organization of cells and an elongated structure (Tagler et al., 2011). The biofabricated tissue encasing the follicles should permit volumetric expansion, either through elasticity or degradation (J. Kim et al., 2016) as human ovarian follicles grow 600-folds during folliculogenesis (Vanacker et al., 2012). Last but not least, the artificial ovary should be designed for an efficient application in the operation rooms. The bioprinted technology needs to provide sterile settings for the aseptic organ biofabrication and the ovarian construct has to be convenient for handling by a surgeon.

2. Scaffolds for Follicle Support

The first prototypes of artificial ovaries were biofabricated using only isolated follicles and different types of scaffolds. It was demonstrated on animal models, that follicles encapsulated into scaffolds can provide growth and function (Xu et al., 2006; Luyckx et al., 2014; Kim et al., 2016; Kniazeva et al., 2016; Laronda et al., 2017). For the successful ovarian construct function the scaffolds have to possess several properties (see for comprehensive review Amorim, 2011). Ideally, the scaffold has to be rigid to provide mechanical support for the follicles, yet it has to be flexible enough to allow construct remodeling for angiogenesis, somatic cell proliferation, and follicle growth. It is of high importance for the scaffold to be biocompatible as immune reactions can lead to follicle loss and artificial organ rejection. It has to be safe for the patient so potentially toxic materials cannot be used for scaffold production. Natural, synthetic and mixed scaffolds can be applied for ovarian tissue biofabrication.

2.1 *Natural Scaffolds*

Natural hydrogels (fibrin, alginate, etc.) are widely used for the support of isolated follicles and *in vitro* culture. (Kniazeva et al., 2016; Xu et al., 2009, 2006; Vanacker et al., 2012). Natural biomaterials are biocompatible, biodegradable and often contain biofunctional molecules essential for cellular attachment, proliferation, and differentiation (Yoon and Fisher, 2009) which makes them suitable for artificial ovary scaffolds. The most common materials for natural scaffolds are collagen, fibrin, and alginate. Collagen is a structural protein that is the major component of the extracellular matrix throughout the ovary with higher concentrations of collagen I in the ovarian surface epithelium and follicular compartments (Berkholtz et al., 2006). It is a natural component of wound healing that carries cell adhesion domains (Yoon and Fisher, 2009). Selected concentrations of collagen hydrogels can provide follicle survival, growth and hormone production of isolated rat follicles (Joo et al., 2016). Fibrin is another natural polymer formed out of fibrinogen and thrombin. It plays a major role in wound healing coagulation. Moreover, fibrin can guide cellular and matrix response and promote angiogenesis (Chiti, Dolmans, Donnez, et al., 2017). It was demonstrated on a murine model that fibrin hydrogel can provide follicle support and growth up to the antral stage after transplantation. Such fibrin-follicle ovarian constructs successfully restored reproductive function in ovariectomized mice (Smith et al., 2014). The adjusted combination of fibrinogen and thrombin can also mimic the human ovarian cortex in terms of rigidity, porosity and fiber thickness (Chiti et al., 2018) and provide survival and proliferation of isolated human ovarian cells (Luyckx et al., 2013).

Unfortunately, fibrin on its own has low mechanical strength and degrades fast. Another concern is that commercially available fibrin is produced with the application of aprotinin, bovine fibrinolytic inhibitor, which might carry the risk of pathogen infection and possible immunoreaction. (Chiti et al.,

2017). Alginate is a water soluble natural polysaccharide. It can be cross-linked to form a hydrogel when exposed to divalent ions (Yoon and Fisher, 2009), such as calcium, strontium or barium. Alginate with matrigel can support the viability of isolated ovarian cells allowing vascularization and natural degradation of graft in mice (Vanacker et al., 2012). It was demonstrated that murine follicles can successfully grow up to the antral stage in an artificial ovary with an alginate scaffold and produce mature oocytes with normal spindle morphology and high developmental potential (Vanacker et al., 2012). Alginate scaffold can be biofabricated in a form with several compartments for different cell types providing immuno-isolation For instance, granulosa and theca cells were encapsulated in an alginate scaffold in a rat model, and such constructs were able to restore endocrine function (Sittadjody et al., 2017).

The major concern with alginate biomaterial is that calcium (Ca2+) and strontium (Sr2+) necessary for alginate cross-linking are not suitable for clinical practice. Calcium might lead to calcification of the construct and most likely result in a decline in estrogen secretion (Sittadjody et al., 2017). Strontium, on the other hand, might lead to the uncontrolled meiosis resumption in oocytes (Fraser, 1987). In general natural scaffolds have a tendency to degrade abruptly (Yoon and Fisher, 2009) which might compromise bioprinted organ function. Moreover, the longevity of a natural scaffold depends on the enzymatic activity of each recipient which makes it difficult to determine its lifespan (Yoon and Fisher, 2009).

2.2 Synthetic Scaffolds

Compared to natural scaffolds synthetic hydrogels can be produced with no limitations in all different shapes and sizes. It is possible to adjust synthetic hydrogels' properties for the desired stiffness which would make the scaffolds easy to manipulate in the operating rooms. Poly(ethylene glycol) vinyl sulfone (PEG-VS) is a widely used synthetic scaffold. PEG-VS belongs to the family of two-component hybrid hydrogels and is structurally similar to natural extracellular matrices (Lutolf and Hubbell, 2003). Because of its non adhesive nature, PEG can benefit from modification with integrin-binding peptides (such as RGD (Arg-Gly-Asp)) to allow biospecific cell adhesion (Hern and Hubbell, 1998). Experiments in mice proved PEG-VS hydrogel to be suitable for *in vivo* folliculogenesis and steroidogenesis (J. Kim et al., 2016). The stiffness of PEG hydrogel was adjusted to mimic the stromal tissue in order to allow follicular expansion. In that study, primordial and primary follicles were encapsulated into PEG hydrogels and transplanted into ovariectomized mice. Ovarian constructs were revascularized with the increasing density of functional blood vessels over time. Restoration of the ovarian constructs function was proven by the presence of corpora lutea, growth of follicles up to the preovulatory stage and normalization of FSH levels. Most importantly selective activation of primordial follicles was demonstrated which imitated the physiological process of follicle recruitment (Kim et al., 2016). Nevertheless, scaffolds formed out of PEG need to be treated with great caution. The main concern about PEG itself is that it is not biodegradable which might compromise the long-term function of a biofabricated organ. Moreover, it might provoke embolism by inducing blood clotting and inducing specific as well as nonspecific recognition by the immune system (Knop et al., 2010) which may lead to transplant rejection and failure.

2.3 Fabrication of Mixed Scaffolds using Electrospun Matrices

In order to improve scaffold properties, natural biomaterials such as gelatin can be blended with polyepsilon caprolactone (PCL) using electrospinning technology (Liverani et al., 2019). This approach is based on the implication of electrostatic forces in order to fabricate ECM-mimicking fibrous scaffolds from biocompatible polymers (Jun et al., 2018). During electrospinning biofabrication, with the increase of electrical potential in the electrospinning apparatus the polymer solution elongates and forms a cone first, and then a hemisphere. The applied electrostatic charge overcomes the surface tension of the polymer solution and a charged polymer jet congregates in a metallic collector. As a result, nanoscale/microscale fibrous structures with interconnecting pores are produced (Jiang et al., 2015; Jun et al., 2018). The combination of PCL/gelatin can reinforce scaffold properties. While the PCL provides a stiff structure essential for follicle support and manipulation during transplantation, the natural polymer gelatin has biofunctional molecules providing cell adhesion, proliferation, and differentiation (Liverani et al., 2019). The addition of PCL can also improve the degradation rate of the scaffold making it controlled and enzymatically independent. Experiments with porcine follicles demonstrated that seeded follicles into PCL/gel fibers form adhesion points on the entire surface of the fibrous scaffold, retaining their spheroidal shape and viability for 30 days (Liverani et al., 2019).

However, like with the synthetic materials, the main concern for artificial ovary application are the cytotoxic chemicals utilized in this technology. Though the glacial acetic acid used to solve PCL for the electrospinning process is less toxic than the common solvents (chloroform, dichloromethane, N,N-dimethylformamide) it is classified as corrosive and still can be hazardouss to health.

2.4 Growth Factor Delivery-based Scaffolds

In order to enhance biofabricated tissue function, it is possible to anchor growth factors into the scaffolds. This delivery strategy by means of incorporation of growth factors (GF) into polymer matrices allows achieving a low degradation rate of GF and controlled concentrations in the tissue (K. Lee et al., 2011). The proximity of GF to the cells can guarantee the targeted effect and adequate cellular response. GF might be delivered by physical, covalent, or bioaffinity immobilization and might be incorporated in synthetic or natural scaffolds (Wang et al., 2017). Natural polymer fibrin can be easily cross-linked with GF (VEGF, bFGF, and others) via heparin as a mediator. RGD (arginine-glycine-aspartate) sequence of the fibrin can bind with heparin which in turn has the ability to associate with GF (Chiti, Dolmans, Donnez, et al., 2017). It was demonstrated that the addition of fibrin-HBP-VEGF to the ovarian tissue during transplantation significantly increased the number of surviving primordial follicles and the number of formed blood vessels (Shikanov et al., 2011). Alginate sulfate (AlgS) carries multiple anionic charges because of the sulfation. As a result, it can interact with reciprocally charged growth factors and signaling proteins (Billings and Pacifici, 2015). Incorporation of AlgS with affinity bound BMP-4 into macroporous alginate scaffold leads to improved follicle growth and endocrine function of a biofabricated ovary in a porcine model with xenotransplantation into ovariectomized mice (Felder et al., 2019).

Nanocomplexes of BMP-4/AlgS do not change the pore structure and physical properties of the scaffold. Felder and coauthors seeded primordial follicles together with stromal ovarian cells into the BMP-4/AlgS alginate scaffold. Compared to the control, fortification of the constructs with affinity-bound BMP-4 increased the number of developing follicles 5-fold, estradiol secretion, and GDF-9/AMH gene expression. Inclusion of affinity-bound vascular endothelial growth factor (VEGF) and platelet-derived growth factor-ββ (PDGF-ββ) enhanced vascularization, and most likely increased viability and follicle development after transplantation of the artificial ovary (Felder et al., 2019). It has been demonstrated on the rat model that in triple factor loaded scaffolds, VEGF, PDGF-BB and TGF-b1 deliver sequentially: first high levels of VEGF are released, then PDGF-ββ and TGF-b1 in the end which mimics the signal cascade acting in angiogenesis. This approach resulted in larger and more mature vessels and a 3-fold increase in blood vessel density over scaffolds with no factor supplementation (Freeman and Cohen, 2009). Taking into consideration that ischemia is the main factor for follicle loss after ovarian tissue transplantation (S. S. Kim et al., 2004), growth factor delivery based ovarian tissue engineering can be very promising for clinical application.

2.5 Decellularized Ovarian Tissue as a Natural Scaffold

Decellularized tissue can serve as an alternative to biofabricated scaffolds. This approach allows removing cells from an organ while maintaining the extracellular matrix (ECM) with the same mechanical and bioactive properties as in the natural ovary. The ECM can provide an optimal microenvironment for homeostatic and regenerative cell development as it has suitable pH and CO_2 levels, cell adhesion spots and has a reservoir of growth factors (Kawecki et al., 2018). Ovarian cells can be reseeded in the decellularized scaffolds. Studies in mice showed that such constructs can restore hormone production in 2-3 weeks and initiate puberty (Laronda et al., 2015). The clear advantage of the decellularized scaffold is that it represents the real skeletal structure of the organ with an appropriate size, biomechanical properties, and compartmentalization. Experiments with the human ovarian tissue demonstrated that within 1 month isolated ovarian stromal cells and preantral follicles can repopulate some parts of the decellularized ovarian tissue (DOT) (Pors et al., 2019). This study confirmed that DOT can support follicle viability and preserve its normal morphology. However, the follicles recovery rate remained low and only 25% of human follicles survived after three weeks grafting to immunodeficient mice and showed no signs of growth. Interestingly, only early preantral follicles were viable and were localized only at the periphery of the construct. Though the protein composition was preserved, preantral follicles were placed not in their original spots but into artificially made lacunas in DOT created with a scalpel; between the layers of DOT; or on top of the DOT surface (Pors et al., 2019).

It is not clear with such static seeding methods if ovarian cells can successfully repopulate the inner part of the DOT (Laronda et al., 2015). Dynamic seeding techniques such as rotational seeding which induces hydrostatic forces or vacuum seeding which creates pressure differentials might increase cell penetration throughout the scaffold (Villalona et al., 2010). It was demonstrated that the low-speed rotational culture system using a spinner flask and stimulates cell repopulation deep into the DOT (Mirzaeian et al., 2019). This approach promoted cell alignment and tissue remodeling and increased the survival rate of seeded cells (Mirzaeian et al., 2019). Nowadays there is still no evidence of the feasibility of full decellularized ovary recellularization. Even if this approach proves its efficiency, it would require the implementation of donor DOT along with patients' ovarian cells and follicles, which would bring the hot topic of the donor organs shortage.

A more promising approach has been recently developed for processing DOT into biomaterial which can be used in the form of gels (Saldin et al., 2017) or tissue papers (Jakus et al., 2017). Tissue papers are formed out of the decellularized organs by means of washing, lyophilizing, and mechanically milling. Tissue papers are very convenient for handling as they can be cut, rolled and folded for long-term storage which might give a patient more time for a donor-recipient match. It was demonstrated that ovarian tissue papers can provide follicles viability, morphology preservation and adhesion (Jakus et al., 2017).

Nevertheless, before the introduction of the decellularization approach into clinical practice, the safety of the technology should be thoroughly evaluated. Chemical decellularization remains the most popular method. While it might be highly efficient for cell dissolvement, applied chemicals are highly risky for medical applications due to cytotoxicity and effect on ECM ultrastructure. For instance, the frequently used sodium dodecyl sulfate (SDS) is a highly toxic chemical that destroys non-covalent interactions of the native protein (Kawecki et al., 2018). Sodium lauryl ester sulfate (SLES) can serve as an alternative decellularizing agent (Hassanpour et al., 2018). Unlike SDS, SLES being a milder anionic detergent provides a lower level of inflammation and better ECM structure with bioactive molecules such as proteoglycans and cytokines preservation (Hassanpour et al., 2018; Kawasaki et al., 2015). However, all kinds of decellularization processing affect the structure and composition of the ECM (Kawecki et al., 2018) leading to the loss of its bioactivity and mechanical properties. Another concern is that after decellularization some cellular and intracellular debris remains in the scaffold which might lead to an inflammatory response and degradation of the transplant (Kawecki et al., 2018). In order to reach the highest safety of technology, other decellularization methods should be tested. Physical methods (freezing, sonication, agitation), biological decellularization methods (enzymatical) or their combination might be better suited for implementation in artificial ovary biofabrication.

3. Scaffold-free Three-dimensional Microtissues Technology

It is also possible to biofabricate artificial ovaries with scaffold-free technology. This method is based on the physical ability of single cells to self-organize into spherical microtissues, and several microtissues to self-segregate to form multilayered three-dimensional structures. The desired architecture of microtissues can be reached by application of micromolded agarose to guide the spontaneous self-assembly of cells and the size of the construct can be regulated by the number of cells seeded (Rago et al., 2009). Micromolds can be designed in different shapes (rod, toroid, loop-ended dog bone or honeycomb). It allows biofabrication of versatile structures of cellular aggregates while the nonadhesive surface of micromolds provides perfect conditions for cell-to-cell binding. The absence of a scaffold allows cells easy access to nutrients and waste exchange (Napolitano et al., 2007).

An artificial ovary can be constructed using three types of self-assembled cell microtissues: theca, granulosa and cumulus-oocyte complexes (COCs). This approach was implemented by Krotz and coauthors. In their work, the majority of cells in the artificial ovary were represented by theca cells which can form stable honeycomb 3-dimensional microtissues containing multiple lumina (Krotz et al., 2010). The honeycomb shape of the micromolded agarose is quite beneficial for artificial ovary biofabrication since its hexagonal geometry provides evenly distributed tension in the structure (Napolitano et al., 2007). In this case, theca cells serve as a natural scaffold, yet providing the endocrine function. The self-assembled granulosa cell spheroids and COCs could be placed in the theca honeycomb openings. The culture of three types of ovarian microtissues leads to complete enveloping of granulosa spheroids and COCs by theca without stromal invasion or disruption maintaining the structural integrity of the artificial ovary (Krotz et al., 2010). Gap junctions remained intact between the oocytes and granulosa cells; however, it was not clear if gap junctions were formed between theca cells. The scaffold-free technology opens new horizons for ovarian biofabrication as this approach provides direct endocrine and paracrine interactions between the ovarian cells required for correct follicular maturation. Since, 90-95% of follicles in an ovary remain at the primary stage (Feher, 2012), it is crucial to demonstrate in future experiments that theca and granulosa microtissues can support *in vitro* growth in such biofabricated constructs of preantral follicles as well.

4. 3D Bioprinting

The first successful results of 3d bioprinting an artificial ovary were achieved using mice as a model organism. An artificial ovary, consisting of a bioprinted scaffold with manually seeded preantral follicles supported oogenesis leading to the live birth of fertile offspring (Laronda et al., 2017). In the described experiments the scaffold was bioprinted using gelatin ink, a bioactive, degradable biomaterial with cell adhesion sites. The optimal physical properties of the gelatin scaffold were achieved by adjusting the temperature regime of bioprinting: 30°C was selected, which is right in between the liquid (>33°C) and fully cross-linked gel (<25°C) state. The 10% gelatin solution was chemically cross-linked with N-(3-dimethylaminopropyl)-N'-ethylcarbodiimide/N-hydroxysuccinimide (EDC/NHS) which improved its mechanical properties and thermal stabilization (Laronda et al., 2017). Interestingly, follicle survival and growth depended on the number of struts contacting it. 30° and 60° scaffolds were more favorable compared to the 90° scaffold as there was always an extra underlying strut contacting a follicle in the pore. Without it, the follicles were not able to maintain their physiological spherical shape; they spread out, resulting in the disconnection of oocytes and granulosa cells from each other (Laronda et al., 2017).

The size of the micropores was adjusted to fit secondary follicles and to allow vascularization. In the course of experiments, 40-50 small preantral follicles were manually seeded in the scaffold following 4 days of in vitro culture. Surgical transplantation in a donor mouse resulted in spontaneous vascularization and folliculogenesis with ovulation and corpus lutea formation as an endpoint. The study described above proved that the bioprinted ovary restored the endocrine and the reproductive functions of a bioprinted ovarian construct (Laronda et al., 2017).

5.   Conclusions and Future Perspectives

The ovary is one of the few organs for which donor organ transplantation is not optional as it is of high importance to preserve the individual genetic material of each patient. Thus, it is of high importance to develop artificial ovary biofabrication. Due to the growing demand and recent success on animal models we believe that artificial ovary technology will be developed for human tissue in the upcoming decade. In order to provide safety and standardization of the technique, the whole process has to be automated including robotic follicles and ovarian cell isolation. There might be no need for the biofabricated scaffold if the required support is provided by ovarian stromal cells and prefabricated autologous blood vessels. With the development of vascular-tissue engineering, it would be possible to minimize the risk of loss of precious follicles due to ischemia. In order to provide long term functioning of a biofabricated ovary several hundreds of preantral follicles should be automatically seeded with an adjusted distance from each other using 3d printing technology. The adapted distance between primordial follicles would allow communication between them and selective physiological follicle activation.

The technological principles underlying the biofabrication of an artificial ovary are the same as those for bioprinting other organs. Nevertheless, higher safety and ethical standards should be applied to this technology. The artificial ovary approach needs to provide not only a functional organ for a patient but should also guarantee the health of future children, conceived with the oocytes developed within a biofabricated ovary. Broad and thorough genetic and epigenetic studies should be carried out for such oocytes. If the 3D printing technology proves to provide high standards of follicle development, long-term function, and safety, the biofabrication technology might substitute ovarian cortex cryopreservation with the subsequent transplantation method. The application of the artificial ovary might go even beyond fertility preservation and be used instead of pharmaceutical hormonal replacement therapy or for delayed motherhood due to social reasons.

References

Amorim, C.A. (2011). Artificial ovary. In Principles and Practice of Fertility Preservation, J. Donnez and S.S. Kim, eds. (Cambridge: Cambridge University Press), pp. 448–458.

Amorim, C.A. and Shikanov, A. (2016). The artificial ovary: current status and future perspectives. Future Oncology *12*, 2323–2332.

Berkholtz, C.B., Shea, L.D. and Woodruff, T.K. (2006). Extracellular Matrix Functions in Follicle Maturation. Semin Reprod Med *24*, 262–269.

Billings, P.C. and Pacifici, M. (2015). Interactions of signaling proteins, growth factors and other proteins with heparin sulfate: mechanisms and mysteries. Connective Tissue Research *56*, 272–280.

Chiti, M.C., Dolmans, M.-M., Hobeika, M., Cernogoraz, A., Donnez, J et al. (2017a). A modified and tailored human follicle isolation procedure improves follicle recovery and survival. J Ovarian Res *10*.

Chiti, M.C., Dolmans, M.M., Lucci, C.M., Paulini, F., Donnez, J et al. (2017b). Further insights into the impact of mouse follicle stage on graft outcome in an artificial ovary environment. MHR: Basic Science of Reproductive Medicine *23*, 381–392.

Chiti, M.C., Dolmans, M.M., Donnez, J. and Amorim, C.A. (2017c). Fibrin in Reproductive Tissue Engineering: A Review on Its Application as a Biomaterial for Fertility Preservation. Annals of Biomedical Engineering *45*, 1650–1663.

Chiti, M.C., Dolmans, M.-M., Mortiaux, L., Zhuge, F., Ouni, E et al. (2018). A novel fibrin-based artificial ovary prototype resembling human ovarian tissue in terms of architecture and rigidity. Journal of Assisted Reproduction and Genetics *35*, 41–48.

Da Silva-Buttkus, P., Marcelli, G., Franks, S., Stark, J. and Hardy, K et al. (2009). Inferring biological mechanisms from spatial analysis: Prediction of a local inhibitor in the ovary. Proceedings of the National Academy of Sciences *106*, 456–461.

Dath, C., Dethy, A., Van Langendonckt, A., Van Eyck, A.S., Amorim, C.A. et al. (2011). Endothelial cells are essential for ovarian stromal tissue restructuring after xenotransplantation of isolated ovarian stromal cells. Human Reproduction *26*, 1431–1439.

Dees, W.L., Hiney, J.K., McArthur, N.H., Johnson, G.A., Dissen, G.A. et al. (2006). Origin and Ontogeny of Mammalian Ovarian Neurons. Endocrinology *147*, 3789–3796.

Donnez, J. and Dolmans, M.-M. (2013). Fertility preservation in women. Nat Rev Endocrinol *9*, 735–749.

Fan, X., Bialecka, M., Moustakas, I., Lam, E., Torrens-Juaneda, V. et al. (2019). Single-cell reconstruction of follicular remodeling in the human adult ovary. Nature Communications *10*.

Feher, J. (2012). Female Reproductive Physiology. In Quantitative Human Physiology, (Elsevier), pp. 846–855.

Felder, S., Masasa, H., Orenbuch, A., Levaot, N., Shachar Goldenberg, M. et al. (2019). Reconstruction of the ovary microenvironment utilizing macroporous scaffold with affinity-bound growth factors. Biomaterials *205*, 11–22.

Fraser, L.R. (1987). Strontium supports capacitation and the acrosome reaction in mouse sperm and rapidly activates mouse eggs. Gamete Research *18*, 363–374.

Freeman, I. and Cohen, S. (2009). The influence of the sequential delivery of angiogenic factors from affinity-binding alginate scaffolds on vascularization. Biomaterials *30*, 2122–2131.

Hassanpour, A., Talaei-Khozani, T., Kargar-Abarghouei, E., Razban, V. and Vojdani, Z. et al. (2018). Decellularized human ovarian scaffold based on a sodium lauryl ester sulfate (SLES)-treated protocol, as a natural three-dimensional scaffold for construction of bioengineered ovaries. Stem Cell Research & Therapy *9*.

Hern, D.L. and Hubbell, J.A. (1998). Incorporation of adhesion peptides into nonadhesive hydrogels useful for tissue resurfacing. Journal of Biomedical Materials Research *39*, 266–276.

Hickey, T.E., Marrocco, D.L., Amato, F., Ritter, L.J., Norman, R.J. et al. (2005). Androgens Augment the Mitogenic Effects of Oocyte-Secreted Factors and Growth Differentiation Factor 9 on Porcine Granulosa Cells1. Biology of Reproduction *73*, 825–832.

Hillier, S.G., Whitelaw, P.F. and Smyth, C.D. (1994). Follicular oestrogen synthesis: the 'two-cell, two-gonadotrophin' model revisited. Molecular and Cellular Endocrinology *100*, 51–54.

Jakus, A.E., Laronda, M.M., Rashedi, A.S., Robinson, C.M., Lee, C. et al. (2017). "Tissue Papers" from Organ-Specific Decellularized Extracellular Matrices. Advanced Functional Materials *27*, 1700992.

Jiang, T., Carbone, E.J., Lo, K.W.-H. and Laurencin, C.T. (2015). Electrospinning of polymer nanofibers for tissue regeneration. Progress in Polymer Science *46*, 1–24.

Joo, S., Oh, S.-H., Sittadjody, S., Opara, E.C., Jackson, J.D. et al. (2016). The effect of collagen hydrogel on 3D culture of ovarian follicles. Biomedical Materials *11*, 065009.

Jun, I., Han, H.-S., Edwards, J. and Jeon, H. (2018). Electrospun Fibrous Scaffolds for Tissue Engineering: Viewpoints on Architecture and Fabrication. International Journal of Molecular Sciences *19*, 745.

Kawasaki, T., Kirita, Y., Kami, D., Kitani, T., Ozaki, C. et al. (2015). Novel detergent for whole organ tissue engineering: Organ Tissue Engineering for Various Organs. Journal of Biomedical Materials Research Part A *103*, 3364–3373.

Kawecki, M., Łabuś, W., Klama-Baryla, A., Kitala, D., Kraut, M. et al. (2018). A review of decellurization methods caused by an urgent need for quality control of cell-free extracellular matrix' scaffolds and their role in regenerative medicine: REVIEW OF DECELLURIZATION METHODS. Journal of Biomedical Materials Research Part B: Applied Biomaterials *106*, 909–923.

Kehm, R.D., Yang, W., Tehranifar, P. and Terry, M.B. (2019). 40 Years of Change in Age- and Stage-Specific Cancer Incidence Rates in US Women and Men. JNCI Cancer Spectrum *3*.

Kim, J., Perez, A.S., Claflin, J., David, A., Zhou, H. et al. (2016). Synthetic hydrogel supports the function and regeneration of artificial ovarian tissue in mice. Npj Regenerative Medicine *1*.

Kim, S.S., Yang, H.W., Kang, H.G., Lee, H.H., Lee, H.C. et al. (2004). Quantitative assessment of ischemic tissue damage in ovarian cortical tissue with or without antioxidant (ascorbic acid) treatment. Fertility and Sterility *82*, 679–685.

Kniazeva, E., Hardy, A.N., Boukaidi, S.A., Woodruff, T.K., Jeruss, J.S. et al. (2016). Primordial Follicle Transplantation within Designer Biomaterial Grafts Produce Live Births in a Mouse Infertility Model. Scientific Reports *5*.

Knop, K., Hoogenboom, R., Fischer, D. and Schubert, U.S. (2010). Poly(ethylene glycol) in Drug Delivery: Pros and Cons as Well as Potential Alternatives. Angewandte Chemie International Edition *49*, 6288–6308.

Krotz, S.P., Robins, J.C., Ferruccio, T.-M., Moore, R., Steinhoff, M.M. et al. (2010). In vitro maturation of oocytes via the pre-fabricated self-assembled artificial human ovary. Journal of Assisted Reproduction and Genetics *27*, 743–750.

Lai, D., Labuz, J.M., Kim, J., Luker, G.D., Shikanov, A et al. (2013). Simple multi-level microchannel fabrication by pseudo-grayscale backside diffused light lithography. RSC Advances *3*, 19467.

Laronda, M.M., Jakus, A.E., Whelan, K.A., Wertheim, J.A., Shah, R.N. et al. (2015). Initiation of puberty in mice following decellularized ovary transplant. Biomaterials *50*, 20–29.

Laronda, M.M., Rutz, A.L., Xiao, S., Whelan, K.A., Duncan, F.E. et al. (2017). A bioprosthetic ovary created using 3D printed microporous scaffolds restores ovarian function in sterilized mice. Nature Communications *8*, 15261.

Lawson, A.K., Klock, S.C., Pavone, M.E., Hirshfeld-Cytron, J., Smith, K.N. et al. (2014). A Prospective Study of Depression and Anxiety in Female Fertility Preservation and Infertility Patients. Fertil Steril *102*, 1377–1384.

Lee, K., Silva, E.A. and Mooney, D.J. (2011). Growth factor delivery-based tissue engineering: general approaches and a review of recent developments. Journal of The Royal Society Interface *8*, 153–170.

Lee, W.-S., Otsuka, F., Moore, R.K. and Shimasaki, S. (2001). Effect of Bone Morphogenetic Protein-7 on Folliculogenesis and Ovulation in the Rat1. Biology of Reproduction *65*, 994–999.

Lee, W.-S., Yoon, S.-J., Yoon, T.-K., Cha, K.-Y., Lee, S.-H. et al. (2004). Effects of bone morphogenetic protein-7 (BMP-7) on primordial follicular growth in the mouse ovary. Mol. Reprod. Dev. *69*, 159–163.

Letourneau, J.M., Melisko, M.E., Cedars, M.I. and Rosen, M.P. (2011). A changing perspective: improving access to fertility preservation. Nat Rev Clin Oncol *8*, 56–60.

Letourneau, J.M., Ebbel, E.E., Katz, P.P., Oktay, K.H., McCulloch, C.E. et al. (2012). Acute ovarian failure underestimates age-specific reproductive impairment for young women undergoing chemotherapy for cancer. Cancer *118*, 1933–1939.

Liverani, L., Raffel, N., Fattahi, A., Preis, A., Hoffmann, I. et al. (2019). Electrospun patterned porous scaffolds for the support of ovarian follicles growth: a feasibility study. Scientific Reports *9*.

Logan, S., Perz, J., Ussher, J.M., Peate, M. and Anazodo, A. et al. (2019). Systematic review of fertility-related psychological distress in cancer patients: Informing on an improved model of care. Psycho-Oncology *28*, 22–30.

Lutolf, M.P. and Hubbell, J.A. (2003). Synthesis and Physicochemical Characterization of End-Linked Poly(ethylene glycol)- *co* -peptide Hydrogels Formed by Michael-Type Addition. Biomacromolecules *4*, 713–722.

Luyckx, V., Dolmans, M.-M., Vanacker, J., Scalercio, S.R., Donnez, J. et al. (2013). First step in developing a 3D biodegradable fibrin scaffold for an artificial ovary. Journal of Ovarian Research *6*, 83.

Luyckx, V., Dolmans, M.-M., Vanacker, J., Legat, C., Fortuño Moya, C. et al. (2014). A new step toward the artificial ovary: survival and proliferation of isolated murine follicles after autologous transplantation in a fibrin scaffold. Fertility and Sterility *101*, 1149–1156.

Martinez, F., Andersen, C.Y., Barri, P.N., Brannigan, R., Cobo, A. et al. (2017). Update on fertility preservation from the Barcelona International Society for Fertility Preservation–ESHRE–ASRM 2015 expert meeting: indications, results and future perspectives. Fertility and Sterility *108*, 407-415.e11.

Medrano, J.V., Andrés, M. del M., García, S., Herraiz, S. et al. (2018). Basic and Clinical Approaches for Fertility Preservation and Restoration in Cancer Patients. Trends in Biotechnology *36*, 199–215.

Mirzaeian, L., Eftekhari-Yazdi, P., Esfandiari, F., Eivazkhani, F., Rezazadeh Valojerdi et al. (2019). Induction of Mouse Peritoneum Mesenchymal Stem Cells into Germ Cell-Like Cells Using Follicular Fluid and Cumulus Cells-Conditioned Media. Stem Cells and Development *28*, 554–564.

Morgan, S., Anderson, R.A., Gourley, C., Wallace, W.H. and Spears, N. et al. (2012). How do chemotherapeutic agents damage the ovary? Human Reproduction Update *18*, 525–535.

Muñoz, M., Santaballa, A., Seguí, M.A., Beato, C., de la Cruz, S. et al (2016). SEOM Clinical Guideline of fertility preservation and reproduction in cancer patients (2016). Clinical and Translational Oncology *18*, 1229–1236.

Napolitano, A.P., Dean, D.M., Man, A.J., Youssef, J., Ho, D.N. et al. (2007). Scaffold-free three-dimensional cell culture utilizing micromolded nonadhesive hydrogels. BioTechniques *43*, 494–500.

Nilsson, E.E. (2003). Bone Morphogenetic Protein-4 Acts as an Ovarian Follicle Survival Factor and Promotes Primordial Follicle Development. Biology of Reproduction *69*, 1265–1272.

Oktay, K., Harvey, B.E., Partridge, A.H., Quinn, G.P., Reinecke, J. et al. (2018). Fertility Preservation in Patients With Cancer: ASCO Clinical Practice Guideline Update. Journal of Clinical Oncology *36*, 1994–2001.

Orisaka, M., Tajima, K., Mizutani, T., Miyamoto, K., Tsang, B.K. et al. (2006). Granulosa Cells Promote Differentiation of Cortical Stromal Cells into Theca Cells in the Bovine Ovary1. Biology of Reproduction *75*, 734–740.

Pacheco, F. and Oktay, K. (2017). Current Success and Efficiency of Autologous Ovarian Transplantation: A Meta-Analysis. Reproductive Sciences *24*, 1111–1120.

Penrose, R., Beatty, L., Mattiske, J. and Koczwara, B. (2013). The Psychosocial Impact of Cancer-Related Infertility on Women: A Review and Comparison. Clinical Journal of Oncology Nursing *17*, 188–193.

Poirot, C., Brugieres, L., Yakouben, K., Prades-Borio, M., Marzouk, F. et al. (2019). Ovarian tissue cryopreservation for fertility preservation in 418 girls and adolescents up to 15 years of age facing highly gonadotoxic treatment. Twenty years of experience at a single center. Acta Obstetricia et Gynecologica Scandinavica *98*, 630–637.

Pors, S.E., Ramløse, M., Nikiforov, D., Lundsgaard, K., Cheng, J et al. (2019). Initial steps in reconstruction of the human ovary: survival of pre-antral stage follicles in a decellularized human ovarian scaffold. Human Reproduction *34*, 1523–1535.

Practice Committee of the American Society for Reproductive Medicine (2019). Fertility preservation in patients undergoing gonadotoxic therapy or gonadectomy: a committee opinion. Fertility and Sterility *112*, 1022–1033.

Rago, A.P., Dean, D.M. and Morgan, J.R. (2009). Controlling cell position in complex heterotypic 3D microtissues by tissue fusion. Biotechnology and Bioengineering *102*, 1231–1241.

Saldin, L.T., Cramer, M.C., Velankar, S.S., White, L.J. and Badylak, S.F. et al. (2017). Extracellular Matrix Hydrogels from Decellularized Tissues: Structure and Function. Acta Biomater *49*, 1–15.

Shahri, P.A.K., Chiti, M.C. and Amorim, C.A. (2019). Isolation and characterization of the human ovarian cell population for transplantation into an artificial ovary. Animal Reproduction *16*, 39–44.

Shikanov, A., Zhang, Z., Xu, M., Smith, R.M., Rajan, A. et al. (2011). Fibrin Encapsulation and Vascular Endothelial Growth Factor Delivery Promotes Ovarian Graft Survival in Mice. Tissue Engineering Part A *17*, 3095–3104.

Sittadjody, S., Saul, J.M., McQuilling, J.P., Joo, S., Register, T.C. et al. (2017). In vivo transplantation of 3D encapsulated ovarian constructs in rats corrects abnormalities of ovarian failure. Nature Communications *8*.

Smith, R.M., Shikanov, A., Kniazeva, E., Ramadurai, D., Woodruff, T.K. et al. (2014). Fibrin-Mediated Delivery of an Ovarian Follicle Pool in a Mouse Model of Infertility. Tissue Engineering Part A *20*, 3021–3030.

Soares, M., Saussoy, P., Maskens, M., Reul, H., Amorim, C.A. et al. (2017). Eliminating malignant cells from cryopreserved ovarian tissue is possible in leukaemia patients. British Journal of Haematology *178*, 231–239.

Tagler, D.J., Shea, L.D. and Woodruff, T.K. (2011). Contributions of ovarian stromal cells to follicle culture. In Principles and Practice of Fertility Preservation, J. Donnez and S.S. Kim, eds. (Cambridge: Cambridge University Press), pp. 409–420.

Tajima, K., Orisaka, M., Mori, T. and Kotsuji, F. (2007). Ovarian theca cells in follicular function. Reproductive BioMedicine Online *15*, 591–609.

Vanacker, J., Luyckx, V., Dolmans, M.-M., Des Rieux, A., Jaeger, J. et al. (2012). Transplantation of an alginate–matrigel matrix containing isolated ovarian cells: First step in developing a biodegradable scaffold to transplant isolated preantral follicles and ovarian cells. Biomaterials *33*, 6079–6085.

Villalona, G.A., Udelsman, B., Duncan, D.R., McGillicuddy, E., Sawh-Martinez, R.F. et al. (2010). Cell-Seeding Techniques in Vascular Tissue Engineering. Tissue Eng Part B Rev *16*, 341–350.

Wallace, W.H.B., Kelsey, T.W. and Anderson, R.A. (2016). Fertility preservation in pre-pubertal girls with cancer: the role of ovarian tissue cryopreservation. Fertility and Sterility *105*, 6–12.

Walters, K.A., Allan, C.M. and Handelsman, D.J. (2008). Androgen Actions and the Ovary. Biology of Reproduction *78*, 380–389.

Wang, Z., Wang, Z., Lu, W.W., Zhen, W., Yang, D. et al. (2017). Novel biomaterial strategies for controlled growth factor delivery for biomedical applications. NPG Asia Materials *9*, e435–e435.

Xu, M., Kreeger, P.K., Shea, L.D. and Woodruff, T.K. (2006). Tissue-Engineered Follicles Produce Live, Fertile Offspring. Tissue Eng *12*, 2739–2746.

Xu, M., Barrett, S.L., West-Farrell, E., Kondapalli, L.A., Kiesewetter, S.E. et al. (2009). In vitro grown human ovarian follicles from cancer patients support oocyte growth. Human Reproduction *24*, 2531–2540.

Yoon, D.M. and Fisher, J.P. (2009). Natural and Synthetic Polymeric Scaffolds. In Biomedical Materials, R. Narayan, ed. (Boston, MA: Springer US), pp. 415–442.

28

3D Bioprinting of Kidney

Chandra Lekha Putta,[1] *Rounik Karmakar*[1]
and *Aravind Kumar Rengan*[1]*

1. Introduction

Long-term impairment of kidney function is known as chronic renal failure, and 697.5 million individuals worldwide were afflicted with it in 2017 (Bikbov et al., 2017; Bülow and Boor, 2019). Kidney fibrosis, which is typified by an upsurge in extracellular matrix (ECM) accumulation, is the characteristic endpoint of chronic renal failure (Bülow, Boor, 2019). As renal failure worsens, individuals are kept waiting for an appropriate donor kidney, and patients with an advanced illness of renal disease are put on life-saving dialysis treatment (Peired et al., 2020; Peloso et al., 2015; Wilm et al., 2016). Humans have 2 kidneys, and although it is possible to survive with just one, kidney donations from living humans are extremely uncommon, and organs from deceased donors now meet the demand for organs. However, the lack of sufficient functional donor kidneys is a limitation of kidney transplantation. Three-dimensional (3D) bioprinting technology presents a significant possibility to supply those much-needed organs. The detailed therapy for kidney transplantation is explained in Figure 1.

The field of organ biofabrication holds great promise. It is anticipated that 3D printing would completely transform the area of regenerative medicine by making it possible to create intricate, precise, and personalised structures. Customised structures may be printed with remarkable precision because of the automation of bioprinting (Hesuani et al., 2016). Medical professionals have already used 3D plastic replicas of complex tumours, or bone fractures created from images obtained from CT (computed tomography) or MRI (magnetic resonance imaging), to train physicians and give them an excellent training platform prior to working on the patient's tissues (Colaco et al., 2018). Nevertheless, live cells provide a new degree of complexity to bioprinted tissues. Simple tissues like cartilage have previously been successfully printed (Colaco et al., 2018). Yet, the formulation and choice of the "printing ink", comprising a blend of cellular components and biomaterials that support cell viability and proliferation, will be pivotal for bioprinting soft tissues or intricate organs like the kidneys (Murphy, Atala, 2014; Skardal, Atala, 2015). Nonetheless, there has already been

[1] Department of Biomedical Engineering, Indian Institute of Technology Hyderabad, Kandi, India.
* Corresponding author: aravind@bme.iith.ac.in

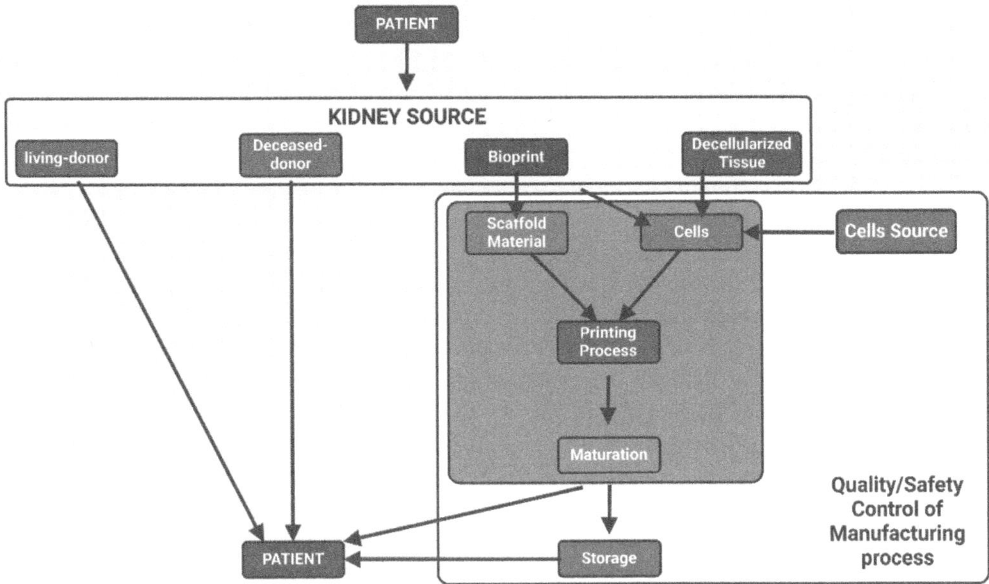

Fig. 1   Timeline therapy for kidney donation

significant success, as seen by the recent revelation of the 3D bioprinting of a functioning thyroid gland (Bulanova et al., 2017).

Significant efforts have been made to produce bioengineered kidney units that could replace or supplement a kidney to improve renal function, particularly to tackle the kidney shortage (Peired et al., 2021). Though the attainment of these units remains distant from reality, academics have worked on building *in vitro* models that can be used to study kidney disease and potential regenerative therapeutics. Bioprinting technology, which enables the construction of 3D structures integrating biomaterials, cells, and other biological components in pre-planned techniques, has produced kidney *in vitro* models. However, there are many obstacles to overcome when bioprinting renal constructs: (i) selecting the right type(s) of renal cells, (ii) selecting the right biomaterial(s), and (iii) finding an approach to build the intricate renal architecture needed to maintain the biological structure while promoting tissue integration after printing (Peired et al., 2020). *In vitro* models are crucial for researching kidney illnesses and developing novel treatments. These *in vitro* models will shed light on the prospect of creating functional organs in the future, a goal scientists pursue. In this chapter, the current state of bioprinted renal models will be investigated, emphasizing kidney cells, biomaterials, and manufacturing processes. In addition, a brief discussion of various models will be given because of their ability to enable increased tissue mimicking, function, and maturation. Lastly, a perspective is given that highlights some important aspects to think about further development.

2.   Renal System: Kidney Anatomy and Physiology

The kidneys are a major component of the urinary system, including the ureters, bladder, and urethra **Figure 2**. They eliminate waste from the blood and the body through urine. The adult kidney filters about 120 milliliters of blood plasma each minute and is located in the peritoneal cavity on either side of the spinal cord (Gueutin et al., 2012). The 11th and 12th pairs of ribs provide partial safeguarding of the kidneys. Since the liver is located above the kidney on the right side, as shown in the **Figure 2**, the left kidney is located slightly higher than the right one. The kidneys perform several additional homeostatic functions, such as: modulating blood pressure, volume, pH, and the equilibrium of electrolytes; erythropoiesis (the process of making red blood cells) stimulation; aiding in the production of vitamin D (Moinuddin, Dhanda et al., 2015).

2.1 *Kidney Anatomy*

The typical dimensions of an adult kidney are 12 cm long, 6 cm broad, and 3 cm deep (Mahadevan, 2019). Typically, the right kidney is approximately 2 mm shorter and weighs around 8 g less than the left kidney. Its position is slightly lower compared to the left kidney, primarily due to the presence and size of the liver beneath the upper right portion of the abdominal cavity (Kalucki et al., 2020).

Three major layers surround each kidney. Following in order of outermost to the innermost layers are: Renal fascia, a delicate covering of connective tissue that gives the kidney structural support by joining it to surrounding tissue, such as the abdominal wall; The perirenal fat, the "adipose capsule," helps keep the kidney within the abdominal cavity and shields it from injury; The connective tissue known as the renal capsule aids in preserving the structural integrity of the kidney.

The renal cortex, renal medulla, and renal pelvis are typically considered as the three primary sections that make up the kidney's internal structure. The highest density of renal corpuscles (Figure 2) at the outermost portion, the cortex, gives the area a granular appearance (Mahadevan, 2019). The renal corpuscles, comprised of Bowman's capsule and glomerulus, serve as the filtration units for the nephrons. Blood arteries that supply the nephrons are analogously highly concentrated in the cortex. Renal pyramids are triangular structures located in the medulla, the centre portion of the kidney, and they are made up of the Henle loops and renal collecting ducts (Figure 2); and vasa recta arteries (Song, Yosypiv, 2012). The filtrate produced by the nephrons drains into the minor calyces, then the major calyces, via the renal papillae, and finally through pyramid-like structures. It is considered as urine when it reaches the minor calyces. The renal pelvis, connected to the deepest part of the kidney, is a structure created by the major calyces joining together, eventually becoming the ureter (Mahadevan, 2019). As a result, the renal pelvis leverages the ureter to transport urine from the main calyces to the bladder. The kidney is penetrated by the ureter, renal artery, vein, nerves, and lymphatic vessels at a location known as the hilum.

2.2 *Kidney Physiology*

Nephron

An adult kidney contains approximately 1 to 1.3 million nephrons, which are vital for the renal system's function (George et al., 2019). Since the majority of them have their structure in the renal cortex, 80–85% of them are referred to as cortical nephrons; the other 15-20% are referred to as juxtamedullary nephrons since they are located on the cortex-medulla boundary (RHickling et al., 2015).

Urine Production

Urine formation occurs in three key stages:

Glomerular filtration results in the production of renal filtrate, which contains blood components that are screened out; The body reabsorbs approximately 99% of the water and electrolytes present in the renal filtrate through tubular reabsorption (Zhuo, Li, 2013). The distal convoluted tubule and collecting duct are used to eliminate waste materials such as urea, uric acid, and metabolites in urine via the secretion process.

Nephrons are comprised of the following five sections (Figure 2).

Renal Corpuscle

The renal corpuscle, which consists of a dense network of glomerular capillaries (glomerulus) and the cup-shaped tubule (Bowman's capsule), filters blood plasma and produces renal filtrate as a byproduct. Blood flows from the renal artery to the glomerulus via the afferent arteriole and exits via the efferent arteriole. The renal corpuscle has several structural components that enable efficient and quick filtration. According to Koeppen and Stanton, the glomerular capillaries have roughly 100 times higher permeability than other body parts for water, tiny ions, and other solutes (Bruce Koeppen, 2018). This ensures effective filtration. The smaller diameter of the efferent arteriole

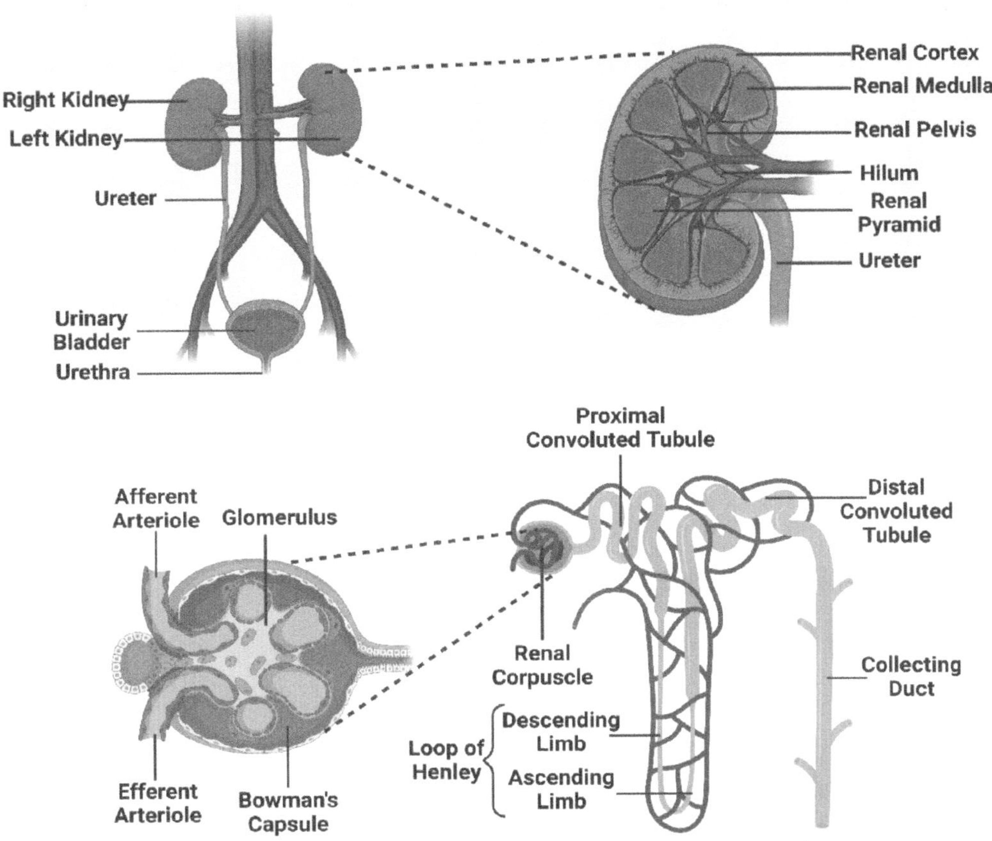

Fig. 2   Anatomy and physiology of kidney and its structural unit; Nephron illustration.

compared to the afferent arteriole restricts outflow and increases resistance, resulting in higher pressure within the glomerular capillaries (Theodorou et al., 2021). Subsequently, a filtration membrane composed of the basement membrane, the glomerular capillary endothelium, and a layer of podocytes is used to filter blood plasma into the internal cavity of the Bowman's capsule from the glomerular capillaries (Theodorou et al., 2021). Together, all three offer a very efficient method of selective permeability that allows only the substances that require filtration to pass through (Figure 2).

Proximal Convoluted Tubule

The renal filtrate enters the proximal convoluted tubule from the Bowman's capsule (Figure 2). One of its main functions is to allow the reabsorption of numerous significant water-soluble electrolytes, such as calcium bicarbonate, sodium chloride, and potassium, in addition to 70% of the filtrate's water (Zhuo, Li, 2013; Feraille et al., 2022). The body reabsorbs about 80% of the filtered bicarbonate from this region (Zhuo, Li, 2013). An additional 15% comes from the Henle's loop, which is primarily the ascending limb of Henle's loop, and 5% comes from the collecting duct and distal convoluted tubule (Zacchia et al., 2018; Hamm et al., 2015).

Loop of Henle

The remaining filtrate moves on to the loop of Henle, a crucial segment of the nephron responsible for the kidney's ability to concentrate urine and facilitate additional reabsorption of water and electrolytes following its passage through the proximal tubule (Chang, Davies, 2019). Consequently, this area is essential for controlling blood pressure, fluid volume, and acid-base balance via bicarbonate reabsorption (Marcoux et al., 2021). Its distinct structure and differential permeability enable the processes occurring in this region. The ascending and descending limbs are the primary sections of the Henle loop (Figure 2). The renal medulla has an osmotic gradient due to the Henle's loop path and the descending and ascending limbs' varying water permeabilities. This determines the kidney's capacity to concentrate urine depending on the countercurrent multiplier system (Price et al., 2023). The descending limb originates at the renal cortex and descends far into the renal medulla. It continues as an ascending limb, which returns to the renal cortex, by means of a hairpin bend (Zacchia et al., 2018). The descending limb is divided into two sections: the thick descending limb, which is the initial segment and shares structural similarities with the proximal convoluted tubule, and the thin descending limb, which narrows towards the end. Similarly, the thin ascending limb comes after the hairpin curve, and the broad ascending limb follows thereafter (Hoehn and Human, 2018). Comprising simple squamous epithelium, the descending limb exhibits high permeability to water. Approximately 20% of the water content in the filtrate is reabsorbed here as it exits the tubule and enters the interstitial fluid surrounding the nephrons (Feraille et al., 2022). Likewise, electrolytes like sodium chloride can pass through this area, facilitating significant reabsorption of these essential solutes. Additionally, urea enters the tubule to be eliminated (Cinnamon VanPutte et al., 2022). The ascending limb, on the other hand, is water impermeable. However, there are several ways in which ions, such as potassium, sodium, and chloride, pass into and out of the ascending limb. Here, ions are transported using active transport mechanisms, such as the utilization of specific transport proteins (Cinnamon VanPutte et al, 2022). The reabsorption of magnesium and calcium by the body is also attributed to the ascending limb (Zacchia et al., 2018). The region's impermeability to water, coupled with active solute transport, greatly enhances the kidney's ability to conserve water and maintain the osmotic gradient in the interstitial fluid surrounding the loop of Henle (Zacchia et al., 2018; Cinnamon VanPutte et al., 2022).

Distal Convoluted Tubule

The distal convoluted tubule, which starts where the thick ascending limb returns to the cortex and passes close to the glomerulus, is important for several processes, including the concentration of the renal filtrate and the reabsorption of water and electrolytes (Frederic et al., 2016). The juxtaglomerular (JG) apparatus is essential to the distal convoluted tubule's ability to regulate blood pressure. This complicated structure is the consequence of a specific interface between three major components at the point where the distal convoluted tubule enters the afferent arteriole (Hoehn and Human, 2018). Effective blood pressure regulation is accomplished by these three structures working together, both locally and more broadly. The JG apparatus is made up of the following three parts: the macula densa, JG cells and extraglomerular mesangial cells. At the juncture where the distal convoluted tubule passes the afferent arteriole, the tall, densely packed epithelial cells are compromised by the macula densa. These specific macula densa cells function as chemoreceptors, able to identify changes in the concentration of the solute (Hoehn and Human, 2018; Frederic et al., 2016). Juxtaglomerular (JG) cells are specialized smooth muscle cells found along the walls of the afferent and efferent arterioles. These cells, which contain secretory granules, produce the aspartic protease renin, an enzyme essential for blood pressure regulation and electrolyte balance as it activates the renin-angiotensin-aldosterone system (RAAS) (Yoshio Takei, Hironori Ando, 2015). When blood pressure decreases at the afferent arteriole, JG cells are stimulated to release renin, acting as mechanoreceptors. Extraglomerular mesangial cells, also called lacis cells, are flat cells situated between the afferent and efferent arterioles and in close proximity to the macula densa within the distal convoluted tubule. Although their precise role is still mostly unknown, it has been demonstrated that they contribute to the renin and erythropoietin production processes, stimulating the formation of red blood cells. Extraglomerular mesangial cells can metaplastically convert into distinct mature cell types that can produce renin when needed (Broeker et al., 2022).

Collecting Duct

The filtrate subsequently enters the collecting ducts, whose main function is to adjust its composition before the minor and major calyces direct it to the renal pelvis. Here, the filtrate can be modulated to regulate blood pressure, extracellular volume, acid-base balance, electrolyte levels, and overall water balance (Leiz, Schmidt-Ott, 2018). The collecting ducts are a crucial area from which the reabsorption of salt and chloride occurs because they employ specialized membrane transport mechanisms supported by hormonal regulation. The reabsorption of these solutes produces a concentration gradient, which facilitates water reabsorption (Leiz, Schmidt-Ott, 2019). The antidiuretic hormone regulates the resorption of about 9% of the water content of the filtrate in the collecting ducts. This is essential for controlling blood pressure (Feraille et al., 2022).

3.   Bioprinting Methods

The scarcity of donor kidneys for transplantation and the limitations of traditional tissue engineering approaches have spurred the development of bioprinting methods for kidney tissue engineering. Extrusion-based, microfluidics, and inkjet bioprinting have emerged as promising techniques for fabricating complex kidney structures. These methods offer unique advantages in terms of scalability, resolution, and cell viability (Li et al., 2016). Additionally, the integration of thermal, piezoelectric, electromagnetic, and acoustic actuation mechanisms has facilitated precise control over the deposition of cells and biomaterials, leading to enhanced structural and functional properties of bioprinted kidney constructs.

Extrusion-based Bioprinting

Extrusion-based bioprinting is one of the most common methods used for creating 3D kidney structures (Zhang et al., 2021; Krishna, Sankar, 2023). In this technique, bioink containing living cells is extruded through a nozzle onto a substrate in a layer-by-layer fashion to build the desired structure. The bioink typically consists of a hydrogel matrix that provides support for the cells.

Advantages

- Extrusion-based bioprinting can use a wide range of bioinks, including those containing different types of cells and biomaterials.
- It allows for the deposition of cells with high viability, as the shear stress on cells during extrusion can be controlled.
- This method offers precise control over the deposition of bioink, enabling the creation of complex kidney structures with defined architecture.

Challenges

- Extrusion-based bioprinting may have limitations in achieving high resolution, which can affect the ability to mimic the intricate structures of the kidney.
- The properties of the bioink, such as viscosity and crosslinking kinetics, must be carefully optimized to ensure proper extrusion and cell viability.

Microfluidics

Microfluidic bioprinting involves the use of microscale channels to manipulate bioink and cells with high precision. In this method, cells are encapsulated within droplets or fibers of bioink and then deposited onto a substrate to create the desired kidney structure (Streets, Huang, 2013; Wioland et al., 2020).

Advantages

- Microfluidic systems offer precise control over the size and placement of bioink droplets or fibers, allowing for the creation of complex kidney structures with microscale resolution.
- Microfluidic bioprinting can be scaled down to create small-scale kidney models or scaled up for mass production.
- This method enables the deposition of single cells or small clusters of cells, which is beneficial for mimicking the cellular composition of the kidney.

Challenges

- Microfluidic bioprinting systems can be complex to design and operate, requiring expertise in microfabrication and fluid dynamics.
- Despite the high precision, microfluidic bioprinting may have limitations in terms of throughput compared to other methods.

Inkjet Bioprinting

Inkjet bioprinting utilizes printheads to deposit tiny droplets of bioink containing cells onto a substrate to create 3D kidney structures. There are several types of inkjet bioprinting based on the energy source used to eject the droplets, including thermal, piezoelectric, electromagnetic, or acoustic energy (Li et al., 2020; Angelopoulos et al., 2020).

Advantages

- Inkjet bioprinting can achieve high printing speeds, making it suitable for high-throughput fabrication of kidney structures.
- Inkjet bioprinting typically involves gentle deposition of bioink droplets, minimizing shear stress on cells and preserving cell viability.
- Different types of inkjet bioprinters can accommodate a variety of bioinks, allowing for the incorporation of various cell types and biomaterials

Challenges

- Inkjet bioprinting works best with low-viscosity bioinks, which may limit the types of biomaterials that can be used.
- Achieving uniform droplet size and spacing can be challenging, affecting the resolution and structural integrity of the printed kidney tissue.
- Inkjet printheads are prone to clogging, particularly when using bioinks containing cells or biomaterials.

4. Biomaterials for Printing

The choice of biomaterial inks and bioinks varies depending on the bioprinting method utilized. Biomaterials fall into two main categories: polymers (such as thermoplastics, elastomers, and hydrogels) and composites. Certain polymers like thermoplastics and elastomers, along with specific composite formulations, are unsuitable for bioink creation due to their high processing temperatures and pressures. Instead, they are often employed to fabricate supportive 3D structures for softer hydrogel materials or as chambers for bioreactors.

Thermoplastic polymers, which soften when heated above their melting point and solidify upon cooling below their crystallization temperature, are useful for bioprinting renal in vitro models. A commonly used thermoplastic polymer is poly(ε-caprolactone) (PCL) due to its relatively low melting point (around 60°C). When used with fused deposition modeling (FDM), PCL serves as a scaffold structure for bioinks or chips utilized for perfusion in bioprinted kidney models. Utilizing elastomers as bioink for kidney bioprinting presents both opportunities and challenges in the field of tissue engineering. Elastomers, known for their flexibility, stretchability, and resilience, offer unique advantages for bioprinting applications. Their mechanical properties closely resemble those of native tissues, making them suitable for constructing soft and deformable structures, such as blood vessels and tubules, which are integral components of the kidney's architecture. Additionally, elastomers can be formulated to mimic the elasticity and compliance of renal tissues, providing a more physiologically relevant microenvironment for encapsulated cells. Hydrogels, consisting of hydrophilic polymer chains dissolved in aqueous solutions, offer numerous advantages such as biocompatibility, adjustable biodegradability, and a highly porous structure. Achieving the ideal hydrogel formulation involves balancing bioprinting resolution with post-bioprinting cellular behavior, which necessitates careful control of processing conditions. Hydrogels can be natural or synthetic, each offering unique benefits. While natural hydrogels mimic the biological microenvironment of native extracellular matrices (ECM), synthetic hydrogels allow for broader modifications such as chemical functionalization and precise control over physicochemical properties.

Decellularized ECM (dECM) is a highly investigated natural-based material for bioprinting due to its ability to form hydrogels with tissue-specific composition and biophysical properties conducive to cell proliferation, adhesion, and maturation. However, challenges include the requirement for donor organs or tissues, multistep processing for decellularization, and limited adjustability of biochemical composition. Chemical modification of dECM through methacrylation has been proposed to improve its bioprinting capabilities.

Biomaterials	Printing method	Advantages	Drawbacks	Ref.
Gelatin	Extrusion bioprinting, Microfluidics	Biocompatible	Limited mechanical strength	(Addario et al., 2020; Kolesky et al., 2018)
Alginate	Extrusion bioprinting	Excellent biocompatibility	Limited control over degradation rate	(Singh et al., 2020; Addario et al., 2020; Ouyang et al., 2015)
Fibrin	Extrusion bioprinting	Promotes cell attachment and migration	Rapid degradation	(King et al., 2017)
Poly(ε-caprolactone) (PCL)	Fused Deposition Modeling	Low melting temperature allows for cell encapsulation	Limited biodegradability	(Baskapan, Callanan, 2022; Pati et al., 2014)
Poly(lactic-co-glycolic acid) (PLGA)	ice particle leaching technique	Tunable degradation rate	Poor cell adhesion	(Cha et al., 2023)
Hyaluronic acid	Extrusion bioprinting	Provides native microenvironment	Requires donor organs or tissues	(Ali et al., 2019)
Hydrogels	Extrusion bioprinting, Inkjet bioprinting, Microfluidics	Highly porous structure for nutrient exchange	Difficulty in achieving mechanical strength	(Chai et al., 2017; Malda et al., 2013)
Pluronic F127	Extrusion bioprinting	Thermoresponsive for sacrificial bioprinting	Limited control over degradation rate	(Shamma et al., 2022)

5. In Vitro Model

In vitro 3D models for the kidney hold immense promise for advancing research and therapeutic strategies in nephrology (Chambers et al., 2023). These models, often constructed using bioprinting techniques and biomimetic materials, aim to recapitulate the intricate architecture and physiological functions of the kidney in a controlled laboratory setting. By faithfully replicating the microenvironment of renal tissues, these models offer researchers a platform to study various aspects of kidney biology, disease mechanisms, drug toxicity, and personalized medicine. One significant advantage of in vitro 3D kidney models is their ability to mimic the complexity of the native tissue, including the spatial arrangement of different cell types and the intricate network of blood vessels and tubules. This level of structural fidelity allows researchers to investigate cell-cell interactions, signaling pathways, and transport mechanisms in a more physiologically relevant context than traditional 2D cell cultures. Moreover, these models can be tailored to represent specific renal diseases or conditions, enabling researchers to explore disease pathogenesis and test potential therapeutic interventions in a controlled and reproducible manner. For example, researchers can use patient-derived cells to create personalized kidney models, allowing for the study of individual variations in drug responses and disease progression.

In addition to their research applications, in vitro 3D kidney models hold promise for clinical translation. They could serve as platforms for drug screening and toxicity testing, potentially reducing the reliance on animal models and accelerating the development of new therapies for kidney diseases. Furthermore, these models could facilitate the testing of novel regenerative medicine approaches, such as tissue engineering and cell-based therapies, by providing a platform for optimizing cell delivery strategies and assessing therapeutic efficacy. In vitro 3D models for the kidney, encompassing diverse methodologies such as renal organoids, microfluidics chips, decellularized scaffolds, and bioprinted constructs, represent a frontier in renal research and therapeutic development.

Type of Model	*Description*	*Ref.*
Renal Organoids	Three-dimensional structures derived from self-organizing renal progenitor cells or pluripotent stem cells that mimic aspects of kidney tissue architecture and function. Renal organoids contain multiple cell types organized in a spatially defined manner, resembling early stages of kidney development. They offer higher physiological relevance compared to traditional 2D cell cultures and allow for the study of kidney development, disease modeling, drug screening, and regenerative medicine applications.	(Lawlor et al., 2021; Takasato et al., 2016)
Kidney-on-a-Chip	Microfluidic devices designed to replicate the physiological conditions of the kidney, including fluid flow, shear stress, and cellular interactions. Kidney-on-a-chip models typically consist of microchannels lined with renal cells, allowing for the study of renal physiology, disease mechanisms, and drug responses in a controlled in vitro environment. These models offer advantages such as real-time monitoring of cellular responses and the ability to mimic complex tissue-tissue interfaces found in the kidney.	(Addario et al., 2020; Homan et al., 2016)
Bioprinted Constructs	Tissue-engineered constructs fabricated using bioprinting technologies, such as extrusion-based or inkjet bioprinting, to deposit renal cells and biomaterials layer-by-layer. Bioprinted kidney constructs enable precise spatial organization of cells and biomaterials, mimicking the native kidney architecture. These constructs can be used for studying tissue development, disease modeling, drug screening, and regenerative medicine applications, offering advantages such as customizable design and the ability to recapitulate complex tissue structures.	(Carreno-Galeano et al., 2020)
Decellularized Scaffolds	At present, renal transplantation stands as the most efficient remedy for end-stage renal disease, a significant contemporary public health concern. However, the scarcity of donor kidneys significantly falls short of meeting the demand, resulting in lengthy waitlists. Consequently, tissue engineering emerges as a promising avenue to augment the pool of available organs for kidney transplantation. This involves seeding cells onto supportive scaffold materials. These biological scaffolds are created by eliminating cellular elements from donor organs through a decellularization process employing detergents, enzymes, or similar solutions. The extracellular matrix constituting the scaffold plays a pivotal role in guiding cell attachment and fostering a conducive environment for cell viability, growth, and differentiation. Currently, researchers are exploring intact scaffolds derived from animal or human kidneys, aiming to preserve extracellular matrix integrity, biological activity, and mechanical stability. The process of recellularization encompasses strategies for cell seeding and selecting the appropriate cell source for repopulating the scaffold, which is deemed the most challenging phase due to the kidney's intricate nature.	(Figliuzzi et al., 2017; Caralt et al., 2015)

The functionality of bioprinted in vitro kidney models has been extensively characterized through various assays, including measurement of metabolic activity, expression of renal markers, and evaluation of physiological responses to stimuli such as nephrotoxic drugs or inflammatory cytokines. These studies have demonstrated that bioprinted kidney models can recapitulate key aspects of renal physiology, including tubular reabsorption, secretion, and barrier function.

6. Vasculature in Kidney Models

The kidney's vasculature network is of particular significance because it plays a major role in maintaining fluid homeostasis and filtering blood from waste materials (Pourhanifeh et al., 2019). The vascular tubule in the *in vitro* models; the proximal convoluted tubule and the vascular channel were first formed by a channel made up of pluronic filaments, as reported earlier (Lin et al., 2019). The co-cultivation of vascular endothelial cells and proximal tubule epithelium in the Lin et al. model results in crosstalk across compartments when subjected to hyperglycemic conditions (Lin et al., 2019). Bioprinting using ink with a layered-structure throughout the length of the tubules is another method for creating a tubular model (Singh et al., 2020). PT epithelial cells were printed using a triple coaxial nozzle, and the cells were added to the bioink formulations encircling a layer of epithelial cells that served as the filament's shell and were then printed around the pluronic core. These preliminary methods demonstrate that vascular lumens as large as hundreds of microns can be constructed; however, further investigation is required to reach the kidney glomerulus and the tubule interstitium's microvessel network's typical diameters of less than 100 microns.

7. Challenges/Limitations

The kidney is a large, intricate organ that must be printed with all its components in one attempt. This task is extremely challenging due to the organ size and the cell variability needed to operate it. Consequently, the only practical strategy is to 3D bioprint tiny fragments which might be assembled to form larger organs after printing. Organoids could be used for printing to address both of these issues—the organ's size and cell diversity. However, more pressing issues must be resolved first, such as the kidney's vascularization and the ductal system's vital role in urine drainage.

Vascularization

The most significant and unresolved issue in 3D bioprinting technologies is vascularization, or the printing of vascularized organs. Evidently, only thick bioprinted tissues and organs with good vascularization could endure after implantation. Many outstanding reviews have been written about the importance of vascularization in 3D bioprinting (Rouwkema et al., 2008; Rouwkema, Khademhosseini, 2016; Lovett et al., 2009; Costa-Almeida et al., 2014; Novosel et al., 2011), which emphasize how important it is to properly perfuse the vascular network and create a sufficiently dense system to keep the capillary distances under a minimum of 200 μm. The proper vasculature in freshly constructed kidneys is crucial for the long-term health of the kidneys because it has also been demonstrated that the development of kidney disease depends on the altering of the vascular structure (Ogunlade et al., 2018). Although there have been several optimistic technological advances over the past ten years, the bioprinted kidney's vascularization ability remains unclear and unattainable. The primary obstacle in our quest to bioprint a functioning human kidney continues to be the unresolved issue of vascularization. The vascularization of the kidney is particularly significant because it is essential to the two primary renal functions of filtration and reabsorption.

Theoretically, there are two main ways of accomplishing kidney vascularization: vasculogenesis from endothelial progenitors in the bioprinted kidney before implantation or emerging angiogenesis from the host organism's pre-existing vasculature after implantation. Indeed, it has been established that following implantation under an extensively vascularized kidney capsule (Xinaris et al., 2012; Xinaris et al., 2016) or subcutaneously (Bantounas et al., 2018), the kidney organoids can be efficiently vascularized and even facilitate glomerulogenesis. Furthermore, it is a common surgical procedure to omentopexy or vascularize an organ by mobilizing it and attaching it to extensively vascularized and angiogenic omentum tissue (Zhang et al., 2011; Hammerman, 2002). Nevertheless, this method works best when transplanting a very modest amount of renal tissue, as the growing metanephros (Hammerman, 2002).

Nonetheless, numerous studies (Bikbov et al., 2017; Halt et al., 2016; Gao et al., 2005; Robert et al., 1998; Hyink et al., 1996) have documented the formation of the renal vasculature from an indigenous group of endothelial progenitors. However, in the absence of blood flow, only the initial stages of renal vascularization-before the glomerular tuft formation could occur (Halt et al., 2016; Rymer et al., 2015). According to an investigation, blood circulation plays a vital role in the development of vascularized glomeruli (Serluca et al., 2002), consistent with observations from studies involving the transplantation of renal organoids (Xinaris et al., 2012; Xinaris et al., 2016; Bantounas et al., 2018). Vascularized mini-tissues can be biofabricated, attributed to the swift advancement of microfluidic technology (Bersini et al., 2015; Song et al., 2015). One successful application of microfluidic technology is the biofabrication of vascularized tumor spheroids (Jeon et al., 2015). It provides a feasible opportunity to employ human endothelial cells to develop vascularized human kidney organoids. Vascularized kidney organoids have the potential to be an effective research tool for real-time, single-cell analysis of human glomerulogenesis and nephrogenesis. Automation and robotization strategies are relatively new, and further research is needed before it can be successfully implemented, particularly on an extensive level.

When sacrificial hydrogels—also known as removable hydrogels—are developed, a novel and intriguing method for vascularizing thick 3D tissues and organs is put forward. This method involves creating passages in 3D tissues that can later be seeded with endothelial cells (Kolesky et al., 2016; Kolesky et al., 2014; Miller et al., 2012). There are two primary drawbacks to this strategy, though. It is highly effective in biofabricating microvascular networks with tiny diameters, but it cannot create large diameter capillaries with relatively thick walls that could be surgically attached to the recipient's primary arteries. Furthermore, it is currently unclear how this method could be used to bioprint the kidney's vascularized parenchyma. The Jennifer Lewis group has most recently bioprinted functioning kidney tubules utilizing the sacrificial hydrogel approach (Homan et al., 2016). Anthony Atala's group has recently presented another sophisticated and perhaps effective method for renal vascularization (Huling et al., 2016). The kidney vascular system was biomimicked by biofabricating a collagen-based hydrogel covering on a tubular scaffold. Mini-tissues or tissue mini-blocks must be placed robotically in an open area; however, this method cannot be used with the current 3D scaffold. Furthermore, it is unclear if the artificial kidney vascular structures or other large diameter segments have strong adequate material for surgical suturing.

Therefore, the primary obstacle to resolving the vascularization of a bioprinted kidney is not merely producing renal tissue modules with a microvascular network or bioprinting several kidney nephrons and tiny kidney pieces. Rather, the primary obstacle is to bioprint a kidney construct that has an integrated intra-organ branched vasculature, complete vascular segments with large diameter that can be sutured surgically.

8. Possible Solutions

The adult kidney is a complicated organ comprising millions of cells that are diversely categorized into hundreds of types. Individual cell bioprinting is currently not feasible due to technical limitations, and printing a complicated morphological structure would be very difficult. We assume the renal development program will be used in the bioprinting process for bioprinting kidneys. The embryonic kidney's capacity for independent development *in vitro* is remarkable (Unbekandt, Davies, 2010; Rak-Raszewska et al., 2012). The ability of primary differentiated cells to develop into renal cells and create functional nephrons through organoids' self-assembly is even more remarkable (Takasato et al., 2014; Takasato et al., 2015; Morizane, Bonventre, 2017). The kidney's general morphology cannot be recapitulated by the renal structures, which limits this potential.

Although there are still certain obstacles to overcome, we firmly think that the kidney may be 3D printed utilizing cell spheroids as the building units; this approach considers all necessary components, including the ductal system, the major kidney mass, and the vasculature. This idea has already been described in some reviews and studies (Mironov et al., 2008; Visconti et al., 2010) regarding printed vasculature. Additionally, many groups have produced bioprinted vascular segments with a large diameter that can be sutured surgically (Kelm et al., 2010; Itoh et al., 2015; Norotte et al., 2009). Large lumenized capillary segments can be bioprinted using sacrificial vascular tissue spheroids. Using lumenized vascular tissue spheroids, vascular segments could be fabricated and bioprinted (Gentile et al., 2008; Fleming et al., 2010). Vascular endothelial growth factor (VEGF) could be used for developing the vascular network from fibrin and collagen hydrogels implanted with endothelial cells (Davis et al., 2002; Kamei et al., 2006; Nunes et al., 2010). Lastly, isolated vascular tree segments or endothelial spheroids can combine to form an *in vivo* and *in vitro* microvascular network (Laschke, Menger, 2015; Alajati et al., 2008).

It is plausible to develop organoids using only patient-derived cells, given the protocols currently in place to differentiate human pluripotent stem cells (HPSCs)/human-induced pluripotent stem cells (HiPSCs) into neural progenitor cells. Furthermore, similar to the organoids developed from primary mouse MM cells, these organoids could fuse together when printed in close proximity, allowing the development of bigger complexes. Another potential method is deriving urinary bladder progenitor cells from HPSCs/HiPSCs, allowing the ureter structures to be printed without non-human cells. A tiny kidney and the vascular units would need to be installed in a microfluidic chamber once they were 3D bioprinted to supply the flow and allow the kidneys to function. The larger vasculature structures would maintain the primary flow. This flow would allow the endothelial cells to reorganize themselves in close proximity to the kidney units, forming capillaries that would reach the renal organoids and vascularize the growing glomeruli.

9. Practical Application

Although the primary objective of regenerative medicine is to facilitate the manufacture of organs free from rejection for transplantation, the smaller 3D bioprinted operational kidney units might currently have applications in pharmacology or other biomedical fields (Figure 3).

Screening of Nephrotoxicity

The detrimental effects of pharmaceutical compounds, homes, industrial, and environmental pollutants, as well as dietary additives and natural substances, are highly sensitive to the kidney (Shirali, Pazhayattil, 2014; Perneger et al., 1994; Kataria et al., 2015; Gutiérrez 2013; Jha, Rathi, 2008; Isnard Bagnis et al., 2004). Glomerular blood filtration is the first step in the renal excretion of hazardous chemicals. Subsequently it passes into the proximal convoluted tubule, which reabsorbs the essential components, and then through the loop of Henle, which concentrates the filtrate. Urine then travels through the collecting duct and distal tubule before being further concentrated and stored in the bladder until the micturition process, which is the last stage of the procedure, removes it from the body. The proximal tubule, where the reabsorption of hazardous substances leads to kidney damage, is the focus of most nephrotoxicity research.

About 90% of potential medications fail in human trials due to the animal models' prediction limitations (Gintant et al., 2016). Furthermore, the *in vitro* models currently used for nephrotoxicity research do not accurately represent the biological processes involved in kidney function. While nephrotoxicity accounts for just 7% of new therapeutic agent failures in pre-clinical trials, pharmacological substances' nephrotoxic effects cause acute kidney injury in 17%–26% of hospital patients (Mehta et al., 2004; Uchino, 2005). The capacity to test the nephrotoxicity of novel substances will be enhanced by even the smallest 3D bioprinted functional kidney units. On the other

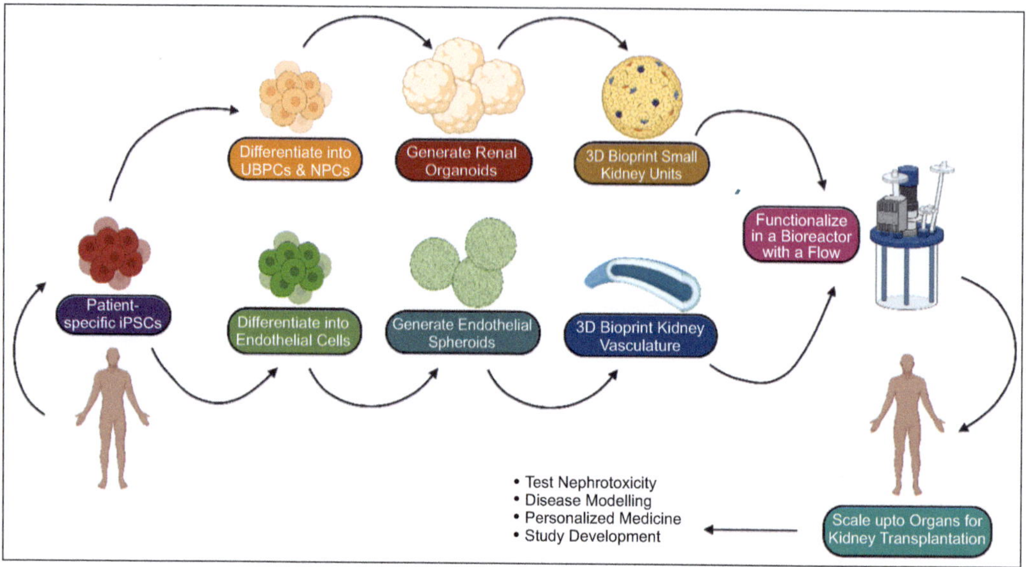

Fig. 3   Schematic workflow of kidney 3D bioprinting

side, this would make it possible to stop using defective medications earlier or change the drugs to make it less harmful to kidney cells. Additionally, this could speed up research and lower the cost of producing new medications by reducing the number of animal tests required during the pre-clinical testing phase (Chu et al., 2013; Greek, Menache, 2013; Olson et al., 2000). Numerous kidney *in vitro* simulations have been designed (Huang et al., 2013; Jang et al., 2011; Sciancalepore et al., 2014), but none have the functionality or the 3D structure closely resembling the genuine nephron *in vivo*. A kidney-on-a-chip enables the culture of renal cells and organoids within 3D networks. This technology replicates the renal filtering, absorption, and excretion of the drug while simulating the physiological environment (Sochol et al., 2016; Lee et al., 2018). Generally, they consist of a single layer of kidney cells within a microfluidic container devoid of the three-dimensional structure found in the actual organ.

Although the hPSC-derived kidney organoids produced by investigators using various techniques were able to react to nephrotoxicity studies (Takasato et al., 2015; Freedman et al., 2015; Morizane et al., 2015), they are still devoid of the collecting duct system and vasculature. Numerous known nephrotoxic and non-nephrotoxic chemicals would need to be tested to validate the concept (Wilmer et al., 2016; Xie et al., 2013). However, a mini-kidney library developed from hPSCs might benefit pharmaceutical companies. In addition to being used as customized testing platforms for nephrotoxicity, these 3D bioprinted kidneys would also be used to customize treatment plans to prevent kidney failure in individuals with pre-existing risk factors like diabetes and lessen kidney damage.

Personalized Medicine and Kidney Disease Model

Another crucial use for the 3D bioprinted kidney would be renal disease modeling. Patient-specific hiPSCs or genetically modified hPSCs with mutations that cause kidney disease would be used to develop the illness-specific kidneys (Cruz, 2018). The kidney disease organoids particular to each patient might then be employed for either genomic repair of the genetic abnormalities or fast ex vivo testing of targeted medication therapy. The model would produce information to improve our knowledge of the disease's pathogenesis and molecular foundation. It would be beneficial as well (Mundel, 2017). 3D cultures of primary cells derived from patients have been used to model polycystic kidney disease (PKD) (Jansson et al., 2022). Freedman et al. have derived induced pluripotent stem cells (iPS cells) from renal disease patients and observed decreased polycystin 2 levels in the cilia of polycystic renal disorder cells. This problem was remedied by overexpression of polycystin 1 (Freedman et al., 2013). The same group has previously investigated gene-modified kidney organoids with PKD (Cruz et al., 2017). In this study, they mutated the kidney organoid to include PKD1, examined cysts' formation, and discovered cystogenesis's modulators. The creation of organoids can supply the latter, and it has previously been suggested that this would make an ideal platform for disease modelling (Freedman, 2015; Clevers, 2016; Garreta, 2018).

Kidney Development Study

The kidney has the most intricate architecture, second only to the central nervous system, and is made up of over 20 distinct specialised cell types. Understanding the development and vascularization of the metanephric kidney would be aided by the utilization of the bioprinted and vascularized kidney. Recently, the differentiation of podocytes has been studied using hPSCs/hiPSC-derived kidney organoids, and the study emphasized the role of podocalyxin in podocyte production (Kim et al., 2017).

Regenerative Medicine

The human kidney lacks the capacity to produce new nephrons after birth, although it can regenerate new tubular cells in an episode of acute renal damage (Little, McMahon, 2012). Thus, dialysis/kidney transplantation are now the only alternatives available for treating individuals with chronic kidney failure. The main objective is to establish methods for repairing and regenerating damaged kidney tissue and producing whole kidneys for transplantation, given the rapidly expanding population of individuals needing new kidneys. It has an excretory system to operate and discharge urine, even if the existing organoid model demonstrates incredible cellular differentiation and tissue design potential. Although creating transplantable kidneys is the ultimate goal of 3D bioprinted kidneys, recapitulating the *in vivo* functional kidney is a more practical and immediate goal. How simple or complex should it be is the question.

10.   Conclusion and Future Scope

Rapid advancements in 3D bioprinting technologies will soon make it feasible to 3D bioprint soft tissues like the kidney and solid ones. Many of the technologies are actually already in use. Our ability to effectively differentiate patient-derived cells into endothelium or kidney lineages will be a great supply of cells for creating organoids. We can build fully formed renal organoids with several functioning cells and nephron structures arranged correctly. Other sphcroids derived from endothelial cells can also be produced, and they could serve as a source of tissue for 3D bioprinting of the vasculature. The innovations that were demonstrated all have the potential to be utilized as building blocks for vascularized tiny kidney units to be printed using 3D bioprinting. It would be necessary to print the kidney structure and the vasculature simultaneously, or to print them separately and then combine them in a bioreactor or microfluidic chamber so that the applied flow could start the kidneys' process of capillarization.

Regarding the bioink material selection for renal bioprinting, kidney-derived decellularized extracellular matrix may present an intriguing substitute to attain enhanced cell capacity, provided that its power-driven integrity is reinforced through other means, such as blending it with another hydrogel. While each type of bioink has advantages and disadvantages of its own, it is possible to combine two or more complimentary bioinks to reach sufficient qualities for successful kidney bioprinting. Alternatively, it's possible that an entirely new bioprinting strategy will be developed to address the drawbacks of the available printing techniques.

Future methods will probably investigate combining several bioprinting techniques on one board, ranging from macro-scale and multi-cellular prototypes to single cell deposition. These models will be crucial for studying renal disorders, and developing drugs *in vitro*. These will also gradually aid in the resolution of numerous upcoming problems that remain unresolved, enabling the gradual production of new knowledge that will undoubtedly support prospective alternative therapies. It will therefore only be a matter of time until we are able to appropriately integrate our understanding of developmental biology and stem cells with 3D bioprinting and microfluidic technologies, assembling the final pieces of the puzzle to successfully 3D bioprint the kidney's functional units.

References

Addario G., Djudjaj S., Farè S., Boor P., Moroni L. et al. Microfluidic bioprinting towards a renal in vitro model. Bioprinting [Internet]. 2020 Dec;20:e00108. Available from: https://linkinghub.elsevier.com/retrieve/pii/S240588662030035X

Alajati A., Laib A.M., Weber H., Boos A.M., Bartol A. et al. Spheroid-based engineering of a human vasculature in mice. Nat Methods. 2008 May; 5(5): 439–45.

Ali M., PR A.K., Yoo J.J., Zahran F., Atala A. et al. A Photo-Crosslinkable Kidney ECM-Derived Bioink Accelerates Renal Tissue Formation. Adv Healthc Mater [Internet]. 2019 Apr 6; 8(7). Available from: https://onlinelibrary.wiley.com/doi/10.1002/adhm.201800992

Angelopoulos I., Allenby M.C., Lim M., Zamorano M. Engineering inkjet bioprinting processes toward translational therapies. Biotechnol Bioeng [Internet]. 2020 Jan 6; 117(1): 272–84. Available from: https://onlinelibrary.wiley.com/doi/10.1002/bit.27176

Bantounas I., Ranjzad P., Tengku F., Silajdžić E., Forster D. et al. Generation of Functioning Nephrons by Implanting Human Pluripotent Stem Cell-Derived Kidney Progenitors. Stem Cell Reports. 2018 Mar; 10(3): 766–79.

Baskapan B., Callanan A. Electrospinning Fabrication Methods to Incorporate Laminin in Polycaprolactone for Kidney Tissue Engineering. Tissue Eng Regen Med [Internet]. 2022 Feb; 19(1): 73–82. Available from: https://link.springer.com/10.1007/s13770-021-00398-1

Bersini S., Moretti M. 3D functional and perfusable microvascular networks for organotypic microfluidic models. J Mater Sci Mater Med. 2015 May; 26(5): 180.

Bikbov B., Purcell C.A., Levey A.S., Smith M., Abdoli A. et al. Global, regional, and national burden of chronic kidney disease, 1990–2017: a systematic analysis for the Global Burden of Disease Study 2017. Lancet. 2020 Feb; 395(10225): 709–33.

Broeker K.A.E., Schrankl J., Fuchs M.A.A., Kurtz A. Flexible and multifaceted: the plasticity of renin-expressing cells. Pflügers Arch - Eur J Physiol. 2022 Aug; 474(8): 799–812.

Bruce M. Koeppen B.A.S. Renal Physiology E-Book. Elsevier Health Sciences; 2018. 272 p.

Bulanova E.A., Koudan E.V., Degosserie J., Heymans C., Pereira F D.A.S. et al. Bioprinting of a functional vascularized mouse thyroid gland construct. Biofabrication. 2017 Aug; 9(3): 034105.

Bülow R.D., Boor P. Extracellular Matrix in Kidney Fibrosis: More Than Just a Scaffold. J Histochem Cytochem. 2019 Sep; 67(9): 643–61.

Caralt M., Uzarski J.S., Iacob S., Obergfell K.P., Berg N. et al. Optimization and Critical Evaluation of Decellularization Strategies to Develop Renal Extracellular Matrix Scaffolds as Biological Templates for Organ Engineering and Transplantation. Am J Transplant [Internet]. 2015 Feb; 15(1): 64–75. Available from: https://linkinghub.elsevier.com/retrieve/pii/S1600613522000855

Carreno-Galeano G., Ali M., Jackson* J., Yoo J., Lee S.J., Atala A. et al. MP52-08 3D BIOPRINTED RENAL TISSUE CONSTRUCTS USING A NOVEL KIDNEY ECM-DERIVED BIOINK. J Urol [Internet]. 2020 Apr; 203 (Supplement 4). Available from: http://www.jurology.com/doi/10.1097/JU.0000000000000914.08

Cha S-G., Rhim W-K., Kim J.Y., Lee E.H., Lee S.Y. et al. Kidney tissue regeneration using bioactive scaffolds incorporated with differentiating extracellular vesicles and intermediate mesoderm cells. Biomater Res [Internet]. 2023 Feb 9; 27(1). Available from: https://spj.science.org/doi/10.1186/s40824-023-00471-x

Chai Q., Jiao Y., Yu X. Hydrogels for Biomedical Applications: Their Characteristics and the Mechanisms behind Them. Gels [Internet]. 2017 Jan 24; 3(1): 6. Available from: http://www.mdpi.com/2310-2861/3/1/6

Chambers B.E., Weaver N.E., Wingert R.A. The "3Ds" of Growing Kidney Organoids: Advances in Nephron Development, Disease Modeling, and Drug Screening. Cells [Internet]. 2023 Feb 8; 12(4): 549. Available from: https://www.mdpi.com/2073-4409/12/4/549

Chang C., Davies J.A. In developing mouse kidneys, orientation of loop of Henle growth is adaptive and guided by long-range cues from medullary collecting ducts. J Anat. 2019 Aug; 235(2): 262–70.

Chu X., Bleasby K., Evers R.. Species differences in drug transporters and implications for translating preclinical findings to humans. Expert Opin Drug Metab Toxicol. 2013 Mar; 9(3): 237–52.

Cinnamon VanPutte, Jennifer Regan, Andrew Russo, Rod Seeley T.S. and P.T. Seeley's Anatomy & Physiology. 13th ed. 2022.

Clevers H. Modeling Development and Disease with Organoids. Cell. 2016 Jun; 165(7): 1586–97.

Colaco M., Igel D.A., Atala A. The potential of 3D printing in urological research and patient care. Nat Rev Urol. 2018 Apr; 15(4): 213–21.

Costa-Almeida R., Granja P., Soares R., Guerreiro S. Cellular strategies to promote vascularisation in tissue engineering applications. Eur Cells Mater. 2014 Jul; 28: 51–67.

Cruz N.M., Freedman B.S. CRISPR Gene Editing in the Kidney. Am J Kidney Dis. 2018 Jun; 71(6): 874–83.

Cruz N.M., Song X., Czerniecki S.M., Gulieva R.E., Churchill A.J. et al. Organoid cystogenesis reveals a critical role of microenvironment in human polycystic kidney disease. Nat Mater. 2017 Nov; 16(11): 1112–1119.

Cui X., Breitenkamp K., Lotz M., D'Lima D. Synergistic action of fibroblast growth factor-2 and transforming growth factor-beta1 enhances bioprinted human neocartilage formation. Biotechnol Bioeng. 2012 Sep; 109(9): 2357–68.

Davis G.E., Bayless K.J., Mavila A. Molecular basis of endothelial cell morphogenesis in three-dimensional extracellular matrices. Anat Rec. 2002 Nov; 268(3): 252–75.

DesRochers T.M., Suter L., Roth A., Kaplan D.L. Bioengineered 3D Human Kidney Tissue, a Platform for the Determination of Nephrotoxicity. Egles C, editor. PLoS One [Internet]. 2013 Mar 14; 8(3): e59219. Available from: https://dx.plos.org/10.1371/journal.pone.0059219

Feraille E., Sassi A., Olivier V., Arnoux G., Martin P-Y. et al. Renal water transport in health and disease. Pflügers Arch - Eur J Physiol. 2022 Aug; 474(8): 841–52.

Figliuzzi M., Bonandrini B., Remuzzi A. Decellularized Kidney Matrix as Functional Material for whole Organ Tissue Engineering. J Appl Biomater Funct Mater [Internet]. 2017 Jan 11; 15(4): e326–33. Available from: http://journals.sagepub.com/doi/10.5301/jabfm.5000393

Fleming P.A., Argraves W.S., Gentile C., Neagu A., Forgacs G. et al. Fusion of uniluminal vascular spheroids: A model for assembly of blood vessels. Dev Dyn. 2010 Feb; 239(2): 398–406.

Frederic H. Martini and Edwin F. Bartholomew. Essentials of Anatomy & Physiology. 7th ed. 2016. 808 p.

Freedman B.S., Brooks C.R., Lam A.Q., Fu H., Morizane R., Agrawal V., et al. Modelling kidney disease with CRISPR-mutant kidney organoids derived from human pluripotent epiblast spheroids. Nat Commun. 2015 Oct; 6(1): 8715.

Freedman B.S., Lam A.Q., Sundsbak J.L., Iatrino R., Su X. et al. Reduced Ciliary Polycystin-2 in Induced Pluripotent Stem Cells from Polycystic Kidney Disease Patients with PKD1 Mutations. J Am Soc Nephrol. 2013 Oct; 24(10): 1571–86.

Freedman B.S. Modeling Kidney Disease with iPS Cells. Biomark Insights. 2015 Jan; 10s1:BMI.S20054.

Gao X., Chen X., Taglienti M., Rumballe B., Little M.H. et al. Angioblast-mesenchyme induction of early kidney development is mediated by Wt1 and Vegfa. Development. 2005 Dec; 132(24): 5437–49.

Garreta E., Montserrat N., Belmonte J.C.I. Kidney organoids for disease modeling. Oncotarget. 2018 Feb; 9(16): 12552–12553.

Gentile C., Fleming P.A., Mironov V., Argraves K.M., Argraves W.S. et al. VEGF-mediated fusion in the generation of uniluminal vascular spheroids. Dev Dyn. 2008 Oct; 237(10): 2918–25.

George S.K., Abolbashari M., Kim T-H., Zhang C., Allickson J. et al. Effect of Human Amniotic Fluid Stem Cells on Kidney Function in a Model of Chronic Kidney Disease. Tissue Eng Part A. 2019 Nov; 25(21–22): 1493–503.

Gintant G., Sager P.T., Stockbridge N. Evolution of strategies to improve preclinical cardiac safety testing. Nat Rev Drug Discov. 2016 Jul; 15(7): 457–71.

Greek R., Menache A. Systematic Reviews of Animal Models: Methodology versus Epistemology. Int J Med Sci. 2013; 10(3): 206–21.

Gueutin V., Deray G., Isnard-Bagnis C. Physiologie rénale. Bull Cancer. 2012 Mar; 99(3): 237–49.

Gutiérrez O.M. Sodium- and Phosphorus-Based Food Additives: Persistent but Surmountable Hurdles in the Management of Nutrition in Chronic Kidney Disease. Adv Chronic Kidney Dis. 2013 Mar; 20(2): 150–6.

Halt K.J., Pärssinen H.E., Junttila S.M., Saarela U., Sims-Lucas S. et al. CD146 + cells are essential for kidney vasculature development. Kidney Int. 2016 Aug; 90(2): 311–24.

Hamm L.L., Nakhoul N., Hering-Smith K.S. Acid-Base Homeostasis. Clin J Am Soc Nephrol. 2015 Dec; 10(12): 2232–42.

Hammerman M.R. Xenotransplantation of developing kidneys. Am J Physiol Physiol. 2002 Oct; 283(4): F601–6.

Hesuani Y.D., Pereira F.D.A.S., Parfenov V., Koudan E., Mitryashkin A. et al. Design and Implementation of Novel Multifunctional 3D Bioprinter. 3D Print Addit Manuf. 2016 Mar; 3(1): 64–68.

Hickling D.R., Sun T-T, Wu X-R. Anatomy and Physiology of the Urinary Tract: Relation to Host Defense and Microbial Infection. Mulvey MA, Stapleton AE, Klumpp DJ, editors. Microbiol Spectr. 2015 Jul; 3(4).

Hoehn E.N.M. and K. Human Anatomy and Physiology. 11th ed. 2018. 1272 p.

Homan K.A., Kolesky D.B., Skylar-Scott M.A., Herrmann J., Obuobi H. et al. Bioprinting of 3D Convoluted Renal Proximal Tubules on Perfusable Chips. Sci Rep. 2016 Oct; 6(1): 34845.

Huang H-C., Chang Y-J., Chen W-C., Harn HI-C., Tang M-J. et al. Enhancement of Renal Epithelial Cell Functions through Microfluidic-Based Coculture with Adipose-Derived Stem Cells. Tissue Eng Part A. 2013 Sep; 19(17–18): 2024–34.

Huling J., Ko I.K., Atala A., Yoo J.J. Fabrication of biomimetic vascular scaffolds for 3D tissue constructs using vascular corrosion casts. Acta Biomater. 2016 Mar; 32: 190–197.

Hyink D.P., Tucker D.C., St John P.L., Leardkamolkarn V., Accavitti M.A. et al. Endogenous origin of glomerular endothelial and mesangial cells in grafts of embryonic kidneys. Am J Physiol Physiol. 1996 May; 270(5): F886–99.

Isnard Bagnis C., Deray G., Baumelou A., Le Quintrec M., Vanherweghem J.L. et al. Herbs and the kidney. Am J Kidney Dis. 2004 Jul; 44(1): 1–11.

Itoh M., Nakayama K., Noguchi R., Kamohara K., Furukawa K. et al. Scaffold-Free Tubular Tissues Created by a Bio-3D Printer Undergo Remodeling and Endothelialization when Implanted in Rat Aortae. Zhu D, editor. PLoS One. 2015 Sep; 10(9): e0136681.

Jang K-J., Cho H.S., Kang D.H., Bae W.G., Kwon T-H. et al. Fluid-shear-stress-induced translocation of aquaporin-2 and reorganization of actin cytoskeleton in renal tubular epithelial cells. Integr Biol. 2011; 3(2): 134–41.

Jansson K., Nguyen A-NT, Magenheimer B.S., Reif G.A., Aramadhaka L.R. et al. Endogenous concentrations of ouabain act as a cofactor to stimulate fluid secretion and cyst growth of in vitro ADPKD models via cAMP and EGFR-Src-MEK pathways. Am J Physiol Physiol. 2012 Oct; 303(7): F982–90.

Jeon J.S., Bersini S., Gilardi M., Dubini G., Charest J.L. et al. Human 3D vascularized organotypic microfluidic assays to study breast cancer cell extravasation. Proc Natl Acad Sci. 2015 Jan; 112(1): 214–219.

Jha V., Rathi M. Natural Medicines Causing Acute Kidney Injury. Semin Nephrol. 2008 Jul; 28(4): 416–28.

Kalucki S.A., Lardi C., Garessus J., Kfoury A., Grabherr S. et al. Reference values and sex differences in absolute and relative kidney size. A Swiss autopsy study. BMC Nephrol. 2020 Dec; 21(1): 289.

Kamei M., Brian Saunders W., Bayless K.J., Dye L., Davis G.E. et al. Endothelial tubes assemble from intracellular vacuoles in vivo. Nature. 2006 Jul; 442(7101): 453–456.

Kataria A., Trasande L., Trachtman H. The effects of environmental chemicals on renal function. Nat Rev Nephrol. 2015 Oct; 11(10): 610–25.

Kelm J.M., Lorber V., Snedeker J.G., Schmidt D., Broggini-Tenzer A. et al. A novel concept for scaffold-free vessel tissue engineering: Self-assembly of microtissue building blocks. J Biotechnol. 2010 Jul; 148(1): 46–55.

Kim Y.K., Refaeli I., Brooks C.R., Jing P., Gulieva R.E. et al. Gene-Edited Human Kidney Organoids Reveal Mechanisms of Disease in Podocyte Development. Stem Cells. 2017 Dec; 35(12): 2366–78.

King S.M., Higgins J.W., Nino C.R., Smith T.R., Paffenroth E.H. et al. 3D Proximal Tubule Tissues Recapitulate Key Aspects of Renal Physiology to Enable Nephrotoxicity Testing. Front Physiol [Internet]. 2017 Mar 8; 8. Available from: http://journal.frontiersin.org/article/10.3389/fphys.2017.00123/full

Kolesky D.B., Homan K.A., Skylar-Scott M., Lewis J.A. In Vitro Human Tissues via Multi-material 3-D Bioprinting. Altern to Lab Anim [Internet]. 2018 Sep 1; 46(4): 209–15. Available from: http://journals.sagepub.com/doi/10.1177/026119291804600404

Kolesky D.B., Homan K.A., Skylar-Scott MA, Lewis JA. Three-dimensional bioprinting of thick vascularized tissues. Proc Natl Acad Sci. 2016 Mar;113(12):3179–84.

Kolesky D.B., Truby R.L., Gladman A.S., Busbee T.A., Homan K.A. et al. 3D Bioprinting of Vascularized, Heterogeneous Cell-Laden Tissue Constructs. Adv Mater. 2014 May; 26(19): 3124–30.

Krishna D.V., Sankar M.R. Extrusion based bioprinting of alginate based multicomponent hydrogels for tissue regeneration applications: State of the art. Mater Today Commun [Internet]. 2023 Jun; 35: 105696. Available from: https://linkinghub.elsevier.com/retrieve/pii/S2352492823003872

Laschke M.W., Menger M.D. Adipose tissue-derived microvascular fragments: natural vascularization units for regenerative medicine. Trends Biotechnol. 2015 Aug; 33(8): 442–448.

Lawlor K.T., Vanslambrouck J.M., Higgins J.W., Chambon A., Bishard K. et al. Cellular extrusion bioprinting improves kidney organoid reproducibility and conformation. Nat Mater [Internet]. 2021 Feb 23; 20(2): 260–71. Available from: https://www.nature.com/articles/s41563-020-00853-9

Lee J., Kim S. Kidney-on-a-Chip: A New Technology for Predicting Drug Efficacy, Interactions, and Drug-induced Nephrotoxicity. Curr Drug Metab. 2018 Jul; 19(7): 577–83.

Leiz J., Schmidt-Ott K.M. Claudins in the Renal Collecting Duct. Int J Mol Sci. 2019 Dec; 21(1): 221.

Li J., Chen M., Fan X., Zhou H. Recent advances in bioprinting techniques: approaches, applications and future prospects. J Transl Med [Internet]. 2016 Dec 20; 14(1): 271. Available from: http://translational-medicine.biomedcentral.com/articles/10.1186/s12967-016-1028-0

Li X., Liu B., Pei B., Chen J., Zhou D. et al. Inkjet Bioprinting of Biomaterials. Chem Rev [Internet]. 2020 Oct 14; 120(19): 10793–833. Available from: https://pubs.acs.org/doi/10.1021/acs.chemrev.0c00008

Lin N.Y.C., Homan K.A., Robinson S.S., Kolesky D.B., Duarte N. et al. Renal reabsorption in 3D vascularized proximal tubule models. Proc Natl Acad Sci. 2019 Mar; 116(12): 5399–404.

Little M.H., McMahon A.P. Mammalian Kidney Development: Principles, Progress, and Projections. Cold Spring Harb Perspect Biol. 2012 May; 4(5): a008300–a008300.

Lovett M., Lee K., Edwards A., Kaplan D.L. Vascularization Strategies for Tissue Engineering. Tissue Eng Part B Rev. 2009 Sep; 15(3): 353–70.

Mahadevan V. Anatomy of the kidney and ureter. Surg. 2019 Jul; 37(7): 359–64.

Malda J., Visser J., Melchels F.P., Jüngst T., Hennink W.E. et al. 25th Anniversary Article: Engineering Hydrogels for Biofabrication. Adv Mater [Internet]. 2013 Sep 23; 25(36): 5011–28. Available from: https://onlinelibrary. wiley.com/doi/10.1002/adma.201302042

Marcoux A., Tremblay L.E., Slimani S., Fiola M., Mac-Way F et al. Anatomophysiology of the Henle's Loop: Emphasis on the Thick Ascending Limb. In: Comprehensive Physiology. Wiley; 2021. p. 3119–39.

Mehta R.L., Pascual M.T., Soroko S., Savage B.R., Himmelfarb J., Ikizler T.A., et al. Spectrum of acute renal failure in the intensive care unit: The PICARD experience. Kidney Int. 2004 Oct; 66(4): 1613–21.

Miller J.S., Stevens K.R., Yang M.T., Baker B.M., Nguyen D-HT. et al. Rapid casting of patterned vascular networks for perfusable engineered three-dimensional tissues. Nat Mater. 2012 Sep; 11(9): 768–74.

Mironov V., Kasyanov V., Drake C., Markwald R.R. Organ printing: promises and challenges. Regen Med. 2008 Jan; 3(1): 93–103.

Moinuddin Z., Dhanda R. Anatomy of the kidney and ureter. Anaesth Intensive Care Med. 2015 Jun; 16(6): 247–52.

Morizane R., Bonventre J.V. Generation of nephron progenitor cells and kidney organoids from human pluripotent stem cells. Nat Protoc. 2017 Jan; 12(1): 195–207.

Morizane R., Lam A.Q., Freedman B.S., Kishi S., Valerius M.T. et al. Nephron organoids derived from human pluripotent stem cells model kidney development and injury. Nat Biotechnol. 2015 Nov; 33(11): 1193–200.

Mundel P. Podocytes and the quest for precision medicines for kidney diseases. Pflügers Arch - Eur J Physiol. 2017 Aug; 469(7–8): 1029–37.

Murphy S.V., Atala A. 3D bioprinting of tissues and organs. Nat Biotechnol. 2014 Aug; 32(8): 773–85.

Norotte C., Marga F.S., Niklason L.E., Forgacs G. Scaffold-free vascular tissue engineering using bioprinting. Biomaterials. 2009 Oct; 30(30): 5910–5917.

Novosel E.C., Kleinhans C., Kluger P.J. Vascularization is the key challenge in tissue engineering. Adv Drug Deliv Rev. 2011 Apr; 63(4–5): 300–11.

Nunes S.S., Krishnan L., Gerard C.S., Dale J.R., Maddie M.A. et al. Angiogenic potential of microvessel fragments is independent of the tissue of origin and can be influenced by the cellular composition of the implants. Microcirculation. 2010 Jul; 557–567.

Ogunlade O., Connell J.J., Huang J.L., Zhang E., Lythgoe M.F. et al. In vivo three-dimensional photoacoustic imaging of the renal vasculature in preclinical rodent models. Am J Physiol Physiol. 2018 Jun; 314(6): F1145–53.

Olson H., Betton G., Robinson D., Thomas K., Monro A. et al. Concordance of the Toxicity of Pharmaceuticals in Humans and in Animals. Regul Toxicol Pharmacol. 2000 Aug; 32(1): 56–67.

Ouyang L., Yao R., Chen X., Na J., Sun W. et al. 3D printing of HEK 293FT cell-laden hydrogel into macroporous constructs with high cell viability and normal biological functions. Biofabrication [Internet]. 2015 Feb 18; 7(1): 015010. Available from: https://iopscience.iop.org/article/10.1088/1758-5090/7/1/015010

Pati F., Jang J., Ha D-H., Won Kim S., Rhie J-W. et al. Printing three-dimensional tissue analogues with decellularized extracellular matrix bioink. Nat Commun [Internet]. 2014 Jun 2; 5(1): 3935. Available from: https://www. nature.com/articles/ncomms4935

Peired A.J., Mazzinghi B., De Chiara L., Guzzi F., Lasagni L et al. Bioengineering strategies for nephrologists: kidney was not built in a day. Expert Opin Biol Ther. 2020 May; 20(5): 467–80.

Peloso A., Katari R., Murphy S.V., Zambon J.P., DeFrancesco A. et al. Prospect for kidney bioengineering: shortcomings of the status quo. Expert Opin Biol Ther. 2015 Apr; 15(4): 547–58.

Perneger T.V., Whelton P.K., Klag M.J. Risk of Kidney Failure Associated with the Use of Acetaminophen, Aspirin, and Nonsteroidal Antiinflammatory Drugs. N Engl J Med. 1994 Dec; 331(25): 1675–1679.

Pourhanifeh M.H., Mohammadi R., Noruzi S., Hosseini S.A., Fanoudi S. et al. The role of fibromodulin in cancer pathogenesis: implications for diagnosis and therapy. Cancer Cell Int. 2019 Dec; 19(1): 157.

Price N., Wood A.F. Acute kidney injury in the critical care setting. Nurs Stand. 2023 Sep; 38(9): 45–50.

Rak-Raszewska A., Wilm B., Edgar D., Kenny S., Woolf A.S. et al. Development of embryonic stem cells in recombinant kidneys. Organogenesis. 2012 Oct; 8(4): 125–36.

Robert B., St. John P.L., Abrahamson D.R. Direct visualization of renal vascular morphogenesis in Flk1 heterozygous mutant mice. Am J Physiol Physiol. 1998 Jul; 275(1): F164–72.

Rouwkema J., Khademhosseini A. Vascularization and Angiogenesis in Tissue Engineering: Beyond Creating Static Networks. Trends Biotechnol. 2016 Sep; 34(9): 733–45.

Rouwkema J., Rivron N.C., van Blitterswijk C.A. Vascularization in tissue engineering. Trends Biotechnol. 2008 Aug; 26(8): 434–41.

Rymer C.C., Sims-Lucas S. In Utero Intra-cardiac Tomato-lectin Injections on Mouse Embryos to Gauge Renal Blood Flow. J. Vis Exp. 2015 Feb; (96).

Sciancalepore A.G., Sallustio F., Girardo S., Gioia Passione L., Camposeo A. et al. A Bioartificial Renal Tubule Device Embedding Human Renal Stem/Progenitor Cells. Camussi G, editor. PLoS One. 2014 Jan; 9(1): e87496.

Serluca F.C., Drummond I.A., Fishman M.C. Endothelial Signaling in Kidney Morphogenesis. Curr Biol. 2002 Mar; 12(6): 492–7.

Shamma R.N., Sayed R.H., Madry H., E.L. Sayed N.S., Cucchiarini M. et al. Triblock Copolymer Bioinks in Hydrogel Three-Dimensional Printing for Regenerative Medicine: A Focus on Pluronic F127. Tissue Eng Part B Rev [Internet]. 2022 Apr 1; 28(2): 451–63. Available from: https://www.liebertpub.com/doi/10.1089/ten. teb.2021.0026

Shirali A., Pazhayattil G.S. Drug-induced impairment of renal function. Int J Nephrol Renovasc Dis. 2014 Dec; 457.

Singh N.K., Han W., Nam S.A., Kim J.W., Kim J.Y. et al. Three-dimensional cell-printing of advanced renal tubular tissue analogue. Biomaterials. 2020 Feb; 232:119734.

Singh N.K., Han W., Nam S.A., Kim J.W., Kim J.Y. et al. Three-dimensional cell-printing of advanced renal tubular tissue analogue. Biomaterials [Internet]. 2020 Feb; 232: 119734. Available from: https://linkinghub.elsevier. com/retrieve/pii/S014296121930852X

Skardal A., Atala A. Biomaterials for Integration with 3-D Bioprinting. Ann Biomed Eng. 2015 Mar; 43(3): 730–46.

Sochol R.D., Gupta N.R., Bonventre J.V. A Role for 3D Printing in Kidney-on-a-Chip Platforms. Curr Transplant Reports. 2016 Mar; 3(1): 82–92.

Song J.W., Bazou D., Munn L.L. Microfluidic Model of Angiogenic Sprouting. In 2015. p. 243–54.

Song R., Yosypiv I.V. Development of the kidney medulla. Organogenesis. 2012 Jan; 8(1): 10–17.

Streets A.M., Huang Y. Chip in a lab: Microfluidics for next generation life science research. Biomicrofluidics [Internet]. 2013 Jan 1; 7(1). Available from: https://pubs.aip.org/bmf/article/7/1/011302/1065237/Chip-in-a-lab-Microfluidics-for-next-generation

Takasato M., Er P.X., Becroft M., Vanslambrouck J.M., Stanley E.G. et al. Directing human embryonic stem cell differentiation towards a renal lineage generates a self-organizing kidney. Nat Cell Biol. 2014 Jan; 16(1): 118–26.

Takasato M., Er P.X., Chiu H.S., Little M.H. Generation of kidney organoids from human pluripotent stem cells. Nat Protoc [Internet]. 2016 Sep 18; 11(9): 1681–92. Available from: https://www.nature.com/articles/nprot.2016.098

Takasato M., Er P.X., Chiu H.S., Maier B., Baillie G.J. et al. Kidney organoids from human iPS cells contain multiple lineages and model human nephrogenesis. Nature. 2015 Oct; 526(7574): 564–8.

Theodorou C, Leatherby R, Dhanda R. Function of the nephron and the formation of urine. Anaesth Intensive Care Med. 2021 Jul; 22(7): 434–438.

Uchino S. Acute Renal Failure in Critically Ill Patients<SUBTITLE>A Multinational, Multicenter Study</SUBTITLE>. JAMA. 2005 Aug; 294(7): 813.

Unbekandt M., Davies J.A. Dissociation of embryonic kidneys followed by reaggregation allows the formation of renal tissues. Kidney Int. 2010 Mar; 77(5): 407–16.

Visconti R.P., Kasyanov V., Gentile C., Zhang J., Markwald R.R. et al . Towards organ printing: engineering an intra-organ branched vascular tree. Expert Opin Biol Ther. 2010 Mar; 10(3): 409–20.

Wilm B., Tamburrini R., Orlando G., Murray P. Autologous Cells for Kidney Bioengineering. Curr Transplant Reports. 2016 Sep; 3(3): 207–20.

Wilmer M.J., Ng C.P., Lanz H.L., Vulto P., Suter-Dick L. et al. Kidney-on-a-Chip Technology for Drug-Induced Nephrotoxicity Screening. Trends Biotechnol. 2016 Feb; 34(2): 156–70.

Wioland H., Suzuki E., Cao L., Romet-Lemonne G., Jegou A. et al. The advantages of microfluidics to study actin biochemistry and biomechanics. J Muscle Res Cell Motil [Internet]. 2020 Mar 20; 41(1): 175–88. Available from: http://link.springer.com/10.1007/s10974-019-09564-4

Xie H-G., Wang S-K., Cao C-C., Harpur E. Qualified kidney biomarkers and their potential significance in drug safety evaluation and prediction. Pharmacol Ther. 2013 Jan; 137(1): 100–107.

Xinaris C., Benedetti V., Novelli R., Abbate M., Rizzo P. et al. Functional Human Podocytes Generated in Organoids from Amniotic Fluid Stem Cells. J Am Soc Nephrol. 2016 May; 27(5): 1400–11.

Xinaris C., Benedetti V., Rizzo P., Abbate M., Corna D. et al. In Vivo Maturation of Functional Renal Organoids Formed from Embryonic Cell Suspensions. J Am Soc Nephrol. 2012 Nov; 23(11): 1857–68.

Yoshio Takei, Hironori Ando K.T. Handbook of Hormones. 1st ed. 2015.

Zacchia, M., Capolongo, G., Rinaldi, L. and Capasso, G. (2018). The importance of the thick ascending limb of Henle's loop in renal physiology and pathophysiology. International journal of nephrology and renovascular disease, 81–92.

Zhang C., Hou J., Zheng S., Zheng Z., Hu S. et al. Vascularized Atrial Tissue Patch Cardiomyoplasty With Omentopexy Improves Cardiac Performance After Myocardial Infarction. Ann Thorac Surg. 2011 Oct; 92(4): 1435–42.

Zhang T., Zhao W., Xiahou Z., Wang X., Zhang K. et al. Bioink design for extrusion-based bioprinting. Appl Mater Today [Internet]. 2021 Dec; 25: 101227. Available from: https://linkinghub.elsevier.com/retrieve/pii/S2352940721002900

Zhuo J.L., Li X.C. Proximal Nephron. In: Comprehensive Physiology. Wiley; 2013. p. 1079–123.

Index

Drugs 36, 52, 89, 90, 106, 117, 118, 170, 223, 226, 233, 247, 274, 275, 316, 332, 337, 338, 341, 369, 370, 386, 389, 451, 453, 472, 482, 491, 492, 494, 496, 498, 529

E

Ethics 41, 116, 121

Extracellular matrix 53-55, 61, 75, 108, 131, 135, 148, 177, 195, 203, 204, 207, 211, 248, 277, 325, 332, 337, 339, 371, 391, 393, 437, 438, 440, 448, 449

Extrusion-based bioprinting 29, 30, 48, 52, 64, 125, 126, 132, 149, 199, 241, 314-316, 400, 402, 445, 448, 451, 459, 460, 465, 474, 525

Eye 15, 108, 137, 166, 227, 228, 230, 263, 341, 464, 482-495, 497-499

F

Fabrication 2, 5, 8, 9, 11, 14, 15, 20, 27, 28, 31, 32, 35, 36, 43, 47, 48, 50, 52, 58, 62, 70, 79, 81, 88, 128, 140, 141, 147, 191, 192, 199, 200, 397, 398, 401-403, 406, 408

FDA 75, 92, 139, 140, 159, 169, 182, 207, 212, 233, 236, 326, 378, 408

Fertility preservation 509, 516

H

Hydrogels 2, 6, 7, 9, 10, 14, 15, 18, 28, 30, 31, 33, 51, 52, 54, 56, 59, 61, 63, 70, 73, 103, 116, 117, 130, 148, 153, 178, 180, 182, 184, 185, 192, 193, 195, 197, 200, 204, 206, 239, 246, 247, 286, 289, 291, 298, 416, 428, 430, 447, 448, 462, 464, 466, 472, 475, 511, 512, 530, 531

I

in vitro models 9, 11, 38, 104, 134, 167, 168, 326, 338, 393, 408, 414, 434, 439, 490, 521, 526, 529, 531

iPSCs 136, 162, 166, 208, 377, 389, 400, 432, 433, 531, 532

K

Keratinocytes 6, 8, 37, 93, 104, 161, 166, 203, 242, 316, 324, 330, 332, 334, 391, 438, 439, 441, 442, 444, 446, 447, 449, 451

Kidney 8, 11, 14, 15, 18, 43, 53, 92, 100, 105, 106, 118, 119, 136, 153, 164, 336, 341, 349, 386, 387, 390, 391, 394, 407, 417, 520-534

L

Liver 2, 6, 7, 9, 11, 13, 14, 15, 17, 18, 34, 36, 41, 51, 53, 59, 61, 87-92, 94, 100, 105, 106, 116, 117, 125, 130, 136, 137, 148, 152, 154, 155, 157, 158, 164, 165, 167, 182, 185, 193, 198, 205, 223, 226, 235, 238, 247, 248, 273, 274-279, 284, 315, 316, 412-418, 500, 512, 513, 521, 522

Lung tissues 104, 424, 427-429, 431, 432

M

Maxillofacial Surgery 249, 457

Medical devices 36, 79, 86, 88, 92, 107, 139, 153, 179, 221, 224, 226, 233, 234, 236, 258, 268, 276, 282, 277, 488, 500

Medicinal products 222

Medicine 1, 2, 7, 9, 13, 14, 17, 20, 21, 28, 29, 31-36, 104-108, 116, 117, 122, 126, 131, 139, 141, 149, 153, 164, 169, 170, 172, 177, 178, 182, 186, 191, 193, 212, 213, 221, 225, 243, 248, 257, 261, 312, 320, 326, 328, 332, 336, 341, 343, 350, 351, 366, 369, 412, 413, 414, 417, 419, 422-427, 432, 433, 449, 452, 457, 458, 463, 473, 478, 509, 520, 527, 528, 531

Microfluidics 17, 57, 104, 154, 337, 338, 389, 391, 406, 407, 510, 525, 527, 528

Microfluidics Natural polymers 177, 180, 183

O

Ocular tissue 485, 486, 498, 499, 500

Oncofertility 509

Organ transplantation 20, 35, 39, 41, 43, 61, 62, 99, 117, 153, 170, 186, 250, 261, 271, 277, 326, 351, 415, 423, 434, 516

Organ-on-a-chip 13, 21, 104-107, 154, 164, 168, 213, 387, 407, 427

Orthopedics 37, 28, 272

P

Printable food inks 291, 294

Prosthetic devices 256, 257, 259, 262, 263, 268, 282, 284

Prosthetics 36, 37, 38, 170, 221, 249, 257, 263-265, 268, 282-284, 425, 487

R

Regenerative medicine 1, 2, 7, 9, 13, 14, 18-21, 28-34, 37, 38, 41, 43, 47, 51, 52, 54, 60-62, 79, 82, 83, 88, 108, 116, 126, 131, 129, 153, 170, 172, 177, 193, 212, 213, 248, 257, 271, 320, 328, 332, 336, 341, 343, 350, 366, 369, 412, 414, 419, 422-424, 426, 427, 433, 449, 452, 457, 458, 473, 478, 482, 483, 488, 492, 520, 528, 531, 533

Retina 108, 166, 358, 487, 488, 490, 491, 492, 496, 499, 500

S

Safety 39-42, 75, 83, 109, 119, 221, 222, 226-235, 268, 280, 281, 294, 301, 326, 337, 343, 378, 386, 389, 407, 419, 450, 451, 459, 491, 497, 498, 514, 516

Scaffolds 5, 6, 10, 13, 14, 17, 19, 21, 34, 35, 37, 39, 48, 52, 59, 61, 72, 88, 95, 98, 101, 125, 126, 128-